Nutrition and Physical Fitness

G6836.25

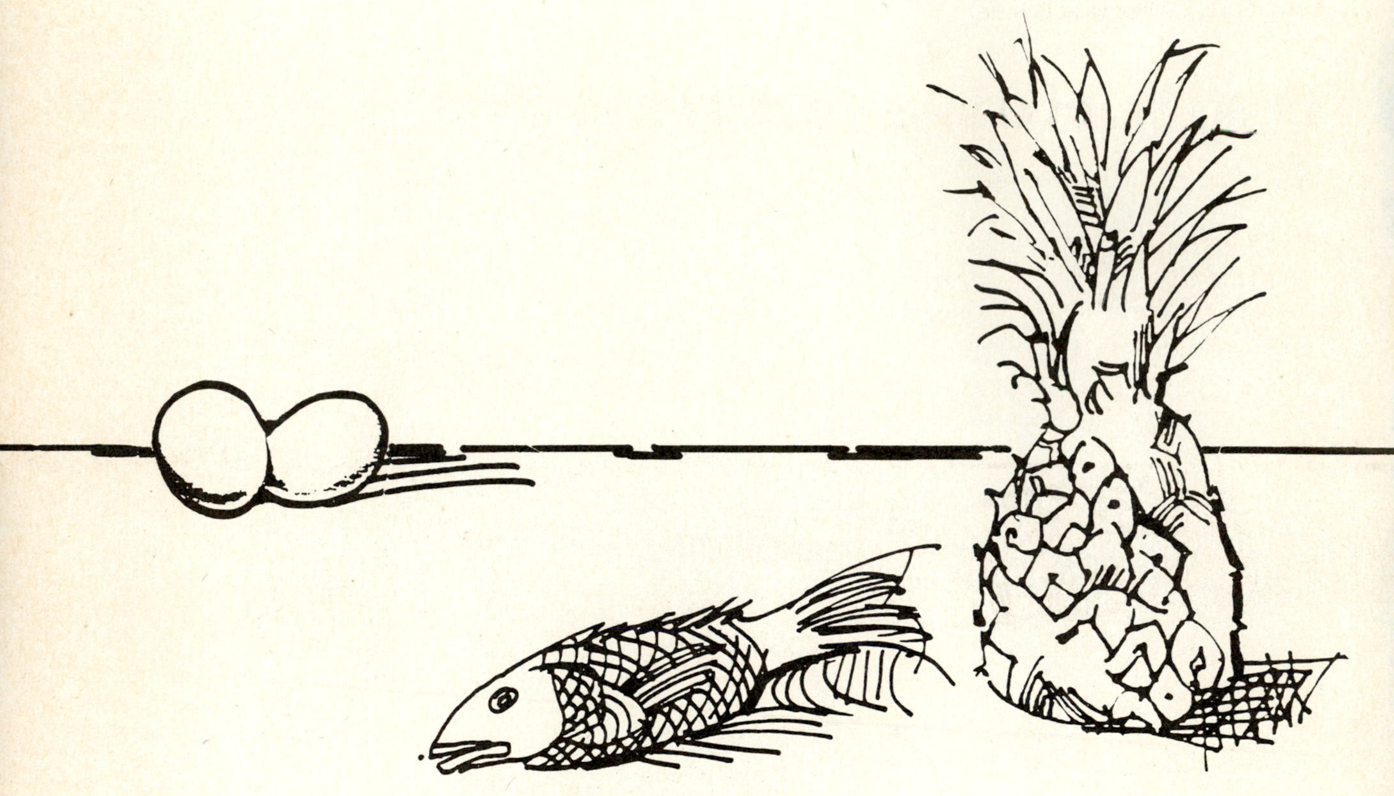

HOLT, RINEHART AND WINSTON

New York Chicago San Francisco Philadelphia Montreal Toronto London
Sydney Tokyo Mexico City Rio de Janeiro Madrid

Nutrition and Physical Fitness

11th EDITION

George M. Briggs

University of California at Berkeley

Doris Howes Calloway

University of California at Berkeley

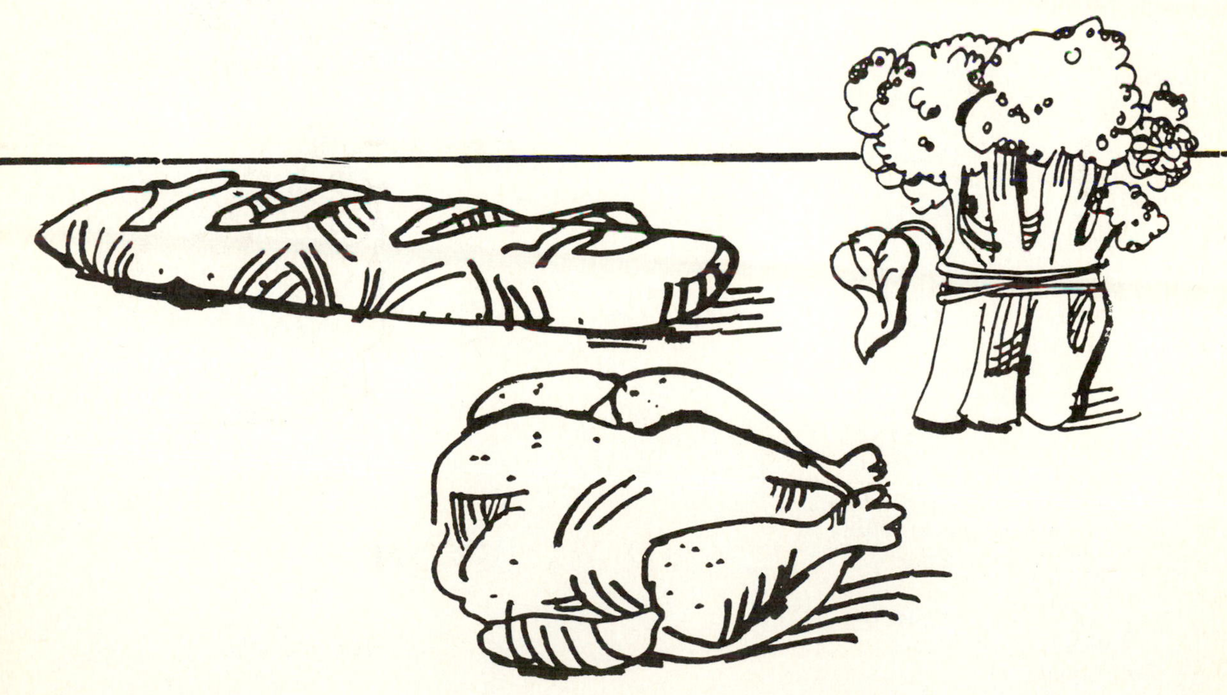

Publisher Susan Katz
Acquiring Editor Karen Dubno
Developmental Editor Herbert Kirk
Special Projects Editor Jeanette Ninas Johnson
Art Director Gloria Gentile
Production Manager Annette Mayeski

Chapter and front matter opening art by **Gloria Gentile.**

Cover photo: Photomicrograph of vitamin C crystal, courtesy Vitamin Nutrition Information Service, Hoffman-La Roche, Inc.

Library of Congress Number: 83-18581
ISBN 0-03-058587-2

Copyright © 1984 by CBS College Publishing
© 1979 by Saunders College Publishing/Holt, Rinehart and Winston under the title *Bogert's Nutrition and Physical Fitness*
Copyright 1931, 1935, 1939, 1943, 1949, 1954, 1960, 1966, and 1973 by W.B. Saunders Company
Address correspondence to:
383 Madison Avenue
New York, N.Y. 10017
All rights reserved
Printed in the United States of America
Published simultaneously in Canada

4 5 6 7 016 9 8 7 6 5 4 3 2

CBS COLLEGE PUBLISHING
Holt, Rinehart and Winston
The Dryden Press
Saunders College Publishing

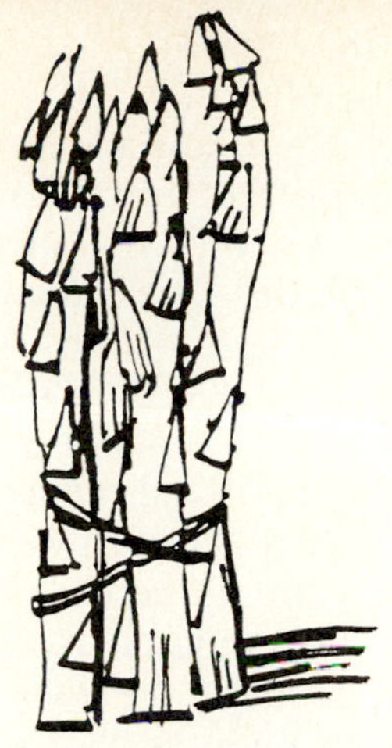

Preface

The overall aim of this eleventh edition is to provide students with sufficient knowledge about foods and nutrition to guide their own eating habits and to provide a sound basis for independent and advanced study. Awareness of good nutrition and good health practices will greatly help one to have a healthy and vigorous life now and over a lifetime. This has been the main purpose of this text since the first edition was written by the late Dr. L. Jean Bogert in 1931, over *fifty* years ago. Each succeeding edition has not only included the years of cumulated experience of, and experimentation by, the authors and the discoveries of nutritionists throughout the world, but also has benefited greatly from suggestions that have come from teachers and students.

The book is primarily for college students taking their first course in nutrition. It is written so that it may be useful and readily understood not only by food, dietetics, and nutrition majors, but also by nonmajor students who are interested in basic nutrition and concerned about what to eat for a healthy life. This includes students majoring in physical education, chemistry, home economics, health sciences, agriculture, or biology. It will be a useful text, as well, for other college students who have had at least high school chemistry and biology, especially with the expert guidance that experienced and informed instructors can give.

Fortunately, as there has been increased emphasis on science in secondary schools, most present-day college students have already acquired some knowledge of fundamental scientific terms and concepts in high school courses or even at grade school levels. Hence, college students may be expected to comprehend a presentation of nutrition that relies on an elementary understanding of science.

We firmly believe that a thorough knowledge of basic facts about foods and nutrition is essential to building a real understanding of applied nutrition topics and the ability to evaluate new developments constantly being discovered in this dynamic field. Only with this level of understanding of basic nutrition can one begin to learn, independently, how to accept or reject new claims, fads, and even frauds presented by the mass media and commercial interests.

An understanding of basic nutrition is not easy. To the uninitiated student it is similar in difficulty to learning the fundamentals of a new language or, for instance, of chemistry or biology. This explains why the first two-thirds or so of the book is primarily a presentation of the "basic facts." However, practical applications of these basic facts are interspersed throughout the book—more than in previous editions. The last third of the book contains practical information about some of the more important applied nutrition topics not covered in the earlier chapters.

The text purposely contains more subject matter than can usually be covered in one introductory course. This provides flexibility in lecture topics and chapter assignments by teachers of various disciplines and with different backgrounds. Experience has demonstrated that many of today's students have a wide spectrum of interests not always shared by other students. Among these interests are obesity and overweight, athletic performance as it relates to nutrition, vegetarianism, pregnancy, cultural nutrition, food composition, infant nutrition, dental health, and solutions to world hunger problems. The inclusion of coverage on these subjects in this text allows students of different backgrounds and interests to pursue these topics in more detail than usually can be offered in any one class. The degree of detail in the text can provide answers to questions of individual students that cannot be always covered in lectures due to time constraints.

Some colleges, we have learned, have preferred to use the text over a two-quarter, or two-semester, sequence of courses, thus allowing coverage of more topics in greater depth.

Research in nutrition in recent years has concentrated more and more on the study of the basic life processes—the chemistry of the cell, the chemical changes that take place in the various tissues, and the role of enzymes, vitamins, and mineral elements in catalyzing these processes. This deeper inquiry into the need for and functions of the various nutrients is often a team effort, involving the collaboration of biochemists with physiologists and microbiologists. Looking at the vast amount of data and numerous fundamental discoveries that have been accumulated by this type of research, it becomes apparent that even though this material may be somewhat difficult to translate into terms that are understandable to less advanced college students, it cannot be ignored; to be as meaningful as it should be, nutrition must be treated in greater depth than was formerly the case.

The dependence on the scientific method for establishing facts about foods and nutrition is often a difficult concept for today's student to accept. Though we could not exist in America without a responsible food industry, the student today has seen evidence of certain segments of the food industry putting the consumer at the low end of the priority list. The student has learned, rightly or wrongly, to distrust certain intentional food additives, highly processed foods, foods treated with "synthetic chemicals," and certain food advertising. We recommend that teachers using this book in classes comprised mainly of students not trained in science spend the first few days or so of class discussing the meaning of science, the scientific method, a controlled experiment, the placebo, and the difference between a true scientific publication (with its system of peer review) and a typical magazine or newspaper article. (The improved Chapter 1 will assist you in this.)

Many improvements have been made in this edition: extensive revisions have been made throughout the text and many of the chapters have been completely rewritten. There is much new material in each chapter and many topics not included before, such as dietary fiber, weight control, megavitamins, cancer and nutrition, vegetarianism, vitamin C in the treatment and prevention of colds and cancer, newer trace elements, vitamin and mineral requirements, excessive salt intake, bottled versus tap water, caffeine and health, nonnutrients and natural toxins in food, exercise and diet, new dietary guidelines, and calcium requirements. There are many new tables and figures. In addition, there has been a major rearrangement of subject matter in order to present a more logical sequence of current nutritional topics. The subject of energy, including both basic and applied aspects, is presented in Chapters 6 and 7, following the discussion of carbohydrates, fats, proteins, and digestion and absorption (Chapters 2–5). Factors affecting food regulation and utilization have been incorporated in the chapters on the macronutrients and energy, earlier than in the previous edition.

On the basis of many suggestions from reviewers and users of the text, a special feature in this new edition is the inclusion of a variety of controversial topics that we have presented as "health considerations" in most of the chapters. These health considerations focus directly on nutrition controversies existing today that will be of special importance to the student's general health and future life. Literature references for these and other related topics are provided.

As an added help to the student and teacher, the coverage of vitamins and minerals, as well as energy, has been divided into several smaller chapters so that approximately one chapter can be covered in no more than one or two lecture periods (in a 40- to 45-hour course).

Because nutrition is a rapidly growing field with a current explosion of research, some topics covered in previous editions have been condensed or left out. For instance, the previous Chapter 17, Food: From the Producer to the Consumer, has been totally omitted, though some essential material from this chapter has been incorporated in the new Chapter 18, Food: Our Source of Nutrients and Nonnutrients. Information on the history of individual nutrients and their biochemical function has been considerably condensed.

Table 2 on food composition in the appendix has been updated according to newer values in the new *USDA Handbook 8* and other sources for traditional foods and for many new foods. In this table, vitamin A values are given as retinol equivalents in agreement with the 1980 RDAs. A column on the polyunsaturated fatty acid content of foods has also been added. Presentation of this information in such detail is generally not provided in other nutrition textbooks.

Supplementary readings have been carefully chosen for use by teachers and motivated students alike and have been placed together in the appendix. These have been completely revised and brought up to date. We consider this collection of readings to be unique, not available elsewhere.

We are pleased that an instructor's manual, prepared by Dr. Kay Franz and Dr. Merrill J. Christensen, both of Brigham Young University, is available for this edition of the textbook.

We have attempted, as in previous editions, not to straddle the fence on controversial issues but to give our informed opinion on such issues when valid information exists. Nevertheless, nutrition as a field is a constantly evolving and controversial subject area, especially because of its essentiality to physical fitness and health, its economic, ecological, and environmental aspects, and because of the use of food to provide political influence. No textbook can contain the latest information on all nutrition and food topics beyond the date of publication. We suggest, therefore, that teachers and students wanting the newest information make use of current literature and of the periodicals and agencies listed at the end of Chapter 1. One will need to keep abreast of information on newer Recommended Dietary/Nutrient Allowances as they appear. We especially recommend current issues of such useful publications as the *Journal of the American Dietetic Association, American Journal of Clinical Nutrition, Journal of Nutrition, Journal of Nutrition Education, Journal of Home Econom-*

ics, New England Journal of Medicine, American Journal of Public Health, and the *Journal of the American Medical Association,* as well as other related quality publications.

We sincerely hope that you will find the book better able to meet your needs than ever before. We would very much appreciate receiving any comments, suggestions, or questions. Send them to either Dr. Briggs, responsible for Chapters 1, 8–18, 23, and 24; or to Dr. Calloway, responsible for Chapters 2–7, 19–22, 25, and for Table 2 of the appendix, on food composition. Comments from our readers are always welcome.

Acknowledgments

The authors are indebted to many persons who have helped in one way or another in making it possible for this eleventh edition to be published. Suggestions from teachers, teaching assistants, and students who have used earlier editions have been especially helpful. We wish to thank especially the following reviewers: Richard Ahrens, University of Maryland; Della Bannister, Virginia State University; Georgene Barte, Oregon State University; Kay Franz, Brigham Young University; Jean Peters, Oregon State University; Dennis Ponton, State University College at Buffalo; Marsha Reed, University of Nevada at Reno. We appreciate, too, the help of a number of persons at Holt, Rinehart and Winston who have worked diligently to produce a publication of the highest possible quality; our thanks especially to Karen Dubno, Herbert Kirk, Jeanette Ninas Johnson, Gloria Gentile, Nelson Smith, and Annette Mayeski.

We are particularly indebted to the following persons who have had the major role in the preparation of certain chapters; Catherine Briggs, M.D., M.P.H. (Chapters 13–15, 23, and 24); Christine Wilson, Ph.D. (Chapter 19); and Gail Butterfield, Ph.D. (Chapter 21).

Our thanks go to those who supplied photographs and other material for the text. We appreciate, too, the help of the persons who typed the manuscripts and references, and those who assisted in other capacities.

Special acknowledgments go to Mrs. Eleanor Briggs and Dr. Robert Nesheim, who have assisted in numerous ways in making this book possible.

George M. Briggs
Doris Howes Calloway

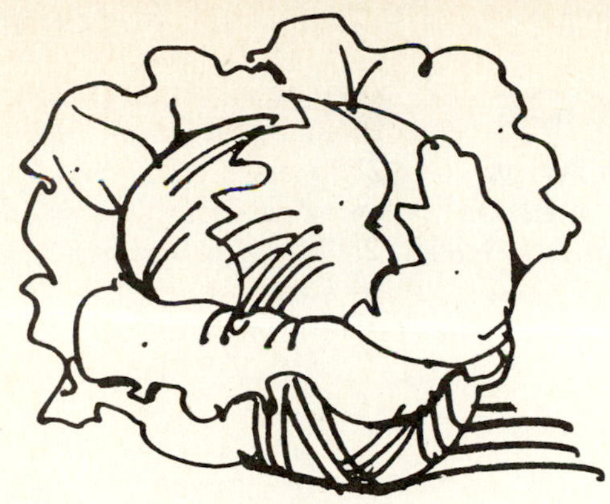

Contents

1 Food and Its Relation to Physical Fitness

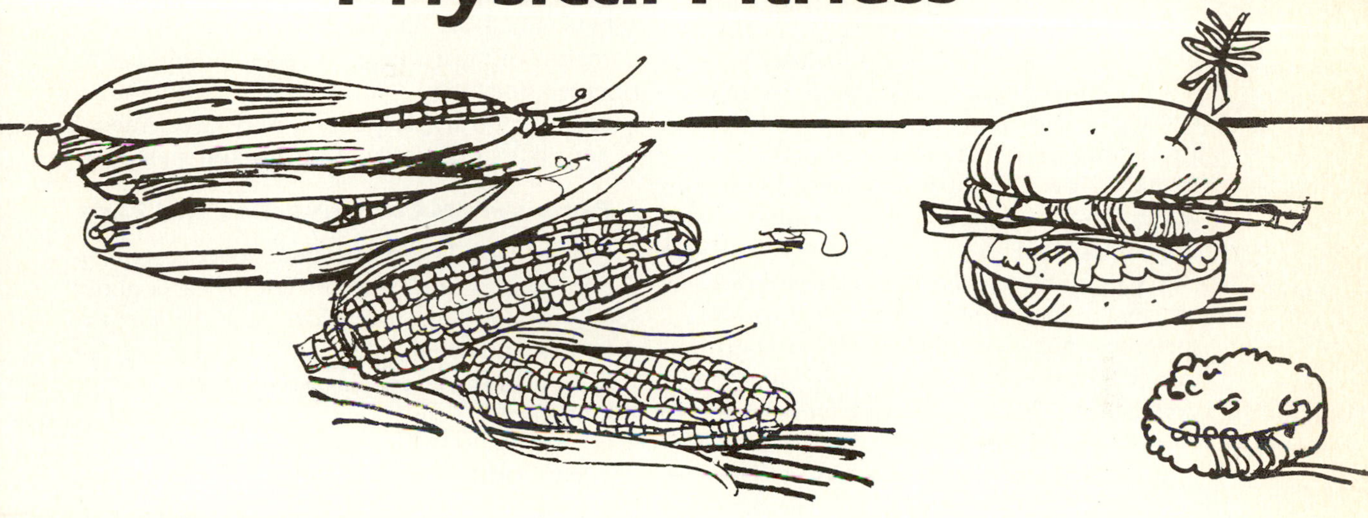

Why do I need to eat?
What should I eat to keep as physically fit as possible?
What is the truth about nutrients in food?
What happens to food in my body after I have eaten it?
How can I save money buying and preparing food and still have a tasty and nutritious meal?
Should I take vitamin and mineral supplements?
What is the best way to keep my weight down?
Do I have special nutritional needs during stressful periods?
Can I reduce my chances of heart disease and cancer by eating the right foods?
Should I eat less salt?
How can I separate fact from fiction when I hear or read about nutrition and reducing diets?
Just what are fats, carbohydrates, fiber, amino acids, protein, vitamins, and minerals?
Why should I study nutrition?
Where can I find more information to answer my questions?

The answers to these and to many other questions are what this book—and the subject of nutrition—is all about.

THE IMPORTANCE OF NUTRITION

The foods we eat contain thousands of compounds, but especially forty-four to forty-seven *nutrients. Nutrients are the highly important substances that each of us must consume in our diets in adequate amounts in order to live, be physically fit, grow, reproduce, and lead a full, healthy life.* Our bodies can not manufacture these nutrients. The *water* we drink, another nutrient, and the *oxygen* of the air we breathe are equally essential to our well-being.

From these relatively few essential nutrients that we must obtain from a source outside the body, our body tissues make literally thousands of substances essential for life and physical fitness. Most substances produced by the body are far more complicated than the few nutrients required in our diets.

If our bodies could manufacture, in some manner, the essential nutrients that we now obtain from our food, we would not have to eat at all. But, of course, that is impossible. In common with green plants and all other forms of life, we must be provided first with water plus seventeen or so minerals and trace elements from some outside source (see Chap. 13 to 17). Our bodies, however, are more specialized than green plants. As with most higher animal species, we must obtain from our food twenty-six or more additional nutrients in order to have normal life and physical fitness. The additional nutrients (the vitamins, amino acids, fats, and probably several carbohydrates for energy and roughage) are, with few exceptions, rather simple organic chemicals.

The essential nutrients are vital to provide the equivalent of fuel, catalysts, and machinery so that we can grow, move about, see, hear, taste, smell, feel, speak, think, learn and remember, walk, run, play, sing, love, innovate and create, avoid many infections, repair our tissues, and regenerate our species. All of these things and more are possible only if we first consume in our food at least minimal amounts of each of the forty-four to forty-seven essential nutrients in some form or another on a regular basis. If we eat an inadequate amount or too much of some, these functions will be impaired. Life itself is dependent on what we eat.

Nutrition, then, may be defined as *the science of food as it relates to optimal health and performance.*

Each of us is, or should be, vitally interested in promoting or protecting our own health, since upon it depends our well-being, our work capacity, and even our length of life. How we choose our food, as well as how and where we choose to eat, also affects our budget, our environment, and our social and cultural life. Nutrition is more than just eating the right nutrients; as a field of study it has chemical, physiological, biochemical, and behavioral aspects, and it reaches into the realms of agriculture, food technology, medicine, sociology, anthropology, economics, ecology, business, politics, and government, as well as international health and stability.

Facts *versus* Controversies and Fads

The rapidly developing science of nutrition has accumulated a mass of facts about how foods are used for building healthy bodies and what constitutes the best type of diet, within budgetary limitations. At the same time, while still producing a mass of new facts, nutritionists are working closely today with other scientists in areas of research on human diseases where facts are often difficult to obtain. These areas often overlap with the interests of clinicians, immunologists, cancer experts, and other specialists. Final conclusions about these diseases may take many years to reach.

Since clear-cut answers are not always available, many differences of opinion exist, even among scientists. The result is a nutrition controversy. When the difference is between scientists as a group and nonscientists who have a product or idea to promote, the topic generally becomes known as a food fad or a health fad. In some instances it is recognized that the nonscientist may turn out to be right in the long run. More rarely, traditional folk remedies have been the basis for later important scientific discoveries. Most fads today, however, are without a scientific basis.

Throughout this book the authors will be discussing—and in many instances, highlighting—the most controversial areas today of nutrition as it is applied to humans. Some of these areas fit well into the "fad" category.

The authors will give what they believe is the best available answer or advice about these controversies. Where no answers are available yet, students will be referred to supplementary readings and reliable sources of nutrition information so they can perhaps judge for themselves with the help of their teachers.

Controversies that will be studied in various degrees of detail are listed in Table 1–1. Many of them are critically examined and highlighted in special sections of the book under the heading of "health considerations." Many others not listed in this table are also discussed in various chapters, as are various current nutrition-related fads. Some of the controversies examined are fad weight-reducing diets, "meganutrition," "forbidden foods," macrobiotics, "hot" and "cold" foods, high vitamin C intake for pro-

Table 1–1 SOME CURRENT CONTROVERSIAL NUTRITION TOPICS TO BE DISCUSSED[a]

Topic	*Primary Chapter(s)*
What constitutes reliable nutrition information?	1 (also see 2–25)
Diseases related to nutrition	1 (and throughout)
Is there malnutrition in North America? (Are deficiencies widespread?)	1, 8–12, 15–17, 20–24
What is the role, if any, of dietary fiber?	2, 20
How much sugar is too much?	2, 20, 23, 24
Lactose intolerance and milk consumption.	2, 5, 20
What is the role, if any, of alcohol in the diet?	3
Are we eating excessive amounts of fat? Is fat toxic? (also fat and heart disease)	3, 20
Are we eating excessive amounts of protein?	4, 20
What is our protein requirement?	4, 20, 22, 23, 25
Is a small degree of overweight harmful? (What is an ideal weight?)	7
What is a sound diet for reducing weight? (Is there a place for "fad" diets?)	7
Is there a role for vitamin supplements?	8–12, 20
Megavitamins. (Can vitamins be toxic?)	8 (also see 9–12)
Vitamin A: acne and cancer	9
Vitamin B-6 in infant foods	11
Vegetarianism—is it harmful or desirable? (or does it make a difference?)	11, 20
Vitamin C and colds (Is vitamin C toxic?)	12
Vitamin C and cancer	12
Mineral supplements—general	13
Bottled vs. tap water	13
Water and the athlete	13, 21
Blood pressure and salt intake	14
What is excessive salt intake?	14
Can osteoporosis be prevented or treated by calcium? By fluorine?	15, 17
Magnesium and heart disease	15
Are "organic foods" superior?	16
Is there a need for mineral supplements?	13, 16, 20

continued

Table 1–1, continued

Topic	*Primary Chapter(s)*
How much iron do people need?	16, 21–23
Hair mineral analysis—a reliable technique?	17
Trace elements and cancer	17
Is caffeine harmful?	18
Are food additives good or bad?	18
Should we enrich our foods with more nutrients?	18
Food fads—what is believable?	19
What is the most important meal?	19, 20
What controls eating habits?	19 (also see 7, 20)
What roles, if any, do snacks have in nutrition? In "empty calorie" foods?	19, 20
What constitutes a good diet? (Should there be one national dietary guideline?)	20
Raw foods—effect of cooking?	20 (also see 8–12)
Do elderly persons have special nutritional needs?	20 (also see 9–12)
Are there special nutritional needs for physically active persons?	21 (also see 7)
What are the special energy and nutrient needs, if any, during pregnancy and lactation?	22
What are the advantages of breast feeding?	22, 23
What about vitamin-mineral supplements for infants and children?	23
Sugar and dental caries	24
Are there advantages to fluoridation of water supplies?	24
What can we do about malnutrition in developing countries?	25

[a]These topics are discussed, and most of them are critically examined and highlighted as "health considerations" in the chapters indicated. Many other controversial areas are described in the text. More research is needed on each of these topics.

tection against colds, and laetrile and pangamic acid.

Why Study Nutrition?

We face many of these controversies and fads often—sometimes every day. To make informed decisions is sufficient reason by itself for college students (as well as the public) to have some basic knowledge about nutrition. There are many other good reasons, however, for anyone who has to make food choices to understand basic nutrition facts.

Nutrition as Vital to Health. Good nutrition is absolutely vital to good health. Although this fact has been known for centuries, it needs constant emphasis because so many conflicting factors affect each of us in our increasingly complex way of life. We are easily influenced to forget the basic need to choose food wisely.

In extensive studies on undernutrition, using human volunteers during World War II, Dr. A. Keys and his colleagues showed that changes in behavior and work capacity result from prolonged underfeeding (1). Today, hundreds of research studies are being conducted in many countries on animals and humans that demonstrate clearly that inadequate nutrition can result in, or is related to, lowered intelligence, abnormal behavior, and impaired mental health (2); damage to nerve and brain tissue (3); loss of resistance to infection (4); inadequate physical development and fitness, problems in pregnancy and infant growth, and many chronic diseases (5–9). (See Fig. 1–1, the next section, other chapters, and supplementary readings in the Appendix.)

Many chronic diseases are related directly or indirectly to what we eat. These diseases cost each nation much money and grief. In listing them, it should be kept in mind that poor nutrition habits alone are not their only cause. Generally, except for obesity, most bear relatively little relation to nutrition—10 percent or less in some diseases to up to 40 percent in others.

The diseases most closely related to what we eat include atherosclerosis and heart disease, high blood pressure (hypertension), stroke, obesity, liver disease, dental diseases, nutritional deficiencies, and certain developmental disorders. Also closely related are food allergies, many digestive diseases, infant mortality, certain cancers, diabetes in adults, certain skin disorders, softening of the bones (osteoporosis), and alcoholism. There are other nutrition-related diseases as well. All of these may be caused, in part, by deficiencies of nutrients or, in many instances, by excessive intake of specific nutrients. The authors cannot promise in this text—nor can anyone—that a person can ward off these diseases by choosing food wisely. Wise eating habits, however, can reduce a person's chances of suffering these diseases at any given age. Eventually, of course, one has to succumb from some cause, if not just from old age. Nevertheless, the value of preventive medicine in lengthening the span of a healthy life has been demonstrated over and over again.

Many chronic diseases start during the college years, if not before. Though their long-term effects are not generally obvious early

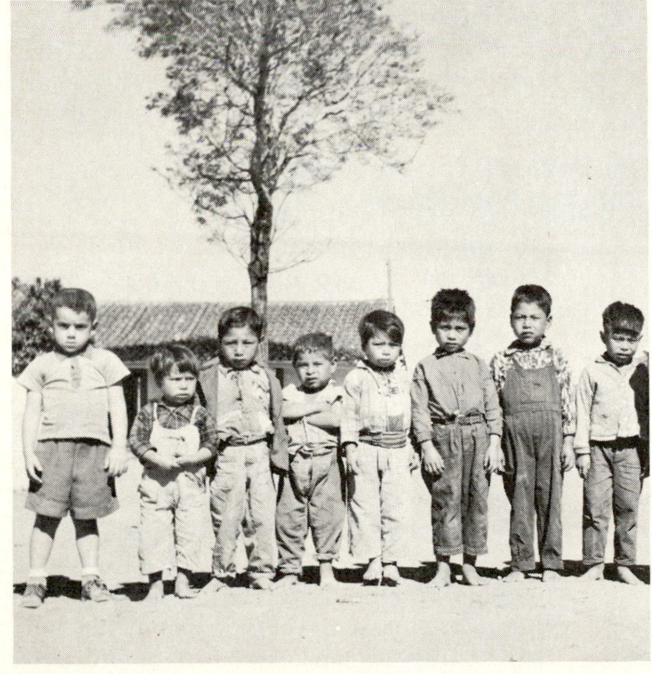

Normal Stunted growth

Figure 1–1 A group of Guatemalan boys, showing stunted growth caused by the inadequate native diet, as compared with a boy of the same racial stock who had a superior diet and is of normal weight and height for his age. The boy at left (normal) is four and a half years old, while the seven boys next to him range from five to eight years of age. (Courtesy Dr. Miguel A. Guzman, Institute of Nutrition for Central America and Panama.)

in life, it is certain that a person at any age without good nutrition and physical activity can not enjoy maximum health. Dental caries, digestive disturbances, skin disorders, alcohol toxicity, and overweight are examples of nutrition-related diseases commonly seen in college-age students. These and other nutrition-related problems will be discussed in the following chapters.

Health Costs of Nutrition-Related Diseases. The high cost of maintaining or recovering our health is another reason why we should study nutrition. In the United States the total national health bill is more than $321 billion per year and still is increasing rapidly. This figure is 10.3 percent of the gross national product.[1] The health bill includes costs of doctors, drugs, health care, hospital stays, dental care, health insurance, and other costs, amounting to an average of about $1,360 per year per person based on a population of 236 million people. This cost per person is far greater than the annual income of each of many hundreds of millions of individuals in the world.

Poor nutrition and the misuse of food and alcohol reflect only a part of these health costs, but they are a very significant part. It was estimated in 1977 that the costs in the United States of poor nutrition and food misuse amounted to at least $40 billion or more a year (10). This estimate was made when the nation's health bill was much less than it was in the 1980s, so it is a conservative figure. Most of this cost is due to the care necessary in long-term diseases and in illness resulting from misuse of alcohol.

Food Costs. Another practical reason why we need to know about obtaining the best nutrition that we can from our food supply is the amount of money we spend unnecessarily on food. In developed countries, people spend on an average at least 16 to 20 percent of their total budget, including time and money, in buying, preparing, and eating food and cleaning up afterwards. In the United States, for instance, people spend more than $380 billion for eating, including food eaten at home and outside the home. This amount averages more than $1,600 per person per year, or $4.50 per day. This sum, however, is much more than is necessary for a nutritious meal. Obviously, Americans prefer to spend considerable money for the social aspects of food, for convenience, and to please their taste buds. They also waste a lot of food. It needs to be remembered that in many parts of the world only $0.10 to $0.20 are available per person per day for food. This low amount can provide only for the basic necessities of a nutritious meal, if that, and the bare minimum of labor-saving devices. Such a diet would be mainly grains (such as corn or rice) and beans and a few low-cost vegetables and fruit. The authors are not suggesting that American students try to get along on this budget unless they wish to experience first hand the difficulties of people in developing countries.

[1]J. Amer. Med. Assoc., *249*:2223, 1983; Chem. Eng. News, *61* (No. 26):6, 1983.

Need for Training Policymakers in Nutrition

People in countries such as the United States, with a plentiful supply of a wide variety of foods, do not necessarily choose the right kind and amount of food to eat. It should be obvious then, with so many health problems associated with poor food choices, that it would benefit everyone to have adequate knowledge of nutrition.

Especially in need of such knowledge are the decision makers, those members of the various health professions and makers of food policy who have the responsibility of feeding others (11). These people include those who participate in health education programs, such as homemakers, nurses, doctors, dentists, elementary school teachers, home economists, social workers, and health and physical education teachers. They also include extension workers in the field of nutrition, public health workers, food scientists, food industry and advertising personnel, and managers of public eating places and school lunchrooms. Complete training and up-to-date knowledge of nutrition is required by nutritionists at all levels, such as teachers of nutrition, public health nutritionists, dietitians, and nutritional scientists in public and private institutions. More medical schools need to incorporate nutrition in the training of physicians.

The United Nations food and health agencies are concerned with attempting to bring more of the right kinds of food to people in developing countries all over the world, many of whom now exist at a semistarvation level. It should be clear to all, including United States leaders, that no country can achieve the vigor essential for economic, social, and political stability without adequate nutrition for all its people.

Nonnutritional Factors and Good Health

Although proper nutrition provides an essential basis for health, good health also depends on one's life-style, heredity, environment, and freedom from disease and accidents. Infection, disease, stress, emotional instability, excessive consumption of drugs and alcohol, smoking, and lack of exercise may counterbalance the effects of a good diet. Persons who do not eat luxuriously but whose mode of life involves more exercise may often be more healthy. Less physical work in the factory and home, together with the almost universal use of the automobile, often results in Americans getting little exercise.

Fortunately, in the past several years the interest of college students and the public in physical fitness has increased. This trend is desirable and is closely related to opportunities for improved nutrition and better health (see Chap. 21).

Malnutrition in the World

Malnutrition is a term widely used to mean faulty or poor nutrition in all of its aspects, whether from inadequate intake of nutrients or overconsumption of foods.

In spite of years of accumulated knowledge of the importance of adequate food and of good nutrition for the health of people, hunger and malnutrition exist throughout the world—even in the so-called developed countries.

In the United States, typical of many highly industrialized countries, the nutritional situation has improved somewhat over what it was ten or twenty years ago. At least 30 percent of the U.S. population, however, have diets that fail to measure up to standards for one or more nutrients, especially iron, calcium, vitamin A, vitamin C, riboflavin, and, in many instances, zinc, magnesium, folacin, calories, and still others (12-14). Especially vulnerable to malnutrition are young children, adolescents, pregnant women, the poor, handicapped persons, alcoholics, and people aged more than sixty-five.

The situation in the United States is not much different from that in most other industrialized countries, such as Canada, the European countries, Australia, and Japan. Hunger and malnutrition are still widespread, however, in most of the nonindustrialized and the developing countries—especially those in the tropical areas of South and Central America, in Africa, in India, and in many other Asian countries, including the islands from the Philippines to the East Indies and New Guinea. In some of these countries there is much hunger. Effects of malnutrition are common, including blindness from vitamin A deficiency, anemia, scurvy, and poor growth of babies and children as a result of deficiencies of protein, calories, and many other nutrients (Fig. 1–2). Eventually chronic malnutrition in a society can be a direct or indirect cause of high mortality figures at all age levels.

Many national and international groups–such as the World Health Organization (WHO), the United Nations Educational, Scientific, and Cultural Organization (UNESCO), and the Food and Agricultural Organization (FAO) of the United Nations—and many public and private groups in many parts of the world are attempting to solve the world malnutrition problem, but the task is immense (15). (See Chap. 25 and the supplementary readings in the Appendix.)

Factors Affecting What We Eat

Our food habits often stem from prejudices acquired in childhood, either from parental examples or from childish whims that are indulged. Education that explains why we should choose foods that will supply all the essentials for an adequate diet can provide the motivation to change old food habits for new ones. This is especially true when food habits in the home are based on cultural or religious practice. Deeply rooted food habits, if bad, can often be overcome by suggesting that larger amounts of certain liked or permitted foods be taken or that new foods be prepared in favorite or familiar styles. Diet fads and advertising may also induce a person to subsist on an unbalanced diet that furnishes too little of certain essential nutrients. The foods we eat are also determined by what we can afford to buy—our economic condition.

Complacency and indifference are also strong factors working against change of food habits. Unless people have a vision of the greater vitality to be attained by improving their food habits, they are apt to believe that they are well enough off as they are. There must be education as to why certain foods are essential for health. Remote goals, including longevity, can strongly influence

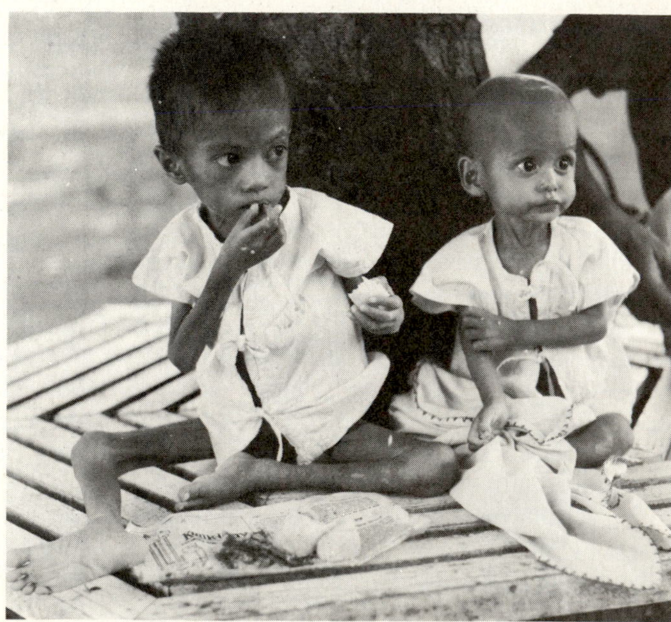

Figure 1–2 Sad and listless, these children show all the signs of advanced malnutrition. Scene is the Southern Islands General Hospital in Cebu, the Philippines. (Courtesy of UNICEF and Mallica Vajrathon. Used with permission.)

choice of foods in the diet. With teenagers and young adults, a more immediate objective, such as the physical prowess, athletic ability, and good looks that are associated with buoyant health, may prove more effective in stimulating interest in good food habits. Young college women, as prospective mothers, should be vitally interested in good diets to safeguard their own health and that of their children: Instead, they are often careless in their eating habits or follow reducing fads in order to retain slender figures.

Still other factors affect what we eat and hence our poor choice of food. Among them are peer pressures to consume poor foods, improper food labeling, lack of home gardens, lack of adequately prepared meals in the home, skipped breakfasts and other meals, and poor snacking habits. Additional factors are lack of physical activity; the widespread availability of inferior, imitation, and fabricated foods and candy; and lack of a national food policy (including inadequate enrichment standards, inadequate control of advertising, and insufficient public service messages on television).

In developing countries many other causes of malnutrition include prevailing poverty, overpopulation, illiteracy, social deprivation, poor sanitation and disease, indifference, and the "inability to cope." Persons working to combat malnutrition in the United States or any place in the world will recognize that working toward the reversal of these causes of malnutrition is necessary if we are ever going to have healthy nations.

Functions of Foods

The primary function of food is providing us with nourishment, but it is useful to us in other ways as well.

The Functions of Nutrients. Nutrition has been defined earlier as the science of food as it relates to optimal health and performance—that is, providing adequately for the body's growth, maintenance, repair, and reproduction. Except for the water we drink and the oxygen we breathe, the needs of the body must be met by the intake of foods. To nourish the body and to qualify as a food, foods must contain nutrients that function in one or more of three ways:

1. furnish body fuel, substances whose oxidation in the body sets free the energy needed for its activities
2. provide materials for the building or maintenance of body tissues
3. supply substances that act to regulate body processes

An individual nutrient may fulfill all three of these functions or only one, but all three functions must be served by the diet as a whole in order to maintain the body in health. Most foods can fulfill more than one function because they are mixtures of a number of nutrients. (See Fig. 1–3.)

Other Uses of Foods. In addition to nourishing us, foods serve less essential purposes such as satisfying our hunger and our individual requirements of taste. They also play a social role. People may eat to ease tension or relieve anxiety and boredom. Consumption of foods often serves as the central focus of celebrations, holidays, anniversaries, and the like; food may even be used as a reward or as a punishment. Students will doubtless be able to think of still other uses. (See Chap. 19.)

THE STUDY OF NUTRITION

Because nutrition is so important to our well-being, we should know as much about it as possible. We need to know the classes of nutrients, their proportions in the composition of various foods, and ways to study foods and choose them wisely.

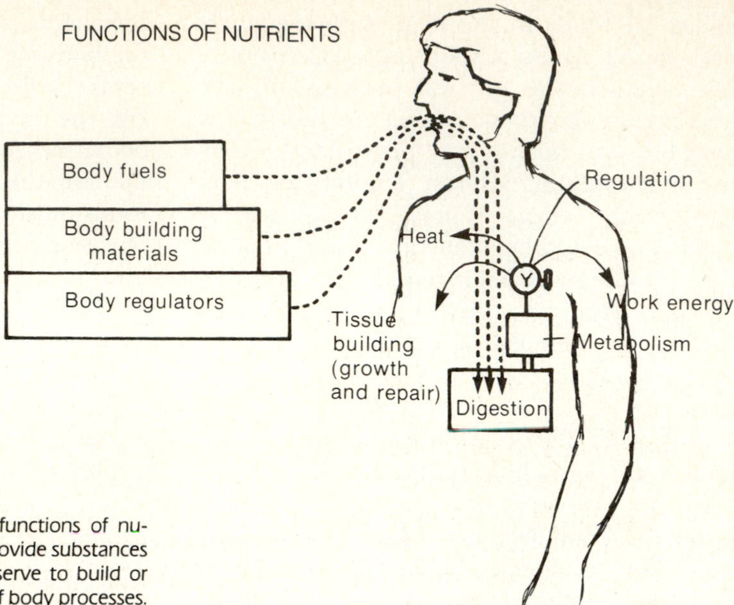

Figure 1–3 Diagram summarizing the functions of nutrients. To qualify as a nutrient food must provide substances that act as body fuel to provide energy, serve to build or maintain body tissues, or act as regulators of body processes. Many foods contain nutrients that serve all three purposes.

Classes of Nutrients

Six general classes, or kinds, of nutrients found in foods that are necessary to the body are as follows:

1. carbohydrates
2. fats
3. proteins (amino acids)
4. vitamins
5. minerals
6. water

Carbohydrates, fats, and *proteins* are often spoken of as the fuel, or energy-yielding nutrients, since they are the only substances that the body can use to supply energy for work and heat. They belong to the great division of chemical substances known as *organic* compounds, which contain carbon and are combustible. The *mineral elements* and *water* are called *inorganic* nutrients, since they do not contain carbon.

Proteins, minerals, and water all enter into the composition of body tissues and hence are necessary for building new tissues or repairing those already built.

Vitamins are chemically diverse organic substances that occur in minute quantities in foods but are essential for normal growth and health. Certain ones may be built into or stored in the tissues, but their chief function is to help regulate body processes. Mineral salts and vitamins act as body regulators by promoting oxidative processes, normal functioning of nerves and muscles, and vitality of tissues. They also assist in many other bodily functions.

Water also serves as an important regulating substance in the body. It holds substances in solution in the digestive juices, blood, and tissues and aids in regulation of body temperature, excretion, circulation, and many other body processes. Vegetable fiber acts along with water to promote intestinal elimination.

The three energy-yielding nutrients—carbohydrates, fats, and proteins—can be used by the body more or less interchangeably to supply energy, depending on which is more abundant in the diet. Next to water, these three classes of substances are the most abundant nutrients in our food; minerals and vitamins make up a relatively small, or even trace, portion.

For building tissues, different proteins are not completely interchangeable, since the "building blocks," or *amino acids,* that compose them vary in kind and relative amounts. Some nine or ten of these amino acids cannot be made in the body and must be supplied in the diet. Also, the fats eaten must supply two essential *fatty acids.* Some seventeen or so different mineral elements must be supplied, in either major or minor amounts, and thirteen different vitamins are known to be needed. Hence, including water and oxygen, there are actually some forty-four to forty-seven different nutrients known to be essential for normal nutrition, and there are probably others not yet identified. (These are all discussed in detail in Chap. 2–6 and 8–17.)

General Composition of Foods and Units of Measurement

It is important that the nutrition student have a basic understanding of the major differences in the distribution of the six classes of nutrients in common foods of distinctly different origins. Table 1–2 shows the composition of fresh and of dried corn (maize), a typical plant, compared with a typical animal body on the same basis. A column also is included for hamburger, a typical animal food. It should become obvious, after study of this table, that a major characteristic of animals that eat largely vegetable material and grain is the conversion within the animal body of plant carbohydrates to body fats (after energy needs). Along with making this conversion, the animal body accumulates minerals and protein. Only small amounts of carbohydrates are present in animal tissues (see Chap. 2). Knowing the figures in Table 1–2, one can estimate, in a rough, general way, the composition of almost all foods, plant or animal.

The detailed composition of many common foods is given in Table 2 of the Appendix for further comparison. In order to understand food composition tables and to have a clear idea of the amounts of foods that we actually need and eat, one must first

Table 1–2 SOME TYPICAL COMPOSITION FIGURES OF PLANTS VERSUS ANIMALS

Classes of Nutrients	*Corn (Maize) Fresh*	*Corn (Maize) Dried*	*Typical Animal Body (Live Basis)*	*Typical Animal Body (Dried)*	*Hamburger (Fresh)*
	%	%	%	%	%
Water	75.0	12.0	60.0	12.0	50.0
Carbohydrates					
Fiber ("dietary")	2.7	9.6	0.0	0.0	0.0
Other carbohydrates[a]	18.3	64.1	trace	0.1	trace
Crude fats	1.1	4.0	19.0	41.7	25.0 to 30.0
Crude proteins[b]	2.5	8.8	17.0	37.0	19.0 to 24.0
Minerals	0.4	1.3	4.0	9.0	1.0
Vitamins[c]	trace	0.2	trace	0.2	trace
Total percent	100.0	100.0	100.0	100.0	100.0
Kcal/100 gm	93	328	(239)	(523)	319 to 346

[a]Primarily starch and sugars.
[b]Including small amounts of other compounds containing nitrogen.
[c]Including choline and inositol, not considered necessary vitamins for humans.

be at home with the various units of weight and measurement commonly used in nutrition. Most countries of the world now use the metric system, which is by far the most useful way to describe and measure vitamins and trace minerals. It makes calculations easier at all levels. A kilogram (kg) equals 2.2 pounds (which can be visualized, roughly, by thinking of slightly more than 2 pounds of butter or margarine, flour or sugar, or a quart of milk). A pencil eraser or one lima bean weighs about 1 gram (gm); a penny weighs nearly 3 gm; and a shelled egg about 50 gm. A milligram (mg) of sugar would be about the size of a small pinhead—just visible. A microgram (μg) of sugar would not be visible to the eye but a microgram of lint, though very small, can generally be seen (because this amount of lint is far less dense than sugar).

Useful conversion figures are shown in Table 1–3. Students' understanding of nutrition will be much more complete if they learn these relationships now.

Table 1–3 COMMON UNITS USED IN NUTRITION AND IN MEASUREMENT OF FOODS[a]

Metric units[b]	1 kilogram (kg) = 1000 grams	
	1 gram (cm) = 1000 milligrams	
	1 milligram (mg) = 1000 micrograms (mcg., μg., or γ)	
	Metric	***U.S. Avoirdupois***
Weight	1 kilogram = 1000 gm	= 2.2 pounds
	0.1 kilogram = 100 gm	= 3.52 ounces (3.5 oz)
	0.454 kilogram = 454 gm (450 gm)	= 1.0 pound = 16 ounces
	0.028 kilogram = 28.4 gm (30 gm)	= 1.0 ounce
Volume, liquid	3.785 liters = 3750 ml (3.8 l)	= 1 gallon = 4 quarts[c]
	1.000 liter = 1000 ml	= 1.06 quarts
	0.946 liter = 946 ml (950 ml)	= 1 quart = 2 pints = 4 cups
	0.473 liter = 473 ml (475 ml)	= 1 pint = 2 cups = 16 fluid ounces
	0.237 liter = 237 ml (240 ml)	= 1 cup = 16 tablespoons (tbsp)
	0.015 liter = 14.8 ml (15 ml)	= 1 tablespoon = 3 teaspoons (tsp)
	4.9 ml (5 ml)	= 1 teaspoon
Weight per volume of water[d]	1 liter = 1 kg	
	1 milliliter = 1 gm = 1 cubic centimeter (cc)	
	1 quart = 946 gm (950 gm)	
	1 cup[e] = 237 gm (240 gm)	= 8 fluid ounces = ½ pound

[a]Many of these are approximations only. See Appendix for more conversion values. (We should use the metric system whenever possible to avoid the confusion demonstrated by the above table, which must be used when we work with two systems.) In cooking and in calculating dietary intakes figures are often "rounded off" as indicated.

[b]Kilo means × 1000; milli, × $\frac{1}{1000}$; micro, × $\frac{1}{1{,}000{,}000}$. Therefore, kilogram means gram × 1000; milligram means gram × $\frac{1}{1000}$; and milliliter means liter × $\frac{1}{1000}$.

[c]British Imperial Gallon = 4.545 liters.

[d]Other liquids may be lighter (e.g., salad oil) or heavier (e.g., honey, corn syrup) than water.

[e]A cup is not an official unit of measurement. The values given here are approximations only to help one visualize sizes and weights. The weight of a "cup" depends on what is being measured, of course.

Ways to Study the Composition of Foods

What nutrients and how much of each are present in our various everyday foods is usually determined by:

1. chemical analysis
2. biological assay (including microbiological assay)
3. physical methods

Chemical Analysis. Chemical analyses provide useful data on the approximate composition of carbohydrates, fats, proteins, minerals, vitamins, and water in any given food. Methods commonly used for determining the relative amounts of the nutrients are briefly discussed as follows.

Water is determined by weighing a sample of the food before and after drying to constant weight. The difference represents the amount of water in the food.

Ash (mineral matter) is determined by weighing after completely burning the combustible residue. Individual *minerals* are readily analyzed by modern chemical and physical methods.

Protein is computed by multiplying the nitrogen content of a food (chemically determined) by 6.25, since proteins are known to consist of about 16 percent (one-sixth) nitrogen by weight. This is the classic "Kjeldahl method." Slight errors result both because other nitrogen-containing substances that may be present in the food are included as proteins and because proteins vary somewhat in the amount of nitrogen they contain. This measure, nitrogen × 6.25, is often referred to as crude protein for this reason.

Fats are determined by extracting a dried sample of the food with ether. With the true fats (weighed after evaporating to dryness the ether extract) will be included small amounts of other ether-soluble substances such as resins, waxes, and coloring matter (pigments). This measure is often called crude fat, or ether-extract.

Carbohydrates are usually calculated "by difference"; that is, the remainder of the weight not accounted for under the total of the above headings is assumed to be carbohydrate in nature and is listed as such. Although this residue undoubtedly does consist largely of carbohydrates, it will also include organic acids (in fruits and vegetables); fiber, or indigestible carbohydrates (cellulose and hemicelluloses, etc.); and various other undetermined substances not carbohydrates.

More accurate figures for individual carbohydrates, such as sucrose or fiber, may be obtained by direct analyses.

Vitamins must be determined individually. Most of the vitamins may be determined by chemical methods: by specific color reactions, by chromatography, or by complicated laboratory equipment using various chemical or physical properties of the vitamins studied.

Tables of food composition, obtained by the above methods, can never be absolutely accurate for several reasons. First, certain errors are inherent in the methods used or in the manner of calculating results. Second, even in the hands of skilled chemists, small errors occur that are magnified on calculating the composition from the basis of a small sample to a percentage basis for the food as a whole. Third, and probably of most importance, foods may vary considerably in composition either in samples from different sections of the country or from soils of different compositions. These factors may affect trace mineral levels in different samples of food, in different parts of the same sample of food, or especially in cooked foods where moisture and fat content are frequently variable. When a large number of samples of some raw food material, such as flour, milk, or eggs, have been analyzed, average values are obtained from which individual specimens probably will not differ much in composition. With cooked foods, fruits, and vegetables, or whenever only a few samples have been analyzed, variations will be larger and figures less accurate.

Biological Assay and Physical Methods. Biological assays involve actual feeding experiments on laboratory animals (usually rats, mice, guinea pigs, or chickens) or bacteria or protozoa under controlled conditions. White rats, whose heredity and previous diet history are known, are considered the best "standardized" animals and hence are likely to give the most accurate results (16). Moreover, the chemistry of their body tissues is, for the most part, reasonably similar to that of humans. Also their life cycle is short enough so that one can watch the effects of some special diet on several generations. Such animals are fed a simple diet of known composition that is planned so as to provide plenty of all the essential nutrients except one. A certain food is added to this basal diet in known amounts to serve as the sole source of the nutrient in which the diet is lacking and for which the special food is being tested. (See Fig. 1–4.)

By such experiments, for example, the existence of vitamins in natural articles of food was established. Likewise it was discovered that numerous different vitamins are necessary in the diet for the well-being of both humans and animals. Also the relative amounts of each vitamin supplied by different foods have been more or less accurately determined. Laboratory feeding experiments also give information, not obtainable by chemical analyses, as to how efficient the protein content of different foods is for growth or maintaining weight, and how well absorbed and utilized the mineral content of certain foods may be. Biological assays show us how effective different foods really are in supplying the needs of the body for each nutrient.

Each of the vitamins may now be deter-

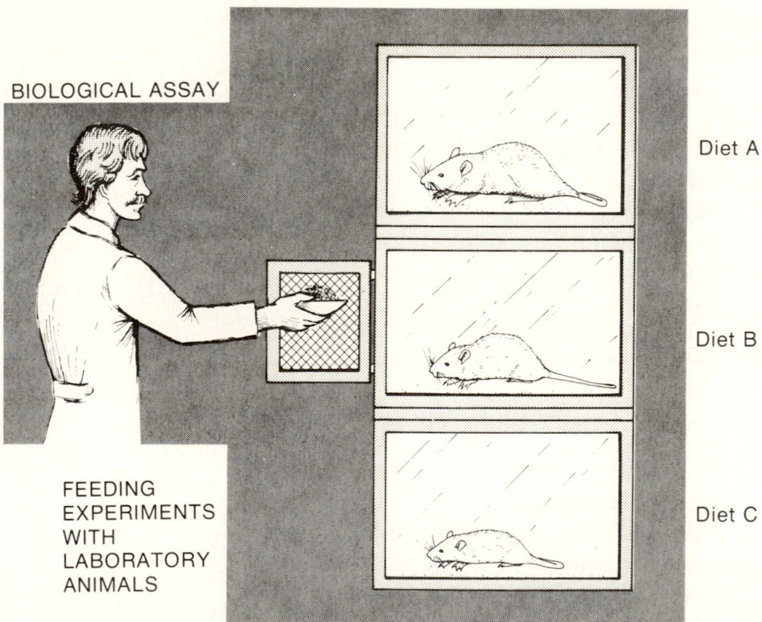

Figure 1–4 A biological assay is used to show how efficient different foods are in supplying body needs for proteins, amino acids, various mineral elements, or vitamins. The rat is a favorite animal for feeding experiments, and the effectiveness of the diet in supplying body needs is gauged by the relative growth and health of animals. In this drawing, the animal fed Diet A obviously got the most complete and adequate diet, while the other two rats fed diets B and C either made less growth or show varying degrees of deficiency of one or more essential nutrients. Normally at least eight to ten rats would be fed each diet. Normal recovery is obtained by adding back the missing nutrient.

mined by physical methods (measurement of absorption spectra, chromatography, fluorescence, turbidity, and so on), by chemical methods (chiefly by color reactions), or by microbiological assay (influence on growth of bacteria). Modern laboratories, to measure small amounts of vitamins, use mass spectrometry, gas chromatography, and, especially, high-performance liquid chromatography procedures. Feeding tests with animals, however, retain their usefulness and in some situations are indispensable.

Experiments with Humans. Experiments with humans are very costly and require great control and care to protect the health and rights of the subjects. Interpretation of the results of human studies is very difficult, partly because of psychic factors which can affect results. The use of *placebos* (pills that, unknown to the subject, contain a completely inactive substance such as sugar), as controls and *double blind tests* (in which neither the investigator nor the persons directly responsible for the giving of diets or supplements or for diagnosing the subjects know the composition of the dietary variables) should be standard procedures in studies of human nutrition. In such studies a code may be used for the various test groups that is disclosed only after the tests are all completed (17). Often studies are reported with incomplete or faulty statistical analysis, if such analysis is used at all.

Peer Review of Scientific Papers

When an experiment about a nutrition topic is completed, it is written in the form of a scientific paper, analyzed statistically, and submitted to a scientific journal to be considered for publication. If the editor considers it possibly suitable, he or she sends the paper to two or more associate editors, or reviewers, who are respected scientists. These *peer reviewers* critically examine the paper and recommend to the editor whether or not it should be published and their reasons. The editor then sends the reviewers' comments anonymously to the author(s) of the paper. This system of review is traditional and of proven value. Peer-review journals in the nutrition area are listed at the end of this chapter.

Unfortunately, many articles about nutrition reach nonscientific journals and magazines, newspapers, books, and pamphlets without peer review.[2] In such situations they just represent someone's opinion and may be right, speculative, or wrong. One needs to examine carefully the source of a piece of nutrition information before accepting the information as fact. Does the journal have an editorial board (a sign of peer review)? Is the author trained in the subject about which he or she is writing? Is the author an authority in the field and/or working at a creditable laboratory? Does the information provided make sense or is it contrary to all established opinion? (Such contradiction is not sufficient reason alone to doubt information but should be considered.) Does the article give sufficient information to allow the reader to evaluate the work, and could it be repeated in another laboratory? Does the author have something to sell?

Because there is lots of money to be made on nutritional products, the field has more than the average number of charlatans. That is another reason for people to learn all they can about nutrition.

A Food Plan Based on Food Groups

The different common foods may be grouped in several classes according to the nutrients they supply most abundantly. Thus, there have been in the past the "seven food groups," the "five food groups," and

[2]*Nutrition Today* and *Nutrition Action* are two well-known nutrition publications that are not peer reviewed in the usual sense. The *Journal of Applied Nutrition* is another example and cannot be considered reliable. There are many more.

more recently the well-known "four food groups." Foods grouped together in this way are similar in general chemical makeup and hence contribute the same types of nutrients to the diet. (See Chap. 20.)

The basis of good nutrition is eating a variety of foods from different food groups. No single food group supplies all the essential nutrients in proper proportions to maintain health, but a food plan that includes a suggested number of servings from different groups furnishes at least a major portion of the proteins, minerals, and vitamins needed for an adequate diet. Additional foods may be required to meet the energy needs, and these may be supplied by selecting extra portions of the foods listed in one of the basic groups or, after nutrient requirements have been satisfied, by choosing foods from the "primarily energy," or "fifth," group of sweets (such as sugars, candies, honey, syrups, cakes, jams) and fatty foods (such as butter, margarine, and salad oils,), items not included in usual food guides. These foods are useful chiefly for their fuel value, for pure sugar and fats contribute little except energy value to the diet. (Fats, however, may carry vitamins A and E and essential fatty acids.)

There are some major disadvantages to a food plan based on food groups. One is that many cultural, religious, and social groups of people in the United States and in most other parts of the world do not, or cannot, have all the foods in any particular group readily available to them. For instance, milk products are not universally used. A second is that today many manufactured foods are available in the market that do not conveniently fit into a single food group (for instance, pizza, hamburger "with the works," imitation cream products, or complete "meal replacements").

Alternate Food Plans

It is now clear that there are many ways possible to learn about good food choices. This is a rapidly developing field. The final selection of food by people depends on the types of foods readily available to and used by them and on their level of understanding about nutrition. In the United States new and improved guides for teaching about good nutrition are now available. Nutrition education in schools is being better supported at local, state, and national levels. There are now better guides for the feeding of infants and children and for different ethnic groups (for instance, Spanish-American and Chinese food guides are now widely available in the United States and elsewhere). Material is also available for pregnant women, for partial and complete vegetarians, for elderly persons living alone, and for people living in, or coming from, different countries and cultures, and for other special groups.

There is no magic or secret way to good nutrition, nor is the path easy. Some degree of nutrition knowledge is essential if an individual is going to ensure good health and physical fitness when so many forces around us today are working against those goals.

Chapter 20 has a more detailed discussion of various foods and their place in the diet for normal adolescents and adults. Chapters 22 and 23 discuss the special food needs of pregnant women and of infants and children, respectively, and Chapter 24 discusses the role of good nutrition in dental health.

Recommended Dietary Allowances as Standards

Throughout this text the authors have used the *Recommended Dietary Allowances* (RDA), published every five years or so by the Food and Nutrition Board of the National Academy of Sciences in the United States, as the major standard for adequacy of nutrient intake (see Appendix, Table 1, and Chap. 8 and 20) (9). Nearly every major country has its own standards, generally differing in some degree from the Academy standards. These differences exist because of differences of opinion; climatic, geographical, and social differences; differences in type of basic foods available; and other factors. Nevertheless, the standards of the various countries show many similarities.

The RDAs are "the levels of intake of essential nutrients considered . . . to be adequate to meet the known nutritional needs of practically all healthy persons." They are established for "healthy populations" and "population groups" rather than for specific individuals. The RDA committee, in its publication, states that "intakes below the recommended allowance for a nutrient are not necessarily inadequate, but the risk of having an inadequate intake increases to the extent that intake is less than the level recommended as safe." The committee also states that the RDAs "are intended to be met by a diet of a wide variety of foods rather than by supplementation or by extensive fortification of single foods." They suggest that the variety of foods be "acceptable, palatable, and economically attainable by the consumer using the RDA as a guide . . ." (9).

The United States Food and Drug Administration (FDA) has devised a simplified version of the allowances based on the older (1968) recommended dietary allowances of the academy. These are the United States Recommended Daily Allowances (USRDAs). They are used in commerce on food labels and vitamin and mineral supplement labels (see Chap. 18)—and have legal ramifications. They are easily confused with the RDAs, but they are not so scientifically accurate or helpful to a nutrition student as the Academy values. That is why the authors use the Academy RDAs as their major standard.

History of Nutrition

Nutrition begins with the beginning of humans on the earth. Many references to food and nutrition exist in the earliest writings. People had to seek the facts for themselves, largely by trial and error, as they chose their food from available plants, berries, nuts, roots, grains, and fruit, and from the plentiful supply of animal life. All history has been greatly influenced by the distribution, availability, and search for foods and spices.

Not until the development of modern science in the eighteenth and nineteenth centuries did an appreciation of the essential nature of certain nutrients begin. Among the first nutrients to be recognized as essential were protein, oxygen, calcium, iodine, and a scurvy-preventing factor (later identified as vitamin C). Most of these early milestones were in the years 1775 to 1825. Many of the early pioneers in nutrition and the more recent discoverers of the various nutrients will be mentioned later in this book.

Students interested particularly in nutrition history will find references on this subject in the supplementary readings in the Appendix. These readings will include the stories of the lives and discoveries of such early nutrition pioneers as Lavoisier, Priestley, Liebig, Bernard, Mulder, Spallanzani, Magendie, Davy, E. Fischer, Abderhalden, Beaumont, Voit, Lusk, Rubner, Chittenden, Lind, Lunin, Takaki, Eijkman, Hopkins, Mellanby, Babcock, Hart, Wills, McCollum, Osborne, Mendel, Funk, Elvehjem, Goldberger, Jansen, R. R. Williams, György, Kleiber, Dam, Steenbock, Mitchell, Evans, Forbes, Morgan, Armsby, Deuel, Best, Kuhn, Murlin, Sherman, Roberts, Atwater, Prout, and many others to whom we owe so much.

Likewise, others living today (though retired) have pioneered in nutrition discoveries that have greatly influenced the course of nutrition history and the health of all of us. Interested students will want to learn more about such nutrition pioneers as King, R. J. Williams, Folkers, Lepkovsky, Burr, C. Williams, Sebrell, Jukes, Stokstad, Snell, Davis, Szent-Györgyi, Rose, Stare, Darby, Todhunter, Norris, Waddell, and Almquist, along with many others.

As far as is known, the first professor of human nutrition in the United States was M. Jaffa, in 1908, at the University of California, Berkeley (18). In 1912 he became chairman of the Department of Nutrition at the Berkeley College of Agriculture. This may also have been the first department of nutrition in the country. Since then, nutrition departments or divisions have prospered in almost all American general colleges and universities and are widely scattered throughout the world. They exist independently at the undergraduate or graduate level or form part of such departments as home economics, public health, animal science, food science, medicine, or biochemistry. Generally the training of dietitians is closely associated with, or a part of, training in nutrition. There are still insufficient nutrition training centers, especially in medical schools.

Approximately 10,000 research papers on food and nutrition are published worldwide each year. The science of nutrition is well established throughout the world, and important discoveries are being made nearly every day. Almost every major country has a nutrition society and publishes its own scientific nutrition journal. The International Union of Nutritional Sciences (IUNS), more active than formerly, is in the process of setting up better international standards for nutrition research, nomenclature, and training.

A list of resource materials on the broader aspects of nutritional sciences may be found at the end of this chapter.

QUESTIONS

1. What is meant by nutrition? A nutrient? An adequate diet?

2. What is the difference between a nutrition controversy and a nutrition fad?

3. How is it possible to improve an apparently adequate diet, and what benefits may be expected as a result? Name the chief motives for making changes in food habits indicated as nutritionally desirable; name some of the factors that stand in the way of changing food habits.

4. What are the three functions of nutrients in the body? What other uses do foods have? Name the six kinds of essential nutrients found in foods. Which of them can serve as body fuel (energy) and why? Which are used in the building and repair of tissues? Which are necessary to regulate body processes?

5. Explain what is meant by the biological assay of foods. What information can be obtained by biological assay and how does it supplement facts obtained by chemical analysis? Describe how a food may be assayed for its content of a certain vitamin.

6. Make a record for two days of the amounts of each food you eat at each meal, including beverages and snacks. Calculate your daily intake of protein, fat, iron, calcium, vitamin A, vitamin C, and riboflavin and the energy that you consumed each day (using Table 2 of the Appendix) and compare with your RDA (inside the front cover). How could you improve your dietary habits?

7. As a special project, write a report on some aspect of the history of nutrition or on one of the nutrition pioneers.

References

1. Keys, A., et al.: *The Biology of Human Starvation.* Minneapolis, University of Minnesota Press, 1950.
2. Scrimshaw, N. S., and Gordon, E. (eds.): *Malnutrition, Learning and Behavior.* Cambridge, Mass., MIT Press, 1968; Read, M. S.: *Malnutrition, Learning, and Behavior.* Nat. Inst. Child Health Human Devel., U.S. Dept. HEW Pub. NIH–76–1036, 1976; Brozek, J.: Malnutrition and behavior. J. Amer. Dietet. Assoc. *72*:17, 1978; Nutrition and behavior. Dairy Council Digest, *50* (Sept.):25, 1979; Energy-protein malnutrition and behavior. Nutr. Rev., *38*:164, 1980; Levitsky, D. A. (ed.): *Malnutrition, Environment, and Behavior: New Perspectives.* Ithaca, Cornell Univ. Press, 1979; Hirsch, J., and Yarrow, M. R. (chairman): Effects of nutritional status on functional states. Amer. J. Clin. Nutr. *35* (Supplement, May):1200–1240 (6 papers), 1982.

3. Rodriguez, R., et al.: Nutrition and development of children from poor rural areas. Nutr. Rept. Internat., *19*:315, 1979; Anderson, G. H.: Diet, neurotransmitters and brain function. Brit. Med. Bull., *37*:95, 1981; Baer, M. T.: Nutrition and developmental disabilities. Nutrition Update, *1*:179, 1983.
4. Gross, R. L., and Newberne, P. M.: Role of nutrition in immunologic function. Physiol. Rev., *60*:188, 1980; Chandra, R. K.: Immunocompetence as a functional index of nutritional status. Brit. Med. Bull., *37*:89, 1981; Beisel, W. R.: Single nutrients and immunology. Amer. J. Clin. Nutr., *35* (Supplement, Feb.):417, 1982.
5. Winick, M. (ed.): *Nutrition and the Killer Diseases.* Vol. 10 in the series on Current Concepts in Nutrition. New York, John Wiley and Sons, 1981 (see other volumes in this series).
6. Goodhart, E. S., and Shils, M. F. (eds.): *Modern Nutrition in Health and Disease.* 6th Ed. Philadelphia, Lea and Febiger, 1980.
7. Hodges, R. E.: *Nutrition in Medical Practice.* Philadelphia, W. B. Saunders Co., 1980.
8. Recheigl, M., Jr.: Reviews relating to food, nutrition and health, a selected bibliography. World Rev. Nutr. Dietet., *16*:398, 1973.
9. Food and Nutrition Board: *Recommended Dietary Allowances.* 9th Ed. Washington D.C., National Research Council, National Academy of Sciences, 1980.
10. Select Committee on Nutrition and Human Needs, United States Senate (McGovern, G., chairman): *Dietary Goals for the United States.* 2nd Ed. Washington, D.C., U.S. Gov't. Printing Office, Dec., 1977.
11. Herbert, V.: Will questionable nutrition overwhelm nutrition science? Amer. J. Clin. Nutr. *34*:2848, 1981; Young, E. A.: Nutrition: An integral aspect of medical education (a review). J. Amer. Dietet. Assoc. *82*:482, 1983.
12. Pao, E. M., and Mickle, S. J.: Problem nutrients in the United States. Food Tech., *35* (Sept.):58, 1981 (also see pp. 40, 50, and 70); See also Chapter 8 (ref. 26) and supplementary readings in Appendix.
13. Consumer Nutrition Center: *Food and Nutrient Intakes of Individuals in One Day in the United States, Spring 1977. Nationwide Food Consumption Survey 1977–78,* Preliminary Rept. No. 2. USDA, Science and Education Administration, Sept. 1980.
14. Simopoulos, A. P. (ed.): Assessment of nutritional status (Conference proceedings). Amer. J. Clin. Nutr., *35* (Supplement, May):1089–1325 (many papers), 1982; Chandra, R. K.: Poverty amidst plenty: The enigma of malnutrition in affluent North America (editorial). Nutr. Res., *2*:211, 1982.
15. Sevenhuysen, G. P., and Burgess, A. P.: Evaluation of nutrition interventions. Food Nutr. (FAO, United Nations), *6* (No. 2):40, 1980 (also see other articles on this topic in this and other issues of this journal, as well as in other United Nations publications); Schuftan, C.: Nutrition intervention programmes for rural areas: African experiences. J. Trop. Pediatr., *27*:177, 1981; Barr, T. N.: The world food situation and global grain prospects. Science, *214*:1089, 1981; Chichester, C. O., and Owen, D. F.: *World Hunger: Debate or Action* (a symposium). Food Tech., *35* (Sept.): 93–119 (5 papers), 1981; Brady, N. C.: Chemistry and world food supplies. Science, 218:847, 1982.
16. Newberne, P. M., et al.: Control of diets in laboratory animal experimentation. ILAR News (National Academy of Sciences), *21* (No. 2):A 1, 1978; Bieri, J. G., et al.: *Report of the AIN ad hoc Committee on Standards for Nutritional Studies.* J. Nutr. *107*:1340, 1977 (also see J. Nutr. *112*:567, 1982); Oser, B. L.: The rat as a model for human toxicological evaluation. J. Tox. Environ. Health, *8*:521, 1981; Clough, G.: Environmental effects on animals used in biomedical research. Biol. Rev., *57*:487, 1982.
17. DerSimonian, R., et al.: Reporting on methods in clinical trials. New Eng. J. Med., *306*:1332, 1982.
18. As cited in the University of California Bulletin of 1908.

Also see supplementary readings in Appendix for additional literature citations.

General Nutrition Resources

Journals (peer reviewed and/or generally reliable)

Agenda (formerly *War on Hunger*) (monthly). Agency for International Development, Department of State, Washington, D.C. 20523.

American Journal of Clinical Nutrition (monthly). American Society for Clinical Nutrition Inc., 9650 Rockville Pike, Bethesda, Maryland 20014.

American Journal of Public Health (monthly). American Public Health Association Inc., 1015 15th Street N.W., Washington, D.C. 20036.

British Journal of Nutrition (with the *Proceedings of the Nutrition Society*) (bimonthly and three times annually, respectively). Cambridge University Press, Bentley House, 200 Euston Road, London NW 1, or 32 East 57th St., New York, N. Y. 10022.

Cereal Science Today (monthly). American Association of Cereals Chemists, 3340 Pilot Knob Rd., St. Paul, Minnesota 55104.

CERES, FAO Review (bimonthly), and *Food and Nutrition* (biannually). Food and Agriculture Organization of the United Nations. Available in major cities of the world, including Rome (Vai delle Terme de Caracalla, 00100) and New York (UNIPUB, Inc., 650 First Ave., P.O. Box 433).

Ecology of Food and Nutrition (quarterly). Gordon and Breach Science Publishers Ltd., One Park Avenue South, New York, N.Y. 10016 or 42 William IV Street, London, W.C. 2.

Federation Proceedings (monthly). Federation of American Societies for Experimental Biology, 9650 Rockville Pike, Bethesda, Maryland 20014 (containing review articles and abstracts of the American Institute of Nutrition, etc.).

Food Technology (monthly). Institute of Food Technologists, Suite 2120, 221 N. LaSalle St., Chicago, Illinois 60601.

Human Nutrition (in two separate sections—*A: Applied Nutrition* and *C: Clinical Nutrition)* (monthly). John Libbey & Co. Ltd., 80/84 Bondway, Vauxhall, London SW81SF.

Indian Journal of Nutrition and Dietetics (monthly). SRE Avinashilingan Home Science College, Coimbatore–11, India.

Journal of the American Dietetic Association (monthly). American Dietetic Association, 620 North Michigan Ave., Chicago, Illinois 60611.

Journal of the American Medical Association (weekly). American Medical Association, 535 North Dearborn St., Chicago, Illinois 60610.

Journal of the Canadian Dietetic Association (quarterly). 385 Yonge St., Suite 304, Toronto, Canada M5B1S1.

Journal of Food Science (monthly). Suite 2120, 221 N. LaSalle St., Chicago, Illinois 60601.

Journal of Home Economics (ten times a year). American Home Economics Association, 1600 20th St., Washington, D.C. 20009 (see also Home Economics Research Review, same address).

Journal of Nutrition (monthly). American Institute of Nutrition, 9650 Rockville Pike, Bethesda, Maryland 20014.

Journal of Nutrition Education (quarterly). Society for Nutrition Education, 1736 Franklin St., Oakland, California 94612.

New England Journal of Medicine (weekly). Massachusetts Medical Association, 10 Shattuck St., Boston, Massachusetts 02115.

Nutrition Abstracts and Reviews, Section A (monthly). Commonwealth Bureau of Animal Nutrition, Rowett Research Institute, Bucksburn, Aberdeen, AB 2 9SB, Scotland.

Nutrition and Cancer (quarterly). Franklin Institute Press, Box 2266, Philadelphia, Pennsylvania 19103.

Nutrition Reports International (monthly). Geron-X, Inc., Box 1108, Los Altos, California 94022.

Nutrition Research (bimonthly). Pergamon Press, Fairview Park, Elmsford, New York 10523. (Vol. 1 in 1981)

Nutrition Reviews (monthly). The Nutrition Foundation, 888 17th St. N.W. Suite 300, Washington, D.C. 20006.

Public Health Reports (monthly). U.S. Dept. Health and Human Services, Rm. 814 Reporter's Bldg., 300 Seventh St., S.W., Washington, D.C. 20201.

(Note: for other peer-reviewed nutrition journals, not quite as available as the above, see Supplementary Readings, Chapter 1, in Appendix.)

Nutrition Review Series Published Annually (usually very reliable)

Advances in Food Research
(Vol. 29 in 1983)

Advances in Nutrition Research
(Vol. 5 in 1983)

Annual Review of Nutrition
(Vol. 3 in 1983)

Current Topics in Nutrition and Disease
(Vol. 7 in 1983)

Nutrition Update
(Vol. 1 in 1983)

Vitamins and Hormones
(Vol. 41 in 1983)

World Review of Nutrition and Dietetics
(Vol. 41 in 1983)

Other Sources of Nutrition and Food Information (generally reliable)*

American Dental Association, 211 E. Chicago Ave., Chicago, Illinois 60611.

American Dietetic Association, 620 North Michigan Ave., Chicago, Illinois 60611.

American Heart Association, 7320 Greenville Ave., Dallas, Texas 75231.

American Home Economics Association, 1600 20th St. N.W., Washington, D.C. 20009.

American Medical Association, 535 North Dearborn St., Chicago, Illinois 60610.

Cereal Institute Inc., Education Department, 135 So. LaSalle St., Chicago, Illinois 60603.

Food and Agriculture Organization, Rome or New York (UNIPUB, Inc., 650 First Ave., P.O. Box 433). (Publishes various nutrition education materials and booklets. Also has a library for nutrition workers in developing countries described in J. Nutr. Educ. *8*:160, 1976.)

Food and Drug Administration, Washington, D.C. (Provides miscellaneous consumer information, including the "FDA Consumer.") Office of Public Affairs, 5600 Fishers Lane, Rockville, Maryland 20852.

General Mills, Inc., P.O. Box 1113, Minneapolis, Minnesota 55440. (Publishes *Contemporary Nutrition* monthly.)

National Academy of Sciences, Food and Nutrition Board, 2101 Constitution Ave., Washington D.C.

National Dairy Council, 6300 North River Rd., Rosemont, Illinois 60018. (Publishes a bimonthly "Dairy Council Digest" and quarterly "Nutrition News." Local Dairy Councils in most large cities are staffed with qualified nutritionists.)

National Live Stock and Meat Board, 444 North Michigan Ave., Chicago, Illinois 60611. (Publishes a monthly "Food and Nutrition News.")

National Nutrition Consortium, 24 Third St. N.E., Suite 200, Washington, D.C. 20002.

Nutrition Foundation, Inc., 489 Fifth Ave., New York, N.Y. 10017.

Nutrition Week (weekly). Community Nutrition Institute, 2001 S St. N.W., Washington, D.C. 20036. (Also publishers of the *Community Nutritionist*, new in 1982.)

*Also see supplementary readings in Appendix.

Society for Nutrition Education, 1736 Franklin St., Oakland, California 94612. (Has a national clearinghouse of nutrition education information.)

U.S. Department of Agriculture (Cooperative Extension Service; Food and Nutrition Service; Consumer Marketing Service; Agricultural Research Service; Office of Information; or National Library of Agriculture), Washington, D.C. 20250.

U.S. Department of Health and Human Services, Washington, D.C. (Children's Bureau; National Institutes of Health; Office of Child Development.)

U.S. Government, Consumer Information Center (free catalog of publications available on request), Pueblo, Colorado 81009.

World Health Organization, P.O. Box 5284, Church Street Station, New York, N.Y. 10249.

2 Carbohydrates: Sugar, Starch, and Fiber

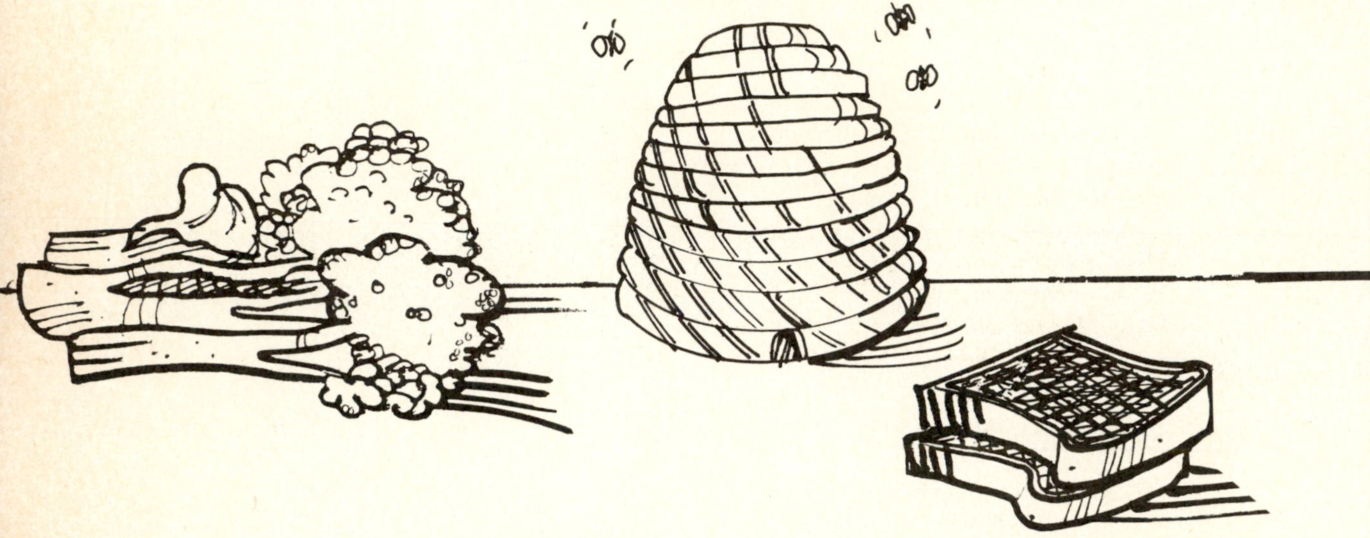

THE ENERGY NUTRIENTS

All living things need energy. In humans and other higher animals, the need for energy is second only to the need for air and water. A critical role of many vitamins and minerals is to facilitate and regulate the utilization of the chief energy-yielding nutrients—carbohydrates, fats, and proteins.

Ultimately, the energy we use comes from the sun. Green plants capture light energy through the process of photosynthesis, storing this solar energy in the form of organic compounds[1] that are used by higher animals for their nutrition.

[1]Organic compounds are substances that contain the element carbon. Most natural products from plant and animal sources are organic in that they contain carbon. Numerous synthetic chemicals, including drugs, pesticides, and plastics, also are organic in the proper sense of the term, that is, they contain carbon.

Classes of Energy Nutrients

By far the most abundant nutrients in foods are carbohydrates, fats, and proteins. Together they constitute about 85 to 99 percent of the dry matter present in foods; the only more abundant constituent of many unprocessed foods is water. Most natural foods contain all three nutrients but in widely varying proportions. The only other significant dietary source of energy is alcohol.

All *carbohydrates* are made up of the elements carbon, hydrogen, and oxygen. The hydrogen and oxygen are almost always present in the same two-to-one proportion as in water. Hence carbohydrate—"carbo" (for carbon) and "hydrate" (for water)—is the class name. Most food carbohydrates are either sugars (such as ordinary table sugar, honey, and corn syrup) or more complex compounds (polysaccharides) formed from the union of many sugar groups, such as the starch in cereals and potatoes.

Fats are also composed of carbon, hydrogen, and oxygen, but these elements are present in relative amounts different from those in carbohydrates. All true fats are alike in chemical nature and physical properties: They have a greasy feel, are insoluble in water, but are soluble in such solvents as alcohol and gasoline.

Proteins consist of carbon, hydrogen, and oxygen (again in proportions different from those in carbohydrates or fats) and, in addition, the element nitrogen. Most proteins also contain some sulfur, and others contain phosphorus, iron, iodine, or other trace elements. Proteins characteristically have a "gluey" consistency and are precipitated or coagulate on heating. The word protein, meaning "to come first," indicates the primacy of protein as an essential nutrient, beyond its role as an energy source.

Alcohol is the class name of chemical compounds containing a particular configuration of oxygen and hydrogen (—OH, a hydroxyl group) linked to carbon. The alcohol present in beer, wine, and whiskey is called ethyl alcohol or ethanol in chemical terms and grain neutral spirits in industry.

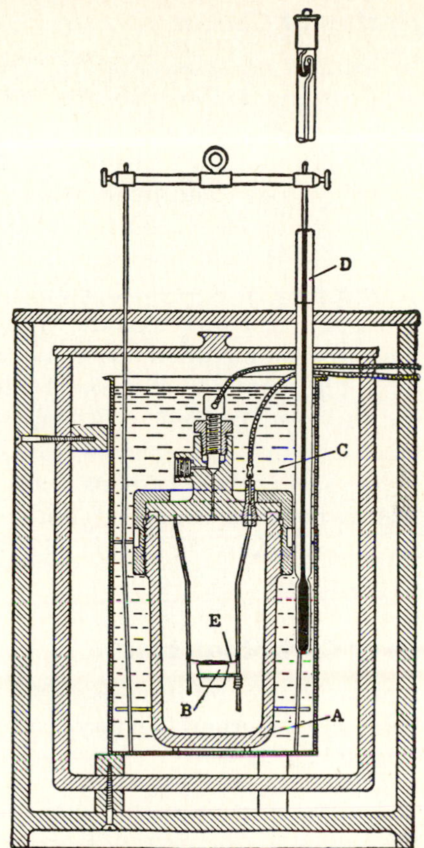

Figure 2–1 Cross-section diagram of the adiabatic bomb calorimeter used for determination of the fuel value of foods. A weighed sample of the food is placed in dish B in the inner chamber, which is charged with oxygen and sealed tight. The burning is set off by an electric spark (passed between the wires), and the heat liberated is measured by the rise in temperature of a known volume of the surrounding water; the outer sections are for insulation to prevent loss of heat to exterior. (Courtesy of Emerson Apparatus Co., Boston, Mass.)

Energy Value of Nutrients

The energy value of a pure nutrient or a natural food may be determined by direct calorimetry, that is, by complete oxidation in a calorimeter (Fig. 2–1). The energy released is measured by the rise in temperature of a known volume of water. The energy unit traditionally used by nutritionists is the kilocalorie (kcal), the amount of heat required to raise 1 kilogram (kg) of water 1° Centigrade; one kilocalorie is equal to 4.18 kiloJoules (kJ).[2] The average heats of combustion of nutrients differ due to differences in chemical composition. The amounts of energy nutrients provide to the body are further affected by completeness of digestion and utilization by the tissues (1). Based on a large number of human feeding studies, it is concluded that rounded figures of 4, 9, and 4 kcal per gram of carbohydrate, fat, and protein, respectively, are acceptable rough estimates of the energy value of nutrients in typical Western diets. Alcohol yields about 7 kcal per gram.

[2]The Joule is the accepted unit of work energy; 1 Joule equals 10^7 ergs.

Description of Carbohydrates

Carbohydrates are subdivided into several groups, according to the size and relative complexity of their molecules.

All simple sugars have a chain of carbons linked with hydrogen and hydroxyl groups, in the configuration H—C—OH or its mirror image HO—C—H, and one carbon doubly bonded with oxygen (C=O, called an aldehyde group when it occurs at the end of a molecule and a ketone when it is in the inner structure). The names of sugars all end in -ose, and they are grouped according to the number of carbons in the chain. For example, a sugar having three carbons is a triose. The chief carbohydrates in foods and in the body are either hexoses (6-carbon sugars) or multiples of hexose sugar groups.

Classes of Carbohydrates

The major classes of carbohydrates are listed below. Important dietary carbohydrates are in bold face.

Monosaccharides, or simple sugars, consist of one sugar unit.
- trioses: glyceraldehyde, dihydroxyacetone . . .
- pentoses: ribose, xylose, arabinose . . .
- hexoses: **glucose** (dextrose)[3]
  fructose (levulose)[3]
  galactose
  mannose, sorbose

Disaccharides are composed of two sugar units.
- **sucrose** (glucose + fructose)
- **lactose** (glucose + galactose)
- **maltose** (glucose + glucose)
- trehalose . . .

Other oligosaccharides have up to ten sugar units.
- raffinose, stachyose, verbascose . . .

Polysaccharides consist of many sugar units.
- dextrin (all glucose)
- plant starches: **amylose** (all glucose)
  amylopectin (all glucose)
  inulin (mainly fructose)
- animal starch: glycogen (all glucose)
- dietary fiber, partially or completely indigestible
  - **cellulose** (all glucose)
  - **pectin, gums,** agar, guar gum . . . (mainly galacturonic acid)
  - **hemicellulose,** pentosans, mannosans . . . (mainly pentoses)

Derivatives of monosaccharides have slightly different structures.
- sugar alcohols: glycerol (3 carbons)
  xylitol (5 carbons)
  sorbitol, mannitol . . . (6 carbons)
- amino sugars: glucosamine, galactosamine . . .
- uronic acids: glucuronic acid, galacturonic acid . . .

[3]A beam of polarized light passing through a solution of glucose is bent to the right—hence the common synonym for glucose, dextrose, from dextro ("on the right" and -ose ("sugar"). A solution of fructose bends light to the left, so fructose is also called levulose from levo ("on the left").

The carbohydrates just named are merely a sample of the wide variety found in nature. Some are not present in nutritionally significant amounts in foods but play important parts in human metabolism—trioses and pentoses, for example. Amino sugars and uronic acids are constituents of important tissue substances, often linked with proteins. The sugar alcohols are reduced forms of sugar, having a hydroxyl group in place of the aldehyde or ketone group. Glycerol is a basic component of fat molecules.

Chemical Structure of Carbohydrates

Each molecule of glucose consists of 6 carbon, 6 oxygen, and 12 hydrogen atoms; in other words, its formula is written as $C_6H_{12}O_6$. The carbon atoms are linked with each other in a chain (Fig. 2–2A) or in a ring form (called pyranose structure) (Fig. 2–2B). The characteristic features that make this sugar glucose (rather than another hexose) are the presence of an aldehyde (terminal C = O) group, and the exact configuration of the hydroxyl (OH) groups at carbons 2 through 6. The other common hexoses—

H
$C^1{=}O$
$H{-}C^2{-}OH$
$OH{-}C^3{-}H$
$H{-}C^4{-}OH$
$H{-}C^5{-}OH$
$H{-}C^6{-}OH$
H

C^6H_2OH, C^5, O, C^4, C^1, C^3, C^2, H, OH

A. STRAIGHT-CHAIN STRUCTURE B. RING OR PYRANOSE STRUCTURE
GLUCOSE

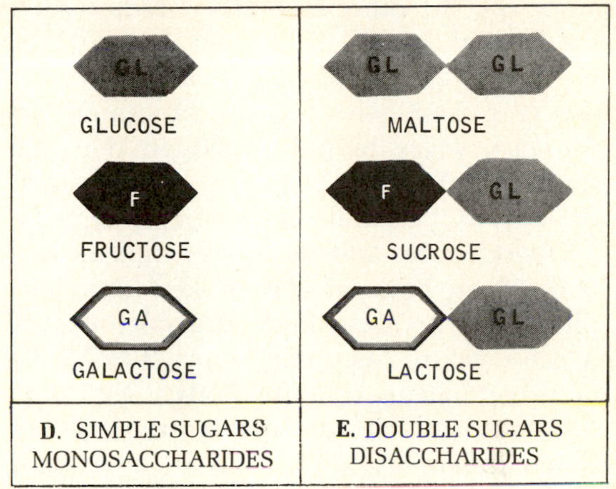

D. SIMPLE SUGARS MONOSACCHARIDES

E. DOUBLE SUGARS DISACCHARIDES

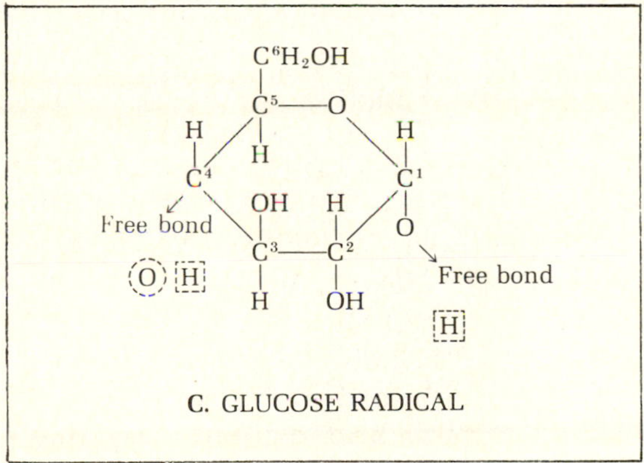

C. GLUCOSE RADICAL

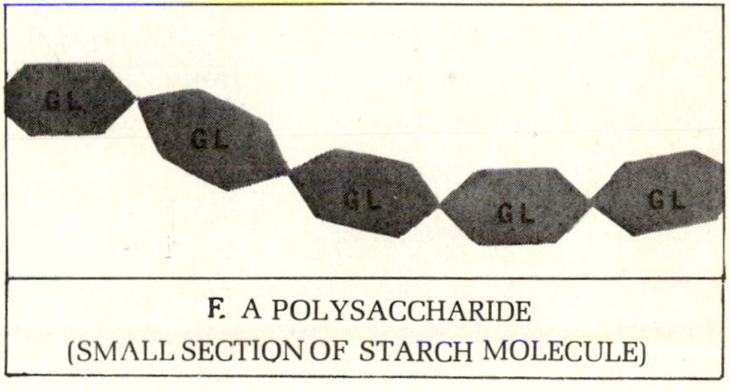

F. A POLYSACCHARIDE (SMALL SECTION OF STARCH MOLECULE)

Figure 2–2 Diagram showing arrangement of the atoms in a molecule of the monosaccharide glucose in (A) a straight-chain configuration and (B) a ring (pyranose) configuration, which are freely interchangeable forms of glucose dissolved in water. The carbon atoms have been numbered to show how the ring is arranged. In (C), a glucose radical is shown with two free bonds, each of which could be linked to another monosaccharide. If only one bonding site is used, the resulting compound will be a disaccharide as in (E); or if both bonds are used and many glucose radicals are linked, the resulting compound will be the polysaccharide starch, as in (F). The glucose group, or radical (C), is represented as having lost a hydrogen atom and a hydroxyl radical (OH) in the process of linking with other sugar groups. When broken apart by hydrolysis, these component parts of water (H and OH) are taken up again, and glucose molecules are split off.

fructose and galactose—both have the same formula ($C_6H_{12}O_6$), but the hydrogen and oxygen atoms are arranged differently, which makes them different substances and gives them their different properties. These properties are the basis for identifying the sugars and determining the amount present in foods.

The linkage of sugar groups to form di- and polysaccharides is shown in Figure

2–2E. When two simple sugars unite to form a disaccharide, one loses a hydrogen atom and the other a hydroxyl radical, and these combine to form water (H—OH or H_2O) (Fig 2–2C). In polysaccharide formation (Fig. 2–2F), one molecule of water is lost for each sugar radical added, so the final formula is always $C_n(H_2O)_{n-1}$, rather than the $C_nH_{2n}O_n$ formula of the simple sugars.

Disaccharides and the more complex carbohydrates must all be broken down by digestion into the simple sugar groups of which they are composed before they can be absorbed and used by the body. (See Chap. 5.) The digestible saccharides are split into monosaccharides by hydrolysis, a reaction with water (hydro-, "water," -lysis, "breaking down"). In this change, the water lost in formation of the complex carbohydrate is added back to yield the same simple sugars as were present initially. In animals and in honeybees, hydrolysis is brought about by the action of digestive enzymes. In cookery and industrial processing, usually the reaction is achieved by the action of acid and heat.

Food Carbohydrates

The two principal categories of food carbohydrates are sugars and polysaccharides (starches, fiber).

Sugars. Sugars are very soluble in water and are the form in which carbohydrate is transported in plant sap or stored in the juices of fruits. Hence, glucose, fructose, and sucrose are found chiefly in plant juices and in fruits[4] (Table 2–1). The sweet taste of corn and peas is due to the presence of sugar that will be converted to starch as the immature seed ripens; in some fruits (for example, bananas) starch is present in the unripe fruit and turns to sugar on ripening. Carrots, beets, onions, winter squash, turnips, and sweet potatoes are vegetables that contain appreciable amounts of sugars.

The "sugar" used at table and in cooking is *sucrose,* a disaccharide made up of glucose and fructose. It comes chiefly from juices of the sugar cane or sugar beet (over one third of our supply is derived from the latter source). The sugar obtained from the sap of the sugar maple tree is also sucrose. Fructose and glucose occur in honey in about 50–50 proportion, as it is a digestion product mainly of sucrose from plant nectar.

The sugar *maltose* is formed as an intermediate product during the digestion of starch in the body and is also found in germinated grains such as "malt," and in products prepared from partly digested starch, such as breakfast foods and malted milk. Maltose contains two glucose molecules.

Acid hydrolysis of corn starch yields *glucose* (and intermediate products, that is, maltose and dextrin) and is the principal industrial source of glucose. Food technologists have developed a method for converting glucose to fructose, a much sweeter sugar. Although little fructose is naturally present in the diet, fructose is increasingly used to replace sucrose in processed foods. Commercial corn syrup usually has some sucrose or fructose added for flavor. Regrettably, foods are sometimes advertised as containing no sugar when, in fact, they have much fructose added.

The sugar *lactose* occurs in the milk of most mammals. On digestion it is broken down into glucose and galactose. All young mammals, except some marine species, can digest lactose, but the enzyme required (lactase) falls to very low levels in most adults. Caucasians of Northern European extraction

[4]Plants form galactose, but only a trace or none is present as the simple sugar; rather, it is linked with glucose and fructose to form the trisaccharide raffinose, the tetrasaccharide stachyose, and other oligosaccharides. The linkage is made differently from that in common disaccharides and starch, and the digestive system of higher animals cannot break the bond formed, so these sugars are not absorbed.

Table 2–1 FREE SUGARS IN UNPROCESSED FOODS,[a,b] gm/100 gm

	Total Solids	*Total Carbo-hydrates*[c]	*Total Sugar*	*Sugars* GLUCOSE	FRUCTOSE	SUCROSE	*Other*
Fruits							
Apple	15	15	11	1.2	6.0	3.8	Maltose, tr.
Apricot	15	13	8	1.9	0.4	5.5	—
Banana, ripe	24	22	20	4.5	3.5	11.9	—
Figs, dried	(80)	74	73	42.0	30.9	0.1	—
Grape	18	16	14	5.4	5.3	1.3	Maltose, 1.6
Orange	14	12	9	2.5	1.8	4.6	—
Peach	13	10	9	0.9	1.2	6.9	Maltose, 0.1
Prunes, dry	72	67	47	30.0	15.0	2.0	—
Strawberry	9	8	6	2.1	2.4	1.0	Maltose, 0.1
Vegetables							
Beet (red, root)	11	9	7	0.2	0.2	6.1	Raffinose/ Stachyose, tr.
Broccoli	12	6	2	0.7	0.7	0.4	—
Lettuce	5	3	1	0.2	0.5	0.1	—
Potato, white	20	17	1	—	—	—	Raffinose/ Stachyose/tr.
Sweet potato	23	22	9	0.3	0.3	3.4	—
Tomato	5	4	2	1.1	1.3	tr.	—
Legumes							
Beans, dry	89	61	7	—	—	2.4	Raffinose, 0.8 Stachyose, 3.4
Green beans	8	5	3	1.1	1.2	0.2	Raffinose, 0.1 Stachyose, 0.2
Peas, fresh	26	14	4	—	0.1	3.0	Raffinose, 0.1 Stachyose, 0.1
dry, split	91	63	14	0.2	—	4.1	Raffinose, 1.8 Stachyose, 8.0
Soybean, dry	90	34	8	—	—	4.5	Raffinose, 0.7 Stachyose, 2.7

[a]Values from Shallenberger, R. S. (2), Hardinge, M., Swarner, J. B., and Crooks, H. J. (3), U.S. Department of Agriculture Handbook No. 8 (4), and Paul, A.A., and Southgate (5). Dash (—) means value unknown; tr means trace amount.

[b]The disaccharide lactose, or milk sugar, makes up 7.5 percent of human breast milk and 4.5 percent of fluid whole cow's milk. Dry skim milk powder is 52 percent lactose, and dry whole milk is 38 percent lactose. Additional values for lactose will be found in Chap. 5, Table 5–3.

[c]By difference; therefore includes fiber and starch.

and some pastoral African groups appear to be an exception to this rule and retain the ability to digest lactose through adulthood. If the digestive enzyme is low or absent, then lactose cannot be digested and absorbed. (See Chap. 5.).

Sugars are not equal in sweetness. Some are barely sweet at all (Table 2–2). Fructose is much sweeter than sucrose but lactose is only one-third as sweet. Other compounds than sugars can evoke the sensation of sweetness; saccharin is a well-known example (sweetness is 500 times that of sucrose). Several of the amino acids also have a very sweet taste. The sugar alcohols sorbitol and mannitol are nearly as sweet as glucose; maltitol and xylitol approach sucrose in sweetness. Sugar alcohols are used to add sweetness to

Table 2–2 SOME SWEET-TASTING SUBSTANCES

Substance	*Relative Sweetness Sucrose = 1.0*
Artificial sweeteners	
Neohesperidin dihydrochalcone[a]	1500
Saccharin (sodium salt)	500
Aspartame(dipeptide)[b]	160
Cyclamate (calcium salt)[c]	100
Sugars	
Fructose	1.7
Invert sugar[d]	1.3
Sucrose	1.0
Glucose	0.7
Maltose	0.4
Lactose	0.2
Sugar alcohols	
Maltitol	0.9
Xylitol	0.9
Mannitol	0.7
Sorbitol	0.6
Amino acids	
Tryptophan	30
Glycine	0.8

[a]New sweetener derived from citrus peel.

[b]Trade name for a synthetic compound made from two amino acids, phenylalanine and aspartic acid.

[c]Cyclamate is not allowed in foods because of the possibility that it can lead to cancer. An end-product of cyclamate that can be formed in the body (cyclohexylamine) also is known to raise blood pressure.

[d]Invert sugar is a hydrolysis product of sucrose, and is half glucose and half fructose. Honey is also hydrolyzed sucrose and has the same sweetness.

"sugarless" chewing gum and some dietetic foods. Sorbitol is absorbed more slowly than glucose but has about the same energy value; mannitol is less completely absorbed and so it has a slightly lower energy value.

Polysaccharides. *Starch* is the carbohydrate found in seeds, tubers, and roots. It is formed by union of many molecules of glucose (from 300 up to many thousands). Starch occurs in two structural forms. One form (amylose) consists of long, unbranched chains (wavy or kinked so as to form a three-dimensional spiral); the other form (amylopectin) has highly branched chains. Such large molecules have no sweet taste.

In plants, starch is laid down in "granules" of characteristic size and shape, so the source of a starch can be determined by microscopic examination. Starch grains commonly have about 15 to 20 percent amylose and 80 to 85 percent amylopectin. (The waxy varieties of rice and maize corn are very low in amylose, which accounts for the difference in texture.) When subjected to moist heat (as in cooking), starch granules absorb water, swell, and rupture. After such treatment, starch is more easily digested. *Dextrins* (and the sugar maltose) are intermediate products formed in the process of breaking down starch to glucose; dextrins are more soluble than starch, and their molecules may average about one fifth the size of those of starch.

Cellulose is also a polysaccharide of glucose, but because the glucose units are linked differently, it is resistant to degradation. *Hemicelluloses* are not, as one might think, a smaller version of cellulose; they are polysaccharides made up of varying proportions of xylose, arabinose, mannose, galactose, other sugars, and uronic acids. *Pectins,* polysaccharides made up of galacturonic acid, galactose, and arabinose units, are found in small quantities in many fruits and some vegetables; pectin is the agent responsible for the setting of jelly and jam. (See Table 2–3.) Cellulose and hemicellulose (and a noncarbohydrate compound, lignin) make up the structural or fibrous part of plants (leaves, stems, roots, and seed and fruit coverings) and also the cell walls. This group of polysaccharides is not digested by humans. It is used by bacteria and thus serves as an energy source for ruminants.[5]

[5]Lignin is very resistant to attack, even by microorganisms, which is the reason that wood and sawdust (very high in lignin) are not used for cattle feed.

Table 2–3 POLYSACCHARIDES AND LIGNIN IN FOODS, gm/100 gm[a]

Food	Total Solids	Total Carbo-hydrate	Starch	Dietary Fiber: Cellulose	Hemi-Cellulose	Pectin	Lignin	Total Dietary Fiber	Crude[b] Fiber
Fruits									
Apple with skin	15	15	—	0.7	0.2	2.6	0.2	3.7	1.0
Apricot	15	13	0.8	—	1.2	1.0	—	2.2	0.6
Banana									
yellow-green	24	22	8.8	—	—	—	—	—	—
yellow	—	—	1.9	0.2	0.1	1.0	0.5	1.8	0.5
Orange, peeled	14	12	0	0.3	0.3	1.3	—	1.9	0.5
Prunes, dry	72	67	0.7	2.8	10.7	0.9	—	14.4	1.6
Vegetables									
Broccoli	12	6	1.3	0.9	0.9	—	—	1.8	1.5
Cabbage, raw	8	5	—	0.8	1.0	0.4	0.1	2.3	0.8
Carrot	12	10	—	1.0	0.5	2.2	0.1	3.8	1.0
Lettuce	5	3	—	0.4	0.6	0.2	0.1	1.3	0.5
Potato, white (no skin)	20	17	15.0	0.4	0.3	1.4	0.1	2.2	0.5
Spinach	9	4	—	0.3	0.2	—	0.1	—	0.6
Sweet potato (no skin)	23	22	16.5	0.6	1.4	2.2	—	4.2	0.9
Tomato	5	4	—	0.2	0.3	0.3	tr.	0.8	0.5
Legumes									
Beans, common dry seed	89	61	35.2	3.1	6.4	—	—	9.5	4.3
Green or snap beans	8	5	2.0	0.5	1.0	0.5	—	2.0	1.0
Peas, green, fresh	26	14	4.1	0.5	1.0	—	0.4	3.7	—
dry, split	91	63	38.0	5.0	5.1	—	—	10.1	1.2
Nuts									
Chestnuts, Virginia	48	42	18.6	0.3	—	—	—	0.3	1.1
Peanuts, no skins	95	18	4.0	2.4	3.8	—	0.2	6.4	1.9
Cereals									
Corn (maize)									
fresh, sweet	27	22	14.5	0.6	0.9	tr.	—	1.5	0.7
Corn, dry, whole	88	74	62.0	4.5	4.9	—	0.2	9.6	1.6
Cornflakes, cereal	96	85	60.0	0.4	0.2	—	0.1	0.7	0.7
Oatmeal	91	64	48.0	1.0	4.8	4.5	1.1	11.4	2.0
Rice, polished, dry	88	80	72.9	0.3	—	—	—	0.3	0.3
Wheat, wholegrain, dry	87	69	59.0	2.0	5.8	—	0.8	8.6	2.3
flour, white	88	76	68.8	0.4	0.7	—	0.1	1.2	0.5
bran[c]	90	65	17.4	(15)	(32)	3.0	3.2	53.2	8.9

[a]Values from Hardinge, M., Swarner, J. B., and Crooks, H. J. and U.S. Department of Agriculture Handbook No. 8 (3). Those in parentheses are estimates from secondary sources. Dietary fiber includes cellulose, hemi-cellulose and pectin. Dash (—) means value is unknown; tr. means trace amount.

[b]Crude fiber refers to material not digested by laboratory methods. Human digestion is not so complete.

[c]Values for wheat bran are from the American Association of Cereal Chemists (Standard bran R07-3691) (4).

Other indigestible or only partially digestible polysaccharides occur less commonly in plant foods. *Inulin,* found in Jerusalem artichokes, is made up of fructose units. Gums, found in some seeds, are viscous in water and contribute, for example, to the characteristic texture of oatmeal porridge. *Agar, alginic acid,* and *carrageenan* are gums present in seaweeds; they are used industrially as thickening agents in ice cream and salad dressing. These carbohydrates plus cellulose, hemicellulose, pectin, and lignin constitute what is generally called roughage or dietary fiber. Plants also contain some nondigestible sugars (raffinose, stachyose). The hard covering of shrimp and crayfish is made of chitin, an indigestible polymer of a type of glucosamine; it also occurs in fungi and insects.

The "crude fiber" value given in most tables of food composition refers to the residue remaining after particular chemical procedures of food analysis; it includes cellulose and lignin but not all the other indigestible carbohydrates. Thus "crude fiber" in ordinary diets is only about one fifth the value of the physiologically significant dietary fiber. Since most of this material remains undigested, it serves to give bulk to the food residues in the intestine.

Glycogen is sometimes called animal starch because it is the polysaccharide stored in animal tissues. Glycogen molecules are large and vary in size. They are similar to those of the branched form of starch (amylopectin), but they have shorter chains of glucose units and hence a more complicated branched structure.

Carbohydrate is an immediate source of energy for animals. For this purpose animals use glucose, which is the only sugar found in substantial amounts in the blood or tissue fluids. In the postabsorptive state, a person has about 30 g of glucose in the body, plus about 300 g of glycogen. Glycogen stored in the liver (about one third of the total) is used as a reserve supply to maintain the blood sugar level; muscle glycogen (two thirds of the total) is used to meet energy needs of exercising muscles.

Carbohydrate Content of Foods

In determining the composition of foods, the amount of water, protein, fat, and mineral (ash) is measured chemically, and the portion of weight not accounted for (the difference between the initial weight and the sum of the four components mentioned) is called carbohydrate. Thus, the portion listed as carbohydrate in most tables of food composition includes true carbohydrates plus organic acids, flavorants, vitamins, and so on.

The *organic acids,* included in the values for "carbohydrate, by difference," do have some energy value but less than the sugars. The common organic acids, citric and malic, provide 2.47 and 2.42 kcal/gm, respectively, in contrast to sugars and starch, which yield about 4 kcal/gm. Organic acids contribute about 3 percent of the energy in many vegetables and about 4 to 6 percent of that in fruits. A notable exception is lemon juice, in which 62 percent of the energy is from organic acids. Citric acid is a common component of manufactured foods; it is used either for its acid quality (many soft drinks are about 2 to 6 percent solutions of citric acid plus sugar, flavoring, and colorant) or to bind metals that cause off flavors to develop in, for example, processed cheese.

Some typical foods including some of relatively high carbohydrate content, together with the approximate amount of carbohydrate each contains, are listed in Tables 2–1, 2–3, and 2–4 and are shown in Figure 2–3.[6] A few highly refined substances—such as refined sugar and corn starch—are pure carbohydrate (99.5 and 88 percent respectively, the rest of the weight being mainly due to small amounts of water). In their natural state foods relatively rich in either sugar or starch contain other substances besides carbohydrates. Sugar cane juice, being a plant sap, contains minerals and some vitamins; when sugar is removed by crystallization, the sugar (sucrose) becomes very pure and the nutrient substances left behind are concentrated in the leftover molasses. Honey con-

[6]Figures for the carbohydrate content of foods used here and elsewhere in the book are for *total* carbohydrate, by difference, as given by the U.S. Department of Agriculture. These figures are apt to be slightly higher than the actual amount of carbohydrates available to the body.

Table 2–4 EXAMPLES OF SUGAR ADDED TO FOODS[a]

Packaged Food	*Serving Size*	*Sugar Added* Grams/Serving	*Sugar Added* Percent of Total kcal
Beverages			
Cola type	12 oz	34	100
Fruit juice drink	8 oz	27	95
Lemonade	8 oz	26	98
Kool-Aid	8 oz	25	98
Chocolate milk	8 oz	15	30
Desserts			
Peaches, light syrup	½ cup	9	48
heavy syrup	½ cup	12	61
Pudding, starch type	5 oz	25	50
Gelatin dessert	5 oz	26	97
Milk chocolate candy	1 oz	13	36
Brownies	1 ea (20 gm)	12	56
Coconut Cream pie	⅐ pie (130 gm)	24	66
Yogurt, fruit-flav. sweetened	8 oz	26	45
Ready-to-eat cereals			
Corn or wheat flakes	1 oz	2–3	11–15
Presweetened, flavored	1 oz	8–14	26–45
100% Natural (Granola)	1 oz	6	18
Condiments			
Catsup	1 T	3	80
Sweet pickle	1 small	4–5	95

[a]Includes cane, beet, and corn sugars, and cornstarch added to foods.

tains very small amounts of some nutrients, but these are not nutritionally significant because of the small amount of honey normally eaten. (In the United States, per capita consumption of honey is about 500 gm per year, or about 1.3 gm/day (¼ tsp), while consumption of refined sugars is about 130gm/day (⅓ lb).

Foods of high sugar content (65 to 99 percent) include table sugars, honey, syrups, candies, cakes, jams, jellies, preserves, and dried fruits (dates, figs, raisins, prunes, apricots); others containing appreciable amounts are fresh fruits (9 to 23 percent) and soft drinks (8 to 10 percent).

Although highly milled dry rice and white flour are more than four-fifths starch (total carbohydrate content of 81 and 76 percent respectively), they also contain significant amounts of protein (6.5 to 10.5 percent). Whole-grain cereals have somewhat more protein and less starch. Dry peas and beans have approximately 60 percent of starch and 20 percent of protein; soybeans differ from other beans in that they contain less starch and more fat. The legumes and whole grains also contain some fiber, and certain minerals and vitamins. Starchy roots of the taro and cassava (manioc), which are staple foods in parts of Africa, South America, and the islands of the South Pacific, have very little protein, minerals, or vitamins.

In contrast to their dry forms, cooked rice, spaghetti, and macaroni are 23 to 32 percent carbohydrate, and white potatoes (boiled or baked in the skin) are about 17 to 22 percent. Cooked breakfast cereals (oatmeal and farina, for example) average about 11 percent carbohydrate.

Animal foods, such as muscle meats, have little carbohydrate because the liver and

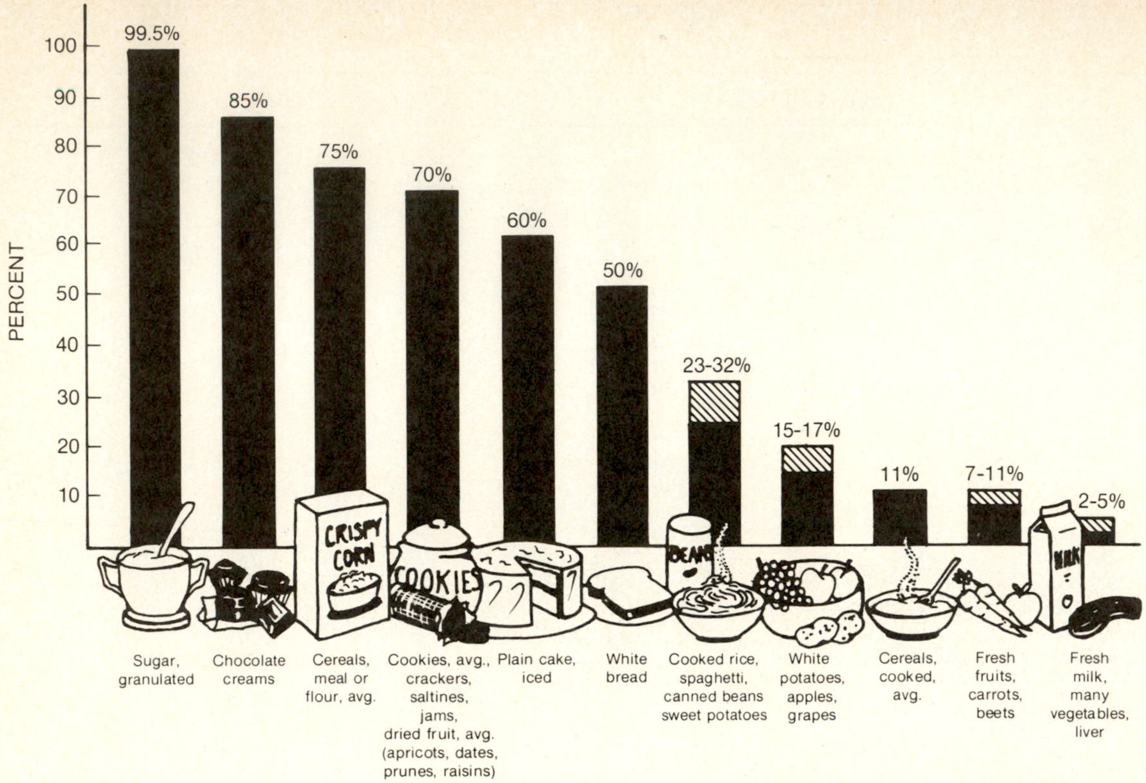

PERCENT
100
90
80
70
60
50
40
30
20
10
99.5%
85%
75%
70%
60%
50%
23-32%
15-17%
11%
7-11%
2-5%
CRISPY CORN
COOKIES
BEANS
MILK
Sugar, granulated
Chocolate creams
Cereals, meal or flour, avg.
Cookies, avg., crackers, saltines, jams, dried fruit, avg. (apricots, dates, prunes, raisins)
Plain cake, iced
White bread
Cooked rice, spaghetti, canned beans sweet potatoes
White potatoes, apples, grapes
Cereals, cooked, avg.
Fresh fruits, carrots, beets
Fresh milk, many vegetables, liver

Figure 2–3 Carbohydrate content of common foods as served.

518
330
275
760 millions
Areas proportional to the population concerned
Gross domestic product per head per year in US $ (logarithmic scale)
2600
2000
1500
1100
800
600
400
300
200
150
90
50
Separated edible fats
Unseparated vegetable fats
Unseparated animal fats
Various carbohydrates (starch)
Sugar
Animal proteins
Vegetable proteins
10%
20%
30%
40%
50%
60%
70%
80%
90%
100%
100%
90%
80%
70%
60%
50%
40%
30%
20%
10%
Percentage of calories provided by various nutrients

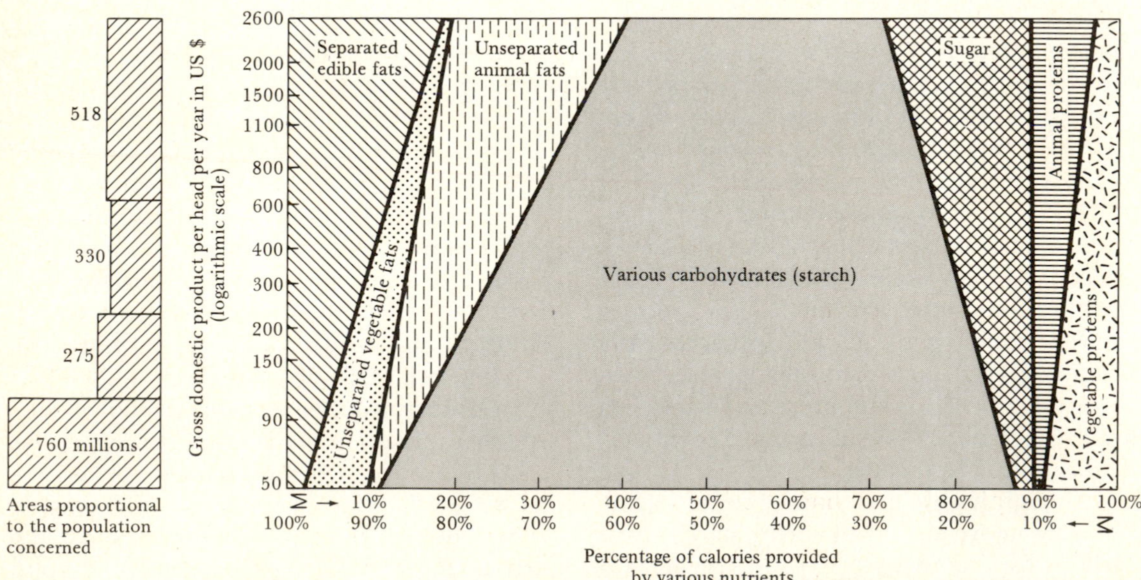

Figure 2–4 Energy derived from fats, carbohydrates, and proteins as percentage of total energy, according to the income of the countries (correlation based on 85 countries). (From Perisse, J., Sizaret, F., and Francois, P.: FAO Nutr. Newsletter, 7:3, 1969.)

Table 2–5 REPRESENTATIVE MENUS HIGH AND LOW IN CARBOHYDRATE, gm per serving

High Carbohydrate				*Low Carbohydrate*	
HIGH FIBER		LOW FIBER			
		—Breakfast—			
Oatmeal, ¾ cup	18	Corn flakes, 1 oz	24	Omelet, 2 eggs,	1
Bread, whole gr., 2 slices	24	Bread, white, 2 slices	26	Cheese, 1 oz	1
Butter, 1 pat		Margarine, 1 pat		Bread, whole gr., 1 slice	12
Jam, 1 Tbsp	14	Jelly, 1 Tbsp	13	Butter, 2 pats	
Milk, low fat, ½ cup	7	Milk, skim, ½ cup	6	Grapefruit, ½	10
Orange, 1 medium	16	Banana, 1 medium	25		
Sugar, 1 tsp	4	Sugar, 1 tsp	5		
		—Lunch—			
Bean soup, 1 cup	22	Chicken-noodle soup, 1 c	8	Consommé, 1 cup	3
Rye crackers, 2	10	Saltine crackers, 2	8	Ritz crackers, 2	9
Sandwich		Sandwich		Tuna salad[a], ½ cup	4
Egg, 1		Bologna, 1 slice		Avocado, ½	7
Bread, whole gr., 2 slices	24	Bread, white, 2 slices	26	Lettuce	
Lettuce		Margarine, 1 pat		Thousand Is. Dressing, 2 Tbsp	4
Mayonnaise, 1 Tbsp		Mustard, 1 tsp		Strawberries, ½ cup	6
Pear, 1 medium	25	Grapes, 20 seedless	18	Cream, heavy, ¼ cup	2
Milk, low fat, 1 cup	14	Milk, whole, 1 cup	11		
		—Dinner—			
Chicken, broiled, ¼		Chicken, fried[b]	14	Tomato juice, ½ cup	5
Baked potato w/skin	35	Rice, white, ½ cup	25	Steak, 12 oz (lean only, 8 oz).	
Winter squash, ½ cup	16	Gravy, 2 Tbsp	4	Green beans, ½ cup	4
Mixed green salad, 1½ cup	3	Peas, canned, ½ cup	14	Butter, 1 pat	
Vinegar, ½ Tbsp		Tomato, 1 medium	6	Mixed green salad 1½ cup	3
Oil, ½ Tbsp		Biscuits, 2	30	Italian dressing, 2 Tbsp	2
Rolls, whole grain, 2	30	Honey, 1 Tbsp	17	Red wine, 7 fl. oz	8
Butter, 3 pats		Margarine, 1 pat		Cheese, brie, 1 oz	1
Blueberry pie, ⅙	55	Ice cream, ½ cup	16	Apple, 1 medium	20
		Chocolate brownie, 1	13		
		—Snacks—			
Apple juice, ½ cup	15	Soda pop, 12 oz	34	Sparkling water	
Yogurt, flavored, 1 cup	42	Potato chips, 1 oz	15	Almonds, roasted, 1 oz	6
TOTAL	374		357		108

[a]Made with 1 Tbsp salad dressing and celery.
[b]Commercial, breaded, one thigh and one leg.

muscle tissues store only limited amounts of glycogen, which are rapidly used up during fasting or muscular work. (Animals are usually not fed before slaughter or are hunted until they are exhausted.) Liver contains about 1.5 to 5 percent glycogen, while shellfish (including oysters) have about 1 to 6 percent.

Consumption of Carbohydrate

The relative prominence of carbohydrate-rich foods in the diet varies widely in different parts of the world. Consumption depends chiefly on the availability and relative cost of fat- and protein-rich foods (animal products such as meats and dairy products) and the amount of money that can be spent for food. Such foods as grains, starchy roots or tubers, and dried peas or beans are usually the cheapest foods for energy value. In poor countries, carbohydrates, mainly starch, contribute 80 percent of the total energy intake, while in the United States, where fats are used more liberally, only 50 percent or less of the energy intake comes from carbohydrates (Fig. 2–4).

Representative menus having high and low levels of carbohydrates are shown in Table 2–5. The two high-carbohydrate menus have about 375 gm, but the first menu features whole-grain cereals, fruits, and vegetables and thus is higher in fiber than the second menu. The third menu, with very few grain products, no potatoes, and mainly low-carbohydrate vegetables and fruits, contains about 100 gm of carbohydrate.

THE ROLE OF CARBOHYDRATE IN THE BODY

Most tissues of the body can use other energy sources, but the central nervous system is dependent on a continuous supply of glucose. If the blood-glucose supply to the brain falls below a critical concentration, unconsciousness will result; if glucose is not provided, death will follow. This is because the brain has no reserve energy supply and cannot use energy substrates other than glucose until after a period of adaptation, when some capacity to use fat products develops.

Regulation of Blood Sugar by the Liver

The products of digestion of carbohydrates—chiefly glucose, with smaller amounts of fructose and galactose—are absorbed from the intestine into the blood, which passes directly to the liver via the portal vein. The liver has the ability to remove excess glucose from the blood and to take up and metabolize fructose and galactose (only glucose is found in significant amounts in the general circulation). Thus, after a meal rich in carbohydrates, a great deal of glucose appears in the portal vein, but the glucose content of the blood in circulation in the rest of the body is only slightly increased and soon returns to its remarkably constant level.

In the liver, simple sugars are combined to form the more complex and less soluble carbohydrate, glycogen. This glycogen can be reconverted into glucose and released into the blood. In this way, the liver acts as a reservoir to keep the body from being flooded with glucose just after meals and from running short at other times. Tissues continually withdraw glucose from the blood for their own uses, and the glycogen in the liver must be reconverted to glucose to maintain blood glucose at the normal level.

Carbohydrate Reserves

The muscles also can store glycogen. Even though muscle glycogen can be readily drawn on for the energy needed for muscular work, liver glycogen is the only reservoir from which the glucose of the blood can be replenished.

The amount of glycogen in the liver and muscles naturally depends somewhat on whether the supply of carbohydrate (or of energy in other forms) in the diet has been liberal or scanty, but there is an upper limit beyond which no more glycogen is normally stored. The liver normally contains about 70 gm of glycogen and the muscles about 200 gm in well-nourished adults. Muscle glycogen can be increased significantly by special diet and exercise practices, a fact of interest to athletes. This procedure is described in Chapter 21.

Dietary carbohydrate in excess of the relatively small amount that can be converted into glycogen is stored as fat in the fatty (adipose) tissues of the body. If the body receives no food, the glycogen stores are practically exhausted in one day, after which the body draws largely on its reserves of fat and muscle protein for energy.

Hormonal Regulation of Blood Sugar

In healthy individuals, the blood-sugar concentration is normally controlled within the range of 70 to 150 milligrams per 100 milliliters of blood (sometimes written as 70 to 150 mg percent). The concentration of blood glucose is the result of the equilibrium between the rate of entry of glucose into the blood and the rate of glucose uptake by the tissues (removal from the blood). This process is regulated by the available supply of glucose, as previously discussed, and by the homeostatic influence of hormonal regulation.

The hormone *insulin* has a central role in the regulation of blood glucose. Insulin is produced by the pancreas and is secreted when the blood-glucose level exceeds 80 to 100 mg per 100 ml. It increases the rate of glucose uptake by insulin-sensitive tissues, such as adipose tissue, and muscle, thereby reducing the level of blood glucose. *Glucagon* is another hormone secreted by the pancreas, but the stimulus for secretion of this hormone is a *lowered* level of blood glucose. The primary function of glucagon is to promote the breakdown of glycogen into glucose in the liver, thus raising the level of blood glucose.

Insulin acts with glucagon to control the extent of the daily fluctuations of blood glucose imposed by the marked changes in glucose supply resulting from the fasting-feeding cycles within the day. The appropriate hormone is secreted and acts within a few minutes of a change in blood glucose to restore the blood concentration to normal. For example, during the overnight fast the liver, under the influence of glucagon, releases sufficient glucose to supply the brain and to maintain the blood-glucose concentration at about 80 mg per 100 ml. Following a meal containing carbohydrates, glucose is absorbed from the intestine, transported to the liver, and overflows to some extent into the general circulation. This rise in blood glucose causes a decrease in glucagon secretion by the pancreas and an increase in insulin secretion, resulting in deposition of glycogen in liver and muscle and an accelerated conversion of glucose to fat in adipose tissue. The blood-glucose concentration does not usually increase above 130 mg per 100. During exercise, glucose uptake and utilization by muscle is increased, but the blood-glucose levels are maintained in an acceptable range by the action of glucagon released from the pancreas.

Other hormones also influence blood glucose concentrations. Under stress conditions, *epinephrine* is immediately released from the adrenal gland and causes blood sugar to rise by stimulating the breakdown of liver glycogen to glucose. Epinephrine, unlike glucagon, also facilitates conversion of muscle glycogen to an intermediate compound, lactic acid, which may be converted to glucose in the liver. *Cortisol,* another hormone from the adrenal gland, acts more slowly than epinephrine to depress glucose utilization by muscle, and to promote formation of glucose in the liver from certain of the amino acids. (See Chap. 4 and 6.) All these actions tend to raise blood glucose levels. *Growth hormone,* secreted from the pituitary, and the thyroid hormones favor elevation of blood glucose by a variety of mechanisms.

The complexity of the blood-glucose–regulating system is apparent. A disturbance in any one of several factors may result in faulty maintenance or adjustment of blood-glucose levels. In the disease *diabetes mellitus* there is a deficiency of or insensitivity to insulin, resulting in excessively high blood-glucose levels. As muscle and other insulin-sensitive tissues are unable to use this glucose, the body must provide fat to meet the energy needs of these tissues. In the absence of adequate carbohydrate metabolism, fat oxidation is not fully completed, and incompletely oxidized products (ketones) accumulate. In severe diabetes, the combination of elevated blood-glucose level and ketones results in a sequence of events leading to coma and death if insulin is not provided. In adults a milder form of diabetes occurs more commonly, usually in association with obesity. Blood-sugar levels are high, but ketosis is rare in this type of diabetes; the disease can usually be controlled by reducing body weight to normal, increasing exercise, and avoiding sugar-rich foods.

While many hormones (glucagon, epinephrine, cortisol, growth hormone, thyroid hormones) act to insure adequate blood levels of glucose, insulin is the only hormone that prevents excess accumulation of glucose. Thus, it is not surprising that hypoglycemia, the state of having abnormally low blood glucose, is relatively rare. The most common form of hypoglycemia occurs in diabetics who accidentally take too much insulin. In other very rare instances (for example, an insulin-producing pancreatic tumor or severe liver disease) hypoglycemia will be present as one symptom in a constellation of symptoms typical of these diseases. Some few individuals have hypoglycemia that has no evident organic basis. This functional hypoglycemia is diagnosed by a finding of very low blood-sugar levels (30 to 40 mg per 100 ml) three to five hours after administration of a test dose of glucose *and* the simultaneous presence of characteristic symptoms (such as tremors). This functional disorder usually responds to simple dietary management, including more frequent, small meals (five or six a day) containing generous amounts of protein-rich foods, and avoidance of free sugars.

The Need for Carbohydrate in the Diet

There is no clear evidence that more than a very small amount of carbohydrate is absolutely required in the diet if substances from which the body can make sugar are sufficient. Through metabolic processes the body can produce carbohydrate from the sugar alcohol glycerol, which makes up 10 percent of the weight of fat. (See Chap. 3.) About half of the amino acids that make up protein can also be converted to carbohydrate. (See Chap. 4.)

There are limits to these metabolic processes, and if carbohydrate intake is very low, fats are not completely utilized and protein is diverted from its essential roles. Under these conditions, body chemistry is disturbed, salts and water are lost excessively, and dehydration results. (See Chap. 14.) To prevent these events, *the diet should include about 70 to 100 gm of preformed carbohydrate.*

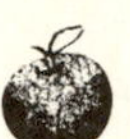

health considerations

Concerns about carbohydrate intake are principally two: that sugar (sucrose and, increasingly, fructose) is bad per se: and that the increasing use of refined carbohydrate foods, especially sugar, impoverishes the diet with respect to essential nutrients and fiber. These are valid concerns, but their importance varies depending on the overall diet and the person's genetic makeup and lifestyle.

Too Much Sugar?

In the United States, between 1910 and 1970, intake of starch declined about 50 percent as a result of decreased consumption of cereals, legumes, and potatoes. Total sugar intake increased about 25 percent between 1910 and 1925, to about 200 gm per person per day (including that in fruits, milk, and other foods). Intake has been fairly constant at this level since 1925, but as total energy consumption has fallen, the percentage contribution of energy from sugar has increased. (See Fig. 2–5.) There was an upturn in the use of refined caloric sweeteners between 1960 and 1970, chiefly because of greater use of manufactured food products, presweetened cereals, and baked goods. Consumption of sweetened carbonated beverages has steadily increased, and the present average U.S. consumption is 14 oz. (400

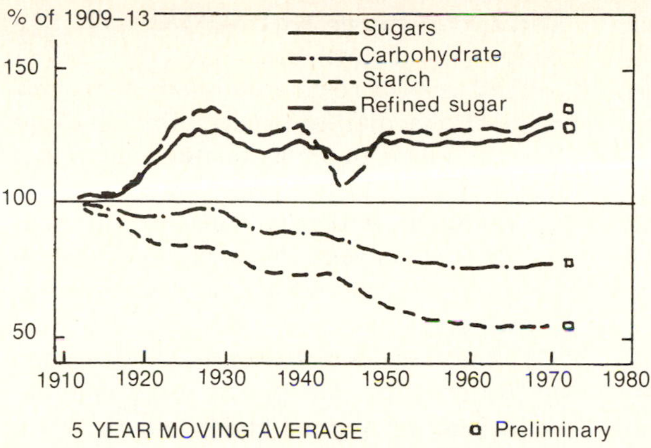

Figure 2–5 Changes in consumption of starch and sugar in the United States between 1910 and 1970. Intake of starch has declined nearly 50 percent, due to decreased consumption of cereals, legumes, and potatoes, while total sugar intake increased about one-fourth between 1910 and 1925. In 1980, U.S. consumption of all caloric sweeteners (including corn syrup solids, honey, and molasses) was 172 gm/day, of which 104 gm was cane and beet sugar. (From Page, L., and Friend, B.: Level of use of sugars in the United States. In *Sugars in Nutrition,* ed. H. L. Sipple and K. W. McNutt, New York, Academic Press, 1974. Used with permission.)

ml) per day. (See Fig. 2–6.) Considering that some people use little or no soda pop, others may drink twice as much as the average. Unless these consumers also have very high energy needs, other more nutritious foods must be displaced from the diet. Failing that, the sugar energy is in excess and will contribute to obesity.

Figure 2–6 About one-third of snacks eaten by children are beverages other than milk. Often the beverage is a refreshing but carbohydrate-rich soft drink. In 1980, Americans consumed 39.6 gal per capita of carbonated beverages, which accounted for 20 percent of all sugar used. (Photo courtesy of D. A. Hobbs, Seattle.)

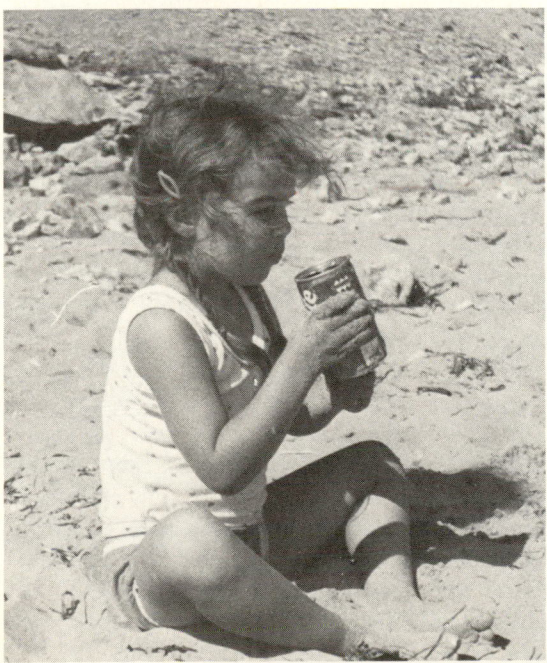

Many believe that sugar does contribute to human obesity, but there is no unequivocal evidence that this is true. In animal studies, food can be rigidly controlled, and a very large portion (60–80 percent) can be fed as a single carbohydrate. Under these conditions, animals fed sucrose have slightly more body fat than those fed starch. Human diets are not that extreme. The problem then is to unravel the separate effects of sugars and fats on total energy intake and energy balance; this is a difficult task because many foods (pastries, candies) and total diets are high in both substances making it almost impossible to have clear evidence related to one factor only. Generally speaking, where supply and income are not limiting, per capita consumption of refined sugar levels off at about 130 gm per day worldwide, and per capita fat intake is high where refined sugar intake is high. Thus, cross-national epidemiologic evidence on this point has not been particularly helpful.

Evidence linking sugar to certain diseases—notably diabetes and heart disease—is mainly through a proposed association with obesity. As we have noted, this is not proved. However, there are two points worth considering. First, the symptoms of diabetes and the level of blood sugar are more readily controlled if refined sugars are eliminated from the diet of persons who have the disease; it is not necessary and may be undesirable to reduce starch intake of diabetics (except as is necessary for correction of body weight). Similarly, persons whose blood sugar rebounds to below-normal levels after meals are advised to omit sugars. Second, in some persons, especially those who have a particular genetic pattern, high-carbohydrate and, often, high-sucrose intakes cause an undesirable increase of fatty substances in the blood, a condition that is, in turn, associated with heart disease. This tendency can be detected by analysis of blood plasma and diagnosed by the physician.

Sugar has been indicted as a cause of hyperactivity in children. Many parents and some clinicians subscribe to this view. Unfortunately, it is almost impossible to conduct an adequate test of this theory. Whenever the outcome under study is readily affected by subjective factors (attitudes, expectations) it is especially important that the test be "blind," that is, that neither the subject nor the observer know what treatment has been given. Many persons can differentiate between artificial and natural sweeteners, so it is difficult to make the treatment blind in this respect. If the observer expects hyperactive behavior, it is likely to be detected. Recent tests conducted with these precautions did not find an association between sugar and erratic behavior; in fact, the boys studied were significantly less active when given sugar blind (6).

As there is no health benefit from habitual consumption of large amounts of sugar, prudence suggests sensible limitation of sugar by children—and adults—whether or not they are hyperactive. At the same time, the evidence does not warrant eliminating all sweets from the diet, providing toothbrushing follows. Sugar, especially "sticky" forms, does contribute to dental caries (see Chap. 24).

Too Little Fiber and Nutrients?

The question of dilution of the nutritional value of the diet is equally difficult to answer, as much depends on the quality and amounts of all the foods that a person consumes. If the diet includes enough high-quality protective foods (such as milk, vegetables, and meat) then it is likely to meet nutritional needs, even with 100 gm of sugar (400 kcal) included. If the diet is poor, simply taking a vitamin pill or using commercially fortified refined foods will not make up the difference because these do not contain the full array of nutrients, especially the trace minerals.

The lack of fiber (contained in unrefined cereals, vegetables, legumes, and fruits) may also be an issue. About fifty years ago, dietary roughage was considered important for promoting laxation to rid the body of toxins presumed to be formed by the bacteria that normally inhabit the intestinal tract. This topic went out of vogue in medical circles until interest was reawakened by observations and hypotheses advanced by Dennis Burkitt and others linking a lack of dietary fiber with chronic intestinal disorders, including constipation, inflammation, and cancer. There is no question concerning laxation; dietary fiber, particularly hemicellulose and cereal brans, does increase fecal bulk. (However, this is not true of all fibers; pectin and gums have little laxative power.) The unabsorbed carbohydrates also provide a rich substrate for the intestinal bacteria, leading to the formation of gas and also, of some other end products that stimulate motility. There is as yet, however, no direct proof that the diseases in question are caused by lack of fiber or that in its presence the numbers or ratios of intestinal bacteria are altered beneficially or that mutagenic effects are lessened. Epidemiologic evidence does indicate that colon cancer is more prevalent among consumers of refined, high-fat

diets than among those who eat a bulkier diet; dietary fiber may be a factor in this association, but it is only one of a number of factors that differ between these diets.
Other beneficial effects of fiber—reduction in the level of blood sugar after meals and a small lowering of blood cholesterol—are due principally to pectin and gums, rather than to dietary fiber in general (6). The effect of fiber in delaying and muting the rise in blood sugar is thought to reflect delayed emptying of the stomach and delayed absorption from the intestine. The effect of fiber on blood lipids is not large and wheat bran is not effective in this regard, being low in content of mucilaginous polysaccharides.

Some caution in the addition of fiber, particularly bran, to the diet is needed because it interferes with the absorption of calcium and the trace elements. (See Chap. 15 and 16.) Pure cellulose does not appear to duplicate the desired properties of dietary fiber. The best way to increase the fiber content of the diet is to eat whole-grain breads and cereals and plenty of vegetables, legumes, and fruits, which provide vitamins and minerals along with the fiber.

In summary, carbohydrate-rich foods contribute to the diet chiefly by

1. providing a ready supply of glucose to the brain and other tissues
2. providing an economical energy supply
3. furnishing some proteins, minerals, and vitamins (whole grains, legumes, and potatoes)
4. providing fiber
5. adding flavor (sugars) to foods and beverages

There need be no health hazard in subsisting chiefly on carbohydrate-rich foods, provided those foods are not lacking in proteins, minerals, or vitamins, or the diet includes enough other food sources of these nutrients. There is no compelling reason to eliminate sugar from the diet, but prudence dictates that intake be kept in reasonable limits. Sugar is sugar and weight-for-weight, the sugar in honey will not improve the outlook over table sugar. For dental health, eschew sticky sweets.

QUESTIONS

1. Define carbohydrates, fats, and proteins. Why are they referred to as the fuel foodstuffs, or energy nutrients? Which element is supplied in utilizable form only by proteins?

2. Explain the chemical basis for the division of carbohydrates into mono-, di-, and polysaccharides. How do the mono- and disaccharides (sugars) differ in properties (taste, solubility, etc.) from polysaccharides (starch, cellulose, etc.)? How are these differences in properties related to the size of the molecules? What are the other classes of carbohydrates?

3. Name three common monosaccharides and some foods in which they are found. Why are they called carbohydrates? Why are the monosaccharides that occur most commonly in nature called hexoses? What is the hexose that occurs in blood and body tissues?

4. When two molecules of monosaccharide link to form a disaccharide (as two glucose molecules link to form one molecule of maltose), what substance is split off at the point of linkage? Does the same thing happen when many molecules of glucose unite to form the polysaccharide starch? What happens when these linkages are broken during digestion or hydrolysis outside the body? Why is this breakdown called hydrolysis?

5. What is the chemical name of common table sugar, and from what sources in nature is it made? Does it carry any other nutrients? What are the disadvantages of using sugar too liberally? Name four common foods of high sugar content.

6. What types or classes of food have a high content of starch? Into what monosaccharide is starch broken down in digestion? What polysaccharides found in foods are poorly digested, and

why is this so? What polysaccharide is stored in the animal body?

7. Make a list of the foods you have consumed in one day, including sugar added at the table and any between-meal snacks. Using the table in the Appendix on Nutritive Values of Foods in Average Servings, calculate your total intake of carbohydrate for the day. At 4 kcal per gram, how much energy did you obtain in the form of carbohydrate? Since the figures for total carbohydrate include indigestible carbohydrate in the form of fiber, how would this affect the total energy actually obtained? Of what use is the fiber in vegetable foods? Do all plant fibers have the same physiological properties?

8. What are the chief uses of carbohydrate-rich foods in the diet? In what countries and under what economic conditions is the consumption of carbohydrates high? Are there any disadvantages of diets that are made up chiefly of carbohydrate-rich foods? Why is it important that whole-grain or enriched bread and cereal be used when grain products make up a large proportion of the diet?

9. Is there a dietary requirement for carbohydrate? Justify your answer. How is the blood-sugar level regulated?

References

1. Merrill, A. L., and Watt, B. K.: Energy value of foods—basis and development. USDA Agric. Handbook No. 74, Washington, D.C., 1955.
2. Shallenberger, R. S., and Birch, G. G.: *Sugar Chemistry.* Westport, Conn., Avi Publishing Co., 1975.
3. Hardinge, M., Swarner, J. B., and Crooks, H.: Carbohydrates in foods. J. Amer. Dietet. Assoc., *46*:197, 1965.
4. Consumer and Food Economics Institute: Composition of foods. USDA Agric. Handbook No. 8, Washington, D.C., 1976–82.
5. Paul, A. A., and Southgate, D. A. T.: *McCance and Widdowson's The Composition of Foods.* 4th rev. ed. London, HMSO, 1978.
6. Rapoport, J.: Unpublished data from the Natl. Institute of Mental Health. Cited in Science, 21:1210, 1982.
7. Food & Agricultural Organization: Carbohydrates in human nutrition. FAO Food and Nutr. Paper No. 15, Rome, 1980; Vahouny, G. V.: Conclusions and recommendations of the symposium on "Dietary fibers in health and disease," Washington, D.C., 1981. Amer. J. Clin. Nutr., *35*:152, 1982.

3 Fats, Other Lipids, and Alcohol

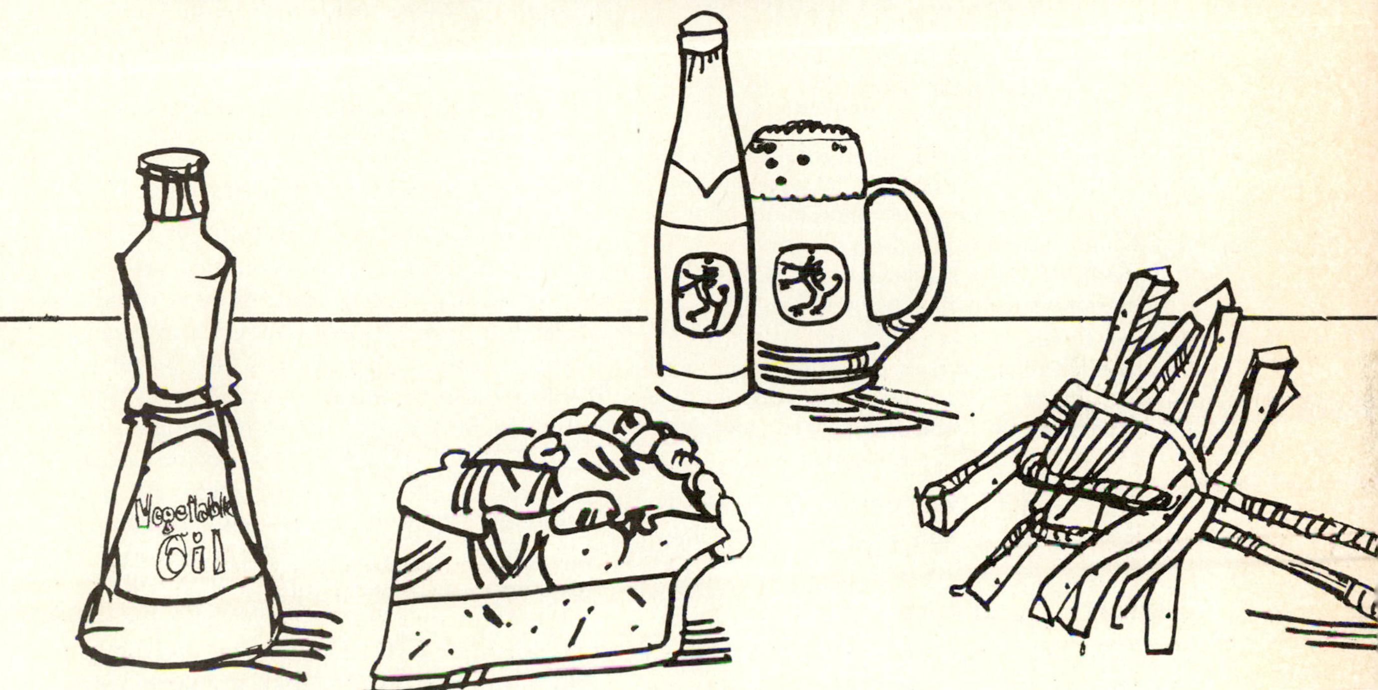

FATS AND OTHER LIPIDS

Fats are part of every meal. They are familiar to everyone—butter, margarine, vegetable oils, lard, salad oils, and suet being examples. These common fats are also, chemically speaking, *lipids,* a less familiar word with a broader meaning than the true chemical meaning of "fats." Lipids include many other related substances such as cholesterol. The two words fat and lipid are often used interchangeably. However, while all fats are lipids, not all lipids are true fats.

A dietary *oil*—say, corn oil or soybean oil—is a food fat that is liquid at room temperature. (It is not to be confused with mineral oil or crude oil used in manufacturing gasoline—they are different chemicals.) It is not wrong to speak of the "fat content of soybeans"; the words oil and fat are interchangeable for fats that are liquid at room temperature.

All fats and most lipids are distinguished from other food components by feeling greasy to the touch, by leaving a translucent spot on paper, and by being insoluble in water. All lipids, in addition, are soluble in "fat solvents," such as ether, alcohol, gasoline, acetone, and the common household cleaning fluids. In fact, lipids may be defined simply as those organic substances that are extracted from biological materials by fat solvents. Some of the vitamins, as well as many natural food pigments, are lipids.

Classification of Lipids

A simplified classification of lipids follows. Only a few of the many lipids are found in nutritionally significant amounts in foods; these are indicated in boldface type.

Simple Lipids
- **fatty acids**
  - **fats** (mono-, di-, and **triacylglycerols** [also called **mono-, di-,** and **triglycerides**] are glycerol esters of fatty acids)
  - **waxes** (esters of fatty acids with alcohols other than glycerol)

Compound Lipids
- **phospholipids** (contain phosphate, fatty acids, glycerol, and usually a nitrogenous compound, for example, phosphatidylcholine, also called lecithin)
- **glycolipids** (contain galactose)
- **lipoproteins** (contain protein)

Derived Lipids
- **sterols** (alcohols of high molecular weight with a characteristic central structure; include **cholesterol,** some hormones, and vitamin D)

All the fat-soluble vitamins (A, D, E, and K) are lipids, but they will be discussed in Chapter 9.

Importance of Fats

Fats yield about 900 kcal (3800kJ) of energy per 100 gm, more than twice the energy value of the same weight of carbohydrate or protein (400 kcal). This amount—100 gm, or about a quarter of a pound—is slightly less fat than the average daily per capita intake in industrial societies. Fat makes up 15 to 20 percent of our food on a weight basis and provides more than 40 percent of our energy. Because so much fat is eaten each day (a practice not without nutritional hazards), fat has tremendous economic value. Many billions of dollars' worth of fat are sold and eaten each year in North America. Because of this large consumption there are many political and advertising pressures to persuade us to eat one kind of fat or another.

Fats are essential to the life of all cells. As will be shown in more detail, fats are made up of glycerol combined with fatty acids. Two of these, linoleic and linolenic acids, are dietary *essential fatty acids* because they cannot be made by our bodies but are needed for critical body functions. A dietary source of these acids, then, is essential for life. Linoleic and linolenic acids are the first specific nutrients that this book will discuss of about twenty-two rather small organic chemicals (including amino acids and vitamins) that the body must obtain from foods.

Chemical Structure of Fats

The principal fatty acids present in food fats are straight-chain compounds with one acid (carboxyl) group and an even number of carbon atoms. There is very simple and precise nomenclature for the fatty acids, but they are still generally referred to by their older, trivial names. For example, the saturated fatty acid having 10 carbon atoms, technically called decanoic acid,[1] is more commonly known as capric acid ("capric" refers to goat and is a hint about the odor of this compound) (see Table 3–1).

The saturated fatty acids all have the general formula $C_nH_{2n}O_2$. Except for the terminal carboxyl group, both available bonds of each carbon in the chain are occupied by hydrogen:

```
      H   H   H      O
      |   |   |     //
R— C — C — C — C
      |   |   |     \
      H   H   H      OH
```

In the unsaturated fatty acids, one hydrogen atom is missing from each of two adjacent carbons, which then share a double bond:

```
      H   H   H   H
      |   |   |   |
R— C—C=C—C—R
      |           |
      H           H
```

[1]In the Genevan system, the first portion of the name indicates the number of carbon atoms in the chain (in the example, "dec" for 10), and the ending indicates whether the fatty acid is saturated (-anoic) or unsaturated (-enoic).

Table 3–1 STRUCTURE AND MELTING POINT OF SOME COMMON FATTY ACIDS

Common Name	*Chemical Abbreviation*[a]	*Melting Point°C*	*Occurrence*
	Saturated		
Butyric	4:0	−7.9	Small amts. in milk fat
Capric	10:0	31.6	Small amts. in plant fats
Lauric	12:0	44.0	Palm oil, coconut oil, laurel
Myristic	14:0	59.0	Palm oil, coconut, myrtle
Palmitic	16:0	62.9	All fats
Stearic	18:0	69.6	All fats
	Unsaturated		
Oleic	18:1,n-9	16.3	All fats
Elaidic	trans 18:2,n-9	44.	Hydrogenated fats
Linoleic	18:2,n-6,9	−5.0	Vegetable oils, smaller amounts in animal fats
Linolenic	18:3,n-3,6,9	−11.0	Vegetable oils
Arachidonic	20:4,n-6,9,12,15	−49.5	Animal fats, human milk
Eicosapentenoic	20:5,n-3,6,9,12,15		Fish oil, human milk

[a]Abbreviated formula indicates the number of carbon atoms, followed by a colon and a number denoting the number of double bonds, followed by designation of the position of the double bonds counted from the CH_3 (methyl) end of the fatty acid. The Greek letter *omega* (ω) is used interchangeably with the symbol n, marking the methyl end of the fatty acid.

The resulting fatty acid lacks two hydrogen atoms and is thus unsaturated. If there is one double bond, the fatty acid is *monounsaturated,* if there are two or more double bonds, the fatty acid is *polyunsaturated* (see Fig. 3–1). The location of the double bond is an important determinant of biological properties. Location of the double bond is indicated by counting from the methyl (CH_3) end of the fatty acid chain.

The spatial arrangement of the portions of the molecule at either side of the double bond pair can differ, yielding substances having different physical and biological properties. In the instance of the C-18 monounsaturated fatty acid, these spatial or stereoisomers may be viewed as follows:

```
         H           H
          \         /
Cis:        C===C
          /         \
CH3(CH2)7            (CH2)7COOH
```

```
        CH3(CH2)7        H
                 \      /
Trans:            C===C
                 /      \
                H        (CH2)7COOH
```

Most naturally occurring fatty acids have the *cis* configuration. In this example, the *cis* form is oleic acid, which is liquid at room temperature. The *trans* form is elaidic acid, which is a solid. Oleic acid is the most common of all fatty acids. Only the *cis* form occurs in natural plant fats; animal fats contain oleic acid and small amounts of the *trans* form also.

Acylglycerols. True fats, or *triacylglycerols,* as they are technically called, are formed by combining three fatty acids with the sugar alcohol glycerol, in an ester linkage (Fig. 3–2). In this linkage the carboxyl (acid) group of the fatty acid unites with the hydroxyl group of glycerol, with the loss of water. Mono- and diacylglycerols contain one

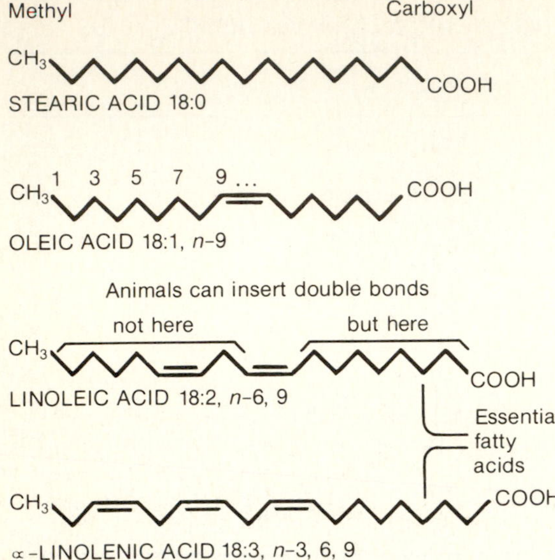

Figure 3–1 Diagrammatic representation of the fatty acids. All shown have 18 carbons in the chain. Stearic acid is saturated; oleic acid has one double bond at the n-9 position. Linoleic acid has two double bonds but the first, at n-6, is in a place where animal cells cannot synthesize a double bond. Similarly, linolenic acid, another polyunsaturated acid, has three double bonds, in positions that cannot be made in the body. Animal cells can convert linoleic and linolenic acids to longer and more highly unsaturated acids. (See Appendix.)

and two fatty acids linked to glycerol, respectively. During digestion, fatty acids are split from the glycerol with the addition of water, that is, by hydrolysis.

Thousands of different triacylglycerols are found in foods because of the many possible combinations of fatty acids that may be linked with glycerol. It has been calculated that butter contains more than 100,000 different triacylglycerols, for example. The physical properties of various fats, such as differences in consistency at room temperature, are due to differences in the kinds and amounts of fatty acids that enter into their composition. Melting points of some of the common fatty acids are given in Table 3–1. The shorter the chain length and the more unsaturated the structure, the lower the melting point of the fatty acids and of the fat of which they are constituents.

Phospholipids. The *phospholipids* are usually glyceryl esters[2] of two fatty acids and a nonlipid component, instead of the third fatty acid present in a true fat. The third ester linkage is with phosphoric acid. Another substance is linked with the phosphoric acid, usually a nitrogenous base. In phosphatidylcholine (lecithin) the nitrogenous base is choline, a vitamin (see Chap. 11); other phospholipids contain different nitrogenous constituents (the amino acid serine, for example) or a nonnitrogenous substance (inositol, see Chap. 11). Usually one of the two fatty acids is saturated and the other is unsaturated. Glyceryl esters of the higher fatty acids are insoluble in water, but the phosphoric ester group of the phospholipids is strongly polar, that is, oriented toward and mixable with water. The fact that phospholipids contain both types of ester linkage allows them to occupy a position between fatty and aqueous surfaces, forming an interface between two substances that would not otherwise be mixable. It is this property that is thought to be important to the biological functions of these compounds and to their use in foods and industrial products as emulsifiers.

Sterols. The *sterols* are complex alcohols of high molecular weight, having a characteristic four-ring structure. (See the appendix.) *Cholesterol* is the most prominent member of this class found in animal tissue, where it occurs free or esterfied with fatty acid. Other sterols are found in plants. Bile acids, such as cholic acid, which are secreted in the intestine in large amounts, belong to the class of sterols, as do hormones from the adrenal gland and the gonads, and the D vitamins.

Fats make up a large part of the diet and

[2]Some phospholipids found in large quantities in brain and nerve tissue, called sphingomyelins, are esters of a different alcohol, sphyngosine, but the common phospholipids are esters of glycerol.

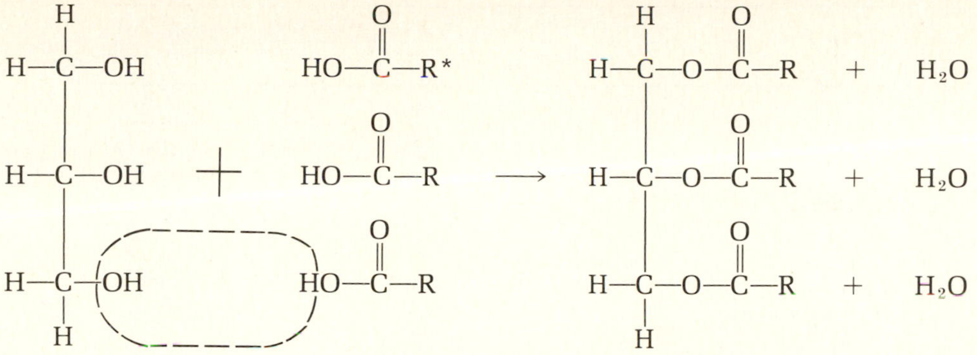

GLYCEROL + 3 FATTY ACIDS $\longrightarrow$ FAT (Triglyceride) + 3 H_2O (Water)

Figure 3–2 Fatty acid molecules have a chain of carbon atoms with hydrogen attached, and at one end of the chain, an organic acid group (COOH, a carboxyl group). In the figure R = the rest of the carbon chain. In the fatty acids that occur most commonly in food fats, there are either 15 or 17 carbon atoms in the chain attached to the carboxyl group, i.e. the fatty acids have 16 or 18 carbon atoms. In forming the ester linkage with glycerol, making a triglyceride, three molecules of water are lost from the three fatty acids combining with one glycerol molecule.

transporting these water-insoluble substances from the intestine to the tissues presents a problem. For transportation, fats and cholesterol are linked with phospholipids to protein, making hydrophylic lipoproteins. Fatty acids released from adipose tissue for use elsewhere in the body are transported as a complex with the plasma protein albumin.

Food Fats

Fatty acids rarely exist in the free state in nature, and most food fats are triacylglycerols. Fat is the chief form in which animals store extra energy for future use, in adipose tissue beneath the skin, around organs, and even within muscle tissue. In nonruminants the composition of the fatty acids in this storage fat is affected to some extent by the animal's diet, being softer if the diet includes plant oils. In cows and sheep the rumen bacteria increase the saturation of fatty acids, so beef and mutton fat are more saturated than fat from pigs and chickens (which are fed corn and other fat-containing items). Animal fats would be more solid at room temperature were it not for an abundant content of oleic acid—from 25 to 45 percent of the fat. Beef fat and pork fat (lard) have about 40 percent of oleic acid, but beef fat has more stearic acid and less linoleic acid and is harder at room temperature (see Table 3–2). The amount of fat in poultry and meats is quite variable, depending on feeding conditions and age. Young animals (calves, broiler chickens) are relatively low in fat (about 5–15 percent).

Shrimp, oysters, crab, and many fishes (tuna, halibut) are very low in fat, which comprises about 1–2 percent of the cooked wet weight. Salmon is quite variable, with fat content increasing with color (pink to red). The fatty fishes such as herring and mackeral have about 13–16 percent fat.

Chicken eggs have about 11 percent fat. All this fat is in the yolk, which is about one-third fat.

Milk varies in fat content with species and breed. Whole cow milk is marketed at about 3.3 to 3.7 percent fat. Goat milk is usually about 4.1 percent fat and that of the water buffalo, about 6.9 percent. Human milk has about 4.4 percent fat, and it is higher in content of polyunsaturated fatty acids than is cow milk (about 0.5 percent versus 0.14 percent). Milk fat is present in cheeses which range from a low of 4 percent in creamed

Table 3–2 FAT CONTENT AND FATTY ACID COMPOSITION OF SELECTED FOODS[a]

	Total Fat %	*Fatty Acids, % of Fat*	
		SATURATED	POLYUNSAT.
Separated Fat			
Safflower oil	100	9	74
Sunflower oil	100	10	66
Linseed oil	100	9	66[b]
Wheat germ oil	100	19	62
Corn oil	100	13	59
Soybean oil	100	14	58
Sesame oil	100	14	42
Rapeseed oil (no erucic)	100	7	33
Peanut oil	100	17	32
Olive oil	100	14	8
Palm oil	100	49	9
Cocoa butter	100	60	3
Palm kernel oil	100	81	2
Coconut oil	100	86	2
Vegetable shortening	100	25–30	12–26
Margarines, first ingredient			
Safflower oil, liquid, tub	80	14	60
Corn oil, liquid, tub	80	18	48
Soybean, cottonseed, hydrog., tub	80	20	16
Corn, soy, cottonseed, hydrog., stick	80	20	28
Butter	81	62	4
Foods			
Walnuts, English	64	11	62
Peanuts	51	18	27
Almonds	54	8	17
Avocado	17	19	12
Chicken, turkey	5–20	30	20
Pork	20–35	39	11
Beef, lamb	10–40	50	4
Salmon, trout	9	17	51
Sardines	10	30	42
Tuna, prawns[c]	2	41	30
Mayonnaise[d]	79	15	52
Egg yolk	33	30	13

[a]Data from United States Department of Agriculture Handbook No. 8.
[b]Contains 54% linolenic acid.
[c]Raw or water-packed.
[d]Varies with oil.

cottage cheese to 30–35 percent in cheddar types.

Some plants store fats in fruits, seeds, seed germ, or nuts, from which we obtain our common vegetable oils (such as olive, coconut, peanut, soybean, corn germ, cottonseed, and palm). Most common nuts contain 50 to 70 percent of fat, and soybeans about 30

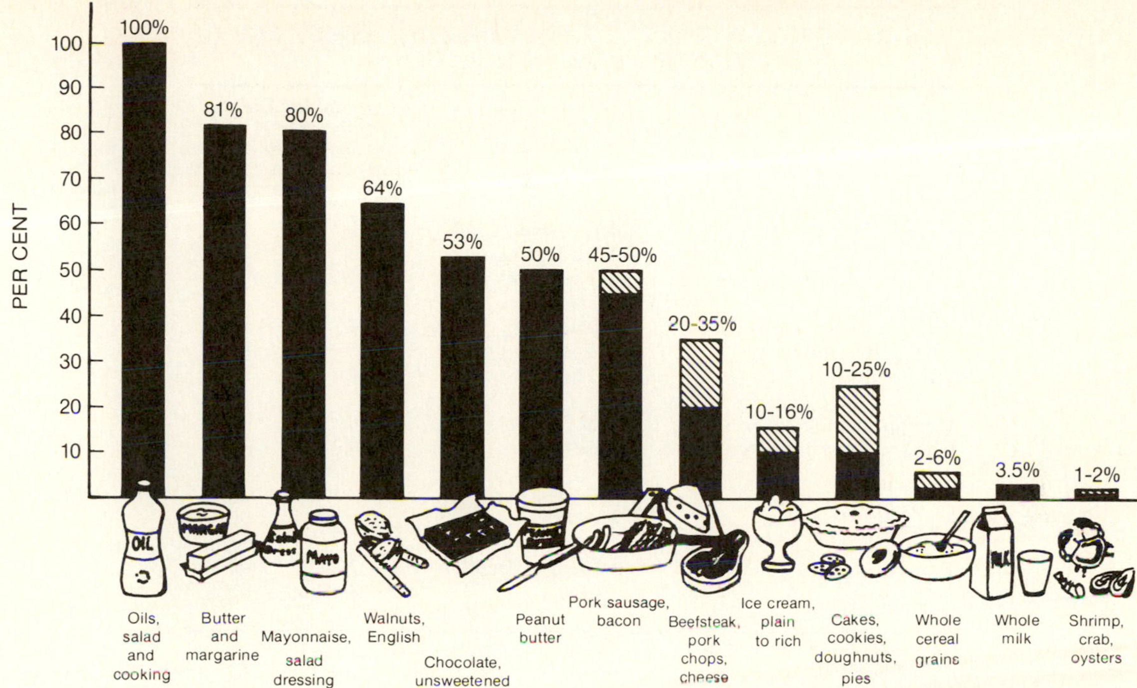

Figure 3–3 Fat content of common foods as served.

percent (dry basis). Avocados and olives range from about 11 to 20 percent fat. Whole cereal grains have 2 to 6 percent fat, mainly in the germ portion. Coconut fat has almost no polyunsaturated fatty acid. Palm and olive oils are relatively low in polyunsaturates compared to the other vegetable oils and are more like animal fats in composition.

With suitable chemical treatment, the double bonds in molecules of unsaturated fatty acids may be reduced to single ones, setting free bonds that enable the compound to take up more hydrogen. It is by *hydrogenation* and other chemical modifications that vegetable oils are converted into a semisolid state for use as margarines, shortening, or peanut butter. During hydrogenation, some *trans* fatty acids are formed. These isomers may be as high as 45 percent in some margarines. Typically, *trans* acids make up about 4 percent of our fat intake.

Much of the fat we eat is invisible. It is present in or added to foods in such a way that it becomes part of the product, as for example, in pie crust. Fat is also added for texture and flavor, and a low-fat food is sometimes converted to a high-fat food when it is prepared for the table. Potatoes, for example, have only traces of fat but when they are made into potato chips, the fat content reaches 40 percent because of the fat used for frying. Other examples of fat addition to foods are given in Table 3–3.

Foods also contain structural and functional lipids, chiefly phospholipids and sterols. The principal dietary phospholipid is phosphatidylcholine, which is abundant in egg yolk and from which it was first isolated. Granular commercial lecithin is extracted from soybeans; it is not simply phosphatidylcholine, but contains about 40 percent of other phospholipids and 35 percent of residual fat. Skeletal muscle contains less than 1 percent phospholipid, heart and lung muscle

Table 3–3 EXAMPLES OF FATS ADDED TO FOODS FOR FLAVOR OR IN PREPARATION

Food	*Serving Size*	*Added Fat* GM PER SERVING	PERCENT OF ENERGY
Coffee whitener, dry	1 tsp (level)(2gm)	1	48
Half-and-half	1 Tbsp (15 gm)	2	78
Whipped topping (pressurized)	1 Tbsp level (3 gm)	1	86
Butter or margarine	1 pat (5 gm)	4	99
French dressing, reg	1 Tbsp (15 gm)	6	83
Mayonnaise	1 Tbsp (14 gm)	11	99
Shrimp, breaded & fried	3 oz (85 gm)	10	47
Chicken leg, commercial fried	2 oz (54 gm)	6	40
Crackers, butter-type	½ oz (14 gm)	3	36
Pie crust, ⅙ shell	1 oz (28 gm)	10	60
Potatoes, french fried	10 strips (50 gm)	7	40
Potato chips	10 (20 gm)	8	63

about 2 percent, the liver and kidney about 3 percent, and the brain about 5 percent. Cholesterol is a normal constituent of all cells but in far lower concentration than that of phospholipids. It makes up about 0.3 percent of body weight in humans and is also present in milk. Cholesterol content tends to parallel the phospholipid distribution in animal tissues, being high in organs and low in muscle (see Table 3–4). Plants do not contain cholesterol but a related compound, sitosterol. Yeast contains ergosterol, which is a precursor of one form of vitamin D. (See Chap. 9).

The physical size of fat particles affects the use of fat. *Homogenized fat* goes through a process that breaks up the fat into fine particles or droplets that remain evenly distributed (an emulsion), as in homogenized milk for example. Fats that are emulsified are generally more readily digested than large amounts of nonemulsified fat because the tiny droplets can be more easily and thoroughly mixed with digestive juices. Fats that are fluid at body temperature also are generally more readily digested than those that have higher melting points. But most common food fats are fully digested, absorbed, and utilized. (See Chap. 5.)

Waxes are normally present in very small amounts in many foods, usually of vegetable origin. Comb honey is an example of a rich source of wax, but it is perhaps of more interest to sculptors and crayon makers than to nutritionists.

Fatty acids linked to long-chain alcohols are not digestible and so are unavailable to the body. An artificial "fat" has been made by uniting fatty acids to sucrose. This polyester of the lipid family is not digestible. It is under consideration but not yet approved for formulation of low-calorie foods with the texture of fat. Mineral oil (not a lipid and devoid of dietary energy value) has from time to time been used for this purpose. Unfortunately, fat-soluble nutrients are excreted in the feces along with the unabsorbed oil, so the practice is ill-advised.

Table 3–4 CHOLESTEROL CONTENT OF COMMON MEASURES OF SELECTED FOODS (IN ASCENDING ORDER)[a]

Food	*Amount*	*Cholesterol (mg)*
Milk, skim, fluid or reconstituted dry	1 cup	4
Cottage cheese, uncreamed	½ cup	8
Mayonnaise	1 Tbsp.	10
Butter	1 pat	11
Lard	1 Tbsp.	12
Cottage cheese, creamed	½ cup	17
Milk, low fat, 2%	1 cup	18
Half and half	¼ cup	23
Ice cream, approx. 10% fat	½ cup	30
Cheese, cheddar	1 oz	30
Milk, whole	1 cup	34
Oysters, salmon	3 oz	40
Clams, halibut, tuna	3 oz	55
Chicken, turkey, light meat	3 oz	67
Beef, pork, lobster, chicken, turkey, dark meat and	3 oz	75
Lamb, veal, crab	3 oz	85
Shrimp	3 oz	130
Heart, beef	3 oz	230
Egg or egg yolk	1 each	270
Liver, beef, calf, hog, lamb	3 oz	370
Kidney	3 oz	680
Brains, raw	3 oz	>1700

[a]From Feeley, R. M., Criner, P. E., and Watt, B. K.: Cholesterol content of foods. J. Amer. Dietet. Assoc., *61*:134, 1972; and Fats in Food and Diets. U.S. Department of Agriculture Information Bulletin No. 361, 1974.

THE ROLE OF FAT IN THE BODY

Fat plays several important roles in maintaining the well-being of the body.

Essential Fatty Acids and Their Functions

Body tissues possess a marked ability to synthesize complex compounds by combining relatively simple ones. It is well known that excess energy from food eaten can be transformed into stored fat. For this purpose, the long carbon chains of saturated fatty acids and oleic acid (with one double bond at the n–9 position) are built by combining simple, 2-carbon groups (acetate radicals) produced in metabolism of carbohydrates, fats, and proteins. The body, however, is not able to introduce a double bond at the n–6 position and so cannot synthesize *linoleic acid* (18:2, n–6,9). Because *linoleic acid* is needed for the growth and well-being of almost all species of higher animals, including humans, it must be obtained from the diet. Arachidonic acid (20:4,n–6,9,12,15), with four double bonds and 20 carbon atoms used to be included as an essential fatty acid, but since it can be made in the body from linoleic acid, it is not actually essential in the diet. (However, linoleic acid will not suffice for cats, which require dietary arachidonic acid.) Newborn children may benefit from having preformed arachidonic acid, and human milk contains it.

The dietary need for linoleic acid was established with the discovery that rats fed fat-free diets failed to grow or lost weight, developed a scaly condition of the skin and tail, and developed kidney damage that eventually led to their death (1). These conditions could be prevented or alleviated by giving the rats linoleic acid. A. E. Hansen and coworkers produced the same symptoms—poor growth and eczematous skin lesions—in infants fed a formula lacking essential fatty acids (2). (See Fig. 3–4.) Hansen and his associates established definitely that adults as well as infants require essential fatty acids (3). The need for dietary linoleic acid by adults has been amply confirmed by recent studies of hospital patients receiving fat-free feeds intravenously. Usually it is difficult to produce a deficiency of essential fatty acids in adults because body fat stores contain some essential fatty acids, which can be used in

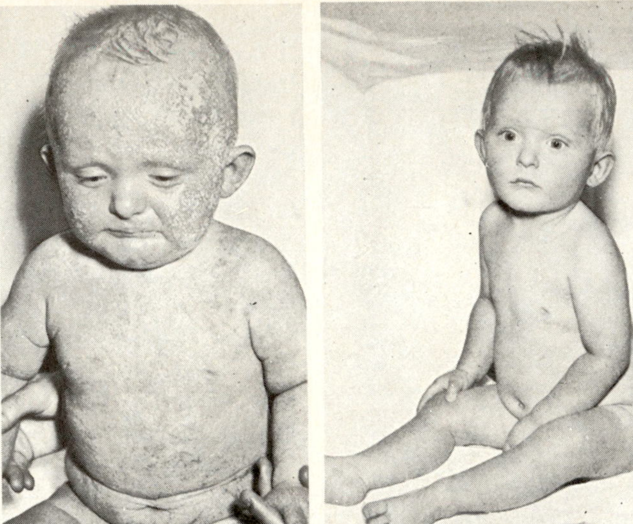

Figure 3–4 The first symptoms identified specifically as being due to essential fatty acid deficiency were skin lesions in rats. Similar lesions were seen in infants given formulas devoid of EFA. This research was carried out before the critical nature of EFAs was known. Ethical considerations would prohibit such research today. *Left,* six-month-old infant with very resistant eczema since two and a half months of age. *Right,* the same child six months later, after a source of linoleic acid had been included in the diet. (Courtesy of the late Dr. A. E. Hansen.)

times of need. However, in patients given very high carbohydrate feedings by vein (called parenteral feeding), augmented insulin activity inhibits release of fatty acids from adipose tissue, resulting in deficiency.

The essentiality for humans of the triply unsaturated fatty acid, *linolenic acid* (18:3, n–3,6,9) was formerly in doubt. The body cannot introduce a double bond at the n–3 position, and fatty acids made from linolenic acid do have specific functions in the brain and retina of the eye, but a deficiency had never been demonstrated in rats or humans. Recently a set of symptoms was identified in a child, being fed parenterally, which were corrected by administration of linolenic acid (4). The symptoms attributed to linolenic acid deficiency are numbness, tingling, and pain in legs and blurred vision.

A number of symptoms have been identified in rats deficient in essential fatty acids; only a few of these symptoms have been demonstrated in humans, probably because depletion has not been so severe. Symptoms of deficiency are as follows:

In both humans and rats
- abnormal skin conditions
- reduced regeneration of injured tissues
- increased susceptibility to infection
- altered ratios of fatty acids in blood[3]

In rats
- decreased weight and growth
- sterility in males and females
- kidney abnormalities
- increased water loss and consumption
- increased fragility of capillaries and red blood cells
- enlargement of the heart
- accumulation of cholesterol in lungs, liver, adrenal glands, and skin

[3]The ratio of triene (20:3,n–9) to tetraene (20:4, n–6) fatty acids is increased. This is because in the absence of adequate amounts of essential fatty acids, cells produce a polyunsaturated series from the n–9 position. These polyunsaturated acids cannot fulfill essential functions. The metabolic basis of these symptoms is still being investigated.

In recent years, nutritionists have learned of the importance of *prostaglandins,* a class of vital hormonelike compounds made in various tissues of the body from arachidonic acid and other derivatives of linoleic acid. The prostaglandins have an important function in regulating such diverse reactions as inhibition of gastric secretion, reduction of blood pressure, antagonism to some hormones and release or activation of others, and contraction of smooth muscle, including the uterus (5). Administration of prostaglandins does not, however, cure skin symptoms in rats made deficient in essential fatty acids. A prominent function of essential fatty acids is in the membrane structure of cells; prostaglandins (and related compounds) do not play a role in this function.

Some odd-numbered synthetic fatty acids have been shown to have essential fatty acid activity. The availability of these compounds may provide a new tool for metabolic research.

Functions of Other Fatty Acids and Lipids

Fat stored in adipose tissue constitutes the major energy reserve of the body. Fat layers beneath the skin provide thermal insulation, and fat surrounds and cushions the internal organs. In these functions, fat is relatively inert. However, the various nonessential fatty acids and lipids also play extremely important roles in many enzyme reactions, in cell membrane structure, in the synthesis and regulation of certain hormones, in the maintenance of the proper structure of blood vessels, and in energy metabolism, digestion, tissue structure, transmission of nerve impulses, memory storage, and other functions.

Cholesterol gives rise to an intermediate substance, 7-dehydrocholesterol, from which vitamin D is formed by ultraviolet light when it penetrates the skin. Certain hormones formed in the adrenal cortex and sex glands (such as *cortisone* and *testosterone*) are sterols, closely related to cholesterol, which serves as a precursor in their synthesis. The *bile acids,* also derivatives of cholesterol, are formed in the liver and excreted by way of the bile into the intestine; a portion of the bile acids are reabsorbed and used again, being excreted in the feces. The same pathway (bile, intestine, feces) serves for the excretion of cholesterol and other related sterols.

Cholesterol is thus seen to be a substance useful to the body. Approximately 2 gm are synthesized, and metabolized, each day within the body of normal adults. The level of cholesterol in the blood is normally kept constant by the body's maintaining a balance between the supply, obtained through the diet and manufactured in the body, and the amount lost, used up in the body and excreted through the intestine. This balance explains why it is so difficult to lower the cholesterol level in the blood simply by restricting cholesterol in the diet.

The Need for Fat in the Diet

Fats and fat-containing foods are of value in the diet for six main reasons:

1. as a source of essential fatty acid (Linoleic and linolenic acids and their metabolic derivatives are essential to all cells and tissues of the body. This is the sole essential use of fat; the others listed below are very important but not essential.)
2. as carriers of fat-soluble vitamins A, D, E, and K and as an aid to their absorption in the intestine (discussed in Chap. 9)
3. as a concentrated source of energy and as a builder of fat stores in the body
4. for satiety value
5. for making foods appetizing and flavorful
6. for providing various "functional properties" to cooked and processed foods

There is no set allowance for essential fatty acids, but the Food and Nutrition Board states that linoleic acid intake equivalent to 2 percent of the total energy in the diet should be sufficient for adults (for example, about 6 gm per day in a diet of 2700 kcal) and 3 percent of energy for infants (6). Most Americans meet this requirement, and many people eat much more than that. Most vegetable oils, such as corn, soybean, cottonseed, safflower, sunflower, and wheat germ oils, are especially rich in linoleic acid. Margarines, vegetable shortenings, nuts, and poultry and fish fat are also good sources.

Other authorities place the minimum requirement of linoleic acid for infants at 1.4 to 4.5 percent of total energy in the diet, the higher requirement being for premature babies. Based on a single case (a six-year-old child), the minimum requirement for linolenic acid is thought to be 0.54 percent of energy, or 0.6 gm per 1000 kcal (4).

Human milk provides a generous allowance of essential fatty acids (4 to 6 percent of total energy), but formulas based on cow's milk just barely meet the minimum requirement. Because the lactating mother must provide the essential fatty acids in her milk, her own needs are increased. The United Nations Food and Agricultural Organization (FAO) and World Health Organization (WHO) estimate the additional requirement to be 4 percent of energy intake.

It is difficult to state how much of the essential fatty acids, beyond the minimum figures just given, it is desirable to have in the diet. The polyunsaturated fatty acids are closely interrelated with other dietary components, and these affect the need for the essential fatty acids. Most of the interactions have been worked out in animals, but at least some are known to be operative in humans. Factors believed to increase the requirement for essential fatty acids are high intakes of saturated fatty acids and of monounsaturated fatty acids (both *trans* and *cis* isomers). Linolenic acid inhibits the conversion of linoleic acid to arachidonic acid; hence, it is important to maintain a balance between these fatty acids in which intake of linoleic acid is several fold higher than that of linolenic acid. This balance is assured by a person's consuming a varied mixture of plant and animal fats. The need for the antioxidant vitamin E is increased when unsaturated fatty acid intake is high. (See Chap. 9.)

There is no specific requirement for consuming phospholipids and cholesterol, even though they are essential components of body cells, because both can be made in the body.

The high energy value of fats (9 kcal/gm) means that relatively small amounts of fat-rich foods decidedly raise the energy value of the diet. Fats are useful when it is desirable to have a higher intake of food energy without adding unduly to the bulk of the diet. A diet very low in fat often either supplies less energy than the body needs, thereby causing weight loss, or is much more bulky than the customary American or European diet. This is a particular problem in meeting the energy needs of very young children where sheer volume of a bulky low-fat diet may limit intake.

The satiety value of fats depends on the fact that fats slow down the emptying time of the stomach; meals that contain considerable fat prevent the early recurrence of hunger. But when too much fat is taken, the result may be a feeling of discomfort.

Fats incorporated and naturally present in foods give prized flavor and make the food more appetizing to most people. The flavor varies somewhat with the kind of fat used, individual preference being largely based on habit, culture, and economic conditions. Since certain fats have become scarcer and more costly, the attitude of American consumers has altered to include a greater acceptance of formerly less used but cheaper fats—for example, corn or cottonseed oil instead of olive oil, and margarine instead of butter.

Fat-Rich Foods in the Diet

The amount of fat in the diet, like the amount of carbohydrate, may be varied widely. How much is used depends on personal tastes, money spent for food, and availability of fat-rich foods. Only about 10 percent of the energy in the average diets of poor Asiatic peoples is furnished by fats. Population pressure in any country requires that land be used primarily for the production of carbohydrate-rich foods that furnish energy at least cost, instead of for the production of less efficient meat and dairy products (though often range lands or waste by-products can be used for farm animals).

Among people of moderate means in many countries, fat intake may account for only 20 to 25 percent of total energy intake. In countries such as the Netherlands, Denmark, New Zealand, Canada, and the United States, meat fats, dairy products, and vegetable oils (or shortenings and spreads made from them) are available at prices most people can afford. Under such conditions, 40 to 45 percent of the energy content of the diet may come from fat-rich foods.

In the United States, the percentage of dietary energy derived from fat has been increasing since the 1920s (Fig. 3–5). A study of students from fifty colleges showed that fat content of meals averaged 126 gm a day, representing 42 percent of total energy(8). This amount was made up of 46 gm saturated fatty acids, 48 grams oleic acid, and 17 gm linoleic acid.

Representative menus deriving different percentages of energy from fat are given in Table 3–5. The high-fiber menu derives 30 percent of its energy from fat; it could easily be made higher in fat by using whole milk rather than low-fat milk, spreading butter on the luncheon sandwich, adding a more generous amount of butter or sour cream to the baked potato, and putting more oil on the dinner salad. The high-fat menu derives 58 percent of its energy from fat. Only the lean portion of the steak is consumed; were all the steak fat eaten, fat intake would increase by 92 gm. National food supply data show a higher "consumption" of food energy than actual food intake surveys reveal, and such practices as discarding visible fat from meat contribute to this difference.

In the United States, about 40 percent of fat comes from fats and oils (including butter); 33 percent from meat, poultry, and fish; 17 percent from dairy products (other than butter); and 4 percent from eggs.

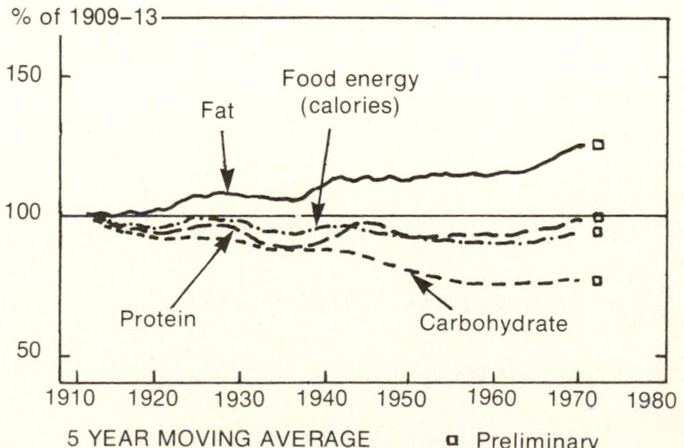

Figure 3–5 Shift in per capita consumption of food energy, protein, fat, and carbohydrate in the United States between 1910 and 1970. Carbohydrate in the national food supply has declined about one-fourth over this period (down from 500 gm to 380 gm per day) and fat intake has risen steadily. In 1970 per capita utilization of fat was 155 gm per day and protein, 100 gm per day. (From Page, L., and Friend, B.: Level of use of sugars in the United States. In *Sugars in Nutrition,* ed. H. L. Sipple and K. W. McNutt, New York, Academic Press, 1974. Used with permission.)

Table 3–5 REPRESENTATIVE MENUS OF HIGH AND MODERATE FAT CONTENT, gm per serving

Moderate Fat				*High Fat*	
HIGH FIBER		LOW FIBER			
		Breakfast			
Oatmeal, ¾ cup	1	Corn flakes, 1 oz		Omelet, 2 eggs	12
Bread, whole gr., 2 slices	2	Bread, white, 2 slices	2	Cheese, 1 oz	9
Butter, 1 pat	4	Margarine, 1 pat	4	Bread, whole gr., 1 slice	1
Jam, 1 Tbsp		Jelly, 1 Tbsp		Butter, 2 pats	8
Milk, low fat, ½ cup	2	Milk, skim, ½ cup		Grapefruit, ½	
Orange, 1 medium		Banana, 1 medium			
Sugar, 1 tsp		Sugar, 1 tsp			
		Luncheon			
Bean soup, 1 cup	6	Chicken-noodle soup, 1 cup	1	Consommé, 1 cup	
Rye crackers, 2		Saltine crackers, 2	1	Ritz crackers, 2	3
Sandwich		Sandwich		Tuna salad[a], ½ cup	11
Egg, 1	6	Bologna, 1 slice	8	Avocado, ½	18
Bread, whole gr., 2 slices	2	Bread, white, 2 slices	2	Lettuce	
Lettuce		Margarine, 1 pat	4	Thousand Is. Dressing, 2 Tbsp	16
Mayonnaise, 1 Tbsp	11	Mustard, 1 tsp		Strawberries, ½ cup	
Pear, 1 medium		Grapes, 20 seedless		Cream, heavy, ¼ cup	22
Milk, low fat, 1 cup	5	Milk, whole, 1 cup	8		
		Dinner			
Chicken, broiled, ¼	3	Chicken, fried[b]	33	Tomato juice, ½ cup	
Baked potato w/ skin		Rice, white, ½ cup		Steak, 12 oz (lean only, 8 oz)	16[c]
Winter squash, ½ cup		Gravy, 2 Tbsp	4	Green beans, ½ cup	
Mixed green salad, 1½ cup		Peas, canned, ½ cup		Butter, 1 pat	4
Vinegar, ½ Tbsp		Tomato, 1 medium		Mixed green salad, 1½ cup	
Oil, ½ Tbsp	7	Biscuits, 2	6	Italian dressing, 2 Tbsp	18
Rolls, whole grain, 2	4	Honey, 1 Tbsp		Red wine, 7 fl. oz	
Butter, 3 pats	12	Margarine, 1 pat	4	Cheese, Brie, 1 oz	8
Blueberry pie, ⅙	17	Ice cream, ½ cup	7	Apple, 1 medium	
		Chocolate brownie, 1	4		
		Snacks			
Apple juice, ½ cup		Soda pop, 12 oz		Sparkling water	
Yogurt, flavored, 1 cup	3	potato chips, 1 oz	11	Almonds, roasted, 1 oz	16
TOTAL	85		99		162

[a]Made with 1 Tbsp salad dressing and celery.
[b]Commercial, breaded, one thigh and one leg.
[c]Fat discarded = 92 gm.

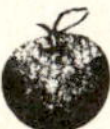

health considerations

Toxicity of Fats

Few fats in foods are toxic, but there are important exceptions. Some varieties of rapeseed oil, castor oil, and impure cottonseed oil contain unusual fatty acids or other lipids that can cause toxic symptoms. Most of these substances can be removed or destroyed by plant breeding and proper processing. (See Chap. 18.) Of probably greater importance is the possibility of toxins—pesticides or other toxins—being inadvertently carried along in the food chain by improperly processed or stored fats.

Rancidity is a chemical reaction in fat caused by oxidation that is hastened by heating or lack of antioxidants. Mildly rancid fats are not particularly toxic but are distasteful to most people. In some cultures, small amounts of rancidity are considered desirable. Fats used over and over in cooking or frying may develop toxic substances.

The *trans* fatty acids, formed during hydrogenation (and to a very small extent in animal tissues), may be of some concern because of their reported inhibiting effects on enzymes involved in essential fatty acid metabolism and prostaglandin synthesis (9). This subject is still being examined and it would be premature to conclude that *trans* acids are a threat to health at levels usually consumed, but a note of caution is in order.

Heart Disease

Atherosclerosis is a disease process in which the diameter of the arteries is narrowed as a result of the development on the interior wall of fibrous lesions rich in cholesterol and fat. Blood clots tend to form in these narrowed spaces occluding the vessel and stopping blood flow (and hence oxygen and nourishment) to the organ it serves. When the vessels affected are in the heart or brain, the result is a coronary heart attack, or a stroke. Although the mortality rate has been on the decline since about 1960, coronary heart disease is still the leading cause of death in the United States.

Atherosclerosis has been associated with dietary fat ever since high levels of blood cholesterol and fat were identified as predisposing or risk factors (along with obesity, high blood pressure, smoking, and family history) in human populations. Supporting evidence has come from animal studies in which experimental feeding of high levels of cholesterol and saturated fat has resulted in deposition of lipids in the arteries. These same animal models have been used to identify protective effects of polyunsaturated fatty acids and, more recently, dietary fiber.

Population studies have ruled out fat intake per se as the principal factor in heart disease, but they do indicate that the type of fat is important. Higher intakes of polyunsaturated fatty acids, a higher ratio of polyunsaturated to saturated fatty acids (P/S) in the diet, and lower cholesterol intake are associated with lower risk of coronary heart disease. Many experimental studies demonstrate that serum cholesterol in humans can be reduced about 15 percent by increasing the dietary P/S ratio, increasing the intake of mucilaginous fiber (gums and pectin, which increase the excretion of fecal sterols), and, sometimes but not always, by reducing dietary cholesterol.

Recently, attention has focused on risk associated with specific forms of cholesterol and fat in the blood. As has been noted, triacylglycerides, phospholipids, and cholesterol are combined with globulin proteins and carried to the tissues as lipoprotein complexes. Chylomicrons are the largest of the lipoprotein complexes and are basically large fat droplets covered with a very thin protein layer. After a meal rich in fats, plasma becomes turbid from the chylomicrons formed in the intestine, which are taken up by the lymph system and released into the blood; but this extra fat leaves the blood and passes into the tissues within a few hours. The liver is the primary site of synthesis of the other lipoproteins. These particles are the means of transporting fat to the tissues from the liver; they are smaller than chylomicrons and contain varying amounts of protein, from 10 to 60 percent of their weight.

Fat is lighter than water (that is, its specific gravity is less than 1.0), and proteins are heavier. The transport lipoproteins are generally classified by weight; the lighter they are, the more lipid they contain in proportion to protein. The very low density lipoproteins (VLDL) formed in the liver and intestines contain less fat but more protein, phospholipid, and cholesterol than chylomicrons. Fatty acids are removed by body tissues from the chylomicrons and VLDLs, which decreases the size of these particles. The low-density lipoproteins (LDL) resulting from these processes thus are smaller and contain still less fat and more protein and cholesterol than the VLDLs. The high-density lipoproteins (HDL) are quite different; they are rich in protein, phospholipids, and cholesterol and appear to be involved in disposal of cholesterol from the tissues.

The LDLs are thought to be the major source of cholesterol deposited in the arteries, and elevated levels of LDLs in the blood are associated with high risk of heart disease. Conversely, high levels of HDLs are associated with reduced risk. Generally, conditions associated with reduced risk of heart disease—high P/S ratio in the diet, adequate physical exercise, moderate consumption of alcohol, and correction of obesity—are accompanied by an increased ratio of HDLs to LDLs in the blood.

Many other physiological variables play a role in heart disease and serve to moderate or intensify the effects of other diseases. How easily the blood tends to clot is thought to be important. Dietary factors that reduce clottability are thus of interest; a fatty acid found in fish fat (eicosapentenoic acid, C20:5), garlic, and onions are all under study in this connection. Predisposing injury to blood vessels (as a result of hypertension, for example) is another variable. Some variables are genetic. Therefore, altered diet may not always be an effective measure. Diet is, however, a matter over which the individual has control, and it is worth serious attention on this and other grounds.

Cancer

Recently a U.S. National Research Council committee has sounded another warning because of epidemiological evidence linking diets consumed in affluent cultures with high incidence of *cancer of the breast, colon, and uterus.* The committee observed that the complexity of modern diets makes it difficult to pinpoint any one factor as causal, but it stated that, of all the components studied, "evidence is most suggestive for a causal relationship between fat intake and the occurrence of cancer." Other dietary factors, identified with lower cancer risk, are greater consumption of fiber-rich and carotene-containing foods and avoidance of alcohol.

Obesity

Evidence linking high fat intake and obesity is stronger than that linking obesity to high intake of sugar. This is not surprising because the higher energy yield from fat makes it possible to obtain much energy in a small volume. A nutrition survey of 300,000 people in Brazil illustrates this association between dietary fat and the conformation of the human body (10). Correlation analysis showed normal weight for height to be associated with diets in which 30–40 percent of the energy came from fat. Diets having 20–30 percent of energy derived from fat were associated with slenderness and those below 12–15 percent with emaciation. As noted in Chapter 2, fat intake is income-related and low consumers of fat are liable to be deprived of food in general. Laboratory animals, however, also are more easily made obese with high-fat diets than with diets lower in fat content.

All of these considerations have led many authorities to recommend a prudent diet that meets the following guidelines.

1. Fat contributes not more than 30 percent of

dietary energy. This means about 33 gm of fat per 1000 kcal.

2. The ratio of polyunsaturated fatty acids (PUFA) to saturated fatty acids is high, about 1:1. Since monounsaturated oleic acid is so very common in fats, this means about 10 percent of dietary energy in each form of fatty acids. As demonstrated, this amount of PUFAs more than meets the specific essential fatty acid requirement.
3. The energy from fat is replaced with complex carbohydrate (starches), in food forms that include dietary fiber.
4. Cholesterol is not more than 300 mg per day. This is a controversial recommendation and is, perhaps, the least well-justified feature of the prudent diet. Eggs are the only high-cholesterol food eaten regularly by many people, and this prescription would limit intake to not more than one egg a day (270 mg cholesterol).

ALCOHOL

Probably one of the best-known food processing techniques is fermentation, the production of potable alcohol by the action of yeast on carbohydrate. Almost all cultural groups (some native American Indian tribes were exceptions) have learned to use and control the process. The starting material may be fruit, palm or cactus juices, molasses or sugar, honey, milk, potatoes, or cereal grains; the flavor of the final product will vary accordingly, but the alcohol produced is the same: the simple compound ethyl alcohol or ethanol, C_2H_5OH.[4] Because fermentation is a metabolic process, a number of intermediate and alternate compounds may be present; carbon dioxide (CO_2) is given off as a by-product. If the process is not stopped before the yeast uses all the available carbohydrate, the yeast will begin to convert ethanol to acetic acid (CH_3COOH), making vinegar instead of wine.

[4]Destructive pyrolysis of wood pulp results in production of another alcohol, methanol or wood alcohol, which is highly poisonous.

Yeast cannot continue to grow if the concentration of alcohol becomes excessive (over about 20 percent), so the hard liquors are produced by distillation, which concentrates the alcohol and separates it from the starting material. Thus, the natural products—beer and wine—contain some nutrients present in the original malted barley and fruit juice, but distilled spirits have no essential nutrients. In terms of dilution of the nutritive quality of the diet, distilled spirits (such as gin, rum, whiskey, and brandy) have the same effect as refined sugar. It is not surprising, then, that habitual overusers of alcoholic beverages often have poor intakes of vitamins and minerals.

Alcohol is metabolized in the liver, but the liver's capacity is limited. Most individuals can metabolize about 0.1 gm/kg body weight/hr (range 0.06–0.2 gm). Alcohol yields 7 kcal/gm, so the hourly capacity of a 70 kg man would be $70 \times 0.1 \times 7$, or about 50 kcal/hr from ethanol. In the course of a day of steady drinking, the total energy from this source could reach 1200 kcal, and many regular drinkers consume that much and more. This would amount to some 18 oz (about 520 ml) of 86 proof hard liquor or 1.7 liters (about ½ gal) of wine (Table 3–6).

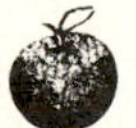

health considerations

Drinking Alcoholic Beverages

If alcohol is consumed at a rate faster than it can be metabolized (that is, for a 70 kg man, 7 gm/hr, or about half a 12 oz can of beer per hour), then the level of alcohol builds up in body tissues; eventually intoxication and, in the extreme, death results.

Table 3–6 SOCIAL BEVERAGES: CALORIC VALUES AND ALCOHOLIC CONTENT OF PORTIONS COMMONLY USED*

	Approximate Measure	*Weight gm*	*Energy kcal*	*Carbohydrate gm*	*Alcohol† gm*
Distilled liquors					
Liqueurs					
Anisette, Sambuca	1 cordial glass	20	75	7.0	7.0
Apricot brandy	1 cordial glass	20	65	6.0	6.0
Benedictine	1 cordial glass	20	70	7.0	6.6
Creme de menthe	1 cordial glass	20	70	6.0	7.0
Curaçao, Triple sec	1 cordial glass	20	65	6.0	6.0
Brandy or cognac	1 brandy glass	30	75		10.5
Gin, dry, 80 proof	1 jigger, 1½ oz.	45	105		15.1
Rum, 80 proof	1 jigger, 1½ oz	45	105		15.1
Whiskey, rye, 90 proof	1 jigger, 1½ oz	45	119		17.2
Whiskey, Scotch, 80 proof	1 jigger, 1½ oz	45	105		15.1
Wines					
California, table wine, red or white	1 wine glass	100	85	4.0	10.5
Champagne, domestic	1 wine glass	120	85	3.0	11.0
Port or muscatel	1 wine glass	100	160	14.0	15.0
Sherry, dry, domestic	1 wine glass	60	85	5.0	9.0
Vermouth, sweet	1 wine glass	100	170	12.0	18.0
Vermouth, dry	1 wine glass	100	105	1.0	15.0
Malt liquors (American)					
Ale, mild	1 bottle, 12 oz	345	150	12.0	13.1
Beer, avg.	Large glass, 8 oz	240	115	10.6	8.9
Beer, avg.	1 bottle, 12 oz	360	175	15.8	13.3
Beer, 'light', avg.	1 bottle, 12 oz	360	100	3.0	12.0
Mixed drinks, cocktails (approx. from recipes)					
Daiquiri	1 cocktail glass	100	125	5.2	15.1
Eggnog, holiday	1 punch cup, 4 oz	123	335	18.0	15.0
High ball	1 glass, 8 oz	240	165		24.0
Manhattan	1 cocktail glass	100	165	8.0	19.2
Martini	1 cocktail glass	100	140	tr.	18.5
Mint julep	1 glass, 10 oz	300	210	3.0	29.2
Old fashioned	1 glass, 4 oz	100	180	4.0	24.0
Planter's punch	1 glass	100	175	8.0	21.5
Rum sour	1 glass	100	165	4.5	21.0
Tom Collins	1 glass, 10 oz	300	180	9.0	21.5
Soft drinks					
Cider, sweet	1 c	250	124	34.4	0
Club soda	12 fl oz	355	0	0	0
Coffee, black	6 fl oz	180	2	tr.	0
Cola type	6 fl oz	180	70	18.5	0
Eggnog	1 c	245	235	18.0	0
Fruit-flavored sodas	12 fl oz	370	170	45.0	0
Ginger ale	6 fl oz	180	55	15.0	0
Hot chocolate, half milk	1 c	220	145	27.1	0
Ice cream soda, chocolate	1 avg.	300	255	46.0	0
Lemonade	10 fl oz	295	105	27.2	0
Postum (cereal-based)	6 fl oz	185	36	8.5	0
Quinine water	6 fl oz	180	55	15.0	0
Root beer	12 fl oz	370	150	39.0	0
Tea, plain	6 fl oz	180	2	tr.	0

*Figure chiefly from Bowes, C. F., and Church, H. N.: *Food Values of Portions Commonly Used*. 12th Ed. Philadelphia, J. B. Lippincott Co., 1975. tr = trace, less than 1 gm.

†The caloric value of alcohol is approximately 7 kcal per gram, but the body has limited capacity to oxidize it. This gives a physiological reason for sipping rather than gulping down such beverages.

Alcohol is damaging to the liver, and chronic users have an increased risk of liver disease (cirrhosis). In high concentration, alcohol is damaging to the lining of the intestinal tract; absorption of nutrients is affected adversely, and the risk of cancer of the esophagus increases with alcohol use. Ultimately, overuse leads to degenerative changes in the nervous system. The U.S. Department of Health and Human Services has estimated that in 1975, there were about 36,000 deaths from cirrhosis, alcoholism, and alcoholic psychosis, and that alcohol was a contributing factor in an additional 51,000 fatalities. In 1977, about 45 percent of all U.S. motor vehicle fatalities involved drinking drivers.

The fetus is especially susceptible to alcohol. A set of malformations called the fetal alcohol syndrome (facial abnormalities, reduced head size, and subnormal mentality) has been described in infants born to women who drink heavily. This syndrome accounts for about 1,400 to 2,000 birth defects annually.

Alcohol abuse is a serious worldwide problem. The World Health Organization reports that in 1970, in the United States, 2.7 percent of persons aged 15 years and older used daily more than 150 ml of alcohol (from all legal beverages consumed); in Canada, the figure is 2.5 percent, and in France it is a staggering 9.0 percent.

On the other hand, there is little evidence that moderate, socially responsible drinking has serious health effects. Alcohol is known to have detrimental effects on the heart and is associated with elevated blood pressure (11). Yet, epidemiologic evidence indicates that death due to cardiovascular causes is higher in teetotalers than in those who drink moderate amounts of alcohol (12). Death from other causes is far higher in heavy drinkers (who consume more than 30 gm daily or about 2 drinks) than in moderate drinkers and nondrinkers (Fig 3–5).

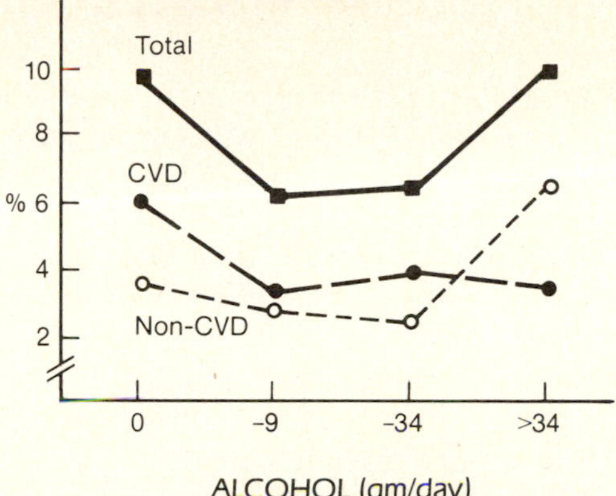

Figure 3–6 Ten-year mortality (age-adjusted %) all causes, cardiovascular (CVD) and noncardiovascular (non-CVD) causes according to daily alcohol consumption. The risk of CVD is higher in heavy drinkers. (From Marmot, M. G., et al., Lancet 1:580, 1981, with permission.)

Conclusion. Alcoholic beverages can have a relaxing effect and stimulate the appetite. As long as beer and wine are used in moderation and with awareness of the risks entailed, there seems no reason, other than any personal beliefs, to deny their occasional consumption by nonpregnant women and adult males. However, the benefits cited with respect to cardiovascular death are not so convincing as to encourage anyone to drink who does not already do so.

QUESTIONS

1. What physical properties are characteristic of fats? What substances does any true fat yield on hydrolysis (in digestion or outside the body)? How many molecules of fatty acid does a molecule of glycerol link with to form one molecule of fat? Do the fatty acids most commonly found in fats consist of long or short chains of carbon atoms? Is the proportion of carbon to the amount of hydrogen and oxygen greater or less in a molecule of fatty acid than in a molecule of glucose? How does this account for the fact that, when fats are burned or oxidized in body tissues, they

yield more than twice as much energy as carbohydrates do?

2. What is the difference between a saturated and an unsaturated fatty acid? What is the difference between a monounsaturated and a polyunsaturated fatty acid? Is oleic acid a polyunsaturated fatty acid? What is the name of the polyunsaturated fatty acid found most abundantly in fatty foods? How do the kinds of fatty acids (saturated or unsaturated) that predominate determine the consistency (solid, semisolid, or liquid) of foods that are almost pure fat?

3. What is meant by an essential fatty acid? What symptoms occur in infants because of insufficient essential fatty acids in their foods? Does a deficiency in essential fatty acids ever occur in adults on normal diets? Why? If one wished to increase the intake of polyunsaturated fatty acids, what foods should be included in moderate amounts in the diet?

4. How can unsaturated fatty acids be made to take on more hydrogen—that is, be converted into saturated ones? Does butter carry any unsaturated fatty acids? When a fluid fat such as corn or cottonseed oil is converted to a semisolid by hydrogenation to make cooking fats or margarine, are all the unsaturated fatty acids converted to saturated ones? Consult Table 3–2 and compare the content of unsaturated fatty acids in butter and the various types of margarine.

5. Define lipids, true fats, phospholipids, and sterols. In what body tissues are phospholipids most abundant? What sterol is found in animal tissues and blood? Can it be formed in the body, and if so, where? Is the level of cholesterol in the blood closely related to the amount that is ingested? Does the intake of total energy, the proportion of the energy intake furnished by fats, or the ratio of saturated to polyunsaturated fats in the diet influence the cholesterol level in the blood? If so, with what results in each instance?

6. What are the chief uses of fats in the body? Of fatty foods in the diet? What percentage of the total energy intake is furnished by fats in the average American diet? What are the disadvantages of too high a level of fat in the diet or of very low fat intake? What foods would you avoid or take in smaller amounts in order to decrease the relative amount of fat in the diet?

7. What is an alcohol? What is ethanol? What nutritional contribution do alcoholic beverages make? How much alcohol can be metabolized per hour? Is it safe to drink alcoholic beverages? Justify your answer.

References

1. Burr, G. O., and Burr, M. M.: A new deficiency disease produced by the rigid exclusion of fat from the diet. J. Biol. Chem., *82*:345, 1929 (reprinted in Nutr. Rev., *32*:19, 1974); Burr, G. O., and Burr, M. M.: On the nature and role of the fatty acids essential in nutrition. J. Biol. Chem., *86*:587, 1930.
2. Hansen, A. E.: Serum lipids in eczema and other pathological conditions. Amer. J. Dis. Child., *53*:933, 1937; Hansen, A. E., et al.: Role of linoleic acid in infant nutrition. Pediatrics, *31*:171, 1963.
3. Wiese, H. F., Gibbs, R. H., and Hansen, A. E.: Essential fatty acids in human nutrition, I and II. J. Nutr., *52*:355 and 367, 1954; Wiese, H. F., Hansen, A. E., and Adams, D. J. D.: Essential fatty acids in human nutrition. J. Nutr., *66*:345, 1955.
4. Holman, R. T., Johnson, S. B., and Hatch, T. F.: A case of human linolenic acid deficiency involving neurological abnormalities. Amer. J. Clin. Nutr., *35*:617, 1982.
5. Samuelsson, B., et al.: Prostaglandins and thromboxanes. Ann. Rev. Biochem. *47*:997, 1978; Lands, W. E. M.: The biosynthesis and metabolism of prostaglandins. Ann. Rev. Physiol. *41*:633, 1979.
6. Food and Nutrition Board: *Recommended Dietary Allowances.* 9th Ed. Washington, D.C., National Research Council, National Academy of Sciences, 1980.
7. Food and Agriculture Organization: Dietary fats and oils in human nutrition. FAO Food and Nutr. Ser. No. 20, Rome, 1980.
8. Walker, M. A., and Page, L.: Nutritive content of college meals. II. Lipids. J. Amer. Dietet. Assoc., *68*:34, 1976.
9. DeSchrijver, R., and Privett, O. S.: Interrelationship between dietary *trans* fatty acids and the 6– and 9–desaturases in the rat. Lipids, *17*:27, 1982; Hwang, D. H., Chanmugam, P., and Anding, R.: Effects of dietary 9–*trans* –12–*trans*–linoleate in arachidonic acid metabolism in rat platelets. Lipids, *17*:307, 1982; Kinsella, J. B., Bruckner, G., Mai, J., and Shrimp, J.: Metabolism of *trans* fatty acids with emphasis on the effects of *trans, trans*-octadecadieonate ion on lipid composition, essential fatty acid, and prostaglandins: an overview. Amer. J. Clin. Nutr. *34*:2307, 1981.

10. Francois, P.: Brazil national nutrition survey, unpublished data. Food & Agricultural Organization, Rome, 1980.
11. Altura, B. M., Chairman: Symposium: Cardiovascular effects of alcohol and alcoholism. Fed. Proc. *41*:2437, 1982; Cooke, K. M., Frost, G. W., Thornell, I. R., and Stokes, G. S.: Alcohol consumption and blood pressure. Med. J. Aust., *1*:65, 1982.
12. Marmot, M. G., Rose, G., Shipley, M. J., and Thomas, B. J., Alcohol and mortality: a U-shaped curve. Lancet *1*:580, 1981.

4 Protein and Amino Acids

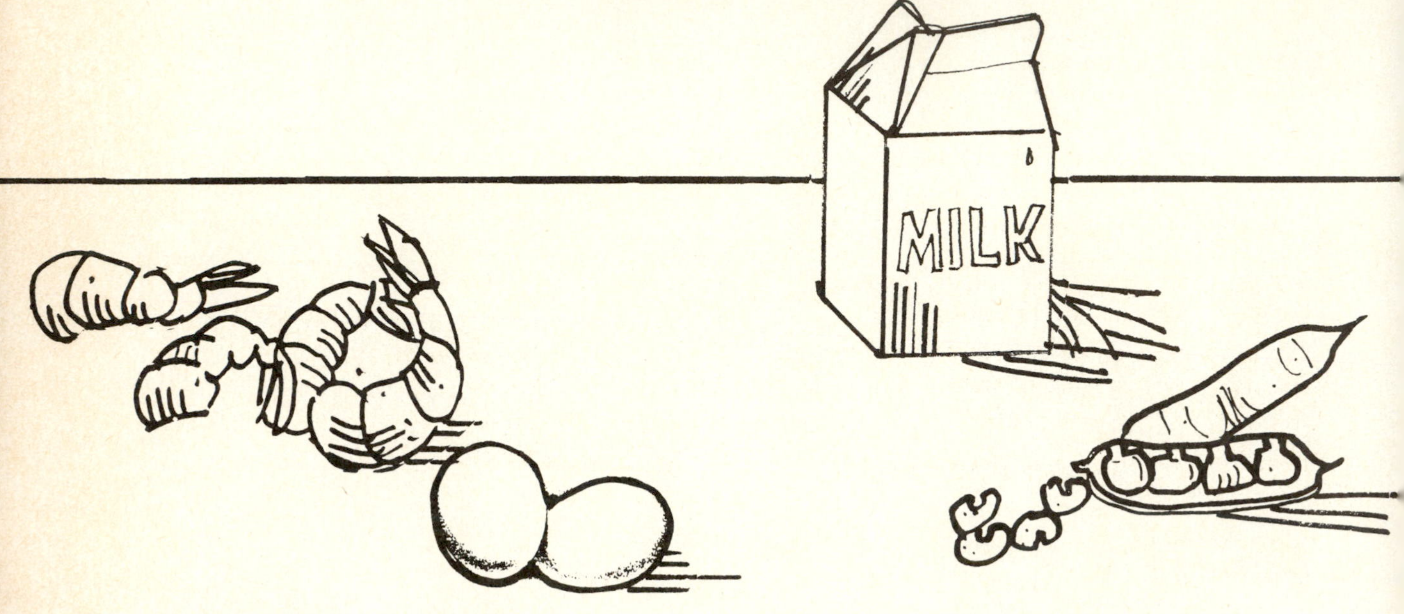

DESCRIPTION OF PROTEIN AND AMINO ACIDS

Protein was recognized very early in the history of nutrition as being not only an energy source but an essential nutrient. Protein-rich foods are generally preferred and command a large share of any food budget. Natural protein-rich foods are also excellent sources of most of the essential nutrients. What accounts for this association of protein and other nutritional factors is that proteins play a vital part in the structural and functional characteristics of every cell in all living tissues, plant and animal. Protein, in a myriad of forms, makes up more than half of all the organic matter in the human body.

The outer layers of skin, the hair, wool and feathers, and nails and horns consist almost entirely of the insoluble protein *keratin.* The most active and abundant tissues of the animal body—the organs and muscles—are very high in protein content. Muscle contains about 20 percent of the proteins *myosin, actin,* and *myoglobin,* by far the most abundant solid constituents of muscles. Blood carries the important iron-containing protein *hemoglobin* in red cells and in the fluid (plasma) portion, *lipoproteins, albumin,* and others. The red marrow of bones is rich in protein, and even adipose tissue, which acts chiefly as a storage depot for excess fat, has some protein. Protein is stored in eggs to provide for the growth of all these tissues in the young bird. Plants similarly store protein in the seed, and the most metabolically active part of a plant, its leaf, also has a relatively high level of protein. (On a dry-weight-basis, spinach is about 40 percent protein, soybeans are 35 percent, eggs are about 50 percent, and lean meat and fish are about 75 percent.) Enzymes and many hormones are protein.

Protein consumption varies widely in different parts of the world according to foods available and income levels. The sparse, mainly vegetarian diets common in tropical and less affluent societies may provide 50 gm daily, or less, whereas the traditional diets of polar regions include about 300 gm. Where a variety of protein-rich foods is abundant, protein consumption is usually determined by personal preferences, cultural habits, and the money available for food. Most people seem to prefer a diet in which 12 to 15 percent of energy is from protein.

Chemical Structure of Proteins

Proteins are composed of larger and more complex molecules than are fats or carbohydrates and differ from other energy nutrients in that they contain nitrogen (in addition to carbon, hydrogen, and oxygen). Most also contain sulfur, and many contain phosphorus, iron, or other minerals. The large molecules of the proteins are made up of great numbers of relatively simple units, the nitrogen-containing compounds called *amino acids.* These basic units all contain at least one organic acid radical (the carboxyl group, COOH) and one amino radical (NH_2) in a typical structure

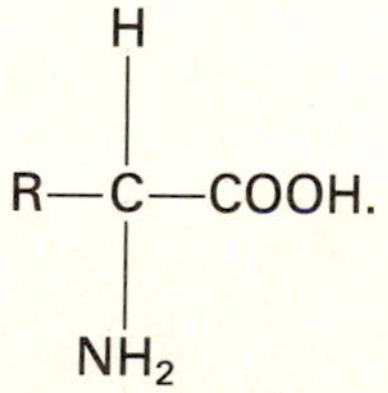

$$\begin{array}{c} H \\ | \\ R\text{—}C\text{—}COOH. \\ | \\ NH_2 \end{array}$$

R may be a chain of different lengths or a ring structure, or simply another H, in which case the amino acid (CH_2NH_2COOH) is glycine. A few amino acids contain two acid or two amino groups, and other amino acids include sulfur in their structures.

Some twenty-two different amino acids are known to be present fairly commonly in proteins that occur in nature. The number of different amino acids in the molecules of individual proteins varies from eight to eighteen. These amino acids are arranged in an intricate pattern characteristic of each individual protein. Because not only the kinds of amino acids may vary but also the relative quantities of each and their arrangement and sequence, the number of individual proteins that are possible is almost infinite. The molecules of protein are so large that their molecular weight varies from several thousand up to several million.

The manner in which the amino acids are joined to form proteins is common to all proteins. This is called *peptide linkage.* Each amino acid has a terminal acid group (COOH) that can react with the basic amino group (NH_2) attached to the carbon atom next to the acid group of a second amino acid. This linkage involves the loss of one H atom and one OH radical, with the formation of a molecule of water, thus:

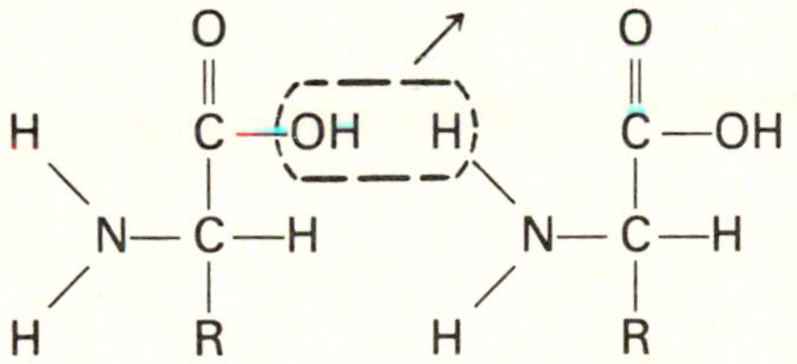

$$\begin{array}{ccccccccc} & & O & & \nearrow & & & O & \\ & & \| & & & & & \| & \\ H & & C & \text{—}(OH & H) & & & C & \text{—}OH \\ & \diagdown & | & & & \diagdown & & | & \\ & & N\text{—}C\text{—}H & & & & N\text{—} & C & \text{—}H \\ & \diagup & | & & & \diagup & & | & \\ H & & R & & H & & & R & \end{array}$$

When proteins are broken down, as happens in digestion, by hydrolysis (reaction with water), the components of water (H and OH) lost when the peptide bond was formed are restored, and the peptide linkage is broken; the protein molecule is broken down into the amino acids from which it was originally formed. Proteins must first be resolved by digestion into their constituent amino acids before they can be absorbed into the blood and utilized by the body cells.

Classification of Proteins

Proteins are divided into two main categories, simple and conjugated. *Simple proteins* contain only amino acids or their derivatives, while *conjugated proteins* are linked to some nonprotein substance.

The simple proteins are all polypeptides, and they are classified according to their solubility and other properties. The most common ones, listed in descending order of solubility, are as follows:

Albumins: (soluble in water) plasma albumin, lactalbumin in milk, albumin in egg white
Globulins: myosin in muscle
Glutelins: abundant in cereal grains, for example, wheat glutenin
Prolamins: common in cereal grains, for example, gliadin in wheat, zein in maize
Scleroproteins: (insoluble in the common solvents, most are resistant to digestive enzymes) common in supporting tissues, for example, collagen, elastin, keratin

Conjugated proteins are subdivided according to their nonprotein component. Protein molecules may be conjugated with fat (lipoproteins in the blood) or carbohydrate (glycoproteins, such as are found in the mucus secreted into the digestive tract). Other important conjugated proteins are formed by linkage with phosphoric acid (phosphoproteins; the milk protein casein is one example); with the lipid phosphatidylcholine (fibrin in clotted blood, vitellin in egg yolk); with an iron-containing compound (heme) to form hemoglobin in the blood; and with nucleic acid to form nucleoproteins, which are essential components of cell nuclei and protoplasm.

Classification of Amino Acids

Amino acids are classified chemically according to their structural features, such as monoamino monocarboxylic, meaning having one amino group and one carboxyl group. They are classified biologically according to whether or not they can be made in the body and are therefore either essential or nonessential in the diet. The common amino acids are listed below; structures will be found in the Appendix. Those in boldface type are essential.

Monoamino, monocarboxylic
- straight-chain
  - glycine
  - alanine
- branched-chain
  - **valine**
  - **leucine**
  - **isoleucine**
- hydroxyl-containing
  - serine
  - **threonine**
- sulfur-containing
  - cystine (and cysteine)
  - **methionine**
- aromatic (contain a benzene ring)
  - tyrosine
  - **phenylalanine**
- heterocyclic (ring contains atoms of different elements)
  - proline
  - hydroxyproline
  - **histidine**
  - **tryptophan**

Diamino, monocarboxylic
- arginine
- **lysine**

Monoamino, dicarboxylic
- glutamic acid
- aspartic acid

Amino Acids, Essential and Nonessential

Certain amino acids are essential—that is, they must be provided preformed in the food. In reality, all amino acids are essential for the building and upkeep of body tissues, but more than half of them can be made in the body. Hence, an amino acid is referred to as nutritionally essential or indispensable only if it cannot be synthesized in the body out of materials ordinarily available, at a speed that will supply the demands for normal growth. W. C. Rose and co-workers at the University of Illinois found that ten different amino acids must be supplied in the food to support normal growth in young rats, whereas his evidence indicated that only eight of these were essential for maintenance of nitrogen equilibrium in fully grown young men. Subsequently it was shown that a ninth amino acid (histidine) is essential.

An amino acid is nonessential (dispensable from the diet) if its carbon skeleton can be formed in the body, and if an amino group can be transferred to it from some donor compound available, a process called *transamination.* In the nonessential amino acid *alanine,* the radical represented by R in the typical amino acid formula $RCHNH_2COOH$ is simply CH_3. The body can make this amino acid readily in any amount needed because the carbon chain is a common metabolic product to which the amino group from another common nonessential amino acid, *glutamic acid,* can be added. In *phenylalanine* R represents a ring, or cyclic group called phenyl radical, consisting of 6 carbon atoms joined in a hexagonal ring with hydrogen atoms attached (C_6H_5) (Fig. 4–1). The carbon skeleton cannot be formed in the human body, so phenylalanine (like several other amino acids) cannot be manufactured but must be supplied preformed in the food. Two other amino acids, *lysine* and *threonine,* are dietary essentials because their carbon skeletons cannot undergo transamination. The nine amino acids that are essential because the body cannot carry out one or another step necessary for their manufacture are listed in Table 4–1.

The nonessential amino acids *tyrosine* and *cystine* are an intermediate class, between amino acids that can easily be formed from a number of precursors and those that cannot be made at all. Tyrosine can be made only from the essential amino acid phenylalanine, and the reverse reaction does not take

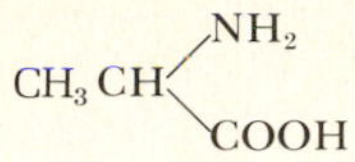

$CH_3\,CH\langle^{NH_2}_{COOH}$

Alanine

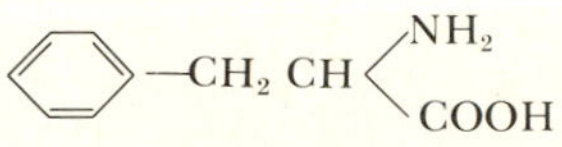

$C_6H_5—CH_2\,CH\langle^{NH_2}_{COOH}$

Phenylalanine

$HO\,C_6H_4—CH_2\,CH\langle^{NH_2}_{COOH}$

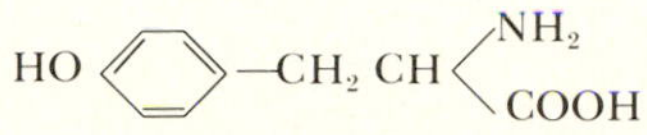

Tyrosine

Figure 4–1 Structures of a nonessential amino acid, alanine, and of an essential one, phenylalanine. The carbon chain of alanine can be synthesized in the human body, but that of phenylalanine cannot be. However, the body can make the amino acid tyrosine from phenylalanine, by adding a hydroxyl (OH) group. Tyrosine is needed to make several regulatory substances in the body. Tyrosine is classed as a semi-essential amino acid because it can be made only from the essential amino acid phenylalanine; when tyrosine is present in the diet, the need for phenylalanine is reduced.

place. Part of the need for phenylalanine in the body is to form tyrosine if the latter is not included in the diet. Thus, the presence of tyrosine will reduce the amount of phenylalanine required in the diet. The nonessential sulfur-containing amino acid cystine can be formed from the essential amino acid *methionine,* and the reaction is not reversible. The cystine needed in the body (to make hair protein, for example) may be supplied in the diet as cystine, or it will be made from methionine.[1] Thus, dietary cystine will spare the need for methionine.

Other nonessential amino acids (such as alanine and glycine) can be assembled from carbon chains derived from the metabolism of carbohydrates, fats, or proteins, and amino groups taken from amino acids or other amino-containing compounds. Proteins of the human body include both the es-

[1]There is some evidence that infants do not have the enzymatic machinery to do this at birth but that the liver develops this capability in the first few weeks of life.

Table 4–1 AVERAGE DAILY REQUIREMENTS OF ESSENTIAL AMINO ACIDS AND ESTIMATED AMOUNTS IN THE US FOOD SUPPLY

	Requirements, mg/kg weight/day[a]				*Per 70-kg Man, g*	
Essential Amino Acids[b]	INFANTS	TODDLERS	CHILDREN	ADULTS	AV. DAILY NEED	IN US FOOD SUPPLY[c]
Histidine	28	?	?	8–12		
Isoleucine	70	31	28	10	0.7	5.3
Leucine	161	73	44	14	1.0	8.2
Lysine	103	64	44	12	0.8	6.7
Methionine						2.1
+ cystine	58	27	22	13	0.9	3.5
Phenylalanine						4.7
+ tyrosine	125	69	22	14	1.0	
Threonine	87	37	28	7	0.5	4.1
Tryptophan	17	12.5	4	3.5	0.2	1.2
Valine	93	38	25	10	0.7	5.7

[a]Values from FAO/WHO pending 1983(1).

[b]The other amino acid required by rats, arginine, can be made in the human body, but some question remains as to whether the rate of synthesis can always keep up with the need.

[c]NAS–NRC, 1970.

sential and nonessential amino acids in their structure, but the nonessential ones can be manufactured, provided the necessary precursors are available.

THE ROLE OF PROTEIN IN THE BODY

Protein is required in the diet to provide essential amino acids and enough additional amino groups to make the nonessential amino acids. The principal uses for amino acids in the body are for

1. building new cells and tissues in growing children, during pregnancy, in athletic training, and after injury
2. maintaining tissues already built
3. manufacturing functional and regulatory substances, such as blood proteins, enzymes, and some hormones
4. forming milk
5. supplying energy

Proteins provide the amino acids from which the bases of the genetic information code are made as well as the substance of the cells. The *nucleoproteins* present in the nucleus of cells consist of proteins linked to *nucleic acids.* These are complex compounds containing phosphoric acid, a 5-carbon sugar, and cyclic nitrogenous bases. The nitrogenous bases are not proteins,[2] but they are made in the body from amino acids. The sugar is either ribose or deoxyribose; accordingly, the two types of nucleic acid are known as *ribonucleic acid* (RNA) and *deoxyribonucleic acid* (DNA).

DNA is found in all cell nuclei and is different for each species (even slightly so for individuals within a species). These differences consist of minor rearrangements of sequences among the nitrogenous bases, which constitute a code containing all the information on the heritable characteristics of cells, tissues, organs, and individuals. Only four nitrogenous bases are found in DNA; these

[2]The nitrogenous bases are classed as purines and pyrimidines according to the nature of the ring. Structures are given in the Appendix.

are adenine, guanine, thymine, and cytosine. The DNA structure is a long, fibrous molecule with two spiral "backbones," consisting of linked sugar and phosphate groups twined about a common axis, forming a double helix (Fig. 4–2). The nitrogenous bases are attached in these spirals so as to extend inward and approach each other in pairs that are joined by a weak hydrogen bond. Of the four bases, adenine can form a pair only with thymine; guanine only with cytosine. The code by which DNA directs the formation and life processes of various cells consists in variations in the kinds and sequences of these pairs.

One type of RNA—*messenger* RNA—transmits the coded information of DNA. RNA differs from DNA in that it has a single-strand structure, the sugar in the chains is ribose (instead of deoxyribose), and a different nitrogenous base, uracil, is substituted for thymine. Messenger RNA, formed in the cell nuclei under the direction of DNA, migrates to the surface of granules (ribosomes) in the fluid portion of the cell (cytoplasm) (see Chap. 6). Another type of RNA—*transfer* RNA—picks up certain amino acids from the cytoplasm and transfers these amino acids to the messenger RNA, where they are lined up in proper order to form specific proteins.

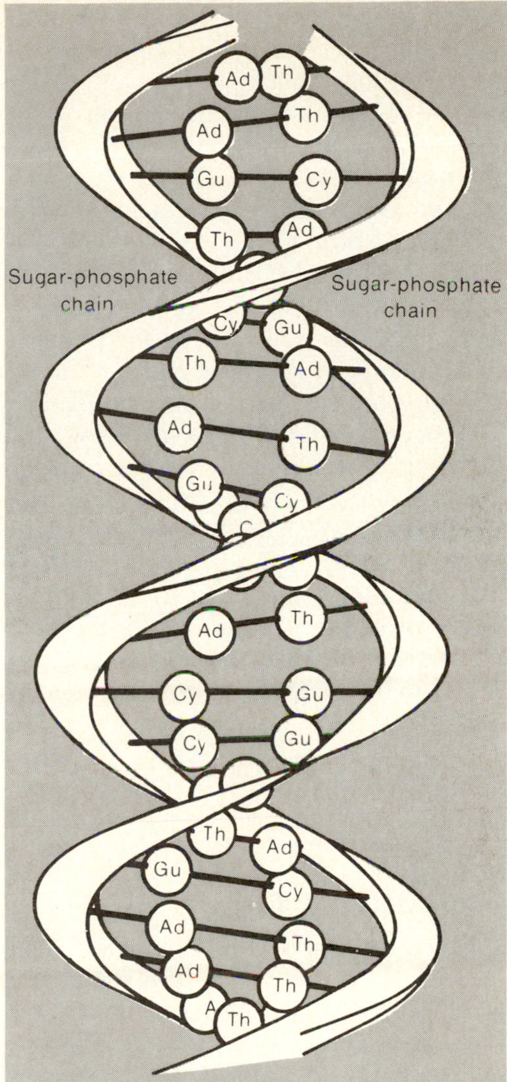

Figure 4–2 The basic building block of life forms is deoxyribonucleic acid, DNA. It transmits the genetic message of reproduction through the chromosome. In this model of the double helix, only a few of the thousands of turns in the hypothetical DNA molecule are illustrated. The sugar-phosphate "backbone" is represented by the two ribbons. The third component of the molecule consists of four bases called adenine (Ad), cytosine (Cy), guanine (Gu), and thymine (Th).

Building New Tissues

The amount of protein needed for building new tissues depends on the extent or rapidity of growth and repair processes. In the rapidly growing infant, as much as one-fourth of the dietary protein may be retained for building new tissue. Tissues and organs do not all grow at an even rate, so depending on the stage of growth, limitation of dietary protein may have its greatest effect on the brain, on the muscle mass, on the blood supply, and so on. As growth becomes less rapid, the proportion of the protein intake retained in the body for tissue building becomes less. An adequate supply of high-quality protein is necessary throughout the growth period to secure the best possible growth and development. Extra protein is needed throughout pregnancy and lactation. An athlete in training, whose muscles strengthen and enlarge as a result of exercise may require some extra protein.

Excessive destruction of body protein occurs in periods of stress. Obviously, after severe hemorrhages, extra protein is needed for regeneration of hemoglobin and other blood proteins. Also, after extensive burns, there is excessive loss of protein from the burn surface, as well as need for protein to rebuild damaged skin and muscle tissues. A slow but prolonged loss of nitrogen from extra breakdown of body protein follows bone fractures, and a similar but brief protein loss occurs even after simple surgical operations. This catabolic reaction to trauma is due to increased output of hormones from the pituitary and adrenal glands. Increased quantities of protein or amino acids are properly given during convalescence, when the metabolic processes become anabolic, to replenish the body protein. A patient who cannot take nourishment by mouth is given intravenous solutions of amino acids with glucose or emulsified fat added to provide energy.

Maintaining Tissues

Although the adult does not build new tissues as a child does, there are some tissues that never stop growing, even in the aged. Skin, hair, and nails are obvious examples. The lining of the intestinal tract is renewed about every day and a half; much of this cellular protein is digested and absorbed, but some cells are lost in the fecal matter. Blood cells have a limited life span of 120 days; and if replacement protein is not adequate for formation of new cells and the hemoglobin that they contain, anemia develops. In fact, all the body proteins are constantly being degraded and resynthesized (turning over) at varying rates. Functional proteins inside and outside cells continuously turn over in carrying out life processes.

Proteins in the cells are in a state of dynamic equilibrium with the plasma amino acids (resulting from digestion of protein in foods and catabolism of body proteins). (See Figure 4–3.) The cells transfer some amino acids to the surrounding fluid and take up others from it for utilization in the tissues. This constant flux involves some net loss of amino acids. Thus, a supply of protein is needed to maintain the body protein pool.

Regulatory Functions

Proteins in tissue cells and in body fluids also serve as regulatory substances. Because of their contribution to osmotic pressure, proteins exert an important influence on the exchange of water between tissue cells and the surrounding body fluids. When the plasma protein (especially albumin) is markedly reduced as a result of severe dietary protein deficiency, extra water is retained in the tissues, which becomes puffy and swol-

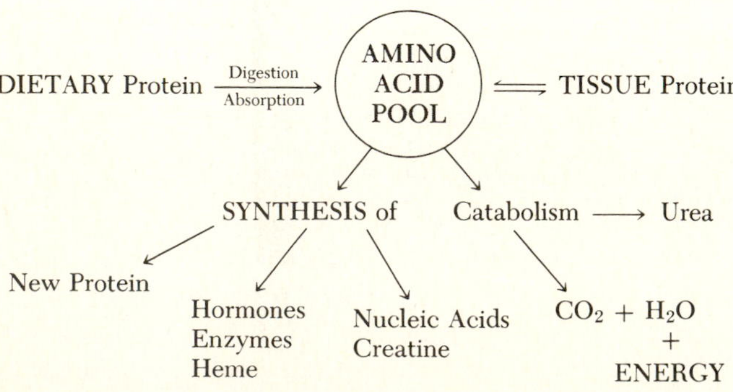

Figure 4–3 Amino acids from food and body tissues enter a common pool, which is drawn upon for synthesis of protein and other compounds or from which amino acids are degraded for energy needs. The word "pool" refers to the total amount of a substance present in the body. "Pool" is a concept, rather than a delineated location, mass, or compartment. (From Routh, Eyman, and Burton: *Essentials of General, Organic and Biochemistry,* Philadelphia, W. B. Saunders Co., 1977.)

len; supply of nutrients to the cells and removal of cellular waste products is then less efficient. This condition is known as *nutritional edema,* to differentiate it from water accumulation due to disease processes. The ingestion of extra protein sufficient to raise the level of plasma protein to normal is followed by excretion of the excess water by the kidneys and disappearance of the edema. Such retention of extra water in the tissues is often seen in persons who have suffered prolonged undernutrition. A plump-looking malnourished baby is often revealed to be pitifully thin when the refeeding regimen restores normal water distribution and edema disappears (Fig. 4–4).

A second regulatory function of proteins is in maintenance of *acid-base balance* of the blood and tissues. The normal, very slightly alkaline condition of blood and tissues (pH7.4) is maintained by the balance between several different factors, one of which is protein content. Through the basic amino groups and the organic acid radicals present in all amino acids, proteins are able to unite with either acidic or alkaline substances arising in the body from metabolic processes. When these substances are bound by protein, they have little effect on the level of tissue acidity. Hemoglobin and oxyhemoglobin in red cells of the blood also help maintain acid-base equilibrium by forming loose

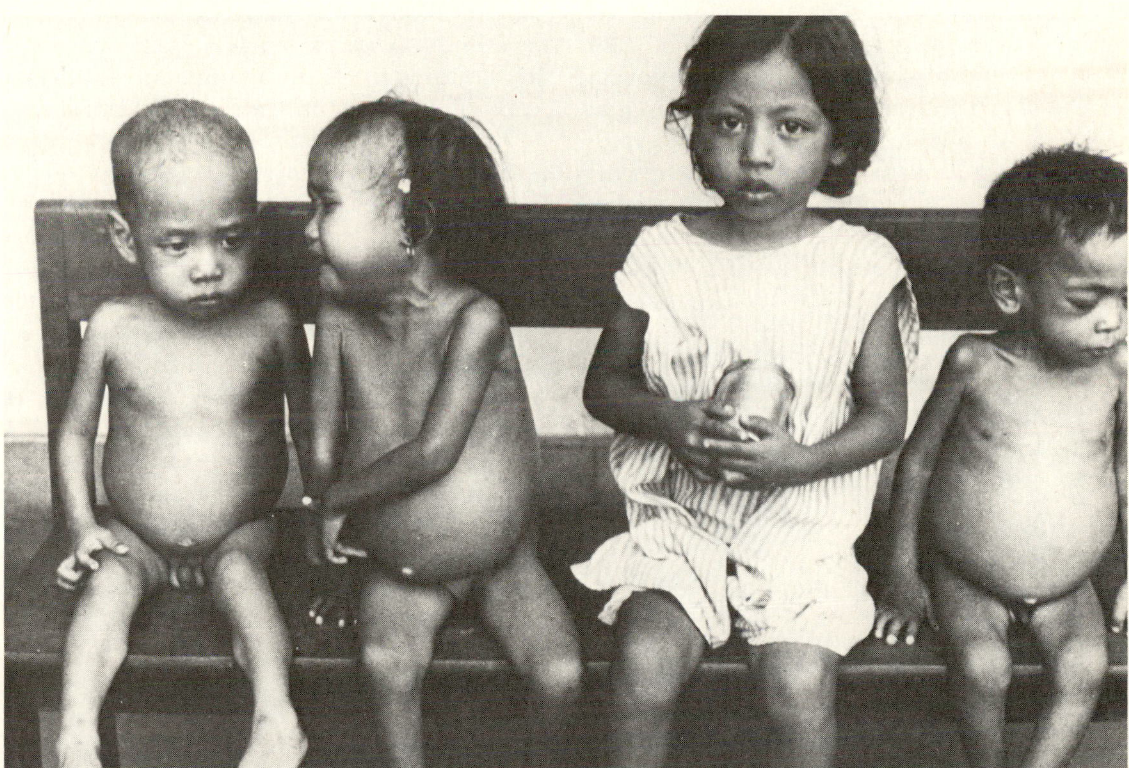

Figure 4–4 One child in this picture is healthy; the other three, all from the same community and of about the same age, are victims of the deficiency disease, kwashiorkor. Note that the faces and abdomens of the two on the left look quite full, due to the accumulation of water as edema. The fact that the children are in reality pitifully thin is apparent from looking at the arms. (Courtesy of WHO, photo by H. Oomen.)

chemical combinations with hydrogen and carbon dioxide from cellular metabolism. (Carbon dioxide in water forms a weak acid, carbonic acid.) Ultimately, carbon dioxide is excreted in expired air.

Smaller but critical amounts of protein are needed for making enzymes that are essential for digestion and metabolic processes in the tissues. Many potent hormones are either proteins (for example, insulin) or smaller peptides (for example, some of the pituitary and gastrointestinal hormones) or are derived from single amino acids (thyroxine, and epinephrine or adrenaline). The amino acid tyrosine is the precursor from which the pigment of skin and hair is made, which is the reason that in severe protein deficiency dark hair often turns to a pale or reddish color (Fig. 4–5). Tryptophan, tyrosine, glutamic acid, and methionine are direct or indirect precursors of substances involved in the transmission of messages in the nervous system. The amino acid tryptophan can act as a precursor of niacin, one of the B complex vitamins. The antibodies that help ward off infectious diseases and the substances responsible for clotting of blood are all proteins.

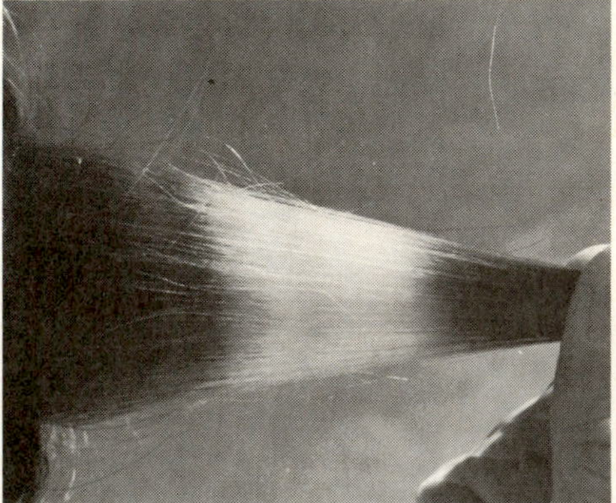

Figure 4–5 So-called "flag sign," often seen during recovery from kwashiorkor, when hair is changing from orange color back to black. (Courtesy of Doctors Scrimshaw and Guzman of the Institute of Nutrition for Central America and Panama, Guatemala City.)

Forming Milk. The proteins of human milk are formed within the mammary glands. During lactation a woman needs as much extra protein in the diet as she secretes in her milk plus the amount required for conversion of dietary amino acids to milk protein. This will be discussed in Chapter 22.

Providing Energy. Amino acids are the ultimate precursors from which the nitrogenous base of adenosine triphosphate (the adenine of ATP) is formed, as well as another nitrogenous substance, creatine phosphate, which is present in muscle. These substances are central to the body's energy metabolism (see Chap. 6), but it is not this aspect that is meant in speaking of protein as an energy source. What is referred to in this connection is utilization of the carbon skeleton of the amino acids in much the same way as dietary carbohydrates or fats, with a yield of 4 kcal (17kJ) per gram of protein.

Nitrogen, which is indispensable as long as protein is used for all other functions, becomes a liability when it is necessary to use protein for energy. Amino groups are split off from the amino acids and formed into simple nitrogen-containing substances (chiefly urea) that are excreted by the kidneys. The nonnitrogenous fragments of amino acids, the carbon chains, are metabolized along the carbohydrate or fat pathways. About half of the amino acids can provide some glucose when necessary (see Chap. 6). As with fat and carbohydrate, protein is converted to body fat if the total energy intake is excessive.

If the energy intake is inadequate, that is, if the diet does not supply carbohydrates and fats in sufficient quantity to meet the energy needs of the body, proteins are used for energy, because energy needs have a higher priority than does maintenance of some of the tissue proteins. In this event, building or repair processes will suffer.

The symptoms of protein deficiency seen in poor people all over the world almost always are due to the fact that these people do not have the means to obtain enough basic food and their diets are too low in energy to make fullest use of whatever protein is eaten. The deficiency state is called protein-calorie malnutrition (PCM, or, more properly, PEM for protein-energy malnutrition) in recognition of its usual origin.

REQUIREMENTS FOR PROTEINS AND AMINO ACIDS

Because of the importance of proteins and amino acids to the body, requirements for their consumption must be established and the value and quality of individual proteins understood.

Establishing Protein Requirements

Protein requirements have been determined principally by two methods. The first is the epidemiologic method, in which the protein intake of healthy populations is accepted to meet requirements. The second method involves laboratory measurement of nitrogen balance in small numbers of representative individuals.

Epidemiologic Evidence. Much of the important early work on protein requirements came out of the German school, beginning with the nineteenth-century French-trained chemist Liebig. He appreciated the importance of protein in the diet but had the erroneous idea that muscle protein was the source of energy for muscular work.

This idea seemed to be confirmed by Playfair's surveys of British diets (ca. 1860) showing intakes varying from 57 gm of protein for bedridden hospital patients to 184 gm for manual laborers. Thus, Voit studied the diets of German workers and, based on their usual consumption of protein, in 1881 suggested 118 gm of protein daily as a desirable allowance. In 1902, Atwater (a student of Voit, and the American pioneer in nutrition) recommended an allowance of 125 gm of protein, based on studies of protein consumption among men. It is now known that these figures are far above the actual *need* for protein but instead reflect the consumption of foods that was customary in the groups surveyed. Today, the consumption of protein is about 100 gm per day in the United States and most other affluent countries.

In 1904 Chittenden was among the first to maintain that such a high intake of protein is not only unnecessary for maintenance of body tissues but might even be disadvantageous to health. For months he studied a volunteer group of athletes and soldiers (men who performed considerable muscular work) given a low-protein diet. He found that 44 to 53 gm of protein daily sufficed to keep them in excellent health, with their physical abilities in no way lessened. Chittenden kept his own protein intake to about 35 gm a day for years and maintained that, as compared with his previous history, he was freer from minor ailments and more vigorous on such a diet. Since he lived to be more than eighty years old, his diet must have been sufficient, if not optimal. Chittenden's findings have been confirmed by modern investigators, who found that men and women could exist for short periods without apparent harm on 25 to 40 gm of protein a day along with generous intakes of energy-producing foods.

Others have offered evidence indicating that liberal consumption of protein is not harmful. The Kroghs found that the Eskimos of Greenland, who subsisted almost entirely on a carnivorous diet, having an average protein intake of 280 gm a day, were healthy, had excellent physical endurance, and were free from liver and kidney disease.

The explorer Stefansson used a nearly all-meat diet in the Arctic for long periods and found it quite satisfactory. Along with his associate, Andersen, he lived for a year under observation by DuBois while eating a diet exclusively of meats and animal fats (daily intake: 100 to 140 gm of protein, 200 to 300 gm of fat, and only 7 to 12 gm of carbohydrate). They showed no high blood pressure or liver or kidney damage during or after the test.

Nitrogen Balance. Balance experiments are carried out to determine if the body is gaining or losing nutrient stores under defined conditions. The body balance of a nutrient is simply the difference between the intake and outgo from the body. For protein, intake and output are measured as the element nitrogen, which makes up, on the average, 16 percent of protein. (Crude protein content of foods is calculated from nitrogen content times 100/16, or the factor 6.25.) Nitrogen in the feces, usually about 1 to 2 gm a day, consists of unabsorbed dietary protein, bacteria, and intestinal residues. The difference between dietary and fecal nitrogen is the net amount absorbed and available for metabolism. Because nitrogen-containing end products of protein metabolism (principally urea) are excreted mainly in the urine, the nitrogen in the urine is a measure of how much protein has been oxidized in the body.[3] When intake and output are practically equal, the body is said to be in *nitrogen* (or protein) *equilibrium* (Fig. 4–6). A *positive* nitrogen balance—intake is greater than output—indicates that new tissue is being built, with consequent retention of nitrogen in the body. A *negative* nitrogen balance—output is greater than intake—indicates that some body protein must have been oxidized in addition to that provided in the food.

[3]Small quantities of nitrogen are also lost in perspiration, menstruation and seminal emissions, nail parings, and hair clippings. Except under conditions in which perspiration is excessive or when unusual accuracy is required, these nitrogen losses, amounting to less than 1 gm daily, are usually disregarded.

Nitrogen balance is usually unrelated to the actual intake of protein, because the body can establish nitrogen equilibrium at any level of protein intake that is above the minimum requirement. It has been noted that protein consumption varies widely (Fig. 4–7). The amount of protein used as an energy source when the energy intake is adequate depends upon the extent to which protein intake exceeds requirement. Adults will be in nitrogen balance with quite different amounts in the excreta, depending on the amount habitually eaten.

On changing from a higher level of protein consumption to a lower level, there is always a lag period during which nitrogen balance is negative. There is also a delay period in adjusting the balance between the amount metabolized and the intake on changing to a higher protein level, and balance is positive for the first several days. Under these conditions the nitrogen pool in the body is decreased or increased, reflecting gradual adjustment to a changed intake of protein.

To determine protein requirement, nitrogen balance is measured in people fed progressively lower levels of protein. Sufficient time is allowed for adjustment at each level, and the amount of protein just sufficient to promote equilibrium is taken to be the minimum requirement. Because some days of negative balance will have occurred at each progressively lower level, the total protein pool in the body will be reduced in conjunction with the estimate of the minimum requirement. At present there is no basis for deciding at what point a decrease in pool size is biologically significant.

Ordinarily a positive nitrogen balance, which indicates protein storage in tissues, is found only in conditions such as growth and pregnancy, when new tissues are being formed. After prolonged undernutrition or

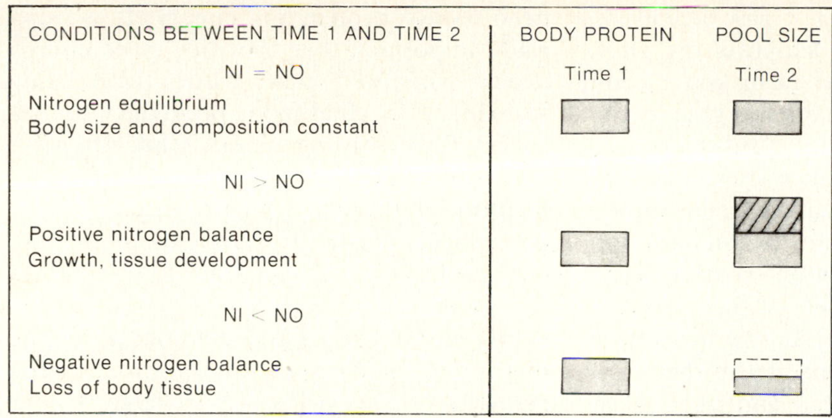

Figure 4–6 The nitrogen balance test is one way to determine an individual's dietary protein requirement. When dietary protein, or nitrogen, intake (NI) equals nitrogen output (NO) amount lost in the urine, feces, sweat, etc., the adult requirement is met and the individual is neither gaining nor losing body protein. Disequilibrium between NI and NO indicates accumulation or loss of body proteins.

serious illness, the protein content of tissues becomes depleted; with a generous intake of protein during recovery, retention of nitrogen continues until the normal protein content of the tissues is restored.

Whether or not the body can build true protein reserves is uncertain. When the intake of protein is liberal, such tissues as the liver and muscles may have a slightly higher content of protein, amino acids, or other nitrogenous products. This might constitute a reserve that could be drawn on in time of need. Studies involving tagging of body proteins by isotopic nitrogen or carbon have shown that part of the body protein is more labile—that is, more readily drawn on for metabolic uses—while the remainder is more firmly fixed. In protein deficiency the liver is the most susceptible to depletion, the muscles are relatively easy to deplete, and the brain is the most difficult. Because of the mass of tissue involved, muscle constitutes the chief reservoir of protein available to sustain critical functions when intake is low.

Opinion is divided concerning the functional importance of this labile protein. Some investigators have reported no benefit from a previous high protein intake in rats subsequently deprived of protein, but others reported that feeding chicks extra protein

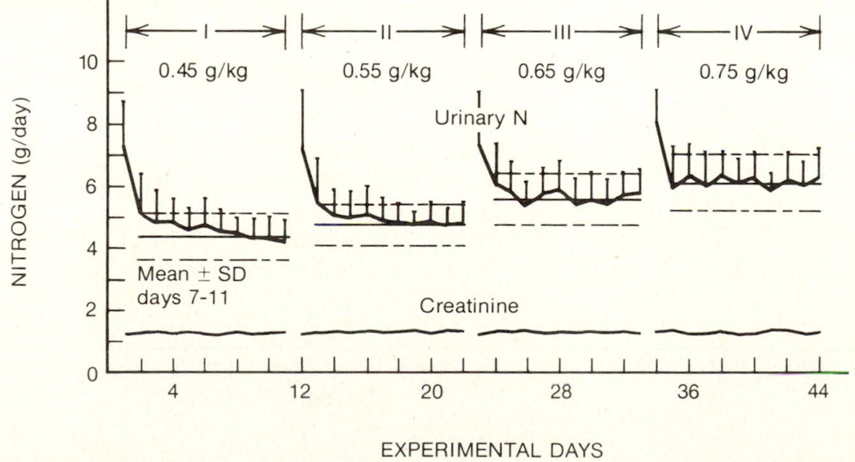

Figure 4–7 Pattern of urinary nitrogen and creatinine excretion of men fed four levels of protein, all below their usual intake of Chinese mixed diet. Note that there is always a period of adjustment before nitrogen excretion reaches a new stable level, during which time the men were losing body nitrogen. Creatinine excretion is essentially constant and reflects the amount of lean muscle tissue in the body. (From Huang, P.C., and Lin, C.P., J. Nutr. 112:897, 1982, with permission.)

before depriving them of it was beneficial. The weight of evidence supports the view that liberal protein intakes favor better condition of tissues and perhaps also greater resistance to infections and toxic substances.

Negative nitrogen balance inevitably occurs when the protein intake is reduced below the amount required for maintenance of body tissues—the minimum requirement. However, negative nitrogen balance may occur at levels of protein intake that are above the minimum requirement, if the diet furnishes too little carbohydrate and fat to meet the energy requirement (Fig. 4–8). Carbohydrate and fat are both regarded as protein sparers, for the presence of an adequate quantity of these foodstuffs eliminates the need to use protein for energy. It is especially important that the diet meet energy needs whenever new tissues are being formed, as in childhood, pregnancy, or recovery from wasting illness. Children grow best when their food supplies both a liberal quantity of protein, which furnishes all the amino acids needed for tissue building, and, enough fat and carbohydrate to cover their energy needs.

Protein requirement is increased when the diet is devoid of carbohydrate—even if large amounts of fatty acids are available. Under these conditions, the carbon chains of some of the amino acids are used to supply essential amounts of glucose to the tissues, a function that fatty acids cannot fulfill.

Figure 4–8 Relationship between nitrogen balance and energy intake during diet period A (●) when the carbohydrate-to-fat ratio was 1 : 1, and during diet period B (o) when the ratio was 2 : 1. Nitrogen intake was low and constant. Nitrogen balance improved with increased energy intake and was less negative with the higher ratio of carbohydrate. (From Richardson, et al., Am. J. Clin. Nutr. 32:2217, 1979, with permission.)

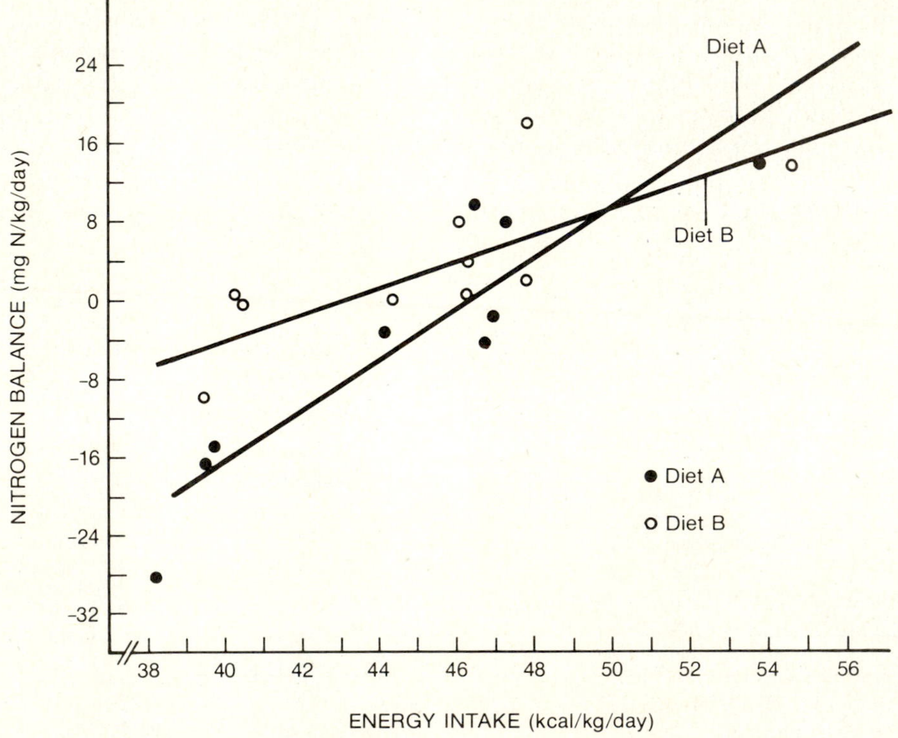

Establishing Requirements for Essential Amino Acids

Rose was the first to determine how much of each essential amino acid was needed to meet the minimum requirement. He fed healthy college men nitrogen in the form of a well-balanced mixture of all the known amino acids in pure form (instead of in proteins) in an otherwise adequate diet (plenty of energy supplied by pure carbohydrate and fat and all recognized essential minerals and vitamins added). In following periods, different amino acids were left out of the mixed solution, one at a time, and the effect on nitrogen balance was observed. If the amino acid omitted could be made in the body, no notable results followed; but if the amino acid was one that must be furnished in the food, nitrogen balance became negative. Histidine and arginine, which were essential for rat growth, did not seem to be essential for maintaining nitrogen balance in young men. Subsequently, histidine was shown to be essential in the diet of infants, and there is evidence from studies of longer duration than those of Rose that it is needed by adults as well. The tenth amino acid, arginine, can be synthesized in the human body, although some doubt remains if it can be manufactured at a sufficiently rapid rate to meet needs under all conditions.

Natural food proteins always contain a spectrum of amino acids, so the total absence of any one amino acid from a normal diet would never occur.[4] For this reason, little direct information exists as to the effects in humans of single amino acid deficiencies. There is biochemical evidence for specific roles of some of the amino acids, and absence of any of the essential amino acids from the diet leads, as has been noted, to a loss of body protein. In animals, absence of any of the essentials also causes a prompt reduction in appetite. Some specific attributes of the amino acids are herewith described.

[4]The availability of relatively inexpensive pure amino acids (made by chemical synthesis or fermentation) has made it practical to give these orally or intravenously for the treatment of some diseases, so the issue of specific requirements and balances has become a practical matter. It was due to such feeding of amino acids to patients with kidney disease that the need for histidine came to be reevaluated.

Histidine. The amino acid histidine is present abundantly in muscle as part of a dipeptide, carnosine (the other portion is alanine), whose exact function is unknown but probably relates to muscle contraction. Hemoglobin is high in histidine content, and in the rat, omission of histidine from the diet leads to severe anemia, as well as to a dry, scaly skin condition, fatigue, and irritability. The acid or carboxyl group can be removed (a process called decarboxylation) by intestinal bacteria and by tissue enzymes, especially when the tissue is injured, and the compound histamine is left. Histamine causes small blood vessels to expand and is responsible for some of the symptoms noted with injury and with allergies like hay fever; it is a powerful stimulant to acid production in the stomach. At high concentrations histidine is toxic, and a genetic disease that results in its accumulation in the blood, called histidinemia, results in increased susceptibility to infections and in speech defects.

Isoleucine, Leucine, Valine. Isoleucine and leucine are metabolized along the same pathway as fat. Leucine is also one of the precursors of cholesterol. Leucine and isoleucine have branched carbon chains and, together with the other branched-chain essential amino acid, valine, share common absorption and excretion mechanisms. The branched-chain amino acids play an important role in energy release during muscular work. A rare genetic disease has been described in which the urine contains partially oxidized acidic end products of the branched-chain amino acids, which have a peculiar maplelike odor. The disease, called "maple syrup urine disease," causes severe impairment of the nervous system and is fatal early in life. The high degree of specificity of the amino acid sequences in a given protein is illustrated by the fact that in sickle cell anemia, the entire defect in the red blood cells is caused by substitution of just one valine for one glutamic acid in one portion of the hemoglobin molecule. This small change allows the hemoglobin molecule to coil up on itself; its volume is thereby reduced, and the red blood cell changes from the usual disc shape to a sickle shape, which is more fragile than normal and breaks down, resulting in anemia.

Lysine. Unlike the other essential amino acids lysine has two amino groups. The second amino group is not bound in peptide linkage. For this reason it is quite susceptible to being damaged by heat in cooking and processing foods. In addition to its presence in tissue and milk proteins, a hydroxylated form of this amino acid is an important constituent of collagen in the skeleton and connective tissues. In humans, its omission from the diet results in negative balances of nitrogen and sulfur and in symptoms that include nausea, dizziness, and increased sensitivity to metallic sounds.

Methionine. Two important characteristics distinguish methionine: the presence in its molecule of sulfur and of a methyl (CH_3) radical that can easily be transferred to form other needed compounds, such as muscle creatine, carnitine (important in fat metabolism), and the vitamin choline. (See Chap. 11.) When choline and methionine are deficient, the liver accumulates an abnormal amount of fat. Methionine is the precursor of numerous important sulfur-containing compounds in the body, including a tripeptide, glutathione, involved in oxidative metabolism, and an amino acid, taurine, needed in bile production. The sulfur-containing amino acid cystine can be made from methionine, so it is not essential in the diet even though it is a major constituent of the hormone insulin (12 percent by weight) and of the protein keratin in hair and nails. Premature babies and the newly born may not have the metabolic machinery fully developed for making cystine from methionine, so it should be included in their diets. Cystine will substitute for about 30 percent of the dietary methionine requirement, and most foods contain both acids.

Phenylalanine. Phenylalanine and its hydroxylated derivative tyrosine are called "aromatic" amino acids in chemical terminology because they contain the phenyl group, a ring structure. About 50 percent of the dietary requirement for phenylalanine is due to the need for tyrosine, and the phenylalanine requirement is accordingly reduced if enough tyrosine is in the diet. Two hormones—thyroxine and epinephrine (adrenaline)—are derivatives of tyrosine; melanin, the dark pigment of skin and hair, is also made from tyrosine. The addition of a second hydroxyl (OH) group forms the compound dihydroxyphenylalanine, called DOPA; DOPA is then decarboxylated to form the neurotransmitter dopamine. Epinephrine and a similar compound also made from DOPA, norepinephrine, also effect transmission of nerve impulses; the three transmitters can all be grouped in the term catecholamines. Phenylalanine is thus the foundation of three of the six known neurotransmitters, and it is little wonder, then, that the brain is seriously affected by derangement in the metabolism of these compounds. This is true in the genetic disease phenylketonuria (PKU), in which untreated cases have severe mental retardation. Fortunately, PKU, like most other inborn errors of metabolism, is an uncommon disorder.

Some psychiatric patients are treated with drugs that alter the way the body handles these neurotransmitters. Because their normal control mechanisms are abridged, such patients are very sensitive to the presence of free amines (decarboxylated amino acids) in foods. Blood pressure can be dangerously elevated when these amines are in excess. Tyramine (from tyrosine) and other free amines occur in aged cheeses owing to action of the bacteria used in cheese manufacture, and in yeast extracts, chianti types of red wine, and less commonly in beer and some legumes.

Threonine. The last one of the essential amino acids to be identified was threonine, which was discovered in 1935, by Rose and his co-workers. Its discovery allowed the work on the amino acid requirements of mammals finally to proceed. A specific role for threonine, other than as a constituent of proteins where it is commonly a point of attachment for phosphate groups, has not been identified.

Tryptophan. Of all the essential amino acids, tryptophan has the lowest quantitative requirement, and its presence in proteins is commensurately low. One of the B vitamins, niacin, can be manufactured from tryptophan but not in sufficient amounts to meet the total requirement for the vitamin. However, the niacin-deficiency disease, pellagra, is most likely to occur when the diet is low both in the vitamin and in proteins that supply tryptophan. (See Chap. 10.)

Tryptophan is the precursor of an important neurotransmitter, serotonin (5-hydroxytryptamine), which functions in counterbalance to the catecholamines. Rats fed a maize (corn) diet, which is naturally low in tryptophan, have reduced levels of serotonin in the brain and show behavioral abnormalities. Serotonin affects a wide range of behaviors, including feeding (see Chap. 7) and sleep. Cats experimentally deprived of brain serotonin become insomniacs. Administration of tryptophan at bedtime has been reported to improve the pattern of sleep in people who have this problem. Consumption of carbohydrate, but not protein, leads to an elevation of brain serotonin.

The explanation of this seeming anomaly lies in the system by which amino acids enter the brain. There is a physiological barrier between the brain (and cerebrospinal fluid) and the blood which amino acids cannot cross unless they are actively transported by carrier molecules. The molecule that transports tryptophan also carries several other amino acids. After a protein-rich meal, amino acid levels in the blood are raised, but levels of the amino acids abundant in food protein are much higher than that of tryptophan. Thus the abundant amino acids compete for carrier molecules and relatively little tryptophan is transported to the brain. When a carbohydrate-rich meal is eaten, insulin is released. This hormone increases the uptake of amino acids into muscle, but the effect on the competing amino acids is large and on tryptophan is negligible. Thus, levels of competing amino acids in the blood are reduced, more tryptophan is able to enter the brain, and more serotonin is produced. Drowsiness results.

Some Nonessential Amino Acids. Some of the nonessential amino acids are of special interest. Arginine, like lysine, has two amino groups. It is essential for growth in the rat and can be made in the human body, but the rate of synthesis is limited. Even though nitrogen balance was maintained in men fed a diet devoid of this amino acid, one group of investigators has reported a sharp decrease in sperm production. This occurrence has not been confirmed, but it is true that the head of the sperm is extraordinarily high in arginine content. Glycine is a precursor for many important compounds, such as the heme portion of hemoglobin, creatine, glutathione, the basis of some nucleic acids (purines), and some compounds present in bile; it is used by the liver to detoxify benzoic acid, a ring-containing organic acid present in some foods (cranberries, plums) and commonly used as a food preservative.

Glutamic acid is one of the most abundant amino acids, especially high in cereal grains; its salt (monosodium glutamate, or MSG) is used to add a "meaty" flavor in cooking. Physiologically, glutamic acid and glutamine play a key role in the metabolism of amino groups, and glutamic acid is the precursor of a neurotransmitter (gamma-aminobutyric acid). Some individuals are especially sensitive to glutamic acid and experience nausea, tremors, and chest and head pain on eating foods, particularly oriental dishes, high in MSG content. Hydroxyproline is the major amino acid component of collagen; gelatin, which is derived from collagen by acid hydrolysis, consequently is very high in hydroxyproline. Alanine has an important function in the energetics of exercising muscle.

Minimum Requirements. Sufficient data have been accumulated so that the minimum human requirements for eight of the amino acids essential in the diet can now be stated with fair accuracy. More information is needed as regards histidine (Table 4–1). The content in the average American diet of these eight amino acids (based on the average consumption of various foods or food groups) has been calculated and is given in Table 4–1. The supply of each of these essential amino acids is well above the required level(1). There is little danger of their shortage when the diet contains as much protein as is customary in the United States, Canada, and most European countries.

To meet the total protein needs, a larger quantity of the dispensable amino acids is needed than of essential ones. If the dispensable amino acids are not available from the diet, they can be synthesized in the body, using amino groups drawn from a pool to which all nonspecific amino nitrogen sources (essential and nonessential amino acids, ammonium salts, and urea) contribute. For this reason, the absolute minimum requirement for essential amino acids cannot be determined under conditions wherein a portion of them must be broken down to provide amino groups needed for the dispensable or, more correctly, nonspecific amino acids. The minimal requirements for the various essential amino acids depend upon the adequacy of nonspecific amino nitrogen sources.

A larger requirement for nonspecific amino nitrogen than for essential amino acids has been demonstrated even in infants; the sum of the dietary essential amino acids is only about 40 percent of the infant's total protein need. In adults, the essential component is less than 15 percent of the total. Most food proteins contain ample amounts of the dispensable amino acids, and ordinarily the concern is to meet the needs of infants and children for essential amino acids from proteins of varying quality.

Nutritional Value of Proteins

The quality of a protein—that is, its relative usefulness for the formation of tissue protein—depends on the amount and proportions of amino acids it provides after digestion and absorption into the blood.

Some of the first information on how the amino acid makeup of a protein determines its biological value came from the pioneer experiments of Osborne and Mendel at Yale in the early 1900s. In one series of experiments they fed young rats diets containing 18 percent protein in the form of either casein (a milk protein), gliadin (a wheat protein), or zein (a protein from maize) (Fig. 4–9). With casein as the sole protein, the rats

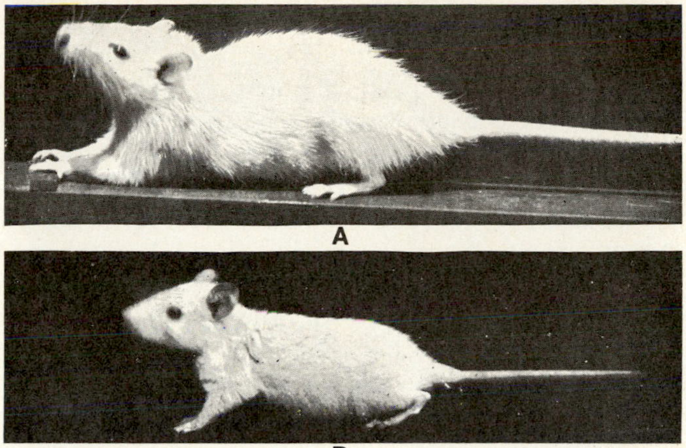

A

B

Figure 4–9 This historically interesting photo illustrates stunting of growth due to feeding poor quality protein as sole source of protein in the diet. Two rats of same age were kept on diets alike except for the protein, which was a good quality protein (casein from milk) in the case of A, and a poor protein in the case of B (gliadin from wheat). (From experiments by Osborne and Mendel, Connecticut Agricultural Experiment Station; pictures reproduced by courtesy of Yale University Press.)

remained healthy and made excellent growth; those fed gliadin were able to maintain their weight but did not grow much; those whose sole source of protein was zein not only could not grow, but also lost weight and eventually died if kept on that diet.

Since casein evidently supplied all the amino acids needed for growth, it was said to be a *complete* protein. Gliadin was found to contain too little lysine to support growth; when lysine was added to the ration, the animals grew normally. Since gliadin provided for maintenance but not growth, it was said to be a *partially incomplete* protein. Zein, on the other hand, proved to be an *incomplete,* or *inadequate,* protein that supported neither growth nor maintenance because it was quite low in lysine and tryptophan. When the diet was supplemented with suitable amounts of these two amino acids, the animals grew and thrived. The terms complete and incomplete still are sometimes used in referring to proteins of good and poor quality, but it should be recognized that a protein almost never is totally lacking in one of the essential amino acids, and in that sense most proteins are not incomplete. Gelatin is an exception because it is produced by treating animal bones with acid, a process that destroys tryptophan completely.

In general, the pattern of amino acids in proteins of animal origin (such as those in eggs, dairy products, and meats) is well balanced in relation to mammalian requirements. All of the essential amino acids are present in significant amounts. Therefore, animal proteins are said to be of higher *biological value* than other proteins. Yet they are not all alike in efficiency for promoting growth. For example, Osborne and Mendel found lactalbumin (one of the proteins in milk) to be quite efficient for promoting growth in rats; only 8 percent of lactalbumin in the diet produced the same weight gain as 12 percent of casein (a second protein in milk). Casein was found to contain relatively small amounts of the sulfur-containing amino acids, and addition of methionine (or cystine) to the diet led to improved growth.

When a protein is low in an essential amino acid, this is said to be *limiting,* for only as much tissue can be built as the smallest amount of necessary amino acid provided. Enough of any protein or mixture of proteins must be taken to furnish the minimum requirement for the amino acid that is in poorest supply. The excess of other essential amino acids, provided at amounts above requirement, serves as a nonspecific nitrogen source and is used for energy.

Protein Quality Ratings

The mixtures of proteins found in egg and milk have been found to be the best quality natural protein for maintenance of tissues; they are arbitrarily rated as "100" for comparison with other natural proteins in human assays of protein quality (1)(2). In standardized feeding tests in the rat (the animal most often used for measuring protein quality), egg protein rates at the top with an observed value of 94, while the proteins of milk and fish rank about 80, those in meats and soybeans rate about 75, and those of other legumes, vegetables, and cereals are in the range of 60 to 40 (Table 4–2). Experience has shown that values obtained in rat assays have good but not perfect predictive value for human feeding. The rat has a much higher proportional requirement for the sulfur-containing amino acids than humans have, so proteins such as milk and meat that are relatively low in methionine plus cystine rank lower in the rat than in humans; values for proteins low in lysine and tryptophan match more closely.

Table 4–2 QUALITY OF SOME COMMON FOOD PROTEINS ESTIMATED BY VARIOUS METHODS[a]

Food	Food Protein: % As Purchased	Food Protein: % of Dry Solids	Food Protein: kcal, % of Total kcal	*Digestibility,[a] %*	*Rat Biological[b] Value, %*	*Net Protein[b] Utilization, %*	*ND_pCal, %[c]*	*PER[d]*	*FAO/WHO Amino Acid Score[e]*
Hen's egg, whole	13	48	33	99	94	94	31	3.92	100
Cow's milk, whole	3.5	27	23	97	84	82	19	3.09	100
Fish	19	72	61	98	83	81	49	3.55	100
Beef	18	45	29	99	74	73	21	2.30	100
Soybeans	38	41	39	90	73	66	26	2.32	100
Dry beans, common	22	25	22	73	58	42	9	1.48	75
Peanuts (groundnuts)	26	27	16	87	54	48	8	1.65	62
Green leaves	1.5–4.5	23–31	18–45	85[f]	64[f]	54[f]	6–24	—	70–90
Yeast, brewer's	39	41	54	84	66	55	30	2.24	100
Wheat, whole grain	12	14	13	91	65	59	8	1.53	50
Wheat, white flour	11	12	12	99	52	51	6	0.60	36
Corn, whole grain	10	11	7	90	59	53	4	1.12	47
Rice, brown	8	9	7	96	73	70	5	—	66
Rice, polished, white	7	8	7	98	64	63	4	2.18	62
Potato, white	2	9	7	89	67	60	4	—	76
Cassava (manioc)	2	2	1	No information				—	59

[a]From FAO Nutrition Studies(3).

[b]Determined by rat feeding studies. Digestibility is the amount of fed protein absorbed, and biological value is the portion of absorbed protein that is retained as body tissue. Net utilization is simply digestibility × biological value.

[c]Net dietary protein calories as percentage of total energy. The percentage of energy from protein in the food is adjusted according to the net utilization, or quality, of the protein, i.e. (gm protein/100 gm food × NPU × 4 kcal) kcal/100 gm food.

[d]Protein Efficiency Ratio is the grams of weight gained per gram of protein eaten by the rat.

[e]Amino acid score is based on amino acid composition. The amount of the most limiting amino acid present is expressed as a percentage of the amount present in the FAO/WHO reference pattern(1) for the preschool child.

[f]Values listed are for kale; net utilization of other leaves may be higher (mustard greens, 60) or lower (cabbage, 35).

Knowledge of the body's quantitative requirements for amino acids and their occurrence in foods now allows evaluation of dietary protein quality on the basis of amino acid composition. In 1957, the Food and Agricultural Organization (FAO) proposed an "ideal or reference pattern" of amino acids for the purpose of rating the nutritive value of the proteins furnished by various foods or combinations of foods in the human diet. This pattern was revised by FAO and the World Health Organization (WHO) in 1973 and again in 1983. The present recommendation is to use amino acid scoring patterns appropriate to each of four age groups: infants to age two years; preschool children aged two to six years; schoolchildren aged six to twelve years; and teenagers and adults of all ages and both sexes (Table 4–3). Practical experience indicates that only four amino acids are likely to be low in mixed diets. These are lysine, tryptophan, threonine, and the sulfur-containing amino acids (methionine plus cystine). Virtually all mixed diets, even vegetarian and low-cost diets, easily meet the essential amino acid patterns of adults, so adjustments are liable to be needed only for younger age groups in the population. Comparing the FAO/WHO pattern with the amino acid composition of one or a mixture of food proteins allows computation of an *amino acid score* that depends on the most limiting amino acid. If the most limiting amino acid (farthest below the level in the reference pattern) is 80 percent of the amount called for in the ideal pattern, then the food or combination of foods in the diet is given a score of 80. Since the reference pattern is based on amino acids that are 100 percent absorbable, the chemical score must be corrected for the factor of digestibility. If digestibility is not known, then for this calculation a figure of 95 percent may be applied to proteins of refined cereals and 85 percent to those of whole-grain cereals, legumes, and coarse vegetables; animal proteins are assumed to be 100 percent digestible.

Complementarity among Proteins

A protein that may in itself be deficient or low in some amino acid can supplement another protein by furnishing one or more of the amino acids that may be present in insufficient amounts in the other protein. This is illustrated in Table 4–3, by comparing the percentage of amino acids in some typical proteins and mixtures of proteins. The proteins of the cereal grains (wheat, rice, maize, sorghum, rye, oats) are low in lysine, but they furnish sulfur-containing amino acids that will supplement the typically low content of these amino acids in legumes and nuts. These foods contain other amino acids in addition to the ones mentioned, and they may supplement each other in numerous respects. For example, protein of white potato is limiting for preschool children in the sulfur-containing amino acids with a score of 76 and is below standard in lysine and leucine as well; a mixture of two-thirds potato protein and one-third egg protein has a score of 95. Substantial improvements in amino acid pattern always result when a high-quality protein source is added to a diet based on cereals, starchy roots, or tubers.

Imbalance of amino acids in the diet has been shown, in the rat, to have deleterious effects. An excess of a certain amino acid may reduce the utilization of, or increase the need for, another amino acid(2), leading to reduced appetite and growth. Such severe imbalances are unlikely to occur with normal human diets. Even so, most nutritionists recommend supplementing a protein low in one or more amino acids with some other food protein. The poorer proteins are usually low in more than one amino acid, so it is more expedient to supplement with proteins than with pure amino acids. If the mixed proteins in the diet are very poor (below a

Table 4–3 CONTENT OF ESSENTIAL AMINO ACIDS (EAA) IN FOOD PROTEINS COMPARED WITH THE FAO/WHO REFERENCE PATTERNS[a,b]

	Most Common Limiting Amino Acids								Amino Acids Usually Adequate in Diets					
	Lysine		Methionine + Cystine		Threonine		Tryptophan		Histidine	Isoleucine	Leucine	Phenylalanine + Tyrosine	Valine	Total EAA
Estimated requirement pattern, mg/gm dietary protein														
Adult, age 12 and above	16		17		9		5		16	13	19	19	13	127
Schoolchild, age 6–12 yr.	44		22		28		9		19	28	44	22	25	241
Preschooler, age 2–6 yr.	58		25		34		11		19	28	66	63	35	339
Infant, to age 2 yr.	66		42		43		17		26	46	93	72	55	460
Composition of food proteins	mg/gm	%[b]	mg/gm	%[b]	mg/gm	%[b]	mg/gm	%[b]	mg/gm	mg/gm	mg/gm	mg/gm	mg/gm	mg/gm
Hen's egg	70	121	58	232	51	150	15	136	24	62	88	99	68	535
Cow's milk	72	124	34	136	44	129	14	127	34	64	125	131	74	592
Beef	89	153	40	160	46	135	12	109	34	48	81	80	50	480
Soybeans	64	110	26	104	39	115	13	118	25	45	78	81	48	419
Peanuts (groundnuts)	36	62	24	96	26	76	10	91	24	34	64	89	42	349
Cassava leaf	62	107	28	112	47	138	14	127	22	48	86	94	57	458
Cassava meal (root)	41	71	27	108	26	76	11	100	21	28	39	41	33	201
Potato, white	48	83	19	76	38	112	16	145	15	38	60	67	47	348
Wheat, whole grain	29	50	40	160	29	85	11	100	23	33	67	75	44	351
Wheat, white flour	21	36	40	160	27	79	11	100	21	36	70	72	41	339
Maize, whole grain	27	47	35	140	36	106	7	64	27	37	125	87	48	429
Rice, brown	38	66	34	136	39	115	12	100	25	38	82	86	55	409
Rice, polished	36	62	37	148	33	97	13	118	23	42	82	80	58	404
⅓ egg, ⅔ potato	55	95	32	128	42	124	16	145	18	46	69	78	54	410
⅓ milk, ⅔ white flour	38	66	38	152	33	97	12	109	25	45	89	92	52	424
⅓ soybean, ⅔ white rice	45	78	33	132	35	103	13	118	23	43	81	80	55	408
⅓ beef, ⅔ maize	38	66	36	144	39	115	8	73	29	41	110	85	49	435
⅓ cassava leaf, ⅔ cassava meal	48	83	27	108	33	97	12	109	21	35	55	58	41	330

[a]FAO, computed from amino acid content per gram of nitrogen × 0.16, i.e. crude protein.

[b]FAO/WHO/UNU(1) requirements patterns are established for specific age categories, so there is no one single "reference pattern." Percentages of adequacy listed are in relation to the requirements pattern for preschool children. Proteins would be less limiting for schoolchildren. The most limiting amino acid is underlined.

score of 60), it is best to add protein of higher value, such as egg, milk, meat, legumes, or nuts. In the American diet, with about 50 percent of the protein from foods of animal origin, the amino acid mixture provided is more than sufficient to satisfy the daily requirement for all essential amino acids.

Other Factors Affecting the Utilization of Proteins in the Diet

Another factor that must be considered in practical dietaries is the amount of protein in a food relative to the amount of energy supplied. Foods such as the starchy roots and tubers (potatoes, cassava, yams) and cereal grains have fairly high energy value, but most of this comes from starch rather than protein (Table 4–2). They may be thought of as "dilute" protein foods, and in order to meet the required amount of protein, so much of them would have to be taken that they would provide energy in excess of body needs. Also, the volume of food that would have to be eaten might well exceed the capacity of young children and some adults. This is why protein malnutrition is most commonly seen where foods of relatively low protein content form the basis of the diet (such as cassava in Africa and rice in the Orient).

It is possible to provide an adequate diet from relatively dilute protein sources (such as rice or potatoes) if supplemented with small amounts of some foods such as milk or eggs or legumes. Taking one example, to meet the requirement for sulfur-containing amino acids, an eleven-year-old child (45 kg) would have to consume 60 gm of potato protein (need 23 mg × 45 kg ÷ 19 mg/gm potato protein, digestibility 90 percent; see Tables 4–1 and 4–3). Potatoes have 2.1 percent of protein, so the daily allowance would amount to 2800 gm of boiled potatoes (6.2 lb) and provide 2100 kcal. A mixture of one-third egg protein plus two-thirds potato protein reduces the amount of protein necessary to meet methionine and cystine requirement to 36 gm (1035 ÷ 32 ÷ 0.9), which would be supplied by two very small eggs (89 gm) plus 1100 gm (2.4 lb) of potatoes, in 980 kcal.

Even when the diet contains only high-quality sources, protein may be inadequate. The total amount of protein or amino nitrogen may be the limiting factor rather than lack of any essential amino acid—that is, it is possible to run out of total amino acids before reaching a limiting amount of essential amino acids. This has been demonstrated in infants fed milk protein and adults fed egg as the only source of protein.

Digestion and absorption are ordinarily not major factors in meeting requirement, unless the diet is very coarse. Proteins that are less completely digested and absorbed than others are less efficient for meeting the body's protein needs on this account. Early experiments of Atwater and Bryant showed that, in an ordinary mixed diet, the proteins from animal foods have a high "coefficient of digestibility"[5] (that is, the net percentage digested and absorbed) of about 95 to 99, while those from cereals, fruits, and vegetables have lower values of 85 to 90, and some legumes have values as low as 75 to 80 (Table 4–2). Nitrogen loss in the feces is increased when the diet is composed chiefly of foods that are high in dietary fiber (as a result principally of the increased intestinal bacterial growth these carbohydrates support). Relative to eggs, meat, and milk (the reference protein standard, arbitrarily 100),

[5]Apparent protein digestibility is calculated as the amount of nitrogen in the feces subtracted from the amount eaten, divided by the amount eaten, times 100. For example, with 75 gm protein in diet (12 gm N) and 1.3 gm N in feces, digestibility is (12 − 1.3) ÷ 12 × 100, or 89 percent. To determine true protein digestibility, fecal nitrogen must be corrected for the amount excreted when no protein is fed.

the digestibility of refined cereals and potatoes and of mixed diets that include animal protein is about 95; diets based on coarse vegetables, whole-grain cereals, and legumes have a relative digestibility of 85 (1).

The percentage of food protein that is absorbed and retained in the body is also influenced by the treatment to which the food may have been subjected in cooking or processing. The protein in legumes is rendered more digestible by cooking, but high heating of cereals (as in toasted or puffed breakfast cereals) and milk (as in processing of some canned and dried products) causes adverse structural changes in the protein. Reactions occur between amino acids and carbohydrates with heating that make a portion of the amino acids (especially lysine) unavailable for their essential functions. Processing with acid and heat, as is done in the manufacture of gelatin, completely degrades one amino acid (tryptophan) and damages others. Careful home cooking and commercial processing techniques are required to preserve maximum protein quality.

The distribution of protein foods in the meals throughout the day is thought to be important. All the amino acids that are needed for a specific protein must be present at the same time in order to build that protein. That is, protein formation is an all-or-none reaction, and if one amino acid is missing, no protein is made. To some extent, partially complete mixtures of amino acids may be adjusted by contributions from the tissues, but for assured maximum utilization, balanced protein mixtures should be included in each meal and taken with sufficient carbohydrate and fat to prevent the use of protein for energy.

The Dietary Protein Requirement

In 1920, Sherman examined requirements data obtained by the nitrogen balance method from forty-seven different persons and, to make them comparable, calculated each to a common basis of 70 kg body weight. Individual values ranged from 21 to 65 gm, but the average was about 44 gm of protein per day as maintenance requirement for a man of this average weight. Sherman estimated that 0.5 gm of protein per kg of body weight would suffice to meet the minimum requirement (35 gm daily for a 70-kg man). A summation of data available sixty years later produced a figure of 0.6 gm, not far different from Sherman's estimate (1). The normal individual variability is ± 12.5 percent of that value.

Although it would be unwise to limit the protein intake over long periods to the average minimum for maintenance, the establishment of such a figure (about 0.6 gm protein per kg body weight) is useful in permitting nutritionists to gauge how much more protein should be included in the diet to provide a suitable margin to cover variations in individual needs. Other factors that have a systematic effect on protein need are *body size* and *age,* and the conditions of *pregnancy* and *lactation.*

Size. The total amount of protein needed for tissue upkeep is dependent in part upon the amount of active tissues in the body; for this reason the protein requirement is stated as so much per unit of body weight. If the average minimum requirement is placed at 0.6 gm per kg, a woman who weighs only 44 kg should consume a minimum of 26 gm of protein daily; a tall and muscular man weighing 80 kg would need to take a minimum of 48 gm. Regardless of sex, a person of small body weight requires less, and one of larger than average lean weight needs more than a standard allowance based on average body weight.

Age. In the younger years extra protein is needed for growth. Rapidly growing young children may need two to three times as much protein per unit of body weight as adults do, to provide for depositing protein in new tissues. The high protein requirement of infants and young children is striking when considered per unit of weight, but the total amount needed by their smaller bodies is, of course, less than the amount needed by an adult. The amount of protein needed for growth falls as growth rate slows. Requirements reach adult level after puberty (age twelve to sixteen for girls and fourteen to eighteen for boys).

Dietary records of older persons sometimes disclose that they are subsisting on considerably less than optimal protein intakes (for example, meats may be mostly eliminated because of low income or difficulty in chewing.) It is now advised that, although energy intake should be somewhat reduced, protein intake of old people should be about the same as in earlier adult life.

Pregnancy and Lactation. Extra protein is needed during pregnancy primarily for the growth of the baby during the second and third trimesters; smaller amounts are needed for the development of maternal supporting tissues and fluids. Additional dietary protein is also required for production of milk. The basis for these recommendations is given in Chapter 22.

Muscular Work Not a Factor. Although muscular work is the largest single factor in determining energy needs, it has no appreciable effect on the protein requirement except during initial periods of training when muscular tissue is developing. A physically active person does require more carbohydrate and fat in order to obtain energy. Since protein is an integral part of many foods, protein intake by an active person usually is increased in proportion to total energy consumption.

Standard Allowances of Protein

The daily allowances of protein recommended by various governmental agencies for adults and teenagers are shown in Table 4–4.

The FAO/WHO has expressed protein allowances in terms of a good quality diet with the understanding that this will be adjusted according to the digestibility of local food supplies (1). The safe level of protein intake

Table 4–4 RECOMMENDED DAILY ALLOWANCES OF PROTEIN FOR HEALTHY ADULTS, in gm per day

Country or Organization	*Men*		*Women*	
	ADOLESCENT[a]	MATURE ADULT	ADOLESCENT	MATURE ADULT
FAO/WHO(1)				
Per kg body weight	0.87	0.75	0.82	0.75
United States(4)				
Per kg body weight	0.85	0.80	0.84	0.80
Per day, avg. weight	56 (66 kg)[b]	56 (70 kg)	46 (55 kg)	44 (55 kg)
Canada(5)				
Per kg body weight	0.87	0.77	0.89	0.69
Per day, avg. weight	54 (62 kg)	57 (74 kg)	43 (48 kg)	41 (59 kg)
United Kingdom(6)				
Percent of energy	10	10	10	10
Per day, for moderately active person	75 (61 kg)	75 (65 kg)	58 (56 kg)	55 (55 kg)

[a]Range 15 to 18 years.
[b]Value in parentheses is average or reference body weight.

for men and women is 0.75 gm per kg, which is the average requirement plus two standard deviations, allowing for population variability in requirement (that is, 0.6 gm + [2 × 12.5 percent]). If the local diet is based on coarse, fibrous foods, a correction for digestibility of 85 percent or 90 percent may be required.

The United States National Research Council (NRC) allowances for normal adults are based on 0.8 gm protein per kg body weight (1). Because variability is substantial, no differentiation was made between allowances for men and women. Authorities agree that such an allowance gives a safety margin of 50 to 100 percent above the normal requirements for maintenance, the margin varying somewhat with individual differences in utilization and body needs. The Canadian Council on nutrition recommends somewhat less protein for women, 0.69 gm per kg of body weight, allowing a smaller margin of safety (5).

The protein allowances just given are for adults of average weight. Adults who are markedly under- or overweight should have protein allowances based on the normal weight for their height, rather than on actual body weight.

The NRC allowances for pregnant and lactating women and for children who are growing and maturing provide more protein per kg body weight. A woman in the second and third trimesters of pregnancy should have an additional 30 gm protein daily, and during lactation 20 gm protein above the normal allowance may be required. Allowances for younger children (which usually range from 1.2 to 2.2 gm protein per kg body weight) are found in Chapter 23.

Using a different philosophy a United Kingdom panel (6) has recommended that the protein intake should furnish 10 percent of the energy intake. In making this recommendation, it was observed that the majority of people in the United Kingdom take between 10 and 45 percent of their energy in the form of protein, that this habitual intake is without apparent harm, and that this level of protein contributes to the palatability of the diet. For persons of normal energy expenditure, an arbitrary allowance of 10 percent of energy intake clearly exceeds minimum requirements by an adequate margin for safety. Care is required in applying this standard in that sedentary and old people may have low energy needs, but their protein needs are not decreased correspondingly.

Meeting the Protein Allowance

For the average adult sufficient protein will be ensured if the daily diet includes three or four average servings of milk, meat, fish, poultry, eggs, or other protein-rich foods (Fig. 4–10). The "other" protein-rich foods may be legumes such as peas, beans or peanuts, other nuts, cheese, or additional servings of the foods listed. The protein furnished by these foods will vary according to the size of the portions and the choice among the protein-rich foods but is likely to average at least 30 gm protein.

Grain products and the vegetables needed to make an adequate diet usually provide about 15 to 20 gm protein, which brings the total protein to 50 gm, which is about the amount now recommended for the average adult. Table 4–5 illustrates these points.

It can be seen that the foods in Table 4–5 provide about 50 gm protein, with about 80 percent of it of animal origin in the mixed diet. A vegetarian diet can be made entirely adequate in quality of proteins by the liberal use of legumes and cereal products, and by supplementing vegetable proteins with milk and milk products or with eggs.

Meats are one of the most expensive sources of protein, but they furnish it in concentrated form: a 3½ oz (100 gm) serving of meat may be depended on to give 18 to 25 gm protein (depending on its fat and mois-

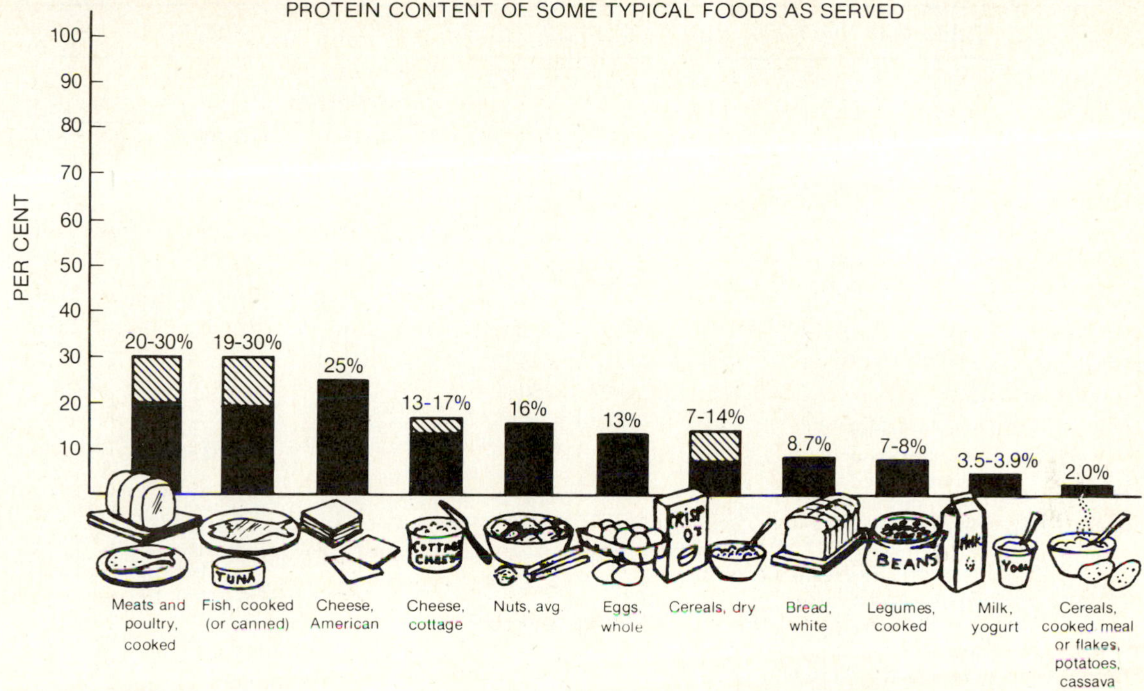

Figure 4–10

ture content), or about one fourth to one third of the adult's daily ration (Table 4–6). Fish, shellfish, and poultry are usually leaner and slightly higher in protein content than the red meats. Among the least expensive foods for protein are dried legumes, cereal products, dark green leafy vegetables, and potatoes. Eggs and milk, especially dried skim milk, are usually low to moderate in cost.

Table 4–5 FOODS THAT PROVIDE THE PROTEIN ALLOWANCE IN DIFFERENT DIETARY PATTERNS

Vegetarian Diet	*gm/serving*	*Mixed Diet*	*gm/serving*
	Protein-Rich Foods Group		
Red beans, ½ cup	8	Cheddar cheese, 1 oz	7
Peanut butter, 2 Tbsp	8	Salmon, 3 oz	17
Milk, 2 cups	16	Egg, 1	6
	Cereal Grains and Vegetables		
Whole-wheat bread, 2 slices	6	Macaroni	7
Rice, white, 1 cup	4	French bread, 2 slices	6
Brussels sprouts, ½ cup	4	Corn, whole kernel, ½ cup	2
Mushrooms, ½ cup	1	Potato, 1 medium	3
Pretzel, twist, 1	2	Spinach, ½ cup	3
Total	49		51

Table 4–6 PROTEIN YIELD OF SOME COMMON FOODS AS SERVED

Food	*Serving Size*	
	HOUSEHOLD MEASURE	COOKED WEIGHT, gm
Protein 20 to 25 gm per serving, or nearly 1/2 the adult daily allowance:		
Meat, fish, poultry	3–3 1/2 oz	90–100
Soybeans	1 c	260
Other dry beans, peas	1 1/2 c	400
Protein 5 to 8 gm per serving, or 1/10 the adult daily allowance:		
Milk	1 glass	200–400
Brick-type cheeses	1 oz	30
Cottage cheese	1/4 c	55
Egg	1	50
Nuts	1–1 1/2 oz	30–40
Peanut butter	2 tbsp	30
Macaroni, noodles	1 c	150
Green peas	3/4 c	120
Bean or pea soup	3/4 c	185
Bacon	3 strips	25
Frankfurter	1 medium	50
Custard and cream pies	1/6–1/8 pie	140–160
Puddings, ice cream	2/3–1 c	120–150
Protein 2 to 4 gm per serving, or 1/20 the adult daily allowance:		
Bread	1 slice	25
Dark green vegetables	1/2–2/3 c	70–120
Ready-to-eat cereals	3/4–1 c	25–30
Potato, white or sweet	1 medium	100
Cakes	2 in slice	50–100
Chocolate candy bar	1 oz	30

Normally we include protein-rich food in each meal, partly for its satiety value. Breakfast may be an exception for those who eat a hurried or light meal in the morning. Inclusion of some high-quality protein in each meal is especially important in periods of growth, pregnancy, or recovery from wasting illnesses. The distribution of protein and energy throughout the day is a much more urgent matter if the diet is borderline than if it is liberal in nutrient content.

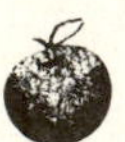

health considerations

Most of us eat far more protein than we need to meet protein requirements per se. The representative menus given in Table 4–7 show typical American intakes. The lowest amount, 78 gm (menu B), is nearly double the allowance for a woman. The high-cost, low-carbohydrate menu C provides 133 gm, with only 11 percent from vegetable sources. Protein in the U.S. food supply is about 100 gm per capita, or twice the amount recommended for adults. In poorer countries, where the total food supply is low, the amount of protein available per capita is half as much, or less, and a large proportion comes from basic cereal grains.

Excess Protein Intake

Questions have arisen about the advisability of high protein intake, since laboratory studies have revealed increased urinary excretion of calcium with high-protein diets. Protein has at least two counterbalancing effects on the body's calcium economy. The

Table 4–7 MENUS SHOWING PROTEIN LEVELS TYPICAL OF AMERICAN DIETS, gm per serving

Moderate Cost				*High Cost*	
A-HOME PREPARED		B-CONVENIENCE FOODS		C-RESTAURANT	
		Breakfast			
Oatmeal, ¾ cup	4	Corn flakes, 1 oz	2	Omelet, 2 eggs,	12
Bread, whole gr., 2 slices	6	Bread, white, 2 slices	4	Cheese, 1 oz	7
Butter, 1 pat		Margarine, 1 pat		Bread, whole gr., 1 slice	3
Jam, 1 Tbsp		Jelly, 1 Tbsp		Butter, 2 pats	
Milk, low fat, ½ cup	5	Milk, skim, ½ cup	4	Grapefruit, ½	1
Orange, 1 medium	1	Banana, 1 medium	1		
Sugar, 1 tsp		Sugar, 1 tsp			
		Luncheon			
Bean soup, 1 cup	8	Chicken-noodle soup, 1 cup	2	Consommé, 1 cup	5
Rye crackers, 2	2	Saltine crackers, 2	1	Ritz crackers, 2	1
Sandwich		Sandwich		Tuna salad[a], ½ cup	15
Egg, 1	6	Bologna, 1 slice	3	Avocado, ½	2
Bread, whole gr., 2 slices	6	Bread, white, 2 slices	4	Lettuce	
Lettuce		Margarine, 1 pat		Thousand Is. Dressing, 2 Tbsp	
Mayonnaise, 1 Tbsp		Mustard, 1 tsp		Strawberries, ½ cup	
Pear, 1 medium	1	Grapes, 20 seedless		Cream, heavy, ¼ cup	1
Milk, low fat, 1 cup	10	Milk, whole, 1 cup	8		
		Dinner			
Chicken, broiled, ¼	20	Chicken, fried[b]	34	Tomato juice, ½ cup	1
Baked potato w/skin	4	Rice, white, ½ cup	2	Steak, 12 oz (lean only, 8 oz)	72
Winter squash, ½ cup	2	Gravy, 2 Tbsp		Green beans, ½ cup	1
Mixed green salad, 1½ cup		Peas, canned, ½ cup	4	Butter, 1 pat	
Vinegar, ½ Tbsp		Tomato, 1 medium	1	Mixed green salad, 1½ cup	
Oil, ½ Tbsp		Biscuits, 2	4	Italian dressing, 2 Tbsp	
Rolls, whole gr., 2	4	Honey, 1 Tbsp		Red wine, 7 fl. oz	
Butter, 3 pats		Margarine, 1 pat		Cheese, Brie, 1 oz	6
Blueberry pie, ⅙	4	Ice cream, ½ cup	2	Apple, 1 medium	
		Chocolate brownie, 1	1		
		Snacks			
Apple juice, ½ cup		Soda pop, 12 oz		Sparkling water	
Yogurt, flavored, 1 cup	10	Potato chips, 1 oz	1	Almonds, roasted, 1 oz	6
TOTAL	93		78		133

[a]Made with 1 Tbsp. salad dressing and celery.
[b]Commercial, breaded, one thigh and one leg.

first is promotion of calcium absorption, which is seen with intakes in the range of no protein up to the minimum requirement level. The second is progressively increased urinary excretion of calcium with increasing dietary protein intakes at and above the requirement. This latter effect is dominant given usual patterns of food consumption in the United States.

Recent research indicates that the source of protein is an important variable. Sulfur-containing amino acids enhance calcium excretion because of the acidic nature of their metabolic end products (sulfate and hydrogen). Phosphorus is also acidic but because of the regulatory relationships between calcium and phosphorus (see Chap. 14), increased intake of phosphorus reduces calcium excretion (7). Thus, intake of proteins rich in highly available phosphorus, such as milk and meat, does not result in loss of body calcium, provided that calcium intake and absorption are adequate. (Other minerals, notably sodium, are involved in this complex regulatory system. See Chap. 13.)

In the past there was concern about the burden placed on the kidneys by the necessity of excreting urea, the principal end product of nitrogen metabolism. This excretory process is not costly, in terms of renal work, but does require sufficient water. About 50 ml of urinary water are needed to excrete one gram of nitrogen in the form of urea. A diet having 100 to 120 gm protein would demand about 750 ml of water for renal excretion of about 15 grams urea nitrogen.

On the other hand, high-protein diets are known to increase the amount of blood passing to and through the kidneys and, ultimately, to increase kidney size (8). These effects are not duplicated by giving urea or acidic loads equivalent to the protein metabolized but are mimicked by administering glycine. It is postulated that increased renal blood flow is mediated by the hormone glucagon, secreted in response to elevated amino acid levels in the blood. Sustained high rates of renal blood flow and filtration may damage the functional units of the kidney. Humans have about 3 to 4 times as much renal capacity as is theoretically required, so these changes may not impair health but simply use up reserve capacity. A generous, protein-rich diet may, however, contribute to the decline in kidney function seen in aging and some diseases.

Uric Acid

The final end product of the metabolism of *purines* present in nucleic acids is uric acid. Uric acid is a fairly insoluble substance that easily precipitates from solution, especially at acidic pH. Crystals of uric acid may form in the joints when the concentration of uric acid in body fluid is raised, causing gout or gouty arthritis. Uric acid may also crystallize in the urine, leading to formation of one type of kidney stone.

Purines are formed in the body from amino acids; nucleic acids present in food also contribute to the body pool. In most instances, high levels of uric acid in the body result from overproduction of purines (due to disease or enzyme defects). Uric acid level in body tissue fluids is also increased if the kidney does not excrete uric acid efficiently. Purine and, hence, uric acid production is increased at high levels of protein intake, but the relatively small excess is usually simply excreted in the urine. Alcohol and fructose also promote formation of uric acid. Thus gout is popularly associated with high living. Ketosis due to fasting or low carbohydrate intake impairs renal ability to excrete uric acid.

Usually the amount of purines in the diet is of little significance, but the very large amount of nucleic acid present in yeast (and other microbial cells) is a bar to their use in large amounts, that is in excess of about 10 gm dry weight daily. Other purine-rich foods (but having far lower concentration) are organ meats, small fishes, and leafy green vegetables. Generous intake of water is important to prevent renal or bladder stones from forming.

Protein-Energy Malnutrition

There are many areas of the world where protein-rich foods, especially those of animal origin, are practically unavailable to the poorer segments of the population (Fig. 4–11). Protein is probably the single essential nutrient most commonly deficient worldwide. This is because protein intake itself is marginal but, more importantly, because total food consumption and, hence, energy intake is so inadequate that the protein eaten is not spared to function as an essential nutrient.

Those most liable to show marked symp-

Distribution of proteins in grams per person per day

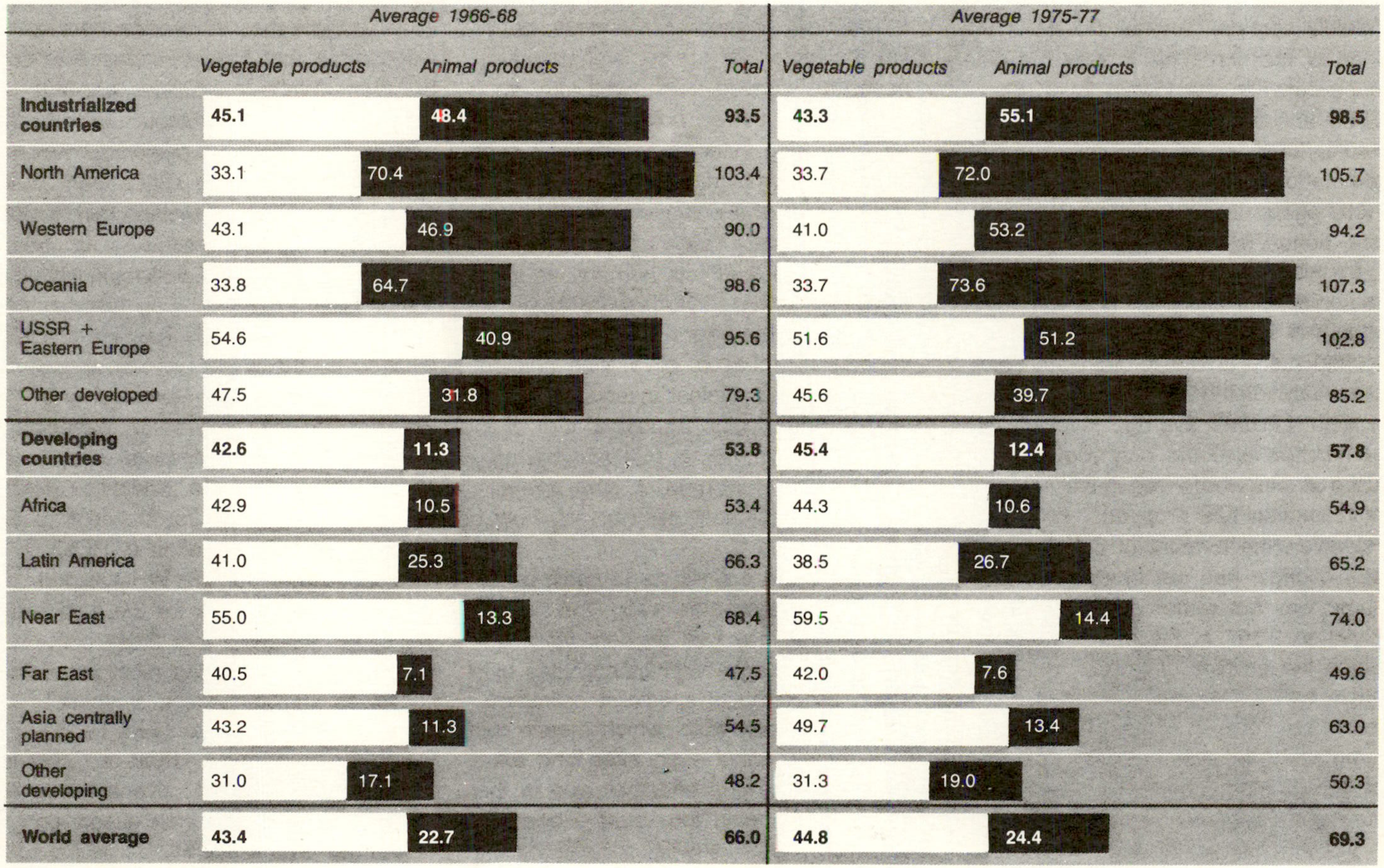

	Average 1966-68			*Average 1975-77*		
	Vegetable products	*Animal products*	*Total*	*Vegetable products*	*Animal products*	*Total*
Industrialized countries	**45.1**	**48.4**	**93.5**	**43.3**	**55.1**	**98.5**
North America	33.1	70.4	103.4	33.7	72.0	105.7
Western Europe	43.1	46.9	90.0	41.0	53.2	94.2
Oceania	33.8	64.7	98.6	33.7	73.6	107.3
USSR + Eastern Europe	54.6	40.9	95.6	51.6	51.2	102.8
Other developed	47.5	31.8	79.3	45.6	39.7	85.2
Developing countries	**42.6**	**11.3**	**53.8**	**45.4**	**12.4**	**57.8**
Africa	42.9	10.5	53.4	44.3	10.6	54.9
Latin America	41.0	25.3	66.3	38.5	26.7	65.2
Near East	55.0	13.3	68.4	59.5	14.4	74.0
Far East	40.5	7.1	47.5	42.0	7.6	49.6
Asia centrally planned	43.2	11.3	54.5	49.7	13.4	63.0
Other developing	31.0	17.1	48.2	31.3	19.0	50.3
World average	**43.4**	**22.7**	**66.0**	**44.8**	**24.4**	**69.3**

Source: FAO

Figure 4–11 Worldwide distribution of protein in gm per capita, 1966–68 and 1975–77. It is evident that world protein supplies are adequate, even in the poor regions, to meet requirements, provided supplies were evenly distributed, which we know they are not. Rich countries can afford and use more total protein and animal protein than do poor countries. Total food intake (energy) is also low where protein supplies are low, so the problem is compounded. The distribution of protein supplies between rich and poor countries has not changed appreciably in the past two decades. (From FAO, 1980.)

toms as a result of too little food, too little protein, or both, are young children in the years immediately after weaning. Naturally, with insufficient amino acids for building tissue protein and with some of the small protein supply burned for energy, children fail to grow and their tissues waste away. In areas where protein-energy malnutrition is endemic, adults do not reach their genetic potential in height. If food deprivation occurs in the adult after growth has ceased, as happened in concentration and prisoner-of-war camps in World War II, severe emaciation is the obvious result. Depending on the relative deficit of protein to energy in the diet and on other factors (such as liver function), both infants and adults may show marked edema, especially of the legs and abdomen. This symptom results from a decline in the level of protein in the plasma and sometimes, disturbance in the salt-regulating system. (See Chap. 14.) Anemia is present because of the failure to form hemoglobin and red blood cells. When people are poor and ill-fed, other public health problems abound, so cases of protein-energy malnutrition are commonly complicated by the presence of infectious diseases and intestinal parasitism; protein deficiency also impairs the ability to resist infections. Because foods carry more than one nutrient, protein-energy deficiency may have superimposed deficiencies of vitamins and minerals. Naturally, a range of different symptoms may be seen in individuals, depending on these other dietary and environmental factors.

The picture in young children may be one of *marasmus*, appropriately named from the Greek word meaning "to waste away," in which the muscles are atrophied and the face has a wizened "old man" look. Others in whom edema is a prominent symptom are said to have *kwashiorkor* (Fig. 4–4). This name comes from the Ga tribe of the African Gold Coast and was popularized by Cecily Williams when she described the condition in Ghanaian children. Some say that the word means "red boy," referring to the odd reddish-orange color of the hair as well as a skin rash characteristic of the disease. Other interpretive meanings suggest displacement or jealousy, from the frequency with which the disease occurs in children who are deprived of breast feeding by the birth of a second infant or by urbanization and employment of the mother. This disease, or gradations between the two types of symptom complexes, has been known by many names over the years (for example, "sugar baby," *dystrophie des farineux, Mehlnahrschaden, distrofia pluricarencial infantile*), but it is one entity caused basically by lack of protein and energy.

Brain growth is impaired by severe protein lack *in utero* and during the first few months of life. Some neurological deficit may be expected to follow deprivation throughout the early years of life, until the nervous system is formed completely, but the probability is lessened with increasing age. A legacy of poor educability and achievement may be one major cost of failure to feed mothers and babies.

For prevention, satisfactory prenatal diets and nutritionally adequate breast-feeding and weaning diets are essential. When milk is not available or is too costly, an assortment of vegetable foods may be used that supplement one another as to amino acids and other essential nutrients. Several special high-protein, low-cost infant foods have been developed by teams of nutritionists and food scientists using locally available foods.

In countries where protein intake is low and most of it is furnished by cereal grains or starchy roots and tubers, some of the essential amino acids are likely to be less than children require. Lysine, tryptophan, methionine, and threonine are the ones most likely to be lacking in such diets. It has been suggested, and experiments have been made, to fortify cereal foods, such as wheat flour, rice, and corn meal, with the limiting amino acids. Attempts also are being made to improve the amino acid pattern of cereal grains by genetic selection. Actually, supplementation of the diet with some available protein-rich food or vegetable protein mixture is more practical because these supply a mixture of supplementary amino acids and other nutrients and energy.

Much effort has been directed by United Nations and governmental aid agencies and by philanthropic organizations toward securing more adequate diets for people in underdeveloped countries. To make sustained improvement in nutritional state, it is evident that general levels of living must be raised, enabling people to produce or purchase enough food and needed amounts of high-quality protein foods.

There appears to be a wide range of protein intake to which adults can adapt and retain good health. Many factors affect the amount of dietary protein retained in the body for tissue building or upkeep, such as the energy supply (quantity of carbohydrate and fat in the diet); the quantity, quality, and digestibility of the proteins ingested; and the distribution of protein over the day's meals. Since conditions for assimilation may be more favorable at one time and less at another, the diet should supply some extra protein over the minimum requirement.

The protein allowance should be liberal in conditions of

1. growth or repair
2. pregnancy and lactation
3. reduced digestion an absorption
4. poor dietary protein quality

A reasonable margin over the minimum requirement is good insurance even under normal conditions, but superabundant intakes (over twice the minimum) provide no added advantage and may be disavantageous. A safe recommendation is that 10 percent of dietary energy should be derived from protein, or up to 15 percent if energy requirement is low, to avoid risks associated with very low or very high intakes.

QUESTIONS

1. What four chemical elements are combined in proteins? Which one of these is furnished in proteins but not in carbohydrates or fats? What other elements are often or sometimes incorporated in protein molecules?

2. Define amino acids. How many different amino acids have been found to occur commonly in proteins? How many are "essential" in the sense that they must be furnished preformed in the food? How many of these are needed for the growth of young rats? To maintain tissue proteins in human adults? Does the body need the other amino acids listed as "nonessential" to build and maintain tissues? If so, why do we not list them as "essential"? What is meant by the statement that a low supply of any essential amino acid may be a "limiting factor"?

3. Define high-quality (in regard to biological value), or complete proteins and low-quality, or incomplete proteins. Which class of proteins is furnished by foods of animal origin? Are there any exceptions? Explain how incomplete proteins may be supplemented by complete proteins in a mixed diet. How do cereals with milk furnish a well-balanced mixture of amino acids?

4. Where is protein found in the body? Why is an adequate supply of protein essential? Can protein be oxidized in the body—that is, does protein serve as an energy nutrient? How does a liberal supply of carbohydrate or fat in the diet "spare" protein for tissue maintenance?

5. What are nucleoproteins and where are they found in the body? What important biologic functions do they perform? How does DNA differ from RNA in composition and function? How do compound or conjugated proteins differ from simple proteins? What important compound protein is found in red blood corpuscles? Name two

other proteins found either in the body or in food that are linked with some nonprotein substance.

6. What foods or types of food contribute the largest amount of protein in the average diet? Which other types of food contribute less, but valuable, amounts of protein? Which foods are the most expensive and which are the least expensive sources of protein? If you were a farmer and had a choice of maize or rice or cassava as the staple crop, which would you choose for protein value? Why? What other factors would you have to consider in deciding which to plant?

7. What proportion of the energy should proteins contribute? List the foods in your diet for one day. From the Table of Nutritive Values of Foods in the Appendix calculate how many gm of protein you consumed and what relative proportion of the total energy this furnished. Compare this with your standard allowance for protein, and if your protein intake was as much as 20 percent lower than that recommended, make suggestions as to how to bring your protein intake up to a desirable level. Does it matter if you are eating more protein than the standard allowance? If so, why; if not, why not? Under what conditions would your answer be different?

8. Plan a day's diet for a vegetarian that excludes meat and eggs but includes milk or cheese, or both, and that furnishes 50 gm protein. Calculate the amount of lysine and sulfur-containing amino acids provided by the diet as you planned it and with legumes replacing the milk and cheese. Do these diets meet adult requirements for these amino acids? Children's requirements?

9. What physical symptoms occur when the diet is deficient in protein? What is marasmus? Kwashiorkor?

References

1. FAO/WHO/UNU: *Energy and Protein Requirements.* FAO Nutr. Rept. No. XX, WHO Tech. Rept. No. XXX. Rome and Geneva, 1983.
2. Committee on Amino Acids, NRC: *Improvement of Protein Nutriture.* Washington D.C., National Academy of Sciences, 1974; Pellett, P. L., and Young, V. R.: Nutritional evaluation of protein foods. UNU World Hunger Prog. Food & Nutr. Bull., Supp. 4, WHTR–3/UNUP–129, United Nations—Univ. Japan, 1980.
3. FAO Nutritional Studies: *Amino Acid Content of Foods and Biological Data on Proteins.* No. 24, Rome, 1970.
4. Food and Nutrition Board: *Recommended Dietary Allowances.* 9th Ed. Washington, D.C., National Research Council, National Academy of Sciences, 1980.
5. Committee for the Revision of the Dietary Standards for Canada, Bureau of Nutritional Sciences, Food Directorate: *Recommended Nutrient Intakes for Canadians.* Ottawa, Dept. of Natl. Health and Welfare, 1983.
6. *Recommended Intakes of Nutrients for the United Kingdom.* Dept. Health and Soc. Sec. Rept. No. 120, 1969.
7. Schuette, S. A., and Linkswiler, H. M.: Effects on Ca and P metabolism in humans by adding meat, meat plus milk, or purified proteins plus Ca and P to a low protein diet. J. Nutr. *112*:338, 1982.
8. Brenner, B. M., Meyer, T. W., and Hostetter, T. H.: Dietary protein intake and the progressive nature of kidney disease: The role of hemodynamically mediated glomerular injury in the pathogenesis of progressive glomerular sclerosis in aging, renal ablation, and intrinsic renal disease. New Eng. J. Med., *307*:652, 1982.

5 Digestion and Absorption

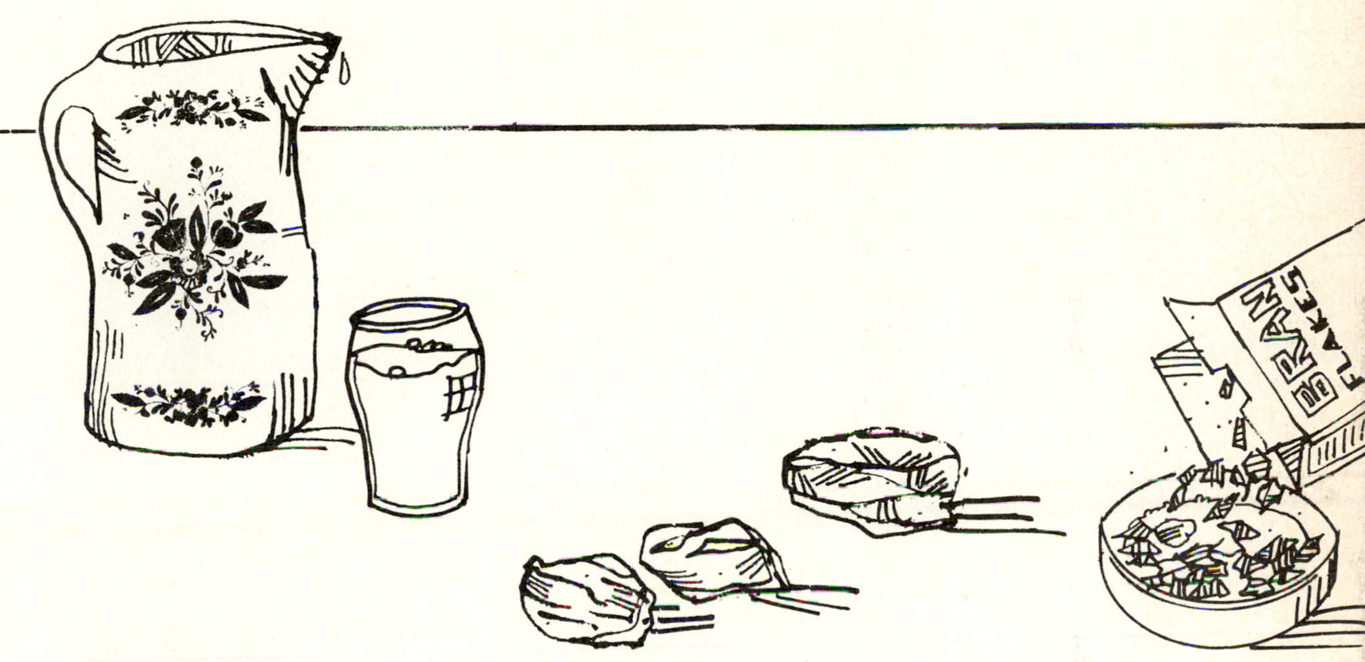

DIGESTION

Digestion, which takes place in a series of organs known collectively as the alimentary tract, is the process by which food is prepared for absorption into the body proper. Most food materials are complex substances, which are either insoluble in water or of such a nature that they cannot cross the membranes that line the digestive organs and cannot be absorbed into the blood and lymph. Moreover, even if the materials could be absorbed most of these complex substances could not be used by the cells.[1]

The alimentary, or gastrointestinal (GI) tract is best understood if it is considered as organized for its main functions: motor, secretory, and absorptive. Muscular activity is required for mixing the food mass with digestive juices and for moving partially digested material from one part of the alimentary tract to another. The GI tract and associated organs (the liver, pancreas, and gallbladder—Fig. 5–1) form the important digestive fluids, which are responsible for bringing about the chemical breakdown of foodstuffs. These fluids contain enzymes, electrolytes, and emulsifiers needed for the digestive process and for promoting the ab-

[1]Tissues can use fat if it is injected into the blood stream, but food fat cannot cross the intestinal barrier without first being broken down into simpler substances. When patients are fed parenterally (bypassing the digestive system and administering nutrients by vein, or intravenously), amino acids, rather than proteins, and glucose, rather than disaccharides or starch, must be given; fat must be very finely emulsified and is not well tolerated. The subject of intravenous alimentation is beyond the scope of this book, but references for individual study are included in the supplementary readings.

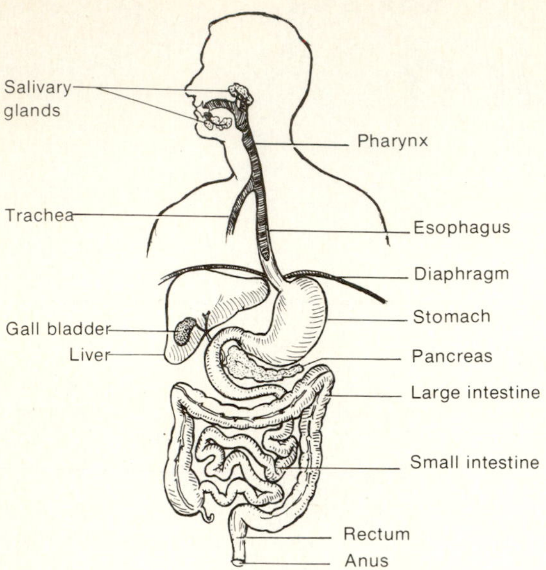

Figure 5–1 Schematic drawing of the digestive system.

sorption of the digestion products. The endocrine cells of the digestive organs secrete hormones that regulate the motor and secretory activities of the GI tract itself and that also participate in blood-sugar regulation and the control of food intake (see Chap. 7). All of the available nutrients are finally absorbed and transferred into a rich network of blood and lymphatic vessels.

The structure of the walls of the alimentary canal is essentially similar throughout its whole length—a mucous membrane lining the cavity, layers of smooth muscular tissue, and a thin covering membrane.

The mucous membrane and its secretion serve to protect and lubricate the more delicate tissues that lie within and below it. The cells of the mucous membrane are constantly renewed. The lining of the small intestine turns over completely about every one and one-half days, which means that this is one of the most rapidly growing tissues of the body. The aged cells are discharged into the digestive tract. These cells (as well as the digestive secretions) are largely recovered in the processes of digestion and absorption, and their constituents are used again by the body just as are nutrients from the diet.

Some of the cells that secrete the digestive enzymes and fluids are located in crypts and glands that lie within the walls of the stomach and intestine; others are located in the pancreas and liver, and their secretions pass through a duct system into the small intestine. Hormone-producing cells are present in the stomach, pancreas, and intestine; the hormones may act locally or be transported by the blood to target tissues elsewhere within and outside the GI tract. The tract also has an extensive network of nerves that both receive and transmit information between the gut and the central nervous system. Motor activity, secretion, and blood flow all are under neural, as well as hormonal, control.

The smooth muscle of the healthy GI tract is never fully relaxed but maintains a steady state of contraction referred to as tonus. When the circular muscle fibers contract, as they do in small, separate segments, they produce a squeezing motion, which presses the contents of the tube closely against its inner wall and churns and mixes the mass in separate segments. When the longitudinal muscle fibers contract, the resulting motion pushes the food mass along the digestive tract. These contractions occur in regular waves that pass along the tract almost always in such a way as to propel the food from the mouth toward the anus. Such rhythmical, recurring waves of contraction are referred to as *peristalsis.* Each wave of contraction is preceded by a wave of relaxation, which allows the sequential gut segment to receive the food bolus.

Progress of Food Material through the GI Tract

In the mouth, food is more or less finely divided by chewing and is mixed with saliva, which moistens the food and also produces a chemical action, and with mucus, which assists in lubricating the food for swallowing. The swallowed food mass is carried down the esophagus by peristalsis.

The stomach acts as a reservoir where food may remain for some time before it is gradually pushed along toward the pylorus (a circular muscle that guards the opening into the intestine). Glands situated in the stomach wall secrete the digestive fluid gastric juice. The food mass is mixed with gastric juice and churned about until, partly by mechanical means and partly by action of the digestive fluid, it is reduced to a semiliquid state (chyme). From time to time, the pylorus opens and a peristaltic wave sends a gush of the more fluid portion of the stomach contents into the first part of the intestine (duodenum); thus the stomach is gradually emptied. As it empties, the stomach contracts upon itself, so that it is relatively small and usually contains only a little fluid between meals. The rate at which the stomach empties is chiefly dependent on the type of foods that compose the meal. Liquids leave the stomach relatively quickly; concentrated foods are retained longer. In general, carbohydrate-rich foods tend to pass out faster than foods high in protein, and proteins faster than fatty foods, while mixtures of proteins and fats leave the stomach more slowly than either alone. The average time for the stomach to discharge an ordinary meal is about three hours. When the stomach is empty for a long period, strong rhythmical contractions occur, the hunger contractions. The inclusion of some fat or fat and protein in a meal delays the onset of these hunger contractions.

In the duodenum chyme is mixed with the digestive juices poured in at that point. The largest part of the processes of digestion and absorption takes place in the small intestine. These processes are aided by contractions of the intestinal muscles: those of the circular muscle fibers, which divide intestinal segments, thus mixing the contents thoroughly and squeezing them against the intestinal walls; and those of longitudinal fibers, whose peristaltic movements gradually pass the intestinal contents along toward the ileocecal valve opening into the large intestine. By the time the large intestine is reached, food material is nearly completely digested and absorbed. The length of time required for food material to pass along the small intestine varies with the relative muscular activity of that organ. Irritating or toxic substances within the intestine, as well as some cathartics, stimulate peristalsis, causing diarrhea, a condition in which intestinal contents pass through so quickly as to be excreted in fluid condition.

The large intestine has about twice the diameter of the small intestine but is much shorter and less muscularly active. It acts as a reservoir in which food and digestive residues are concentrated by absorption of the large volume of water added in the digestive process. Propulsive motion moves the progressively drier mass into the descending colon and rectum. These propulsive waves are strongest after eating and are enhanced by physical activity. Final evacuation through the anus, an opening guarded by a double ring of circular muscle fibers, is voluntarily controlled in healthy older children and adults and housebroken animals. Food residues and excretory material remain in the colon from eighteen to ninety-six hours, and conditions for bacteria to grow are more favorable here than in any other part of the GI tract. Some of these bacteria are beneficial, such as those that manufacture vitamins; others form products that may be absorbed and must be detoxified elsewhere in the body.

Chemical Processes in Digestion

The chemical processes by which foodstuffs are broken down in preparation for absorption and use by the tissues constitute digestion in the narrower, correct use of the term.

In digestion, complex food materials are cleaved into simpler components. This chemical breakdown takes place gradually, so that many intermediate compounds are created before the original material is reduced to absorbable forms. The long chains of glucose units that constitute starch molecules are gradually broken down by splitting off two sugar groups at a time (maltose molecules), the intermediate compounds being dextrins. Eventually the dextrins are completely converted to maltose, and the maltose is broken down into the simple sugar, glucose (Fig. 5–2). The disaccharides (sucrose, lactose, and maltose) are broken up at a single step into their components—the simple sugars (glucose, fructose, and galactose).

The very large molecules of proteins are broken down in orderly fashion into those of gradually decreasing size (polypeptides, tripeptides, dipeptides). Most are completely reduced to amino acids, but a small amount of dipeptides is also absorbed.

Fats are also broken down in a series of steps. The fatty acids are split off one at a time, forming di- and monoacylglycerols. A good portion of fat is absorbed in the form of monoacylglycerols; only 40 to 50 percent of the fat is completely broken down into fatty acids and glycerol.

The simplest constituents of the diet do not need to be broken down by digestion.

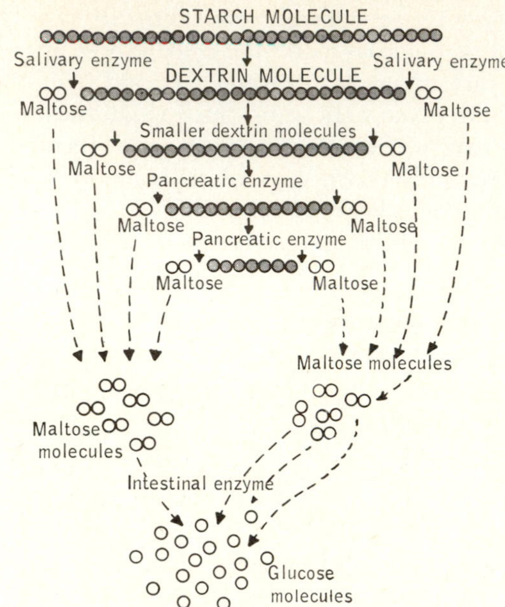

Figure 5–2 Gradual breaking down of large starch molecules by enzymes in digestion. The disaccharide maltose is split off by enzymes in the saliva and pancreatic juice, with smaller and smaller dextrin molecules formed as intermediate products, until the starch has been completely reduced to maltose. An intestinal enzyme then acts on the maltose molecules, splitting them into molecules of the monosaccharide glucose.

This is true of simple sugars, alcohol, and water, which are absorbed in the form in which they are consumed.

The gradual breakdown of proteins and of starch through various intermediate stages until they are finally reduced to their simplest units, and the simpler cleavage of fats and disaccharides into their components during digestion, are summarized in Table 5–1.

Enzymes. In each instance the splitting of a larger molecule into a number of smaller ones is brought about by means of the chemical process of hydrolysis through the agency of *enzymes,* which are catalysts formed by living cells. The same chemical changes take place if proteins, starch, fats, or disaccharides are subjected, outside the body, to prolonged heating with water and

Table 5–1 SUMMARY OF DIGESTION AND ABSORPTION OF THE ENERGY-YIELDING NUTRIENTS

Substrate	*Enzyme Activity*	*Final Products Formed*	*Products Absorbed*
Starch and glycogen	Salivary amylase (ptyalin)	Dextrins, maltose	
	Pancreatic amylase	Maltose	
Disaccharides	Intestinal disaccharidases	Monosaccharides	
Maltose	Maltase	Glucose	In small intestine via blood vessels to liver
Sucrose	Sucrase (invertase)	Glucose and fructose	
Lactose	Lactase	Glucose and galactose	
Monosaccharides			
Hexoses	None		In small intestine via blood vessels to liver
Pentoses			
Protein	Rennin (gastric)	Precipitate of casein	
	Pepsins (gastric)	Polypeptides	
Protein and polypeptides	Trypsin (pancreatic)	Small polypeptides	
	Chymotrypsin (pancreatic)	Small polypeptides	In small intestine via blood vessels to liver
Polypeptides	Carboxypeptidase (pancreatic)	Amino acid (and peptide residue)	
	Aminopeptidase (intestinal)	Amino acid (and peptide residue)	
Dipeptides	Intestinal dipeptidases	Amino acids	
Fats	Lingual lipase	Diacylglycerols, fatty acids	In small intestine, glycerol and fatty acids of < 10 C atoms via blood to liver; of > 10 C atoms via lymphatics, thoracic duct to blood.
Fats emulsified with bile	Pancreatic lipase	Mono- and diacylglycerols, fatty acids	
Monoacylglycerols	Intestinal lipase	Glycerol and fatty acids	
Ethanol	None		In stomach and small intestine via blood to liver and tissues

acid or alkali. In the body, digestive enzymes bring about these chemical changes more rapidly and at lower temperatures.

As catalysts, the enzymes do not themselves take part in the chemical processes by which foodstuffs are broken down, but their presence facilitates these processes. The digestive enzymes are formed by the secreting cells of the digestive tract. To protect the cells themselves, the powerful proteolytic enzymes within the cells are in an inactive form, called a zymogen (or specifically pepsinogen, for example). The enzymes become active under the influence of other factors present in the stomach and intestine, such as acid and other enzymes.

Enzymes are typical proteins, although of relatively small molecular size. Their enzymatic activity is lost if they are exposed to any chemical that renders protein insoluble or to a degree of heat sufficient to coagulate protein. All enzymes are sensitive to heat and cold; they are destroyed by high temperatures, and their activity is suspended by cold. The digestive enzymes all seem to work best at about body temperature (37°C).

Enzymes are specific in that each one acts only on a certain type of substance (called a substrate) and brings about only one specific chemical reaction. Thus, when a digestive fluid has the ability to act on two or more kinds of foodstuffs, we know that there must be separate enzymes in it for the performance of each of these chemical reactions. Nor are the enzymes in different digestive juices that act on the same kind of foodstuff identical—we know this because they require different conditions to act. The proteolytic enzyme in the gastric juice requires quite a high degree of acidity to be effective, whereas a protein-splitting enzyme in the pancreatic juice works well in either a slightly acid or an alkaline medium. Each of the digestive enzymes has some optimum pH at which it works best and a certain range outside which it will not work at all. Cells located in the stomach secrete strong hydrochloric acid, which after a time acidifies the mixture of saliva and food present, reducing the pH below the optimum for the starch-splitting enzyme present in saliva but optimizing conditions for the action of the proteolytic gastric enzymes. Secretions of the pancreas and intestine are rich in bicarbonate and are therefore alkaline, which neutralizes the acid in the chyme as it leaves the stomach and provides the pH needed for the pancreatic and intestinal enzymes.

In addition to optimum temperature and pH, two other conditions are required for the action of digestive enzymes. One is surface contact with the substance acted on, and for this reason intimate mixing of digestive juices with finely divided food material and getting the food material ultimately into solution or colloidal dispersion (as with fats) are important. Also important is the removal of the products formed by the reaction. Hence it is only in the small intestine, where the products of digestion are continuously removed by absorption, that conditions are favorable for digestive processes to run to completion.

Kinds of Enzymes. Enzymes are usually named to indicate the substances on which they act. To this substrate root is added the suffix *-ase,* which indicates that it is an enzyme, and often an adjective is prefixed to show the source of the enzyme. Thus, all protein-splitting enzymes are *proteases;* fat-splitting enzymes are *lipases* (from the word lipids, for fats); and starch-splitting enzymes are *amylases* (from the Latin name *amylum,* for starch). To distinguish between the different enzymes, the starch-splitting enzyme found in saliva is called *salivary amylase* and the one secreted by the pancreas is known as *pancreatic amylase.*

Although this system of naming is more descriptive, many enzymes have other names which are well established. For instance, the salivary amylase is well known by the name of *ptyalin,* while almost everyone is familiar with the names of *pepsin* and *trypsin,* which are respectively gastric and pancreatic proteases. Some of the more recently identified enzymes, such as lingual lipase, have no such common names (Table 5–1).

Enzymes secreted into the intestine carry on the digestive processes started by those in saliva and gastric juice. Thus, any of the foodstuff that escapes digestion by the action of one enzyme is subjected to digestion by others secreted lower in the digestive tract, which makes for very efficient utilization.

Bile, which is formed by the liver and discharged from the gallbladder and liver into the intestine, is important for good digestion of fats, even though it contains no enzymes. Bile acts to emulsify fats and assists in the absorption of the fatty acids formed by digestion so that they are removed from the intestinal contents and digestion goes to completion.

Rennin, contained in the gastric juice, is an enzyme that precipitates milk in solid form (curds). It is different from digestive enzymes in that it does not control hydrolysis. Rennin is especially abundant in gastric juice of young animals fed on milk; it is less important in adults.

Regulation

Secretory and motor activity of the GI tract are carefully regulated by a complex system of neural and hormonal signals. The systems are interactive and have some degree of redundancy (that is, they provide more than one way to control a given process). The intricacies of the systems are still being worked out, and only the highlights are presented here. Additional information will be found in Table 5–2.

Small amounts of saliva and gastric juice are secreted all the time, but their flow is stimulated when food is present. Factors that stimulate the flow of saliva are chewing, and the taste, sight, smell, or even the thought of food. The latter type of stimulus causes what is known as *psychic secretion,* not only "watering of the mouth" but also secretion of gastric juice in preparation for receiving food. *Appetite* (a psychic factor) thus initiates the secretion of digestive juices. Appetite is influenced by one's state of mind, by companionship, and by the attractiveness of the table service and food, so that all these factors may have an influence on digestion. Fear, anger, worry, other strong emotions, and fatigue all produce undesirable effects on the secretion of gastric juice and on the muscular movements of the GI tract.

The strongest stimulus to the secretion of gastric juice results from the presence of food in the stomach; it is mediated by discharge of the vagus nerve and the formation and release of the hormone *gastrin* from the pyloric glands of the stomach. These agents stimulate the muscular activity of the stomach and the secretion of gastric acid. One of the signals to which the neuroendocrine controls respond is distention of the stomach with food or fluid, and some foods elicit a more copious secretion of gastric juice than others. Meats and meat extract (as in soups made from meat) and dilute alcoholic beverages are thought to have an especially stimulating effect.

The chief stimulus to the secretion of the pancreatic juice and bile comes from the hormones *secretin* and *cholecystokinin.* These are hormones formed in the duodenum in response to substances (acid and the partially digested proteins and fats) present in the chyme discharged from the stomach into the duodenum. Secretin stimulates the formation of pancreatic bicarbonate, the secretion of bile, and the gastric enzyme pepsin. Cholecystokinin stimulates the secretion of pancreatic enzymes, augments the action of secretin, and causes the emptying of stored bile from the gallbladder. The presence of fatty food residues and glucose in the small intestine leads to formation of another hormone, *gastric inhibitory peptide* (GIP, formerly enterogastrone), which, as the name implies, inhibits gastric acid production but also stimulates the production of the hormone insulin.

Some GI hormones also have trophic action; that is, they stimulate the growth of their target tissues. Gastrin stimulates growth of the gastric mucosa, and cholecystokinin stimulates growth of the exocrine pancreatic tissue. Secretin counteracts the trophic effect of gastrin but augments that of cholecystokinin. When GI hormone secretion is low, as in food deprivation or when patients are fed by vein rather than by mouth, there is thinning or deterioration of these tissues.

There are a number of other GI hormones whose specific roles are only partially known. Some have effects on food intake. (See Chap. 7.)

ABSORPTION

Absorption is the process by which the products of digestion pass through the lining of

Table 5–2 GASTROINTESTINAL ACTIONS OF GASTROINTESTINAL HORMONES

Hormone	*Stimulus*	*Principal Actions*
Gastrin	Distention of stomach, protein, esp. aromatic amino acids	Stimulates gastric acid and enzyme secretion, contraction of lower esophageal sphincter and stomach. Trophic to gastric mucosa.
Cholecystokinin pancreozymin (CCK-PZ)	Fat, protein and digestion products in intestine	Stimulates gall bladder contraction and pancreatic enzyme secretion. Inhibits gastric emptying. Trophic to pancreas.
Secretin	Low pH in duodenum	Stimulates pancreatic and biliary bicarbonate secretion and augments action of CCK on enzyme secretion; contraction of pyloric sphincter and gall bladder. Inhibits contraction of esophageal sphincter, stomach, and intestine. Stimulates insulin release, inhibits gastrin.
Gastric inhibitory polypeptide (GIP) "enterogastrone"	Standard meal, glucose, amino acids, fat	Inhibits gastric acid and enzyme secretion and motility and gastrin release. Stimulates intestinal secretion, release of insulin and glucagon.
Enteroglucagon	Glucose, fat in intestine	Inhibits gastric acid and enzyme and pancreatic enzyme secretion and contraction of stomach and intestine. Stimulates bile formation, secretion of insulin, and glycogenolysis.
Vasoactive intestinal polypeptide (VIP)	?	Inhibits gastric acid and enzyme secretion, motility and gastrin release. Stimulates pancreatic bicarbonate and water secretion, augments bile flow, stimulates intestinal secretion of water and salts. (Pronounced effects on blood pressure, etc.)
Motilin	?	Stimulates gastric and colonic motility.
Bombesin	?	Stimulates gastrin release, gastric acid secretion, contraction of gall bladder, release of CCK, motilin, VIP, pancreatic enzyme secretion. Inhibits intestinal motility. Stimulates release insulin, glucagon.
Somatostatin	?	Stimulates intestinal motility, inhibits gastric acid secretion. Inhibits release of insulin, glucagon. (Principal hypothalamic and metabolic role.)

the intestine into the blood and lymph. Simple sugars, amino acids, and short-chain fatty acids are absorbed directly into the blood stream, but the products of fat digestion pass chiefly into the lymph, which is collected through tiny lymph vessels and finally emptied into the blood.

The absorption of food material takes place almost entirely in the small intestine and is favored by the fact that the area of the inner surface of this part of the digestive tract is much increased by being formed into tiny projections, or *villi* (Fig. 5–3). Each of these villi contains numerous small blood vessels and a lymph space and is covered with still smaller units (microvilli). Both the blood and lymph are brought very close to the intestinal membrane, and the muscular contractions of the intestine serve to bring its contents into close contact with its wall and to squeeze blood and lymph into and out of the villi. Because chyme is emptied from the stomach gradually and the products of digestion are absorbed as they are formed, the intestine is not overwhelmed with a great surplus of food material to be absorbed at one time.

Anything that makes for either more intimate contact of the intestinal contents with the lining membrane or slower passage of food through the small intestine favors more complete absorption. Incomplete absorption may be the result of an irritated, highly motile intestine through which food passes too rapidly, of the formation of insoluble compounds in the intestine, or in the case of fat absorption, of lack of bile.

Water-soluble substances can be absorbed by the passive process of diffusion, but in most instances transport is carried out by active or facilitated processes. Active transport processes enable absorption of a large amount of nutrient in a much shorter time than would be possible by simple diffusion. In active transport, the absorbing cells perform metabolic work and require energy. Active transport mechanisms have been described for all essential and some nonessential amino acids, for most simple sugars (fructose is an exception), and for some micronutrients. For active transport of sugars and amino acids, sodium is required as well as oxygen, energy sources, and carrier substances within the cell.

Absorption of some nutrients (calcium, for example) depends on the presence of spe-

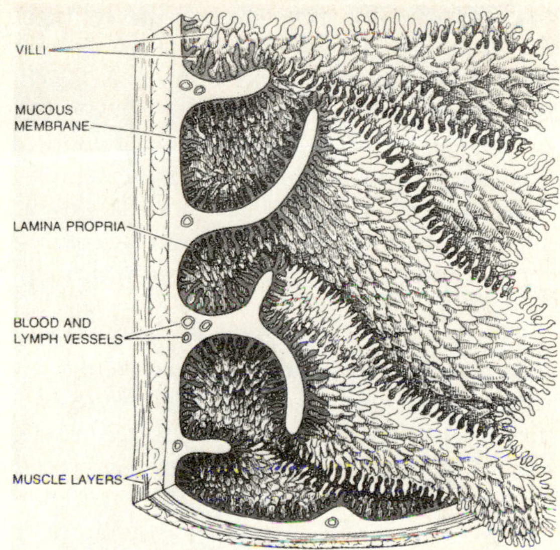

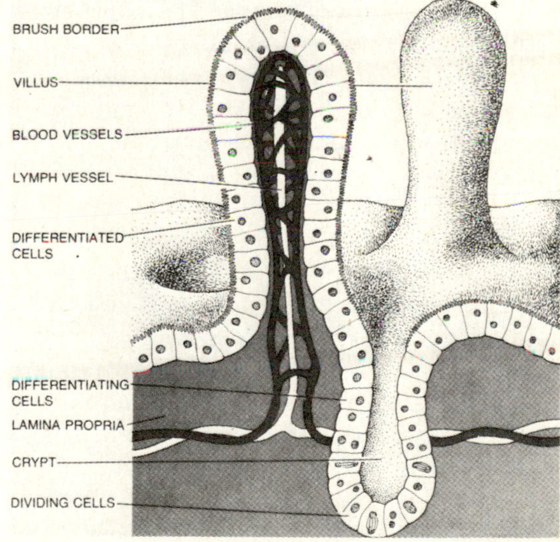

Figure 5–3 Wall of small intestine, seen in longitudinal section (*top*), has outer muscle layers, a submucosa layer, and an inner mucous membrane. The mucous membrane (*bottom*) has a connective-tissue layer (lamina propria), which contains blood and lymph capillaries, and an inner surface of epithelial cells. The cells multiply and differentiate in the crypts and migrate to the villi. At what stage the lactase is manufactured is not known; it is found primarily in the microvilli, which constitute the brush border of the differentiated cells. (From Kretchmer, W., "Lactose and Lactase." Scientific American 227(4):3, 1972. Copyright © 1972 by Scientific American, Inc. All rights reserved.)

cific carrier substances, usually proteins, in the intestinal wall. Absorption of vitamin B-12 is uniquely dependent on the stomach. In order for vitamin B-12 to be absorbed in the intestine, the vitamin must be bound to intrinsic factor, a specific glycoprotein secreted by cells in the stomach wall. A specific intestinal enzyme (a deconjugase) is required for absorption of most food forms of folacin. (See Chap. 11.)

Bile plays an essential role in enabling products of fat digestion and fat-soluble vitamins, which are insoluble in water, to pass through the membrane lining the intestine. Bile salts combine with monoacylglycerols formed during fat digestion to make compounds that are able to bind with both water and lipids, acting much in the same way as dishwashing detergents, which bind greasy food residues in dishwater. The short-chain fatty acids (10 carbon atoms or fewer) may pass directly into the blood, but those with larger molecules (chains of 16 and 18 or more carbon atoms) pass into the lymph. Fatty acids of intermediate size may enter either system. Rather than being transported in the blood as free fatty acids, however, most fatty acids are re-formed by the cells of the intestine into fats, which are then carried in loose combination with protein.

Normal amounts of mixed food fats are well digested and absorbed by healthy persons. In diseases with associated impairment of lipid digestion and absorption and in experimental studies, differences in the absorbability of various forms have been demonstrated. In general, short-chain fatty acids appear to be better absorbed than those of long-chain length, and unsaturated acids are absorbed better than saturated acids of the same length. Fatty acids may unite with calcium and magnesium ions to form insoluble compounds, resulting in failure to absorb both the mineral and the lipid. This is usually of little significance unless either the diet contains very large amounts of hard fat or absorption is impaired.

Absorption of both calcium and iron (and of some of the other minerals) is adversely affected when the diet includes large amounts of substances that form highly insoluble compounds with these metals. For example, iron and calcium form insoluble salts with phytic acid, which is found in whole-grain cereals; and calcium reacts with oxalic acid found in rhubarb, spinach, and beet tops to form the insoluble calcium oxalate (see Chap. 15). Normally, the diet does not contain enough of these interfering substances to impair nutrition, but these can assume importance if the diet provides only marginal amounts of the nutrients or if absorptive processes are impaired by disease.

Dietary factors can also influence absorption favorably. Iron is more readily absorbed in reduced (ferrous) state than when oxidized (ferric form). Thus, the presence in the diet of factors that promote reduction or prevent oxidation—such as vitamins C and E and antioxidants that are added to fats—favors absorption of iron. Calcium absorption requires an adequate supply of vitamin D.

Absorption is usually very efficient and complete; the energy nutrients (carbohydrates, fats, and proteins) are about 90 percent digested and absorbed in a mixed diet and under normal conditions. Absorption is less complete when the diet has a very high content of coarse cereal grains, legumes, and other vegetable matter.

EXCRETION THROUGH THE INTESTINE

The intestinal waste, feces, consists of the following:

1. indigestible, undigested, and unabsorbed food residues
2. residues from digestive secretions, mucus, and cell debris from the lining of the alimentary tract
3. small amounts of material secreted into the digestive tract

4. bacteria and the products of their action
5. water

The bulk of the feces is made up of water and food and digestive residues. The factor that most affects the volume of feces passed by normal persons is the amount of water retained in the feces. Indigestible substances consumed (chiefly cellulose and other complex carbohydrates) and the growth of intestinal bacteria contribute to fecal dry matter. A combination of these influences accounts for the increased bulk of feces formed when the diet contains large quantities of vegetables and fruits, unrefined cereals, and milk, in contrast to large amounts of meat and refined cereals.

When the diet has large amounts of animal products and refined cereals, fecal weight is about 100 to 150 gm per day; with coarse diets, fecal weight may be as much as 300 to 400 gm per day. In either instance the fecal matter is about 60 to 80 percent water. This reflects the remarkable ability of the intestine to reabsorb water, considering that the daily fluid intake is of the order of 1500 to 2000 ml and that the digestive fluids add up to some 7 liters a day. The water content is higher when the fecal material is hurried through the alimentary tract and lower when its excretion is long delayed, owing to further absorption of water in the colon.

Some mineral salts (notably salts of calcium and phosphorus) are excreted through the intestinal wall into the lower digestive tract; the main pathway for excretion of excess or unutilized calcium and iron is by way of the intestine. Some of the substances present in bile (for example, bile salts) are partially reabsorbed and recirculated in the bile; others are degraded in the intestine and excreted in the feces or reabsorbed and excreted in the urine. The pigment that gives the feces their brown color is formed from the bile pigment, which in turn comes from hemoglobin. Bile is the major excretory route for cholesterol and is used as a disposal system for some heavy metals and drugs.

About one-tenth to one-third of the feces consists of bacteria (both living and dead), and the number excreted per day has been estimated to vary between 50 and 500 billion. The presence of bacteria in the intestinal contents is entirely normal, and some of them may even be beneficial in that they synthesize certain vitamins. (See Chap. 9 and 11.)

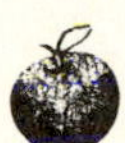

health considerations

The chief factors that affect digestion act either by affecting the motor functions of the digestive organs, by exerting an influence on the flow of the digestive juices, or by altering the health of the digestive tract itself.

Psychological Factors

Fear, worry, anger, irritation, and stress all exert unfavorable influences on secretion and motility. Prolonged tension or stress is common in the life experiences of people who develop peptic ulcers. In these people, emotionality is accompanied by increased acid secretion and gastric blood flow. Others react to fear or sadness with decreased acid production and blood flow. Peace and quiet, cheerful companionship, appetizing food, and attractive surroundings all favor good digestion.

Nutritive Factors

Because the lining of the digestive tract is continuously and rapidly being renewed, and because secretions and enzymes are formed constantly and in large volume, the digestive system is particularly susceptible to the effects of poor nutrition. Lack of thiamin is especially likely to be associated with lack of appetite, and diarrhea is one of the typical symptoms of pellagra, a niacin-deficiency disease. Iron deficiency and failure to secrete gastric acid occur together. Protein is needed for formation of digestive enzymes and intestinal cells, as are other vitamins and minerals. Deficiencies of protein and of the B vitamin folacin often result in failure of absorption. Through these effects on the digestive system, deficiency of one nutrient can impair the utilization of virtually all other nutrients.

Food Factors

The healthy GI tract can digest any ordinary food or combination of foods without trouble. A few people are unquestionably sensitive to certain foods and are made ill by them, but food allergy is not very common and needs to be confirmed by the tests of a physician. The reason many people experience digestive distress when they eat foods or combinations of foods that they believe will give them trouble is that the apprehension of "indigestion" is sufficient in itself to alter gastrointestinal motility and blood flow.

Some types of food are digested more slowly than others, and such foods are often spoken of as being "hard to digest." In general, liquids and finely divided foods are those most rapidly handled by the digestive tract. Fats and foods rich in fats (especially mixtures of proteins with fats), foods that are introduced into the stomach in large pieces (and especially in chunks coated with fat), and protein-rich foods that have been made tough in texture by overcooking are digested more slowly but not less completely than other foods.

The influence of cooking operates more through making the food palatable and appetizing than through any effect on the nutritive properties or digestibility of the food. Most raw foods are easily digested, but starchy foods (especially potatoes) and those that contain tough fiber need thorough cooking in order to rupture the starch granules and to soften the fiber so that the digestive juices can penetrate them. There is seldom more than 5 percent difference between the extent to which raw or poorly cooked foods are ultimately digested and absorbed, and the degree of utilization of the same foods when properly cooked.

Incomplete digestion results in the formation of gases (through bacterial action on food residues in the intestine), which may cause pain and distention. (Nervous swallowing of air, chewing gum, and smoking may also cause gaseousness of nondietary origin.) Some foods, such as legumes, have carbohydrates that are not digested by human enzymes but that are used by bacteria, with formation of gas (chiefly CO_2 and H_2, and sometimes methane, CH_4) and other end products. The intestinal bacteria will attack almost any foodstuff that is not absorbed in the small intestine, so gas formation (and, in severe cases, cramping pain and diarrhea) always accompany malabsorption.

Raw legumes contain a number of antinutritional substances, including some that inhibit digestive enzymes. An enterprising firm has marketed a bean antiamylase (referred to as a "starch blocker") as a weight-control agent. It claims that taking this preparation with meals prevents starch digestion and leads to avoidance of a significant amount of food energy. While a starch blocker sounds like a painless way to diet, evidence casts doubt on its efficacy. As has been noted, even small amounts of undigested carbohydrate lead to bloating and flatulence, so if the treatment worked there would be socially unacceptable side effects. In fact, symptoms of carbohydrate malabsorption were encountered in earlier medical trials with another enzyme inhibitor (acarbose, an α-glucoside hydrolase inhibitor that blocks both starch and sugar digestion) intended for treatment of diabetics. How much of the substrate remains undigested is unknown, but the evidence indicates that digestion is at least slowed with acarbose treatment and that some carbohydrate reaches the colon. Studies with rats fed raw beans show, however, that the pancreas responds to the presence of antienzymes by secreting more digestive enzymes, so digestion proceeds fairly well. Ultimately the rats' health and growth are impaired by consumption of large amounts of raw beans. At the present time there is no evidence on this point in humans.

In recent years it has been discovered that many adults and some youngsters have little or no lactase enzyme in the intestine and experience flatulence and softening of stools when they drink large amounts of milk or other products containing the milk sugar, lactose. The incidence of this lactase deficiency is higher in American Indian, Asiatic, Mediterranean, and African populations than in Caucasians of northern European extraction. The incidence increases with age and also occurs temporarily or permanently as a result of severe protein malnutrition and of diseases that damage the intestine. People who have this problem can eat cheese without any distress, proving conclusively that sugar absorption is at fault. Almost all preschool children of any stock have adequate intestinal lactase, and most children and young adults can tolerate milk and milk products in amounts normally consumed, even with reduced enzyme levels. Some traditional dairy foods whose preparation involves microbial treatment (yogurt and kefir, for example) have reduced lactose content (Table 5–3). Milk can also be processed with commercial enzymes (usually from yeast or mold) that split the lactose into glucose and galactose, thereby eliminating lactose and increasing sweetness as a side effect. Simply swallowing lactase enzyme with milk has not proved very effective, as would be expected if the enzyme (a protein) were not protected from peptic digestion or resistant to it.

Table 5–3 LACTOSE CONTENT OF DAIRY FOODS[a]

Food	*gm/cup*
Regular milk	12
Buttermilk	9
Yogurt, traditional (no added milk solids)	6
Yogurt, commercial, low-fat	12
Kefir	8
Acidophilus milk	6
Ice cream (150 gm/cup)	17

[a]Values except US yogurt and ice cream from Alm, L., J. Dairy Sci. (65:346, 1982).

Some foods stimulate intestinal motility in the same way laxative drugs do. Prune juice is especially effective in this respect. Similar but less potent effects are produced by acid fruit juices and cooked pulp of dried fruits. Little information is available concerning the active factors in these foods. Mineral oil softens the feces and is often used as a mild laxative, but its regular use is to be avoided because fat-soluble nutrients are also soluble in mineral oil and are excreted along with this nonabsorbable substance.

Frequency. Stimuli produced by feces in the rectum result in the desire and ability to defecate. Psychic influences, such as hurry and overanxiety to have a movement daily, have the effect of inhibiting these stimuli and preventing the normal reflex, which causes the colon to contract and expel its contents. Thus, a good many people either have, or think they have, trouble in producing bowel movements with sufficient frequency or regularity. This problem may persist at intervals throughout life, and it is perhaps especially frequent among elderly people. Constipation can usually be corrected by establishing a regular time for going to the toilet, preferably shortly after breakfast; drinking one or two glasses of water half an hour before breakfast; and increasing consumption of prunes, figs, unrefined cereals, fibrous vegetables, fruits, and milk, as well as taking some brisk physical activity. (For discussion of fiber, see Chap. 2.)

Diarrhea is another commonly encountered symptom that may be due to many causes: irritant substances or toxins in food, infectious disease, allergy, and so on. Mild, transient cases of diarrhea usually respond favorably to severe restriction of dietary fat, fruits, and vegetables, and to increased consumption of tea in preference to coffee. The loss of fluids and minerals is potentially *very* dangerous, particularly in infants and children. Dehydration and finally death result from severe diarrhea, owing to the loss of water, sodium, and potassium. Many victims can be saved by oral administration of a simple solution of the following composition as recommended by the World Health Organization (WHO) and the United Nations International Children's Emergency Fund (UNICEF):

sodium chloride (table salt)	3.5 gm
sodium bicarbonate (baking soda)	2.5 gm
potassium chloride	1.5 gm
glucose (or honey)	20.0 gm
boiled water to make a total of	1000.0 gm

A simple formula suitable for emergency conditions contains 1 teaspoon salt, 8 teaspoons sugar, 1 liter boiled water.

A child should receive about 1 tsp (5 ml) per minute.

If possible, a physician should be consulted if the condition persists beyond a few hours in infants and more than a few days in adults, or if there are accompanying symptoms such as fever or vomiting.

QUESTIONS

1. What is digestion? Why is it necessary? Describe the GI tract and show how it is especially adapted for carrying out the process of digestion.

2. What are the end products of digestion of proteins, starch, table sugar, and fats? Name the principal digestive fluids that bring about the chemical breakdown of these foodstuffs into their simplest components. Tell where each of these digestive fluids is formed, and give the main functions of each.

3. Chemical changes involved in digestion are brought about or facilitated by the presence of enzymes in the digestive fluids. What is an enzyme? What is meant by saying that enzymes are specific in their action? Name the different enzymes (and substances on which they act) in gastric juice and in pancreatic juice and those formed in the intestinal mucosa. What is the chemical nature of enzymes? What are the optimum conditions for activity of the enzymes in saliva, in gastric juice, and in the digestive fluids in the intestine?

4. What are the chief factors that stimulate or inhibit the secretion of saliva and gastric juice? Explain the action of hormones in stimulating the flow of the digestive fluids that act on food in the small intestine. What happens to food residues in the large intestine or colon?

5. Describe how absorption of amino acids, simple sugars, and end products of fat digestion takes place in the intestine. What substances taken in food can be absorbed without being chemically changed in digestion? Explain how bile helps in the digestion and absorption of fats. What substances are found in the residues at the end of the digestive tract—the feces—and what factors alter the consistency and composition of the feces?

6. Discuss the effects that nervous factors, general nutritive condition of the individual, and different types of food eaten have on gastric secretion and emptying time; upon the completeness of digestion.

7. What are the main constituents of the feces? Which of these may be described as residues from the contents of the digestive tract? What waste products of metabolism are excreted through the intestine?

6 Energy I: Basics

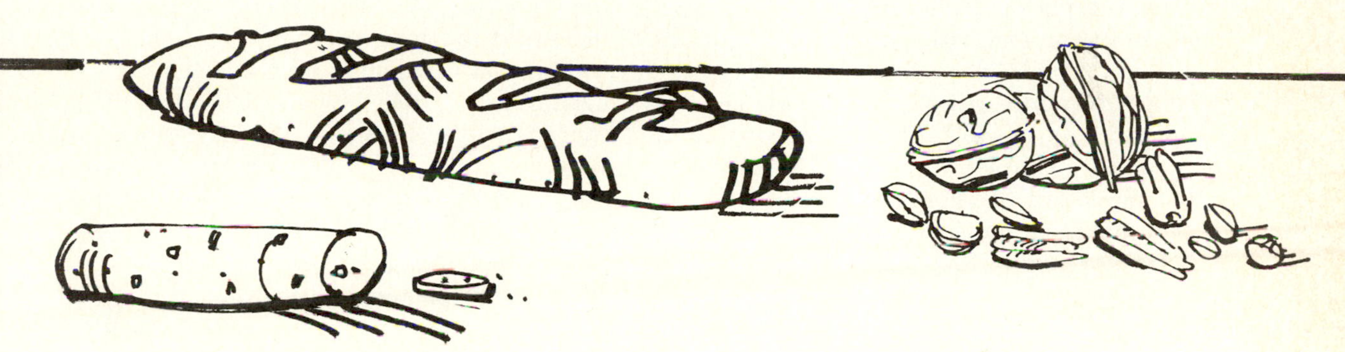

Energy is defined as the power to do work. Energy exists in many different forms, all of which are interconvertible. Heat, light, sound, and electricity are familiar forms of energy; the fact that electricity is converted to heat and light in a lamp and to mechanical action and sound in an alarm clock is evidence of its interconvertibility. Energy also is stored in chemical forms, as in an automobile battery. Whenever change takes place in a system, energy must be transferred from one part of the system to another to effect the change, but the total amount of energy in the system remains the same. Only its form may be different. It may seem difficult to believe that energy is not simply "used up" in, for instance, riding a bicycle. But if the bicycle wheel is fitted to an electrical generator, it can easily be proved that energy remains and can be used to light a lamp or charge a battery. The fact that energy is neither created nor destroyed during any chemical or physical process is one of the most fundamental tenets of science, the *law of the conservation of energy*.

The body needs energy because it has indispensable work to perform. Internal work is carried out to maintain life processes, even during sleep, in the uncounted numbers of chemical and physical activities of the cells and organs. Muscular work is required for a person to sit and stand erect and to move the body or objects. Energy is also needed to form new tissues during growth and pregnancy or after an injury, to produce milk, and sometimes to heat the body.

METABOLISM AND ENERGY

Metabolism is all the chemical changes that occur in living things in the course of their vital activities.

Metabolic Change

The changes that constitute metabolism are of two kinds—anabolic and catabolic. *Anabolism* includes all chemical changes by which the absorbed products of digestion are used to replace substances broken down during life processes and to build new tissues in growth. *Catabolism* refers to processes by which nutrients, reserve tissue material, and cellular substances are broken down into chemically simpler compounds resulting in the liberation of energy. In catabolism, energy-yielding nutrient and tissue components are oxidized by a series of biochemical reactions, ultimately yielding carbon dioxide, water, some nitrogen compounds (from protein catabolism), and energy (Fig. 6–1). Part of the energy released by catabolism is used as the source of energy for anabolism, and the remainder is used to accomplish the chemical and physical work of the organism. Heat, used to maintain body temperature, is the final product of this energy expenditure, but it is the adenosine triphosphate (ATP) formed during oxidation of nutrients that sustains life processes.

Measurement of Energy

This linkage of heat production, oxygen utilization, and carbon dioxide formation forms the basis for the two principal methods used to measure human expenditure of energy—direct and indirect calorimetry. *Direct calorimetry* measures the amount of heat given off as a by-product of energy metabolism. This method was elucidated in 1761 by the Scottish physician Joseph Black, who measured the heat resulting from chemical combustion by melting ice under controlled conditions. During the period 1782 to 1784, the French scientists A. L. Lavoisier and P. S. de Laplace used this principle to demonstrate that animal metabolism is a kind of combustion in which heat is given off, oxygen is used, and carbon dioxide is produced. With much further refinement, the exact relationships of oxygen usage and heat production were quantified, enabling measurement of energy metabolism indirectly from oxygen utilization, that is, by *indirect calorimetry*.

Proof of these relationships in humans was quite a feat. Such experiments had actually been undertaken by Lavoisier, but his re-

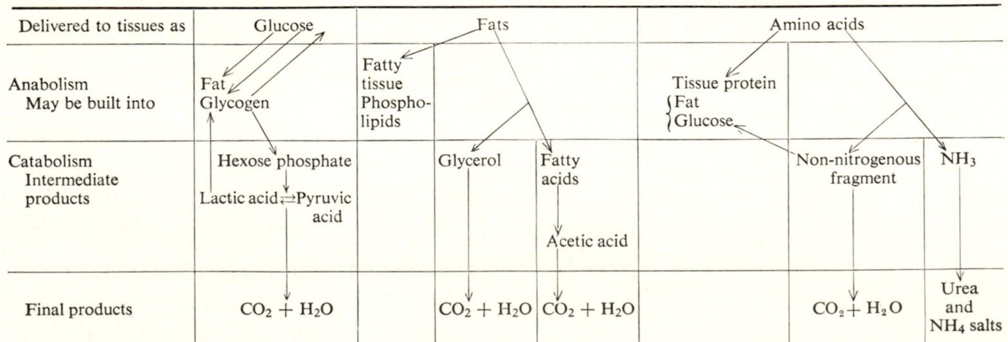

Figure 6–1 A simplified summary of metabolism of the three energy nutrients. This diagram shows graphically that the final products of oxidation of all three are the same—*carbon dioxide and water*—with the exception of those substances derived from the amino groups of proteins.

search was cut short when he was sent to the guillotine by the French Revolutionary tribunal. More than a century passed before Atwater, Benedict, and Rosa constructed the first human respiration calorimeter, at Wesleyan University in Connecticut. This device, a few of which are still in use, is called a respiration calorimeter because it can measure not only the respiratory exchange (amounts of oxygen used and carbon dioxide produced) but also the amount of heat given off by the human subject.

The calorimeter portion of the apparatus consists primarily of a chamber large enough to hold a person comfortably, encased and insulated to prevent any loss of heat through the walls. The heat generated by the subject is carried away by circulating water, so that the inner temperature is maintained constant. The heat that is transferred to the water and the heat required to vaporize water in the subject's breath (and perspiration) together represent the total heat production of the body in a given time (direct calorimetry). At the same time, by devices included in the closed circuit of air which the subject breathes, the quantities of oxygen consumed and carbon dioxide given out are measured. From these values, the amount of energy that would have been set free by oxidations within the body can be calculated (indirect calorimetry). Values obtained by the two methods differ by only a fraction of 1 percent.

Today, human energy expenditure usually is measured by means of any of several devices (Figs. 6–2 and 6–3) that collect part or all of the air exhaled by a subject during a given time period. By determining the volume of air breathed and the amount of oxygen and carbon dioxide present in the inhaled and exhaled air, the amount of oxygen used and carbon dioxide produced can be computed and, from these values, the amount of energy expended and the nature of the fuels burned.

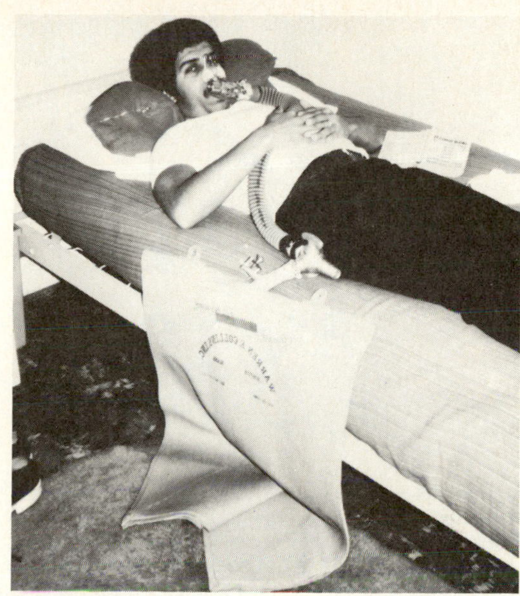

Figure 6–2 Measurement of basal metabolism using a Douglas bag for the collection of expired air. The nasal passages are occluded by a clamp; the subject breathes in room air through a one-way valve while exhaled air passes into the collection bag. Exhaled air is collected within an exact time period, and the volume collected is measured by evacuating the bag through a gas flowmeter. The oxygen and carbon dioxide concentrations in the expired air are measured, and as the composition of the room air is known, the amount of oxygen used and carbon dioxide produced per unit of time can be determined. By using tables previously developed from direct calorimetry, the energy equivalent of the gases exchanged can be calculated. (Courtesy of D. Armstrong, the University of California, Berkeley.)

The energy value assigned to the oxygen utilized differs according to the material being oxidized. If carbohydrate is being metabolized, one molecule of carbon dioxide is formed for every molecule of oxygen used, according to the following equation for glucose:

$$C_6H_{12}O_6 + 6\ O_2 \rightarrow 6\ CO_2 + 6\ H_2O$$

The ratio of carbon dioxide produced to oxygen used is the *respiratory quotient,* which is abbreviated to RQ. In the glucose example, $6\ CO_2/6\ O_2$ equals an RQ of 1.0. For complete metabolism of fat, the RQ is about 0.7, as illustrated for stearic acid:

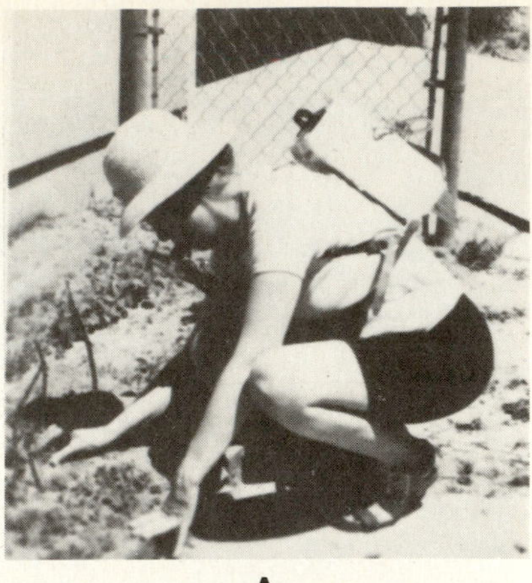

A

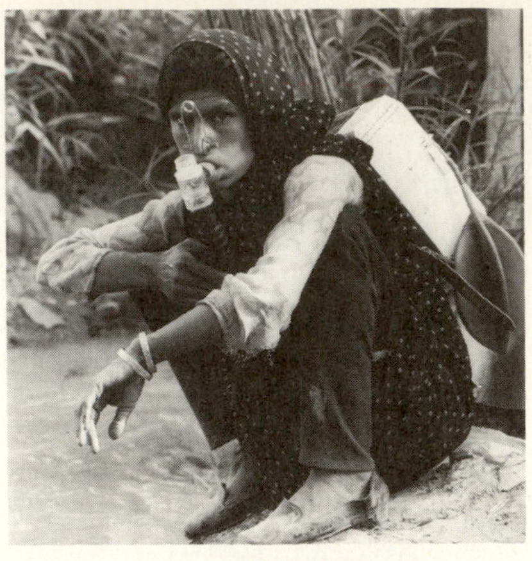

B

Figure 6–3 Energy cost of activities being measured in the United States (A) and in Iran (B) by use of a portable respiration apparatus. The Kofranyi-Michaelis apparatus consists of a lightweight box, which contains a meter that records the volume of expired air. Samples of the expired air are automatically taken at intervals and stored in a small bag attached to the meter. Analysis of the gas in this bag for carbon dioxide and oxygen content gives the necessary data for calculating energy expenditure. (A, courtesy of D. H. Calloway; B, courtesy of C. Geissler-Brun and T. Brun, University of California, Berkeley.)

$$C_{18}H_{36}O_2 + 26\ O_2 \rightarrow 18\ CO_2 + 18\ H_2O$$

and 18 CO_2/26 O_2 equals 0.7. When protein is oxidized, RQ is about 0.8. The energy values of a liter of oxygen at RQs of 1.0, 0.8, and 0.7 are 5.0, 4.8, and 4.7 kcal per liter, respectively. The figure of 4.8 kcal (20 kJ) per liter is a good approximation when, as is usual, a mixture of carbohydrate, fat, and protein is being used.

BASAL METABOLISM

In a living organism, cells must be continually active to maintain life processes. Energy is necessary to maintain these vital processes. The nervous system never stops working, and the activity of the brain alone accounts for about one-fifth of the energy expended by the body at rest. The liver and kidneys constantly work at a high rate. Other activities go on at a somewhat lower rate during rest—for example, the beating of the heart, the work of the lungs and of the chest and diaphragm in breathing, the peristaltic movements of the stomach and intestines, and the work of digestive glands in forming their secretions. Even when a person is completely in repose, the tone of the skeletal muscles is maintained.

This internal work of the body is known as *basal* metabolism because upon it are superimposed the other energy needs of the body—the amount of energy needed for food intake and muscular work and at times for adjustment to climate and for the formation of new tissues. *Basal metabolism,* or metabolism at rest, is defined as the amount of energy expended by a person when lying quietly in a comfortable environmental temperature, relaxed but awake and without food (twelve to fifteen hours after the last meal). Energy expenditure measured under the same conditions but at different intervals after eating is *resting* metabolism. Basal metabolism of adults amounts to about 1200 to 1800 kcal (5000 to 7500 kJ) per day. The basal energy need is comparatively constant for the same individual but varies slightly at different times and more widely between different persons.

Factors That Influence Basal Metabolism

The main factors that determine the basal metabolic energy requirement are the following:

1. body size
2. age
3. sex
4. secretions of endocrine glands, especially the thyroid

The *basal metabolic rate* (BMR) is higher in young people than in older individuals; it increases for some months after birth, then decreases (at first fairly rapidly, but later more gradually) up to and through adolescence. In adults, there is a still slower decline in BMR with increasing age. Metabolic rate is higher in males than in females.

Basal metabolic expenditure varies as a function of body size, but not precisely with weight. When expressed as energy per square meter of body surface area[1] (or per kilogram of body weight raised to the three-fourths power[2]), basal metabolic rate of warm-blooded animals ranging in size from mice to elephants is nearly the same. Why these relationships exist is not certain. The close correlation between internal work and surface area, or the three-fourths power of body weight, may be due to a mathematical relationship these measurements have to the active cellular mass of the body. Basal metabolism reflects the activity of all body functions carried on in the resting state (including maintenance of body temperature), and these functions reside in the soft, lean tissues.[3]

Attempts have been made to explain the differences in BMR between people as being due entirely to differences in the amount of lean body mass. This concept has a certain plausibility when one considers that men have more lean body mass in proportion to fat than do women of the same age, and men have higher BMR than do women. (See Fig. 6–4.) Also, the percentage of body fat rises with age in both sexes, and metabolic rate declines with age. However, while total basal energy expenditure does increase with increasing lean body mass, the increase is not linear, because the body tissues do not increase in size proportionately. (See Table 6–1.) In the adult, skeletal muscle is the largest component of the nonbone lean mass, and muscle has a relatively low resting rate of metabolism; the brain, a very active tissue, increases little in weight from infancy to adulthood. Other tissues, such as the liver and kidneys, increase less in size than does the muscle mass during the growth years and constitute about the same percentage of body weight in muscularly well-developed adults as in those who are less fit. Even adipose tissue is not inert metabolically; it has about the same rate of oxidation per unit of protein as does kidney tissue. Of course, adipose tissue, when filled with fat, has only one-third to one-fourth as much protein as does kidney tissue; but fatty tissue may make up about half of the body weight in many adults, so its total contribution to the BMR is not inconsiderable.

For purposes of nutritional planning it is sufficient to remember that the total basal

[1]Because of the difficulty of actually measuring the body surface area, it is usually computed for man from the body weight and height by means of a mathematical equation. Body surface area (m^2) = Weight $(kg)^{0.425} \times$ Height $(cm)^{0.725} \times 0.007184$ or from a nomogram constructed from DuBois' chart by Boothby and Sandiford (Fig. 6–5).

[2]This weight, often called metabolic body weight, is determined by multiplying the log of body weight by 0.75 and converting to the antilog. Other estimates of the metabolic size may be computed from body weight according to formulas of Brody in *Bioenergetics and Growth* (New York: Reinhold, 1945) or Kleiber in *The Fire of Life* (New York: John Wiley & Sons, 1961).

[3]A specialized brown adipose tissue functions as a source of body heat to maintain body temperature in some animals and human infants. (See later in this chapter.)

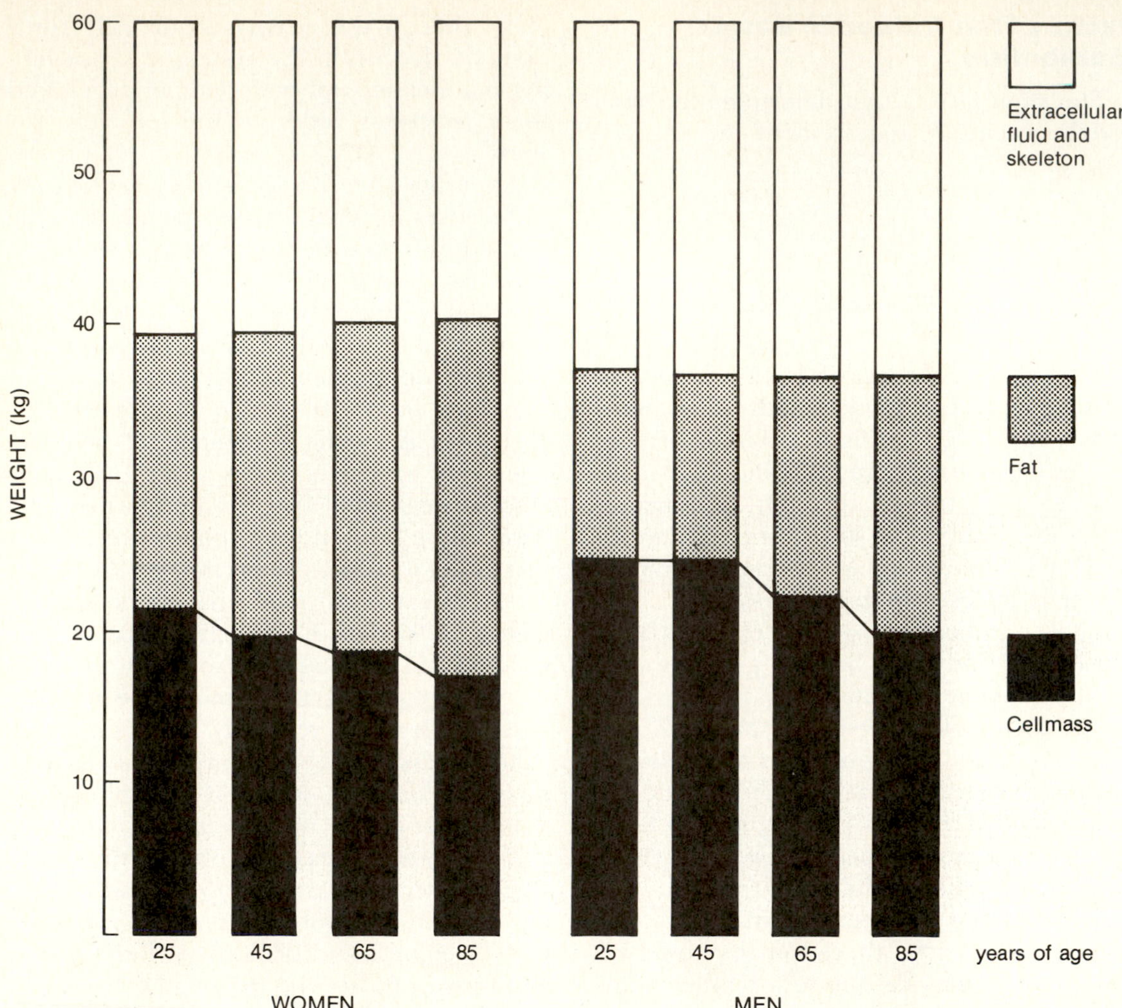

Figure 6–4 Typical body composition of 60 kg women and men aged 25 to 85 years. Even if body weight is kept constant throughout adult life, lean tissue decreases and fat increases with advancing age. Men have a greater proportion of lean tissue and less fat than women of the same age. Body composition can be estimated by a number of indirect methods that rely on constant relationships of water and potassium to body cells and tissues, or by determining body density (fat being lighter than lean tissues), or by width of skin-folds. (See Chap. 7.) (The values shown here were obtained from whole body potassium data, reported by Moore, F. D., et al., *The Body Cell Mass and Its Supporting Environment.* W. B. Saunders Co., Philadelphia, 1963.)

energy requirement is greater in persons of larger size than in smaller persons of the same age and sex; and that the *rate* of basal metabolism is higher in men than in women and decreases with age. Basal metabolism of healthy men requires about 1600 to 1800 kcal (6500 to 7500 kJ) daily; basal expenditure of women is about 1200 to 1450 kcal (5000 to 6000 kJ) (Fig. 6–5).

Role of the Thyroid Hormones

The secretions of the *endocrine glands* are the primary regulators of the rate of metabolism of the cells. The overall rate of cellular

Table 6–1 PERCENTAGE OF BASAL METABOLIC RATE (BMR) DUE TO FIVE MAJOR ORGANS AND THE REST OF THE BODY IN AN INFANT WHOSE BMR IS 540 KCAL PER DAY AND AN ADULT WHOSE BMR IS 1780 KCAL PER DAY*

	10 kg (22 lb) Infant			*70 kg (154 lb) man*		
	Organ Weight	*Organ Metabolism*		*Organ Weight*	*Organ Metabolism*	
Organ	(KG)	KCAL/DAY	% OF BMR	(KG)	KCAL/DAY	% OF BMR
Brain	0.92	240	45	1.4	365	21
Heart	0.05	30	6	0.3	180	10
Kidney	0.07	28	5	0.3	120	7
Liver	0.30	105	19	1.6	560	32
Lung	0.12	24	4	0.8	160	9
Total of above	1.46	427	79	4.4	1385	79
All other	8.64	113	21	65.6	395	21

* In the infant the organs constitute 15 percent of body weight and account for 79 percent of BMR. These organs still account for 79 percent of BMR in an adult of normal weight and leanness but make up only 6 percent of body weight. Thus, BMR does not increase linearly with lean body mass or with total body weight. (Adapted from Holliday, M. et al. The relation of metabolic rate to body weight and organ size. Pediat. Res., 1:185, 1967.

oxidation is under the control of the thyroid gland. The iodine-containing hormones thyroxine (T_4) and triiodothyronine (T_3) affect the metabolism of virtually all the tissues of the body. Essential for normal rates of protein synthesis and most other metabolic processes, they increase the rates of reactions such that the rate of energy utilization is increased. As little as a single milligram of thyroxine raises basal metabolism 3 percent above normal. Apparently only about one-third of a milligram needs to be released daily from storage in the thyroid into the blood to keep basal metabolism at a normal level. The specific sites of action of these hormones have not been fully elucidated at this time.

The regulation of thyroid hormone synthesis is complex. The pituitary gland synthesizes a protein, thyroid-stimulating hormone (TSH, or thyrotropin), which is responsible for stimulating the thyroid gland to synthesize and release thyroid hormones. In addition, the hypothalamus in the brain secretes a peptide, thyrotropin-releasing hormone, which has some regulatory effects on the pituitary TSH production. This system is then subject to *feedback inhibition* by thyroid hormones.[4] (See Fig. 6–6.)

Hypothyroidism, or underactivity of the thyroid, results in a condition known as *myxedema,* which is characterized by puffiness of the hands and face, low basal metabolism, dulling of mental activity, sluggishness of body processes, and a tendency to put on weight. However, the commonly held belief that underactivity of the thyroid gland leads to fatness is erroneous. The greater proportion of weight gained when the thyroid is underactive results from water held because of faulty protein structure in the tissues. Animals in which the thyroid gland is removed actually have a lower percentage of body fat than do normal animals. Basal metabolism can be restored to normal by giving thyroxine, which also improves the other symptoms.

Hyperthyroidism, or overactivity of the thy-

[4]The process, a very important one in biological systems, whereby the responder component creates a substance or change in conditions (in this example, heat) that turns off the response, is called negative feedback or feedback inhibition.

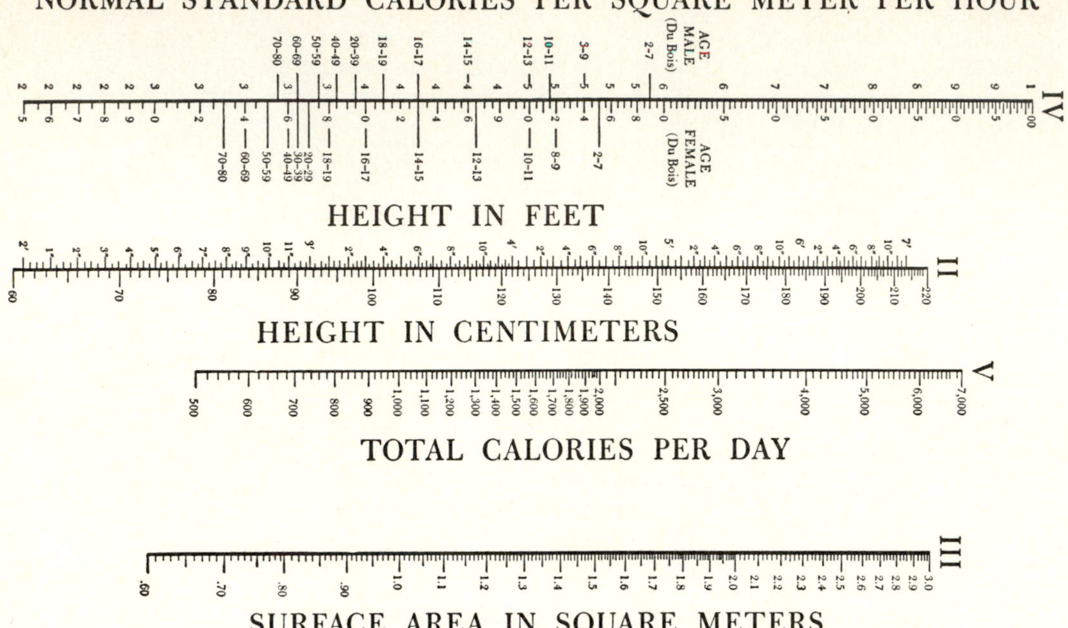

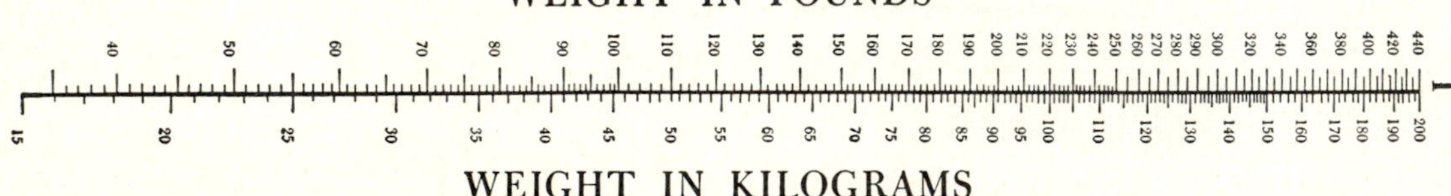

Figure 6–5 This nomogram can be used to derive the basal metabolic expenditure (Scale V, labeled "Total Calories per Day") of normal adults whose height and weight are known. Use only a ruler with a true straight edge. Do not draw lines on the chart but merely indicate their positions by the straight edge of the ruler. Locate the various points by means of needles (pin stuck through the eraser of a lead pencil). Locate the person's normal weight on Scale I and his height on Scale II. The ruler joining these two points intersects Scale III at the person's surface area. Locate the age and sex of the person on Scale IV. A ruler joining this point with the person's surface area on Scale III crosses Scale V at the basal energy requirement. To convert Calories (kcal) to kJ, multiply by 4.184. (Nomogram of Boothby and Sandiford, adapted by the Mayo Clinic and reprinted with their permission.)

roid with excessive secretion of thyroxine, is evidenced by an abnormally high rate of basal metabolism, emaciation, rapid heartbeat, nervousness, and frequently by protruding eyes. The energy need may be increased to two or three times normal, causing loss of weight in spite of increased consumption of food. The overactive gland usually becomes enlarged, and such a condition is known as toxic or exophthalmic goiter (the latter name because of the eye involvement).

Simple goiter is a nutritional disease, brought about by an insufficient supply of iodine, and is discussed in Chapter 16. The gland enlarges because the pituitary continues to form TSH owing to inadequate feedback inhibition in the absence of sufficient

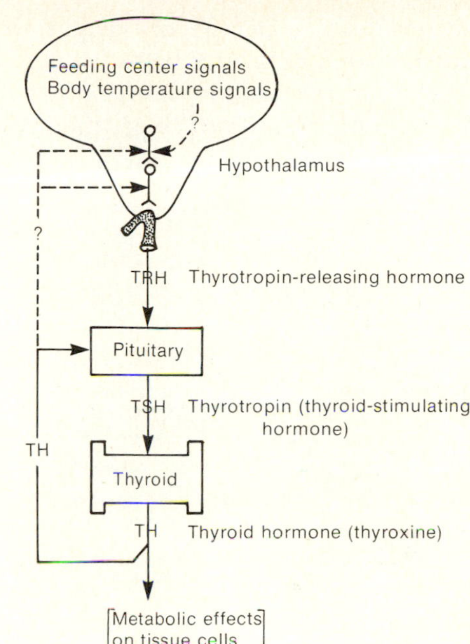

Figure 6–6 Hypothalamic-pituitary-thyroid system for the control of thyroid hormone secretion. Pituitary formation of thyroid-stimulating hormone (TSH) is controlled by two opposing factors: (1) inhibition by the thyroid hormone thyroxine (classical negative feedback) and (2) release by thyrotropin-releasing hormone (TRH). Secretion of TRH is controlled by nerve cells; it has been suggested that formation of TRH may be responsive to the presence of thyroxine or to signals from others centers in the hypothalamus that relate to feeding drive and body temperature regulations, or to both factors. (See Chapter 7.) (Adapted from Reichlin, S., et al.: Recent Progr. Horm. Res. *28*:229, 1972.)

thyroid hormone. Basal metabolism may or may not be affected, depending on how severe the deficiency is, but the symptoms of excessive thyroxine seen in toxic goiter are absent.

Role of Other Hormones

The hormone epinephrine (adrenalin) produced by the adrenal glands also exerts an influence on basal metabolism, although not so markedly as does the thyroid hormone. Stimulation of the adrenal glands (such as happens in fright, excitement, and other emotions) causes a temporary rise in the metabolic rate. It has been shown that cats have a fall of about 25 percent in basal metabolism after an operation to remove these glands.

The sex difference in metabolism is brought about by the activity of the male and female hormones. The difference in BMR is due partly to the effect these hormones have on body composition, since women have more fatty tissues than do men, and partly to their effects on cell metabolism. BMR varies with menstrual cycle, rising just before or at the time of ovulation, reaching a peak with the onset of the menses, and then falling sharply. During pregnancy the BMR increases about 20 percent; this increase is roughly proportional to the increase in body weight of the healthy pregnant woman.

Influence of Other Factors

Several factors may affect the metabolism of a person at rest and, thus, the accuracy of determination of basal metabolic rate, which is why the standardized conditions of measurement include the stipulation that the subject must be awake, but physically and mentally relaxed, in a post-absorptive state (twelve to fifteen hours after eating), in a comfortable environment, and free from fever.

Sleep. Individual sleep patterns vary. Some people rest quietly for about an hour and are restless for the remainder of the night, while others rest completely all night. It is not surprising, then, that energy expenditures during a period of sleep may be about the same as in the basal (resting quietly but awake) state, or more or less than that. During the hours of sleep, the internal processes gradually slow down, and may reach a minimum that is 10 percent below basal rate after about five to six hours (Fig. 6–7). During an 8 hour period of sleep, most adults expend about 400 to 600 kcal (1600 to 2500 kJ).

Muscle Tone. Most people do not realize that the muscles are never completely relaxed, but that a certain amount of tension (muscular tone) is maintained even in sleep. The amount of energy required for muscular tension varies with the degree of tenseness or relaxation of the individual; it is significant because the total amount of muscle tissue is so great. People are most relaxed on first waking, and muscular tension increases

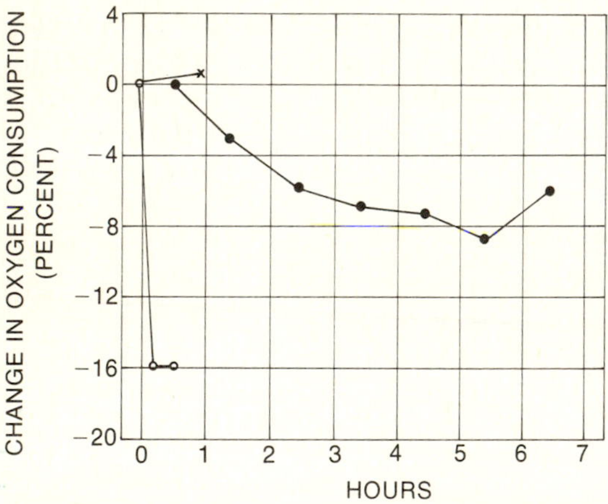

Figure 6–7 Comparison of metabolic rates, measured by consumption of oxygen, that occur during hypnosis, sleep, and meditation. No significant change occurs during hypnosis (which is therefore not represented on the graph). One study shows that oxygen consumption is reduced by about 8 percent after 5 hours of sleep. Meditation causes twice the reduction in a fraction of the time. The "x" represents hypnosis, the solid circles indicate sleep, and the open circles signify meditation. (Redrawn from Wallace, R. D., and Benson, H.: The physiology of meditation. Copyright © 1972 by Scientific American, Inc. All rights reserved.)

as the day advances. For this reason, it is best to determine BMR early in the morning.

Emotions and Mental States. Stimulation of the sympathetic nervous system and the adrenal glands, such as takes place under emotional stress, results in an increased rate of metabolism. In adults such stimulation may increase the BMR by 25 percent or less, but in infants the BMR may be doubled. Another effect of mental strain seems to be an increase in muscle tone; the tenseness of the muscles during suspense, anxiety, or excitement, or even during mental work, is a familiar phenomenon.

Transcendental meditation induces a number of physiological changes, including a lowering of the metabolic rate below the resting level. Studies conducted at the University of California and at Harvard showed a 16 percent fall in oxygen utilization during meditation, accompanying a reduced rate of breathing and a fall in blood pressure. This reduction occurred within a few minutes and was twice the magnitude of the decline that followed several hours of sleep in similar individuals (Fig. 6–7). These effects are probably due to a lowered activity of the nervous system, which is, in a sense, the direct opposite of stress reactions.

In measuring metabolism, relaxation is aided by reassurance that the test will not cause discomfort. Even so, a second test will often give lower figures than the first, and therefore will more truly represent "basal" metabolism.

Exercise. Of course in talking of *basal* metabolism, exercise is ruled out, since basal metabolism always means metabolism at rest. The aftereffects of severe muscular work persist, however, and the metabolic rate during the night that follows a day of strenuous exercise is higher than after an inactive day. The oxidative recovery processes keep going on in the body for hours after severe muscular effort and for shorter periods after less strenuous work.

Food. The immediate influence of food is ruled out in measuring basal metabolism, which is always taken twelve to fifteen hours after a meal, but the aftereffects of food, like those of exercise, sometimes linger on into the resting period. This is especially true if the food eaten is rich in protein.

Fasting. The internal processes slow, and the basal energy requirement is lower after a long fast or in an adult whose food supply has been insufficient for some time. This adjustment does not occur in a short period of food deprivation.

During World War I, Benedict studied a group of twelve young male students who volunteered for a prolonged period of underfeeding. When they had sustained an average weight loss of 12 percent, basal metabolism was reduced by 18 to 20 percent. During World War II at the University of Minnesota, conscientious objectors were fed diets simulating conditions in occupied countries. After twenty-two weeks, the men showed an average 18 percent reduction in the metabolic rate (together with a lowered expenditure of energy for exercise) on a daily energy intake of 1550 kcal. In undernourished children, however, basal metabolism per unit of weight usually is normal and the BMR is increased during recovery.

Fever. In fevers, or when heat loss from the surface of the body is prevented, the temperature of the body rises. Because the rate of the internal processes is elevated, the basal metabolism is increased. It has been calculated that the increase in energy expenditure is about 7 percent for every degree Fahrenheit rise in body temperature. A rise in body temperature of 4° F from 98.6° to 102.6° F (or from 37° to 39° C) would increase the basal metabolism by 28 percent, or by 400 to 500 kcal per day for an average-sized person.

ENERGY REQUIREMENTS OF MUSCULAR WORK

No person could live for long at the basal level of energy. The ordinary activities of life necessitate moving about, which involves muscular work. Even holding the body in sitting or standing posture requires some muscular work, as do the minor movements that all of us are constantly making even when sitting at rest or during sleep. Some people take active exercise or must do physical work in earning their living. What is more, everyone must eat, and the internal processing of food requires energy.

Muscular work is by far the most important of those factors that raise the energy requirement of adults above the BMR. Whenever muscular work is done, energy is used, and the amount required is proportional to the work done. Smaller quantities of energy are needed for maintaining the body in sitting or standing position, while active work, such as walking, climbing stairs, and pushing or lifting objects, requires much more energy. The heavier the person moving about and the greater number or size of muscles involved, the larger the amount of energy that is required. Thus walking, even at a moderate pace, requires more energy than typing rapidly. There is a two- to sixfold increase in metabolism with common, everyday activities.

Very hard work with high energy output cannot be kept up for very long at a time, so the total increase in energy requirement for the day (working eight hours) may not be more than 100 percent over the maintenance requirement even for active workers. In an inactive (sedentary) man or woman, the distribution of the energy used is about two-thirds for the internal work of the body and one-third for physical activity. For example, a small woman might spend a total of 1800 kcal (7500 kJ), with 1200 kcal for basal metabolism and only 600 kcal above that for body movement. As soon as more exercise is taken, however, the energy required for external work mounts rapidly, and the proportion used for physical activity may come to be as much as a half to three-fourths of the whole. (See Fig. 6–8.) A young college man during football training, for instance, might have a basal metabolic rate of 1800 kcal per day but use a total of 4000 kcal (17,000 kJ) or more per day because of his vigorous activity.

It is difficult to generalize concerning energy needs at various occupations or trades, since not only do the workers vary in body weight and rate of working, but under modern conditions, jobs in the same industry often involve widely different amounts of physical exertion. In an automobile factory, a 68-kg man who sits and operates a machine (which does the real work) may require no more than 2500 kcal per day, while an 80-kg man whose job calls for much walking and some lifting obviously uses much more energy—3700 kcal or even more. Both men belong to the same union and are classed as factory or industrial workers. Furthermore, the way one employs leisure time affects the total energy need. A sedentary worker, such as an office clerk, by working "out-of-hours" at home (carpentry, painting,

Figure 6–8 Components of the energy requirement of 65-kg adult. Basal metabolism, or internal work of the body, is uniform but accounts for two-thirds of the total need of a sedentary person and only one-half or less for the active individual. Physical activity is the most variable component both day-to-day and between persons. The energy cost of processing food (called DIT or SDA) is a very small component. Variation between seemingly like individuals is substantial; the standard deviation is about 15 percent of the average. Climate and age also affect requirement (see text).

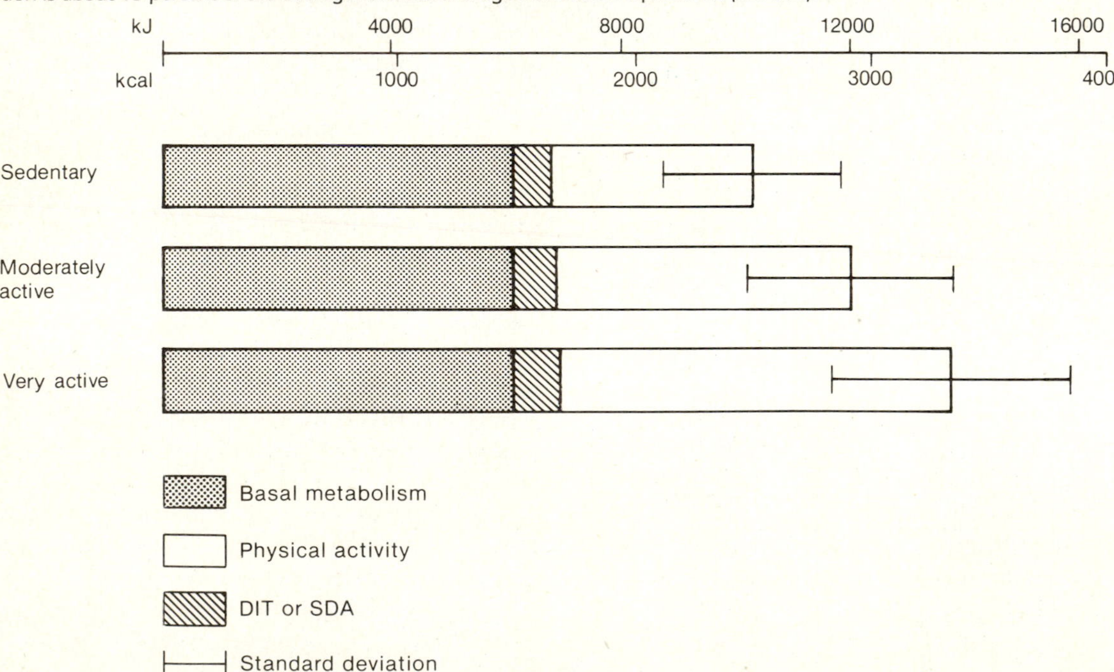

gardening) or going in for some active sport, may raise total energy requirement to that of a person whose working day involves more physical exertion but who spends most evenings viewing television or reading.

EFFECT OF FOOD ON ENERGY REQUIREMENTS

DuBois compared the effect of food on metabolism to a tax, deducted at the source, which thus reduces the amount of a person's income; we do not derive the full energy value of the foods eaten because the metabolic rate rises as a consequence of eating. Part of the increase in metabolism, which begins in a matter of minutes after eating, is due to the energy costs of digestive and absorptive processes, and the remainder is due to effects of the absorbed digestion products on cellular metabolism. The elevation of metabolism is greatest in the first two hours after a meal, and values return to the basal level after three to four hours. The stimulating effect of food on energy production is called *dietary induced thermogenesis* (DIT), or *specific dynamic action* (SDA), or simply, the thermic effect of food.

The rise in metabolism after eating 100 kcal of carbohydrate or fat is about 6 percent, while the rise in metabolism after eating protein is much greater, amounting to about 30 percent. The greater thermogenic effect of protein than the other energy nutrients is thought to be due to the additional processes required to rearrange or remove the nitrogen-containing portion of its components, processes that are carried out primarily in the liver.

If the diet contains a great deal of meat, the day's increase over the basal metabolism may amount to 18 percent. On the ordinary mixed diet, however, the usual allowance to cover the stimulating effects of the food itself is about 6 to 10 percent, averaged over twenty-four hours. Thus, in order to have energy intake equal to output so that weight is maintained, a person whose energy needs for the day amount to 2200 kcal would probably be spending about 200 kcal to cover the effects of the food.

The energy cost of physical activity usually is measured in individuals who have eaten normal mixed meals within the past several hours. Hence, these values reflect the sum of all processes going on at the same time—work, basal metabolism, and DIT. As has been pointed out in preceding discussion, "basal metabolism" is arbitrarily defined as energy expended under precise conditions of measurement, conditions that exist only briefly and infrequently. For these reasons, it is customary to determine energy expenditure from oxygen utilization of persons resting quietly at various times of the day, that is *resting metabolic rate,* or RMR (in contrast to BMR), and carrying out representative or actual work tasks at various times of the day. When the RMR is measured three to four hours after a meal, it is not, of course, significantly different from the BMR(1). If these practical values are used to estimate energy requirements, there need be no extra allowance for DIT of healthy people eating mixed diets; any error introduced thereby (at the most 6 to 10 percent) is less than the variation in energy expenditure for a given activity measured at different times in different people.

ENERGY REQUIREMENTS OF REGULATING BODY TEMPERATURE

Cold-blooded animals have no ability to regulate their body temperature, which accordingly rises and falls as the temperature of their environment changes. Humans (and the other warm-blooded animals) possess a heat-regulating apparatus that keeps the body temperature almost constant at a point usually considerably higher than that of the surroundings. Small variations of body temperature are normal; but variations from the average 98.6°F (37°C) rarely exceed 1°F.

Temperature regulation is ordinarily accomplished without effect on the basal metabolism or total energy needs. Excessive heat loss in a cool environment is prevented by insulation (clothing, shelter), and the heat produced as a by-product of body processes and muscular work is more than sufficient under these circumstances. Heat regulation is usually a problem of getting rid of the surplus heat produced. About 80 percent of this excess heat is dissipated by loss at the body surface, or through the skin. Some also is lost through the lungs by evaporation of moisture in the expired air. About 0.6 kcal is removed by evaporation of 1 gm of water at body temperature, or 600 kcal per liter of sweat.

Heat is lost from the skin (1) by radiation or conduction and (2) by evaporation of moisture (invisible or visible perspiration). The amount of heat removed by these means depends on the surrounding conditions. Low temperature of the air promotes heat loss by radiation and conduction, whereas high temperature of the air cuts down heat loss by this means and increases loss by evaporation. Low humidity aids evaporation, and high humidity reduces it. Wind or circulating currents of air favor heat loss by both conduction and evaporation. A further regulatory mechanism is to increase or decrease the amount of blood sent to the body surface under conditions of heat and cold.

Under only two conditions do changes in the temperature of the environment have any effect on metabolism. First, if the body surface is insufficiently protected from heat loss and the temperature of the air is sufficiently low, extra fuel must be burned to keep body temperature up to normal. In such a situation, there is likely to be shivering (involuntary muscular activity) and increased oxidative processes in the tissues to generate the extra heat needed, so that the rate of metabolism increases. Conversely, under conditions of extreme heat, some energy is required for body cooling because of increased work of the heart and circulatory system and the secretion of sweat.

The main factors that affect the rate at which heat is lost from the body surface are the amount of body surface, the presence or absence of a layer of fat under the skin, and insulation provided from clothing and shelter.

Body Surface

A child has a larger amount of body surface in relation to its total size than an adult has, the tiny infant having the largest relative amount of surface for its size. The shape of the body also influences the amount of surface. A tall, thin person possesses about one and one-half times as much surface area as a short, fat person of the same body weight. Since heat loss takes place through the surface, the body with a large amount of surface must generate more heat to maintain its normal temperature under conditions of cold than one with a relatively smaller surface exposure.

Subcutaneous Fat

A layer of white fatty tissue, directly under the skin, is normally present in well-nourished individuals, but the thickness of this layer of subcutaneous fat can vary considerably. Fat is a very poor conductor of heat, so that people with a well-developed layer of fat under the skin lose heat to the exterior much less readily than do those who have little subcutaneous fat. Thin people radiate about 50 percent more heat per unit of weight than fat people. This may be an advantage in winter but may not be in hot weather when, because the heat is held within by this layer of insulation, fat people are likely to experience discomfort, especially if they generate extra heat by exercise.

The subcutaneous white fat has no specific role in warming the body; it simply acts as insulation. In contrast, in many animals including humans (but not pigs or cattle), there is a second type of fat, brown adipose tissue, that plays a metabolic role in response to exposure to cold. Brown adipose tissue is fairly abundant in the newborn and is gradually replaced with white fat in adulthood. This specialized fat is located between the shoulder blades, around the neck, in the armpits, around the kidneys, and in the abdomen. Brown fat is the source of nonshivering thermogenesis, which is accomplished by oxidation of fat uncoupled from phosphorylation (see p. 135), thus greatly increasing the amount of heat generated. The rich blood supply of brown adipose tissue carries the heat to the rest of the body. In some species brown adipose tissue is found in adults that are adapted to cold. The question of its retention or regeneration in human adults is under study.

Clothing and Shelter

In summer, we leave some of the body freely exposed and wear loose clothing of porous weave and light color, which allows heat to escape readily. In cold weather we cover the body with several layers of clothing usually of thicker, less porous material, and we use blankets at night. Winter clothing usually helps considerably in conserving body heat. Exposure to cold water involves great heat loss, and even the heat generated by vigorous swimming may be insufficient to maintain body temperature. Scuba divers have learned to wear protective suits, and distance swimmers often apply grease to the body as insulation, but prolonged chilling will increase energy needs.

Primitive housing conditions protect the inhabitants somewhat from extremes of temperature and from exposure to the elements. With modern conditions of heating houses and suitable indoor clothing, energy is seldom needed to maintain body temperature. Air conditioning, which permits homes and public buildings to be kept at constant temperatures both winter and summer, is a further factor in ruling out a direct influence of the seasons on body temperature.

Net Effects of Climate

In cold climates, a small extra expenditure of energy (2 to 5 percent) may be incurred by reason of the extra weight and hobbling effect of cold-weather clothing. If the body is inadequately clothed, body cooling will occur and energy needs will increase. In this situation, the heat production with exercise and DIT are useful in sustaining body temperature. Comfort is maintained longer during sleep in the cold (as for example, outdoors in a sleeping bag) if a small meal is taken at bedtime.

People who live and perform necessary physical work at a temperature range of 30 to 40° Celsius (86 to 104°F) may require an extra dietary allowance to compensate for the energy expenditure at such high temperatures (increased metabolic rate, lower mechanical efficiency, and efforts to rid the body of excess heat, such as profuse sweating). Under these conditions, energy allowance should be increased at least 0.5 percent for every degree of temperature rise between 30° and 40°C.

OTHER FACTORS AFFECTING ENERGY REQUIREMENTS

Mental work, physical growth, and pregnancy and lactation also affect the body's energy requirements.

Mental Work

Because the brain is always active, specific mental work does not affect the energy requirement appreciably except as it may be accompanied by muscular tension. Although the metabolism of nervous tissue is increased slightly by activity, the amount of extra energy required is so small that the influence of this activity is insignificant. Benedict and Benedict, who found that the effort of complicated mental arithmetic increased metabolism 3 to 4 percent during the short periods it was carried on, compare the relative effects of mental and muscular work as follows: "The professor absorbed in intense mental effort for an hour has an extra demand for food or for calories during the entire hour not greater than the extra need of the maid who dusts off his desk for five minutes"(2).

Growth, Pregnancy, and Lactation

Children need extra energy for increasing the body weight in growth. Rapidly growing infants, three to six months of age, store about 15 percent of the energy from the food they eat in the form of newly built tissues. As growth rate diminishes, although the total food requirement is more because of the increased size, the allowance needed per unit of body weight becomes smaller. Adults recovering from a wasting illness also require extra energy for rebuilding tissue. In pregnancy energy is needed for growth of the fetus and the increased size of the uterus and mammary glands. In lactation energy is needed to provide for the milk secreted. Information concerning the energy needs of children and pregnant or lactating women is contained in Chapters 22 and 23.

ESTIMATION OF ENERGY REQUIREMENTS

Human energy requirements may be estimated for men and women in general according to their habitual pattern of activities and for individuals according to specific activities during the day.

General

The total requirement for energy includes amounts needed for resting metabolism and physical activity and the lesser factors of temperature regulation, growth, and lactation.

Basal metabolism determinations on healthy adults have shown the following normal ranges:

Men
1600–1900 kcal (6500–8000 kJ)
Women
1200–1500 kcal (5000–6000 kJ)

Resting metabolism of healthy adults throughout the day is nearly the same as the BMR in the interval three to four hours after a meal, but soon after eating it is up to 10 percent greater than the basal level. RMR ranges from 1.1 to 1.4 kcal per minute for men and 0.8 to 1.1 kcal per minute for women (Table 6–2). A rough estimate of the resting metabolic rate of adults of either sex is about 1 kcal per kg of ideal body weight per hour, with values for women ranging to about 10 percent below this figure and those for men 10 percent above it.[4] Resting metabolism of a man of average body build and weight (70 kg) is about 1.21 kcal per minute, 73 kcal per hour, or 1742 kcal (7.3MJ) per day. The resting metabolism of an average woman (55 kg) is about 1310 kcal (5.5MJ) per day.

A quick and approximate estimation of an

[4]These values are only approximations. Technically, there should be a small deduction in the day's basal metabolism to allow for the slightly lower metabolic rate during sleep. However, this correction amounts to only 0.1 kcal/kg/hr, or for eight hours sleep for a 70-kg man, about 56 kcal. Also, the correction for sleep varies with the soundness of sleep and amount of body movement during sleep. Hence, it is ignored in the rough estimation of energy requirement.

Table 6–2 RESTING ENERGY METABOLISM OF ADULTS[a] ACCORDING TO BODY WEIGHT AND COMPOSITION

Body Build: Men	Body Build: Women	Body Fat, %	50 (110)	55 (121)	60 (132)	65 (143)	70 (154)	75 (165)	80 (176)
						kcal/minute[b]			
Thin		5	0.99	1.06	1.12	1.19	1.26	1.32	1.39
Average		10	0.94	1.01	1.08	1.14	1.21	1.28	1.34
Plump	Thin	15	0.89	0.96	1.03	1.09	1.16	1.23	1.30
Fat	Average	20	0.84	0.91	0.98	1.05	1.11	1.18	1.25
	Plump	25	0.80	0.86	0.93	1.00	1.07	1.13	1.20
	Fat	30	—	0.81	0.88	0.95	1.02	1.08	1.15
						kcal/kg/day[b]			
Thin		5	28	28	27	26	26	25	25
Average		10	27	26	26	25	25	25	24
Plump	Thin	15	26	25	25	24	24	24	23
Fat	Average	20	24	24	24	23	23	23	22
	Plump	25	23	23	22	22	22	22	22
	Fat	30	—	21	21	21	21	21	21

Weight, kg (lb) applies to columns 50 (110) through 80 (176).

[a]Values for young adults. Metabolic rate declines about 2 to 3 percent per decade over age 30 years, and by age 70 it is about 85 to 90 percent of the BMR of younger adults.

[b]These values are slightly higher than basal because the subject is not in the strictly postabsorptive conditions (12 hours or more from the last meal). Adapted from Durnin and Passmore(1).

adult's energy requirement may be made, based on resting metabolism (which is based on body weight and age) and the degree of physical activity as the two variables. The increase above resting is proportional to the degree of activity in the usual life-style, as follows: For sedentary or maintenance activity, add 50 percent of the resting; for light activity, 60 percent; for moderate activity, 70 to 80 percent; for strenuous activity, 100 percent or more. A brief description of what is meant by these varying degrees of activity follows:

Maintenance:[5]
: sitting most of day: about two hours moving about slowly or standing

Light activity:
: typing, teaching, shop work, laboratory work; some walking but no strenuous exercise

Moderate activity:
: walking, housework, gardening, carpentry, light industry, little sitting

Strenuous activity:
: unskilled labor, forestry work, skating, outdoor games, dancing; little sitting

Very strenuous activity:
: tennis, swimming, basketball, football, running, lumbering; little sitting

On this basis, a 70-kg male secretary engaged in "light activity" would expend 1.6 times his resting metabolism of 1765 kcal, or a total of about 2820 kcal per day. A 58-kg female gardener, in the "moderate activity" class, would expend 1.7 times her resting rate of 1350 kcal, or about 2300 kcal per day. This method of estimating energy needs gives only a rough approximation. Individuals may vary considerably from the average because of differences in the vigor

[5]Experimental data indicate that the average maintenance energy requirement (for constant body weight and composition without any work demanded) of many species (humans, rats, cows, sheep, pigs) is about 1.5 times BMR or 105 kcal per kg of body weight to the 0.75 power.

with which one works, and the amounts of time devoted to the different activities. However, the two factors that have the most influence in determining energy requirement (resting metabolism and level of occupational physical activity) have been taken into account. For application to older age groups, the rate of resting metabolism would have to be adjusted downward by 2 to 3 percent per decade of age, and any decreased vigor of effort due to infirmity would need to be considered.

Individual

To obtain a more exact idea of an individual's need for energy it is necessary to have a detailed record of the time spent at different types of activity throughout a representative day. The energy used in each activity can be computed from figures such as those listed in Table 6–3. Values for the energy cost of specific tasks (sedentary occupations, walking at different speeds, standing jobs such as ironing or dishwashing, and sports such as tennis or horseback riding) have been determined by numerous research workers.(1,3) In Table 6–3, these figures are grouped according to levels of activity, ranging from sleeping, through sitting tasks, to those that require moderate or more severe physical exertion, in terms of the elevation above the RMR. As the exertion increases, the energy cost increases gradually from 1.2 times the RMR while sitting at ease, to 10 times the RMR, or more, for tasks or sports that involve strenuous muscular activity (such as swimming, rowing, track events). In some activities, body weight is an important factor; for example, a 64-kg man spends 5.2 kcal per minute in walking at 4 mph (7.4 km/hr); but an 82-kg man must move an additional 18 kg and uses 6.4 kcal per minute (Table 6–4). The men's energy requirement for this activity, which is markedly affected by weight, differs by 1.2 kcal/min; but the difference in their RMR's (calculated from Table 6–2) is only about 0.24 kcal/min. Energy cost of a given activity also varies among people according to their body conformation, skill, tension, and the like. Even for sleep there is a 20 percent variation. The values assembled in Table 6–3 are representative of the average young adult, but the range of observed energy costs is substantial (Fig. 6–9). To improve on these estimates would require numerous measurements of the actual energy expenditure of the individual concerned.

The rate of energy expenditure is less for women than for men because of the smaller body weight involved. Not only is basal metabolism less at lower body weight, but in all activities that require moving the body about (such as walking, climbing stairs, active exercise), the expenditure required increases as the body mass to be moved increases in size. This means that when the rates of energy expenditure for various activities are given as a combined amount (a single factor that includes basal metabolism, influence of food, and cost of the specific activity), this factor should vary slightly according to sex and body weight. The differences are small enough, however, that they are ignored in the table.

In calculating the energy cost of the day's activities, the time accounted for must, of course, add up to twenty-four hours, and the energy factor for activity must then be multiplied by the time spent at each activity. Two examples of computation of individual energy requirements are given in Table 6–5. Both are for students—one, a student most of whose day is spent in sedentary occupations (meals, classes, study, watching movies or television); the other, a student whose day is spent fairly similarly except for about one and one half hours of moderately strenuous exercise, which markedly increases the energy requirement. Both spend three hours in the classroom; one drives in a car between home and campus, both walk some about the

Table 6–3 ENERGY COST OF ACTIVITIES IN RELATION TO RESTING METABOLIC RATE*

Energy Cost Activity ÷ RMR	*Activity*
	RESTING
0.9–1.0	Sleeping, nightly average.
1.0	Lying at ease, 3 to 4 hours after a meal.
	VERY LIGHT WORK
1.2	Sitting at ease, listening to music, reading, hand sewing, knitting.
1.4	Sitting and writing, doing office desk work, repairing watches. Piloting an aircraft, milking by machine.
1.7	Sitting, typing using electric typewriter or using desk calculator; standing and moving around an office. Playing cards; playing woodwind instruments.
1.9	Lower range of domestic and light industrial work, e.g., cleaning shoes, paring vegetables and cooking, painting inside, typing using a mechanical typewriter.
2.1	Sitting and eating. General laboratory work.
	LIGHT WORK
2.3	Lower range of work in transportation, building trades, and mechanized agriculture and forestry, e.g., driving a car or truck with manual shift, or a combine harvester; planting by machine, sharpening a saw. Playing piano or stringed instrument; playing billiards.
2.5	Upper range of light industrial work, e.g., assembly work, machine sewing, bakery tasks. Canoeing 2.5 mph (4.0 km/hr). Horse riding at a walk.
2.7	Walking 2.0 mph (3.2 km/hr) on the level. Dusting, setting a dinner table, washing dishes. Hanging wallpaper.
2.9	Walking 2.0 mph (3.2 km/hr), level, with 22 lb (10 kg) load. Walking 2.5 mph (4.0 km/hr) on the level. Personal care, e.g., dressing, bathing. Lowest range of manual agricultural work, e.g., troweling, transplanting. Repairing shoes, operating a lathe. Playing a pipe organ.
3.1	Milking by hand; weeding and raking. Playing volleyball.
	MODERATE WORK
3.5	Walking 3.1 mph (5.0 km/hr) on the level, usual pace. Light janitorial work, industrial laundry.
3.5 (cont.)	Garage mechanics, washing a car. Bowling.
3.7	Walking 3.1 mph (5.0 km/hr), level, with 22 lb (10 kg) load. Bed-making, vacuuming, scrubbing (kneeling). Cutting wood with power saw.
4.0	Hoeing and weeding, window-cleaning. Cycling at 5.5 mph (8.8 km/hr). Playing with children; table tennis.
4.5	Cutting hedge by hand. Painting outside, plastering. Swimming leisurely, golf, archery.
5.0	Walking 2.0 mph (3.2 km/hr) up a 10% grade. Dancing a waltz.
6.0–6.5	Climbing stairs (70 to 80 kg person) Shoveling, 18 lb (8 kg) load thrown 3.28 ft (1 m) ten times per minute. Canoeing 4.0 mph (6.4 km/hr). Tennis; skiing downhill and using tow-bar uphill. Cycling 10 mph (16 km/hr), usual pace.
6.5–7.0	Walking 2 mph (3.2 km/hr) up a 20% grade. Cutting hard wood with hand saw.
	HEAVY WORK
7.0–7.5	Digging pit in soil; felling, trimming, and barking trees. Weight lifting. Swimming leisurely underwater wearing fins and suit.
7.5–8.0	Upper range of manual work in peasant agriculture and in building, mining, and steel industries. Hockey, basketball, football (game average).
8.0–9.0	Chopping with axe, 1.25 kg head, 35 blows/min. Skiing on the level over hard snow, 3.7 mph (6.0 km/hr). Horse riding at a gallop. Dancing actively, country or folk style.
9.0–10.0	Cross-country running. Climbing, light load and slope. Swimming strenuously. Boxing.
10.0–15.0	Climbing, heavy load and slope. Heaviest occupational work. Football and squash during play.
Over 15.0	Walking in loose snow with a heavy pack. Skiing uphill at maximum speed. Swimming strenuously underwater with full gear. Bicycle racing.

*Derived mainly from energy expenditure data collated by Durnin, J. V. G. A., and Passmore, R. (1,3).

Table 6–4 ENERGY COST OF WALKING AS AFFECTED BY BODY WEIGHT AND SPEED OF MOVEMENT*

Speed/hr		*Body Weight*					
		KG: 46	55	64	73	82	91
MI	KM	LB: 100	120	140	160	180	200
		kcal per minute†					
2	3.7	2.2	2.6	2.9	3.2	3.5	3.8
3	5.6	3.1	3.6	4.0	4.4	4.8	5.3
4	7.4	4.1	4.7	5.2	5.8	6.4	7.0

*Adapted from Durnin, J. V. G. A., and Passmore, R. (3). Work is defined as the overcoming of force. In walking, man is using his biological machinery to move his body mass against the force of gravity, and the work done is equal to force × distance. If a mass of 1 gm is accelerated at a speed of 1 cm per second per second, then 1 erg has been expended. One Joule is 10^7 ergs, and 1 kcal is 4.184 kJoules. A woman weighing 55 kg and walking over level ground at a rate of 3.7 km per hour actually expends energy at the rate of 2.6 kcal per minute (equal to 10.9 kJoule or 1×10^{11} ergs). However, only part of this cost is reflected in mechanical work because the body operates with only 20 percent efficiency and internal processes continue during work.

†To convert to kJ, multiply by 4.184.

campus, and the second walks to and from home. In spite of similar class schedules, the energy cost of one's activities is one-fourth less than the other's. For 70-kg men total energy requirements are 3223 kcal (13.5 MJ) and 2508 kcal (10.5 MJ) and for 55-kg women, 2424 kcal (10.1 MJ) and 1886 kcal (7.9 MJ).

Keeping accurate diary records of one's activities is difficult; the recording itself becomes a significant "activity," and constant attention may change how time is spent. Also, it is tempting to note that forty minutes were spent sitting at a desk studying when actually the person may have moved about twice in the interval to consult a dictionary and to use the toilet. In sports, much time spent in getting ready to play, waiting for the ball, and so on, is often recorded as play. The figures in Table 6–3 take some account of this in setting the values for tennis, golf, and the like; but the accuracy is obviously limited. For most purposes, however, no better estimates can be derived for total energy needs, and these values will serve.

The influence of mechanization on energy costs is interesting. For instance, typing forty words per minute using an electric typewriter is 70 percent above the resting rate (RMR × 1.7), but manual typing at the same rate is 90 percent over the RMR. Milking a cow by machine involves only 1.4 times the farmer's RMR, while hand milking is much more energetic, costing 3.1 times the RMR. Walking on the level at 2 miles per hour takes more than twice as much energy as the average man (70 kg) spends sitting at ease. Modern athletic-type and old-fashioned country dancing are about on a level with other active sports, such as rapid swimming, football, skiing (on level), or cross-country running. For some of the activities, there is a wide range in energy costs, depending on the conditions under which they are performed (such as speed or whether on level or on incline).

POPULATION STANDARDS FOR ENERGY REQUIREMENTS

In setting international standards for energy requirements the Food and Agricultural Organization (FAO) and the World Health Organization (WHO) recognize that there are

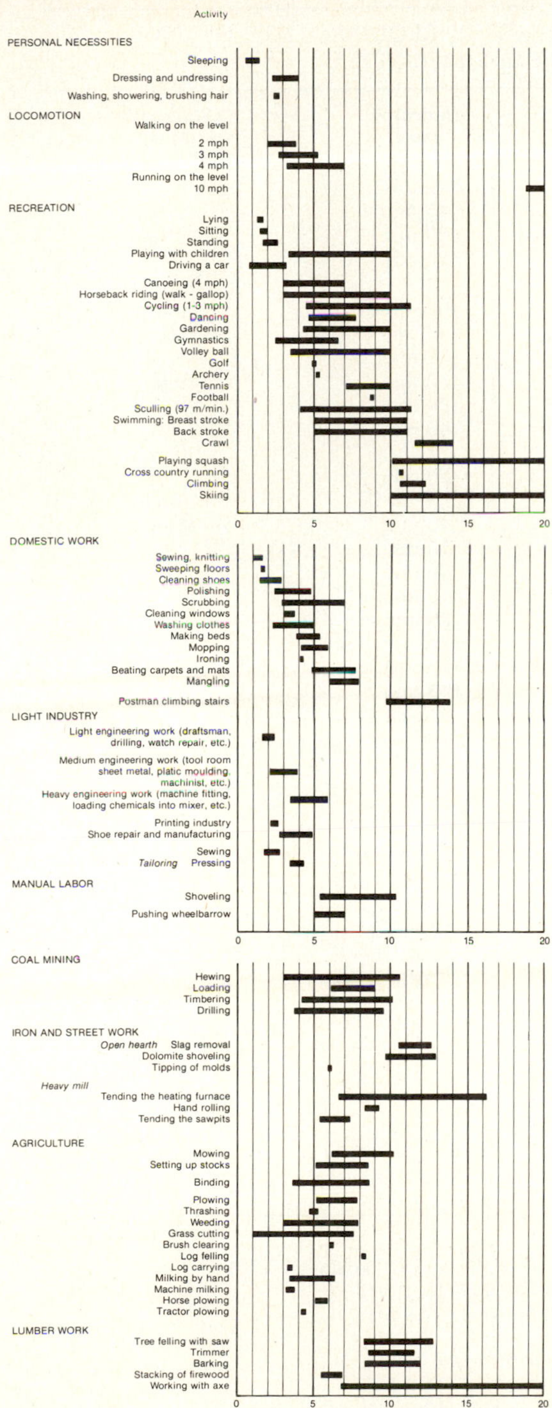

great differences in body size and activity patterns between and within countries.(4) They recommend computation of energy needs in a manner similar to the method illustrated in Table 6–5 but not to that level of detail. An allowance is made for BMR in relation to ideal weight for height and to that is added a factor based on activity pattern (Table 6–6). The FAO/WHO stipulate that all people should exercise enough to maintain fitness, and they make allowance for that in developing the activity factor. They also observe that intake should be generous enough to allow people to be as active in their leisure time as they wish, that is, discretionary (nonoccupational) activity should not be limited by insufficient energy intake. The daily energy requirements of adults whose physical activity is classified as light, moderate, or heavy, expressed as a multiple of BMR are, respectively: for women, 1.56, 1.64, and 1.82; and for men, 1.55, 1.78, and 2.10.

The United States Recommended Dietary Allowances of the Food and Nutrition Board, are presented as average figures with the expectation that normal variation is ± 400 kcal (1.6 MJ) per day. The reference adults are twenty-three through fifty years of age. Allowances are 2700 kcal for 70-kg reference men and 2000 kcal for 55-kg women (Table 6–7). It is suggested that during the postadolescent period the intake should gradually be adjusted downward from the high allowances for growing boys (fifteen to eighteen years, 2800 kcal) and girls (eleven to fourteen years, 2200 kcal) (Fig. 6–10). The downward adjustment (to cover decreased activity and basal metabolism) beyond age fifty years should reach 90 percent of the typical adult value; greater reductions

Figure 6–9 Energy expenditure of different activities can be quite variable. Bars denote range of data presented in the literature. (From Astrand, P. and Rodahl, K.: *Textbook of Work Physiology.* 2d ed. New York, McGraw-Hill, 1977.)

Table 6–5 CALCULATION OF TOTAL ENERGY REQUIREMENTS OF TWO STUDENTS WITH DIFFERENT LIFE-STYLES

Activity Diary Record	*Approximate Energy Cost/RMR*	*Student A Time*	*Student B Time*
Sleep (basal)	1.0	450 min	480 min
Dressing, washing, shaving	2.9	15 min	20 min
Eating breakfast	2.1	20 min	30 min
Walking to campus	3.5	20 min	
Driving to campus	2.3		10 min
Sitting in classrooms	1.4	180 min	180 min
Walking to and from classes	3.5	40 min	40 min
Eating lunch	2.1	30 min	45 min
Studying in library	1.2	180 min	180 min
Walking between locations	3.5	30 min	20 min
Playing tennis	6.2	40 min	
Playing cards	1.7		50 min
Walking home	3.5	20 min	
Driving home	2.3		10 min
Eating dinner	2.1	40 min	45 min
Ironing shirt	3.5	15 min	
Driving to and from date	2.3	20 min	
Dancing, active	8.5	40 min	
Eating snack	2.1	30 min	30 min
Sitting and talking to date	1.2	120 min	
Group discussion, watching television	1.2		150 min
Studying	1.2	120 min	120 min
Undressing, showering, etc.	2.9	30 min	30 min

Summation

Energy Cost Level	*Student A Total Time* MIN	HR	LEVEL × TIME	*Student B Total Time* MIN	HR	LEVEL × TIME
1.0	450	7.5	7.5	480	8.0	8.0
1.2	420	7.0	8.4	450	7.5	9.0
1.4	180	3.0	4.2	180	3.0	4.2
1.7				50	0.83	1.41
2.1	120	2.0	4.20	150	2.5	5.25
2.3	20	0.33	0.76	20	0.33	0.76
2.9	45	0.75	2.18	50	0.84	2.44
3.5	125	2.08	7.28	60	1.0	3.5
6.2	40	0.67	4.15	—	—	—
8.5	40	0.67	5.70	—	—	—
		24	44.4		24	34.6
			÷24			÷24
Avg. energy level, RMR ×			1.85			1.44

If the students are average 55-kg women:
RMR (from Table 6.2) 0.91 kcal/min × 60 min × 24 hr = 1310 kcal
Total energy requirement A = 1310 × 1.85 = 2424 kcal (10.1 MJ)
B = 1310 × 1.44 = 1886 kcal (7.9 MJ)
If the students are average 70-kg men:
RMR (from Table 6.2) 1.21 kcal/min × 60 min × 24 hr = 1742 kcal
Total energy requirement A = 1742 × 1.85 = 3223 kcal (13.5 MJ)
B = 1742 × 1.44 = 2508 kcal (10.5 MJ)
Note that an *active* 55 kg woman and a *sedentary* 70 kg man have almost exactly the same energy requirement, in spite of weight and sex difference.

Table 6–6 EXAMPLE COMPUTATION OF ENERGY REQUIREMENT FOR 25-YEAR-OLD PERSONS IN LIGHT OCCUPATIONS IN AN INDUSTRIALIZED COUNTRY, AS RECOMMENDED BY INTERNATIONAL AGENCIES (4)

Energy Component	*Female Homemaker 55 kg*	*Male Office Worker 65 kg*
Sleep-basal metabolism, 8 h[a]	435	560
Occupational activities		
M—6 h @ 1.7 BMR[b]		710
F—1 h @ 2.7 BMR[c]	150	
Discretionary activities[d] (M,F)		
Socially desirable, 2 h @ 3.0 BMR	330	420
Fitness maintenance, 0.33 h @ 6.0 BMR	110	140
Maintenance activities		
M—7.67 h @ 1.4 BMR		750
F—12.67 h @ 1.4 BMR	965	
TOTAL kcal/day	1990	2580
kcal/kg body weight	36	40
÷ BMR	1.52	1.54

[a]Calculated from formulas (developed in kJ/min) ages 18–30 yr. (4):
Male: BMR, kcal/d = (0.04436 Wt, kg + 1.9705) × 1440 ÷ 4.184
Female: BMR, kcal/d = (0.04256 Wt, kg + 1.4412) × 1440 ÷ 4.184

[b]Weekly work at 8 h/d, 5 d/week ≅ 6 h/d on a weekly basis.

[c]All persons are expected to spend 1 h/d in household activities included with "socially desirable discretionary activities," such as gardening, home decorating and repair, etc. Homemakers are expected to spend an additional 7 h/week doing moderately active household work.

[d]Discretionary activities that benefit the household and community are called "socially desirable." Persons in light and moderate occupations are expected to spend 35–45 min, 3 or 4 times per week in physical activity sufficient to maintain cardiovascular and respiratory fitness; this would not be required of people in heavy work occupations.

Table 6–7 REPRESENTATIVE ENERGY ALLOWANCES FOR HEALTHY ADULTS ACCORDING TO AGE, WEIGHT, AND PHYSICAL ACTIVITY

Conditions Specified	*kcal[a]/day (Weight)*		*kcal/kg/day*		*Standard ÷ RMR*	
	MEN	WOMEN	MEN	WOMEN	MEN	WOMEN
United States (5)						
Light activity	(70 kg)	(55 kg)				
Ages 19 to 22 yr	2900	2100	41.4	38.2	1.62	1.61
Ages 23 to 50 yr	2700	2000	38.6	36.4	1.51	1.53
Canada (6)						
Characteristic activity pattern	(71g)	(58 kg)				
Ages 19 to 24 yr	3000	2100	42	36	1.68	1.50
	(74 kg)	(59 kg)				
Ages 25 to 49 yr	2700	1900	36	32	1.50	1.39
Central America and Panama(7)						
Moderate activity	(62.9 kg)	(51.5 kg)				
Ages 19 to 40 yr	2900	2050	46.1	39.8	1.74	1.49

[a]1 kcal = 4.184 kJ.

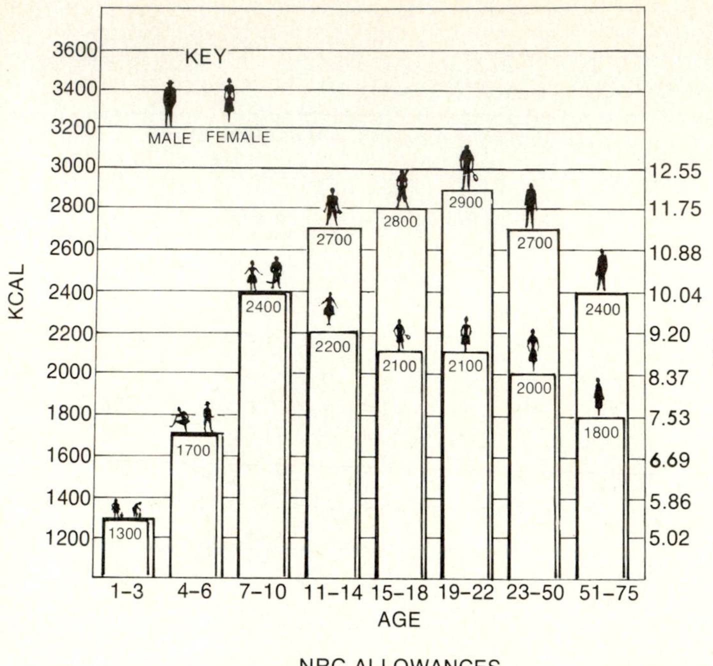

Figure 6–10 Age makes a difference in energy needs. MJ = mega Joule. (Modified from Food and Nutrition Board: *Recommended Dietary Allowances.* 9th ed. Washington, D.C., National Research Council, National Academy of Sciences, 1980.)

will be needed if there is a marked decline in activity with advancing age. Additional requirements for pregnancy and lactation and needs of children are discussed in Chapters 22 and 23.

The daily energy allowances in Table 6–7 are for men and women whose weight is desirable and suitable for height. (The weight attained at twenty-five years of age should be maintained throughout later life.) Overweight persons should use the energy allowance appropriate for their ideal weight for height rather than for their actual weight (which has obviously been too high).

The NRC energy allowances (in Table 6–7) are based on the assumption of typical activity patterns and life-styles.(5) Because physical activity is the most important single factor in altering energy requirements, adjustments need to be made for those who take more or less exercise than that assumed as standard. For these allowances the FAO/WHO examples are illustrative (Table 6–6). The international levels are stipulated according to activity and indicate a range from 2030 kcal per day for a woman in the light activity category to 2370 kcal for an exceptionally active person weighing 55 kg. Similar ranges for a 65-kg man are 2590 and 3510 kcal.

Except for U.S. recommendations, energy allowances are higher, in relation to the resting metabolic rate, for men than for women. Partly this difference is due to the fact that at equal fitness, men have a larger proportion of body weight as muscle than women do, and this has a relatively small effect on resting metabolism but will add to the cost of work involving the movement of body mass. Also, occupational work levels of active men may exceed those of women. This seems unlikely to be the situation, however, as regards sedentary or light activity levels. Studies of young men and women conducted at the University of California, in fact, indicate that little disparity exists under light activity conditions, and the total energy need relative to the resting or basal metabolism is fairly uniform for both sexes. Thus the difference in allowances and standards may reflect a biased view of female work patterns.

The FAO/WHO, in discussing the effects of climate, note that the impact will vary according to occupation and conditions of clothing and shelter. Agricultural workers in the open have some ability to protect themselves against cold, if they are not too poor to purchase clothing, but little opportunity to escape heat. Rich executives may avoid both. Considering all factors, the FAO-WHO concludes that there is no valid basis for adjusting resting and exercise energy requirements according to the climate. If physical activity is restricted by environmental factors, allowances should be selected according to activity level.

It should be evident that the energy allowances set by the various national and international committees are estimates intended for general use and based on the energy needs of so-called average men and women living and working in a comfortable environment (definite weight and arbitrary degree of muscular activity). For persons who vary much from this norm, the energy requirement really needs to be measured individually to achieve any degree of accuracy. The recommended allowances for most other nutrients are purposely set higher than the actual needs (about 30 to 50 percent above), but in respect to energy, the intake should be in balance with the output in order to avoid a loss or gain in body weight. Many persons do not reduce their energy intake sufficiently to compensate for the slightly lower basal metabolism and the far greater influence of decreased activity in later life. Even a relatively small excess of energy foods over the amount needed leads to an accretion of weight over a period of years. Considering the variation in activity from day to day, it is remarkable that body weight can be maintained fairly constant for long periods. The regulatory mechanisms that adjust intake to output and the consequences of failing to adjust adequately are discussed in the next chapter.

ENERGY VALUE OF FOODS

The average heats of combustion of the pure energy nutrients are, in kcal per gm, as follows: carbohydrate, 4.15; fat, 9.45; protein, 5.65; and alcohol, 7.1. The differences in energy yield are due to differences in chemical composition, principally the ratio of hydrogen to oxygen. Molecules such as a long-chain fatty acid (for example, stearic acid, $C_{17}H_{35}COOH$) contain a large proportion of hydrogen and carbon in relation to oxygen; they require a large amount of oxygen for their combustion and give off much heat. Carbohydrates (for example, glucose, $C_6H_{12}O_6$) have a low ratio of hydrogen and carbon to oxygen; they require relatively little oxygen for combustion and produce less heat. Proteins are intermediate between fats and carbohydrates in energy value when completely oxidized in a combustion chamber, but proteins are not completely oxidized in the body. The nitrogen-containing products excreted in the urine represent, on the average, 1.25 kcal for each gram of protein. There is also a small loss of potential energy as a result of incomplete digestion and absorption from the intestine (see Table 6–8).

As has been noted, there are many different carbohydrates, fats, and proteins. Their chemical composition and digestibility differ somewhat, and so does the amount of energy they yield. The average values of 4, 9, and 4 kcal per gm of carbohydrate, fat, and protein, respectively, that are usually applied for rough calculation of energy content of a food or diet were worked out by the pioneer American nutritionist, Atwater, after many

Table 6–8 PHYSIOLOGICAL ENERGY VALUES OF NUTRIENTS (per gm)

Nutrient Class	*Calorimeter Value, kcal*	*Reduction Due to*	*Physiological Energy Value, kcal (kJ)*
Sugars and starches	4.15	3% loss in digestion	4.02 (17)
Fats	9.45	5% loss in digestion	8.98 (38)
Proteins	5.65	2% loss in digestion 22% loss in urine	4.20 (17)
Alcohol	7.10	1–2% loss in urine and breath	7.0 (29)

feeding studies. He also published specific energy values to be applied to a given food; these are used in calculating the energy content of foods listed in most modern tables of food composition, including those given in the Appendix.

The rounded average figures significantly overestimate the energy yield from foods that contain large amounts of nonabsorbable dietary fiber or organic acids such as citric and malic acids (which yield 2.45 kcal per gm on the average). The rounded values, however, are sufficiently accurate for practical estimates of the energy values of foods whose composition is known. The value is computed by multiplying the number of grams of each energy nutrient in a given quantity by the energy values per gram of carbohydrate, fat, protein, and alcohol. For example, the energy value of milk is calculated as follows:

Milk contains 4.9 gm carbohydrate, 3.5 gm protein, and 3.7 gm fat for every 100 gm.

Each gram of carbohydrate and of protein has a value of 4 kcal, and each gram of fat furnishes 9 kcal.

100 gm of whole milk will have a caloric value of

carbohydrate	$4.9 \times 4 =$	19.6
protein	$3.5 \times 4 =$	14.0
fat	$3.7 \times 9 =$	33.3
total		66.9 kcal

A glass of milk (8oz) weights 244 gm, and hence has an energy value of 66.9×2.44, or 163 kcal.

Foods of High and Low Energy Yield

Foods vary widely in their energy value. In general, the foods with *high energy* density are those that are either rich in fat or low in water content. Thus, all the fatty foods (such as butter, nuts, cream cheese, mayonnaise, bacon) are relatively high in energy value, as are foods low in moisture content (dried fruits, cookies, candy bars, and the like) (Table 6–9).

Foods of *low energy* density include most fresh fruits and vegetables, especially green leafy vegetables, since these foods have a high content of both water and fiber. Lean meats, cereal foods, and starchy vegetables are intermediate in energy value.

The amount of the food eaten (portion size) also makes a difference. Twenty-eight gm (one ounce) of energy-dense nuts would be 180 to 200 kcal, but a portion of pie a la mode, made up of somewhat less concentrated energy foods, would add up to about 500 kcal (Table 6–10). But unless a food is fatty or relatively dry it is almost impossible to eat enough to reach high energy levels. A large portion of watermelon—1/6th of a melon, about 1 kg as purchased—yields only about 110 kcal, for example.

Table 6–9 ENERGY DENSITY OF FOOD AS CONSUMED

Per gm KCAL	KJ	*Food*
9	38	Pure fats and oils
8	33	Butter, margarine, mayonnaise; Pure alcohol
7	29	Salad dressing; Walnuts; Almonds, peanuts, and peanut butter
6	25	Milk chocolate candy; Sandwich, chocolate chip and oatmeal cookies, pie crust; Coconut macaroons
5	21	Hard and cheddar cheeses; Sugar, doughnuts; Beef steak with fat
4	17	Dry cereals with or without added sugar; Whiskey, cakes with icing, whipping cream; Frankfurter, luncheon meat
3	13	"Kentucky-fried" chicken; Dates, raisins, table syrup; Pies, ice cream; Turkey and chicken dark meat, beef steak without fat
2	8	Turkey and chicken white meat; Macaroni, noodles (plain), olives; Baked sweet potato, milk shakes
1	4	Cottage cheese; Lima beans, bread, baked white potato; Banana, grapes, peas, apples, pears; Milk, eggs, oatmeal, grits, fresh corn; Fruit juices, carrots, beets, melons
		Leafy vegetables, tomatoes
0		

Energy in the Diet

More exact tables of the energy value of foods are required for a fairly accurate check on the amount of energy furnished by the diet. These have been provided for a wide variety of foods in 100-gm portions and common serving sizes in the series of Handbooks No. 8 published by the United States Department of Agriculture. (Tables of food composition that provide values for foods eaten in other parts of the world are listed in the Appendix.) The energy values of average servings of foods commonly eaten by Americans are given in Table 2 of the Appendix.

The menus examined in Chapters 2 through 4 represent quite different food selections and have different amounts of the three energy nutrients and alcohol. Yet, all supply about 2550 kcal (Table 6–11). This amount would meet the needs of an active woman or a sedentary man. It is not difficult to adjust these diets upward or downward in energy content without appreciably changing the menus. If the consumer were an average twenty-year-old woman those energy requirement was 2100 kcal, for example, she would need only to omit jam from the breakfast toast and skip the pie at dinner. She could also omit the between-meal snacks and have the pie (Table 6–11, Menu A). A young man, with needs of 2900 kcal, might add a second sandwich at lunch or have larger portions of several items.

With the abundance and sophistication of foods available in most Western countries (the average U.S. supermarket offers about 15,000 different items) the only problems in meeting one's energy needs are knowing what to choose and having a sufficient budget. Selecting foods to meet essential nutrient allowances is discussed in Chapter 20.

HOW ENERGY IS DERIVED FROM NUTRIENTS

In the body, oxidation is a controlled process during which energy is released slowly in a

Table 6–10 ENERGY VALUE OF COMMON PORTIONS OF FOODS

Energy/ Serving kcal (kJ)	*Food, in Common Measures*	
	"Kentucky Fried Extra Crispy" Dinner, entire	950
	"Dairy Queen" Chocolate malt, large, 21 oz	840
	Hamburger and hot dog sandwiches, large, various toppings	400–600
	TV dinners, frozen, entire	350–600
400+	Hot cakes with butter and syrup, one order	
(1670+)	Burritos	
	Fried fish sandwich, commercial	
	Chicken à la king, home recipe, 1 cup	
	Macaroni and cheese, home recipe, 1 cup	
300–400	Milk shakes (no ice cream), 11 oz container	
	Most pies, 1/6–1/7 of pie	
(1250–1670)	Beef rib, steaks; pork chops, roast, including fat, 3 oz	
	Chili with beans, canned, 1 cup	
	Beans canned with sweet or tomato sauce, 1 cup	
	Enchiladas, 2	
	Spaghetti with meat balls, 1 cup	
200–300	Danish pastry, yellow or chocolate cake with icing, 1 piece	
	Sandwich, choc. chip, oatmeal cookies, about 5	
(835–1250)	Waffle, 1	
	Hot dog, regular size, on bun, 1	
	Ice cream, flavored yogurt, 1 cup	
	Ground beef (21% fat), lean ham, 3 oz	
	Broiled chicken, ½	
	Rice, noodles, macaroni, 1 cup+	
100–200	Plain pound cake, angel food cake, cupcake, 1 piece	
	Bagel, muffin, sandwich bun, 1	
(420–835)	Hot cereal or presweetened dry cereal, 1 cup	
	Taco, tostada, commercial, 1	
	Soda pop, beer, 12 oz	
	Milk (all but skim), plain yogurt, 1 cup	
	Cheeses, 1 oz cheddar types, ½ cup cottage	
	Most soups, 1 cup	
	Chocolate candies, 1 oz	
	Most fruit juices, 1 cup	
	Tuna (canned in oil), salmon, turkey, 3 oz	
	Peanut butter, 2 Tbsp	
	Baked white or sweet potato, 1 fairly large	
50–100	Egg, 1	
	Skim milk, 1 cup	
(210–420)	Apple, banana, orange, pear, 1; berries, 1 cup; grapefruit, ½	
	Lima beans, peas, corn, ½ cup	
	Breads, 1 slice	
	Ready-to-eat cereals, puffs, and flakes, 1 cup	
	Salad dressings, 1 Tbsp	
<50	Most vegetables, ½ cup	
	Peach, 1	
	Apricots, prunes, 2	
	Raisins, ½ oz	
	Butter or margarine, 1 pat or tsp	
	Jam or jelly, 1 Tbsp	
	Saltine crackers, 2	
	Popcorn (no oil), 1 cup	

Table 6–11 REPRESENTATIVE MENUS HAVING THE SAME ENERGY VALUE BUT QUITE DIFFERENT FOODS

Menu A		*Menu B* Kcal per Serving		*Menu C*	
		Breakfast			
Oatmeal, ¾ cup	98	Corn flakes, 1 oz	106	Omelet, 2 eggs	160
Bread, whole gr, 2 slices	120	Bread, white, 2 slices	140	Cheese, 1 oz	115
Butter, 1 pat	35	Margarine, 1 pat	35	Bread, whole gr, 1 slice	60
Jam, 1 Tbsp	55	Jelly, 1 Tbsp	50	Butter, 2 pats	70
Milk, low fat, ½ cup	68	Milk, skim, ½ cup	42	Grapefruit, ½	38
Orange, 1 medium	55	Banana, 1 medium	97		
Sugar, 1 tsp	15	Sugar, 1 tsp	15		
		Luncheon			
Bean soup, 1 cup	170	Chicken-noodle soup, 1 cup	55	Consommé, 1 cup	30
Rye crackers, 2	45	Saltine crackers, 2	50	Ritz crackers, 2	60
Sandwich		Sandwich		Tuna salad[a], ½ cup	175
Egg, 1	80	Bologna, 1 slice	85	Avocado, ½	190
Bread, whole gr, 2 slices	120	Bread, white, 2 slices	140	Lettuce	neg.
Lettuce	neg.	Margarine, 1 pat	35	Thousand Is. Dressing, 2 Tbsp	160
Mayonnaise, 1 Tbsp	100	Mustard, 1 tsp	5	Strawberries, ½ cup	27
Pear, 1 medium	100	Grapes, 20 seedless	70	Cream, heavy, ¼ cup	210
Milk, low fat, 1 cup	135	Milk, whole, 1 cup	155		
		Dinner			
Chicken, broiled, ¼	115	Chicken, fried[b]	412	Tomato juice, ½ cup	22
Baked potato w/skin	140	Rice, white, ½ cup	112	Steak, 12 oz (lean only, 8 oz)	460
Winter squash, ½ cup	65	Gravy, 2 Tbsp	54	Green beans, ½ cup	15
Mixed green salad, 1½ cup	15	Peas, canned, ½ cup	75	Butter, 1 pat	35
Vinegar, ½ Tbsp	neg.	Tomato, 1 medium	25	Mixed green salad, 1½ cup	15
Oil, ½ Tbsp	60	Biscuits, 2	180	Italian dressing, 2 Tbsp	170
Rolls, whole gr, 2	170	Honey, 1 Tbsp	65	Red wine, 7 fl. oz	170
Butter, 3 pats	105	Margarine, 1 pat	35	Cheese, brie, 1 oz	100
Blueberry pie, ⅙	380	Ice cream, ½ cup	135	Apple, 1 medium	80
		Chocolate brownie, 1	85		
		Snacks			
Apple juice, ½ cup	60	Soda pop, 12 oz	170	Sparkling water	0
Yogurt, flavored, 1 cup	230	Potato chips, 1 oz	160	Almonds, roasted, 1 oz	180
TOTAL	2536		2588		2542

[a]Made with 1 Tbsp salad dressing and celery. neg. = negligible amount
[b]Commercial, breaded, one thigh and one leg.

number of steps rather than in a single instantaneous combustion. Discussion in this chapter is limited to the metabolism of the three main nutrients in food—proteins, carbohydrates, and fats. Much is known about the intermediate compounds formed in the catabolism of these three nutrients, the enzymes and coenzymes involved in bringing about these chemical changes, and the ways in which intermediate products may be built into other substances as needed by the body. This chapter presents a simplified version of this information.

The body constituents are in a dynamic state, with both diet and body tissues contributing to a common metabolic pool in which the chemical compounds from each source are functionally indistinguishable. Thus, when the fate of glucose is being discussed, for example, it includes both the glucose coming from the diet and that coming from the tissues.

Cells: Functional Units of Metabolism

All living matter is composed of cells and cell products. Metabolism of carbohydrate, fat, and amino acids derived from protein takes place within the cells of the body. The structural components of the cell are important functional elements in this process. (See Fig. 6–11.)

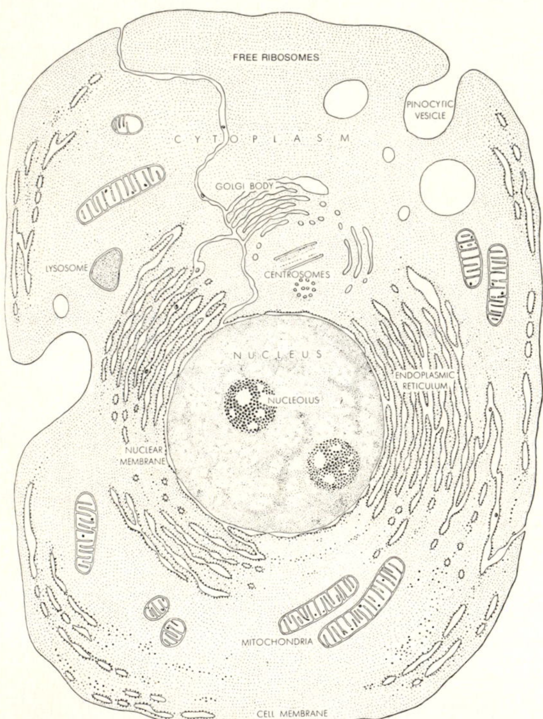

Figure 6–11 A typical cell. Cells are highly variable in structure and function. Within the human body there are many different cell types, such as the striated muscle cell, the smooth muscle cell, the nerve cell, the liver cell, and the sperm cell. However, all cells have certain structural constituents in common, though they may vary in appearance and quantity. These similarities give rise to the concept of the typical cell. (Modified from *The Living Cell*, by Jean Brachet. Copyright © 1961 by Scientific American, Inc. All rights reserved.)

Membranes subdivide the cell into compartments and regulate the passage of substances into, out of, and within the cell. The membranes include those of the endoplasmic reticulum, the mitochondria, the golgi body, and the lysosomes, as well as those surrounding the nucleus and the cell itself. For example, the cell membrane separates the cell from the external environment and selectively controls the rate of movement of nutrient and waste material into and out of the cell. Generally, large molecules do not pass directly through the cell membrane; however, they may be taken into the cytoplasm by being engulfed in a pinocytic vesicle. The endoplasmic reticulum acts, in part, to transport substances through the cell to the exterior (for example, the secretion of plasma proteins). All the cell membranes (including those surrounding organelles) are composed of lipid and protein arranged in such a fashion that both water-soluble and lipid-soluble substances can pass through the membranes. Often the membranes contain specific receptor molecules, which permit hormones to act. Enzymes important in mediating such hormone action, as well as those facilitating the transport of nutrients and wastes, are located within the membranes of the cell.

Simply, most cells consist of a nucleus and a surrounding cytoplasm with its organelles. The nucleus plays a coordinating role in the organization and perpetuation of the cell. The deoxyribonucleic acid (DNA) within the nucleus directs the synthesis of all cell proteins by means of messenger ribonucleic acid (RNA), which carries the information to the protein-synthesizing sites in the cytoplasm, the ribosomes. The DNA duplicates itself during cell division so that each cell of an organism obtains identical genetic information in the form of chromosomes containing the DNA. Thus, an intimate link exists between genetic inheritance and the capacity of the cell to synthesize specific proteins, such as enzymes, which will permit specific reactions to occur in the cells. The nucleolus is the site of origin of the ribosomes, which also contain RNA.

In the cytoplasm, the messenger RNA becomes attached to ribosomes. Amino acids are then linked together according to the genetically determined composition of the messenger RNA, and a protein is made. Proteins for intracellular use are made by ribosomes present in the cytoplasm. Some of the ribosomes are attached to the endoplasmic reticulum, and the proteins made by these ribosomes are secreted from the cell. In some cells much of the endoplasmic reticulum is free of ribosomes (called the smooth endoplasmic reticulum) and is thought to be involved in synthesis of complex lipids (for example, cholesterol) and glycogen as well as in the detoxification of a variety of compounds. The golgi body stores cell products prior to their secretion and appears to participate in the synthesis of complex carbohydrates (for example, glycoproteins) for secretion.

The membrane-rich *mitochondria* are the sites of the final oxidation of nutrients into carbon dioxide and water with the generation of energy. Because of inefficiency of energy transfer, only about 40 to 60 percent of the energy released can be used to synthesize

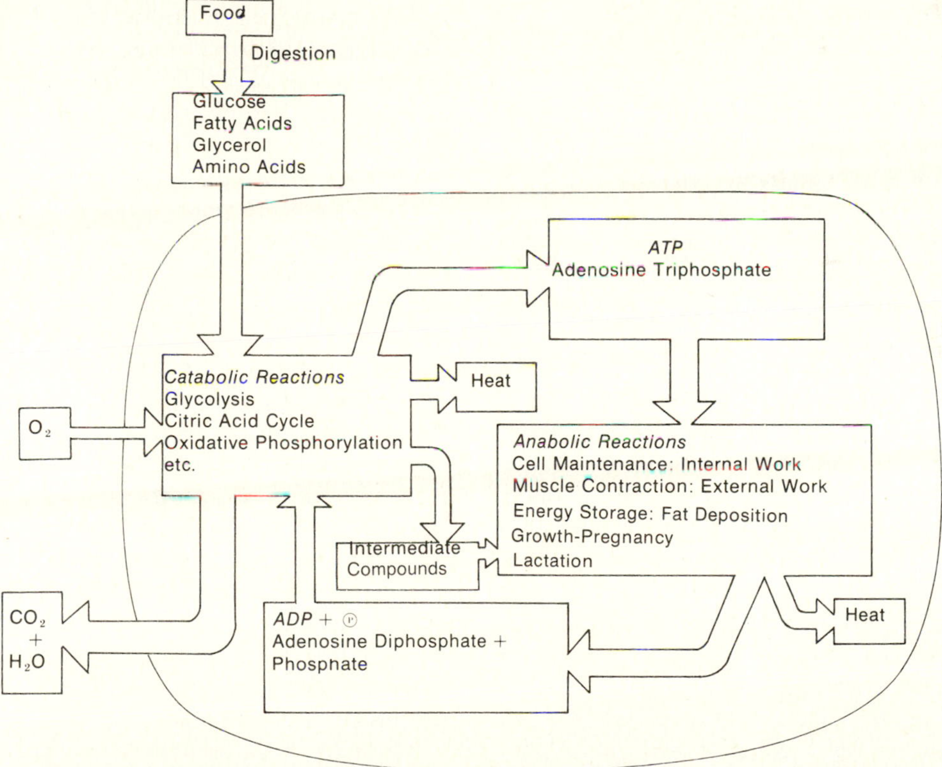

Figure 6–12 Diagrammatic interpretation of the role of adenosine triphosphate (ATP) in the cell. Whenever energy-producing reactions take place, such as the oxidation of glucose to carbon dioxide and water, some of the energy set free goes into forming ATP by the addition of a high-energy phosphate bond to adenosine diphosphate (ADP). The energy for anabolic reactions, whereby simpler groups or compounds are built into larger, more complex molecules, is supplied by the splitting of a high-energy phosphate bond of ATP, leaving ADP plus a free phosphate group. Thus, in the cell ATP acts as a messenger between those reactions that supply energy and those that utilize energy. Heat is a by-product of metabolism; it warms the body but is of no value as a source of internal or external work.

the high-energy phosphate bonds of adenosine triphosphate (ATP) (see Fig. 6–12). The remainder of the energy is released as heat. The ATP formed provides energy for the anabolic reactions in the cell, for internal work, and for muscle contraction (external work). The mechanical efficiency of the body is low (but as good as a gasoline engine), about 20 to 25 percent.[6]

The lysosomes contain, within a membrane, enzymes capable of splitting complex compounds such as proteins, nucleic acids, and polysaccharides. Disruption of the membrane frees the enzymes, and the cell digests itself. In the body, the death of individual cells and their replacement by means of cell replication occur in the normal course of events.

Metabolic Pathways

The initial phases of carbohydrate, fat, and amino acid catabolism proceed more or less independently of each other to yield identical 2- and 3-carbon intermediates. From this common metabolic pool of intermediates, carbohydrate, fat, and protein can be synthesized, or the intermediates can be further oxidized to carbon dioxide and hydrogen atoms by the enzymes of the citric acid cycle. It is the oxidation of the hydrogen atoms to water by a series of enyzmes called the electron transport system that is the primary source of ATP production for the cell (see Fig. 6–13).

Each metabolic reaction is catalyzed by a specific enzyme. Often cofactors are required for the reactions to proceed. These nonprotein substances are usually common to a number of enzymes. Cofactors frequently contain vitamins, such as pantothenic acid, thiamin, riboflavin, and niacin, as part of their structure. Thus, deficiencies of the vitamins may profoundly change the course of metabolism. Mineral elements, such as iron, copper, and magnesium, are also cofactors for some metabolic enzymes. The enzymes required for the chemical reactions shown in Figure 6–14 are not necessarily present in all cells. Furthermore, the entry of nutrients into cells and their subsequent metabolism are often regulated by hormones.

The Citric Acid Cycle. The *citric acid cycle* is the common final oxidative pathway for the intermediate compounds of carbohydrate, fat, and protein catabolism. It is also known as the tricarboxylic acid cycle or the Krebs cycle (named after the man who first worked it out). The carbon compound to be oxidized as the end product in all three pathways is acetic acid, which is presented to the citric acid cycle in the form of acetyl-CoA (Fig. 6–13). For example, pyruvic acid from the breakdown of carbohydrates must enter the mitochondria and be converted to acetyl-coenzyme A before entering the citric acid cycle. The formation of acetyl-CoA from pyruvic acid requires five enzymes and five coenzymes, four of which each contain a different vitamin (pantothenic acid, thiamin, niacin, and riboflavin). The coenzyme A (CoA) contains pantothenic acid as part of its structure. The CoA is released when the 2-carbon acetic acid combines with the 4-carbon oxaloacetic acid to begin the cycle with the formation of citric acid, a 6-carbon compound.

The citric acid cycle is represented in Figure 6–13. The diagram omits a few intermediate substances but includes all steps at which hydrogen atoms, carbon dioxide, or ATP is formed. The reactions by which carbohydrate, glycerol, fatty acids, and amino acids enter the cycle are shown in abbrevi-

[6]This means that to do a given amount of work, about five times as much body fuel must be oxidized as would be represented by the work alone. Since only about one-fifth of the energy of the fuel is transformed into work energy while about four-fifths of it appears as heat, strenuous work has a warming effect on the body.

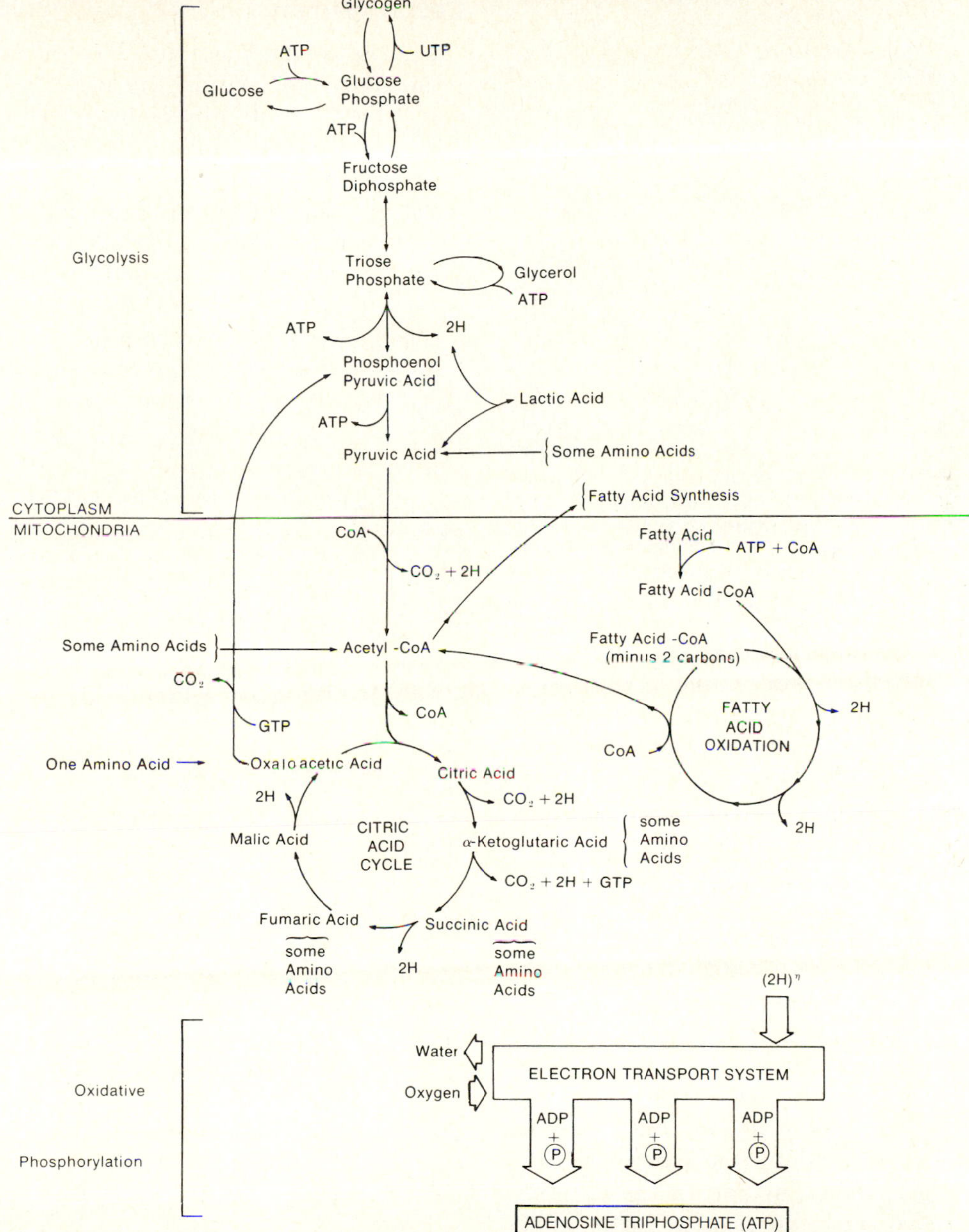

Figure 6–13 This is a simplified illustration of some of the interactions in carbohydrate, fat, and protein metabolism. Acetyl-CoA (CoA contains the vitamin pantothenic acid) serves as an important central compound in the metabolism of these nutrients. ATP acts as an intermediary between the energy-producing and the energy-consuming reactions of the cell. (See Fig. 6–12; the end-products of the use and the precursors of the synthesis of ATP are not shown in order to simplify the diagram.) GTP (guanosine triphosphate) and UTP (uridine triphosphate) are compounds with high-energy phosphate bonds similar to ATP. The hydrogen atoms (2H) produced in metabolism (these are carried by coenzymes containing riboflavin or niacin) are generally oxidized by the electron transport system, which is the major site of ATP production for the cell. Cell compartmentalization of the various sequences of reactions is essential for the life of the cell.

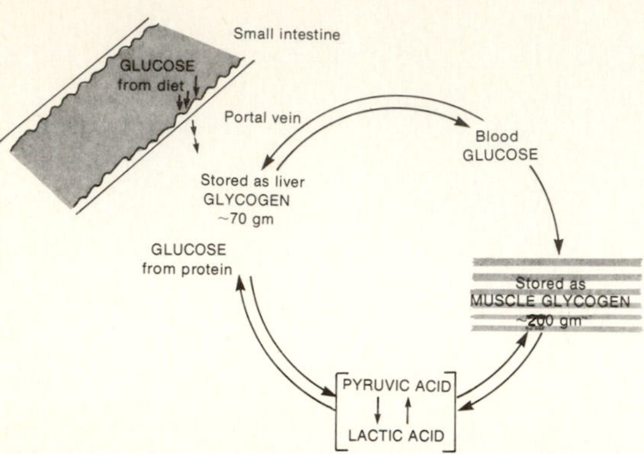

Figure 6–14 General scheme of anaerobic carbohydrate metabolism. This provides for the production of some ATP even though the oxygen supply to the body is limited. When the oxygen supply is adequate, pyruvic acid is oxidized completely via the citric acid cycle to provide energy for metabolism. The lactic acid that is produced during short-term oxygen shortage is largely (80 percent) converted to glycogen on restoration of an adequate oxygen supply.

ated form. The cycle moves only clockwise, starting with citric acid and ending with oxaloacetic acid. Each revolution accomplishes the degradation of one molecule of acetic acid to carbon dioxide and water. At the end, a molecule of oxaloacetic acid is left, free to combine with another acetyl-CoA to form citric acid and start the cycle again.

Oxidative Phosphorylation. The hydrogen atoms formed in the citric acid cycle are transported as coenzymes (containing either niacin or riboflavin) to a nearby set of enzymes called the electron transport system. The hydrogen is oxidized to water with oxygen by this system of enzymes. Some of the energy released by the oxidation of a pair of hydrogen atoms can be used to synthesize three high-energy phosphate bonds of ATP. This process is referred to as *oxidative phosphorylation* and is the major source of the ATP needed as the driving force in many anabolic reactions in cells. The complete set of citric acid cycle enzymes is found in proximity to the electron transport enzymes within the mitochondria of the cell.

Carbohydrates

Glucose is the main product of carbohydrate digestion. Within the tissue cells, the first phase of the breakdown of glucose takes place in the cytoplasm of the cell. This series of ten chemical reactions is known as *glycolysis*,[7] the anaerobic stage of carbohydrate catabolism. It consists of the conversion of glycogen (the storage form of glucose in the body) or glucose to pyruvic acid, which under conditions of adequate oxygen is converted to carbon dioxide and water. In anaerobic conditions (limited oxygen supply), the conversion of pyruvic acid to lactic acid is necessary for the regeneration of a niacin-containing coenzyme (NAD), so that glycolysis can continue to produce ATP. (See Fig. 6–14.)

During glycolysis only a small amount of the potential energy of glucose is set free, but it is sufficient to permit a muscle to operate temporarily when oxygen is not brought to it fast enough by the blood. When an adequate oxygen supply is restored, only about a fifth of the accumulated lactic acid is converted into pyruvic acid and then further catabolized by the citric acid cycle; the rest is conserved by resynthesis into glycogen (Fig. 6–14).

The anabolic formation of glucose from the intermediate compounds of metabolism is called *gluconeogenesis*. In addition to lactic acid, the glycerol moiety of fat and some of the amino acid intermediates can be used to make glucose and glycogen in the body (see Fig. 6–13).

[7]There are several other pathways through which carbohydrates may pass. The amount of traffic over a given pathway varies, depending on hormonal influences, tissue conditions, and the need for specific intermediate compounds. For example, glucose is oxidized to a variable extent by a shunt pathway in which pentoses are formed (such as ribose needed for building nucleic acids and ATP), as well as a coenzyme (containing niacin) required in several steps of fatty acid and steroid synthesis.

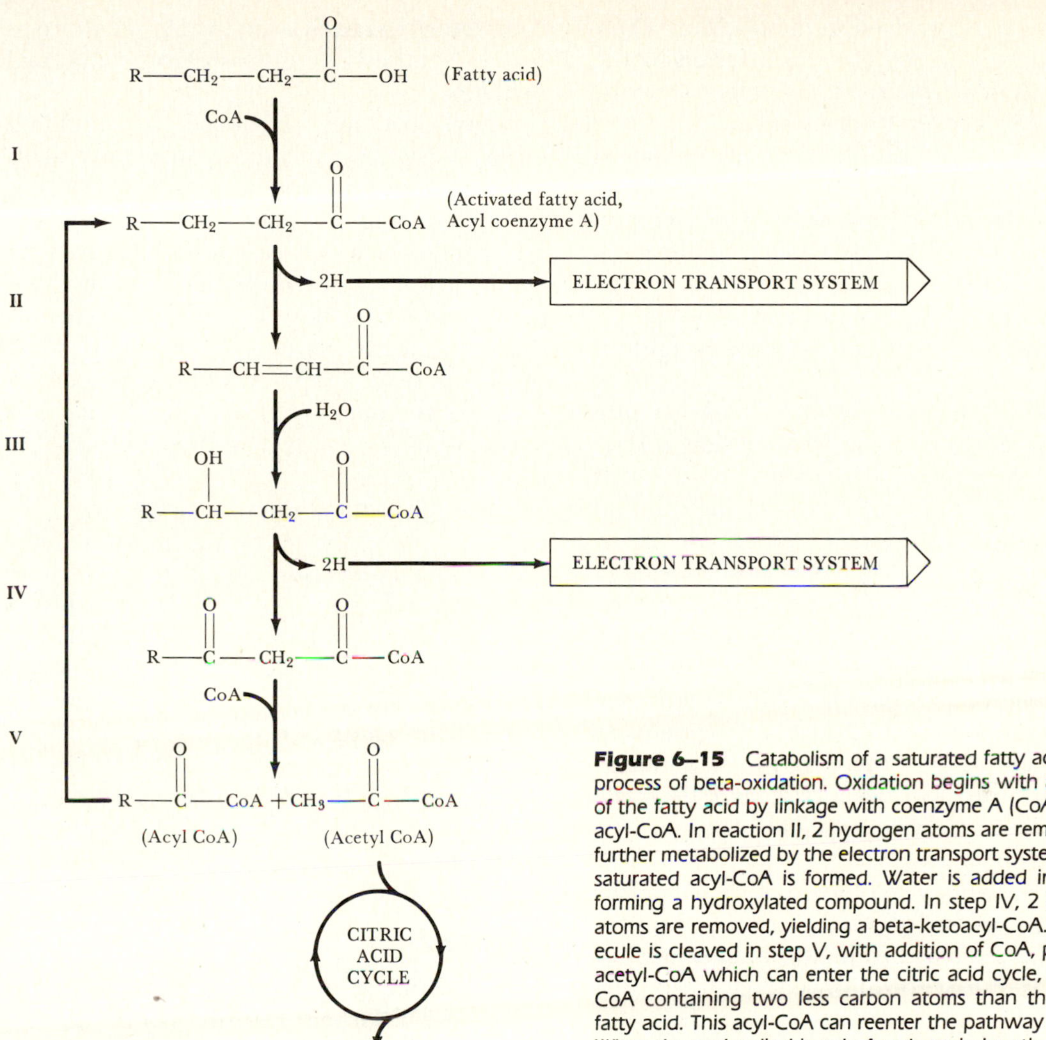

Figure 6–15 Catabolism of a saturated fatty acid by the process of beta-oxidation. Oxidation begins with activation of the fatty acid by linkage with coenzyme A (CoA) to form acyl-CoA. In reaction II, 2 hydrogen atoms are removed and further metabolized by the electron transport system; an unsaturated acyl-CoA is formed. Water is added in step III, forming a hydroxylated compound. In step IV, 2 hydrogen atoms are removed, yielding a beta-ketoacyl-CoA. The molecule is cleaved in step V, with addition of CoA, producing acetyl-CoA which can enter the citric acid cycle, and acyl-CoA containing two less carbon atoms than the original fatty acid. This acyl-CoA can reenter the pathway at step II. When the acyl radical is only 4 carbons in length, two molecules of acetyl-CoA are formed at step V.

These biochemical reactions must be carefully regulated in the body in order to insure the maintenance of an adequate concentration of glucose in the blood as is discussed in Chapter 2.

Fats

Most of the fat ingested is used as body fuel. Formerly it was thought that carbohydrate was the main source of energy used by the tissues, but it is now known that fat also performs this function. In fact, even the brain and other nervous tissues are not totally dependent on glucose for energy.[8] Free fatty acids are thought to be the most active

[8]Fatty acids cannot enter the brain, but their intermediate metabolic products classed as ketone bodies (acetoacetic acid, beta-hydroxybutyric acid, acetone) can. When carbohydrate is deficient, these ketone bodies build up in the blood, and after a lag period (one to two days) brain metabolism shifts principally to utilization of ketone bodies for energy.

form of lipids involved in metabolism. Their concentration in the blood is affected by the mobilization of fat from fat depots and by the action of several hormones.

The final end products of fat oxidation are the same as those formed by the complete oxidation of glucose—namely, carbon dioxide and water. The intermediate steps are very different, and the amount of energy liberated is 2.25 times as great as would be produced by oxidizing an equal weight of glucose.

Initially, fats must be broken down into glycerol and fatty acids, which follow different chemical paths of catabolism. Glycerol is transformed in the cytoplasm of the cell into a triose (3-carbon sugar) phosphate intermediate of glycolysis. The triose phosphate can be used to make glucose, or it can be oxidized to carbon dioxide and water via the citric acid cycle (Fig. 6–13). The fatty acids, with their long chains of carbon atoms, are oxidized stepwise into 2-carbon fragments in the form of acetyl-CoA, which is then metabolized by the citric acid cycle and the electron transport system in the manner described previously.

The breakdown of fatty acids takes place in the mitochondria of the cell, by the process of β-*oxidation*. Initially, a molecule of ATP is required to supply energy to convert the 2-carbon units of fatty acid to the coenzyme A intermediate necessary for further catabolism (Fig. 6–15). This reaction is followed sequentially by hydrogen removal (by means of a coenzyme containing riboflavin), addition of water, removal of another hydrogen atom (with a niacin-containing coenzyme), and finally the addition of another CoA. Acetyl-CoA is split off, and a fatty acid (minus 2 carbons)-CoA is formed, which then goes through the series of reactions again. For a fatty acid like stearic acid, which has a chain of 18 carbon atoms, this series of reactions would have to be repeated eight times in order to produce the nine 2-carbon molecules of acetyl-CoA. The citric acid cycle completely oxidizes acetyl-CoA, so there is no net synthesis of glucose from fatty acid oxidation.

Acetyl-CoA may be used for building other substances, including new fatty acids and cholesterol. As acetyl-CoA is also formed during catabolism of both glucose and amino acids, it is easy to explain how fat can be synthesized from either carbohydrate or protein when these are eaten in excess of the body needs for energy. The deposit of fat in the tissues represents energy taken in excess of the needs of the body, whether it is taken as fat or made from excess carbohydrate or protein.

Although white adipose tissue was formerly thought to be rather inert, experiments with fatty acids tagged by containing an isotopic element indicate that there is a more active interchange of fatty acids between these tissues and the blood than was previously supposed. Stored fat can, of course, be withdrawn from adipose tissue and oxidized to provide energy, whenever energy intake is insufficient for current body needs. Brown fat is broken down only to supply heat, its fatty acids being used within the tissue itself.

Proteins

The products of protein digestion—amino acids—are absorbed into the blood and carried to the liver, and the amino acids released from the liver into the blood are taken up rapidly by the other tissues of the body. The amino acids that are absorbed by the tissues following a meal disappear within a few hours. The primary and unique function of amino acids is to provide the components for synthesis of tissue proteins (including the important proteins of the blood) as needed for maintenance and growth, and to serve as precursors of antibodies, some hormones, and a vitamin. (See Chap. 4.) However, the carbon chain of amino acids can be used to provide energy.

Amino acids are very labile compounds capable of being converted one into another and into substances other than tissue proteins. The first step in this conversion is deamination, or the loss of the nitrogen-containing amino group (—NH_2). Deamination can occur by a transamination reaction in which the amino group is transferred to an acceptor keto-acid to form a new amino acid and leaving a new keto-acid:

$$\mathrm{R{-}\underset{\underset{\displaystyle O}{\|}}{C}{-}COOH}$$

The enzymes catalyzing these reactions, called aminotransferases, usually require a vitamin B-6-containing coenzyme for activity. This is the way the body makes many of the amino acids described as nonessential. The formation of ammonia and a keto-acid from amino acid is another type of deamination. The enzymes catalyzing these reactions, called amino acid oxidases, generally require riboflavin-containing enzymes for activity. Most deamination occurs in the liver, but the kidneys also have enzymes that can perform this function, if needed.

The keto-acid intermediates of amino acids are subject to oxidation, either directly or after transformation into other compounds, depending on the composition of the different amino acids. For instance, the simple amino acid alanine on deamination becomes pyruvic acid, which can readily be oxidized to carbon dioxide and water or used to synthesize glucose. Some amino acids, including alanine, are said to be *glucogenic* because the deaminized fragment may be converted into some intermediate of glucose synthesis. Other amino acids are said to be *ketogenic,* because on deamination compounds that are oxidized like fatty acids are produced. All of the deaminated intermediates can enter the citric acid cycle and be completely oxidized to carbon dioxide and water with ATP production by the electron transport system.

As an example, the metabolic pathway of the amino acid leucine is given in Figure 6–16. The amino group is first removed by transamination to glutamic acid. Successive steps result in the formation of acetyl-CoA, which can be metabolized via the citric acid cycle, and acetoacetic acid, which can be further metabolized by various pathways. The second reaction in this pathway is common to all branched-chain amino acids. This reaction is blocked in "maple syrup urine disease" as a result of the absence of the required enzyme (an oxidative decarboxylase); the maple syrup odor of the urine is caused by accumulation of the alpha-keto acids corresponding to leucine, isoleucine and valine. The third reaction is blocked in isovaleric acidemia, another inborn error of metabolism. The specificity of reactions in the amino acid (and other) metabolic pathways provides the basis for an enormous potential range of metabolic blocks. How serious these are depends on the essentiality of compounds beyond the point of blockage, the toxicity of metabolic products that accumulate before it, and whether or not alternative pathways are available.

The fate of the nitrogen-containing groups split off from the amino acids presents a special metabolic problem. Most of this nitrogen (70 to 90 percent of the nitrogen excreted) is transformed into urea in the liver and excreted in the urine (see Fig. 6–16). Other nitrogen-containing products excreted from the body are uric acid, creatinine, and ammonia.

In summary, the amount of energy a person needs in the diet is determined by the total energy expended. Energy is required to cover the costs of resting metabolism (such as work of the brain and heart) and physical activity, plus a small allowance for the effect of food itself. Activity patterns typical of industrialized countries require energy intake of the order of 1.5 to 2.0 times the basal metabolic rate.

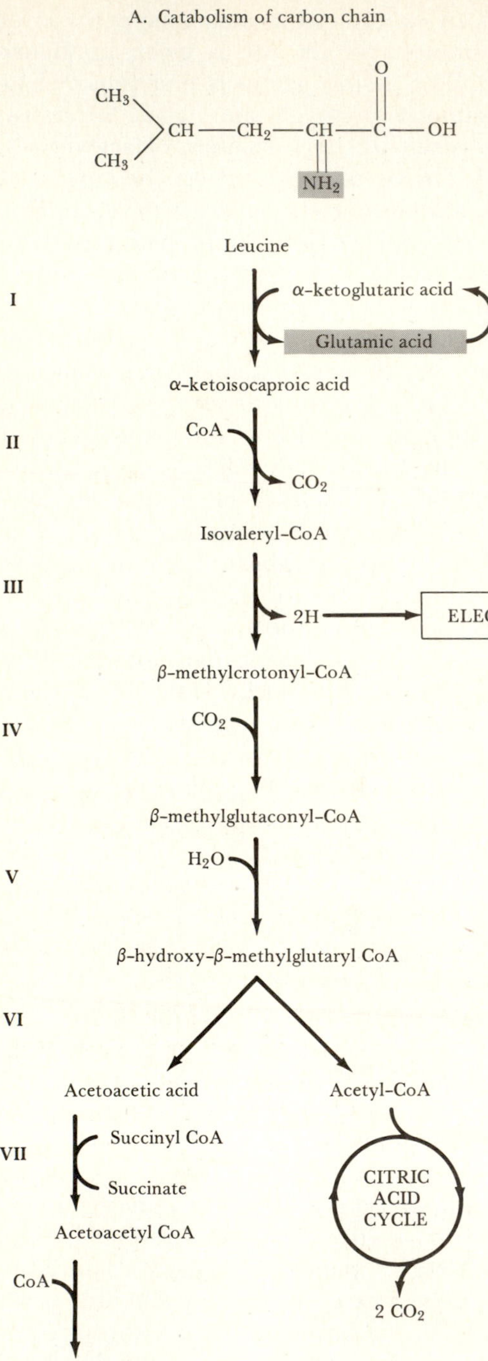

Figure 6–16 Catabolism of the carbon chain and amino group of the amino acid leucine. Step I, dependent on vitamin B-6, is transamination with alpha-ketoglutaric acid, yielding glutamic acid (allowing the amino group to enter the degradative pathway to urea; see below) and alpha-ketoisocaproic acid. Step II is a decarboxylation (removal of CO_2) and linkage with coenzyme A (CoA), forming an acyl derivative similar to an activated fatty acid (see Fig. 6–15). Oxidation in step III delivers 2 hydrogen atoms to the electron transport system. Addition of CO_2 in step IV is dependent on biotin, and yields a CoA-ester of a dicarboxylic acid. This is hydroxylated in step V. Cleavage at step VI yields acetyl-CoA and acetoacetic acid (a ketone body). Acetyl-CoA can enter the citric acid cycle. Acetoacetic acid yields 2 molecules of acetyl-CoA by the scheme shown in step VII, which takes place in muscle but not in liver.

The amino group transferred to glutamic acid can enter the urea cycle by several routes. Shown is a transfer of the amino group to aspartic acid, which contributes one nitrogen to the formation of urea. The other nitrogen and the carbon atom come from NH_3 and CO_2 via the compound carbamyl phosphate. This second, ammonia nitrogen, also comes from amino acids, from transamination and deamination processes in the tissues. Ammonia is quite toxic and is taken up and transported as glutamine or glutamic acid, to the liver where urea is formed.

For clarity, reactions are shown as unidirectional, actually many steps are reversible.

All the energy nutrients (including alcohol) enter a common final metabolic pathway, the citric acid cycle. Hydrogen generated from this cycle undergoes oxidative phosphorylation, yielding ATP, the substance that actually fuels anabolism and the body's internal and external work. The final products of energy metabolism are CO_2, H_2O, and heat. Amino acids used for energy are first deaminated, the nitrogenous end products being excreted in the urine. Amino acids that are built into tissue protein yield no immediate energy to the body.

If the food supplies energy in excess of body needs, the excess is formed into glycogen or fat for storage. If the food supplies less energy than the body needs, the insufficiency is made up by destruction of some body materials—that is, by oxidizing first the stored glycogen, then adipose and muscle tissue, and finally the essential tissue proteins. The law of the conservation of energy holds true for the human body. How intake and expenditure are regulated to maintain energy balance is a subject discussed in Chapter 7.

QUESTIONS

1. Define metabolism. Why is digestion not included in metabolism? What happens when the intake of energy is in excess of body needs? When it is inadequate for body needs?

2. Define basal metabolism. Describe briefly the methods by which it may be determined. How closely do results obtained by the methods compare? Name four main factors that have an influence in determining basal metabolism, explaining how and why each has the effect that it does. If a 70-kg man gains 10 kg of adipose tissue, how will his original and final resting metabolic rate differ? Suppose he goes into training and gains 5 kg of muscle, but his weight does not change; what will be his resting metabolic rate?

3. Name the categories of energy needs that together make up the total energy requirement of a normal adult. What factor has the greatest effect quantitatively in raising energy expenditure? Why does mental work have such an insignificant effect on the total energy expended? Under what circumstances will an adult need an extra allowance of energy for building new tissues?

4. The amount of energy required for muscular work is proportional to the amount and severity of the work done, as illustrated by the following problem: If a man lying quietly requires 77 kcal per hour and his energy need for sitting in a chair is 20 percent higher, how much energy per hour will he need while sitting at rest? If typewriting rapidly increases the energy need by 90 percent over that required for lying down, how many calories will he use per hour in sitting and typing?

5. Make a record of your own activities for a sample day, classifying them as nearly as possible under the headings of activities given in Table 6–3. Group the sitting activities, those that involve standing or walking about the room, and those that require light or moderate exercise; select the nearest comparable figure in Table 6–3 for energy expenditure for each, and multiply by the time involved. Compute energy required for all activities for twenty-four hours. How does this compare with your resting metabolic rate?

6. What is the energy allowance given in the revised 1980 recommended allowances of the Food and Nutrition Board for your weight (without clothing) and age? Would you classify your degree of physical activity as sedentary or moderately active? How does your individual energy requirement, as computed in Question 6, compare with the general recommendation for your age, weight, and the standard of activity? If your specific requirement differs much from the average, explain what factors cause it to differ (for example, variations from average in size and degree of muscular activity).

7. Describe the metabolism of carbohydrate, covering the following points: the form in which

it is absorbed from the intestine into the blood, the form in which it is carried in the blood to the tissues, the role of the liver in carbohydrate metabolism, the fate of glucose in the tissues (both that needed to supply energy and that in excess of immediate needs), and the final products of carbohydrate metabolism.

8. Describe the metabolism of fats, covering the same general points listed in Question 7 for carbohydrate metabolism. Describe the chemical changes that amino acids undergo in the tissues, including the fate of both the nitrogenous and the nonnitrogenous parts of the molecule. What are the chief end products of the metabolism of the three energy-yielding nutrients?

9. What common pathway do all three energy-yielding nutrients follow in the final stages of oxidation to carbon dioxide and water? Why is this route called a cycle? Why the citric or carboxylic acid cycle? What makes acetyl-CoA such an important intermediate compound in the cycle? What are the advantages of having a common pool of lower metabolites from all three energy-yielding nutrients?

References

1. Durnin, J. V. G. A., and Passmore, R.: *Energy, Work and Leisure*. London, Heinemann Educational Books Ltd., 1967.
2. Benedict, F. G., and Benedict, C. G.: The energy requirement of intense mental effort. Science, *71*:567, 1930.
3. Passmore, R., and Durnin, J. V. G. A.: Human energy expenditure. Physiol. Rev., *35*:801, 1955.
4. FAO/WHO/UNU: *Energy and Protein Requirements*. Rome, in press, 1983.
5. Food and Nutrition Board: *Recommended Dietary Allowances*. 9th Ed. Washington, D.C., National Research Council, National Academy of Sciences, 1980.
6. Committee for the Revision of the Dietary Standards for Canada, Bureau of Nutritional Sciences, Food Directorate: *Recommended Nutrient Intakes for Canadians*. Ontario, Dept. of National Health and Welfare, 1983.
7. Institute of Nutrition of Central America and Panama: *Daily Dietary Recommendations for Central America and Panama*. INCAP Pub. E–709, 1973.

7 Energy II: Regulation, Obesity, and Undernutrition

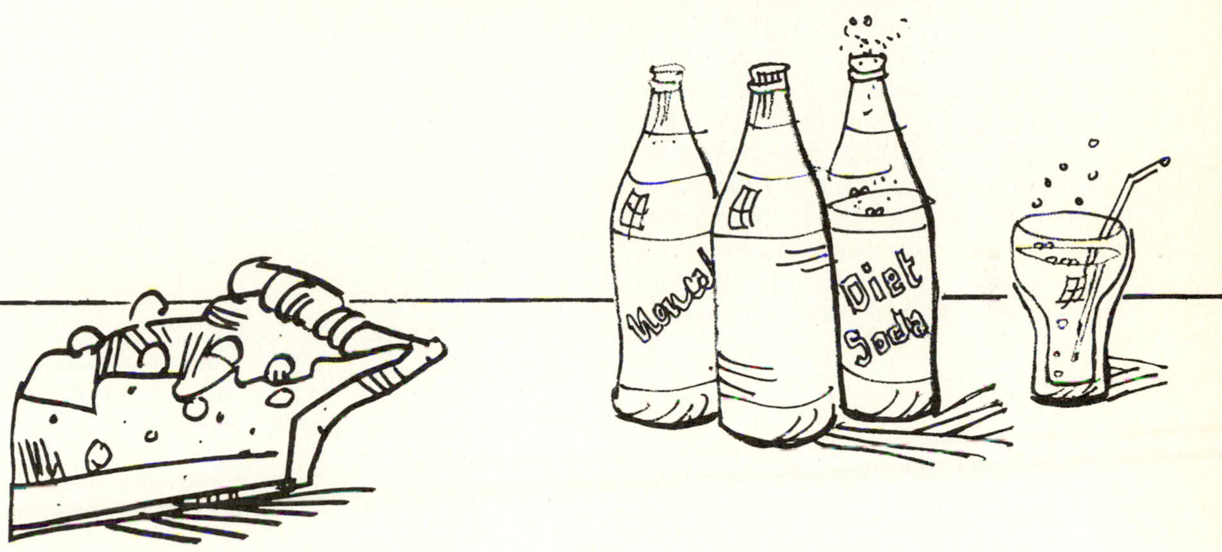

Most people maintain their weight reasonably well in spite of large day-to-day variations in physical activity and, thus, energy need. A person may sit in an office or classroom for the better part of five days a week and then spend almost the entire weekend in active recreation. Or a person may work in heavy construction all week and spend the weekend watching baseball in front of the television set. People do not necessarily eat sufficiently more food on days of increased activity, perhaps even the contrary, yet body weight shifts but little from week to week. Experiments with animals have shown that food intake is regulated each day, approximately according to the day's energy output. Superimposed on the daily regulation is a fine adjustment that corrects for small errors in the daily balance over a longer period of days or weeks. Humans show the same general regulatory pattern except that the daily regulation is less precise than in laboratory animals.

At very low levels of energy output, neither animals nor humans are able to regulate energy balance precisely, with the result that both become fat. Similarly, at very high levels of forced work output, regulation of intake is inadequate to maintain constant body weight. Miraculously, over broad ranges of physical activity and food availability, input and output are nearly balanced. An average adult consumes about a million calories a year. Average Americans gain about 9 kg (20 lb) between ages twenty-five and forty-five, or about 0.45 kg (1 lb) a year. This yearly fat gain represents about 3600 kcal, which means that the error in balance is less than 0.5 percent of intake, or out of adjustment by only 10 kcal per day. Regulation is 99.5 percent accurate.

Far more scientific and popular attention has focused on failures of regulation leading to obesity than on the correlates of thinness. Fatness is the form of disregulation common in industrialized societies, and the self-imposed emaciation of anorexia nervosa is thought to stem from a psychological aversion to body fatness. This disorder, recognized increasingly in young women and some men, represents an extreme manifestation of predominant cultural norm, that there is no such thing as being too rich, or too thin. Worldwide there are far more thin than fat people, living chronically on low planes of food intake. This thinness might be thought to fall outside the scope of the topic of biological regulation, resulting principally from social and economic factors, but examination of the strategies for coping with chronic underfeeding illuminates some aspects of regulation.

The balance of energy can be controlled in three ways: regulation of intake, of physical activity, and of metabolism. It is likely that all three mechanisms act harmoniously to achieve adequate regulation in most people.

REGULATION OF INTAKE

How much food one eats is affected by both physiological regulators and sensory or psychological factors, acting to cause or suppress hunger and satiety. Hunger and appetite are not synonymous terms. *Hunger* refers to the unpleasant group of sensations that are experienced when there is an urgent need for food. *Appetite,* on the other hand, means a desire for food whether or not the individual is hungry. Hunger is a physiologic condition, and while appetite has physiologic components, it is basically an affective state. *Satiety* refers to the set of conditions that exist when the individual stops eating because his or her hunger is satisfied.

Gastrointestinal Factors

Hunger sensations occur simultaneously with contractions of the stomach. These contractions are forceful and recur in groups lasting for varying periods of time from a half-hour to an hour and a half. A common experience is to feel hunger contractions that subside whether or not one eats, only to reappear later in greater intensity unless food is taken. Contractions are inhibited by a number of things, including simply tightening the belt (which probably gives rise to the use of that expression as denoting straitened financial circumstances). Eating food, of course, inhibits the contractions but so does tasting or chewing food without swallowing it, drinking cold water or alcoholic beverages, smoking, or experiencing the emotions of fear or hate. Contractions are enhanced by administration of insulin and inhibited by glucagon, hormones that respectively lower and raise the blood sugar level (Chap. 2). Hunger contractions continue even when the main nerve to the stomach (the vagus nerve) is severed,[1] but the sensation, the hunger pang, is no longer perceived. Severing the vagus nerve does not stop a person from eating the needed amount of food, so the awareness of hunger contractions is apparently not a necessary feature for regulating food intake.

Animals stop eating long before the full metabolic impact of a meal can be felt, so the gastrointestinal (GI) tract must participate in events that lead to cessation of eating. The act of eating and swallowing food is one possibility, but if food is prevented from reaching the stomach (by cutting through the esophagus), animals eat for a longer than normal period of time before stopping, and they begin eating again in a short period of time. If food is placed directly into the stom-

[1]This nerve is sometimes cut surgically to stop acid secretion in persons with ulcers.

ach by means of a tube (intragastrically), so that the animal does not taste, chew, or swallow the food, some lowering of oral intake occurs. This depends on the volume of material administered by tube. In animals, intragastric volumes less than 20 percent of the normal intake are without effect on oral intake, but volumes of the order of 50 percent cause a compensatory reduction of intake. This happens no matter if the material given intragastrically is food or a bulk material without energy value. Young men also are reported to reduce their oral intake of a formula diet if 40 percent or more of their usual oral energy intake is given intragastrically. Even then they consistently took more total energy (oral plus tube) during the day of combined feeding than when they ate only by mouth. When the men were not allowed any food by mouth and were required to administer their own intragastric feedings, however, they did consume an adequate amount of energy (1).

Several stimuli are involved in the GI contribution to cessation of eating. As the preceding discussion suggests, one is distention or stretch resulting from the presence of bulk, which triggers neural responses. Another is osmotic concentration; hypertonicity decreases meal size and inhibits food intake by rats and may do so in humans. Nutrient substances cause release of hormones that act to alter secretion in the alimentary tract (Chap. 5) and that also affect other hormonal systems, specifically those of insulin and glucagon. The GI hormone cholecystokinin acts centrally to inhibit food intake. Bombesin may also be inhibitory. Thus, the GI system anticipates and initiates the integrated mechanisms that ultimately stop one from eating.

The Hypothalamus

Attention was focused on a specific portion of the brain as containing a regulatory feeding center when French pathologists observed at autopsy that very obese people had lesions in that area (Fig. 7–1). Because of their anatomic proximity there was some question whether the regulatory center was in the pituitary gland or in the hypothalamus, with which the pituitary is intimately connected. Development of an instrument capable of destroying a minute area in the brain of a living animal made possible experiments that proved that the center is in the hypothalamus. In the early 1940's Hetherington at Chicago and Brobeck at Yale reported that destruction of two small areas located in the central portion of the hypothalamus (the ventromedial portion) caused rats to eat voraciously and become obese. That is, the rats became hyperphagic because the satiety center had been destroyed. Later, it was discovered that destruction of

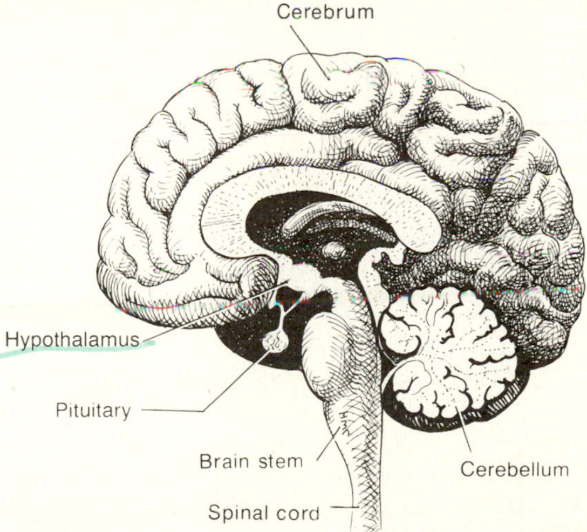

Figure 7–1 The brain has three main divisions: brain stem, cerebellum, and cerebrum. All nerve fibers from the spinal cord pass through the brain stem to the higher brain centers, and nerves that control the muscles of the head and muscles and glands of the abdominal organs arise there. Unconscious coordination of muscle movements is the function of the cerebellum. The hypothalamus, a small area (5 to 6 cm^3) in the base of the cerebrum, is an important integrating center for reflexes that regulate body temperature and control eating and drinking. Note that the hypothalamus is adjacent to and exerts control over the pituitary gland.

two areas in the side region of the hypothalamus (the lateral portion) caused just the opposite effect: The rats refused water and food, and some of them starved to death unless forcibly fed. This meant that they had destroyed the center that causes an animal to eat and drink.

Mayer and his colleagues at Harvard proved that the failure of animals to eat after destruction of the lateral centers was not due to the failure to take in water, and subsequent research has shown that the eating and drinking centers are separate but quite near each other in the rat. Since then, lesions have been made in chickens, cats, dogs, monkeys, and goats, and all show similar anatomic locations and feeding responses. Electrical stimulation of the feeding and satiety centers causes the reactions that would be expected. Stimulation of the satiety center causes animals to stop eating, and stimulation of the feeding center causes them to eat. Precise location of the drinking center is easier in some animals—the goat, for instance—than others, and stimulation of this area of the hypothalamus causes an animal to drink whether or not it is thirsty, thus disproving an old adage; as Mayer has said, you can now lead a (goat) to water and you *can* make him drink.

Further study of the hypothalamic centers has shown that the satiety center is dominant in regulating eating behavior. It is thought to act like a brake on the feeding center. The nerve fibers in the hypothalamus have been mapped out and connections found between the two centers. Once the control center was located, further research uncovered the major signals to which it responds.

The most enduring concept has been that a signal is generated in response to the utilization of glucose, the so-called *glucostatic theory of regulation*. This theory, proposed by Mayer, postulates that there are receptors in the satiety center that are especially sensitive to glucose and are activated according to the rate at which it is being utilized. When food is taken, blood sugar rises and the rate of glucose utilization in the tissues rises. The receptors are stimulated, and the satiety center signals the responses to stop eating. Conversely, some hours later, blood glucose falls, and the receptors detect low utilization rate; the brake is released and eating begins. An important distinction is that the hypothalamic receptors are responsive to utilization of glucose rather than to the level of glucose per se. In the disease diabetes, appetite is great even though blood-sugar levels are elevated.

It is known that the central feeding circuit is integrated with the autonomic nervous system leading to postulation of an *autonomic theory* of *regulation* (2). Injection of the neurotransmitter norepinephrine into the hypothalamus elicits eating in food-satiated animals.[2] In the rat, and probably in humans, synthesis in the brain of the catecholamines (from tyrosine) and serotonin (from tryptophan) is subject to precursor control. Thus the amount of amino acids entering the brain affects the amount of these neurotransmitters. The large neutral amino acids (NAA, namely tyrosine, tryptophan, phenylalanine, valine, leucine, isoleucine, methionine, histidine, and threonine) share a common transport system and compete for entry into the brain. More tyrosine and tryptophan will enter the brain if their concentrations are raised relative to the level of the other NAAs. The tryptophan to NAA ratio is inversely related to the amount of protein in meals, which follows logically from its relatively low concentration in proteins. (See Chap. 4.) The tryptophan/NAA ratio is ele-

[2]The amphetamines, drugs commonly prescribed to suppress appetite, affect the DOPA system, which counterbalances the norepinephrine transmitter. Some psychotropic drugs (chlorpromazine, cyproheptadine) have the opposite effect of increasing food intake, again by affecting the balance among transmitters and allied compounds.

vated by carbohydrate feeding. The ratio of tyrosine to NAAs is inversely related to energy intake (3). A high intake of energy would lead to a reduced ratio of tyrosine to NAA and, presumably, to lessened entry of tyrosine into the brain and lower catecholamine formation and reduced impetus to eating.

The drinking circuit is part of the parasympathetic system and is triggered by application of another neurotransmitter, acetylcholine. Thus in normal animals, these anatomically overlapping systems react to separate and distinct signals, even though eating and drinking are paired behaviors and are both reactive to changes in the osmolality of body fluids. While the various hormones that affect food intake—primarily insulin and growth hormone and, to a lesser extent, estrogen—affect the blood level and tissue utilization of glucose, so do they influence the level and utilization of amino acids and lipids. Severe imbalances of amino acids in the diet lead immediately to cessation of eating, and dietary lack of single nutrients usually causes loss of appetite as an early symptom of deficiency. All of this suggests that regulation of the most vital animal processes is even more complex and interrelated than we now appreciate and that there is participation of higher brain centers in all these functions.

Animals with lesions in the hypothalamus have alterations in behavior other than those relating simply to the amount of food eaten. Rats that have been operated on are less active, have diminished libido, and have altered responses to test situations involving food. They are more encephalized. Placed in a situation in which they must risk a shock to obtain food, they are less responsive to hunger than is the normal animal. The animal with a lesion is also more prone than the normal one to reject food that has an unpleasant taste (for instance, with quinine added to it).

Animals appreciate novelty in the feeding situation. One of the ways obesity is induced experimentally in rats is by "cafeteria" feeding, providing a choice and variety of several preferred foods in addition to the basic diet. Given this opportunity to satisfy sensory cravings, rats eat about 25 to 50 percent more of energy-yielding foods. The shape and size of food pellets also affect the amount of food rats will eat.

Humans, too, like sensory stimulation from food. Hunger can be overcome without having satisfied the appetite. Rolls and her colleagues found that people ate 14 percent more pasta with tomato sauce when they were presented with three different shapes of pasta than when they were given only one shape of their own choosing (4). These investigators have also described "sensory specific satiety" in which palatability of a food declines with consumption of that food in a meal, whereas pleasantness of foods not yet tasted remains unchanged. This implies that more food will be consumed from a varied meal than from a monotonous one. Habit and belief also govern intake. Most of us have taken a sweet after our true hunger has been satisfied because that is how a meal "ought" to end.

Obese people may be more responsive to these external stimuli or perhaps less responsive to the internal cues that tell a body when food is needed and when it has had enough. One study showed that overweight college students would eat more of three sandwiches put before them in a test situation than would students who were thin or of normal weight. If the subjects had to go to a refrigerator to obtain the sandwiches, however, the overweight ones ate less than did those of normal weight. This suggests that the overweight students did not recognize biologically how hungry they were or even if they were hungry at all. The obese also approach the process of eating differently; they eat faster and take fewer bites than do persons of normal weight. Palatability is another factor. Hashim and Van Itallie made freely available a bland and not distasteful formula diet to adults of normal weight and to overweight ones; the normal adults soon learned to take enough to maintain their body weight constant, but the overweight ones did not meet their needs and lost weight (5).

Interesting new research points to another central regulator, beta-endorphin, which may relate to these intake variables. This peptide is an endogenous opiate that acts like morphine. Injection of endorphin into the brain, like dosage with morphine and heroin, inhibits food intake. When the opioid receptors in the brain are blocked chemically, food intake by rats approximately doubles. These results suggest that the food-reward system involved in satiety may contain opioid receptors (2). Physical exercise increases the secretion of endorphin, particularly in people conditioned to activity (6); this may contribute to effects of activity on energy balance.

Long-Term Regulation of Intake

Up to this point we have been discussing immediate or short-term regulation of intake. Little is known about the mechanism whereby the daily small errors in energy regulation are compensated so that body weight remains nearly constant (if that is appropriate) or so that weight is regained after an illness or period of food deprivation. A *lipostatic theory of regulation* is currently the most accepted. This theory suggests that precise information on the current level of fat stores is relayed from the adipose tissue to the nervous control center. If the stores are filled, the animal is directed to stop eating; but if the stores are low, eating continues past the point at which the satiety center is usually activated. Several observations provide general support for this theory. One is that animals with lesions in the satiety center do not go on gaining indefinitely but stop at some degree of obesity. If the obese, lesioned animal is then starved, when food is again available it regains its original obese weight, not some other degree of fatness. Also, when rats are made fat by forced feeding, they subsequently reduce their voluntary food intake until the excess weight is lost. Animals with lesions in the lateral hypothalamus similarly preserve a stable, reduced body weight.

What this adipose tissue sensor might be is unknown. The probability of a humoral substance is suggested by an observation made about animals that are joined surgically so that their blood interchanges but their organs remain separate (parabiotic preparation). If one member of the pair has the satiety center destroyed, it becomes obese; the other member of the pair becomes thin. Presumably this happens because some message is transmitted from the large adipose stores of the fat partner through the blood to the regulatory center of the normal member of the pair; energy intake by the normal partner is then reduced because excessive fat stores have been sensed. By whatever mechanism, the organism apparently is able to detect whether fat stores are being filled or emptied and to adapt food intake accordingly.

REGULATION OF ACTIVITY

Behavioral regulation of the output side of the energy balance equation has been a neglected subject of scientific study until fairly recent times. Almost no one has spoken of a drive to physical activity in the same sense as of a drive to eat or to reproduce. Such firm evidence as we have comes principally from studies of adjustment to low energy intake.

In one experimental model, activity patterns were recorded when subjects were changed from normal to lower intakes. Both obese men following a slimming diet and healthy university students, whose intake was only marginally lowered, reduced their voluntary activity from pretest levels (7). In both situations the reduction in activity was significant but not sufficient to prevent body weight loss in the short term. Another experimental model reverses the situation by giving supplementary food to people habituated to a low level of intake. Three outcomes have been reported. In one study, men increased their wage-labor output in response to feeding. A second group studied did not change their wage-labor performance but did increase their nonoccupational activity, forming a village soccer team. A third study found no change in activity but rather an increase in body weight. This array of responses supports a general concept of physiological regulation but suggests that motivation and future expectations (will feeding continue or not? is change in body weight desirable?) are important variables.

Studies of obese children and adults have revealed that most of them ate about as much as individuals of normal weight but that they were much less active physically. Inactivity is not accompanied by a commensurate decrease in appetite at very low levels of work output in animals or people (Fig. 7–2). Rats become obese if confined to small cages where their movement is restricted, and the standard way for a farmer to finish a steer or fatten a goose for a pâté de foie gras is to limit exercise by penning the animal and to provide plenty of food. These same animals—rats, cattle, and fowl—adjust intake to output better when they are free to range and must forage for food. Control of activity alone, for example, by forcing a rat to run in an activity wheel, allows the animal to remain lean while eating to satisfy its appetite from freely available food.

In commenting on this issue, R. Passmore has said that since his retirement:

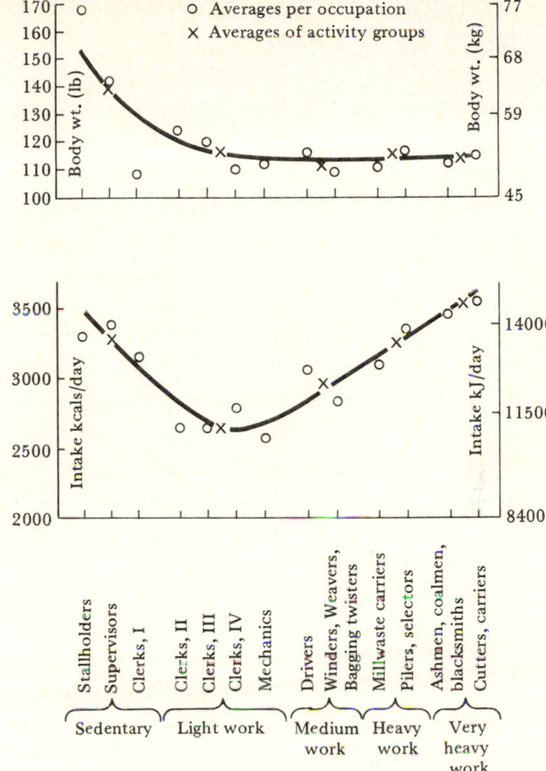

Figure 7–2 Body weight and energy intake as a function of physical activity. (Courtesy of Mayer and Bullen; reprinted from Physiological Reviews.)

> I readily become conscious of a feeling of discomfort after a day or two of sitting and reading and I go out to cultivate my potato patch or to hit a hundred golfballs....It is possible now to give a natural drive for physical activity, obvious in childhood, a free rein.... In early childhood we eat and play naturally, each in varying amounts on different days. I guess that play with its physical activity, rather than appetite with consequent food intake, is the control that regulates energy balance. In other words, in childhood we eat and then play, rather than play and then eat. In adult life work, nowadays mainly sedentary, obstructs a rhythm of life, and over the years a natural drive to physical activity may atrophy...In physiological terms this drive must arise somewhere in the central nervous system and be activated by cumulative information reaching the brain from the stores of nutrients in peripheral tissues...(8).

REGULATION OF METABOLISM

There is no doubt that some people need more food to maintain energy balance than others do. Twenty years ago, Widdowson pointed out the large variation in intake among people of like age, sex, and occupation, noting that the highest consumer in such a group eats twice as much as the lowest. Some people are better adapters than others, being able to maintain weight (or to gain or lose less than is commensurate) in spite of large changes in intake of energy-yielding foods. Difference in the metabolic efficiency with which food is utilized is thought to be a principal cause of these differences among people. In simplest terms this means there is diversion of metabolic traffic over pathways that are more or less exothermic, where more or less adenosine triphosphate (ATP) is generated in relation to heat lost. The least efficient system is one where *no* ATP (or other useful product) is formed; these are called futile cycles.

The most convincing evidence that these differences among people have a metabolic basis—rather than being due, for example, to unnoticed differences in muscle tension, hours of sleep and rest, and the like— comes from studies of animals. Some strains of animals have slimmer or fatter body conformation (lard hogs versus bacon hogs, for example) and gain weight with different feed efficiency, an important economic factor in animal production. Inbreeding has also produced genetically obese rats and mice, which have provided many useful clues in research concerning obesity.

Before the development of agricultural technology, a tendency to store fat might have had survival value, protecting the individual against starvation during the "hungry" season. Environmental and cultural selection may have led to accumulation of a "thrifty" trait in the gene pool, more noticeable in some family lines and racial groups than others. Exposure to cold is the only environmental situation in which built-in inefficiency would be advantageous, favoring a well-developed system for nonshivering thermogenesis. A thicker layer of subcutaneous fat would also be beneficial for insulation against the cold, so efficient energy-storage systems would not be inconsistent with the presence of specialized cold-responsive tissue (brown adipose tissue). Inefficiency in other nonspecialized tissues would, however, be inconsistent with survival in food-limited societies, a human condition for millenia of evolution.

The concept of wasteful metabolism is not new. In 1902, Neuman put forward the theory of *luxuskonsumption* to explain maintenance of energy balance without change in body weight despite dietary excess. Over the years this theory has had its advocates (9) and opponents (10). Chief criticisms of experiments purporting to prove induced thermogenesis center on validity of measures of food intake and on energetics of tissue synthesis. For example, Sims and coworkers fed Vermont prisoners enormously and found large discrepancies between excess food given and weight gain, but critics questioned the control of intake and activity. A later study by this same group featured better control (prisoners were confined to a hospital ward) but still could not assure that all of the food given was consumed. Critics note that computed energy balances did not figure the energy cost of converting carbohydrate to tissue fat, and when this cost is allowed for the remaining discrepancy is small. No real discrepancy between energy fed and gained by Vermont prisoners was found when the extra energy was given in the form of fat. Earlier studies by Miller and Mumford also indicate that the divergence between intake and weight change is greatest when the diet is very high in carbohydrate and low in protein. Body fat is more efficiently laid down from dietary fat than carbohydrate.

In the final analysis, the crux of the argument centers on a small discrepancy in the energy account. Critics believe the discrepancy is within the range of experimental error; proponents believe the discrepancy represents excess thermogenesis, luxuskonsumption. The weight of evidence indicates that metabolism does rise and fall with sustained increases and decreases in intake of energy-yielding foods. Carefully controlled studies at the University of California in which intake of nonobese men was increased by only 15 percent show a gradual rise in basal metabolism rate (BMR) per kg body weight (an important consideration in studies where body mass is changing) amounting to 5 percent or less of the initial value (11). This difference would be undetectable in a normal population study and could be proved in the case cited only by having a very large number of measurements. Animal studies, and some but not all human studies, find increased thermogenesis in relation to eating (dietary induced thermogenesis, or DIT) in habitually overfed individuals. In some human studies, the increase in DIT was augmented by exercise. The site and pathways of increased thermogenesis are unknown. Possibilities are brown adipose tissue, thyroid hormone, and/or insulin. Much is yet to be learned from this active field of research.

A few other observations are worth noting. The frequency of eating affects nutrient utilization in experimental animals, and similar conclusions have been drawn from observations of weight changes in humans. Administration of large meals at infrequent intervals is associated with decreased energy need for weight maintenance, increased deposition of body fat, and decreased deposition of body protein, as compared with a "nibbling" pattern of food intake (frequent, small meals). It is known that the body adapts to long-term food deprivation (days) in such a way that a second period of fasting causes less loss of weight and acidosis than does the first fasting experience. It may be that the altered use of nutrients by animals fed large meals infrequently represents comparable adaptation to short-term food deprivation (hours).

Two commonly used drugs, caffeine (12) and tobacco (13), are known to be stimulants of metabolism. Energy expenditure was found to be 16 percent higher in a two-hour period following consumption of regular coffee (100 mg caffeine) than after consumption of decaffeinated coffee (6 mg caffeine). The effect of smoking is disputed, but reliable evidence indicates that metabolism is elevated about 10 percent in the thirty- to forty-five-minute period after smoking a cigarette. It is well known that smokers gain weight when they stop smoking, usually leveling off at about 3 to 4 kg above previous weight. At the new stable weight, intake of energy-yielding foods is usually somewhat lower than previously, suggesting a true difference in metabolism. Women who smoke gain less weight during pregnancy than nonsmokers and have smaller babies.

INFLUENCE OF ENERGY STATUS IN EARLY LIFE

There is even a possibility that obesity may relate to prenatal food availability. A study of nineteen-year-old men born during the Dutch famine of World War I shows that obesity rates depend upon the time of exposure to food deprivation. Deprivation during the last trimester of pregnancy and the first few months of life is associated with a low incidence of adult obesity, indicating that this may be a critical period for development of adipose cells. Obesity rates are higher for those whose deprivation occurred during the first half of pregnancy, the period of hypothalamic differentiation. The degree or duration of deprivation in utero is not known, nor is the later dietary history of these men; nevertheless, the results of this study warrant further study in animals.

Yet another theory may have important implications for the problem that obese people have in staying lean once they have reduced and for the need for a preventive approach to obesity. Studies of adipose tissue of normal, fat, and formerly fat people show that the tissue of the obese has more cells than normal. It is thought that these cells, when lacking in fat, send chemical messages that elicit eating behavior. Thus, if fewer cells were formed—that is, if children were not allowed to become fat by overeating in infancy and the early years of childhood—there would not be a reservoir of demanding adipose cells.

IDEAL WEIGHT

Everyone should check his or her body weight occasionally with some tables that show normal weight for height. Tables based on the actual average weights of the population at various ages are not good for this purpose, because so many otherwise normal people show some degree of overweight that these figures do not represent the optimum weight so far as health is concerned. (Fig. 7–3). Physicians and life insurance companies now think that, for the sake of health and longevity, it is best to weigh no more in the years after age twenty-five or thirty than is normal for height and body build at that age. Table 7–1 gives desirable weights that men and women should maintain at twenty-five years of age and in later life. An individual who weighs more than 20 percent above the norm for his or her height is classed as *obese.*

Weight tables provide a convenient guide to desirable body weight, but what is of real concern is the amount of fat in the body. A football player may be distinctly overweight for height, yet he may be not in the least obese in terms of having excess adipose tissue. Others who are underweight for height may have a larger percentage of adipose tissue than heavier people who are more physically fit. The goal of any reducing program is not to normalize body weight arbitrarily but to reduce to normal the amount of stored fat in the body.

Body fat is stored mainly in the specialized cells of *adipose tissue.* When filled with fat, adipose tissue has about 85 to 90 percent fat, 2 percent protein, and 10 percent water. This fat is formed in the cells from precursors brought in the blood, and fatty acids are released from the cells when there is a demand for energy. Excess fat may be stored in adipose tissue cells that are not yet filled, or new cells will be made if necessary. Insulin is required to store fat, and adrenal and pituitary hormones are involved in mobilizing it in response to need. The energy value of adipose tissue is about 8 kcal per gram or 3600 kcal per pound (33.5 MJ per kg).

A number of ways to measure body fatness have been developed. Many of these are complex, involving use of radioisotopes or elaborate equipment, but others are relatively simple and ingenious. Fat has a lower specific gravity than water; hence, excess tissue fat tends to buoy up the body when immersed in water. This principle has been used to determine the ratio of lean to fatty tissues in the body. The body weight, taken when immersed in water and divided by the weight of the water displaced, is a true index of the relative amount of body fat. Obviously, a low specific gravity of the body indicates a relatively large proportion of body fat, and vice versa.

Estimates of the amount of subcutaneous fat in various parts of the body may also be made from the thickness of folds of skin and

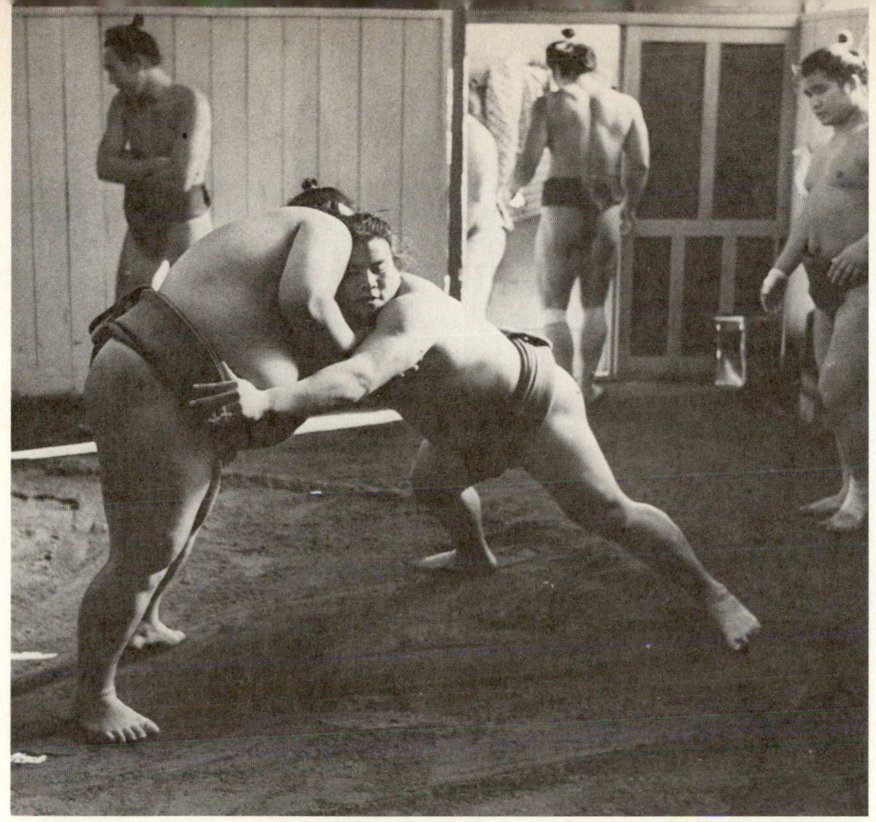

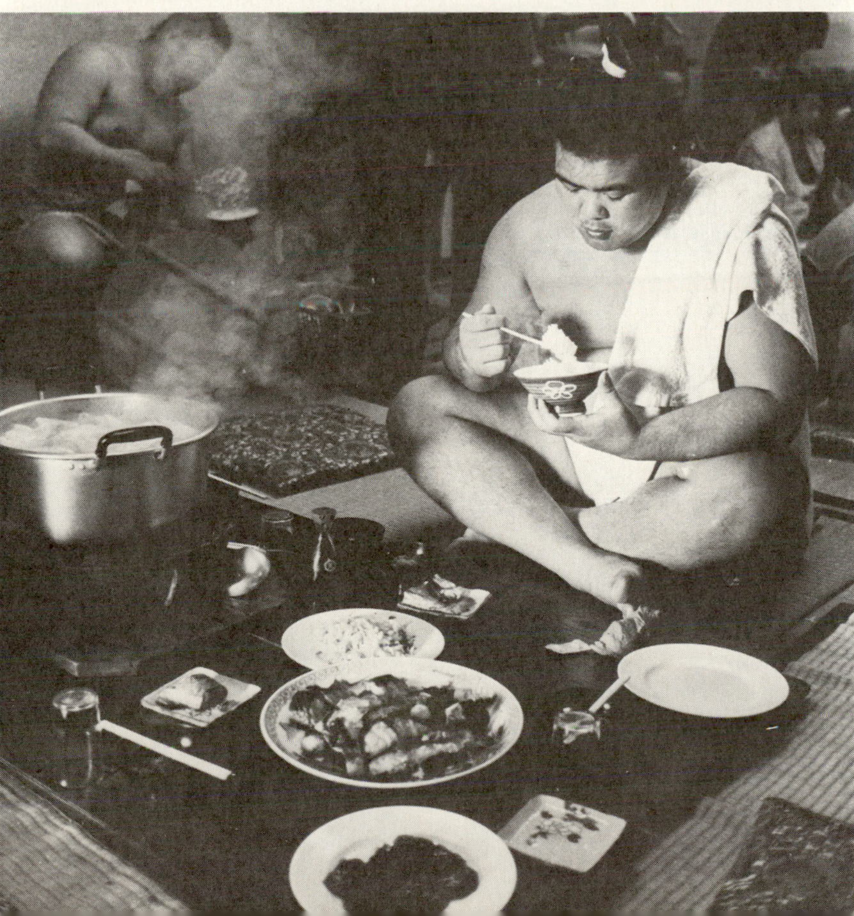

Figure 7–3 What weight is regarded as ideal or optimal depends on the definition of those terms. Usually we mean best mortality and morbidity. But powerful Sumo wrestlers in Japan may struggle for hours at a stretch; afterwards they replace the energy with a no less powerful meal. (Photo courtesy of WHO/E. Schwab.)

Table 7–1 GUIDELINES FOR BODY WEIGHT

Metric

	Men Weight (kg)[a]			Women Weight (kg)[a]		
Height[a] (m)	Average	Acceptable weight		Average	Acceptable weight	
1.45				46.0	41	53
1.48				46.5	42	54
1.50				47.0	43	55
1.52				48.5	44	57
1.54				49.5	44	58
1.56				50.4	45	58
1.58	55.8	51	64	51.3	46	59
1.60	57.6	52	65	52.6	48	61
1.62	58.6	53	66	54.0	49	62
1.64	59.6	54	67	55.4	50	64
1.66	60.6	55	69	56.8	51	65
1.68	61.7	56	71	58.1	52	66
1.70	63.5	58	73	60.0	53	67
1.72	65.0	59	74	61.3	55	69
1.74	66.5	60	75	62.6	56	70
1.76	68.0	62	77	64.0	58	72
1.78	69.4	64	79	65.3	59	74
1.80	71.0	65	80			
1.82	72.6	66	82			
1.84	74.2	67	84			
1.86	75.8	69	86			
1.88	77.6	71	88			
1.90	79.3	73	90			
1.92	81.0	75	93			

Nonmetric

	Men Weight (lb)[a]			Women Weight (lb)[a]		
Height[a] (ft, in)	Average	Acceptable weight		Average	Acceptable weight	
4 10				102	92	119
4 11				104	94	122
5 0				107	96	125
5 1				110	99	128
5 2	123	112	141	113	102	131
5 3	127	115	144	116	105	134
5 4	130	118	148	120	108	138
5 5	133	121	152	123	111	142
5 6	136	124	156	128	114	146
5 7	140	128	161	132	118	150
5 8	145	132	166	136	122	154
5 9	149	136	170	140	126	158
5 10	153	140	174	144	130	163
5 11	158	144	179	148	134	168
6 0	162	148	184	152	138	173
6 1	166	152	189			
6 2	171	156	194			
6 3	176	160	199			
6 4	181	164	204			

[a]Height without shoes, weight without clothes.
Adapted from the recommendations of the Fogarty Center conference on obesity, 1973.

fat pinched up in several places (the upper back, abdomen, chest, arms, or legs), as measured accurately by calipers (Fig. 7–4). By mathematical equations, body fat may be estimated from skinfold measurements. Skin measurement can also be used to diagnose obesity (and undernutrition) by using an arbitrary cutoff point for thickness. For example, a nineteen-year-old male may be classed as obese if a value greater than 100 is obtained when triceps fatfold (mm) is divided by body weight (lbs) and multiplied by 1000. The "educated pinch" has even been suggested for the ordinary layman as a general guide in judging overweight (obesity). If such a skinfold proves to be over an inch (25 mm) in thickness, weight reduction is indicated. Body fatness may also be calculated from "envelope measurements" of the body (torso, legs, and arms, especially circumference of thigh and buttocks).

Probably the simplest method devised for rating accurately the degree of obesity is the Body Mass Index. This index is easily computed by dividing the body weight by the square of height (W/H^2) (Fig. 7–5).

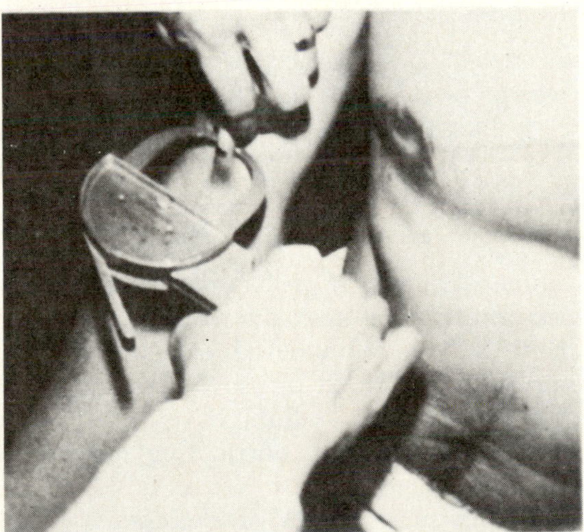

Figure 7–4 Measurement of skinfold thickness. The amount of fat in the body can be estimated reliably from precise measurements of the thickness of the layer of fatty tissue beneath the skin. (Courtesy of Department of Nutritional Sciences, University of California, Berkeley.)

OVERWEIGHT

Obesity is prevalent in all affluent societies. Many people accept as normal the gradual accumulation of weight that so often comes in the later years of life. Not all those overweight are middle-aged—some young people, children, and even babies are overweight. The fact that there are obese nutritionists and physicians indicates that neither nutrition information nor knowledge of health risks guarantees adequate control of body weight. Obesity has proved resistant to efforts aimed at either prevention or cure.

Disadvantages and Dangers

Obesity carries with it increased risk of illness and death from a number of diseases: heart disease, high blood pressure, stroke, kidney disease, gallstones, cirrhosis of the liver, and diabetes. Overweight people have difficulties with their feet and back because of the added burden of weight on the skeleton, and they have, as well, an increased incidence of gout and arthritis. They suffer from shortness of breath, especially on exertion, and have increased surgical risk. Western culture favors a lean look, so the obese are handicapped socially, in employment, and in school admission.

The health hazards that accompany overweight—greater incidence of heart and circulatory diseases and of diabetes—are naturally increased as weight increases and with advancing years (Fig. 7–6). The best mortality statistics overall are for people whose weight is between 90 and 120 percent of the ideal weight for their height.

Several of the diseases associated with obesity are related to one another. The circulatory disorder atherosclerosis (see Chap. 3), is common in diabetics; people with atheroscle-

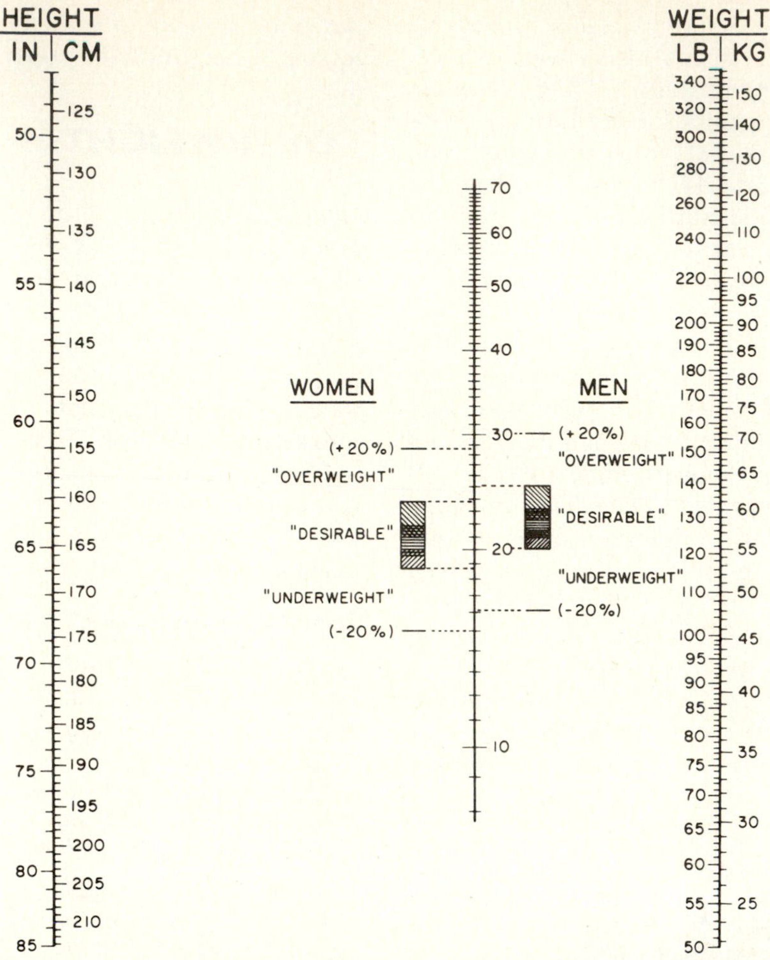

Figure 7–5 Nomograph for body mass index (kg/m^2). The ratio weight/height^2 is read from the central scale. The ranges suggested as "desirable" are from life insurance data. (From Thomas, A. E., McKay, D. A., and Cutlip, M. B.: Amer. J. Clin. Nutr., 29:302, 304, 1976.)

rotic heart disease often have high blood pressure (hypertension); and in both instances they are likely to be obese. Not all people who have these disorders are obese, however, and not all people who are obese will inevitably develop these diseases.

High blood pressure is thought to have several causes, mainly renal and endocrine in origin. Some hypertensive patients are thin, but the incidence is markedly increased in persons who are obese, for reasons that are obscure. The trait is familial, and environmental factors probably play a role in permitting the potential tendency to become manifest. Epidemiological evidence linking salt and high blood pressure is discussed in Chapter 14, but sodium is only one of a number of possible contributing factors, as has been noted.

Factors such as lack of exercise, overeating, and stress and strain of life decidedly affect the incidence of high blood pressure and heart disease. This was strikingly shown in a joint study by investigators at Harvard

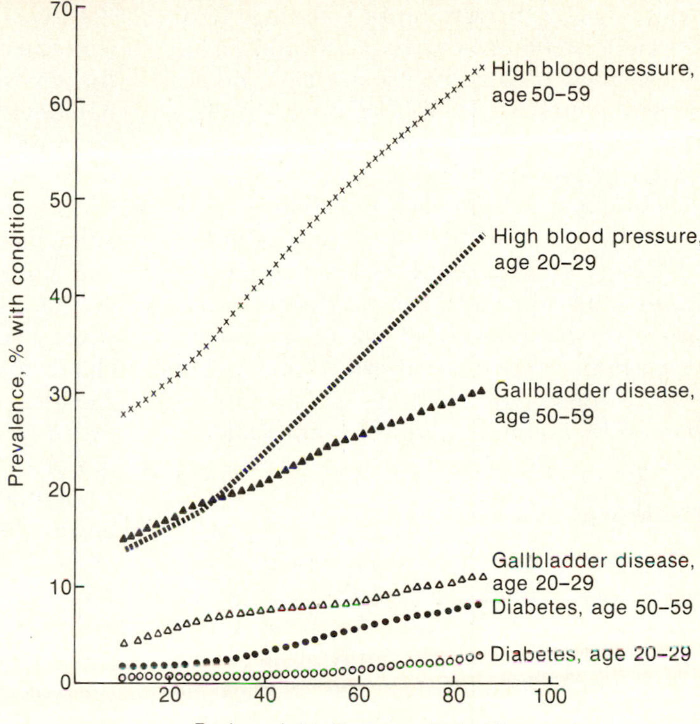

Figure 7–6 Obesity and age-specific occurrence in women with diabetes, gallbladder disease, and high blood pressure. Data are for many thousands of weight-conscious women enrolled in a therapeutic TOPS program. (From Rimm, A. A., et al.: Public Health Rpt., 90:44–51, 1975.)

University and at Trinity College, Dublin. They collected data on Irish-born men who had emigrated to the Boston area and their brothers who had remained in Ireland, chiefly engaged in agriculture. Although the diet of those in Ireland was higher in total energy-yielding foods, starchy foods, and animal fats (almost twice as much butter), the incidence of heart disease was considerably higher among the urbanized, sedentary American residents than among their paired brothers, who had been living a more active life. Several other studies involving comparisons of occupational groups within a country emphasize the importance of physical activity and energy balance: San Francisco longshoremen have a lower incidence of heart disease than do warehouse workers, London bus conductors than drivers, and British postmen than bank clerks.

Diabetes, as it occurs in young people, is a severe disorder. (See Chap. 2.) Juvenile diabetes is quite different from the condition that develops at or past middle age, most commonly in obese people. The reason obesity causes or accompanies maturity-onset diabetes in genetically predisposed individuals is uncertain. It is known that the disorder is less likely to occur in people who remain lean, and the mild form may be controlled simply by reducing weight to normal and increasing the amount of physical exercise. There is no clear evidence that dietary carbohydrate in general or sucrose in particular is causally related to diabetes, although that relation has been suggested. Normalization of body weight and restriction of sugar in the diet are important aspects of dietary treatment.

Obesity in children is common and presents special problems. It handicaps a child socially and in games or sports that involve moving mass in running or jumping. If overweight is not corrected and children are not trained to practice dietary and physical activity patterns that will keep weight down to normal for their height, they will very likely go on to become obese adults. A weight-control regimen for a child must be carefully planned to decrease the intake of energy-yielding foods while liberally furnishing all nutrients needed for growth—proteins, minerals, and vitamins. Dietary restriction cannot be drastic, and weight readjustment for children is best accomplished by holding weight constant while linear growth proceeds.

Principal Cause

Probably the chief causes of moderate obesity are overeating and inactivity, usually in combination. This is what Mayer has termed "regulatory obesity" (in contrast to "metabolic obesity" of genetic or biochemical nature). Most Americans exercise little. They tend toward spectator sports, riding in cars, and sitting while they work. They tend to adjust the temperature of their homes and places of work and entertainment and to dress in a way that minimizes the amount of energy used in body temperature regulation. They don't like cold showers. If appetite and former food habits encourage one to take more food than needed, fat accumulates. Only a relatively small excess of food daily will in time add considerable weight. Excessive portions of food or fat and sugar added to foods may add up to several kilograms in a few months, or 9 to 13 kg extra weight in a few years. For instance, the addition of one martini or 28 gm milk chocolate a day adds the energy equivalent of 0.45 kilograms of adipose tissue in three weeks. But, of the two factors—food and exercise—exercise is probably the more important. The difference need not be large: just thirty minutes of walking each day in three weeks equals the energy content of 0.45 kilograms of adipose tissue.

Fatness does run in families, but the cause is not necessarily genetic. The dominance of the environmental factors over heredity is demonstrated by S. Garn's analysis of data from the extensive studies of the population of Tecumseh, Michigan (14). Garn and his colleagues found essentially the same correlation between skinfold thickness of related and unrelated persons living together (biological and adoptive siblings, husbands and wives, parents and biological and adoptive children). On genetic grounds, the correspondence between dizygotic twins and between twins and siblings should be the same; but the correlation between the twins was much higher (0.7 vs. 0.3), suggesting that the more closely shared environment of the twins altered the expected relationship. Garn concludes that "given fatness similarities between pet-owners and their pets or the far greater fatness similarities between dizygotic twins as compared with siblings, we need not search long for putative control mechanisms of cellular, endocrine, or neurohumoral origin."

Psychologists have concluded that some persons overeat to compensate for emotional insecurity or frustration. Such people need to have the cause of their craving for food resolved and to be made aware of the nature and disadvantages of their behavior. People must recognize the advantages to be gained from changing food habits before they are willing to do so, and they must learn to control those aspects of their own behavior that lead to an imbalance between intake and output.

Modern research suggests that obesity may not be a single entity but, rather, one symptom that has many causes. Knowledge of these causes may one day yield effective methods of therapy. Whatever the contributing causes, the final one is always the same: The food intake of that individual is greater than his or her need. Prevention shows more promise than therapy in dealing with the problem.

UNDERWEIGHT

Being underweight carries its own risks, especially if it is accompanied by deficiency in essential nutrients.

Malnutrition versus Underweight

The terms malnutrition and underweight are not synonymous, though the two conditions often occur together. Underweight results from an intake of energy-yielding foods insufficient to meet the body's needs, just as overweight results from a surplus intake of such foods in relation to need. *Malnutrition* is a broader term: It means, literally, "bad" (from *mal*) nutrition," whether as a result of deficiency or excess of one or more nutrients in relation to the tissue needs. The obese person is overnourished with respect to energy; the emaciated person is undernourished. Either may also be malnourished relative to other nutrients.

Overweight malnourished persons, either children or adults, usually have enough subcutaneous fat so that they may look well nourished to the superficial observer. This combination of fatness and poor vitamin-mineral status may be found among the poor, whose low income forces them to fill up on the cheap, high-energy foods (white flour, sugar, and lard) and does not allow them to buy enough of the body-building foods (milk, fruits, and vegetables). Such malnourished individuals are also found among the well-to-do who simply prefer to eat the wrong types of food.

Undernutrition may result from many different causes. Generally, inadequate food intake is the main reason, but there may be a number of contributing factors. Digestion and absorption may be poor. There may be physical injury or organic disease or infection, which affects nutrient utilization, loss, or requirements, or any combination of these.

A pathological fear of being fat leads to severe self-imposed dieting and weight loss in the emotional disorder *anorexia nervosa.* This disorder has been diagnosed in both men and women, but is most prevalent in young women, about age sixteen to eighteen years or slightly older. It used to be regarded as a rare eating disorder, but either it is on the rise or it is being detected more often than in the past. In London, prevalence has been reported to be 1 out of 550 girls aged sixteen to eighteen in state-supported schools and 1 out of 100 in private schools. A Canadian study of ballet students found 6.5 percent to be anorectic. Social pressures toward thinness appear to be particularly troubling to adolescents, and large numbers of them believe themselves to be fat when, in fact, they are not. Pressures are particularly severe for those whose career interests lie in occupations where extreme thinness is now regarded as the ideal such as dancing and modeling. Anorectics are preoccupied with food and often spend a great deal of time cooking food that they may give away or feed to pets. Some victims go on eating binges, which they then follow with self-induced vomiting or overdosage with laxatives or enemas. This severe condition requires medical intervention, and like obesity, it is resistant to treatment.

In summary, anything that interferes with the intake of some essential material, makes the total amount of intake low, or hinders the normal processes by which food is utilized in the body tends to bring about a condition of undernourishment, which will be more or less severe depending on the extent and duration of the conditions.

Underweight and Health Status

Simply being underweight, without lack of minerals and vitamins, may or may not be serious, depending on the degree of underweight and the age at which it occurs. Life insurance statistics show that for older adults a slight degree of underweight relative to the population average weight (which, as has been noted, is heavier than the ideal weight) increases health and life expectancy. This does not mean underweight to the point of emaciation. Some older people, especially those of small means, live on such abstemious diets that serious malnutrition results. It is with children and young adults, however, that marked underweight is almost sure to be a disadvantage. In general, it may be said that to be more than 10 percent below the standard range of weight for one's height and type of body build[3] usually means lowered vigor.

It is advantageous to have some stores of fatty tissue, as well as reserves of the other nutrients, to draw on in times of extra stress. The very thin person tends to chill easily, owing to lack of a normal layer of subcutaneous fat and lowered basal metabolism. Such persons are more susceptible to infections, and they are disinclined to physical exertion, for their bodies are conserving energy. This state is what is called living on a lower plane of nutrition.

Chronic Energy Shortage and Starvation

The disadvantages of living on a low level of energy intake were evident in experiments on otherwise healthy people. Benedict and Keys studied the effect of sharply reduced intake (1950 kcal in Benedict's group, 1550 kcal in Keys's experiments) on healthy young men who had previously taken well over 3000 kcal daily. Benedict's men reported that they felt well but had less energy and had to drive themselves to do their accustomed tasks, and they tired sooner in various work tests. Keys's subjects subsisted on the low level of intake for six months and developed more serious symptoms—depression, anemia, edema, slowing of heartbeat, and others. They showed marked lack of endurance, tired easily, and reduced unnecessary movements to a minimum. Both groups reported lowered libido, and the sperm quality was poor in Keys's subjects. (With severe weight loss, women become amenorrheic.) When returned to their former level of energy consumption they recovered their vitality, but it took considerable time to restore them to buoyant health (15).

Severe undernutrition in previously well-nourished people comes about when there is famine because of crop failure or war, or it may result from serious diseases of the gastrointestinal tract that impair digestion or absorption of food, or from anorexia nervosa. Loss of about 25 percent of body weight is without serious permanent damage in healthy adults of normal weight, but recovery from losses on the order of 50 percent is difficult or impossible. In Europe, during and after the long period of underfeeding in World War II, there was an increase of stillbirths and of babies who died soon after birth (Chap. 22). Wastage of muscle, edema, and lessened digestive capacity were seen in the severe cases. Tuberculosis and other infectious diseases flared up among both young mothers and children during the postwar years. Even today, among the poor populations of Asia, the Middle East, Africa, and South America, there are millions who exist on a very low nutritional level, and we see the results in general misery and disease (Fig. 7–7).

Undernutrition and Infection

Well-nourished people do not escape infection just because they are well nourished; good nutrition does not confer any sort of immunity. It is true, though, that nutrition must be satisfactory to maintain the skin and internal membranes that are the first barrier to invading organisms, and that secondary infections do follow deficiency (of vitamin A, for example, as discussed in Chap. 9). In

[3]The average weight and height of boys and girls at given ages are found in the Appendix.

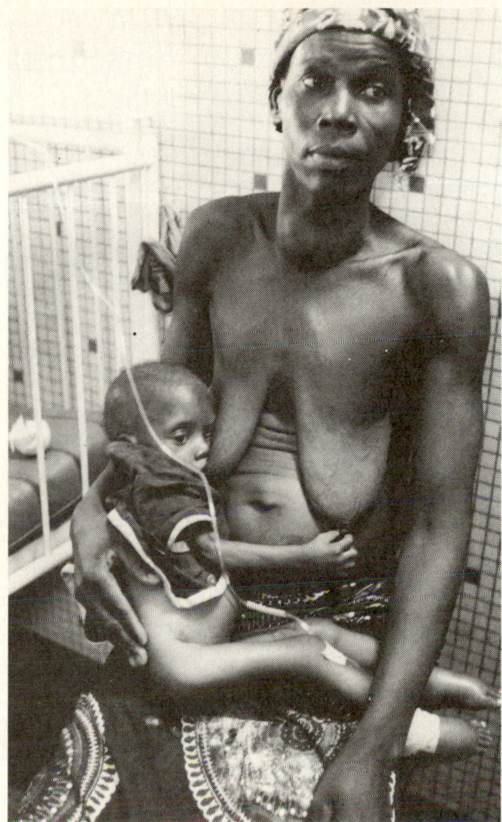

Figure 7–7 Nutrition and infection. These two conditions are a deadly combination. Each aggravates the other, resulting in alarming mortality and morbidity patterns among children in developing countries. Common diseases like diarrhea, respiratory infections, and measles can be fatal for malnourished children. On the other hand, these infections are frequently the main cause of severe malnutrition in children living on a bare subsistence diet, but one that could be adequate for their health if they were not frequently suffering from them. Promotion of nutrition and control of communicable diseases, implemented together, reinforce each other. (From *Guide to Family Health,* Aug.-Sept., 1976. Courtesy of WHO/E. Mandelmann.)

addition, specific nutrients are needed for formation of the antibodies that are the body's internal protection, and suppression of the immune system has been reported in malnourished children and adults, both in those from poor communities where disease is rampant and in hospitalized patients whose disease process has led to malnutrition.[4]

When the infection is established, nutritional status consistently affects the outcome. Persons who are well nourished are more likely to survive an infection than are those who are undernourished, because the latter's reserves are too low to support them during a prolonged illness involving diminished intake and increased need. In the tropics, seemingly healthy individuals often have malaria parasites in the blood or a large population of worms in the intestine. The people are able to cope with these parasites, almost to live symbiotically, as long as diets are adequate. But when nutritional status falls, the disease overwhelms them.

Infection also conditions nutritional deficiency. Little children whose diets are barely adequate develop obvious cases of marasmus or kwashiorkor as a result of contracting some ordinary childhood disease such as measles, whooping cough, or a nonspecific diarrhea. Their reserves are so low that they cannot tolerate the least additional loss from the intestine, the accelerated metabolism of a mild fever, or a few days of nausea or poor intake of food. The child may die of malnutrition consequent to an infection.

PLANNING THE REDUCING REGIMEN

For the ordinary overweight individual, by far the most satisfactory way to effect weight reduction is simply to cut down sharply on the concentrated energy foods (fats, alcohol, sugars), while maintaining an otherwise well-balanced and adequate diet. Such a diet does

[4]Exceptions to this generalization occur in the case of some viruses, including the leukemia virus. It has been found that animals deficient in some specific nutrients are more, not less, resistant to invasion. See Chapter 11.

not involve actually going hungry. It can be used over fairly long periods without harm, and it can be continued into the postreducing period (by adding limited amounts of the foods of higher energy value) in order to hold the lower weight one has attained by reducing. It should be *inadequate* for body needs *in only one respect*—its *energy* content.

Requirements of a Reducing Diet

The main things to plan for in any reducing diet are the following:

1. low energy content
2. adequate protein, minerals, and vitamins
3. good satiety value

Low Intake of Energy Foods. Obviously, a reducing diet must have relatively low energy content. The rate at which stored fat is lost will depend on the magnitude of the difference between energy intake and expenditure of energy. For best results it is desirable to increase the need for energy by increasing physical activity at the same time as lowering intake. If the diet furnishes 500 to 1000 kcal (2000 to 4000 kJ) less than needed, this should effect a weight loss of about 1.5 to 3 kg a month. The same rate of weight loss could be brought about by swimming a whole hour every day, without altering food intake. A combination of diet low in energy foods plus activity accelerates weight reduction, promotes fitness, and prevents tissues from becoming flabby as fat is lost. Contrary to popular belief, increased activity on the part of sedentary persons does not lead to a counterbalancing increase in food intake.

More drastic reduction of energy intake, of course, causes more rapid weight loss. Diets below 1000 kcal (4000 kJ) are not recommended because they too severely limit the sources of essential nutrients in the diet. Diets above 1600 kcal (6400 kJ) give such slow results that they are discouraging to the average adult woman, although men may show good weight loss at that level of intake.

Not only must the choice of foods be right (avoidance of concentrated energy foods), but the size of portions must be limited. For instance, consider a woman dieting zealously but fitfully who announced she was having a low-energy breakfast of fruit. She consumed a large glass of orange juice (285 gm), two large pears, and a bunch of grapes, which meant an intake of at least 500 kcal. One slice of toast with a *small* portion of butter, one egg, and a small glass of juice (114 gm) would have meant only half as much energy. Thus, even foods described as moderately low in energy can raise the energy intake considerably when taken in large portions.

All between-meal snacks or extras (such as cream, sugar, and salad dressings) taken in or on foods must be counted. This includes cocktails or other alcoholic beverages, because both alcohol and sugar in such drinks furnish energy. A table of approximate caloric content of alcoholic beverages is given in Chapter 3.

The exact distribution of energy among protein, carbohydrate, and fat is not critical, except that protein must be adequate and a certain amount of carbohydrate is desirable. Diets high in protein or fat, or low in carbohydrate, have been suggested as particularly successful in causing weight reduction, but there is no agreement among experts that any of these has special efficacy in the long run. As a practical matter, fats are usually sharply limited. They are such concentrated sources of energy that only a small quantity can be included without raising the energy supply too high.

On a diet inadequate in energy to meet body needs, the body is constantly burning some of its stored fat. Under these conditions, fats may not be completely oxidized, and the acid intermediate products of their metabolism (ketone bodies) may accumulate in the body and cause an acidosis, or ketosis. In a typical study, healthy humans, fed a diet exclusively of protein and fat, lost about 1 kg

(2 lb) daily, but there were large losses of nitrogen and salt in the urine and the subjects experienced symptoms resulting from acidosis (ketosis). These symptoms disappeared promptly when carbohydrate was included in the diet. A recent study involved teenagers fed a diet undesirably low in energy food (about 10 kcal/kg) and 1.5 gm protein per kg body weight in the form of lean beef. The subjects lost 7.4 kg and 6.4 kg during twenty-one-day periods when the diet contained protein plus fat (no carbohydrate) and protein plus carbohydrate, respectively. The small difference in weight lost, 1 kg, was due principally to increased loss of lean body tissue with the fat diet. Lean tissue lost was 0.9 kg with the fat diet and 0.2 kg with the carbohydrate diet (16).

Others seem to have better success with a high-protein, low-carbohydrate diet. Weight loss may be more rapid at first on a low carbohydrate diet, but it makes little difference in the end whether reduction of energy-food intake is brought about by restriction of carbohydrate or fat, in long-term reduction programs.

If small amounts of carbohydrate are included in the reducing diet, acidosis is prevented. An intake of 70 to 100 gm of carbohydrate will suffice. Practically all the energy value of fruits and vegetables and more than half that of skim milk comes from the carbohydrates they contain, so that not very much of the more concentrated carbohydrate foods (bread, cereals) is needed.

Foods that are high in dietary fiber content are lower in energy yield than the more completely absorbed foods, and they are beneficial in maintaining bowel regularity. Unrefined cereals, legumes, potatoes, and other vegetables provide an excellent variety of nutrients, and the carbohydrate allowance should be derived mainly from these sources.

Adequate Nutrients. It is important that the reducing diet provide enough protein for the maintenance and upkeep of body tissues and that the mixture of proteins taken provide all essential amino acids. Adults following a slimming diet should have 1 gm of protein per kilogram of ideal weight and not less than 50 gm daily. Children need a more liberal protein allowance. Naturally, if one cuts down on the foods that are high in refined carbohydrates and fats, a greater proportion of the energy tends to be taken as protein. A reducing diet may well include one liberal serving of fish, poultry, or lean meat per day, with either a small second serving of one of these or eggs or cheese. This, together with milk, cereal grains, and vegetables, provides liberal protein.

The reducing diet should provide the recommended allowance of minerals and vitamins to keep the body in condition. This means that any reducing diet should provide liberally for milk, meat or meat substitutes, and vegetables. The reduced amounts of bread and cereals taken should be whole-grain. Skim milk may be substituted for whole milk (it has only about half the energy value). It will furnish calcium and B vitamins but no fat-soluble vitamins. Vitamin A may come from eggs, liver, and the provitamins in green, leafy, and yellow vegetables. These same foods, plus meats, may also serve to meet the need for iron. Many persons who have half starved themselves in order to lose weight rapidly, or who have followed very one-sided diets, show the bad effects of this mistake in the form of vitamin deficiencies or anemia.

Satiety Value. The satiety value of the diet is important if hunger is to be avoided. Meat, poultry, fish, cheese, and eggs have a high satiety value and should be distributed throughout the three meals of the day. Fatty foods, which leave the stomach most slowly and hence have the highest satiety value, must be kept down to small amounts, but a little oil in salad dressing or a piece of cheese may be included. A small portion of fruit taken at the end of a meal often does much toward making one feel well fed. Imaginative use of herbs and spices enhances appetite appeal. Some people are less troubled with hunger if they have a snack between meals or at bedtime (such as an apple or orange, a few crackers, or skim milk), but these must of course be counted in the total day's energy allowance.

Lists of foods to use in the reducing diet and those that must be avoided if the energy intake is to be kept low enough to cause appreciable weight loss are given in Table 7–2.

Basic Pattern for a Reducing Diet

It is entirely satisfactory to construct one's own reducing diet, using whatever foods are preferred in amounts limited to keep the energy content of the diet down to a level at which satisfactory weight loss will be obtained. In practice, it seems to place too much responsibility on the individual and to be too confusing to leave him or her entirely without guidance in the selection of foods for a reducing diet. Therefore, we believe it advisable to suggest a definite type of meal plan for those who desire to reduce, leaving considerable latitude for variety and choice of foods in making up individual menus. Table 7–3 presents a basic pattern for the reducing diet, with many of the details on how the pattern may be met left open to choice. The acceptance of a diet built around a smaller number of simple foods is of great help in making one contented on a more or less restricted diet. To be always in quest of new food combinations is likely to keep one's mind on food to such an extent that one becomes discontented even with a fairly elaborate diet. The use of a basic food pattern in planning reducing diets may be advantageous in three ways.

1. It permits choice.
2. It guides food selection.
3. It teaches desirable food habits.

All sorts of different menu combinations can be made, if desired, either by altering the foods selected from a given food group or by varying the size of servings as needed to raise or lower the resulting level of energy. Two sample menus for a day, which conform to the basic food pattern, are given in Table 7–4; these are planned to meet the needs of young adults who must eat at least some meals away from home.

If the basic food pattern can be adapted to fit the energy level required to produce satisfactory weight loss, it will help to guard the intake of all nutrients other than energy foods, but it need not be followed slavishly. There will be wide variations among individuals in the restriction needed to produce weight loss, according to the body weight

Table 7–2 FOODS FROM WHICH THE REDUCING DIET SHOULD BE BUILT

Foods To Emphasize	*Foods To Minimize*
Clear soups	Alcoholic beverages
Tea and coffee (without sugar or cream)	Soft drinks with added sugar
Milk (especially skim milk or buttermilk)	Fried foods
Fruits without added sugar	Fatty meats
Watery and fibrous vegetables (especially leafy, green, and yellow vegetables)	Rich dressings, sauces, and gravy
Lean meats, fish, and cottage cheese	Nuts and dried fruits
Plain yogurt	Sugar and sweets
	Cream, fats, and oils

Table 7–3 BASIC PATTERN FOR REDUCING DIET APPROXIMATELY 1100 TO 1400 KCAL (4600–5800 KJ)

Total allowance for the day:

2 cups of milk. Each cup of skim milk provides about 85 kcal (350 kJ). Whole milk yields 165 kcal (690 kJ) per cup. 1 oz of Cheddar cheese substitutes for 1 c of milk.

5 oz of lean meat, fish, or poultry, broiled, boiled, or roasted but not fried. All visible fat should be trimmed. Each ounce supplies about 60 to 80 kcal (250–340 kJ); 1 oz of meat equals 1 egg: 3 sardines; 5 shrimp, clams, or oysters; 1/4 c tuna fish, salmon, crabmeat, or lobster.

2 or more servings of fruit without added sugar. One serving should be citrus or other fruit high in vitamin C. Each portion listed counts as one serving and provides about 40 to 50 kcal (170–200 kJ).

1	Small apple (2 in diameter)	1/2	Small mango
1/2	c Applesauce	1	Medium nectarine
2	Fresh apricots or 4 halves dried	1	Small orange or scant 1/2 c juice
1/2	Small banana	1/3	Papaya
1	c Berries (blackberries, raspberries, strawberries)	1	Medium peach
		1	Small pear
2/3	c Blueberries	1/2	c Cubed pineapple or 1/3 c juice
1/4	Cantaloupe (6 in diameter)		
10	Large cherries	2	Medium plums or prunes
2	Dates	2	Level tbsp raisins
1	Small dried fig	1	Large tangerine
1/2	Grapefruit or 1/2 c juice	1	c Cubed watermelon or one slice 3 in × 1 1/2 in
12	Grapes or 1/4 c juice		
1/4	Honeydew melon (7 in diameter)	2	Tomatoes or 1 c juice

2 or more servings of vegetables. At least one serving should be dark green, leafy vegetable. An average (1/2 c) serving yields 10 to 50 kcal (40–200 kJ). Any vegetable may be used, except peas, corn, and dried beans, which must be substituted for bread. No butter, margarine, salad oil, or regular salad dressing may be added except that included in the total allowance for the day. Lemon juice, vinegar, and low-calorie dressings are acceptable.

3 or 4 servings of whole-grain or enriched bread, or ***substitutes.*** One serving, providing 60 to 80 kcal (250–340 kJ), equals: one slice of bread; one muffin or biscuit (2 in diameter); 1/2 c cooked cereal, rice, macaroni, spaghetti, or noodles; scant 3/4 c dry cereal; 5 saltine crackers; 2 graham crackers; scant 1/2 c peas or cooked dried beans; 1/2 ear corn; small potato (2 in diameter) or 1/2 c mashed; 1 1/2 in cube of sponge or angel food cake without icing.

3 or 4 ***small*** servings of fat. One 50 kcal (200 kJ) serving equals: 1/2 tbsp butter, margarine, vegetable oil, or other clear fat; 1 slice of drained, crisp bacon; 2 level tbsp light cream (sweet or sour); 1 level tbsp cream cheese or French dressing; 5 olives.

Coffee, tea, lemon juice, herbs, bouillon, and other food items of negligible energy content may be used as desired.

and degree of muscular activity. For a 75-kg (165 lb) man who is moderately active, the 1400 kcal (about 5800 kJ) level would represent a severe reduction below estimated energy needed for weight maintenance, while for an elderly sedentary woman 1400 kcal would be nearly all she needed for maintaining weight and she would probably need to curtail intake even below the 1100 kcal (4600 kJ) level.

To decide on an appropriate energy level for the reducing diet, one should first determine how much energy would be needed to maintain weight at the ideal weight for height. The minimum maintenance figure would be about 1.5 times the basal metabolic rate or, roughly, 33 kcal per kilogram of *ideal* weight (15 kcal/lb). To lose weight at the rate of 0.5 to 1.0 kg (1½ lb) per week, this figure should be reduced by 500 kcal/day.

Varying the Energy Level of the Reducing Diet

The diet may be adjusted to any required energy level by reducing or using more of the foods of high or moderate energy value.

Table 7–4 SAMPLE MENU PATTERNS FROM THE BASIC REDUCING DIET

Pattern I		Pattern II
	BREAKFAST	
Orange juice (1/2 c) Poached egg (1) on Whole-wheat toast (1 slice) Coffee, with skim milk (1/2 c)		Branflakes (3/4 c) with Sliced banana (1/2) and Milk (1/2 c)
	LUNCHEON	
Consommé Shrimp Louis (6 shrimp on large bed of mixed greens with 1 tbsp dressing) Small muffin (1) Canteloupe (1/4) Iced tea with lemon		Tuna fish sandwich (1/4 c tuna fish with 2 tsp salad dressing and lettuce on 2 slices whole-wheat bread) Hard-cooked egg Dill pickle, green pepper, celery strips Radish roses Milk (1 c)
	DINNER	
Broiled lamb chop (3 oz) Small baked potato with sour cream (1 tbsp) and chives Buttered (1/2 tsp) green beans Sliced tomatoes Cheese (1 oz) with saltine crackers (5) Coffee, with skim milk (1/2 c)		Frankfurters (2) with Sauerkraut Buttered (1/2 tsp) carrots Strawberries (1 c) with Sponge cake (1 1/2 inch cube) Coffee with evaporated milk (2 tbsp)

(Consult the Table of Nutritive Values of Foods in Average Servings in the Appendix.) Foods should be selected from the different food groups as recommended in the basic pattern for a reducing diet given in Table 7–3, limiting the size or number of servings to attain the desired level of intake of energy foods. The menus given in Table 7–4 illustrate diets ranging from 1100 to 1400 kcal (4600 to 5800 kJ). Even with such limited intake, the meals can be made attractive and hunger-satisfying. They will also meet body needs for most essential nutrients (except energy and iron for women).

The actual twenty-four-hour intake of a weight-conscious physician is presented in Table 7–5. This diet provided 1520 kcal and conformed to present recommendations regarding fat intake. Note, however, that the diet was below the Recommended Dietary Allowances (RDA) in a number of nutrients. The reason for this is evident: The diet included 200 kcal in the form of alcohol, 190 kcal from sucrose in the sweetened fruits in the luncheon salad, and about 250 kcal from salad dressing. More than one-third of the total daily intake of energy foods was derived from these three sources, which make little contribution to vitamin and mineral intake. Significant improvement could have been made by simple changes such as substitution of whole-grain cereal for half of the orange juice at breakfast, a bran muffin and glass of skim milk for the saltines and beer at lunch, and a potato for half of the salad dressing at dinner.

Some people may prefer to take a lighter breakfast, or lunch, or both, and use the energy foods thus saved for a more normal meal with the family at noon or at night. Others may be better able to adhere to the slimming diet if the day's food allowance is

Table 7–5 NUTRIENT CONTENT OF A POORLY SELECTED ENERGY-CONTROLLED DIET

Menu	*Nutrient Yield*	
Breakfast:		
Large glass of orange juice	Energy	1520 kcal
Skim milk	Protein	60 gm
Tea	Fat	50 gm
	Cholesterol	80 mg
	Sucrose	50 gm
Luncheon:		
Split pea soup	Vitamin A	6000 IU
Saltine crackers	Vitamin E	6 mg*
Fruit and cottage cheese salad	Vitamin C	170 mg
Beer (one can)	Thiamin	0.9 mg*
	Riboflavin	1.3 mg*
	Niacin	12 mg*
Dinner:	Vitamin B-6	1.2 mg*
Lean beef steak, small serving	Vitamin B-12	3.5 mcg
Mixed vegetables, seasoned	Folacin, free	0.27 mg
Green salad with dressing (3 tbsp)	Pantothenic acid	3.7 mg
Glass of red wine		
	Sodium	2.5 g
Snack:	Calcium	500 mg*
Small apple	Phosphorus	1000 mg
	Magnesium	200 mg*
	Iron	8 mg*
	Copper	1 mg
	Zinc	10 mg*

*Nutrient is below the RDA for an adult male. Copper and pantothenic acid are also substandard and the Ca/P ratio is 0.5.

divided into five smaller meals (or some reserved for snacks). Care must be taken that the total food taken does not exceed the day's allowance. Some regular system of meals should be adopted and adhered to, for only thus does a reducing diet yield the desired results. Although the level of intake does not have to be *absolutely* the same each day, it is desirable that the meal plan be such that the fluctuations made by choice in foods cause it to vary only within narrow limits, probably not more than 100 to 200 kcal (about 400 to 800 kJ) variations.

When the normal weight is achieved, foods should be added back very gradually, one at a time. Minor increase in weight that is sustained for several days indicates that the additions have been made too rapidly, and the last addition should be deleted. Regular recording of weight is essential as motivation for keeping slim. Experience indicates that very few people who have been truly obese manage to hold to their reduced weight; rather they creep back to the same weight, or more, than they had before they began the reducing regimen. Success is greater if the weight is corrected all the way to the ideal rather than stopping short at some intermediate weight that neither satisfies the ego nor noticeably improves the health status. A vigorous exercise program should be of help, provided the person has found an activity he or she enjoys. No one knows if the common pattern of weight gain-weight loss-weight regain (the pattern that Mayer has called the "rhythm method of girth control") is harmful to humans. A famine-feast regimen does shorten the life span of genetically obese mice more than if they are allowed to remain obese. In the mice, life span is prolonged by sustained weight reduction.

Adjuncts and Fad Diets

Probably no type of quackery is more profitable at present than the special remedies sold to effect weight reduction and various adjuncts supposed to make weight loss easy and safe. They flourish because the American public has become conscious of the need to do something about overweight but still hopes to do it as painlessly as possible. So the public is credulous about remedies and fad diets that promise "You can eat all you want and still lose weight." A manufacturer that makes this promise for a product is usually banking on the fact that the product contains something that reduces appetite. This may be a substance such as cellulose that provides little or no available energy but that helps fill the stomach and satisfy the craving to eat. This type of product is harmless but is expensive and probably ineffective. Other products may contain one of the drugs that depress appetite. There are several that may be prescribed by physicians, but only one or two are allowed to be used without a doctor's prescription. The appetite-depressing drugs in preparations sold on the open market are not potent enough to have any marked effect on appetite, but perhaps taking them has some psychological effect. Truly effective products can be prescribed only by a physician. Administration of "rainbow pills" (usually three—a thyroid hormone, a diuretic agent, and an appetite suppressant) is hazardous to health, and injection of chorionic gonadotropin (CG) derived from the human placenta is ineffective in promoting weight loss.

Remedies that promise to reduce weight merely by the patient's lying on a vibrating "couch," or to reduce weight in special places so that unsightly bulges will disappear, are suspect. The government holds that there is no evidence to show that general weight reduction can be effected by such means alone or that fatty tissue in certain areas can be broken down and gotten rid of by such means as massage. Systematic exercises for certain muscles may firm the muscles and, if accompanied by dietary control, may get rid of extra fat. However, indiscriminate exercising for an overweight individual who is unused to it and may have back troubles or other ailments can do harm. Baths, including steam baths, can effect little weight reduction except through loss of water from the body, and this can quickly be regained merely by drinking water. The only type of bath that can be a useful adjunct to weight reduction is the cold shower or plunge. It increases the basal metabolism considerably for some time, provided the individual reacts well after a cold shower, but it is rather heroic treatment for an overweight person to undergo. Swimming in cold water is an effective way of increasing heat loss and of providing beneficial exercise to improve muscular tone.

Although it is possible to obtain all the nutrients needed in a well-planned reducing diet, without care in planning iron intake will be below the recommended allowance for women. Iron and other supplementary vitamins and minerals may well be a safeguard for persons on drastic or long-continued reducing diets. This is especially true of the fat-soluble vitamins, because fats are sharply curtailed and some persons will not take large amounts of leafy vegetables. In this situation, it is better to buy a reputable vitamin preparation, so that the dosage may be known and controlled. Current faddist publications suggest "orthomolecular aids" for dieting, including pseudonutrients and metabolites such as carnitine, high-chromium yeast, and primrose oil. These recommendations are not scientifically justifiable, and the money spent for them would be better spent on nutritious foods.

Special diets for reducing are quite in vogue. Many popular magazines carry such planned diets, with menus for a week to a full month. It seems remarkable that people should be so eager to follow menu plans made out by someone who cannot know their food preferences or circumstances or what foods can be obtained readily in local markets. Such diets may be relatively expensive and cause extra work, especially if the rest of the family does not wish to eat the same foods as the reducer. The best of these diets are no more effective than any well-planned reducing diet, though they may suggest variety and avoid monotony in the diet.

For other people, there is a special appeal in diets that involve a minimum of preparation, such as the "formula diets," which can be bought already mixed in drugstores and food shops. One may lose weight fairly rapidly by subsisting entirely on such a formula (chiefly milk and/or soy protein), or the formula diet may be substituted for one or two meals a day. With a bit of planning, however, one may select a less monotonous and less expensive diet that has the additional advantage of encouraging the improved food habits so necessary for long-term weight control. A breakfast consisting of an ordinary serving of cereal or a slice of toast, a glass of skim milk, and a small glass of fruit juice is easily prepared, is sound nutritionally, and yields no more energy than does one can or package of most of the formula preparations.

There are also the peculiar diets based on only a few foods, such as the all-fruit diet, the green vegetable diet, the pineapple and lamb chop diet, the raw tomato and hard-boiled egg diet. These appeal to some people either because they are short cuts to reducing or because they are unusual. Such diets are not only monotonous but also are so one-sided that they are sure to be too low in some of the various nutrients.

The "all-protein, modified fast" is the latest entrant in the fad field. Originally, this diet consisted solely of lean meat (supplemented with minerals and vitamins), 400 kcal per day, and was prescribed only under close medical supervision. The theory behind this regimen is that carbohydrate should be avoided so that there is minimal stimulus to insulin secretion and thus less propensity to retain fat and to degrade tissue protein. Many liquid and powdered protein products flooded the market, and their indiscriminate, unsupervised use has led to serious health problems, including several deaths. The Food and Drug Administration has recommended that these products not be used for weight reduction and has asked for their voluntary withdrawal from the market.

Total fasting[5] has been used as a therapeutic measure for grossly obese patients, but it is not to be recommended. Even with large energy reserves available in the body, total lack of food has serious risks. There is loss of potassium and marked loss of sodium with depletion of extracellular fluids, and the kidneys do not adequately remove the nitrogenous end product, uric acid. Some patients have developed gout, and a few have died of heart and liver failure in the course of such treatment.

[5]Fasting means abstention but usually not total food deprivation. Most often the religious injunction is to abstain from meals before a specified time of day or to omit one component (for example, meat). During his fasts, Gandhi took fruit juices and sometimes dried fruits, a sensible procedure because some carbohydrate offsets the more serious effects of fasting.

TREATMENT OF UNDERWEIGHT

In order to be effective, treatment of serious undernutrition must follow two courses:

1. location and removal of the contributory causes
2. improvement of the diet

Under the first heading comes a thorough study of the person's daily program to discover whatever faulty food and health habits there may be, and a general medical examination to see if there are any physical defects that need to be corrected. Often, considerable persistence may be needed to determine all the causes. Overfatigue is one of the most common causes and is easily corrected by longer hours of sleep, rest periods during the day, and reducing the activities that cause fatigue. Poverty is an important contributory factor, especially among the working poor who may have hard physical work to perform and often many mouths to feed from a limited supply of food. Mothers of small children are often overtired, and they do not eat if their children are hungry. Persons with more severe undernutrition often require study by a physician so that the factors responsible for keeping them below par physically may be located and treated.

Providing a suitable diet is perhaps the most important single measure for correcting undernutrition—certainly an adequate food supply is indispensable. Supplements may be prescribed if specific deficiencies of vitamins and minerals exist.

The body may not be able to take full advantage of the diet until all adverse factors are remedied, and the diet given in the meantime should be suited to the physical condition of the individual. Administration of large amounts of food to starved or semistarved persons can have disastrous consequences. The refeeding of concentration camp victims showed that small, frequent feeding of soft, nutritious foods is essential if vomiting, intestinal disturbances, and shock are to be avoided. The weakened organism cannot handle a large metabolic load. The same is true for severely undernourished children.

A body that has been depleted by prolonged underfeeding requires gradually increased feeding and building up in numerous respects. Not only should new deposits of fat be laid down, but also the muscles are in need of protein for repair and enlargement. Reserve stores of vitamins and minerals are used up or lost from the body during semistarvation, and an abundance of nutrients in the diet is a help in the processes necessary for repair after a period of undernutrition. The diet should be designed to promote gain of any needed lean tissue and a desirable amount of fat according to satisfactory health and aesthetic standards. As soon as the physical condition permits, a controlled exercise program should be instituted to increase anabolism and improve the person's sense of well-being.

A diet suitable for building up a body that has suffered for some time from deprivation of food should be planned to provide the following:

1. a high intake of energy-yielding foods—in excess of body needs
2. liberal quantities of high-quality protein
3. an abundant supply of minerals and vitamins

The first requirement is met by including in the diet high-energy foods, especially foods rich in fats and starches, such as butter or margarine, cream, salad dressings, bacon, cereals, bread, cream soups, legumes, nuts, and dried fruits—in short, all foods forbidden to overweight individuals. Filling foods that carry little nourishment (for example, clear soups) should be avoided. Protein of high quality for tissue building and repair is provided by including milk, eggs, and meats as freely as costs permit. Organ meats, such as liver, which are excellent sources of minerals and vitamins, should be eaten frequently. Even though they may seem to increase the bulk of the diet, plenty of fruits and vegetables should be included for their content of minerals and vitamins. Milk, eggs, and whole-grain bread and cereals are also valuable sources of minerals and vitamins.

The diet should provide energy in excess of body needs by at least 500 to 1000 kcal (2000 to 4000 kJ). The intake should exceed body needs by one-half to one-third the energy required for maintenance—for example, a person who needs 2100 kcal for maintenance should consume approximately 2600 to 3100 kcal when trying to gain weight. It is often necessary to force oneself to take food in excess of appetite. It is probably easier to accomplish this if the food is divided into more frequent meals, about five to seven a day, taken by clock time rather than by hunger or appetite.

It is easy to increase the energy intake considerably by such devices as an extra square of butter or fortified margarine at each meal (about 220 kcal), liberal use of cream, bacon, and salad dressings (1 Tbsp mayonnaise, 2 Tbsp thick cream, or 2 heaping Tbsp whipped cream each furnishes about 100 kcal), and supplementary nourishment between meals and at bedtime.

The best foods to use for the midmorning or midafternoon lunch are dairy products and fruit juices. These can be served in many combinations—for example, plain cold milk enriched with cream, hot malted milk or milk flavored with chocolate or cocoa, egg-nog, or beaten egg in fruit juice, and plain fruit juices with high-energy content (apple, grape, nectars).

An illustrative menu is given in Table 7–6. The approximate amount of energy furnished is included to show how rapidly the energy value of the diet mounts when fats and concentrated starchy foods are included. The meals alone, as planned in this diet, furnish over 3100 kcal, or 1000 kcal in excess of the energy needs of a 55-kg young woman (2100 kcal) without seeming unduly bulky. Supplementary nourishment between meals (as indicated) may be used to increase intake by another 500 kcal.

The success of any regimen for increasing weight depends chiefly on persuading the individual to accept a high-energy diet, extra rest, and relaxation. Those who have little appetite or have developed fears that foods cause digestive distress must often force themselves to take food in excess of their natural desires at first. If they do so, the general condition usually improves to such an extent that both the appetite and digestion return to normal. Taking vitamins in tablet form may stimulate appetite and improve well-being if the diet has previously been deficient in those nutrients.

Rapid gains in weight should not be the main objective of the program, because such gains are usually due solely to the deposition of fat. Muscle development is favored by a more gradual gain in weight on a diet containing plenty of protein (milk, eggs, and meat). Some form of regular exercise is the best way to build muscles.

QUESTIONS

1. Over what periods of time is energy balance regulated? Where is the regulatory center located? How was this proved to be the regulatory center? What changes in the body activate the center? What mechanisms are involved in long-term regulation of energy balance? How does the GI tract participate in regulation of energy balance?

2. If you were a nutritionist or a physiologist, what question relating to regulation of food intake would you wish to investigate? What factors do you think might affect a person's preference for specific foods, other than the ones discussed

Table 7–6 SAMPLE MENU FOR A WOMAN WHO WISHES TO GAIN WEIGHT

	kcal
Breakfast	
Orange juice 6 oz	80
Oatmeal (2/3–3/4 c cooked), with sliced banana (1/2)	115
Cream, (half-and-half) 1/4 c	80
Poached or soft-boiled egg	80
Bacon, 3 slices	155
Whole-wheat toast, 2 slices	120
Butter or margarine, 1 tbsp	100
Jam, 1 tbsp	55
Coffee, with sugar	45
	830
Midmorning	
Apple, 1 (medium)	90
Lunch	
Lettuce wedge, with sliced tomato and avacado (1/4)	95
French dressing, 1 tbsp	60
Creamed chicken (3/4 c), on slice of toast (1)	370
Hard roll, whole-wheat, 1	60
Butter or margarine, 2 tsp	65
Ice cream, 1/2 c	135
Sweetened strawberries	50
Milk, 8 oz	165
	1000
Midafternoon	
Chocolate milk, 1 c	190
Dinner	
Cream of asparagus soup, 3/4 c	130
Crackers, 2	45
Cottage cheese (1/4 c) and fruit cocktail (1/2 c) salad, with 2 tsp mayonnaise	165
Roast lamb, 4 oz	210
Mint jelly, 1 tbsp	55
Baked potato (1 medium)	95
Butter, 1 tbsp	100
Peas, 1/2 c	55
Lemon meringue pie (1/6 of 9 in pie)	360
Coffee, with sugar	45
	1260
Evening	
Milk	165
Sugar cookie	90
	255
Total—approximately	3600

in this chapter? What factors might affect his or her intake of food?

3. How may the energy value of foods be determined? Why is the physiological energy value of the nutrients somewhat less than their value as determined in the bomb calorimeter? (Refer to Chap. 2.) What types of food are high in energy value? Low in energy value?

4. Give the general energy value per gram of pure protein, carbohydrate, and fat. Calculate the energy value of 100 grams of each of the foods whose composition is given below (by multiplying the grams of protein, fat, and carbohydrate each by the proper energy value per gram and adding these figures).

	Protein gm	*Fat gm*	*Carbo-hydrate gm*
100 gm of white bread contains	*8.7*	*3.2*	*50.5*
100 gm of butter or margarine contains	*0.6*	*81.0*	*0.4*
100 gm of raw cabbage contains	*1.3*	*0.2*	*5.4*

5. Using the food-energy values in Appendix 2, plan a one-day menu that has as much energy as your own twenty-four-hour resting metabolism. (Refer to Chap. 6.) What can you add if you sit for sixteen hours and sleep eight hours in a day? What activity could you add to earn a piece of pie?

6. Give four reasons why persons become overweight. How do you tell how much overweight a person is, and what are the dangers and difficulties of excess weight?

7. Is there any way (or ways) to reduce weight except by restriction of calories in the diet? What foods should be avoided or used only in small amounts in a reducing diet, and why? What foods may be used in quantity, and why? In which nutritive factor (or factors) must the reducing diet be low, and in which should it be adequate or better than adequate? Why? What food groups in the diet assure its adequacy?

8. Following the general meal pattern in Table 7–3, plan a reducing diet that furnishes about 1400 kcal. Revise this diet to drop out 400 kcal.

9. What are the health hazards associated with obesity? With underweight? Are fat people all well nourished? Explain your answer.

10. What are the essential requirements for an effective diet for putting on weight? What kind of a regimen reinforces the good effects of the diet? What benefits may be expected from such a diet and regimen?

11. Plan a fattening and body-building diet that furnishes 3500 kcal for a person with good appetite and digestion. Modify it to give the same energy value for a person whose appetite is poor.

12. Compare your weight with the values given in Table 7–1. What percentage over- or underweight are you? How much will your weight change if you hold all other factors constant but add one 12-oz can of beer each day? Play tennis for thirty minutes?

References

1. Jordan, H.: Voluntary intragastric feeding: oral and gastric contributions to food intake and hunger in man. J. Comp. Physiol. Psychol., *68:*498, 1969.
2. Bray, G. A.: Regulation of energy balance: studies on genetic, hypothalamic and dietary obesity. Proc. Nutr. Soc., *41:*95, 1982.
3. Anderson, G. H., and Blendis, L. M.: Plasma neutral amino acid ratios in normal man and in patients with hepatic encephalopathy: correlations with self-selected protein and energy consumption. Amer. J. Clin. Nutr., *34:*377, 1981.
4. Rolls, B. J., Rowe, E. A., and Rolls, E. T.: How flavour and appearance affect human feeding. Proc. Nutr. Soc., *41:*109, 1982.
5. Hashim, S. A., and Van Itallie, T. B.: Studies in normal and obese subjects with a monitored food dispensing device. Ann. N.Y. Acad. Sci., *131:*654, 1965.
6. Carr, D. B., et al.: Physical conditioning facilitates the exercise-induced secretion of beta-endorphin and beta-lipotropin in women. New Eng. J. Med., *305:*560, 1981.
7. Gorsky, R. D. and Calloway, D. H.: Activity pattern changes with decreases in food energy intake. Human Biol., 55: in press, Sept. 1983.
8. Passmore, R.: Reflexions on energy balance. Proc. Nutr. Soc., *41:*161, 1982.
9. Miller, D. S.: Factors affecting energy expenditure. Proc. Nutr. Soc. *41:*193, 1982.
10. Hervey, G. R., and Tobin, G.: The part played by variation of energy expenditure in the regulation of energy balance. Proc. Nutr. Soc., *41:*137, 1982.
11. Butterfield, G., and Calloway, D. H.: Protein and energy utilization in young men under two conditions of energy balance and work. Doctoral dissertation. Univ. of California, Berkeley, 1980.
12. Hollands, M. A., Arch, J. R. S., and Cawthorne, M. A.: A simple apparatus for comparative measurements of energy expenditure in human subjects: the thermic effect of caffeine. Amer. J. Clin. Nutr., *34:*2291, 1981.

13. Wack, J. T., and Rodin, J.: Smoking and its effects on body weight and the systems of caloric regulation. Amer. J. Clin. Nutr., *35:*366, 1982.
14. Garn, S., et al.: Parent-child, sibling and twin comparisons in the study of fatness. Presented at the meeting of the AIN, ASCN, and NSC, Michigan State Univ., 1976.
15. Keys, A. B., et al.: *The Biology of Human Starvation.* 2 vols. Minneapolis, Univ. of Minnesota Press, 1950.
16. Dietz, W. H., Jr., and Schoeller, D. A.: Optimal dietary therapy for obese adolescents: comparison of protein plus glucose and protein plus fat. J. Pediat., *100:*638, 1982.

8 Vitamins

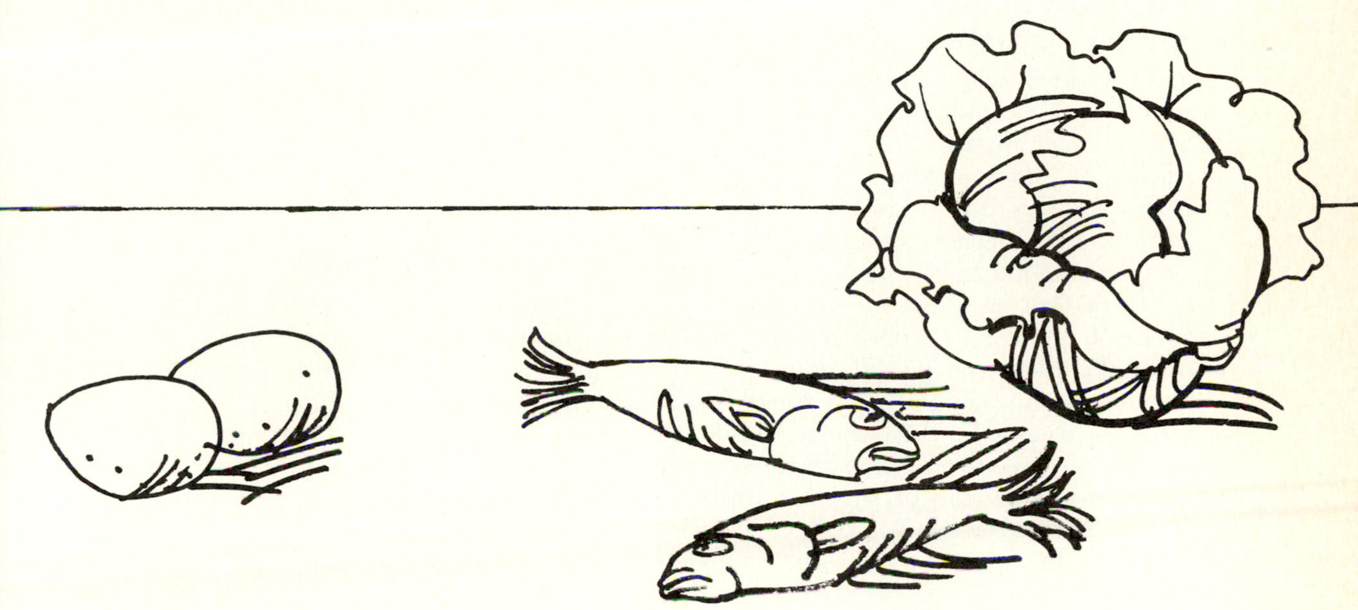

The most dramatic element in the study of nutrition deals with the discovery of the group of body regulators called vitamins. Until the early 1900s it was generally considered that only carbohydrates, protein, mineral elements, water, and possibly fat were needed for normal nutrition of humans and experimental animals (1–3). Most investigators had paid little attention to, or had missed completely, some of the early hints of the existence of vitamins. Among the first such hints were the experiments in Estonia of N. Lunin. In 1880 he found that mice died if fed an artificial mixture of all the then known constituents of milk, whereas they lived if given milk itself (4). Lunin concluded, "A natural food, such as milk, must therefore contain besides these known principal ingredients small quantities of unknown substances essential to life."

After decades of experimental work by thousands of scientists of many specialties and in many countries, these "small quantities of unknown substances essential to life" turned out to be rather simple organic compounds present in small amounts in most all basic foods. They bear little relation to one another, but they have the common characteristic that they cannot be made by tissues of the human body and must be obtained from food or another outside source.

The purpose of this chapter is to make the student better acquainted with vitamins in general before studying them in detail in Chapters 9 to 12.

DESCRIPTION OF VITAMINS

Each of thirteen vitamins is absolutely vital in the diet for a person's optimal health and well-being. They are essential not only for the formation and use of energy, as mentioned in Chapters 6 and 7, but also for the normal, everyday functioning of the body.

Definition of Vitamins

Vitamins may be defined as organic compounds, other than any of the amino acids, fatty acids, or carbohydrates, that are necessary in small amounts in the diet of higher animals for normal growth, maintenance of health, and reproduction.

All animals need vitamins, but not every vitamin that has been discovered is needed in the diet of each animal species. For example, humans and guinea pigs get scurvy when fed diets that provide no vitamin C; but dogs, cats, rats, and many other species make this vitamin in their bodies and do not need it in their food. Some of the vitamin needs of animals can be supplied from microorganisms growing in the digestive tract, especially in animals with a rumen (cows, sheep, and goats, for instance) or with a large cecum (horses or rabbits, for example).

Differences exist between the vitamin requirements of human beings and those of other animal species, but interestingly there are more similarities than differences. The invertebrates, from the protozoa through the insect kingdom, largely depend also on dietary or microbial sources of vitamins. By convention, however, because these organisms often require still other organic substances not required by vertebrates, they are lumped together and called growth factors. All higher plants can manufacture whatever vitamins they require.[1]

The action of vitamins is not unlike that of trace inorganic elements, such as iodine and copper, in that the presence or absence of very small amounts of them in the food means the difference between normal and abnormal functioning of the body. The potent effects of very small quantities in regulating body processes also remind us somewhat of the action of the hormones (thyroxine, epinephrine, and others) that are formed by various endocrine glands. Vitamins differ from hormones in that vitamins are not formed within the body but must be supplied from a dietary source. (In animals, especially in ruminants but also in humans, certain vitamins may be synthesized by microorganisms in the digestive tract.)

[1]A few lower plant forms, such as some bacteria and yeast, need an external source of certain vitamins.

Functions of Vitamins

Individual vitamins have special functions, which are taken up in the following chapters. As a group of body regulators, however, most of them share in certain functions, such as the following:

1. the promotion of growth
2. the promotion of ability to produce healthy offspring
3. the maintenance of health, vigor, and long life through promoting
    a. normal nutrition, especially utilization of mineral elements, amino acids, fatty acids, and metabolism of energy sources
    b. normal functioning of appetite and the digestive tract
    c. mental alertness
    d. health of tissues and resistance to bacterial infections.

It is worthwhile to keep in mind the above general uses of vitamins, since they recur constantly in the study of the functions of individual vitamins (see Fig. 8–1). Also, it should be emphasized that when several vitamins participate in promoting some function of the body, lack of any one of them can inhibit this function. For example, almost all vitamins have a direct influence in stimulating growth. When any one of these vitamins is supplied in inadequate amounts, growth will be stunted, even though the food contains plenty of the other vitamins needed for growth. In similar manner, damage to re-

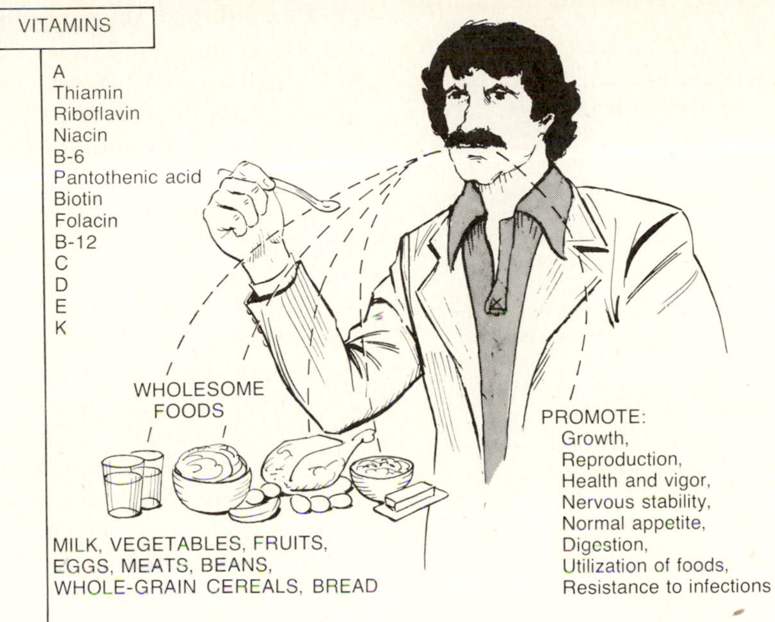

Figure 8–1 Different vitamins found in wholesome foods and their general functions in the body.

productive ability, to functioning of the digestive tract, and to the health of various tissues may result from lack of any one of several vitamins that are needed for the welfare of these organs or tissues.

It should also be remembered that stunting of growth, lack of appetite, poor utilization of food, and so on may be caused by an insufficiency of nutrients other than vitamins or by medical problems unrelated to the food intake. So some of the more general symptoms of vitamin deficiency are not specific—that is, are not due always or solely to vitamin shortages.

The Thirteen Vitamins Required by Humans, and Nonvitamins

The thirteen vitamins recognized by nutrition authorities as being required in the diet of humans are listed in Table 8–1. The names are the official terms used by international agencies and the American Institute of Nutrition, the most important scientific body of nutritionists in the United States (5). Generally, these are generic names for a group or family of compounds having vitamin activity, because for most vitamins more than one related natural compound will fulfill the vitamin requirement. For example, vitamin B-6 is listed in the table as the required vitamin since three compounds including pyridoxine are in food and have full "vitamin B-6 activity," and each will protect against a vitamin B-6 deficiency. To speak of a "pyridoxine deficiency" would be wrong, therefore. In the case of thiamin, only one compound exists in nature with thiamin activity, hence the old name, vitamin B-1, is now obsolete. (See Chap. 9–12 for more details.) Other compounds, such as choline, are needed as vitamins by certain animals but apparently not by humans, as will be explained later and in the footnote of the table. Hence, these are not listed in the table.

Each of these thirteen vitamins is readily available in our food supply if we choose a diet with reasonable care and knowledge. In addition, all the vitamins are now obtainable

Table 8–1 THE THIRTEEN KNOWN VITAMINS REQUIRED BY HUMANS[a]

Vitamin (or Vitamin Group Name)	
FAT-SOLUBLE	WATER-SOLUBLE
	Vitamin B complex
1. Vitamin A	5. Thiamin
2. Vitamin D	6. Riboflavin
3. Vitamin E	7. Pantothenic acid
4. Vitamin K	8. Niacin
	9. Vitamin B-6
	10. Biotin
	11. Folacin
	12. Vitamin B-12
	13. Vitamin C

[a]The need of choline by humans has not been proved. Choline, however, is a vitamin for various animals (see Chap. 11). We have not included taurine, carnitine, or inositol in this listing, evidently required in the diet of several species of vertebrate animals, since their status as vitamins is still not clear. Humans apparently synthesize all they need of these compounds under normal conditions. Claims have been made, generally by commercial interests, for the need of a number of other so-called "vitamins." (See Chap. 9–12 and text of this chapter.) However, these are all the vitamins needed by humans.

either in concentrated preparations or as pure chemical substances at pharmacies or various retail stores at prices that vary considerably according to the firm that puts out the preparation (As will be seen, however, there is no reason to buy pure vitamins if people practice good nutrition habits.)

The thirteen vitamins shown in Table 8–1 have been isolated as chemical compounds or groups of compounds, the composition and structure of which are known. Each of them can be synthesized in the laboratory, though synthesis of vitamin B-12 is very difficult and not a commercial practice. Most of the vitamins are white in color, but three are yellow and one is red; one is an oil and is liquid at room temperature in the pure form. As organic chemicals, many vitamins are subject to destruction by heat (as in cooking), air, light, storage, and blanching. (See supplementary readings in Appendix and see Chap. 9–12.) Many are manufactured in very large amounts by the chemical industry for fortification of foods and for vitamin preparations.

Overzealous promoters of "health foods" often speak of certain other substances as being "vitamins," such as "vitamin B-15" (pangamic acid), para-aminobenzoic acid, bioflavonoids, chlorophyll, orotic acid, lecithin, rutin, hesperidin, and "vitamin B-17" (laetrile). But only those listed in Table 8–1 are recognized by nutritional authorities today. Other vitamins may yet be discovered, though the possibility that any now unidentified vitamin plays more than a minor role remains quite slim (see end of Chap. 11).

Over the years of vitamin discovery a number of other "vitamins" have been proposed by well-meaning nutritionists, although the claims have not held up with time. Thus, there have been proposals for additional B vitamins (see Chap. 11) as well as "vitamin F" (for fatty acids), "vitamin G" (an old name for riboflavin), "vitamin H" (for biotin), "vitamin I" (a pigeon growth factor), "vitamin J" (an antipneumonia factor), "vitamin L" (for lactation), "vitamin M" (an old name for folic acid), "vitamin P" (for certain flavonoids affecting *permeability* of cells), "vitamin P-P" (pellagra-preventive), "vitamin Q" (for blood clotting, named after Dr. Quick), "vitamin T" (for termites), and "vitamin U" (S-methylmethionine, a postulated ulcer-preventive factor found in cabbage and other related vegetables). These terms are all obsolete.

Some of the terms are still quite widely used in the European literature, especially by Soviet scientists (for example, "vitamin P" and "vitamin U"). Such terms are not accepted by Western scientists.

Quantities of Vitamins Needed

The actual amount of each vitamin needed in the diet per day by adults is different from each vitamin. The amounts are measured in micrograms (μg) and milligrams (mg). They range from as little as 2 to 3 μg for vitamin B-12 to as much as 40 to 60 mg of vitamin C per day. This is roughly a 20,000-fold difference, but it has no physiological significance. Thus, it is a useless exercise to try to compare the requirement of one vitamin with that of another except to test one's ability to use the metric system. The specific daily requirement, or allowance, of a vitamin is an important value to learn, however. As will be seen in Chapters 16 and 17, for purposes of comparison, the requirements for vitamins are generally similar, quantitatively, to the requirements for trace inorganic elements—a fact with little physiological significance.

The actual daily requirement of individual vitamins for humans varies somewhat from individual to individual, although approximations can be made. Because of differences of inheritance, of differences in activity of the microbiological flora in the intestine, of greatly different food and eating patterns, of stresses and disease, and other factors, the minimum requirement of normal individuals within large populations might vary as much as up to twofold. As will be seen in the next section, these and still other factors that require reasonable safety margins are considered in setting recommended daily standards of vitamin intake.

Recommended Dietary Allowances

Various national and international groups that establish standards of vitamin intakes generally allow a considerable additional quantity of intake for any recommended dietary allowances (RDA). This allows for a wide safety margin to cover all but a very few persons of any population, and sometimes to allow for losses in preparation and storage of food. Recommended allowances for individual vitamins, then, are generally a generous yardstick and range from 25 to as much as 100 percent higher than the actual requirement of most of a population. Thus, intakes below an allowance do not necessarily mean that a person is receiving insufficient vitamins. On the other hand, recommended allowances are not necessarily sufficient for persons depleted of vitamins because of prior dietary inadequacies, disease, or traumatic stresses (6).

It is to be hoped that some uniformity of national standards can eventually be attained by international nutrition bodies. In the meantime, the different standards for the United States, Canada, the Food and Agriculture Organization (FAO), and several other countries are given inside the front and back covers for comparison. In developing countries, the recommended levels of intake must often be set very close to the minimum because of the impracticality of obtaining safer amounts in most people's diets.

The RDA in the United States represent the most authoritative estimates in the country. They are revised every five years by the Food and Nutrition Board of the National Academy of Sciences as new research becomes available (6). The latest available values are given inside the front and back covers and include daily recommendations not only for vitamins but also for minerals and other nutrients. Where international standards have not been agreed upon, these RDA values are the vitamin allowances most commonly cited in this book, not because they are necessarily "better" than those set by other countries but for uniformity.[2] The levels are not too unlike those of other countries, with vitamin C being a major exception.

In the United States, for legal purposes of the Food and Drug Administration (such as for labeling of food products), a slightly different standard exists. The detailed RDAs

[2]As revisions of the RDAs become available in the future (the next one is expected in 1985), we recommend that the new allowances be used to supplement this edition of the textbook. Generally the changes, if any, are not expected to be greatly different from the present figures, thus not invalidating current information appreciably.

for vitamins have been condensed (giving rise to some artificially inflated values in some instances) in the form of United States recommended daily allowances, known as the USRDA (see Chap. 18). Because these are not as specific as the RDAs, they are useful mainly for food labeling purposes and are not generally referred to in the following chapters.

THE ROLE OF VITAMINS IN THE BODY

Vitamins are highly perishable substances that may be lost before they ever reach the body without normal care to protect against such loss. Once they are ingested, they are quite well absorbed, in general. In the body there are many more functions that they perform than there are vitamins. Some individual vitamins have dozens of roles to play in a healthy body, for example.

Absorption of Vitamins from the Intestine

Each vitamin is absorbed into the body in its own unique way. In general, the fat-soluble vitamins, A, D, E, and K, consumed in a meal are absorbed along with fats and other lipids mainly in the lymphatic system(7). Absorption of the fat-soluble vitamins is aided by bile acids and fatty acids. Although the process is mainly one of simple diffusion, it is sometimes hastened by specific proteins, called *carriers*.

The water-soluble vitamins, B-complex and C, are efficiently absorbed, generally by diffusion but at least sometimes with the assistance of various carriers or electrical gradients associated with the intestinal wall(8). They go directly to the blood stream. Since the B vitamins are generally present in a diet in their natural coenzyme (catalyst) forms and/or combined with proteins, it is important to know that they are split off to the free form in the intestine before absorption. Thus, there is no advantage to taking the coenzyme form of a vitamin, say thiamin phosphate (sometimes put in "vitamin supplements") since the phosphate group or groups are split off in the intestine anyway.

Today much research is being conducted on exact mechanisms of absorption of each of the individual vitamins. Specific information about the absorption of individual vitamins where an unique mechanism is known, for example, B-12, will be discussed with the individual vitamin information in Chapter 11.

Mode of Action of Vitamins

How do vitamins bring about their effects, and why are small amounts of them so indispensable for life? Most of the B vitamins act as a coenzyme or part of a coenzyme. A *coenzyme* is a rather small, non-protein substance that speeds up the reaction of an enzyme without itself taking part in it. In other words, it acts as an "organic catalyst." Most of the hundreds of chemical reactions taking place in plant and animal tissues, which are essential to the life of the organisms, require coenzymes to cause them to occur. For instance, as was explained in Chapter 6, cells derive much of the energy required for their life processes through oxidation of glucose. This takes place in many intermediate steps, so that energy is set free very gradually instead of all at once. The absence of any one of these enzymes means a failure of some indispensable link in the chain of tissue oxidations. Hence the lack of a vitamin that is an essential part of such an enzyme can cripple vital oxidation processes in cells so that tissues all over the body may suffer. Since vitamins, as catalysts, are not generally used up in the reactions they promote, naturally only small amounts of them are needed.

Some of the vitamins occur in enzymes concerned with protein, fat, or mineral metabolism. At least two vitamins are involved in the control of oxidation and reduction (reactions of oxygen and hydrogen) within cells. Although not all vitamins play their role through enzyme action, all act in some manner to promote chemical reactions that are essential for healthy tissues. One vitamin (vitamin D) functions by being converted into a vital hormone, and at least one (vitamin E) serves to prevent abnormal oxidation of fatty acids in the body. The exact biochemical role of some of the vitamins is still a matter of research.

Immunology and Vitamins

Vitamins play an important role in immunological systems and hence in the protection of the body from a wide variety of infectious diseases(9). This is a very active field of research today. Among the more important vitamins in this regard are vitamin B-6, pantothenic acid, folic acid, and vitamins A, C, and E (see chapters on the individual vitamins).

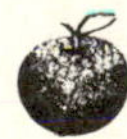

health considerations

Being an Informed Consumer

Nonspecialists should be informed about the importance of vitamins in promoting good physical fitness. They can learn many facts about vitamins that will assist them in deciding what to eat and how to spend their food money. The need for vitamins begins before birth, since it is important that the diet of a pregnant woman have ample vitamins if the infant is to start life with a liberal store of these substances in its body. Children must be sufficiently supplied with numerous vitamins in order to build healthy tissues and to achieve maximum growth. In adult life, good health and a long life cannot be obtained without an adequate supply of all needed vitamins. In all of these instances, however, excessive amounts above the "optimal" confer no further benefits.

Much information about vitamins is available to the general public from a variety of sources, some of it good and, unfortunately, some unreliable. The same may be said for the wide variety of vitamin supplements on the market in Western countries today which, surveys show, are purchased by many millions of people (up to 40 percent or more of the population). It is a desirable trait to want to keep one's body as healthy as possible, but it should be done with knowledge and with the help of reliable physicians or qualified nutritionists in order to avoid fraud, waste of money, and possible damage to oneself.

Because there is money to be made in selling vitamins, they have become big business, involving several billions of dollars of sales in the United States (including vitamin supplements and special vitamin-fortified food products). Again some of this is legitimate use of vitamins and some is not. A total of about 18 million kilograms (kg), or 40 million pounds (lb), of vitamins for pharmaceutical purposes was used in the United States in 1980 with an expected 50 percent increase by 1985(10). These figures show about as much as anything could why the student needs to be an informed consumer. (Also see the discussion on nutrition supplements in Chap. 20, the discussion of individual vitamins in the next four chapters, and the discussion in the Health Consideration section of this chapter on "megavitamins").

THE HISTORY OF VITAMINS

In retrospect, the discovery of the nature of vitamins had to wait until the chemical nature of carbohydrates, fats, and proteins was reasonably well established, which did not occur until the early 1900s. Only then, when chemistry had become a mature science, could proof be provided that food contained unidentified organic substances, other than the amino acids, that were necessary for the life of animals; that is, the vitamins. It had been known for centuries that certain foods such as liver (which was advocated as a cure for night blindness by Hippocrates), citrus fruits and fresh vegetables, and cod liver oil were able to prevent or cure specific human disorders.

Credit for the discovery of vitamins cannot be given to any one person. Instead the honor goes to a rather small group of foresighted chemists and physiologists, working independently in several countries, who had the curiosity and ability to study *why* diets made of purified food ingredients were not able to support life in experimental animals.

The pioneers in vitamin discovery used chemical techniques to make concentrates of the then unknown essential substances in food that could overcome deficiency signs in animals. The Dutch physician G. Grijns reported in 1901 that the water and alcohol extract of the outer layer of rice and other grains contain an unknown substance that prevented a deficiency disease in humans and animals (11). C. A. Pekelharing, also Dutch, fed small amounts of whey from milk to mice and concluded in 1905 that milk had an unknown essential substance (12). He stated, "My intention is to point out that there is still an unknown substance in milk which even in very small quantities is of paramount importance to nourishment. If this substance is absent, the organism loses its power to assimilate properly the well-known principal parts of food, the appetite is lost and with apparent abundance the animals die of want. Undoubtedly this substance not only occurs in milk but in all sorts of foodstuffs, both of vegetable and animal origin."

In England, from 1906 to 1912, F. G. Hopkins established by careful experiments that rats sickened and died when fed diets of pure protein, fat, and carbohydrates to which all the presumably necessary mineral matter had been added (13). Less than one-third of a teaspoonful of milk per day, added to the purified diet, made all the difference between life and death for the experimental animals. An alcoholic extract of dried milk or of certain vegetables also enabled the animals on purified diets to live and grow, but the *ash* of milk or vegetables was ineffectual. Thus, Hopkins showed that the essential unknowns that existed in foods in the natural state were organic (rather than inorganic) substances that could be dissolved in alcohol. For his part in establishing the existence of the substances we now call vitamins, Hopkins later was awarded a Nobel Prize.

In 1907, A. Holst and J. Frolich of Oslo developed the first experimental test in guinea pigs for what we now know to be vitamin C (14). At the University of Wisconsin in 1911 E. B. Hart and his colleagues made independent pioneering studies, using whole grains in experiments with cattle that demonstrated the essential nature of unknown substances in corn (maize) (15). Hart, chairman of the then Department of Agricultural Chemistry, had a special genius for attracting good persons on his staff to work on identifying the essential substances in food. In 1909, E. V. McCollum, then a young chemist, was hired,[3] and in just four years (1913) McCollum and M. Davis had proved the existence of an essential food factor in butter and egg yolk (16). Davis was a young

[3]Other persons now famous for their discoveries in the vitamin field and whom Hart placed on the Wisconsin staff were H. Steenbock, C. A. Elvehjem, S. Lepkovsky, E. E. Snell, D. Woolley, F. M. Strong, K. P. Link, and many others.

biologist who had just obtained her bachelor's degree from the University of California and who volunteered to do the rat work for McCollum without a salary.

In 1916, McCollum and C. Kennedy proposed the terms "fat-soluble A" and "water-soluble B" to distinguish between the essential substances in butterfat and in milk whey (17). So it was proved that at least one of these organic dietary essentials was soluble in water, while another was insoluble in water but soluble in fats and fat solvents. Thus, it became evident that there must be two or more of these mysterious but potent "accessory food substances" carried by natural food.

Research in the field was stimulated greatly by a young biologist, Casimir Funk, who in 1912 at the age of twenty-eight coined the word "vitamine" and who, in 1914, wrote the first book on "The Vitamines" (18). He proposed that the then known dietary deficiency diseases of beriberi, scurvy, pellagra, and rickets were caused by a lack in the diet of "special substances which are of the nature of organic bases, which we will call vitamines," short for "vital amines" (an amine is an organic form of nitrogen). This name caught the popular fancy and has persisted, despite the fact that not all the vital substances turned out to be amines.[4] At the suggestion of J. C. Drummond in 1920, the final "e" was dropped to avoid any chemical significance (19). Also, Drummond suggested that the different vitamins "be spoken of as vitamin A, B, C, etc." thus combining the "fat-soluble A" and "water-soluble B" nomenclature of McCollum with Funk's proposal. These changes were quickly accepted.

The vitamins, we now know, turned out to be a heterogeneous group of substances that differ widely in their chemical nature and in their physiological action.

Numbering and Naming of Vitamins

In the 1920s and early 1930s it became clear, after much painstaking research, that water-soluble vitamin B was in reality a mixture of at least several unrelated vitamins. The term vitamin B complex was suggested by W. D. Salmon of Alabama in 1927. It is used today to describe, collectively, the eight water-soluble vitamins for humans other than vitamin C. The B complex vitamins are distinguished by a combination of traits: being soluble in water, containing nitrogen as part of their chemical structure, and being present in large amounts in liver (used in the early studies made with animals as the major source).

The naming of individual vitamins at first presented a problem, since little was known about their chemistry. As the vitamins became differentiated, they were designated by the letters of the alphabet, usually in order of their discovery. As the fraction originally known as vitamin B became subdivided into many different chemical substances, they were called vitamin B-1, B-2, and so forth[5] or by their chemical names. As the chemical identity of the different vitamins was established, chemical names gradually supplanted the earlier designation for specific chemical

[4]Funk was not, as some have called him, the "father of vitamins," although he can properly be credited for coining the word and for being one of the early vitamin pioneers. He was born in Poland in 1884 and moved to London in 1910. Funk became an American citizen in 1920 and remained active in research in New York City (with interim positions in Europe) until his death in 1967.

[5]Following nomenclature suggestions of the American Institute of Nutrition and the International Union of Nutritional Sciences, the formerly common use of a subscript, as in "B_1" is abandoned in this text (in connection with the different B vitamins only) (5). This has obvious advantages in typing and printing.

compounds found to have vitamin activity. The letter system is still used, however, in referring to groups of closely related substances that show a common vitamin activity (15, 20). For example, one speaks of the "vitamin A activity" of several active chemicals, and of a "deficiency of vitamin A" when the deficiency can be of more than one vitamin A–active substance in food. Most of the individual vitamins exist in several different chemical forms in nature.

Isolation and Synthesis of Vitamins

Once vitamin researchers knew that vitamins were present in a food, or foods, the long and difficult task of isolating them began. Once they were isolated, next came the task of finding out what the vitamin unknowns consisted of chemically. This work was followed by learning how to make them in the laboratory (by chemical synthesis). At first these steps seemed impossible tasks, since vitamins were present in foods in such minute traces. The dry weight of a man's food intake for a day is about 500 grams (gm), whereas the total vitamins in his food, if separated, would weigh about 200 mg (about the size of a very small garden pea), or about one part per 2500 parts of dry food.

To add to the difficulty, vitamins are organic substances and hence liable to destruction by heat, oxidation, and chemical processes used in their extraction. The magnitude of the task and the interesting role of vitamins in nutrition, however, constituted a challenge to chemists and early biochemists, who continued their painstaking labors sometimes for many years before the goal was attained. R. R. Williams, for example, first became interested in the deficiency disease beriberi and the antiberiberi factor in 1910 while with the Philippine Bureau of Science. He continued his research in his free time while head of the American Telephone Laboratories in New York City and more than twenty years later isolated vitamin B-1, and determined its chemical structure. In 1936 he announced its synthesis and gave it the chemical name of thiamin, a sulfur-containing amine. Other scientists in all parts of the world participated in the effort to transform vitamins from unknown mysterious substances found only as traces in foods into known, pure chemical compounds that could be made at will.

The first step was to obtain concentrated preparations of vitamins from materials where they occurred in nature in the largest amounts. Vitamins A and D were extracted from fish-liver oils, and the early B-complex vitamins from rice polishings, liver, and dried yeast. Vitamin C was first obtained in concentrated form from citrus fruits and red peppers. These crude extracts were further concentrated and purified until small quantities of apparently pure substances (usually crystals) were obtained. These were then tested for vitamin activity in animals or microorganisms and analyzed chemically. Finally, the chemical groupings in the molecule of the pure substance were determined and put together to make the substance in the laboratory by chemical synthesis.

Losses of Vitamins in Food

In general, all the vitamins, being natural organic molecules, are subject to destruction by food processing methods (in the factory or the home); by storage; by exposure to heat, light, and oxidation; by blanching; or by still other mechanisms. The fat-soluble vitamins tend to be more resistant to destruction and losses, partially because they are not removed by preparations of food in water. A section in Chapter 20 describes the effects of cooking on the nutritive value of foods, and information is given about specific vitamins in Chapters 9 to 12. Losses or direct inactivation of vitamins can occur not only by processing procedures but also by various antagonists in certain foods; by the consumption of various drugs; to some extent by environmental contaminants; by inadequate absorption and by still other mechanisms.

Current Vitamin Research

Research on vitamins at present is centered on six major concerns. (1) How do vitamins bring about their characteristic effects on body tissues and other aspects of cellular metabolism? (2) Exactly how much is needed of each of the individual vitamins in the various stages of life? (3) What is their distribution in, and addition to, individual diets and foods according to special recent analytical methods? (4) What is the effect of deficiencies on pregnancy, growth and development, learning ability, behavior, metabolic diseases, and aging? (5) What are the possible relations among different vitamins and among vitamins and other nutrient substances, such as proteins, carbohydrates, and minerals? (6) What are the relationships of vitamins to nonfood factors (such as hormones, environmental contaminants, and drugs)? (7) What are the relationships of vitamins to various diseases, whether of infectious origin or of still unknown origin (such as cancer, heart disease, diabetes, and other chronic diseases)?

Such research, although difficult and slow, offers the same challenge to present-day nutritionists that determination of the chemical nature of the vitamins offered in former years.

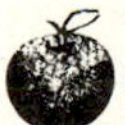

health considerations

Megavitamins

The term *megavitamins* is not officially recognized by nutrition or legal authorities. It is, however, used by the general public in various senses. To some people, megavitamins are large, supplemental doses of vitamins, usually at levels well over 10 times the RDA, which are usually considered by nutritional scientists, including the authors of this text, to be nutritionally worthless, a waste of money, and liable to be toxic if taken over a long period (21,22). To a few advocates, megavitamins are not only high levels of vitamins consumed but also the inclusion of compounds that are not nutritionally essential but "which serve biochemically essential vitamin-like cofactor functions" (such as carnitine, coenzyme Q, biopterin, lipoic acid, and taurine) (23). The use of the term in any sense is illogical.

All vitamins, as with most nutrients, are potentially toxic (24). When taken in the body in amounts much larger than are needed and larger than are normally ingested in basic foods, they are no longer serving their vitamin functions and therefore become pharmaceutical agents, or drugs. There are legitimate uses for drugs in the treatment or prevention of diseases, but they should be used only when the person is under the care of a physician. Besides, vitamins make poor drugs; any possible medical benefit a vitamin may offer can usually be obtained much more efficiently from other drugs.

Exceptions exist to the caution against the therapeutic use of megavitamins. When a patient is under the care of a physician, high levels of certain vitamins may be legitimately used in treating certain rare, vitamin-dependent genetic diseases and rare intestinal absorption defects and as an antidote to certain antivitamins used in curing diseases (21, 22).

The problems associated with the use of megavitamins, however, are far more likely to outweigh any possible benefits. The authors are especially concerned about their use by people who try to prescribe for themselves or when they are suggested by "othomolecular psychiatrists" or similar persons generally poorly trained in nutritional sciences. A recent survey of 2,450 adults in seven western states showed that 11 percent of the population sampled were consuming 2 to 8 gm of vitamin C per day, a level considered by the authors and others as possibly at risk (25). In this same study it was found that 0.3 percent of the people surveyed were taking quite potentially harmful levels of vitamin A, or more than 40 times the RDA. The need for education about vitamin use and safety is evident.

Vitamin concentrates or supplements (along with the presence of key minerals and trace elements) are of course used by physicians for the treatment of deficiencies of these nutrients. Vitamin supplements may also serve a useful purpose in providing nutrients for persons not receiving adequate amounts (RDA levels) of any of the nutrients in a variety of circumstances (26).

Examples are children who are not eating well, growing children existing on poor diets, pregnant and lactating women, alcoholics, persons of all ages and conditions on low-calorie diets, and many older individuals who may be physically, medically, or economically unable to consume adequate diets. Under these conditions, where vitamin supplements are often taken for "nutritional insurance," there is no need to take expensive supplements or much higher levels than the recommended dietary allowances (25,27). Such supplements, if needed, are of little use unless a wide spectrum of minerals and trace elements (especially iron and zinc) are also present.

One objective of normal nutrition is to have enough of all the needed vitamins in the diet to prevent disease and promote health. Moreover, when we obtain our vitamins from eating a wide variety of nutritious foods, we obtain in addition all the various other nutrients essential to health. This is the best way to "get our vitamins" under normal circumstances.

QUESTIONS

1. Why are essential amino acids and fatty acids not classed as vitamins? Why are the trace elements, which are needed in very small amounts and must be supplied in food for normal body functioning, not included with the vitamins? Why are hormones, such as epinephrine and thyroxine, not called vitamins?

2. The rat and dog do not have to have vitamin C (ascorbic acid) supplied in their food because they can make it in their own body tissues; humans, monkeys, and guinea pigs cannot make this substance within their bodies and hence must obtain it from foods. Could you say that ascorbic acid is a hormone for rats and a vitamin for humans? Why or why not?

3. When was it first known that animals could not be maintained in health, or even survive, on diets of purified nutrients that provided plenty of calories, protein, and all necessary mineral elements? Approximately how long was it before it was recognized that natural foods provided traces of definite organic substances that were absent from the purified foodstuffs? When were these substances first called vitamines? Who first distinguished between two groups of these substances and called them fat-soluble A and water-soluble B?

4. What is meant by the following terms that are used in connection with vitamins: biological assay, vitamin concentrates, synthetic vitamins, a milligram, a microgram, minimum requirement, recommended allowance?

5. Why were the vitamins designated by letters of the alphabet? In general, is it better to call a vitamin by its chemical name, when it has been given one, or by a letter, and why?

6. How can the vitamin content of foods be measured? In what types of food are fat-soluble vitamins found? What classes of food are good sources of water-soluble vitamins? Name three foods that furnish considerable amounts of some water-soluble and fat-soluble vitamins together. Name five foods that carry few or no vitamins.

7. Give the general uses of vitamins as a whole in the body. Would rats grow on a diet that furnished adequate energy, proteins, fat, minerals, and all of the vitamins except vitamin A? Why? If it is true that vitamins A and C help to prevent infections, would you expect to raise bacterial resistance satisfactorily by taking a diet rich in one of these vitamins and poor in the other? Would taking 10 times the recommended allowance of vitamin A be any more effective in raising bacterial resistance than taking the adequate level?

8. Why is it normally advantageous to obtain vitamins in natural foods instead of eating a vitamin-poor diet and taking vitamins in pills or capsules?

9. Will an adequate intake of vitamins insure good health? Why or why not?

References

1. McCollum, E. V.: *A History of Nutrition.* Boston, Houghton Mifflin Co., 1957 (Chapters 14–20, 27).
2. Goldblith, S. A., and Joslyn, M. A.: *Milestones in Nutrition.* Westport, Conn., Avi Publishing Co., 1964.
3. Guggenheim, K. Y.: *Nutrition and Nutritional Diseases—The Evolution of Concepts.* Lexington, Mass., The Collamore Press, D. C. Heath and Co., 1981.
4. Lunin, N.: Dissertation, Univ. Dorpat, 1880 (see page 204 of ref. 1); Zeit. Physiol. Chemie, 5:31, 1881 (see reprint of this paper on page 99 of ref. 2).
5. IUNS Committee on Nomenclature: J. Nutr., *101*:133, 1971; *112*:7, 1982, Nutr. Abstr. Rev., *48*:831, 1978.
6. Food and Nutrition Board: *Recommended Dietary Allowances.* 9th Ed. Washington, D.C., National Research Council, National Academy of Sciences, 1980.
7. Hollander, D.: J. Lab. Clin. Med., *97*:449, 1981.
8. Rose, R. C.: Amer. J. Physiol., *240*:G97, 1981.
9. Symposium Proceedings, Amer. J. Clin. Nutr., *35* (Supplement 2):417, 1982.
10. Anderson, W.: Feedstuffs, *53* (Nov. 16): 8, 1981.
11. Grijns, G.: Geneesk. Tijdschr. v. Ned. Ind. 1, 1901 (see page 216 of ref. 1). Also see Eijkman, C.: Arch. Hygiene, *58*:150, 1906.
12. Pekelharing, C. A.: Nederlandsch. Tijdschr. N. Geneesk., *2*:3, 1905, (see page 207 of ref. 1).
13. Hopkins, F. G.: The Analyst, *31*:385, 1906, J. Physiol. (London), *44*:425, 1912 (see reprint of the latter paper on page 109 of ref. 2. Also see excerpts in Nutr. Rev., *31*:19, 1973).
14. Holst, A., and Frolich, J.: J. Hygiene, *7*:634, 1907 (see pages 217 and 255 of ref. 1).
15. Hart, E. B., McCollum, E. V., Steenbock, H., and Humphrey, G. C.: Res. Bull. 17, Wisconsin Agric. Expt. Station, 1911.
16. McCollum, E. V.: *From Kansas Farm Boy to Scientist.* Lawrence, University of Kansas Press, 1964; McCollum, E. V., and Davis, M.: J. Biol. Chem., *15*:167, 1913; *19*:245, 1914.
17. McCollum, E. V., and Kennedy, C.: J. Biol. Chem., *24*:491, 1916.
18. Funk, C.: J. State Med., *20*:341, 1912 (see reprint of this paper on page 145 of ref. 2 and excerpts from the paper in Nutr. Rev., *33*:176, 1975); Funk, C.: *Die Vitamine.* Wiesbaden, 1914 (republished in English in 1922. This is the first complete treatise on the subject of vitamins). Also see Todhunter, E. N.: J. Amer. Dietet. Assoc., *52*:432, 1968.
19. Drummond, J. C.: Biochem. J., *14*:660, 1920 (see reprint on page 177 of ref. 2 and in Nutr. Rev., *32*:209, 1974).
20. Todhunter, E. N.: *A Guide to Nutrition Terminology for Indexing and Retrieval.* Washington, D. C., U.S. Department of Health, Education and Welfare, Public Health Service, 1970.
21. Herbert, V.: Arch. Inter. Med., *140*:173, 1980; DiPalma, J. R., and McMichael, R.: Bull. N.Y. Acad. Med., *58*:254, 1982.
22. Rosenberg, I. H., et al.: Report of FDA Panel on Vitamin and Mineral Drug Products for Over-the-Counter Human Use. Federal Register, *44* (No. 53): 16126, March 16, 1979.
23. McCarty, M. F.: Medical Hypotheses, *7*:515, 1981.
24. Kirkendall, W. M., and Hammond, J. J.: J. Amer. Med. Assoc., *239*:2658, 1978; Mayer, J.: Family Health, *12*:48, 1980; Herbert, V.: Arch. Inter. Med., *140*:173, 1980; Silverman, S. H., and Lecks, H. I.: Clin. Pediatr., *21*:172, 1982; Wason, S., and Lovejoy, F. H.: Amer. J. Dis. Children, *136*:174, 1982. (All on megavitamins).
25. Read, M. H., et al.: Nutr. Rept. Internat., *24*:1113, 1981.
26. Baker, H., et al.: J. Amer. Geriatr. Soc., *27*:444, 1979; Committee on Nutrition: Pediatrics, *66*:1015, 1980; Pao, E. M., and Mickle, S. J.: Food Tech., *35*(Sept.):58, 1981; Koh, E. T., and Chi, M. S.: Amer. J. Clin. Nutr., *34*:1562, 1981; Kerr, G. R., et al.: Amer. J. Clin. Nutr., *35*:294, 1982; Sempos, C. T., et al.: J. Amer. Dietet. Assoc., *81*:35, 1982. (All on dietary surveys and instances of inadequate diets.)
27. Bootman, J. L., and Wertheimer, A. I.: J. Amer. Dietet. Assoc., *77*:58, 1980; Sneed, S. M., Zane, C., and Thomas, M. R.: Amer. J. Clin. Nutr., *34*:1338, 1981; Willet, W., et al.: Amer. J. Clin. Nutr.,

34:1121, 1981; Hale, W. E., et al.: J. Amer. Geriatr. Soc., *30*:401, 1982; Garry, P. J., et al.: Amer. J. Clin. Nutr., *36*:319, 1982. (All on vitamin supplement usage.)

Also see supplementary reading in the Appendix.

For additional up-to-date vitamin references (since this is a very active research field), see current issues of such publications as:

Amer. J. Clin. Nutr.
Ann. Rev. Nutr.
Ann. Nutr. Metab. (Switzerland)
Archivos Latinoamer. Nutr.
Brit. J. Nutr.
FDA Consumer
Human Nutr. (U.K.)
Indian J. Nutr. Diet.
Int. J. Vit. Nutr. Res.
J. Amer. Dietet. Assoc.
J. Amer. Med. Assoc.
J. Biol. Chem.
J. Canad. Dietet. Assoc.
J. Nutr.
J. Nutr. Sci. Vitam. (Japan)
J. Nutr. Educ.
New Eng. J. Med.
Nutr. Abstr. Rev.
Nutr. Rev.
Nutr. Update

Biographies of Early Vitamin Workers in the Journal of Nutrition:

Researcher	*Volume, page, and year*
Best, C. H.	*110*:14, 1980
Cowgill, G. R.	*106*:1227, 1976
Drummond, J. C.	*82*:1, 1964
du Vigneaud, V.	*112*:1465, 1982
Eijkman, C.	*42*:3, 1950
Elvehjem, C. A.	*101*:569, 1971
Evans, H. M.	*113*:929, 1983
Funk, C.	*102*:1105, 1972
Goldberger, J.	*55*:3, 1955
Grijns, G.	*62*:1, 1957
György, P.	*109*:14, 1979
Hart, E. B.	*51*:3, 1953
Hogan, A. G.	*97*:1, 1969
Holst, A.	*53*:3, 1954
Hopkins, F. G.	*40*:3, 1950
Jansen, B. C. P.	*100*:483, 1970
Lind, J.	*50*:3, 1953
McCollum, E. V.	*100*:1, 1970
Mendel, L. B.	*60*:3, 1956
Osborne, T. B.	*59*:3, 1956
Pekelharing, C. A.	*83*:1, 1964
Salmon, W. D.	*108*:17, 1978
Spies, T. D.	*102*:1395, 1972
Steenbock, H.	*103*:1233, 1973
Takaki, K.	*106*:583, 1976
Williams, R. R.	*105*:1, 1975
Wills, L.	*108*:1377, 1978
Woolley, D. W.	*104*:507, 1974

9 Vitamins A, D, E, and K (Fat-Soluble)

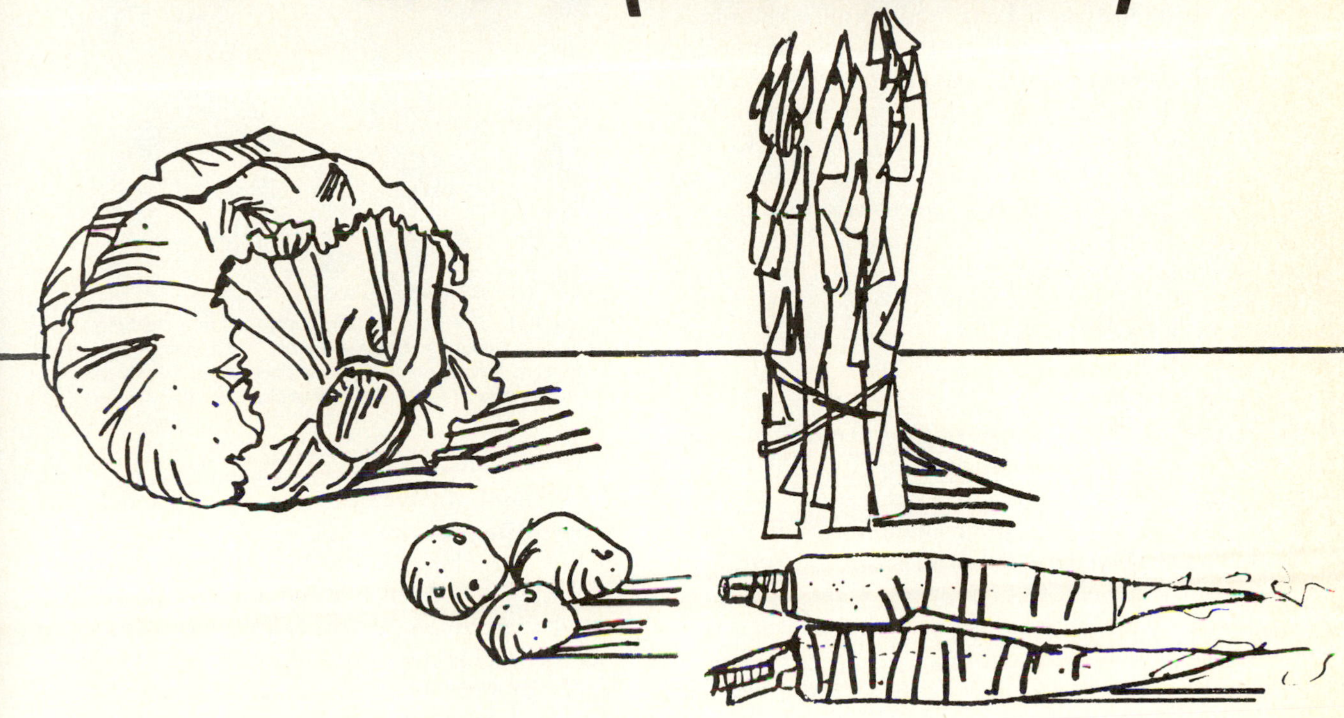

The vitamins A, D, E, and K are organic compounds of carbon, hydrogen, and oxygen (see the Appendix for their structure). Unlike the B vitamins, which contain nitrogen and are soluble in water, these four vitamins contain no nitrogen and are soluble in fat and fat solvents such as ether or cleaning fluid. They are generally found in nature associated with fatty foods such as butter, cream, vegetable oils, and the fats of meat and fish. The precursors of vitamins A and K are present also in yellow and green vegetables.

In addition to their lack of nitrogen and solubility in fat, these vitamins have other similarities.

1. They are more resistant to heat than the B vitamins and therefore less likely to be lost in the cooking and processing of foods.
2. They are generally absorbed from the intestine along with fats in foods, so that if anything interferes with fat absorption, absorption of these vitamins can also be lowered.
3. Because they are not water-soluble, they are not excreted in the urine but are stored to a considerable extent in the body. Hence deficiency symptoms may be slow to develop and hard to detect. Also because the body can store large amounts of vitamins A and D, problems of toxicity can develop in persons taking too much of these vitamins.

Beyond these similarities, each of these four vitamins has quite different chemical and physiological properties.

Between 1910 and 1925, scientists proved that there were at least several vitamins in foods. Of the several types found, some were closely associated with certain natural fats and oils. The first to be discovered was designated by the letter of the alphabet as "fat-soluble A," soon called vitamin A (1920). Vitamin A was also the first to have its chemical structure determined, in 1931. Because of these historical facts, and because vitamin A plays a prime role in the vitamin hierarchy, discussion of the vitamins starts with vitamin A. It is logical to include in this chapter the other fat-soluble vitamins, D, E, and K. The fact that they were not discovered in chronological order and so not named in alphabetical sequence does not matter.

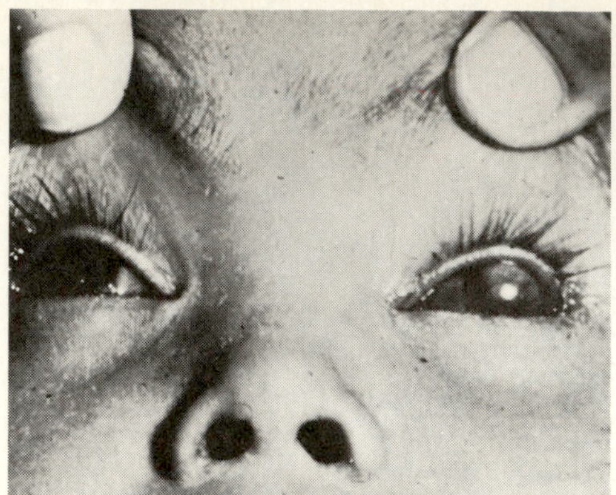

Figure 9–1 Eye changes (xerophthalmia) in a child from a developing country, being examined by a member of a survey team. It costs only a few cents per year to supply this child with adequate amounts of vitamin A. (From NIH Record.)

VITAMIN A

Vitamin A is probably the most important of all vitamins, if any single vitamin can be so distinguished from another. Its great importance is demonstrated dramatically in that, more than any other vitamin, deficiencies of vitamin A are still widespread throughout most developing countries of the world and involve millions of people, especially children.

A deficiency of vitamin A causes a weakening of body tissues resulting in less resistance to infection; poor tooth development; a stunting of growth; faulty reproduction; a disorder of eye tissue resulting in "night blindness;" and weakened epithelial tissues. Unfortunately, these conditions are quite common in many areas of the world in spite of the fact that the cure can be so easily and cheaply obtained (Fig. 9–1).

Discovery

Hippocrates, in ancient Greece, knew that the eating of liver was a treatment for night blindness, now known to be caused by a lack of vitamin A (1). There are many other references to the disease throughout the centuries (as far back as 1500 B.C.). In 1904 M. Mori, of Japan, found that the night blindness-preventing substance was in fatty foods and suggested the use of cod-liver oil and chicken liver for its treatment in children (1). He thought the disease was due to a deficiency of fat.

The fact that certain fats contained the substance now known as vitamin A was detected experimentally by using growth tests with rats. This discovery was made independently in 1913 by E. V. McCollum and M. Davis and by T. B. Osborne and L. B. Mendel (2). Fed on purified foodstuffs with lard as the only fat, the rats ceased to grow and eventually died. With butterfat, egg yolk, or cod-liver oil in the diet, the rats were protected from these ill effects. Eventually, in 1931, the structure of vitamin A was determined by P. Karrer, a Swiss chemist, who received the Nobel Prize for this and for his work with riboflavin, a B vitamin (3). Several years later the most common form of vitamin A in animal tissues, known for years simply as vitamin A, was isolated in crystalline form and synthesized in the laboratory. It is today called retinol, as will be explained in the next section. Today pure, inexpensive, synthetic forms of vitamin A are readily available; they have long replaced cod-liver oils as the primary source of supply in food enrichment and vitamin supplements. (See structural formula in the Appendix.)

Properties of Vitamin A from Animal Sources

Several slightly different chemical forms of vitamin A are found in foods of animal origin. The most common form is *retinol,* formerly called just vitamin A or vitamin A alcohol. Less common is *dehydroretinol,* formerly known as vitamin A_2 (4).

Retinol, with its derivatives, is the traditional type commonly found in most all the animal kingdom (but not in plants). In pure form it is pale yellow, insoluble in water, soluble in fats and fat solvents, and fairly resistant to heat. It may be destroyed by oxidation, such as by exposure to ultraviolet light or to air at high temperatures. Thus, fats and oils may lose vitamin A by oxidation caused by active forms of oxygen or by light. Substances that inhibit this oxidation (antioxidants) are often present in unrefined oils and are often replaced when oils are refined for food.

Dehydroretinol occurs mainly in freshwater fish and in birds that feed on these fish. It has recently been found to occur in human skin in small amounts. Since both types of the vitamin have similar physiological effects, we need make little distinction between them.

Vitamin A exists in animal tissues in alcohol ($—CH_2OH$), aldehyde ($—CHO$), and acid ($—COOH$) forms. Retinol, the alcohol form, is most abundant. The natural aldehyde form (formally called vitamin A aldehyde, retinal, or retinene) is now properly termed *retinaldehyde,* and the corresponding acid form is *retinoic acid* (4). Retinoic acid and various synthetic derivatives have gained lots of attention in recent years as a major ingredient in many pharmaceutical products used in the treatment of acne and as a possible cancer-preventive nutrient, as will be discussed later in this chapter.

Several other active forms of vitamin A exist in animal tissues or as synthetic isomers. In the body, vitamin A exists largely in the form of esters with fatty acids, known as retinyl esters. When fed to humans or animals, the different forms of vitamin A are not necessarily interchangeable in protecting against a deficiency. Retinoic acid, for instance, will not completely prevent all symptoms of vitamin A deficiency such as faulty reproduction or eye disorders.

Provitamins A from Plant Sources versus "True" Vitamin A

"True vitamin A," or retinol, is unique in that, technically speaking, it is present only in animal foods. It can be made in the body, however, from yellow-orange *provitamins A* such as *carotene,* a pigment made naturally only by plants. Hence, strictly speaking, pure vegetarians do not eat any "true" vitamin A but eat foods that have *provitamin A activity*—a term that includes all forms of the vitamin from plant sources. This use of vitamin A nomenclature is a result of historical convention in scientific literature (4). It could be confusing, however, to the student or layperson who has been taught at home or in grade school that carrots, yams, melons, and similar plant foods are good sources of vitamin A. Therefore, in the rest of the discussion of this vitamin, the authors will use the term vitamin A in the broad sense to mean all sources of vitamin A activity. This is also the legal use of the term required in the United States on food labels by the Food and Drug Administration and in most food-composition tables including the one in the appendix of this book (under the heading "total vitamin A activity"). Practically speaking, the term vitamin A deficiency used in this book and elsewhere, generally refers to a dietary deficiency of either "true" vitamin A (retinol) or of provitamins A or both (see Fig. 9–2). Thus, either form of vitamin A or combinations of both can satisfy the requirements by humans. (It is of interest that carotene cannot satisfy the vitamin A require-

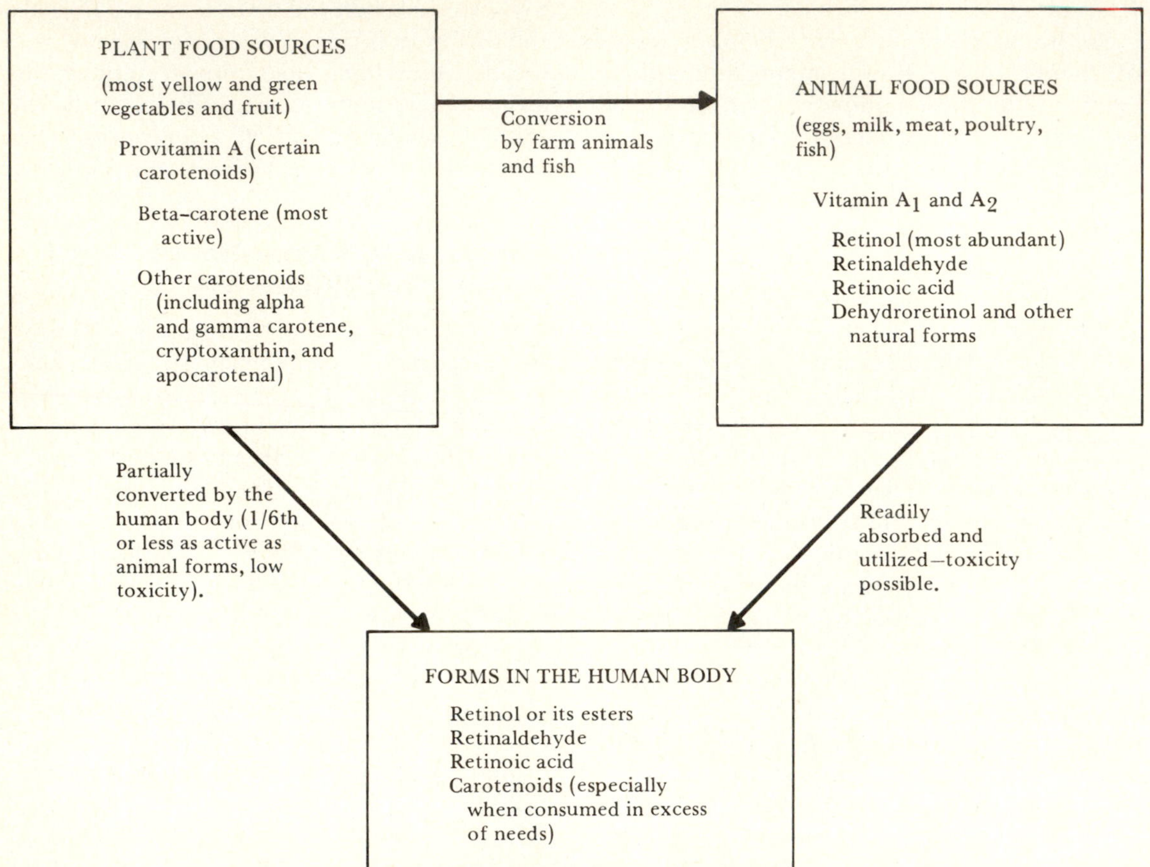

Figure 9–2 The relationship of the major different forms of compounds in foods with vitamin A activity in humans. Note that no retinol or other forms of vitamin A_1 or A_2 are found in plant food sources—only the carotenoids.

ment of members of the cat family—they must obtain it from foods of animal origin. There can be no vegetarian cats!)

Precursors of Vitamin A, the Carotenoids

Carotene is but one kind of several hundred naturally occurring members of the *carotenoid family* of compounds. Only relatively few have vitamin A activity. They are found mainly in plants but also in many animals that consume such plants (since animals cannot manufacture carotenoids in the body). The carotenoids are common bright yellow, orange, and red pigments that give the color to such foods as carrots, sweet potatoes, yams, melons, squash, pumpkins, apricots, oranges, peaches, and yellow corn (maize). Oranges, for example, contain about fifty different carotenoids. Many different carotenoids are also present in most green vegetables such as spinach, broccoli, collards, kale, celery, parsley, and green beans. Their color is masked, however, by that of the common green pigment chlorophyll (not a carotenoid) essential in sugar formation in the plant. Chlorophyll has no vitamin A activity.

The carotenoids make up most of the color of such foods as salmon, shrimp, egg yolk, milk, and butterfat, though all such pigments in these animal foods originally came from plant sources. Carotenoids also provide many of the brilliant colors of flowers, autumn leaves, birds, insects, and exotic animals.

Carotenoids and the Food Industry. It is interesting and important that thousands of pounds of carotene and several other carotenoids, natural and synthetic, are used by the U.S. food industry each year to provide or intensify the color of such foods as margarine, butter, cheese, snacks, pastries, frostings, artificial fruit drinks, salad dressings, popcorn, and frozen desserts. In most instances, these colors provide significant amounts of vitamin A activity. Also segments of the food industry make frequent use of natural sources of carotenoids such as palm oil, paprika (dried red pepper), saffron, and annatto seeds (from a tropical tree) to color food. Palm oil and paprika are rich sources of carotene and other carotenoids. Annatto oil has no vitamin A activity but is used especially to color cheese products, "winter" butter, and baked goods. The safety of natural carotenoid colors, after centuries of use, should be unquestioned.

Cartenoid sources provide color to the skin of poultry and to egg yolks so they are routinely added to poultry feeds—generally as some type of natural *xanthophyll concentrates.* "Xanthophyll" is a group name for a number of common *hydroxycarotenoids* present in most green plants. Some of them have vitamin A activity (5). The concentrates added to poultry feeds satisfy the eye of the consumer but do little to nourish the chicken. Alfalfa, which has more than forty different carotenoids, is often used as a source of these pigments, as are various corn byproducts.

Other Carotenoids in Food. The yellow color of corn (maize) is made up primarily of three types of xanthophylls: *lutein* (over 50 percent of the color), *zeaxanthine* (about 25 percent) and *cryptoxanthin* (about 8 percent). (Cryptoxanthin is a vitamin A-active carotenoid about one-half as active as carotene.) Yellow corn (maize) also contains small amounts of carotene and still other carotenoids. The red color of tomatoes, watermelon, and pink grapefruit, for example, is provided mainly by *lycopene,* a red carotenoid. This pigment has no vitamin A activity, though carotene and other vitamin A precursors are generally present in these fruits to a lesser extent.

In developed countries, an average individual will consume about half of his or her vitamin A needs from carotenoid sources, that is, around 3 to 6 mg of vitamin A-active carotenoids a day. Complete vegetarians might regularly eat at least 4 times as much. The total amount of all carotenoids consumed per day would be at least 2 or 3 times more than this. They are not toxic, even at 200 mg a day, a large dose.

In summary, the carotenoids are substances that we commonly consume each day, providing us not only with food of a pleasing color but in many instances with vitamin A activity. It has been speculated that the carotenoids from plants might play an important role in vision, since they are present in the eyes of all primates including humans, but this remains to be tested (6). It is unlikely that an essential physiological role exists for dietary carotenoids in humans other than as a source of vitamin A.

Variation of Vitamin A Activity of Carotenoids. Only about twenty of the several hundred carotenoids in nature have vitamin A activity in the animal body (5). Three of the most common ones are different forms of carotene itself. These are *beta-carotene* (one of the most common as well as most active carotenoids—see structure in the Appendix), *alpha-carotene,* and *gamma-carotene,* both with half the vitamin A activity of beta-carotene. The two other common carotenoids in plants with vitamin A activity are cryptoxanthin, one of the yellow pigments of corn already mentioned, and orange-colored *apocarotenal.* Apocarotenal is about 25 percent more active than carotene as a source of vitamin A activity, but there is much less of it in natural foods. It is widely used as a food additive.

Carotene was first isolated from carrots in 1831. Not until about 1930, however, when the structure of the several carotene compounds became known, was it clear that they had vitamin A activity (7). They are readily destroyed in foods by oxidation, by heat, by light, and by long periods of storage. It is of interest that about the only vitamin that we can see directly in food is the yellow carotene of carrots and other yellow foods. Carrots can contain up to 0.01 percent or more of carotene, which contributes most of their color. (Riboflavin is another vitamin that one can see, but less easily, in skim milk.)

Conversion of Carotenoids to Retinol in the Body. When the carotenes and other provitamin A carotenoids are taken into the body, their molecules are split, giving rise to "true" vitamin A (retinol). Although beta-carotene is theoretically capable of being split to give two molecules of retinol (twice as much as the other carotenes and cryptoxanthin), this is not done very efficiently in the human body. The amount utilized or absorbed depends on the species and many other factors.

The chief sites of conversion of the provitamins to retinol in humans are in the intestinal wall and, in some animals, in the liver. The site of conversion and the ability to utilize carotenes differ from one animal species to another. It is conservatively estimated that in humans about 1/6 of the beta-carotene intake may be expected to be transformed into retinol by the body (8). This is determined on the basis of the fact that only about 1/3 of the beta-carotene is absorbed and that only about 1/2 of this (or a total of only 1/6) has vitamin A activity for humans. The less active forms of carotenoids have approximately 1/12 of the activity of retinol.

The cow and the hen are efficient in converting the provitamins A from plant foods into the retinol of milk fat, eggs, and tissues. However, since some provitamin A activity in the diet escapes this conversion, milk fat, egg yolk, and other animal products generally contain a mixture of *total vitamin A activity.* The relative amounts of each depend partly on the food of the animal and partly on its species, or even breed. For instance, milk from Holstein cows contains a high proportion of retinol, and that from Guernsey cows carries less retinol and more of the provitamin A, which explains why Guernsey milk is more golden in color. Both milks have about the same amount of total vitamin A activity, however.

Deficiency Symptoms

A diet that contains insufficient amounts of total vitamin A activity will in time cause stunting of growth, and/or lack of ability to see well in dim light (night blindness), or more serious eye trouble. A deficiency also results in diseased conditions of the skin and mucous membranes lining the respiratory passages and the digestive and genitourinary tracts and in abnormalities in the enamel-forming cells of the teeth.

Eye. The eye is one of the first organs to show effects of vitamin A deficiency because the vitamin is a constituent of a pigment in the retina. When light falls on the normal retina, this pigment, called visual purple (rhodopsin), is bleached to another pigment known as visual yellow (retinaldehyde). As a result of this change, images are transmitted to the brain through the optic nerve. In the dark, the retinol-containing visual purple is rebuilt, but there is always some loss of degradation products, which necessitates new supplies of retinol brought by the blood (Fig. 9–3). A Nobel Prize in medicine was awarded in 1967 to George Wald of Harvard University, who is primarily responsible for these studies on the role of vitamin A in vision (9).

If retinol is at a low level in the blood, normal vision will be restored slowly and the adaptation of the eyes to the dark will be faulty. Such adaptation is influenced by too many other factors to be an infallible index of the adequacy of vitamin A in the diet. But lack of vitamin A is one of the common causes of night blindness, and a good many people with this disorder respond favorably to supplementary doses of this vitamin. If a person is suffering from vitamin A deficiency, night driving could prove to be hazardous because vision would be impaired after exposure to the bright headlights of oncoming cars.

A prolonged lack of vitamin A in the eye results in the disease known as *xerophthalmia* (see Figs. 9–1 and 9–4). The secretion of tears is stopped, the eyes are sensitive to light, the lids become swollen and sticky with pus, and bacteria may invade the eye itself and cause ulcers of the cornea, which lead to blindness if the disease is not arrested. Xerophthalmia is a very common disease in infants or undernourished children in those parts of the world where vitamin A deficiency is prevalent. The disease can be prevented completely and cheaply by including in the diet a good source of vitamin A. (For an interesting recent account of the history of night blindness, see Guggenheim [10].)

Epithelial Tissue and Infection. One of the other chief functions of vitamin A is to maintain the health of epithelial tissues, namely the skin and membranes that line all passages that open to the exterior of the body, as well as glands and their ducts. When deprived of an adequate supply of vitamin A, these tissues undergo changes that lead to a peculiar type of degeneration called *keratinization.* In the skin a prolonged lack of vitamin A results in *follicular hyperkeratosis,* a dry, scaly condition in which the skin feels like coarse sandpaper.

Damage to the mucous membranes lining the mouth, throat, nose, and respiratory passages is one of the earlier effects of vitamin A deficiency. In addition to general deterioration of the cells, these membranes lack their normal secretion of mucus. Also there is loss of the little filaments called cilia, which by constant movement aid in keeping the membrane surface clean. As bacteria have easy access to these parts, susceptibility to infections, such as sinus trouble, sore throat,

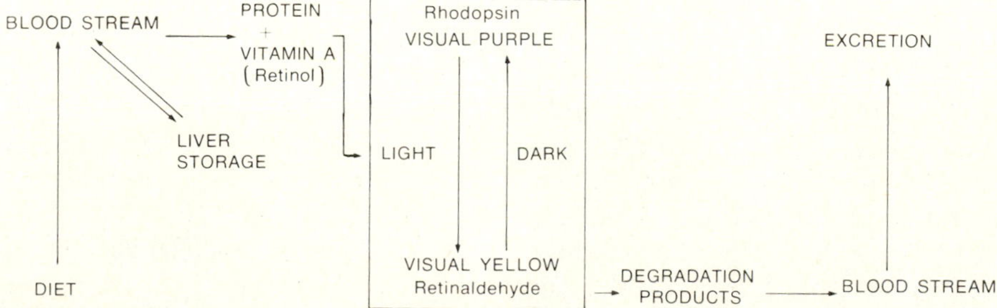

Figure 9–3 Diagram of visual cycle, showing why vitamin A (retinol) from the blood stream is needed to rebuild the pigment, visual purple, in the eye after exposure to light. (From Gordon, E. S., and Sevringhaus, E. L.: *Vitamin Therapy in General Practice,* Chicago, Year Book Publishers, Inc., 1942.)

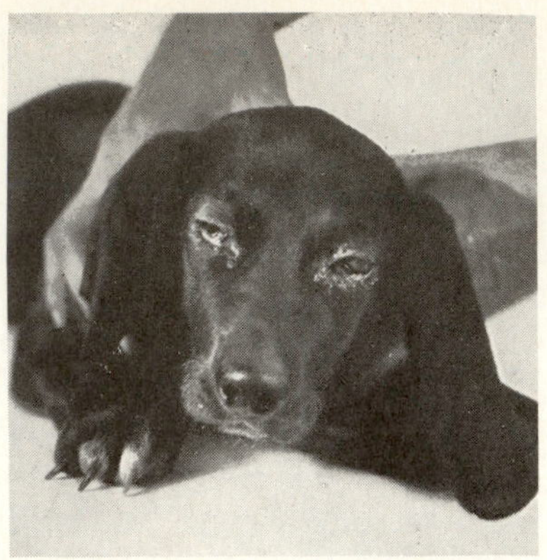

A

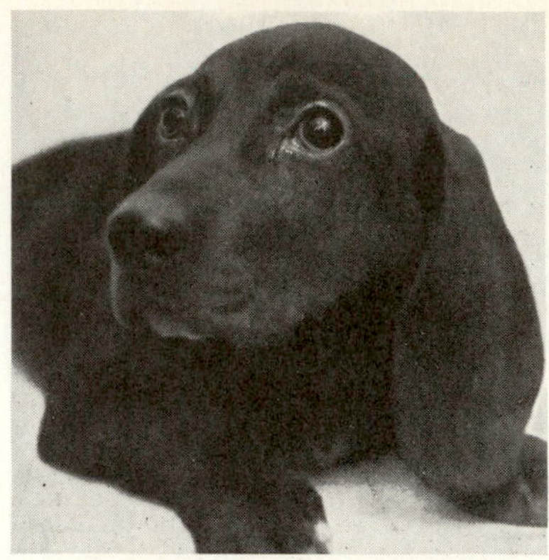

B

Figure 9–4 Xerophthalmia in a puppy due to feeding it a vitamin A-deficient diet. A, Note the swollen lids and sticky discharge from the eyes. B, Full recovery after administration of vitamin A. (Courtesy of Doctors Steenbock, Nelson, and Hart.)

and abscesses in ears, mouth, or salivary glands, is a common manifestation of insufficient vitamin A in the diet. Similar damage to membranes lining the alimentary tract may allow bacteria to penetrate into the stomach or intestinal wall, whence they may be carried in the blood stream to other parts of the body.

Other Tissues. Vitamin A is essential for proper formation and maintenance of tooth enamel and health of gums. It also is vital for the normal health of sex glands, the uterus, and the membranes that line the bladder and urinary passages. Hearing disorders have been observed in vitamin A deficient persons in recent studies (11), but this is not to say that vitamin A will control deafness.

Vitamin A is useful in preventing or treating the conditions described above only when they are due to a deficiency or low intake of this vitamin. Vitamin A shares with many other vitamins the role of protecting the health of tissues. It is anti-infective only in the sense that it helps to keep healthy the lining membranes that are the first line of defense in preventing entrance of bacteria into the body. If there has been a previous low intake of this vitamin in the diet, extra amounts of it, say 5 times the recommended daily allowance (RDA) for a few weeks, are helpful in restoring damaged epithelial tissues to health.

Animals. Animals deficient in vitamin A show most, if not all, of the same symptoms that are described in humans. Reduced growth is an early sign of deficiency in all animals (see Fig. 9–5). Eventually death will occur unless vitamin A is given. Abnormalities in nerve tissue, bone changes, loss of taste, slowness of wounds to heal, and disorders of the ear have also been observed in vitamin A-deficient animals. Reproductive disorders are readily observed, such as poor fertilization, abnormal embryonic growth, placental injury, and, in severe deficiency, death of the fetus. Deficiencies have been obtained in all animal species studies—rat, fowl, pig, cow, sheep, dog, cat, guinea pig, and others.

Vitamin A in the Body

Absorption. Most of the retinol in foods occurs in ester form (generally with a fatty acid), which is split in the intestine. Retinol

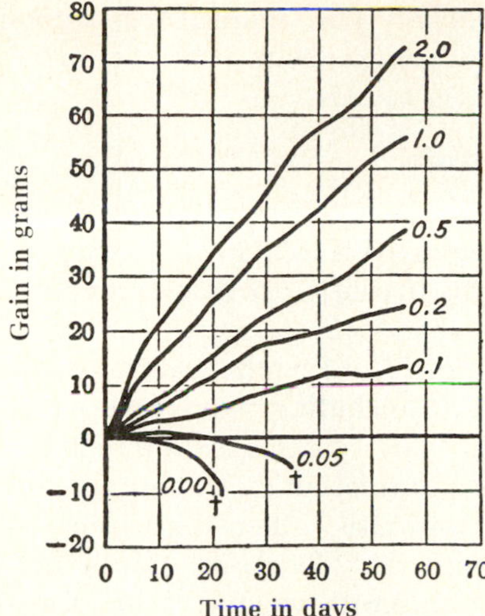

Figure 9–5 Curves of rat growth in pioneer nutrition studies show results due to differences in intake of vitamin A. Figure at end of each curve indicates amount of tomato (in grams) fed to them daily as the sole source of vitamin A. (Courtesy of Dr. H. C. Sherman, Dr. H. E. Munsell, and the *Journal of the American Chemical Society.*)

is absorbed (generally as *retinyl palmitate*) along with fats into the lymph systems before entering the blood with the aid of bile salts and fatty acids. Those vitamin A-active carotenoids that are not converted to vitamin A in the intestinal wall are absorbed in part and are present normally in the blood, liver, and various tissues. Any factor that lowers fat absorption may lower the absorption of fat-soluble vitamins. In certain clinical conditions such as jaundice and celiac disease, much of the vitamin A value of the diet may fail to be absorbed from the intestine.

The presence of significant amounts of mineral oil in the intestine interferes with the absorption of vitamin A, carotenes, and other fat-soluble vitamins. That is because they dissolve in this oil, which is nonabsorbable, and thus are excreted in the feces (12). Therefore, mineral oil should not be incorporated in foods (such as salad dressings) or taken as a laxative too close to mealtimes for many days at a time.

Storage. The liver takes up any excess of vitamin A from the blood and stores it. Nearly 95 percent of the body reserves are in the liver. Under normal conditions they last many months in adults (even if one does not eat foods containing vitamin A). These reserves can be released into the blood as retinol, attached to a specific retinol-binding protein (RBP), an albumin-type protein of low molecular weight, and carried to the tissues as needed. The level of vitamin A in the blood is thus kept fairly constant and is not affected by a diet poor in vitamin A until the body reserves are nearly exhausted. How much vitamin A is stored in the liver depends, of course, on whether the habitual diet has been rich or poor in vitamin A and its precursors. Liver reserves of vitamin A are usually lowest at birth and are built up with advancing years. In diseases of the liver—notably cirrhosis—these stores are markedly reduced. No vitamin A is excreted in the urine because it is not water-soluble, but considerable unabsorbed carotene and other carotenoids are normally found in the feces.

During lactation, a considerable amount of vitamin A is in the milk secreted, so that the need for extra quantities of this vitamin is even greater at this time than during pregnancy.

Function. The exact function of vitamin A in the body, other than its role in vision, is not clearly understood. Because animals die without vitamin A it obviously performs at least one or more essential function in cellular systems. Workers in this field no longer believe that vitamin A is involved directly in the formation of the mucopolysaccharides involved in membrane function, as was suggested in the 1970s. No coenzyme role is known yet for vitamin A.

One of the major functions of vitamin A is in regulation of growth of epithelial cells. This function has been known for a long time, but the exact mechanism is just being worked out. For instance, there is good evidence that vitamin A is necessary for the formation of normal glycoproteins in epithelial cells (13).

There is some evidence that retinol or one of its metabolites (compounds formed from retinol in the body) has a direct role in the replication of epithelial cells. Also, recently there is an indication that, when bound with RBP in epithelial cell nuclei, vitamin A governs the level of ribonucleic acid (RNA) for specific synthesis of the protein keratin(14). It is known, also, that vitamin A deficiency results in major lesions of the testes including atrophy and loss of cells in the "germinal" epithelial tissues (15). Vitamin A-deficient animals also show loss of the male hormone testosterone.

One of the most functionally active forms of vitamin A is its acid form, *retinoic acid.* One of the normal metabolites of vitamin A, it affects many tissue reactions (but not vision or, apparently, reproduction). For instance, it has recently been suggested that retinoic acid is important in regulating vitamin D metabolism in the kidney (16). Retinoic acid cannot be converted back to retinol in the body and is not stored, appreciably, in the liver.

Much popular interest has been shown lately in the apparent therapeutic role, not yet fully clarified, of retinoic acid and various related compounds in the prevention and possible treatment of certain immunological disorders, acne (17), and various forms of cancer. (See Health Considerations and Chapter 20.) Other information about retinoic acid may be found in the references (18) and the list of supplementary readings in the Appendix.

Another normal metabolite of retinol, *5,6-epoxyretinoic acid,* has been recently discovered in body tissues. It is known to have vitamin A activity in cellular systems of plants (19). It is also found in animal tissues and probably has vitamin A activity similar to that of retinoic acid. Still other metabolites are known to exist.

Retinoids

Vitamin A is one of the most active areas of nutrition research in the 1980s. One of the terms that appears frequently in that research is *retinoids.* A retinoid is any one of many natural and synthetic derivatives of retinoic acid, including vitamin A-active compounds, that are being experimentally studied for pharmaceutical action against acne, cancer, psoriasis, other skin disorders, and other diseases. "Retinoid" is not, however, synonymous with vitamin A because only a limited number of retinoids have vitamin A activity. Certain retinoids, like vitamin A, can be very toxic if taken in excessive amounts (20).

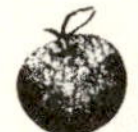

health considerations

Use of Retinoids in Acne

It has been known since the 1940s that vitamin A is useful in treating acne. In recent years a synthetic retinoid, *isotretinoin* (13-*cis*-retinoic acid), has been found to be more effective and possibly less toxic than vitamin A in treating most common forms of acne as well as certain types of persistent acne ("cystic" acne) (21). It is said to help virtually all affected persons to some extent. At this time, it is available only with a physician's prescription because of harmful side effects. The drug is generally taken orally but may also be used in a skin cream. Isotretinoin is known to dry up the sebaceous glands of the skin and is a strong anti-inflammatory agent.

The various synthetic retinoids are also being tested in a number of skin diseases including more severe types of acne, psoriasis, and certain types of inherited skin lesions, with various degrees of success (22).

An easy cure for common acne is not likely to be suddenly upon us, but clinical tests look very encouraging. No one should try to treat any type of acne with any drug without the advice of a physician. The student interested in learning more about acne will find a number of informative and helpful current reviews and popular articles available on this topic (23).

One piece of advice for acne sufferers, and for potential sufferers of skin ailments is to make certain that they receive their recommended allowance not only of vitamin A in their diet but also of zinc and linoleic acid (both known to be important to the skin), along with all the nutrients.

Vitamin A, Other Retinoids, and Cancer

Often college students may be more concerned with acne or any problem that affects them directly than with a topic such as cancer. Yet cancer in all of its various forms, especially lung cancer and breast cancer, is now the second leading cause of death in older adults. Until the 1970s most physicians believed that nutrients in the diet, or their lack, had little or nothing to do with the incidence of cancer in humans. This view has changed considerably. The relationship between cancer and the food we eat is a rapidly growing field of research. It has now become recognized that the nutrients we eat or do not eat play an important role in the prevention of at least several types of cancer (24). Vitamins A, C, and E, fatty acids, proteins, fiber, and selenium are the major nutrients being studied. It can be estimated that these nutrients and others may affect from 10 to 40 percent of the incidence of cancer in humans in the United States. It should be clearly understood that there is no evidence in humans that more than the recommended allowances of any of the nutrients is necessary in order to obtain the maximum protective effect.

It has been long known that vitamin A affects the growth of epithelial tissues and is related to the development of cancer in such tissues. Also, it is well known that most of the persons who die of cancer do so with tumors of epithelial tissues. Currently, there can be no doubt whatsoever that in mice, rats, and other experimental animals normal levels of vitamin A are necessary to protect against various kinds of experimental cancer (certain tumors of the bladder, skin, mammary glands, lung, colon, esophagus, and others) (24,25). Hence the current strong interest in the relationship of vitamin A and cancer in humans.

Much less is known, understandably, about vitamin A in various cancers of humans than in experimental animals. A sufficient number of impressive studies, however, have been published in the past few years on vitamin A in human cancers to conclude that a deficiency of the vitamin increases the chances of having certain kinds of cancers (24,26). It is not clear as yet which retinoids are most effective and safe in humans, which levels are most useful, and, specifically, which cancers are most affected and how and why. Considerable progress is being made by researchers in obtaining some of these answers, though no long-term human studies have been made with vitamin A as the only variable. It is of interest that carotenes from green and yellow vegetables appear, at least under some conditions, to be more active than animal forms of vitamin A in the prevention and treatment of certain animal and human cancers (27). This is not proven yet, however. The carotenes have the advantage of being less toxic than retinol.

Greater understanding exists now for the use of synthetic retinoids in the pharmaceutical treatment of certain cancers in humans and animals (28), but this is clearly a matter of concern for medically trained specialists.

High levels of some of these agents in experimental situations have sometimes promoted certain cancers instead of protecting against them. Much work needs to be done before there is a clear understanding of what the synthetic retinoids can do in routine cancer treatment. At high levels they no longer act as vitamins but as drugs. Again, as with acne, the bottom line of nutrition for a person interested in total health is to eat adequate amounts of foods rich in vitamin A and other essential nutrients as part of a balanced diet to supply the recommended allowances. There is no evidence that under normal conditions excessive vitamin A intakes will result in any added benefit, and such intakes are most likely to be toxic in the long run. A basic, well-balanced diet will, of course, not keep one free of all types of cancer but only those caused by an inadequate intake of vitamin A or any other nutrient. The cause of most cancers is either smoking, environmental toxins, excessive sunlight, natural toxins in food, or other factors not necessarily related to what we eat.

Recommended Allowances

The (RDAs) of the Food and Nutrition Board (8) for vitamin A are given in Table 9–1. They are given in terms of micrograms (μg) of *retinol equivalents* (RE) per day, but for comparison, here, they are also given as *international units* (IU) of vitamin A (see the next section). Additional allowances for different age groups are given in the complete RDA table. Allowances for infants and children are liberal in terms of minimum requirements in order to provide extra vitamin A for growth and to ensure adequate stores. An intake of vitamin A beyond these amounts provides no added benefit in normal persons.

Retinol Equivalents and International Units. As has been stated, the various forms of vitamin A have quite different biological activities. Therefore, to list dietary allowances or food distribution values of total vitamin A activity simply in terms of micrograms or milligrams (mg) retinol and/or carotenes and so on would be quite meaningless. The IU has been used in past years as a summary value for total vitamin A activity based on differences in the rat. This was very helpful in the years before good human studies could be made with newer, pure compounds. The new retinol equivalency values, however, are much more accurate in terms of human nutrition. Hence, we have two systems to use during this transition period.

Vitamin A values are still listed on food labels (and on vitamin supplement labels) in terms of the IU as required by government regulations. Also many tables of food composition still list vitamin A just in terms of IU activity or both as IU activity and, when values are available, as RE. This is done because it takes many years to work out fully the new RE values of all plant and animal foods

Table 9–1 RECOMMENDED DIETARY ALLOWANCE FOR TOTAL VITAMIN A ACTIVITY*

Sex	*Age*	*μg Retinol Equivalents*	*IU Vitamin A*
Females†	11 years and over	800	4000
Males	11 years and over	1000	5000

*From Food and Nutrition Board, 1980(8).

†The allowance during pregnancy is 1000 retinol equivalents (5000 IU/day) and during lactation 1200 retinol equivalents (6000 IU/day).

based on human activity (rather than rat activity) of all forms of vitamin A present in the food including the different active carotenoids. Fortunately, the listing as RE rather than IU values will not make much practical difference in the relative vitamin A value of many foods. In general, however, yellow and green vegetables will show a much lower value for vitamin A activity when expressed as RE values. This is because the carotenoids in these foods, as previously explained, are much less active for humans than for rats.

Vitamin A Standards. An IU of vitamin A is defined on the basis of rat studies as equal to 0.344 μg of crystalline retinylacetate (which is equivalent to 0.300 μg of retinol and to 0.60 μg of beta-carotene). These standards were based on older experiments in rats that showed that about 50 percent of beta-carotene is converted to vitamin A—about 3 times as much as in humans.

In humans, beta-carotene is not as available as in rats owing to poorer absorption in the intestine, poor utilization, and other factors (29). The following relationships hold in humans:

1 μg RE = {
- 1 μg retinol
- 1.15 μg retinylacetate
- 6 μg beta-carotene
- 12 μg other provitamin A carotenoids
- 3.33 IU of retinol
- 10 IU of beta-carotene
- 5 IU of a mixture of both forms.

Extent of Intakes below Allowances. In developed countries it is not difficult or expensive for people to obtain the recommended allowances of total vitamin A activity in daily foods, if good foods are available and are wisely chosen. Although surveys show that it is not uncommon for the intake of vulnerable populations often to fall somewhat below the recommended allowances, marked symptoms of vitamin A deficiency are not seen commonly in developed countries (30,31). In the United States and Canada the allowances provide a 20 to 40 percent margin of safety above basic minimum requirements, so intakes a little below the allowance figure are not necessarily inadequate for body needs. Nevertheless, persons consuming less than the allowance for extended periods of time have increased risk of developing a deficiency, as is true with all nutrients (8).

The intakes of vitamin A by children, teenagers, pregnant women, persons on low-calorie diets, and older persons who do not choose their foods with care may often be too low to allow for a proper margin of safety. E. M. Poa and S. J. Mickle reported, for example, that of more than 37,700 persons in the United States who gave a three-day dietary history in the National Food Consumption Survey, 1977–78, more than 30 percent had an intake of less than 70 percent of the RDA. Many of these people reported eating very few yellow and green leafy vegetables. On the other hand, the *average* daily intake of vitamin A was 7,520 IU (about 1,500 RE), indicating that many people eat much more than their allowance for this vitamin (more than 50 percent of the people studied ate over the RDA level, obviously in quite substantial amounts).

In developing countries, where fat supplies are low and where there are few yellow and green vegetables in the diet it is, unfortunately, very common for populations to receive less than the recommended allowances of vitamin A. It is one of the most serious health problems related to inadequate diets in the world. Night blindness, xerophthalmia, impaired vision, and blindness as a result of vitamin A deficiency are prevalent throughout parts of the Far East, the Middle East, India, Malaysia, Africa, South America, and Central America (32). The deficiency is generally associated with other deficiencies as well—protein, iron, calcium, B vitamins, and sufficient good food in general.

A. Sommer, I. Tarwotjo, and co-workers have recently stated that half a million Asian children develop potentially blinding corneal (of the eye) problems every year as a result of vitamin A deficiency in the vast majority of cases (33). They further state that about half of these children will become blind, or about 250,000 children a year—a tragic figure when, theoretically, it is all preventable with a few cents worth of vitamin A per year. It is known that many of the blind children—as many as half—will eventually die, to say nothing of the untold grief and misery for parents and lifetime disability for most of the survivors. (See the suggested reading list in the Appendix for references about some procedures underway to try to correct this situation in the next several decades. It is a high-priority project for the United Nations and other international health agencies.)

To add to the problem, too low an intake of vitamin A and other nutrients in children and young adults makes them far more susceptible to the damages of various infectious diseases (such as measles and bacterial infections), parasites, fever, and lack of other nutrients. Persons with liver disease, such as seen in alcoholism and hepatitis, are likely to have vitamin A problems also.

Measuring Intake of Vitamin A. It is not easy to determine when a person is deficient in vitamin A unless the deficiency is severe. Night blindness or tests for adaptation to dark are not always successful in diagnosing a deficiency. Most useful are measurements of liver stores and/or serum vitamin A and carotene values in comparison with known standards. Serum levels of 10 to 19 μg of vitamin A per 100 ml are considered low, as are 20 to 39 μg or less of carotene. This is an active field of research (34). (Also see references 32, 33, and the supplementary reading list.)

Vitamin A Activity in Food

Food Sources. Liver, carrots, sweet potatoes, yams, other deep yellow vegetables, and green leafy vegetables are by far the best sources of vitamin A activity in food. One serving of any one of these per day supplies fully all the vitamin A that one needs. This fact may be difficult to believe when we consider all the suffering there is from vitamin A deficiency in the world.

Table 9–2 lists the approximate vitamin A activity in typical foods based on the new RE values (35). The foods are arranged in the order of the most to the least vitamin A supplied per serving. As with all tables of food composition one must understand that these are approximate figures for an average sample of food. Many factors affect the vitamin composition of food—the variety, climate, environment, soil, storage, processing, blanching, cooking procedures, and still others (36).

It is clear that the yellow and green leafy vegetables are the best plant sources of vitamin A. As the vitamin A activity of plants is due entirely to yellow carotenoid pigments, either alone or found with chlorophyll, the depth of yellow or green color is a rough index of their potential vitamin A activity. Most thin green leaves, such as spinach, kale, and turnip greens, have a vitamin A value from 500 to 1500 RE (average about 800 RE) per 100 gm. Bleached inner leaves of cabbage and lettuce, as well as bleached asparagus, have low vitamin A activity. Carrots may vary in vitamin A activity from 200 to 1200 RE per 100 gm, and sweet potatoes also vary widely in vitamin A activity (150 to 770 RE) according to the depth of their color.

Grains, except for yellow corn (maize), white flour, sugar, and the common colorless

Table 9–2 APPROXIMATE VITAMIN A ACTIVITY IN TYPICAL FOODS[a]
(in terms of Retinol Equivalents, RE)

Food	*Approximate μg RE per Serving*
EXCELLENT SOURCES (800 RE OR MORE)	
Liver, fried, beef, 2 slices, 2.6 oz	5000 (4000–9000)
Liver, fried, calf, 3 oz	2800
Liver, chicken, 1 oz	1760
Liver sausage, pork 1½ slices, 1 oz	1200
Carrots, cooked, 3.5 oz (deep color)	1140
Sweet potatoes, 4 oz (deep color, 1 medium)	900
Green leafy vegetables, mixed, cooked, ½ cup, 3.5 oz	800
GOOD SOURCES (300–800 RE)	
Dandelion greens, ½ cup	600
Soup, vegetable, 1 cup	580
Soup, minestrone, 1 cup	430
Apricots, dried, ½ cup, cooked	420
Pumpkin, cooked, ½ cup	380
Squash, winter, yellow, ½ cup cooked	350
Cantaloupe melon ¼	340
Pepper, red, 1 medium, raw	330
FAIR TO GOOD SOURCES (100–300 RE)	
Broccoli, cooked ⅔ cup, 3½ oz (tips)	250
Apricots, fresh, 2–3 medium	240
Eggnog, 1 cup	200
Nectarines, 2 medium	165
Eggs, 2 medium	155
Watermelon, red, 1 cup	150
Milk, skim, fortified, 1 cup	140
Milk, low-fat, fortified, 1 cup	140
Papaya, ¼	135
Peaches, 1 medium	135
Ice cream, vanilla, 1 cup	135
Paprika, 1 tsp	125
Cream cheese, 1 oz	125
Cream, 20%, 2 oz	110
Tomatoes, 1 medium, 5 oz	110
Lettuce, 1 salad, small	100
MEDIUM TO LOW SOURCES (20–100 RE)	
Asparagus, 6 stalks	85
Cheese (various types) 1 oz	70–85
Milk, whole, 1 cup	85
Milk, shake, 1 cup	70
Yogurt, 1 cup	70
Milk, low-fat, (not fortified) 1 cup	65
Soup, pea, 1 cup	60
Grapefruit, ½	55
Peas, fresh or canned, ½ cup	50
Prunes, dried, 4, cooked	50
Brussel sprouts, 4, large	45
Orange juice frozen, ¾ cup	40
Beans, green, ½ cup	35
Corn, sweet yellow, 1 cup	35
Margarine, 10 gm (enriched)	30
Butter, 10 gm (not enriched)	30
Pepper, green, 1 medium	30
Lima beans, green, cooked, ½ cup	25
Chicken, with skin, 100 gm	25
Cottage cheese (various types) 4 oz	25–50
Fish, salmon and similar types, 4 oz	20
POOR SOURCES (0–20 RE)	
Celery, green, 2 stalks	20
Corn bread, 1 piece, 2 oz	15
Beans, canned (red, etc.), ½ cup	15
Apples, 1 medium	10
Hamburger, 1 medium	9
Yellow grits, ½ cup	7
Strawberries, ¾ cup	7
Pears, 1 medium	3
Frankfurter, beef or chicken	3
Nuts, 1 oz	2
Soybeans, ½ cup	2
Potatoes, 4 oz	1
FOODS WITH NO VITAMIN A (OR PRACTICALLY NONE)	
Bread, cookies, nuts, peanut butter, pretzels, rice, sugar, white flour, whole grain wheat, tofu, and similar foods	

[a]These values are approximate and subject to change, as newer and better values become available. The RE values are adapted from both the new and old editions of Handbook 8 (35) since the new edition is still incomplete. To approximate the RE values of plant products for this table the IU values in the 1963 edition were divided by 10 as is done in the new Handbook 8 (see text). See Appendix and Handbook 8 for the vitamin A activity of foods not listed here. Do not be concerned about differences that may exist between these values and those in the appendix. They come from different data bases and illustrate the point that more study of RE values of food is needed.

vegetable oils carry little or no vitamin A activity. Lean muscle meats, nuts, and many common fruits and vegetables provide only minor quantities. The body fat of animals is usually low in vitamin A, but that of certain kinds of fish may contain considerable amounts. Swordfish provides about 200 RE per serving—much higher than other fish.

The yellowness of egg yolk and butterfat is not an infallible guide to their vitamin A value, because they contain both yellow carotenoids and colorless vitamin A. Margarine has been fortified by addition of carotene or vitamin A (also vitamin D) up to the level equal to a year-round average in butter.

Combinations of foods that provide the standard daily allowance of total vitamin A activity for an adult are given in Table 9–3. Each combination combines animal and plant sources, and furnishes somewhat more than 1,000 RE of vitamin A.

There is danger that the diet will provide less than optimum amounts of total vitamin A activity unless green and yellow vegetables are used frequently. In addition, they are inexpensive sources of vitamin A for low-cost diets. This danger of inadequacy of the diet is illustrated by the list of foods in Table 9–4, which might seem to constitute the basis of a normal diet for one day, but which falls considerably short of the 1,000 RE daily vitamin A allowance.

If one of the vegetables listed in Table 9–4 were of the green or yellow variety, the vitamin A value of this diet would be raised decidedly, usually up to the 1000 RE level or more, provided the vegetable chosen was strongly colored and an average-sized serving (100 gm) was eaten. Figure 9–6 shows sources of vitamin A in average American diets.

Vitamin A levels of diets can be raised by using foods enriched with this vitamin. Such enrichment is routine in the United States, Canada, and many other countries (37). Vitamin A, in various purified and/or crystalline forms, is added to such foods as margarines, skim milk, low-fat milk and other milk products, imitation cheese, and certain cereal products. In India, vitamin A is added to most all commercially processed cooking oils. The addition of vitamin A to tea, rice, salt, cooking oils, and even monosodiumglutamate (MSG), used widely as a flavoring agent, is being considered in some countries (37). Special chemical forms of vitamin A,

Table 9–3 FOOD COMBINATIONS THAT PROVIDE THE RECOMMENDED DAILY ALLOWANCE OF TOTAL VITAMIN A ACTIVITY FOR AN ADULT*

	Food	*Amount*
1.	Whole milk	1 pt (480 gm)
	Pumpkin pie	4 in wedge (150 gm)
	Vegetable beef soup	1 c
2.	Margarine or butter	2 tbsp
	Spinach, cooked	2/3 c
	Nectarines	2
3.	Eggs	2
	Carrots, cooked	3 oz
	Tomato juice	6 oz

*Each of these food combinations furnishes somewhat more than 1000 RE of total vitamin A activity.

Table 9–4 A FOOD COMBINATION SUPPLYING AN **INADEQUATE** AMOUNT OF VITAMIN A ACTIVITY FOR DAILY ADULT DIET*

Food	*Amount*
Whole milk	1 pt
Butter or margarine	2 squares
Egg	1
Orange juice	4 oz
Apple	1 medium
Green beans	1/2 c (3–4 oz)
Coleslaw (cabbage salad)	1/2 c
Beets	1/2 c

*This diet contains only about 300 RE instead of 1000 RE of total vitamin activity.

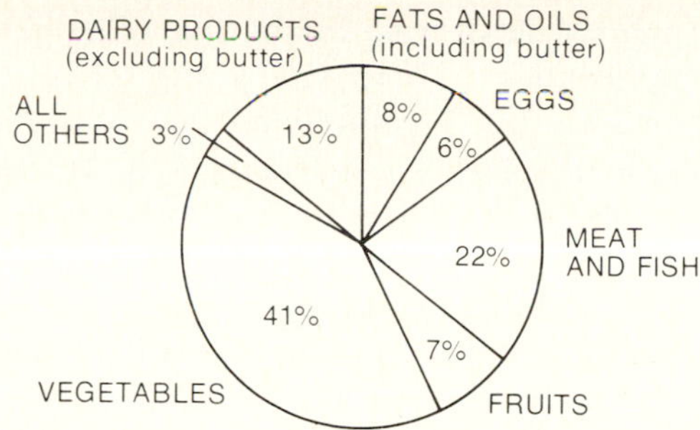

Figure 9–6 Percentages of vitamin A value contributed by various food groups in the average American diet. (From information supplied by U.S. Department of Agriculture, 1978.)

which are very resistant to destruction, are used for fortification.

Of practical interest in supplying vitamin A to children in low-income countries is the use of table sugar as the base food for vitamin A fortification. Sugar is used because in these countries it is one of the few foods bought by almost all families, and it is easily adapted to the addition of vitamin A. It is also widely used in preparation of foods at home and is widely consumed by children. Experiments with fortified sugar in Latin America and elsewhere have proven to be quite successful so far (38). Nutrition students in the United States question a practice that seems to encourage sugar consumption in countries with much malnutrition, but it does not in fact increase consumption and seems to be the best of several possibilities. Nevertheless the practice is not without its potential nutritional problems.

Effect of Cooking or Processing. Because vitamin A and its precursors (the carotenoids) are insoluble in water and resistant to heat at ordinary cooking temperatures, most foods lose little of their total vitamin A activity in normal cooking or processing, unless they are exposed to air. Considerable losses can occur, however, in canning, other processing procedures, and storage unless proper methods of processing are used (36,39). The use of palm oil as a frying medium, for example, is very destructive to the carotene content of food.

Serious losses of vitamin A activity generally result upon the drying of leafy greens, other vegetables, and fruits when exposed to air, sunlight, and high temperatures (see supplementary readings in the Appendix). Dehydration under modern commercial procedures usually prevents such loss, although usual home drying can be very destructive to vitamin A activity. Vegetables should be stored at low temperatures to conserve all their vitamins including vitamin A.

Vitamin A activity of common processed vegetables may be reduced 15 to 20 percent in green vegetables and as high as 30 to 35 percent in common yellow vegetables because of chemical changes in the carotene molecule (some *trans* forms are changed to other isomers with less, or no, activity). Evaporation, pasteurization, or irradiation of milk has little or no effect on its vitamin A content.

Toxicity of Retinol and Carotenoids

Large, long-continued doses of retinol (the animal form of vitamin A) are toxic. Toxic symptoms known as *hypervitaminosis A* may occur in children one to three years of age after they have received 15,000 RE (75,000 IU) or more of retinol daily for at least six months (or less of the water-soluble forms of retinol). Such symptoms—which include excessive irritability, swellings over the long bones, and dry and itching skin—are relieved by discontinuing the dosages of supplementary retinol. In the treatment or prevention of vitamin A deficiency very large doses of A may be given several times a year. These large doses are not toxic when given in this manner (40).

In adults, the early symptoms of toxicity are confusion, headache, nausea, rough skin, and diarrhea; a great excess of retinol may also lead to liver damage and decalcification of bones with consequent bone fragility. The toxicity of retinol has been known for decades, yet examples of high intakes and of toxicity are abundant in the current medical literature (41). The level of retinol that is toxic depends on the condition of the individual, the length of time it has been consumed, the presence of liver disease, and many other factors. A total of 8,000 to 10,000 RE per day (40,000 to 50,000 IU) over a period of seven years, for example, should be considered a toxic level for adults. Generally, levels about 20 times the RDA are considered toxic over shorter periods.

Livers of animals concentrate vitamin A in large amounts over long periods. Eating pork, chicken, or beef liver several times a week is of nutritional benefit and poses no hazards for adults. Liver should not be eaten daily in large amounts, however, unless a person is under the care of a physician. Early explorers in the Arctic, it is said, learned to avoid eating the liver of the polar bear because symptoms of toxicity were observed. These were later found to be due to excessive vitamin A. Carotene and other natural carotenoids, in contrast to retinol, are not considered very toxic even when consumed at high levels. In humans, the only abnormal sign that might be seen when large amounts of carotene are eaten is a yellow skin (as is seen in some persons who consume large amounts of carrots or red palm oil, for example) (42).

VITAMIN D

Vitamin D has long been known as the "sunshine vitamin" because either sunlight or food sources can take care of our needs. As long as persons living the year around in sunny climates receive regular and adequate exposure to the sun no food source of vitamin D is needed.

The importance of vitamin D to humans lies mainly in its role in the use of calcium and phosphorus, both vital for growth, development, and maintenance of bones in persons of all ages. A deficiency of vitamin D results in rickets, a disease characterized by softening of the bones, bowlegs, and other skeletal deformities. Vitamin D deficiencies are still often seen in people in many countries, whether in sunshine belts or not.

Vitamin D has certain unique properties that stand out in comparison with most other vitamins. They are as follows:

1. It can be obtained by the action of sunlight (ultraviolet light) on the skin, even if there is no food source.
2. It changes into a hormone (calcitriol) by the kidney before it performs its role in the body.
3. It is very potent—only a few micrograms (5 to 10) are needed per day. This makes it one of the most biologically active substances known (similar in this respect to vitamin B-12, biotin, and a few very potent hormones and toxins)
4. In large amounts it is very toxic because (like vitamin A) it is fat-soluble and not readily excreted when taken in excess.

For additional information about aspects of vitamin D not covered in the following section see the reviews and other supplementary reading in the Appendix. Vitamin D is an extremely active area of research—only some highlights can be covered here.

Deficiency Symptoms

The effects of a lack of vitamin D, as seen most strikingly in children and young animals, are poor growth and rickets. In rickets, the metabolism of calcium and phosphorus is disturbed in such a way that these minerals, necessary for bone rigidity, can not be normally deposited in the bone. Hence, rickets is characterized by weak bones, which readily develop curvatures when compelled to carry the weight of the body, and by overgrowth of the softer tissues (cartilage) at the ends of the bones. Rachitic deformities develop, such as bowlegs, knock-knees, enlargement of bones about the joints, and a narrow, distorted chest with beading of the ribs (Figs. 9–7 and 9–8).

These deformities, although they do not cause death, may persist into adult life, at which time the shrunken chest may predispose a person to lung diseases, and a narrow pelvis may make childbearing difficult for women.

Milder cases of rickets, associated with less severe lack of vitamin D, may be detected by low blood levels of vitamin D and its metabolites; by failure of bones to grow properly in length; and by x-ray pictures, which show the characteristic failure of normal deposition of calcium phosphate in the ends of the bones. When healing takes place, as a result of giving vitamin D, new deposits of calcium phosphate are laid down in the cartilage along the line of demarcation between the head of the bone (epiphysis) and the main part (shaft) of the long bone. This increase of mineral deposit near the ends of the bones is indicated by increased density in x-ray pictures (Fig. 9–9).

Though vitamin D deficiency is not common today in adults, it does occur in the United States and elsewhere especially during pregnancy (43), lactation, old age (44), and in adults eating foods low in vitamin D who do not receive any sunshine (45). Examples of the latter condition are certain women in the Middle East and North Africa who, by the custom of *purdah,* are confined indoors or are heavily clothed when outdoors (see Fig. 9–10). Rickets in adults, or *osteomalacia* (a form of softening of the bone; see also Chap. 15), is caused by depletion of bone stores of calcium and phosphorus. This may be from poor utilization of these mineral elements associated with vitamin D deficiency—or lack of sunshine—over very long periods, from faulty absorption, from kidney defects, or possibly in old age from changes in activity of certain hormone-producing glands (especially the parathyroid and thyroid glands).

It should be obvious that rickets at any age may be caused also by lack of either calcium or phosphorus, since these are the building

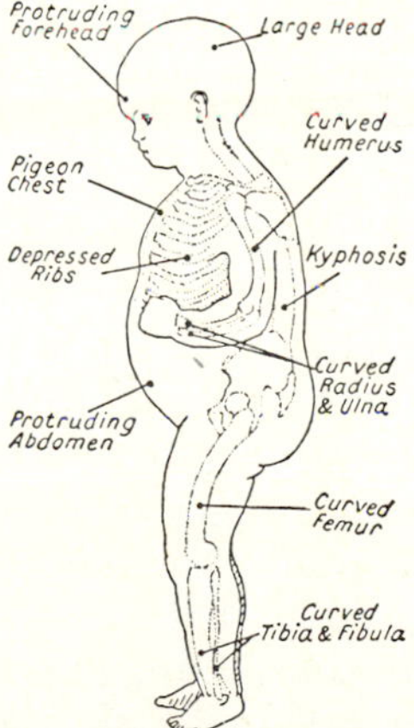

Figure 9–7 Diagram showing deformities that are symptoms of severe cases of rickets. (From Harris, L. J.: *Vitamins in Theory and Practice.* 4th Ed. London, Cambridge University Press, 1955.)

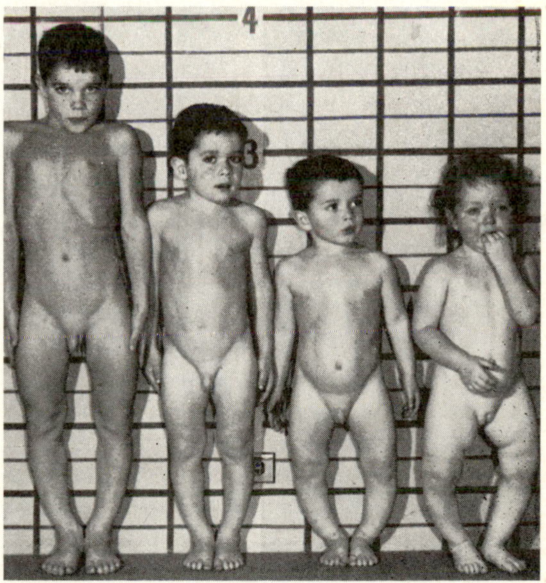

Figure 9–8 Three brothers and a female first cousin with rickets. (These cases were not due to a simple vitamin D deficiency, but the photo illustrates what vitamin D deficiency looks like in children.) (From Fraser, D., and Salter, R. B.: Pediatr. Clin. North Amer. May 1958.)

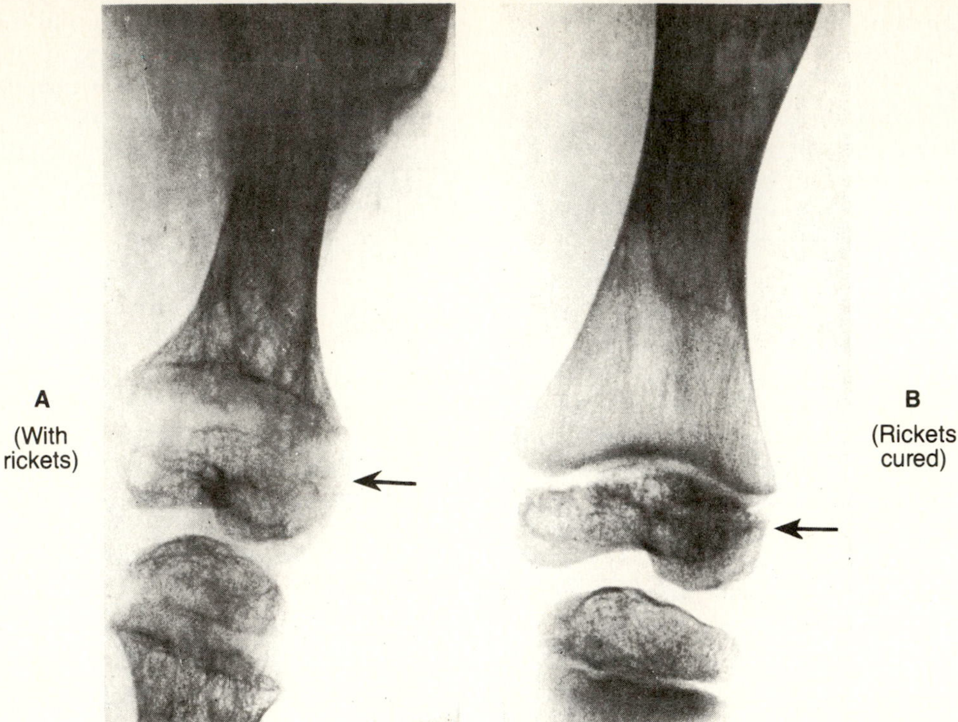

Figure 9–9 X-ray pictures of same joint in a 10-year-old Mexican boy, before and after treatment for rickets. A, Rarefication at ends of bones due to failure of normal deposition of calcium phosphate in rickets. B, One month later, showing increased density of bones and rapid healing of rachitic changes as the result of very large doses of vitamin D. (From McCune. In Whol, M. S. (ed.): *Dietotherapy*. Philadelphia, W. B. Saunders Co., 1945.)

materials for the calcium phosphate upon which the rigidity and strength of bone depend. No amount of vitamin D will promote normal bone development unless the mineral elements necessary for building strong bones are provided in the diet in adequate quantities. Conversely, if vitamin D is lacking, rickets may develop in persons on diets that supply plenty of calcium and phosphorus (for example, in infants on milk diet). The vitamin D may be supplied in food, it may be generated in the body by exposure to sunlight, or some may be obtained from each source. The best *protection* against this disease and the most favorable bone growth are secured when calcium and phosphorus are supplied in approximately equal amounts (as in milk) and when liberal quantities of vitamin D are available.

Vitamin D deficiency may also result in poor tooth development, muscular weakness, a protruding abdomen, listlessness, and an enlarged skull.

Recommended Allowances

Crystalline Standards. Vitamin D need no longer be measured in IU amounts now that crystalline standards are available. Crystalline *cholecalciferol* (vitamin D_3) has been adopted as the standard reference material. One IU equals the vitamin activity of 0.025 μg of this pure substance, and 400 IU equals 10 μg, a day's allowance, a very small amount indeed. Though the Food and Nutrition Board and other authorities give allowance figures only in terms of micrograms of total cholecalciferol, the IU term is still

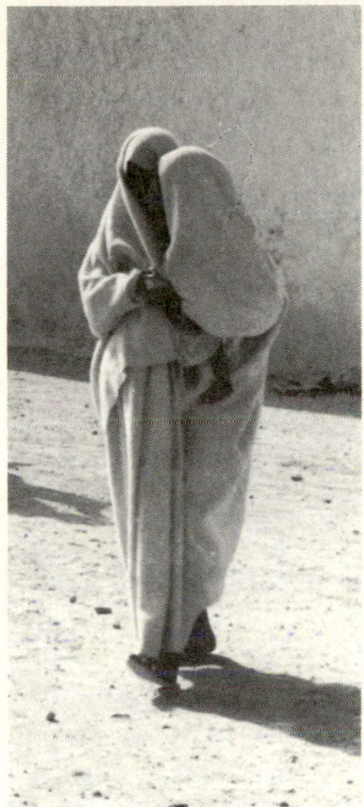

Figure 9–10 An example of *purdah,* a custom of being heavily wrapped in clothes, thus effectively blocking out the sunshine in a land of abundant sunshine. (From World Health, March 1977, p. 20. Courtesy of WHO.)

used by the Food and Drug Administration (FDA) for labeling purposes as the standard for food products and vitamin supplements. Thus both types of units should be kept in mind during this transition period. (At least, it's much easier to understand than a "retinol equivalent.")

Determining Allowances. The Food and Nutrition Board in its 1980 report gave estimated allowances for adults, for the first time, in recognition of their known need for vitamin D (8). Allowances were increased, also, for women during pregnancy and lactation up through twenty-two years of age. Details are given in Table 9–5 showing the requirements in the new (μg) and the old (IU) systems for comparison.

Exact requirements for vitamin D have not been determined, so the RDA values should be considered the best possible allowance figures based on all the evidence available. The amount of extra vitamin D from sunlight and how to measure it is a complicating factor.

Intensive studies of vitamin D requirements of infants show the daily need to be approximately the same as for adults (see Chap. 23). Less is known about the vitamin D requirements of older children than of infants. P. C. Jeans and G. Stearns showed that 7.5 to 10 μg daily of vitamin D (300 to 400 IU) favored calcium retention in children from one to twelve years of age (46). They state that in adolescence the need for this vitamin becomes "as universal and as great as in infancy."

During pregnancy and lactation, extra amounts of vitamin D (5 μg daily, or 200 IU) should be provided. A liberal supply at these periods is undoubtedly wise, because even though transmission to the fetus and milk is relatively low, the stores of vitamin D in the baby's body and the vitamin D content of milk are appreciably increased by vitamin D in the diet of the mother. In addition, optimum amounts of this vitamin promote the most efficient utilization by the mother of the calcium and phosphorus in her diet.

The Importance of Sunlight. The amount of vitamin D that is made in the body through exposure to sunlight varies according to the season, the locality in which one lives, one's habits, and the degree of pigmentation of the skin (47). In the tropics bright sunlight is available the year round; nevertheless, rickets is still possible. In other parts of the world, sunlight is scarce during the winter months. Sunlight also is richer in ultraviolet rays (light of short wavelength and high frequency) in summer, and more of these rays get through to the "consumer" when the sun is directly overhead—between 10 A.M. and 2 P.M. On cloudy or foggy days and in cities troubled with smog, almost all the ultraviolet rays are screened out before light penetrates to the people. Window glass and layers of clothing also effectively prevent ultraviolet rays from reaching the skin.

Table 9–5 RECOMMENDED DIETARY ALLOWANCE FOR VITAMIN D ACTIVITY[a]

Group	*Age in Years*	*Allowance μg/day of Cholecalciferol*	*IU/day*
Infants and children	0 to 10	10	400
Females	11–18	10	400
	19–22	7.5	300
	23 and older	5	200
	Pregnant	+5	+200
	Lactating	+5	+200
Males	11–18	10	400
	19–22	7.5	300
	23 and older	5	200

[a]From the latest Food and Nutrition Board report (8). IU values are given for comparison.

Only the ultraviolet rays have the ability to bring about the chemical change in the skin by which vitamin D is formed. Persons who live and work outdoors in sunny regions manufacture a considerable amount of vitamin D with the aid of sunlight and hence are less dependent on food for it. (See Fig. 9–11.)

Meeting the Recommended Allowances. Because of the widespread use of fortified milk and other foods, intakes of at least 10 RE daily appear to be common for most people plus an unknown amount from sunlight. In fact, medical authorities are probably more concerned about overconsumption of vitamin D than about deficiencies (see section on vitamin D toxicity). Nevertheless, vitamin D deficiency does occur in the United States to a limited extent in people of all ages. This is unnecessary and tragic and should be prevented as much as humanly possible. Public-health nutritionists, nutrition educators, and people who give nutrition advice to normal individuals must always be alert to the possibilities of indifference and forgetfulness concerning food and nutrition habits. Vitamin D supplementation of infant diets is a case in point and has become so routine that the importance of it might readily be forgotten.

Fortification of milk and other foods with vitamin D along with nutrition education programs has helped overcome deficiency in the United States and elsewhere. A classic example of the value of milk enrichment programs is that of preschool children in Chicago from 1926 to 1932. Examination of the children before milk fortification showed 16 to 21 percent with definite evidence of rickets. But by 1935, after vitamin D fortification of milk, the percentage had fallen to 7, with only 0.03 percent having severe rickets. The incidence of severe rickets, on the basis of these 1935 figures, had been reduced to three cases per 10,000 children. The American Academy of Pediatrics made a survey in 1962 and found only four cases of rickets in every 10,000 pediatric admissions to hospitals (48). Some of these may have been caused by mineral deficiencies or metabolic disorders, rather than by lack of vitamin D. It is clear that rickets as a disease could be eradicated in the United States. Many children do not achieve full growth and proper development of bones and teeth,

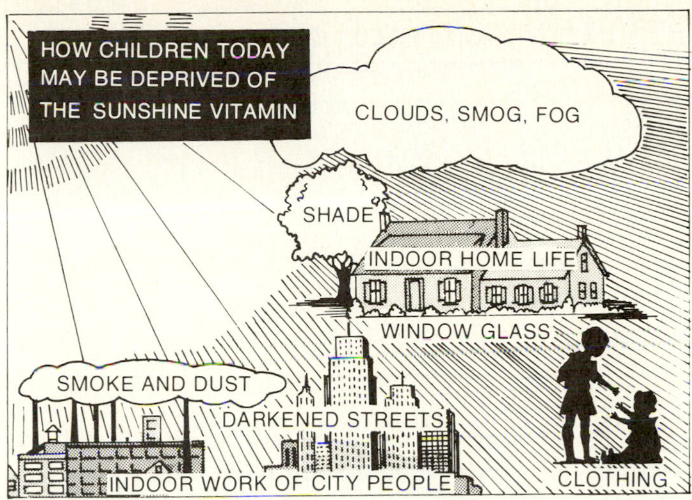
HOW CHILDREN TODAY
MAY BE DEPRIVED OF
THE SUNSHINE VITAMIN
CLOUDS, SMOG, FOG
SHADE
INDOOR HOME LIFE
WINDOW GLASS
SMOKE AND DUST
DARKENED STREETS
INDOOR WORK OF CITY PEOPLE
CLOTHING

Figure 9–11 People in country districts and in the tropics can make vitamin D in their bodies through the agency of direct sunlight. This drawing shows some of the factors of modern life that screen out ultraviolet light and prevent people from exposure to sunlight, thus at least partially depriving them of the chance of making this vitamin in their bodies. (Courtesy of the Wisconsin Alumni Research Foundation.)

however, because of lack of optimum amounts of calcium, phosphorus, vitamin D, or all three nutrients (as well as lack of knowledge, ability, or concern of their parents) (49). The situation in regard to vitamin D deficiency of children appears worse now than it was in the early 1960s.

Vitamin D in Foods

Nature's plan seems to be that humans should generate most of their supply of vitamin D from sunlight, for vitamin D is contained in foods more sparsely than any other vitamin.

Natural Foods. Vitamin D occurs with other fat-soluble vitamins in such foods of animal origin as egg yolk, butter fat, fatty fishes and fish livers, and of course in liver of other animals, since that is the organ that stores it. The amounts found in these foods are small and vary widely according to the diet of the animal and the extent to which it has been exposed to sunlight.

Vegetables, grains, and fruits are generally considered to have little or no vitamin D activity. An important exception is certain shrubs and plants recently found to contain such large amounts of forms of compounds with vitamin D activity that toxic symptoms (extensive calcification) may be seen in farm animals eating an overabundance of such plants (50).

Because vitamin D is resistant to heat and insoluble in water, there is little loss of it in the cooking or processing of those few foods that contain it.

Table 9-6 lists some typical food sources of vitamin D with the amount that may be counted on from an average serving. The content in egg yolk and butter is higher, however, if some rich source of vitamin D has been incorporated in the animals' feed, as is a common practice today. Eggs and dairy products furnish vitamin D in small quantities. Liver and fatty fish (sardines, salmon, mackeral) are good sources, but they are too infrequently used in the United States diets. If the daily diet contains 1 egg, 3 tablespoons (35 gm) of butter, and 1 pint (450 ml) of unenriched milk, one would receive only about 1.6 μg cholecalciferol (vitamin D_3) or 65 IU from natural foods. Three ounces (oz) of salmon (90 gm) would provide about 7.5 μg of vitamin D (300 IU). Most adults, although it is clear they need vitamin D, seem to get along at least fairly well on the small amounts furnished in foods, supplemented with the amounts generated under the influence of sunlight.

Table 9–6 VITAMIN D ACTIVITY OF TYPICAL FOODS

Food	*Size of Serving*	*Amount of Vitamin D (average)*	
		μg	IU
Fatty fish, canned:			
Herring	1 small fish (100 gm)	8.3	330
Salmon	100 gm	7.9	314
Tuna	⅝ c solid (100 gm)	5.0–8.0	200–300
Eggs	1 medium	0.7	27
Butter	1 oz or 3 avg. pats (30 gm)	0.7	28
Liver, raw	2 large slices (100 gm)	0.4–1.1	15–45
Cream, light to heavy	1 oz or 2 Tbsp	0.1–0.2	4–8
Milk, whole, fresh (enriched)	1 pt	5.0	200

Human milk has only about 0.5 μg of vitamin D activity (20 IU) per liter, an insufficient amount to prevent rickets, even though calcium intake is adequate. Breast-fed infants require supplementation with vitamin D or exposure to ample sunlight. Reports in the last few years from England suggesting that human and unenriched cow's milk have a high level of vitamin D activity could not be verified (51).

Enriched and Fortified Foods. Synthetic vitamin D can now be purchased in large wholesale lots for only a few cents, sufficient for one person for seven years. Thus, vitamin D is almost as cheap as sunshine itself and much more dependable. The cost of fortifying a quart of milk is therefore negligible (less than 1/100 cent). Other foods are quite commonly fortified with vitamin D today, so much so that under certain situations there could be danger of getting too much vitamin D (see next section). Nearly all fresh milk sold in North America is fortified with 10 μg of vitamin D activity (400 IU) per quart, as is all evaporated milk. Many breakfast foods are fortified, as are various margarines.

Toxicity of Vitamin D

Enough is better than too much as far as vitamin D is concerned, and parents (especially parents who believe in the practice of "overinsurance") should be warned of this fact in the event that they are giving high-potency vitamin D preparations to their children. There is evidence that certain infants are especially sensitive to the toxic action of vitamin D and may be adversely affected by intakes as low as 75 to 100 μg (3,000 to 4,000 IU) per day, as shown by abnormally high calcium levels in the blood, loss of appetite, and retarded growth (48). This is only about 10 times, or more, of their allowance—a very narrow range indeed. More studies are needed about this subject. With regular daily doses of 0.5 to 1.0 mg of vitamin D_3 (20,000 to 40,000 IU) for infants, or 1.3 to 2.5 mg (50,000 to 100,000 IU) for adults, serious toxic symptoms may develop. (These levels are about 50 to 250 times the recommended levels). These symptoms include vomiting, diarrhea, weakness, loss of weight, and kidney damage. The serum calcium is elevated to such a degree that deposits of calcium salts may be found in various organs.

Adults should be warned against taking massive doses of vitamin D or vitamin A over long periods, unless under the direct supervision of a physician (see ref. 22, Chap. 8).

Discovery of Vitamin D

Rickets has been known since 500 B.C., when it was described by Hippocrates (10). In the industrial towns of nineteenth-century England, rickets was very common in children in the crowded slums, and it became known as the "English disease." In 1824, cod-liver oil, long used as a folk medicine, was found to be important in the treatment of rickets, though it was not used universally for this purpose until nearly a century later (10).

The importance of sunshine for good health was known by ancient civilizations and is probably one of the bases for sun worship by early societies. In the 1890s it was found that sunshine was a specific cure for rickets (52)—though the exact reason for this was not known until the discovery of the vitamin itself in the 1920s.

In 1918, Dr. Mellanby of London, in studies with puppies, provided the first experimental proof that rickets was a disease of vitamin deficiency. He was able to cure it by feeding the puppies cod-liver oil. E. V. McCollum and his co-workers found in 1922 that after destruction (by oxidation) of all the vitamin A in cod-liver oil, it still retained its rickets-preventing potency (1,53). This discovery proved the existence of a second fat-soluble vitamin, carried in liver oils and certain other fats, which he called the calcium-depositing vitamin. It is of interest that although McCollum discovered the existence of vitamin D, he did not call it by that name until after the name was in common use by others.

The first crystalline vitamin D was obtained by Dutch chemists in 1931, and it was synthesized shortly thereafter. Soon, workers in this field thought that there were at least ten natural substances that produce vitamin D-like activity in varying degrees. Allowing for some duplication, only two of these are of practical importance today from the standpoint of their occurrence in foods—*ergocalciferol* (vitamin D_2, from plant tissues) and cholecalciferol (vitamin D_3, mainly found in animal tissues). (See formula in the Appendix for vitamin D_3, the common animal form.) Because these various forms are closely related chemically and produce a like effect on the body, the term vitamin D is used collectively to indicate the group of substances that show this vitamin activity.

The vitamin D group belongs to the class of organic substances known as *sterols*—fairly large lipid molecules in plants and animals containing an alcohol group and having the same solubilities as fats. They are very stable compounds, resisting destruction by heat and oxidation, as well as by acids and alkalis. The sterols, except vitamin D, are synthesized in the body and are the precursors of many important hormones, including several hormones made in the body from vitamin D and the sex hormones. Other common sterols are cholesterol and the several bile acids.

Precursors of Vitamin D

H. Steenbock and A. F. Hess, in the 1920s, discovered independently that when certain foods are exposed to ultraviolet light, their ability to protect animals against rickets is increased. This meant that some foods must contain precursors of vitamin D—substances that are altered chemically by light of certain wavelengths (including sunlight) so that they become capable of functioning as vitamins in the body. We now know that there are two major precursors of vitamin D in nature and that each gives rise to a slightly different vitamin D-active substance when activated by light. In plants, a substance known as *ergosterol*[1] is converted by light into ergocalciferol (vitamin D_2). In animals, and possibly in some plants, a derivative of cholesterol—*7-dehydrocholesterol*—is the precursor in the skin of cholecalciferol, or vitamin D_3.

Formation by Sunlight. The precursor (7-dehydrocholesterol) of vitamin D_3 is present in humans and animals in the oily lubri-

[1]The German chemist Adolph Windhaus received the Nobel Prize in 1928 for his studies on the vitamin activity of irradiated ergosterol. The compound was named from ergot, a black fungus that grows on the rye plant, from which ergosterol was first isolated in 1889.

cating material in the skin and on its surface. When sunlight, in which there is ultraviolet light, falls directly on the skin, some of the provitamin is converted into cholecalciferol, the major animal form of vitamin D (52). An intermediate, also in the skin, is known to be present and is called previtamin D (54). The vitamin thus formed in or on the skin is readily taken into the local circulation and carried by the blood to all parts of the body. Amounts formed in excess of immediate body needs can be stored in considerable amounts in the liver and may be found also in the fatty tissues, lungs, spleen, and brain.

Hess found that rickets could be prevented or cured by exposing children (without clothing) to sunlight or the rays of an ultraviolet lamp, since they thus were enabled to manufacture vitamin D in their own bodies. Ultraviolet lamps used to be much in vogue for this purpose. Today, however, with the availability of foods enriched with vitamin D and of other low-cost food supplements, ultraviolet lamps are not the most practical way of obtaining this vitamin.

The discovery of cheap dietary sources of vitamin D for farm animals (as substitutes for sunshine) was a major factor in the ability to raise swine, cattle, and poultry indoors and the year around (see Fig. 9–12). This resulted in the wide availability of low-cost eggs, milk, and meat in developed countries.

The Role of Vitamin D in the Body

Vitamin D, being fat-soluble, is absorbed from the intestine along with fats. Bile salts aid in this process, and conditions unfavorable to fat absorption (lack of bile, disorders such as sprue and celiac disease, etc.) may result in poor utilization of vitamin D. (See Fig. 9–13.)

Function. The overall function of vitamin D is to produce the vital hormone *1,25-dihydroxycholecalciferol,* known for short as *1,25-dihydroxy* D_3, or *calcitriol.* It was discov-

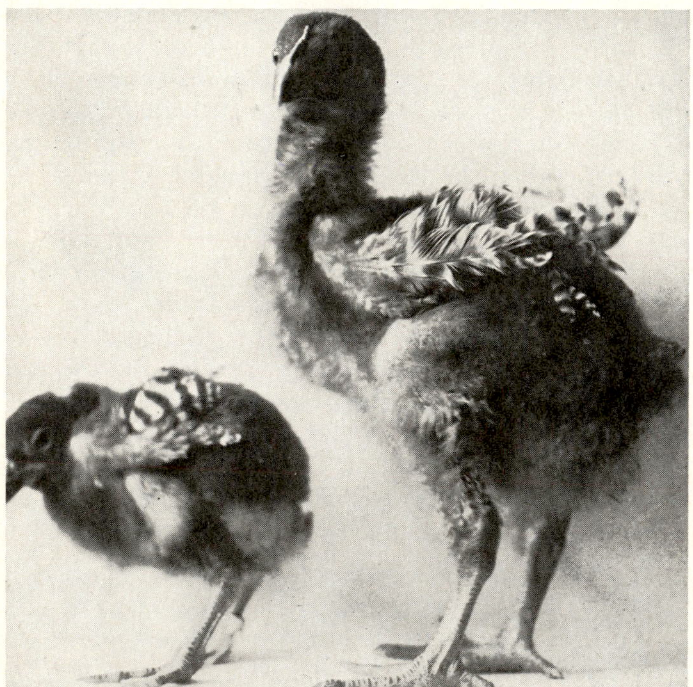

Figure 9–12 Effect of exposure to sunlight in stimulating growth. Both chicks received the same ration, which was poor in vitamin D, but the one on the right was exposed to sunlight one-half hour daily. This permitted generation of the needed vitamin D in its body. (Courtesy of Dr. H. Steenbock, University of Wisconsin.)

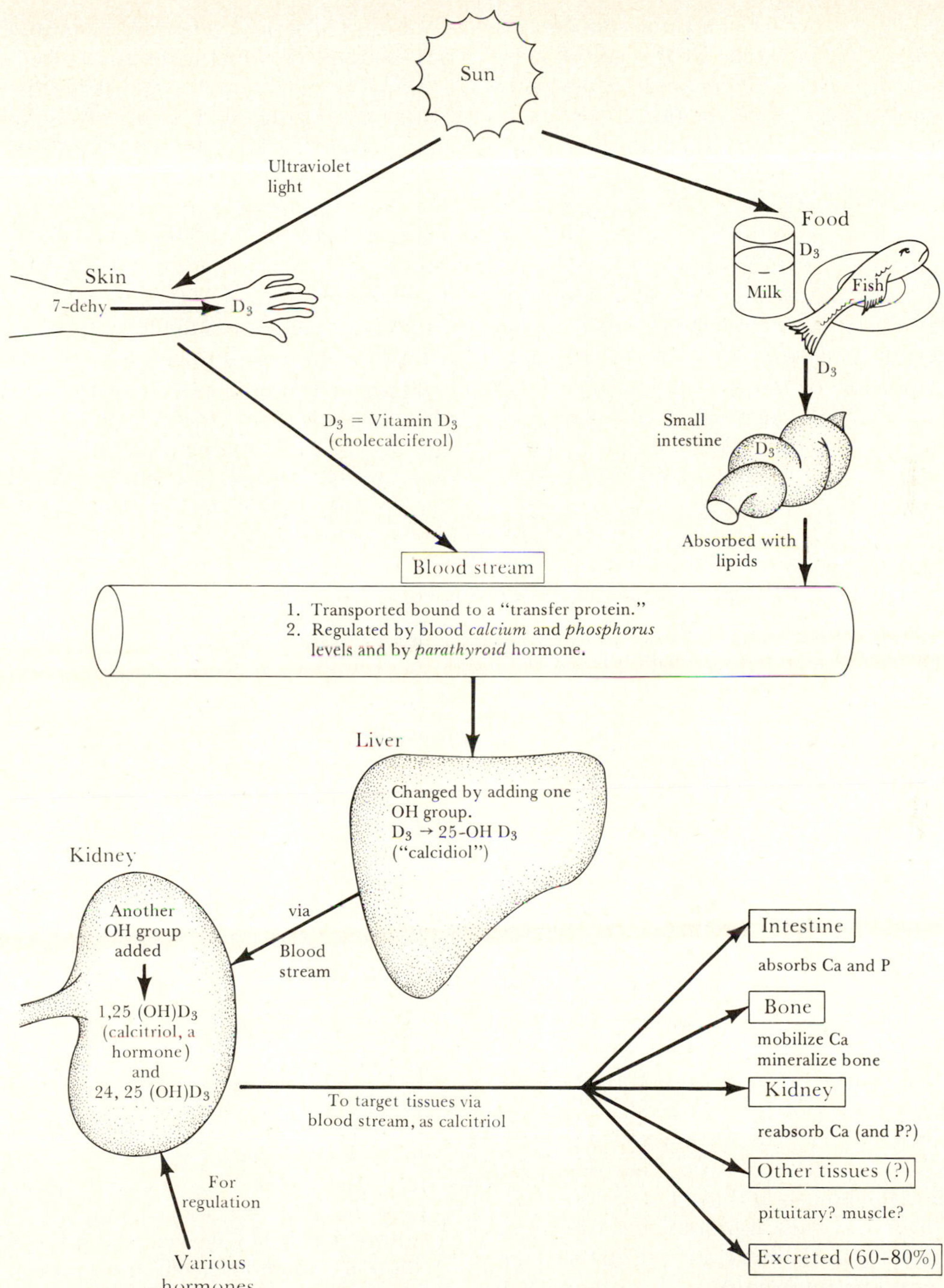

Figure 9–13 Vitamin D Metabolism. Simplified diagram of the paths of travel in the body of vitamin D from skin (sunlight) and/or from food to blood. Then in successive steps it is transferred to the liver (and receives a hydroxy group), then to the kidney (where the addition of another hydroxy group forms the hormone calcitriol), and back to the blood stream to various target tissues (adapted from DeLuca and others).

ered in 1971 by H. F. DeLuca and others. Made in successive steps by the addition of −OH groups by the liver and kidney, this hormone is essential for the overall effects of dietary vitamin D. They include promotion of growth and proper mineralization of the bones and teeth. There is general agreement that the main result of its action is the improvement of the body's use of calcium and phosphorus supplied in the food. Vitamin D, through the action of calcitriol, increases the absorption of calcium, and secondarily also of phosphorus, from the intestinal tract. It is also involved with calcium mobilization from bones and with the preservation of phosphate by control of its excretion from the kidney (see Fig. 9–13). All these reactions help to keep the content of these two elements in the blood up to levels favorable to the deposition of calcium phosphate in the bones. It appears at this time that the only function of dietary forms of vitamin D, such as cholecalciferol, is to serve as a precursor of the hormone form. As far as is known now, vitamin D itself does not function until the two additional OH groups are added in the body.

Considerable interest today exists in the possible clinical use of calcitriol, the vitamin D hormone, in the treatment and/or prevention (often with other agents) of various diseases such as renal osteodystrophy, failure of the parathyroid gland, and softening of the bones in adults (osteoporosis). These clinical applications are mainly beyond the scope of this book. There are many other areas of research of great potential interest to the student, for example, the possible relation of vitamin D to certain cancers, atherosclerosis, diabetes, alcoholism and alcohol metabolism, other liver diseases, immunological defects, increased requirements in premature infants, hypoparathyroidism, drug use and vitamin D requirements, kidney diseases, various bone diseases, and inherited diseases such as vitamin D-resistant rickets. These are important diseases; whether vitamin D will help in their treatment remains to be seen.

Many new metabolites and derivatives are being discovered and their effect on the body studied. Many hundreds of research papers are being published each year in this one exciting field. The authors hope that this small review of the basic nutritional knowledge about vitamin D will help students understand, at least a little better, new findings as they see them in present and future nutrition literature.

Again the authors point out that students who want additional information about vitamin D (or other vitamins) will find many answers in the references at the end of the chapter (17,55) and the supplementary readings in the Appendix.

VITAMIN E

Vitamin E is a common household word. Interest in it is based largely upon many unjustifiable claims being made for it. These claims, including those for sexual potency and superior athletic performance, are made in the public media, in health-food literature, and on store shelves. Recommendations for taking extra amounts of vitamin E, beyond the amount we obtain in our food, are without experimental justification. Nevertheless, vitamin E is an important vitamin for humans as well as for animals.

Vitamin E has a few distinctive properties.

1. Few clinical symptoms of deficiency are ever seen in humans except in premature infants. In normal adults many months of time are required to deplete tissue stores of vitamin E.
2. It is the most efficient, natural antioxidant known. Unlike other vitamins it apparently functions in the body only as an antioxidant, not as a coenzyme or as a hormone.
3. It is fairly widely used in larger amounts than necessary, or even safe, by individuals who treat themselves.

4. It is an oil at room temperature and has not been crystallized. It exists in foods in eight different active forms, each with a different potency.
5. It is very closely related metabolically to selenium, an essential trace element.

These points are discussed in more detail later in this chapter. If any students happen to be vitamin E enthusiasts, they are urged to keep an open mind until they have studied the basic facts as they are presented here, in the references at the end of the chapter, and in the supplementary reading lists in the Appendix.

Deficiency Symptoms

Vitamin E is widely distributed in basic foods such as beans, rice, eggs, meat, green vegetables, fats and oils, and grains. Therefore, strange as it may seem to vitamin E enthusiasts, deficiencies of this vitamin are practically never seen in normal children and adults eating all combinations of food. This is true even in countries where food supplies are scarce. In such conditions other deficiencies will develop long before stores of vitamin E are depleted.

In a classic study lasting six years, even when volunteer humans consumed meals with only about 3.3 mg (5.0 IU) of vitamin E per day, efforts to induce clinical symptoms proved futile (56,57). In these volunteers, however, after five years, changes were noted in the red blood cells, which became more fragile when removed from the body and given a standard hemolysis test. Increased excretion of creatine, indicating muscle loss, and deposition of a ceroid pigment in the muscle of the small intestine have been seen in other studies in vitamin E-deficient patients with long-standing inability to absorb fat (58). No specific clinical symptoms were seen in these studies either.

The point of describing these studies in detail is to show how difficult it is for normal people to develop a vitamin E deficiency (and how easy it is to prevent it with a normal diet).

Symptoms in Premature Infants. Premature infants are born with low concentrations of vitamin E and often have fat-absorption problems. Under these conditions, the feeding of extra polyunsaturated fatty acids, or any factor that might cause vitamin E losses, can result in deficiency signs such as edema, anemia, and low blood levels of vitamin E (8). A serious eye problem *(retrolental fibroplasia)* in premature infants, which can result in blindness, is known to occur and is associated with oxygen treatment of these infants. A number of studies have been made on the possible prevention of this condition with vitamin E (or with vitamin E and selenium together). It appears that very high levels of the vitamin (such as 150 mg a day) might have a beneficial effect. This is one of the few active areas of research on this vitamin, but it is still very controversial (59). Deficiencies of vitamin E along with other fat-soluble vitamins are possible in children with cystic fibrosis or with bile problems.

Lack of Symptoms in Adults. With so many popular claims about benefits from vitamin E, one should know that there has been no convincing evidence put forward in peer-review scientific journals that vitamin E deficiency in normal humans causes reduced athletic performance, heart disease, weakened sex drive, impotence, cancer, muscular weakness or muscular dystrophy, leg cramps, sterility, premature aging, or similar problems, as is often claimed. Nor would the reverse be true. In other words, extra amounts of vitamin E in a diet would not be expected to improve these conditions. For instance, a Canadian study, in 1979, reported "no differences in sexual arousal, or behavior" between two groups of people given 100 IU (about 67 mg) of vitamin E per day in a "double-blind placebo" study (60).

The lack of effect of vitamin E in improving all these conditions is not to deny that high levels of vitamin E might have some pharmacological effects beyond vitamin effects in the treatment of certain other diseases (see later discussion). After all, it is a chemical as are other drugs. It is a strong antioxidant (and hence has the potential of being toxic) and should never be taken without professional advice. It should be kept in mind, however, that no beneficial effects of even high levels of vitamin E, let alone normal levels, have been seen in the above kinds of conditions in reliable studies (61).

Symptoms in Animals. In contrast to the rarity of deficiency signs in humans, a wide variety of deficiency signs are readily obtained in experimental animals. The deficient rat, for instance, fails to grow normally and develops weakness and degeneration of the skeletal muscles. Lesions have also been found in heart muscle. Death results eventually. Deficiencies of vitamin E have been obtained in many species other than the rat. In the chick, brain lesions, muscular dystrophy, and weakened capillaries occur. Liver damage and a number of other muscular symptoms have been seen in deficient mice, pigs, dogs, and other animals.

Recommended Allowances for Vitamin E

The Food and Nutrition Board's recommended allowances for vitamin E activity for young men and women and for older persons are given in Table 9–7. The allowance is 10 mg per day for college age men and 8 mg per day for women. Figures for other ages are given in the complete RDA table. These values are considerably lower than earlier recommendations on which the current U.S. food labeling regulations are based. Until this discrepancy is corrected, food labels show about half of the correct percentage of the vitamin E allowance.

The requirement of vitamin E for humans is known to vary with other ingredients in the diet, as it does for animals. The presence of unusually large amounts of linoleic acid or other polyunsaturated fatty acids in the diet *increases the requirement* up to, say, 15 to 20 mg a day (62). This fact has significance in today's dietary pattern, in which large amounts of vegetable oils may be widely used. Most oils, however, are rich sources of

Table 9–7 RECOMMENDED DIETARY ALLOWANCE FOR VITAMIN E ACTIVITY

		Allowance[a]	
	Age	ALPHA-TOCOPHEROL EQUIVALENTS/DAY (in mg)	IU/DAY
Males	11–14 years old	8	12
	15 years and over	10	15
Females	11 years and over	8	12
	Pregnant	10	15
	Lactating	11	16.5

[a]From Food and Nutrition Board (8). For additional values see inside front cover. These values are lower than the vitamin E values listed on food packages. The U.S. RDA is based on older (1968) estimates. Values are given also in terms of IU/day for convenience during this transition period. The alpha-tocopherol used as the standard is the natural dextro (d) form, the most active form of this vitamin (see text).

vitamin E, so there need be no concern of not getting enough when eating large amounts of these oils (8). The presence of rancid fats, oxidizing substances, and selenium would be expected to modify the requirement for vitamin E. The recommended level is generous and should cover all contingencies for practical purposes.

Tocopherol Equivalents, Units, and Nomenclature. In 1936 the people who first isolated pure vitamin E, thinking it was one compound, called it *tocopherol.* It was isolated from wheat germ oil at the University of California by Herbert Evans and his co-workers, O.H. Emerson and G. A. Emerson[2] (63). The name tocopherol is derived from Greek words meaning "to bear offspring." The "ol" ending signifies it is an alcohol. In fact, vitamin E consists of eight compounds—four tocopherols and four *tocotrienols.* They are light yellow, viscous oils, insoluble in water and resistant to heat but readily destroyed by severe oxidation and ultraviolet light. They are all excellent antioxidants, though their antioxidant activity does not correlate directly with their differences in biological activity because of differences in their availability to the cell.

The structures of the four natural forms of the tocopherols (alpha [α]-, beta [β]-, gamma [γ]-, and delta [δ]-) were soon determined, and synthesis was accomplished in the laboratory (see formula of *alpha-tocopherol* in the Appendix). Alpha-tocopherol (α-tocopherol) is, biologically, the most active natural form of the eight vitamin E compounds. However, there is 2 to 4 times as much gamma-tocopherol, a less active form, in many foods than there is alpha-tocopherol.

[2]Gladys Emerson received her Ph.D. degree in nutrition at California and later became head of the nutritional sciences department at U.C.L.A. where she stayed for many years. When she was asked recently how much vitamin E she consumed per day, she answered, "Just the recommended allowance."

The four other compounds, closely related to the four tocopherols, but with lesser degrees of vitamin E activity (from 1 to 30 percent), occur in food and, hence, in the body: the alpha-, beta-, gamma-, and delta-tocotrienols. Thus, the word tocopherol is not synonymous with the group name, vitamin E. This fact explains why we use alpha-tocopherol equivalents as a summation term for requirement values and for amounts of the vitamin in food and body tissues for measuring total vitamin E activity.

These relationships seem simple enough until we learn that in order to provide vitamin E for the food, animal feed, and vitamin industry, at least forty different isomers and derivatives of alpha-tocopherol with different degrees of activity are manufactured, many in very large amounts. (Some of these are added to food for their antioxidant value, helping to stabilize other valuable nutrients.) Alpha-tocopherol has 3 isomeric carbon atoms and exists in the *d*-form (the natural form) and *dl*-form (a synthetic form, which has about 74 percent of the vitamin activity as the natural *d*-alpha-tocopherol). The natural *d*-form is also called by the trivial name R, R, R-alpha-tocopherol, using today's international nomenclature.[3] Table 9–8 shows the relationship between the various vitamin E-active compounds in terms of

[3]The major vitamin E of commerce today is a mixture of all eight isomers of dl-α-tocopherol acetate with the trivial name of all-rac-α-tocopherol acetate. This appears on food and vitamin supplement labels as "vitamin E acetate," generally. It has 67 percent of the activity of the natural form and, very conveniently, it happens that each milligram of this commercial form has one IU of vitamin E activity. When expressed in terms of milligrams of *d*-alpha-tocopherol equivalents it would be wrong to imply, as is done commonly in vitamin advertisements, that "natural" forms of vitamin E are more active than synthetic forms. They may well be more potent per milligram, for whatever use that may be, but not more active per alpha-tocopherol equivalent.

Table 9–8 RELATIONSHIPS BETWEEN ALPHA-TOCOPHEROL EQUIVALENTS AND INTERNATIONAL UNITS (IU) FOR VITAMIN E-ACTIVE COMPOUNDS

Common Name (1 mg)	*d-Alpha-Tocopherol Equivalents per 1 mg (Approx.)*	*IU Activity per 1 mg (Approx.)*
d-alpha-tocopherol[a]	1 mg	1.49 IU
d-alpha-tocopheryl acetate	0.91 mg	1.36 IU
d-alpha-tocopheryl acid succinate	0.81 mg	1.21 IU
dl-alpha-tocopherol	0.74 mg	1.10 IU
dl-alpha-tocopheryl acetate[b]	0.67 mg	1.00 IU
dl-alpha-tocopherol acid succinate	0.60 mg	0.90 IU
Beta-tocopherol	0.40 mg	0.60 IU
Gamma-tocopherol[c]	0.10 mg	0.15 IU
Delta-tocopherol	0.01 mg	0.02 IU
Alpha-tocotrienol	0.30 mg	0.45 IU
Beta-tocotrienol	0.05 mg	0.08 IU
Gamma-tocotrienol	0.01 mg	0.02 IU
Delta-tocotrienol	0.01 mg	0.02 IU

[a]The natural form in foods and the standard for alpha-tocopherol equivalents. Usually just called alpha-tocopherol but in commerce also called RRR-alpha-tocopherol (the RRR refers to the presence of methyl groups at three asymmetrical centers); see Ames, S.R.: IUNS-AIN nomenclature for vitamin E. J. Assoc. Offic. Anal. Chem. *55*:625, 1972. Also see refs. 29 and 64 for more recent information.

[b]The form of vitamin E most generally used in commerce—a synthetic but more stable form. It is also called all-rac-alpha tocopherol (rac = racemic mixture). This is the standard for International Units.

[c]The form most abundant in most common food oils in terms of weight, not in activity (see Table 9–9).

the new alpha-tocopherol equivalents and the old IU activity (still used today in labeling food products) (4,8,64). These details are given here for background information. Fortunately, the total contribution of all forms in food with vitamin E activity can be expressed in the one term alpha-tocopherol equivalents.

Estimates of Intake. Estimates of daily vitamin E intake in the United States appear to average about 8 to 11 mg alpha-tocopherol equivalents (12 to 16 IU) (8) slightly higher than recommended intakes. These levels should present no problems since the vitamin E allowance is set at about twice the minimum need.

Blood levels of vitamin E activity, often in relation to the total amount of lipids present, are used in order to indicate when a population is deficient in vitamin E. Levels in adults below 0.5 mg per 100 ml of blood are considered too low (8). Few people in any country have levels much below this.

Vitamin E in Foods

In a typical American diet, about 66 percent of the intake of vitamin E comes from salad oils, shortening, margarines, and other fats and oils. The tocopherols are the chief antioxidants in natural fats and oils and act to prevent fats from becoming rancid. Normally, then, persons eating extra polyunsaturated fats, who have a higher requirement for vitamin E, will also consume extra vitamin E. The rest of the vitamin E in the American diet comes mainly from whole grains, liver, beans, and fruits and vegetables (65).

Only in recent years has it been possible to measure with reasonable accuracy the specific amounts of the various forms of vitamin E in foods (see Table 9–9 for representative values). However, there is not sufficient knowledge as yet to know the vitamin E activity of many of these various forms, but, generally, non-alpha-tocopherol forms of vitamin E in a mixed diet are considered to

Table 9–9 SEVERAL COMMON FORMS OF VITAMIN E IN REPRESENTATIVE OILS[a]

	Alpha-tocopherol	*Beta-tocopherol*	*Gamma-tocopherol*	*Delta-tocopherol*	*Alpha-tocotrienol*	*Total alpha-tocopherol equivalents*
	Relative Biological Potency					
	1.00	0.40	0.10	0.01	0.30	1.00
Food Sources	mg/100 gm					
Corn oil	14	0.4	65	8.0	0.6	21
Cottonseed oil	35	0	30	0	0	38
Palm oil	18	0	0	0	11.0	22
Peanut oil	12	—	13	0.3	0	13
Safflower oil	34	—	4	0.5	—	34
Soybean oil	11	—	62	20.4	0	17
Wheat-germ oil	150	81.0	—	—	—	183

[a]Values from McLaughlin, P. J., and Weihrauch, J. L.: J. Amer. Dietet. Assoc., *75*:647, 1979. (See table 4 of this paper for values obtained in last column representing vitamin E *activity*. The values listed in all the other tables of this paper for "total vitamin E" have no biological meaning. They do not reflect vitamin E *activity*, but just the total amount, in milligrams, of the different forms.)

supply about 20 percent of the total vitamin E activity.

Because of the lack of general availability of figures for vitamin E in food, Table 9–10 gives the alpha-tocopherol content of representative foods as determined by recent methods. Use of these figures in calculating one's intake will give a conservative value (somewhat lower, in most instances, than the total vitamin E activity), since other, lower potency forms of the vitamin are disregarded. In mixed diets the total milligrams of alpha-tocopherol may be multiplied by a factor of 1.2 to give an approximation of total vitamin E activity in terms of alpha-tocopherol equivalents (8).

In general, most seeds and oils from these seeds are the best sources of vitamin E. Some vegetables are also good sources, especially green, leafy vegetables. Wheat-germ oil is one of the richest natural sources. Synthetic forms of vitamin E are the least expensive sources, although the authors recommend that vitamin E be consumed in a regular diet as much as possible, in order to obtain all the other essential nutrients also.

The vitamin E activity of foods may be considerably reduced in processing, milling, storage, and packaging (65,66). For instance, as much as 80 percent or more may be lost in converting whole wheat to white bread. Freezing of vegetables is also known to cause some destruction of vitamin E—a finding unique among the vitamins. Vitamin E activity is not destroyed to any great extent by normal temperatures used in cooking in the home. There are appreciable losses of vitamin E activity in oils heated long periods of times at high temperature, such as in deep-fat frying, because rancidity develops (67).

Toxicity and Use as a Drug

Although vitamin E is not considered especially toxic in comparison with vitamins A and D, recent literature suggests precautions in regard to taking very large amounts of vitamin E from nonfood sources. "Very large" amounts would be 300 mg or more per day. Beyond this amount, frequent incidences of toxicity have been observed in humans (8,57,68) as well as in experimental animals.

In spite of these precautions, many people are taking "megadose" amounts of supplements containing vitamin E (see Chap. 8). A recent study made of more than 1,700 registered female nurses in ten states found that

Table 9–10 ALPHA-TOCOPHEROL CONTENT OF REPRESENTATIVE FOODS*

Food	*mg/100 gm*	*Food*	*mg/100 gm*
Seeds		*Vegetables and fruits*	
Almond	27.0	Asparagus, fresh	1.8
Barley	0.5	Carrots, fresh	0.5
Corn	0.6	Beans, dry	0.1 to 0.7
Oat	0.5	Mango, ripe	1.0
Rice, white	0.1	Potatoes	0.1
Rice, whole	0.3	Green leafy (most)	1 to 10
Wheat	1.4	Corn, fresh	0.1
Peanuts	10.0	Most fruits, fresh	0.1 to 1.0
Peas	0.5		
		Other foods	
Oils		Potato chips	2.1
Coconut	0.5	Sugar cookie	2.0 to 5.0
Cod-liver	29.0	Eggs	1.0
Corn	11.0	Liver	2.0
Cottonseed	39.0	Codfish	0.2 to 1.2
Olive	5.0	Beef	1.0
Palm	26.0	Lobster	1.7
Peanut	13.0	Butter	2.0
Rapeseed	18.4	Lard	1.2
Safflower	39.0	Margarine	10.0
Soybean	10.0	Shortening (vegetable)	10.0
Sunflower	49.0	Milk (cow's)	0.1
Walnut	56.0	Yeast	0
Wheat germ	133.0	Infant cereals	0.1 to 1.0
		Wheat flour	0.2
		Wheat germ	13.0
		Bread, white	0.2

*Most values adapted from Dicks (40) and Slover (Lipids, *6*:291, 1971). (Values are for alpha-tocopherol only.) Also see Koehler, H. H., Lee, H. C., and Jacobson, M.: J. Amer. Dietet. Assoc., *70*:616, 1977, for values of canned entrees and vended sandwiches. For a detailed listing of many more foods, including levels of all eight forms of vitamin E (values to be used in the new Handbook 8 of the U.S.D.A.), see McLaughlin, P. J., and Weihrauch, J. L.: J. Amer. Dietet. Assoc., *75*:647, 1979. These authors list "total vitamin E" in all of the tables in their paper. As explained in the text, such a value has no biological meaning and should not be used for vitamin E activity (see footnote, Table 9–9). The values above have not been updated to the 1979 values.

38 percent were taking multiple vitamins and 15 percent were taking special vitamin E preparations—most of them at many times the RDA levels (69). Another recent study reported that more than 16 percent of 2,450 adults surveyed in seven western states took vitamin E regularly in amounts 10 times the RDA (70). The authors of the study, eight nutritionists in four western universities, considered these amounts potentially toxic. (The authors of this book would not suggest taking high levels of *any vitamins* without a *very* good reason. It seems to them unwise, unnecessary, unnatural, and costly. Anyone taking, say, 900 mg of vitamin E per day is taking the equivalent of the vitamin E in 1.1 lb of wheat-germ oil per day, a very unnatural amount.) H. J. Roberts lists about 20 case histories of clinical disorders attributed to high levels of vitamin E plus a number of "laboratory abnormalities" (68). This paper should be "must reading" for anyone considering taking large amounts of vitamin E.

Besides the interest in the use of vitamin E in protecting against anemia and retrolental fibroplasia in premature infants, there may be conditions where a physician would prescribe large amounts of vitamin E for its pharmacological properties in spite of the toxicity risk. Vitamin E is used in patients, for example, with malabsorption problems and in certain genetic diseases. Because of its strong antioxidant activity, vitamin E is being used by physicians, with some degree of success, in protecting against certain experimental immunological disorders, blood clotting abnormalities, and certain types of cancers (24). Studies of these and other clinical disorders (71) are in progress (also see supplementary readings in the Appendix).

The Function of Vitamin E in the Body

The existence of a dietary factor necessary for reproduction in rats, what we now know as the vitamin E group, has been known since 1922 (72). The *antioxidant properties* of the compounds were discovered in 1931, by H. S. Olcott and H. A. Matill (73).

Antioxidant Function. The major function of vitamin E, if not the only function, in the body is reasonably explained by its antioxidant properties, reaching almost every body cell including muscles, membranes, blood cells, and nerve tissue (74).

Vitamin E is highly efficient in preventing cell membrane damage from naturally occurring *free radicals* (varieties of peroxides formed from fatty acids in the cells)—substances that have been suggested as playing a role in the aging process.

Most of the vitamin E in the body is associated with the fat content of cells. Vitamin E is carried in the blood stream mainly attached to lipoproteins. The level in the blood is closely associated with the total plasma lipids and hence is influenced greatly by diet and other factors affecting levels of lipids in the blood.

Vitamin E protects both vitamin A and carotene from destruction by oxidation, especially in the alimentary tract. In this way, vitamin E spares the supply of vitamin A available to the body. This fact may be of importance if the intake of vitamin A is barely adequate for body needs.

Vitamin E deficiency presents such a wide variety of symptoms in so many animals that one might assume that it would be a part of many enzyme systems. However, there is no known specific coenzyme form of the vitamin in tissues (in spite of claims to the contrary), nor does it seem to play a specific role in any enzymatic reaction. Symptoms of a deficiency may be prevented in experimental animals by other antioxidants or by much lower amounts of the trace mineral *selenium*.

Several generations of animals have been reared without any vitamin E in the diet but with selenium and any of several synthetic antioxidants present. Vitamin E compounds, however, are the most active antioxidants in natural foods and belong to the vitamin family by long tradition even without a coenzyme role.

Relation to Selenium. In 1957, K. Schwarz and C. M. Folz discovered a very interesting dietary relationship of vitamin E to the trace mineral selenium (75). They found that extremely low levels of selenium could replace the vitamin E needs of animals under certain conditions. The full significance of this discovery for humans has not been worked out as yet. There are large geographic areas in the United States and in other countries, however, with soils deficient in selenium, where farm animals (usually sheep or cattle) with "white muscle disease" are cured only by combinations of selenium and vitamin E (see Chap. 17), which are either injected into the animals or fed to them. Fortunately, normal foods of mixed origin have sufficient selenium and vitamin E present so that humans do not have to worry about this problem.

VITAMIN K

The fourth, but not the least, of the fat-soluble vitamins was discovered in studies of chickens by H. Dam[4] of Copenhagen in 1935 and a few months later independently by H. J. Almquist and E. L. R. Stokstad of the University of California (76). Because the vitamin is essential for the proper coagulation of blood, Dam proposed that it be called the *Koagulation vitamin* (the Danish and German spelling of the word), from which the term vitamin K was derived.[5] Vitamin K was isolated in pure form in 1939, and shortly thereafter it was synthesized and its chemical structure determined.

The most unusual feature about this vitamin from a nutritional point of view is that unlike other fat-soluble vitamins, considerable amounts are produced by bacteria in the intestine of humans and animals. Generally, sufficient amounts are made each day to take care of most of, if not all, human requirements. (The only other two vitamins synthesized in the intestine by bacteria at, or near, sufficient amounts are vitamin B-12 and biotin.)

Deficiency Symptoms

Vitamin K is essential for blood clotting so that hemorrhages (heavy bleeding) will not occur. If not controlled, such bleeding can result in death. Bleeding from a lack of vitamin K is rarely seen in adults except under special circumstances to be explained. A low level of vitamin K in new-born infants is possible during the first week before the intestinal bacteria have become established. Many physicians routinely give vitamin K, by injection, to infants as a precaution to prevent bleeding. This is especially important if the mother has been given anticoagulants, drugs that prevent blood from clotting.

[4]Dam, who died in 1976, received the Nobel Prize for this in 1943 with Dr. Doisey of St. Louis (who first determined the structure of vitamin K_2).

[5]Vitamins I and J, now obsolete terms for other vitamins, were proposed also in 1935, so that the use of the letter K was in alphabetical order.

Provisional Allowances

The Food and Nutrition Board has suggested a range of recommended intakes in its last report for twelve new nutrients, including vitamin K (8). These are given as "estimated safe and adequate dietary intakes" until more information is available on which to base allowances (see provisional allowance table inside back cover).

The provisional allowance for adults eighteen years and over is 70 to 140 μg per day. An average mixed diet, along with active intestinal flora, appears to provide about 3 times as much each day under normal conditions—300 to 500 μg (8).

Clinical Applications of Vitamin K

A deficiency in infants, children, or adults can occur wherever intestinal synthesis of the vitamin is depressed. This can occur in new-born babies or in any person taking antibiotics or other intestinal sterilizing agents for extended periods. For example, deficiencies have been seen in infants receiving drugs for diarrhea or intestinal infections. A normal infant's requirement is about 12 to 20 μg per day, the amount present in 1 liter of human milk. Larger amounts than this are put in milk formulas for infants to allow for extra needs during diarrhea or intestinal medication.

Vitamin K deficiency, as evidenced by internal hemorrhages, has occurred in humans under conditions in which absorption of the vitamin is hindered or prevented. This can happen in any condition in which bile flow is disturbed, such as obstructive jaundice, or after injuries or surgical operations (as with the other fat-soluble vitamins). In such situations, extra doses of vitamin K given with bile salts have proved effective in raising the level of certain proteins necessary for coagulation of the blood. *Prothrombin* is the best known of these. Prothrombin is a protein necessary for blood clotting that requires vitamin K for its manufacture. Thus, the normal clotting ability of the blood is restored with vitamin K.

Considerable clinical use is made of synthetic substances that act as antagonists of vitamin K (such as dicoumarol, an anticoagulant) to prevent clotting of the blood in patients with certain circulatory disorders. The antagonists are also, interestingly enough, used as very potent rat killers (such as Warfarin), which destroy the rat by preventing its blood from clotting without the rat tasting it in its food.

Except for these abnormal conditions, vitamin K deficiency would seldom be seen in humans. There appears to be no reason for a normal individual eating a varied diet of traditional foods to feel that his or her diet does not contain an adequate supply of this vitamin. Vitamin K has not proved effective in treating hemophilia, an inherited condition causing abnormal hemorrhaging in humans.

Vitamin K in Foods

Food sources of vitamin K include all the green leafy vegetables, cheese, and liver. Lettuce, spinach, kale, turnip greens, broccoli, cauliflower, and cabbage are excellent sources; the inner leaves of cabbage have about one-fourth as much as the outer leaves. Green tea is reported to be an excellent source. Very little vitamin K is present in most cereals, fruits, carrots, peas, meats, oils, potatoes, or highly refined foods (77,78).

This information is rather academic since, as has been stated, unless we have been diagnosed by a physician to be at risk of a vitamin K deficiency for one of the above reasons, we do not need to worry about obtaining enough of this nutrient in our diet. We obtain 2 or 3 times our need each day.

Nomenclature and Properties

Vitamin K_1 and K_2,[6] the major forms of the vitamin in nature, are chemicals known as *quinones* (see the formula of vitamin K_1 in Appendix). Vitamin K_1 is now called by its chemical name *phylloquinone* (4). Vitamin K_2, made by bacteria, actually is a series of similar compounds called *menaquinones*. Vitamin K_1 and K_2 are present in the body (mainly stored in the liver) in about equal amounts. They are not particularly toxic even if taken in large amounts for pharmaceutical purposes.

Several synthetic forms, such as *menadione* (formerly called vitamin K_3) and its various water-soluble derivatives, are converted to vitamin K_2 in the body, and thus have similar vitamin K activity. But, unlike the natural forms, they are toxic when given in large amounts.

All forms of the vitamin are yellow and are quite resistant to heat, air, and moisture, but not to light. Cooking destroys very little of the vitamin because it is not water-soluble.

The Role of Vitamin K in the Body

A primary function of vitamin K is the formation in the liver of at least six different proteins, essential in blood clotting, working directly with calcium in this respect. To do this vitamin K functions as an essential cofactor with several enzymes[7] that change molecules of the amino acid *glutamic acid* in protein to the newly discovered derivative *carboxyglutamic acid*. The enzyme does this with the essential help of vitamin K in trans-

[6]The numbered subscripts for the fat-soluble vitamins, such as K_1 and K_2 signify different forms of the same vitamin. For the B vitamins, subscripts are no longer used since each of the numbers, as in vitamin B-6 and B-12, signifies an entirely different vitamin.

[7]Three enzymes that require vitamin K for their activity are reductase, epoxidase (carboxylase-epoxidase), and epoxidase reductase. See supplemental readings in the Appendix for more information.

fering an extra carboxy group (—COOH, an organic acid) to glutamic acid residues, thus forming vital carboxyglutamic acid residues. Without this compound in several proteins they can not work in making blood clot (17,77).

As previously mentioned, the best known of these proteins required for clotting of blood is prothrombin. Prothrombin is converted to its active form, *thrombin,* which in turn is necessary for the formation of *fibrin,* a protein that is the basis for a blood clot, as is illustrated by Figure 9–14.

Recently several other proteins have been discovered requiring carboxyglutamic acid for their formation (and hence vitamin K). One of these is *osteocalcin* (also called Gla protein) found in the bone. This protein is required along with vitamin D for calcium deposition (79). Other proteins requiring vitamin K for their synthesis (either vitamin K_1 or K_2 work equally well) are thought to be present in other organs of the body.

OTHER FAT-SOLUBLE SUBSTANCES

No other fat-soluble vitamins for humans are recognized by nutritional science groups in the United States or by international agencies (4,8). (See Fig. 9–15.) Certain fat-soluble substances in food are growth factors for lower forms of life, such as cholesterol and other sterols for insects. "Lecithin," containing choline (see Chap. 3 and 11), is fat-soluble but is not a vitamin in itself or a necessary dietary ingredient. Various fatty acids serve as growth factors for lower organisms and two or more fatty acids are essential (see Chap. 3) for humans, but since they are fatty acids they are not vitamins, by definition.

This is not to say that other health-promoting agents do not occur in natural fats. New facts in this field are difficult to obtain and to confirm. The proposal by the late Armand Quick, a pioneer in the study of clotting factors, for the existence of a vitamin Q is interesting but its need in the diet has never been confirmed (80).

The proposed vitamin Q (in honor of its discoverer) was reported to be a phospholipid of unknown composition present in soybeans and, in addition to vitamin K, essential for proper functioning of blood clotting mechanisms in humans. Whether or not it is required in the diet of normal individuals for this purpose, a basic tenet of vitamin identification, remains to be proved. It is widely distributed in food, and a deficiency in normal persons, if it is a vitamin, would no doubt be difficult to obtain. (For other proposed vitamins, see the end of Chap. 11 and 12.)

QUESTIONS

1. Tell in a general way how fat-soluble vitamins differ from water-soluble ones in each of the following respects: solubilities, types of food in which they are carried, losses in cooking and

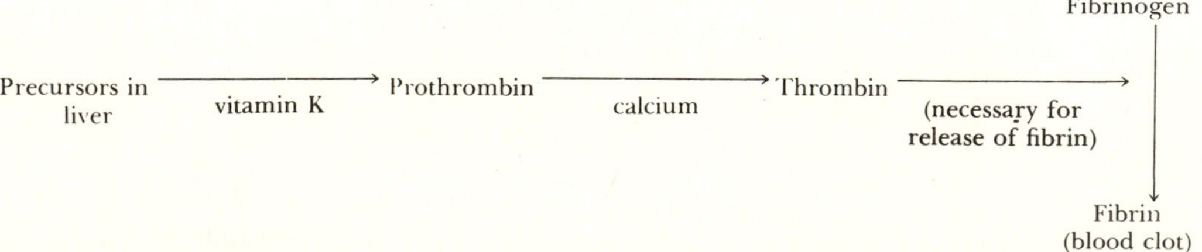

Figure 9–14 A major function of vitamin K is to allow for the production of prothrombin. This is essential for the clotting of blood as shown in the above simplified diagram.

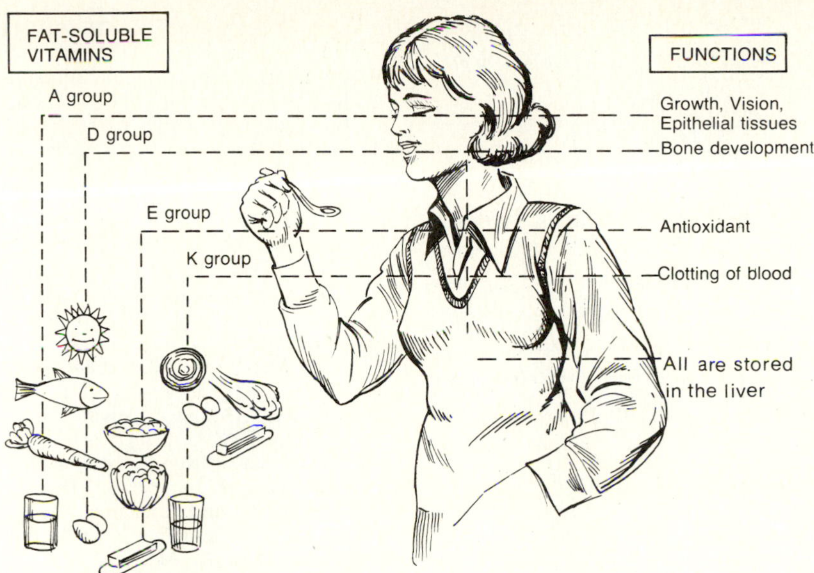

Figure 9–15 Fat-soluble vitamins and their functions.

processing of foods, conditions necessary for good absorption from intestine, path or paths of excretion, and ability to be stored in the body.

2. Name four fat-soluble vitamins and give for each one its chief use, or uses, in the body and the effects of moderate and severe lack of it in the diet. How does its function in nutrition account for the type of symptoms that result from an insufficient supply?

3. What is meant by provitamins? Name the major provitamins of vitamin A, and tell in what classes of foods they are found. How and to what extent are they made into vitamin A in the body? What foods contain both the provitamins A and vitamin A? Which contain only provitamins A? What determines whether the vitamin A value of eggs, milk, and butter is high or low? Is the depth of color of egg yolk and milk fat a reliable index of their vitamin A value. Why? Does the depth of color of green and yellow vegetables indicate their relative vitamin A value, and why?

4. How does changing to the new retinol equivalent units affect what we know about the relative vitamin A contribution of carrots and deep greens to a daily diet? Why?

5. Plan a diet that will furnish 500 RE of vitamin A. Modify this diet so that it provides 1000 RE of vitamin A. Substitute foods or add some rich sources of vitamin A, so that the diet as modified supplies 2000 RE (or more) of vitamin A. Is it difficult to obtain as much as 1000 RE (recommended daily allowance for adult males) in the diet? What will happen if the diet supplies 500 RE one day and 2000 RE the next day? Of what advantage is it to have an intake of vitamin A considerably in excess of the minimum requirement?

6. What are the earliest symptoms of vitamin A deficiency? What course would you recommend for getting rid of such symptoms? How common are these symptoms in the United States? In the world?

7. What are the precursors of vitamin D, and where are they found? By what means are they transformed into vitamin D? Under what circumstances can this vitamin be made in the body? Under what conditions will persons make insufficient amounts of this vitamin in their bodies and so be dependent almost entirely on food sources for their supply? What foods contain small and

variable amounts of vitamin D? How may the natural low content of vitamin D in foods be increased? Give some examples.

8. At what periods of life is the need for vitamins A and D relatively high, and why? What rich source (or sources) of these vitamins is usually given at these periods to insure a plentiful supply of vitamins A and D? Why does a baby that is breast-fed derive more benefit if supplementary vitamins A and D are given to it directly than if they are given to its mother?

9. How can rickets be prevented? How can it be cured? Discuss why rickets is no longer a common disease.

10. What are the chief symptoms of deficiency of vitamin E? Of vitamin K? How often are such deficiencies seen in humans? Why? What are the chief functions of vitamins E and K in the body?

11. Which fat-soluble vitamins may be toxic if taken over long periods in large doses?

12. Describe some important research now under way with any of the fat-soluble vitamins.

References

Vitamin A

1. McCollum, E. V.: *History of Nutrition.* Boston, Houghton Mifflin Co., 1957.
2. McCollum, E. V., and Davis, M.: J. Biol. Chem., *15*:167, 1913; *19*:245, 1914; *23*:181, 1915; Osborne, T. B., and Mendel, L. B.: J. Biol. Chem. *15*:311, 1913, *16*:423, 1913–1914; Becker, S. L.: Connecticut Agric Expt. Stat. Bul., No. 767, 1977.
3. Karrer, P., et al.: Helv. Chim. Acta., *14*:1036, 1431, 1931; Chem. Rev., *14*:17, 1934.
4. Nomenclature policy: J. Nutr., *112*:7, 1982; Nutr. Abst. Rev., *48*:831, 1978.
5. Bauernfeind, J. C.: J. Agric. Food Chem., *20*:456, 1972; Simpson, K. L., and Chichester, C. O.: Ann. Rev. Nutr., *1*:351, 1981.
6. Nutr. Rev., *38*:384, 1980.
7. Karrer, P., et al.: Helv. Chim. Acta., *12*:1142, 1929; Moore, T.: Biochem. J., *24*:692, 1930.
8. Food and Nutrition Board: *Recommended Dietary Allowances.* 9th Ed. Washington, D.C., National Research Council, National Academy of Sciences, 1980.
9. Wald, G., et al.: Vitam. Horm., *1*:195, 1943; *18*:417, 1960; Fed. Proc., *12*:607, 1953; Nature, *219*:800, 1968; Science, *162*:230, 1968.
10. Guggenheim, K. Y.: *Nutrition and Nutritional Diseases—The Evolution of Concepts.* Lexington, Mass., D.C. Heath and Co., 1981.
11. Löhle, E.: Arch. Otorhinolaryngol., *234*:167, 1982.
12. Rowntree, J. L.: J. Nutr., *3*:345, 1931; Dutcher, R. A., et al.: J. Nutr., *8*:269, 1934; Smith, M.C. and Spector, H.: Ariz. Agric. Expt. Stat. Tech. Bull., *84*:375, 1940; Becker, G. L.: Amer. J. Dig. Dis., *19*:344, 1952.
13. Adamo, S., et al.: J. Biol. Chem., *254*:3279, 1979; Kiorpes, T. C., Anderson, R. S., and Wolf, G.: J. Nutr., *111*:2059, 1981.
14. Zile, M. H., Bunge, E. C., and DeLuca, H. F.: J. Nutr., *109*:1787, 1979; Nutr. Rev., *40*:154, 1982.
15. Steinberg, K. K., and Sgoutas, D. S.: Proc. Soc. Exp. Biol. Med., *167*:110, 1981; Nutr. Rev., *40*:187, 1982.
16. Trechsel, U., and Fleisch, H.: F.E.B.S. Letters, *135*:115, 1981.
17. Dairy Council Digest, National Dairy Council, Rosemont, Illinois, *53*(#3):13, 1982.
18. Ott, D. B., and Lachance, P. A.: Amer. J. Clin. Nutr., *32*:2522, 1979; Nutr. Rev., *40*:251, 1982.
19. McCormick, A. M., and Napoli, J. L.: J. Biol. Chem., *257*:1730, 1982; Napoli, J. L., Khalil, H., and McCormick, A. M.: Biochemistry, *21*:1942, 1982; McCormick, A. M., et al.: Biochem. J., *186*:475, 1980.
20. Newell-Morris, L., et al.: Teratology, *22*:87, 1980; Meeks, R. G., Zaharevitz, D., and Chen, R.F.: Arch. Biochem. Biophy., *207*:141, 1981; Yoder, F. W..: J. Amer. Med. Assoc., *249*:348, 1983.
21. Peck, G. L., et al.: New Eng. J. Med., *300*:329, 1979; Jones, H., Blanc, D., and Cunliffe, W. J.: Lancet, *2*:1048, 1980; Macek, C.: J. Amer. Med. Assoc. *247*:1800, 1982.
22. Chang-Sing-Pang, A. F. I., et al.: Arch. Dermatol., *117*:225, 1981; Voorhees, J. J., and Orfanos, C. E.: Arch. Dermatol., *117*:418, 1981; Strauss, J. S. (Chairman of workshop—35 papers on oral retinoids): J. Amer. Acad. Dermatol., *6* (No. 4, Part 2):573–831, 1982.
23. Esterly, N. B., and Furey, N. L.: Pediatrics, *62*:1044, 1978; Hurwitz, S.: Amer. J. Dis. Children, *133*:536, 1979; FDA Consumer, *14*(May):14, 1980; Michaëlsson, G.: Nutr. Rev., *39*:104, 1981; Consumer's Rept., 46(Aug.):472, 1981; Kligman, A. M., et al.: Dermatology, *20*:278, 1981; Pochi, P. E.: New Eng. J. Med., *308*:1024, 1983.
24. Dairy Council Dig., *51*(No. 5):25, 1980; Fink D. J., and Kritchevsky, D. (eds.); Cancer Res., *41*:(No. 9, Part 2):3684–3825, 1981; Kisnek, D. L., and DeWys, W. D. (eds.):Cancer Treatment Rept., *65*(Suppl. 5):1–158, 1981; Gunby, P.: J. Amer. Med. Assoc., *247*:1799, 1982; National Research Council, Washington, D. C., *Report on Diet, Nutrition, and Cancer,* 1982; Gori, G. B.: Food Tech., *33*:(no. 12):48, 1979; van Rensburg, S. J.: J. Nat. Cancer Inst., *67*:243, 1981; Kolonel, L. N., et al.: Brit. J. Cancer, *44*:332, 1981; Jansen, J. D.: World Rev. Nutr. Dietet., *39*:1, 1982. (All on nutrition and cancer, in general.)

25. See the review by Hill, D. L., and Grubbs, C. J.: Anticancer Res., *2*:111, 1982. Also see examples of individual studies: Sporn, M. B.: Science, *195*:487, 1977; Morré, D. M., et al.: J. Nutr. *110*:1629, 1980; McCormick, D. L., Burns, F. J., and Albert, R.E.: Cancer Res., *40*:1140, 1980; Ip, C., and Ip, M. M.: Carcinogenesis, *2*:915, 1981; Morrison, D. G.: Nutr. Cancer, *3*:81, 1981; Longnecker, D. S., et al.: Cancer Res., *42*:19, 1982. (All on vitamin A and cancer.)
26. See reviews: Lancet (March 15): 575, 1980, and Gray, M.A.: Food Chem. Toxic., *20*:333, 1982. Also see Mettlin, C., Graham, S., and Swanson, M.: J. Nat. Cancer Inst., *62*:1435, 1979 (on lung cancer); Kark, J. D., et al.: J. Nat. Cancer Inst., *66*:7, 1981 (3102 individuals); Graham, S., et al.: Amer. J. Epidem., *113*:675, 1981 (on cancer of the larynx); Nomura, A., et al.: J. Nat. Cancer Inst., *68*:401, 1982 (on intestinal metaplasia); Graham, S., et al.: Amer. J. Epidem., *116*:68, 1982 (on minor differences in breast cancer). (All on various types of experimental cancer and vitamin A.)
27. Peto, R., et al.: Nature, *290*:201, 1981; Shekelle, R. B., et al.: Lancet, *2*:1185, 1982; Wolf, G.: Nutr. Rev., *40*:257, 1982.
28. See the reviews by Sporn, M. B., and Newton, D. L.: Fed. Proc., *38*:2528, 1979; Nutr. Rev., *37*:153, 1979; Nettesheim, P.: Canad. Med. J., *122*:757, 1980; Meyskens, F. L., Jr.: Life Sciences, *28*:2323, 1981; Lower, G. M., Jr., and Kanarek, M. S.: Nutr. Cancer, *3*:109, 1981. Also see papers by Verma, A. K., et al.: Cancer Res., *40*:2367, 1980; Jetten, A. M.: Nature, *284*:626, 1980; Gouveia, J., et al.: Lancet, *1*:710, 1982. (All on synthetic retinoids and cancer.)
29. Bieri, J. G., and McKenna, M. C.: Amer. J. Clin. Nutr. *34*:289, 1981.
30. Pao, E. M., and Mickle, S. J.: Food Technol., *35*:58, 1981; U.S. Dept. of Agriculture: *Food and Nutrient Intakes of Individuals in One Day in the U.S., Spring, 1977.* USDA Consumer Nutrition Center, Hyattsville, Maryland, Prelim. Rept. No. 2, 1980.
31. Lee, C. J.: Amer. J. Clin. Nutr., *31*:1453, 1978; Yearick, E. S., Wang, M. L., and Pisias, S. J.: J. Gerontology, *35*:663, 1980; Haider, S. Q., and Wheeler, M., Sr.: J. Amer. Dietet. Assoc., *77*:677, 1980; Chase, H. P., et al.: Amer. J. Clin. Nutr., *33*:2346, 1980.
32. Périssé, J., and Polacchi, W.: Food Nutr. (FAO), *6*(No. 1):21, 1980; Brink, E. W., et al.: Amer. J Clin. Nutr., *32*:84, 1979; Olson, J. A.: Archivos Latinoamer, Nutricion, *29*:521, 1979; Solon, F. S., et al.: Amer. J. Clin. Nutr., *31*:360, 1978; Devadas, R., and Saroja, S.: Indian J. Nutr. Dietet., *17*:401, 1980; Kusin, J. A., et al.: Trop. Geograph. Med., *32*:30, 1980; Le Francois, P., et al.: Internat. J. Vit. Nutr. Res., *50*:352, 1982. (All on world-wide vitamin A deficiency.)
33. Sommer, A., et al.: Lancet, *1*:1407, 1981; Tarwotjo, I., et al.: Amer. J. Clin. Nutr., *35*:544, 1982; Sommer, A.: Compreh. Ther., *9*(April):67, 1983.
34. Carney, E. A., and Russell, R. M.: J. Nutr., *110*:552, 1980; Sommer, A., et al.: Amer. J. Clin. Nutr., *33*:887, 1980; Pitt, G. A. J.: Proc. Nutr. Soc., *40*:173, 1981; Mobarhan, S.: Amer. J. Clin. Nutr., *34*:2264, 1981; Huque, T.: Brit. J Nutr., *47*:165, 1982.
35. U.S. Dept. of Agriculture: *Composition of Foods: Raw, Processed, Prepared.* Agriculture Handbook, No. 8, 1963 (partially republished—Sections 1–9, 1976 to 1982).
36. Lee, C. Y., McCoon, P. E., LeBowitz, J. M.: J. Agric. Food Chem., *29*:1294, 1981 (on four varieties of processed sweet corn); Klein, B. P., and Perry, A. K.: J. Food Sci., *47*:941, 1982 (on selected vegetables from six cities).
37. Solon, F. S., et al.: J. Amer. Dietet. Assoc., *74*:112, 1979; Solon, F. S., et al.: Amer. J. Clin. Nutr., *32*:1445, 1979; Paden, C. A.: Lebensm.-Wiss. Techol., *12*:183, 1979; Parrish, D. B., et al.: Cereal Chem., *57*:284, 1980 and J. Food Sci., *45*:1438, 1980; Bauernfeind, J. C.: Food Nutr. (FAO), *6* (No. 1):10, 1980.
38. Arroyave, G., et al.: Archivos Latinoamer. Nutr., *24*:155, 1974 and *24*:485, 1974; Toro, O.: Archivos Latinoamer. Nutr., *27*:169, 1977; Araujo, R. L., et al.: Nutr. Rept. Internat., *17*:307, 1978 and *18*:429, 1978; Mejía, L. A., and Arroyave, G.: Amer. J. Clin. Nutr., *36*:87, 1982.
39. Holmes, Z. A., et al.: Home Econ. Res. J., *7*:259, 1979; Parrish, D. B., and coworkers: J. Agric. Food Chem., *27*:1134, 1979; J. Food Sci., *45*:1438, 1980; Cereal Chem., *57*:284, 1980; de Man, J. M.: J. Dairy Sci., *64*:2031, 1981 (effect of light); Wilkinson, S. A., Earle, M. D., and Cleland, A. C.: J. Food Sci., *47*:844, 1982.
40. Pirie, A., and Anbunathan, M. B. B. S.: Amer. J. Clin. Nutr., *34*:34, 1981; Reddy, V., and Mohanram, M.: Brit. J. Nutr., *45*:229, 1981; Sommer, A., et al.: Lancet, *1*:558, 1980.
41. Mahoney, C. P., et al.: Pediatrics, *65*:893, 1980; Read, M. H., et al.: Nutr. Rept. Internat., *24*:1133, 1981; Lippe, B., et al.: Amer. J. Dis. Children, *135*:634, 1981; Hatoff, D. E., et al.: Gastroenterology, *82*:124, 1982; Farris, W. A., et al.: J. Amer. Med. Assoc., *247*:1317, 1982; Herbert, V.: Amer. J. Clin. Nutr., *36*:185, 1982; James, M. B., et al.: Pediatrics, *69*:112, 1982. (All on vitamin A toxicity.)
42. Mathews-Roth, M. M.: J. Amer. Med. Assoc., *241*:1835, 1979; Massam, M., et al.: J. Human Nutr., *35*:218, 1981.

Vitamin D

43. Biale, Y.: Amer. J. Clin. Nutr., *32*:2380, 1979; Bashir, T., MacDonald, H. N., and Peacock, M.: J. Human Nutr., *35*:49, 1981; Maxwell, J. D., et al.: Brit. J. Obst. Gyn., *88*:987, 1981.
44. Vir, S. C., and Love, A. H. G.: Internat. J. Vit. Nutr. Res.: *48*:123, 1978; Corless, D., et al.: Gerontology, *25*:350, 1979; Guggenheim, K., et al.: Nutr. Metab., *23*:172, 1979; Weisman, Y., et al.: Israel J. Med. Sci., *17*:19, 1981.

45. Koh, E. T., and Chi, M. S.:Amer. J. Clin. Nutr., *34*:1562, 1981; Compston, J. E., et al.: Amer. J. Clin. Nutr., *34*:2359, 1981; Woodhouse, N. J. Y., and Norton, W. L.: King Faisal Specialist Hosp. Med. J., *2*:127, 1982.
46. Jeans, P. C., and Stearns, G.: J. Pediatr., *13*:730, 1938; J. Amer. Med. Assoc., *11*:703, 1938; Jeans, P. C.: J. Amer. Med. Assoc., *143*:177, 1950.
47. Lawson, D. E. M., et al.: Brit. Med. J., *11*(Aug. 4):303, 1979; Devgun, M. S., et al.: Amer. J. Clin. Nutr., *34*:1501, 1981; Clemens, T. L., et al.: Lancet, *1* (Jan. 9):74, 1982.
48. American Academy of Pediatrics, Committee on Nutrition: Pediatrics, *29*:646, 1962; *31*:512, 1963; and *40*:1050, 1967.
49. Bachrach, S., Fisher, J., and Parks, J. S.: Pediatrics, *64*:871, 1979; Lovinger, R. D.: Pediatrics, *66*:359, 1980.
50. Morris, K. M. L., and Levack, V. M.: Life Sci., *30*:1255, 1982.
51. Leerbeck, E., and Søndergaard, H.: Brit. J. Nutr., *44*:7, 1980; Hollis, B. W., et al.: J. Nutr., *111*:1240, 1981; Reeve, L. E., Jorgensen, N. A., and DeLuca, H. F.: J. Nutr., *112*:667, 1982.
52. See reviews by Chick, H.: Lancet, (Aug. 13 and 20):325 and 377, 1932; Powers, G. V., et al.: J. Amer. Med. Assoc., *78*:159, 1922; Stein, H. B., and Lewis, R. C.: Amer. J. Dis. Children, *41*:62, 1931.
53. McCollum, E. V., et al.: J. Biol. Chem., *53*:293, 1922.
54. Holick, M. F., et al.: Biochemistry, *18*:1003, 1979 (also see Science, *216*:1001, 1982).
55. Lawson, D. E. M., and Davie, M.: Vitam. Horm., *37*:1, 1979; Fraser, D. R.: Physiol. Rev., *60*:551, 1980; Wecksler, W. R., and Norman, A. W.: J. Steroid Biochem., *13*:977, 1980; Schnoes, H. K., and DeLuca, H. F.: Fed. Proc., *39*:2723, 1980; DeLuca, H. F.: Nutr. Rev., *38*:169, 1980; DeLuca, H. F.: Contemp. Nutr. (General Mills), *6*(No. 2):1, 1981; DeLuca, H. F.: Harvey Lectures, *75*:333, 1981; Stanbury, S. W.: Proc. Nutr. Soc., *40*:179, 1981; Haussler, M. R., and Cordy, P. E.: J. Amer. Med. Assoc., *247*:841, 1982; Koshy, K. T.: J. Pharmaceut. Sci., *71*:137, 1982; Bikle, D. D.: Adv. Int. Med., *27*:45, 1982. (Each of these is a good review on some aspect of vitamin D.)

Vitamin E

56. Horwitt, M. L.: Amer. J. Clin. Nutr., *4*:408, 1956; *8*:451, 1960; *12*:99, 1963; and *27*:939, 1974; J. Amer. Dietet. Assoc., *38*:231, 1961; Fed. Proc., *24*:68, 1964; J. Nutr., *108*:1208, 1978.
57. Phelps, D. L.: Pediatrics, *63*:933, 1979 (a review).
58. Binder, H. J., et al.: New Eng. J. Med., *273*:1289, 1965.
59. Hittner, H. M., et al.: New Eng. J. Med., *305*:1365, 1981; and *306*:866, 1982; Nutr. Rev., *39*:121, 1981; Bell, E. F., and Filer, L. J., Jr.: Amer. J. Clin. Nutr., *34*:414, 1981; and *34*:2600, 1981; Finer, N. N., et al.: Lancet *1*:1087, 1982; Puklin, J. E., Simon, R. M. M., and Ehrenkranz, R. A.: Ophthalmology, *89*:96, 1982; Phelps, D. L.: Pediatrics, *70*:420, 1982.
60. Herold, E.: Arch. Sexual Behav., *8*:397, 1979.
61. Committee on Public Information, IFT.: Nutr. Rev., *35*:57, 1977.
62. Horwitt, M. K.: Amer. J. Clin. Nutr., *27*:1182, 1974; Lehmann, J., et al.: J. Nutr. *107*:1006, 1977.
63. Evans, H. M., Emerson, O. H., and Emerson, G. A.: J. Biol. Chem., *113*:319, 1936 (reprinted in part in Nutr. Rev., *32*:80, 1974).
64. Bieri, J. G.: Nutr. Rev., *33*:161, 1975; Amer, S. R.: J. Nutr., *109*:2198, 1979; Machlin, L. J., and Brin, M.: Amer. J. Clin. Nutr., *34*:1633, 1981; Horwitt, M. K.: Amer. J. Clin. Nutr., *34*:1664, 1981; Weiser, H., and Vecchi, M.: Internat. J. Vit. Res., *51*:100, 1981; Machlin, L. J., Gabriel, E., and Brin, M.: J. Nutr., *112*:1437, 1982.
65. Dicks-Bushnell, M. W., and Davis, K. C.: Amer. J. Clin. Nutr., *20*:262, 1967; McLaughlin, P. J., and Weihrauch, J. L.: J. Amer. Dietet. Assoc., *75*:647, 1979; Gertz, C., and Herrmann, K.: Z Lebensm. Unters. Forsch., *174*:390, 1982.
66. Koehler, H. H., Lee, H. C., and Jacobson, M.: J. Amer. Dietet. Assoc., *70*:616, 1977; Kanner, J., Harrel, S., and Mendel, H.: J. Agric. Food Chem., *27*:1316, 1979; Widicus, W. A., Kirk, J. R., and Gregory, J. F.: J. Food Sci., *45*:1015, 1980; Widicus, W. A., and Kirk, J. R.: J. Food Sci., *46*:813, 1981. (All on stability of vitamin E.)
67. Yuki, E., and Ishikawa, Y.: J. Amer. Oil Chem. Soc., *53*:673, 1976.
68. Nutr. Rev., *33*:269, 1975; Tsai, A. C., et al.: Amer. J. Clin. Nutr., *31*:831, 1978; Prasad, J. S.: Amer. J. Clin. Nutr., *33*:606, 1980; Roberts, H. J.: J. Amer. Med. Assoc., *246*:129, 1981.
69. Willett, W., et al.: Amer. J. Clin. Nutr., *34*:1121, 1981.
70. Read, M. H., et al.: Nutr. Rept. Internat., *24*:1133, 1981.
71. Higashi, A., et al.: Pediatr. Pharm., *1*:129, 1980 (in anti-convulsant use); Nutr. Rev., *38*:120, 1980 (in glutathione peroxidase deficiency); Drake, J. R., and Fitch, C. D.: Amer. J. Clin. Nutr., *33*:2386, 1980 (in red blood cell formation); Dion, P. W.: Mutation Res., *102*:27, 1982 (in fecal mutagenicity); Elias, E., and Muller, D. P. R.: Compreh. Ther., *9*(April): 56, 1983 (in nerve disorders).
72. Evans, H. M., and Bishop, K. S.: Science, *56*:650, 1922.
73. Olcott, H. S., and Matill, H. A.: J. Biol. Chem., *93*:59, 1931; Olcott, H. S.: J. Biol. Chem., *110*:695, 1935.
74. Nutr. Rev., *36*:84, 1978; Kornbrust, D. J., and Mavis, R. D.: Lipids, *15*:315, 1980; Hicks, M.: Arch. Biochem. Biophy., *210*:56, 1981; Steiner, M.: Biochem. Biophy. Acta., *640*:100, 1981.
75. Schwarz, K., and Folz, C. M.: J. Amer. Chem. Soc., *79*:3292, 1957.

Vitamin K

76. Dam, H.: Nature, *135*:652, 1935; Biochem. J., *29*:1273, 1935; Almquist, H. J., and Stokstad, E. L. R.: Nature, *136*:31, 1935; J. Biol. Chem., *111*:105, 1935; Almquist, H. J.: Amer. J. Clin. Nutr., *28*:656, 1975.
77. Olson, R. E.: Vitamin K (Chapter 6C), in Goodhart, R. S., and Shils, M. E. (eds.): *Modern Nutrition in Health and Disease,* Philadelphia, Lea and Febiger, 1980.
78. Seifert, R. M.: J. Agric. Food Chem, *27*:1301, 1979; Parrish, D. B.: *Determination of vitamin K in foods: a review,* C. R. C. Crit. Rev. Food Sci., Nutr., *13*:337, 1980; Haroon, Y., et al.: J. Nutr., *112*:1105, 1982.
79. Nutr. Rev., *37*:54, 1979; and *40*:249, 1982 (both on "osteocalcin").
80. Quick, A. J.: Life Sci., *16*:1017, 1975; Wis. Med. J., *74*(Aug.):85, 1975.

10 Vitamin B Complex I: Thiamin, Riboflavin, Pantothenic Acid, and Niacin

Originally the B vitamins were grouped together because they were found in liver and yeast and thought to be just one vitamin—vitamin B. Proof for the existence of more than one "vitamin B" came about in the early 1920s. Within a few years, the group of different water-soluble vitamins found in liver and other natural products became known as the *vitamin B complex.* The process of identification was very slow until the pure substance could be isolated, or at least concentrated. Then it could be added routinely to experimental diets—a step necessary for proving the existence of still other unknown vitamins.

Much progress was made in the 1930s with the identification of thiamin (vitamin B-1), then riboflavin (vitamin B-2), pantothenic acid, niacin, and later, vitamin B-6. During the early 1940s, biotin was discovered. The last two B vitamins to be identified were folacin, in 1945, and vitamin B-12, in 1948.

The B-complex vitamins, which will be described in this chapter and the next, have many characteristics in common.

1. Most function as coenzymes for the release of energy (calories/joules) from food and for nearly every cellular reaction taking place in the body. Thus, they are essential for normal development, growth, reproduction and lactation, maximum physical fitness, and optimal overall good health (although, of course, they cannot guarantee these benefits). Many if not all are essential for normal skin and hair, brain and nerve functioning, blood formation, and normal defense against infections and disease. In the total absence of any B vitamin for sufficient length of time, death will result.

2. They are widely distributed (although not in equal amounts) in almost all basic foods (except vitamin B-12, which is not found in foods of plant origin).
3. They are readily destroyed upon milling, heating and canning, blanching, other excessive modes of processing, and storing. Some are sensitive to light.
4. They are water-soluble, readily absorbed from the intestine (with exceptions), quite free of toxic effects even at reasonably high levels, and readily excreted from the body.
5. They supply no energy (calories/joules) in themselves to the body, although most of them are necessary for forming energy from food.

In addition to these similarities, the B vitamins are all made of carbon, hydrogen, oxygen, and nitrogen (C,H,O,N), and they are all readily crystallized.

Aside from these common features, each of the B-complex vitamins has a different chemical structure and properties. Two contain additional sulfur (S), and one contains phosphorus (P) and cobalt (Co). Five are white, two are yellow, and one is bright red.

These chapters will concentrate on pointing out the differences among the B vitamins. They have little in common so far as recommended allowances—which range from 3 micrograms (μg) a day for vitamin B-12 to 14 to 19 milligrams (mg) for niacin—a difference of an average of about 5,500 fold. Some of their allowances are based on how much energy we utilize each day; some are based on more complicated relationships (1).

These chapters will use the latest recommended nomenclature of the B-complex vitamins (2), the most recently recommended allowances of the Food and Nutrition Board (1), and in so far as possible the latest figures on food distribution (3) and on nutrient intake in the United States (4,5). The authors have cited a number of articles for further study in Chapters 8 and 9 and in the supplementary reading in the Appendix on the vitamin intake of populations, on vitamin supplement intakes (both usual levels and "megadoses"), and on losses of vitamins in processing and cooking. Also, they have cited review articles on the relationship of B vitamins to cancer (ref. 24 in Chap. 9). These references will not be repeated here unless some specific point needs to be made.

For information on other general vitamin topics see the supplementary reading suggestions in the Appendix and the references at the end of Chapters 1 and 8.

THIAMIN

Thiamin was the first of the B complex vitamins to be obtained in pure form, hence the name vitamin B-1, a term proposed by the British in 1927 (but now no longer used.) Various other names were used for short periods, including "antineuritic factor," "antiberiberi factor," "water-soluble B," and simply "vitamin B." The correct spelling is "thiamin," but the old spelling, "thiamine," is still used by the Food and Drug Administration (FDA) and some other authorities.

Deficiency Symptoms

Thiamin deficiency causes the disease traditionally known as *beriberi* (6–8).

Humans. The symptoms of beriberi in humans are numbness or tingling in toes and feet, stiffness of ankles and absence of the ankle jerk reflex, cramping pains in legs, difficulty in walking, and finally paralysis of legs with atrophy of leg muscles (see Fig. 10–1). In later stages various nerves may be affected (which gave rise to the terms antineuritic vitamin, and aneurin in the early literature), and disturbances of heart function are common. In the form known as *wet beriberi,* dropsical bloating or edema (especially of the legs) is a complicating factor as a

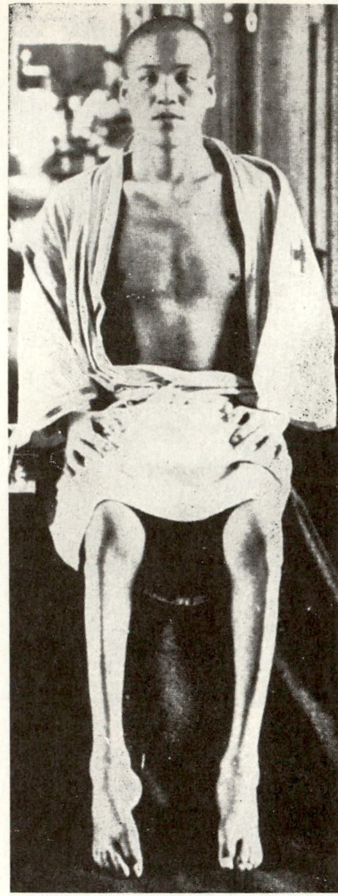

Figure 10–1 Case of "dry" beriberi, showing atrophy of the muscles due to paralysis of the legs. (Courtesy of Herzog and the *Philippine Journal of Sciences.*)

result probably of cardiac disturbances (Fig. 10–2). Although the endemic beriberi, so prevalent in the Orient in years past, was probably due to a deficiency of several nutrients, there is no doubt that the primary deficiency was that of thiamin. The extensive tissue damage that occurs in beriberi, because of lack of thiamin, makes us realize how important a role this vitamin plays in normal nutrition.

Thiamin plays a part in promoting appetite and better functioning of the digestive tract, effects that have an indirect influence in promoting growth. The emptying time of the stomach and intestines is nearly twice as slow in thiamin-deficient animals as in normal ones. Most authorities agree, however, that thiamin is not the only vitamin that produces a lack of appetite with a deficiency; other factors may be responsible. Upon reversal of the deficiency, normal appetite is restored. Large quantities of thiamin, however, do not promote a voracious appetite.

Thiamin has been called "the morale vitamin," because one of the earliest signs of its lack is a lowering of stamina. Studies of people who volunteered to follow a diet moderately low in thiamin demonstrated that after a short time on such a diet (as early as in ten days) the subjects became depressed and irritable, lacking the ability to concentrate on and to take an interest in their work. In three to seven weeks such symptoms as fatigue, lack of appetite, loss of weight, constipation, muscle cramps, and various pains appeared. The subjects promptly recovered normal health and morale when given larger amounts of thiamin (9).

Experimental Animals. Without experimental animals to use in studying the counterpart of human deficiencies, it is likely that the discovery of many of the vitamins would have been postponed many years, and the metabolic function of vitamins would be most difficult to study.

In young experimental animals made deficient in thiamin, symptoms may be seen as early as three to six days after withholding the vitamin. They show poor growth, nervous symptoms, and death in severe cases. Pigeons and fowl develop a severe and characteristic head retraction, a form of polyneuritis (Fig. 10–3). Swine develop generalized weakness, vomiting, and dizziness. Rats show reduced growth (Fig. 10–4), convulsions, slowing of the heartbeat, and a loss of appetite.

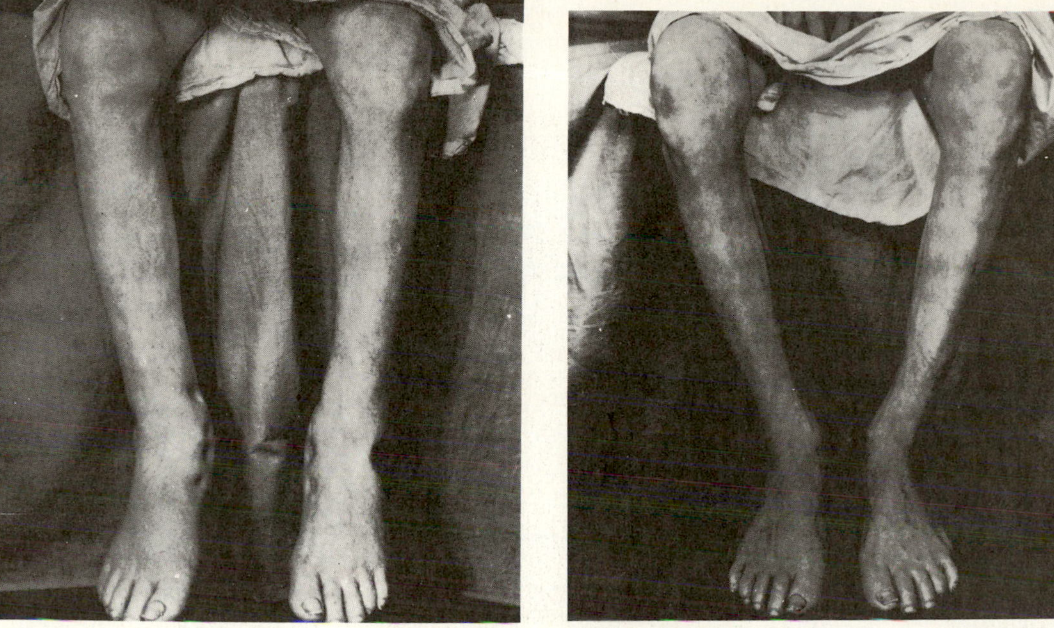

Figure 10–2 Patient before and after treatment for thiamin deficiency (so-called "wet" beriberi). A, Swelling of the legs and marked pitting edema in the ankle region. B, Ten days after initiation of thiamin therapy, during which the patient lost 40 pounds. Presumably this weight loss was due to the loss of fluid because the general nutritive state was greatly improved. (From Spies: *Rehabilitation through Better Nutrition.* Philadelphia, W.B. Saunders, 1947.)

Thiamin Intakes

American diets provide enough thiamin to prevent the appearance of beriberi. A good many diets, however, may provide less than optimal amounts, especially in times of body stress caused by poor nutrition habits and by growth, pregnancy, lactation, fevers, or surgical operations. Nervous symptoms resulting from a lack of thiamin are seen often in chronic alcoholic persons, since their diet is often inadequate. Their high intake of energy in the form of alcohol still further decreases their intake of thiamin, allowing serious deficiency signs to occur. Much research is being done on this problem (10). Alcohol also reduces thiamin absorption from the intestine.

The presence of a thiamin deficiency, as well as the extent of the deficiency, is determined by measuring urinary levels of thiamin or, more specifically, tissue levels of either *thiamin pyrophosphate,* the coenzyme form of thiamin, or *transketolase,* one of the enzymes requiring thiamin pyrophosphate as a cofactor.

Recommended Allowances

The amount of thiamin required by adults varies according to their size, degree of activity, dietary habits, and individual differences in how food is utilized. Since this vitamin takes part in the metabolism of carbohydrate, more of it is needed when the rate of carbohydrate metabolism is high. Persons who do considerable muscular work burn up more energy foods and usually obtain much of this extra energy in the form of starchy

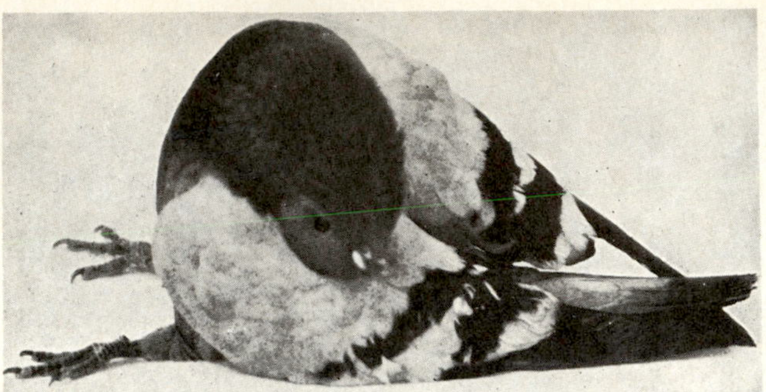

Figure 10–3 Characteristic behavior of a pigeon with polyneuritis (avian beriberi) after 3 weeks' feeding with a diet of polished rice. The pigeon was used year after year as a class demonstration, and the extreme effect passed off within a few hours after feeding foods rich in thiamin. (From Morse: *Applied Biochemistry*. Philadelphia, W.B. Saunders, 1927.)

foods; hence, they need more thiamin than those who are muscularly inactive. The requirement for thiamin is usually stated in terms of the caloric intake (so much for every 1000 kcal), particularly of the nonfat calories of the diet; with more fat and a lower proportion of calories from carbohydrate, slightly less thiamin is needed. Growing children have higher energy needs and therefore have higher thiamin needs per unit of body weight than adults. Women during pregnancy have an increased need for thiamin, and nursing mothers should have approximately 1½ times as much thiamin as under normal conditions.

The current recommendations of the U.S. Food and Nutrition Board(1) provide a moderately liberal daily intake of thiamin for normal adults, varying according to the caloric intake recommended for the different age groups, which is greater in younger adults. The values are based on an allowance of 0.5 mg thiamin per 1,000 kcal. For college-age women the recommended intake is 1.1 milligrams (mg) per day and for college-age men, 1.5 mg. See Table 10–1 for thiamin allowances of selected age groups (and see inside front cover for complete details for all age groups).

The Food and Nutrition Board cautions that older adults who subsist on an intake of less than 2000 kcal should not have less than 1.0 mg of thiamin per day, which is recognized as about the minimum daily requirement. There is no evidence that larger intakes than the recommended allowance will be of any benefit to normal, healthy adults.

Dietary surveys have shown that the average intake of thiamin in the United States is not much higher than the recommended allowance. Americans are indebted to the enrichment program for keeping the level as high as it is (see Chap. 18). For example, R. R. Williams and co-workers concluded in 1942 that the average American diet, prior to the introduction of enriched bread and cereal foods, provided only about 0.8 mg of thiamin per 2500 kcal, which was dangerously near the minimum requirement. The enrichment of bread and cereals, started

Table 10–1 RECOMMENDED ALLOWANCES FOR THIAMIN*

	Age	*Allowance, mg/day*
Males	11–18 years	1.4
	19–22 years	1.5
	23–50 years	1.4
	51 years and over	1.2
Females	11–14 years	1.1
	15–22 years	1.1
	23 years and older	1.0
	Pregnant	+0.4
	Lactating	+0.5

*From the Food and Nutrition Board, 1980.
See Appendix Table 1 for recommendations of FAO and various countries.

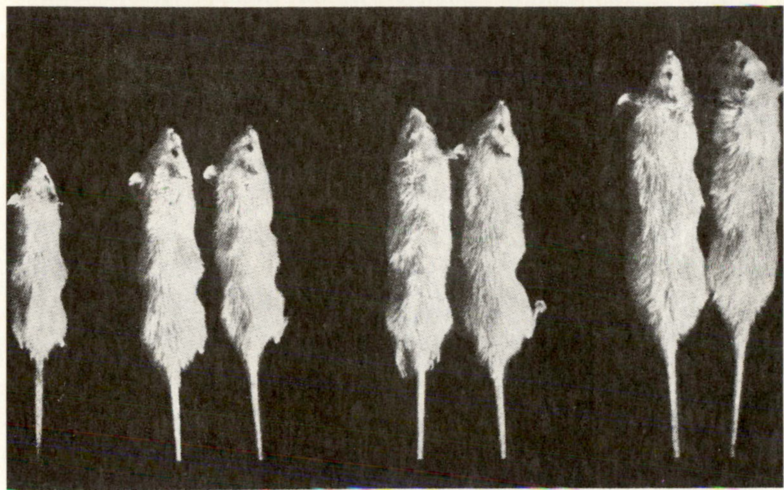

Figure 10–4 Effects on growth of rats of feeding for different levels of thiamin, ranging from none on the left to optimal amounts on the right. (From experiments of Dr. Bertha Bisbey.)

during World War II, has increased by about one-third the amount of thiamin available for the average person, most all of it coming from synthetic thiamin at a negligible cost.

As with all vitamins there are large differences between amounts "available per day" and actual intakes. Intake figures for thiamin are actually 30 to 50 percent lower than "available" figures because of wastage and spoilage of food, use in pet foods, or destruction of thiamin during storage, preparation, cooking, or canning of foods.

It is apparent that many individuals consume levels of thiamin very close to, or even less than, the recommended allowance as shown by recent nutrition surveys (4,5,11,12). In spite of intakes of excessively high amounts of carbohydrate and only borderline amounts of thiamin in some segments of the population, few, if any, clinical signs of thiamin deficiency are apparent in the United States except in alcoholics. Intakes of thiamin in the United States today range from an average of about 1.0 to 1.1 mg per day for females and about 1.4 to 1.5 mg for males. These values are within the range of amounts needed to protect against a deficiency. Unfortunately, these are only averages. Many persons are consuming amounts well below recommended allowances, which, for thiamin, are quite conservative and leave little room for safety.

Thiamin in Foods

Sources. Few foods relatively rich in thiamin are used in quantity in modern diets unless they are enriched with the synthetic vitamin. All natural foods contain thiamin (see Table 10–2), but many are processed heavily, carry only minor amounts, or are not eaten in sufficient quantities. The levels may be still further reduced by cooking or processing. From available figures (see Appendix) it may be seen that the thiamin content of most fruits and vegetables, eggs, milk, and cheese does not generally exceed 0.1 mg per 100 gm. In plants it is concentrated chiefly in seeds (whole grains, legumes, and nuts); in animals it is abundant in the organs (liver, heart, kidneys). Pork flesh is much higher in thiamin content that other meats, but meats and leafy vegetables are moderately good sources. In certain processed or refined foods, such as highly milled cereals and sulfured dried fruits, thiamin is present in traces or entirely absent

Table 10–2 GOOD THIAMIN VALUES IN EXAMPLES OF NATURAL PRODUCTS BEFORE PROCESSING

Food Source	*Thiamin, mg/100 gm*	*Food Source*	*Thiamin, mg/100 gm*
Bacon, Canadian	0.83	Pork	0.50
Beans, Pinto	0.84	Rice polish	1.84
Buckwheat flour (dark)	0.58	Rye, whole grain	0.43
Cornflakes with added nutrients	0.43	Sesame seeds	0.98
Heart, beef	0.53	Soybeans	1.10
Kidneys, hog	0.58	Sunflower seed	1.96
Lentils	0.37	Whole wheat flour	0.55
Liver, lamb	0.40	Wheat flour, enriched	0.44
Oatmeal (dry)	0.60	Wheat germ	2.01
Peanuts (with skins)†	1.11	Yeast	
Peas	0.35	Baker's, dry	2.33
Pecans	0.86	Brewer's	15.61
Piñon nuts	1.28	Torula	14.01

*From U.S. Dept. of Agriculture handbooks. Based on fresh, raw, edible portion, before cooking or roasting. Hence, these values are not meant to show the thiamin content of common prepared foods ready to serve. We eat very little, if any, of these items. If you compare these figures with cooked foods, ready to serve, in the Appendix you will get a good idea of the extent of thiamin losses due to food milling and processing. It can be very considerable.

unless these foods have been enriched with added thiamin. A useful recent report from M. H. Dong and co-workers lists the thiamin content of more than eighty food items sampled from serving lines of military dining halls (13).

The best sources of thiamin—whole grains, organ meats, pork, and legumes—are not used in quantity in the American diet. Foods of more moderate content and thiamin-enriched foods can, however, be used in sufficient amounts to provide this vitamin at a fairly safe level. Of our total thiamin intake about 42 percent comes from bread and cereals; 28 percent from meats, fish, and poultry; 2 percent from eggs; 5 percent from beans, legumes, and nuts; 7 percent from milk and other dairy products; and 16 percent from vegetables and fruits. In low-cost diets, of which grain products and potatoes furnish a high proportion, it is especially important that bread and cereals be whole-grain or enriched. Such foods as oatmeal and dried legumes can be an economical source of thiamin.

Beriberi seldom, if ever, develops in countries where meats, dairy products, whole-grain products, fruits, and vegetables are freely used. It should be noted that sucrose, salad oils, and other fats supply more than 35 percent of the energy intake of an average American diet and yet provide no thiamin or other water-soluble vitamins.

Effects of Cooking and Processing. Thiamin in food suffers little destruction on exposure to air at ordinary temperatures. Thiamin, however, is one of the vitamins that may be most easily lost in food preservation and cooking, depending on the methods used (14).

Dry heating at high temperatures, as in preparation of ready-cooked cereals or in toasting bread, can cause considerable loss. Moist heat (boiling for not more than an hour) causes little destruction of this vitamin, but its solubility in water means that as much as one-third of the original thiamin content may be lost if cooking water is liberal and is discarded. Thiamin is very unstable in an alkaline medium and is largely destroyed if soda is added in the cooking of vegetables. Meats lose about 20 to 60 percent of thiamin in roasting, depending on the extent of roasting, 30 percent in broiling, and only 15 percent in frying. In baking bread, only 5 to 15 percent of the original thiamin content is lost, while there is no significant loss in cooking cereals in a double boiler. Prolonged cooking, as of dried legumes, results in relatively high losses of their thiamin content. Fresh frozen vegetables maintain as much thiamin as is left in the product after blanching to destroy enzyme activity. Canned vegetables suffer a loss owing to solubility of the vitamin in the canning fluid, which is drained away.

Antithiamin Substances in Food. Certain raw fish and seafood, particularly carp, herring, clams, and shrimp, contain the enzyme *thiaminase,* which is capable of splitting the thiamin molecule into its two major chemical groups, thus making it inactive. This effect has been seen in fox farms where the animals were fed raw fish, resulting in severe economic losses. The effect can also be produced in laboratory animals (such as cats and chickens) by feeding them raw fish at a level of 10 to 25 percent. This action can be prevented by heating the fish first and destroying the enzyme. In most countries, humans do not normally eat sufficient raw fish or seafood to produce a thiamin deficiency, but it is known that this may be a contributory factor in producing beriberi in certain populations of the world, especially in the Orient.

Other agents are known to affect thiamin levels in the body. For instance, a large amount of live yeast in the human diet reduces the amount of thiamin absorbed from the intestine. Signs of thiamin deficiency have been seen in Asia in persons who drink large amounts of tea or chew fermented tea leaves or betel nuts, a very common practice. This suggests the presence of antithiamin factors in these substances (15). Alcohol, as has been mentioned, acts as an antithiamin substance.

Discovery and Properties

It took more than fifty-five years, from 1880 to 1936, to unravel the mystery of the nature of thiamin and to synthesize it in the chemical laboratory (6,7). The first synthesis, along with the establishment of its chemical identity, was made in 1936 by R. R. Williams and coworkers, who gave it the name thiamine (from *thio,* meaning "sulfur-containing," and *amine*)(16). (See Fig. 10–5.)

The cause of beriberi was not known to be related to the diet until late in the nineteenth century. In 1880, a Dutch naval doctor, F. S. van Leent, reported that death from beriberi was greatly reduced in Indian naval crews when they ate European-type meals instead of meals consisting primarily of rice. In 1885, K. Takaki, chief medical officer of the Japanese navy, reported that beriberi had been eradicated among the sailors as a result of adding extra meat, fish, and vegetables to the regular diet. Before this time, the disease was so common that three out of every ten sailors were likely to have it, and there were many deaths.

G. Grijns, a Dutch physician assigned to a prison hospital in Java, concluded in 1901 that beriberi was caused by the absence in the diet of some unknown substance present in the germ or outer coat of grains, as well as in beans, but not in highly milled grains (17). His conclusions, based in part on work of his predecessor, Eijkman, were historically important because they led to the discovery not only of thiamin but also of other B vitamins through studies of deficiencies produced in animals. Shortly thereafter, many other scientists in Java, the Philippines, and elsewhere repeated these studies and also found that the disease could be prevented by feeding subjects concentrates from yeast, wheat germ, and milk.

The first pure preparation of what is now

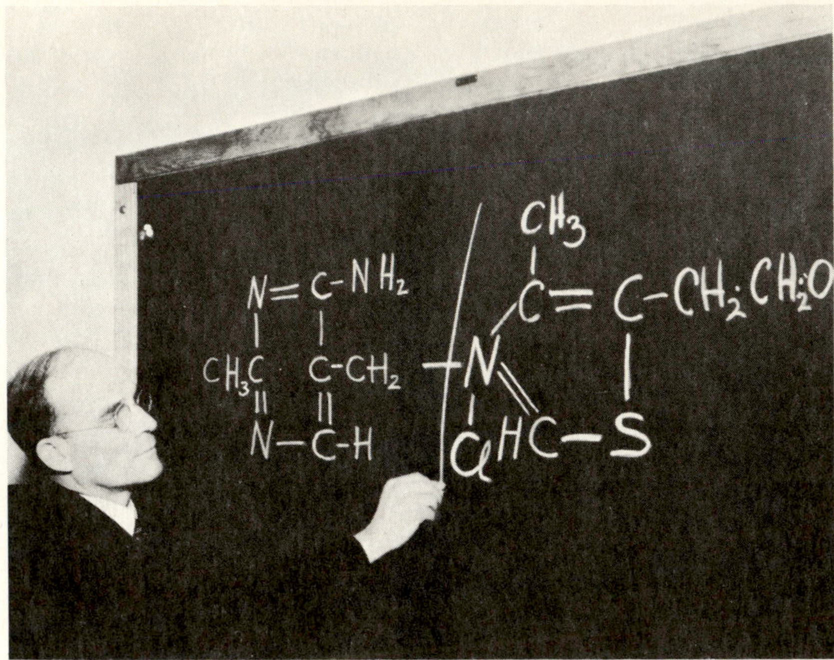

Figure 10–5 Dr. R. R. Williams writing the structural formula of thiamin on blackboard and indicating where the molecule splits on certain chemical treatment. The important sulfur atom is seen in the right-hand part and the amino group (NH_2) in the left-hand part of the molecule. (Courtesy of the late Dr. Williams.)

known as thiamin was isolated from rice polishings in 1926 by B. C. P. Jansen and W. F. Donath of the Dutch East Indian Medical Service in Java in the same laboratory where Eijkman and Grijns did their pioneer work on beriberi in humans and polyneuritis in fowl (18). They isolated 100 mg of crystals from 100 kilograms (kg) of rice polishings. This was an important event since it was the first time any vitamin was obtained from food in crystalline form, thus taking vitamins out of the class of "mysterious substances." It was ten years later, however, before Williams was able to announce its structure and synthesis (16).

Thiamin is a crystalline substance (Fig. 10–6), made up of carbon, hydrogen, oxygen, and sulfur (see formula in Appendix). It is readily soluble in water, slightly soluble in alcohol, and insoluble in fat solvents. It is quite stable (not readily destroyed) in the dry state. Synthetic thiamin is usually prepared in the form of one of its salts, such as thiamin hydrochloride or thiamin mononitrate, which are more stable than the free vitamin.

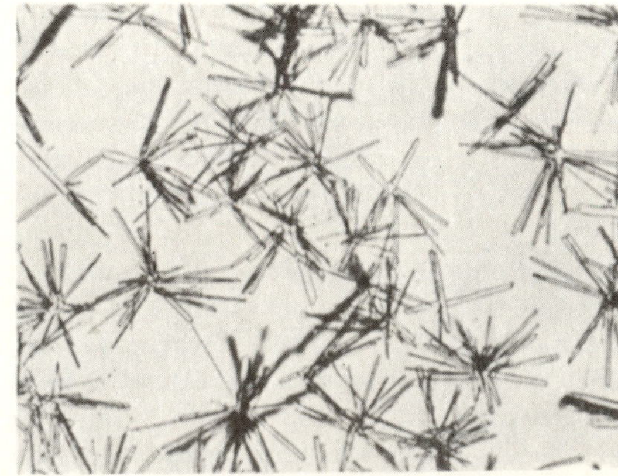

Figure 10–6 Photomicrograph of thiamin hydrochloride, crystalline form. (Courtesy of Merck & Company, Inc.)

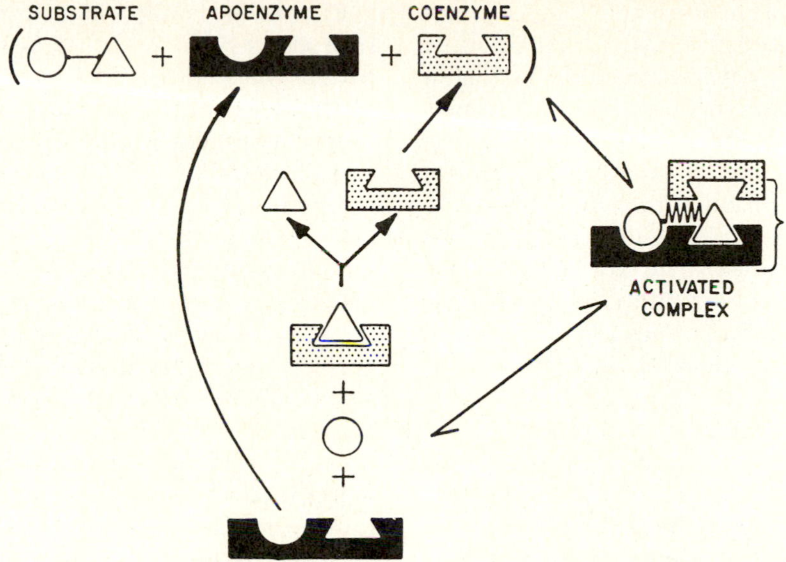

Figure 10–7 Diagram to show function of a coenzyme. The main enzyme (apoenzyme) absorbs the substance to be acted upon on its molecular surface but is unable to complete the reaction until the coenzyme (which is attracted to one part of the substrate molecule) is added to form an "activated complex." Tension is created between the two parts of the substrate and it is disrupted, with one part attached to the coenzyme. Both the apoenzyme and coenzyme release the portions of the disrupted substrate molecule and are free to act over again. (From Cantarow, A., and Shepartz, B.: *Biochemistry,* 3rd ed. Philadelphia, W. B. Saunders, 1962.)

Metabolism of Thiamin

Metabolic Fate. In humans, after thiamin is absorbed it is distributed widely by the blood throughout the body in all tissues and in somewhat higher concentrations in such organs as the heart, liver, and kidneys. The body has limited ability to store thiamin. Tissues are depleted of their normal content of the vitamin in just one or two weeks if the diet is deficient, so fresh supplies are needed regularly to provide for maintenance of tissue levels. The tissues take up only as much as they need, and because thiamin is freely soluble in water, most of the thiamin intake not required for day-to-day use is excreted in the urine, either as the intact molecule or as split halves.

Metabolic Function. Of foremost importance is the part thiamin plays in the life processes of individual cells throughout the body. As was seen in Chapter 6, a large part of the energy for the life processes of body tissues comes from the oxidation of carbohydrate. Oxidation takes place gradually through the formation of intermediate products and requires enzymes to bring about or catalyze each step of the intricate process. Many enzymes require coenzymes to render them active or make them capable of bringing about a certain chemical change (Fig. 10–7). Thiamin is known to be the active part of the coenzyme thiamin pyrophosphate, made in tissue cells by the combining of thiamin with two phosphate groups or radicals.[1]

This very important coenzyme is known to be necessary for at least four different enzyme systems that are needed for the complete oxidation of carbohydrate. Two of

[1]The mono- and tri-phosphate esters of thiamin are found in brain and nerve tissues (19). Whether they play a coenzymatic role is not clear.

these enzymes function by splitting off carbon dioxide in the course of oxidation in the body or in reverse reactions adding it onto some fragment of metabolism. Hence, thiamin pyrophosphate constitutes an essential link in the chain of the complete oxidation of carbohydrate, thus providing energy to the body. Without a dietary source of thiamin, intermediate compounds may build up in the blood and tissues to a toxic level, and these compounds are presumed to be an important cause of deficiency symptoms.

Thiamin pyrophosphate serves also as a coenzyme in reactions leading to the production of ribose, the important pentose sugar needed by all cells of the body. It also serves in the formation of coenzyme A and in the metabolism of leucine, isoleucine, and valine.

Essential cofactors in these actions of thiamin pyrophosphate are the coenzymes of several other B vitamins, such as pantothenic acid and niacin, as well as of magnesium, demonstrating the essential interrelationship in the body of the various vitamins and minerals.

RIBOFLAVIN

Riboflavin is an orange-yellow substance, first found to be a vitamin in the 1920s. It was synthesized in 1935 and proven to be needed by humans shortly thereafter. In the early 1940s riboflavin was made widely available for enriching food, feeding animals, and for vitamin supplements.

Riboflavin, the second of the B-complex vitamins to be discovered, was formerly known as vitamin B-2 (2). For a while it was also called vitamin G and lactoflavin. Only the one compound has "riboflavin activity" (see formula in the Appendix). It consists of a 3-ring nitrogen compound (a flavonoid) attached to *ribitol,* a derivative of the 5-carbon sugar *ribose*—hence the name riboflavin.

Riboflavin is quite widely distributed in nature along with the other B vitamins; milk products are an especially good source. Because of its wide distribution and its use in food-enrichment programs, severe deficiencies of riboflavin are very rare today in developed countries. A person with poor dietary habits would be likely to have low intakes of many B vitamins and other nutrients as well, not just riboflavin alone. (No doubt, the classical deficiency diseases of beriberi and pellagra involved low intakes of riboflavin and other B vitamins as well as thiamin and niacin.) Nevertheless, low intakes of riboflavin are seen in the United States in all age groups, especially among infants and children whose intake of milk products is very low. Riboflavin deficiency can be quite common in developing countries where there are no food-enrichment programs.

Deficiency Symptoms

In animals in which severe deficiencies can be studied, a source of riboflavin in the diet is essential for growth, reproduction, and prevention of a variety of deficiency signs.

In experimental animals (rats), a long-continued insufficiency of riboflavin leads to sore mouth and nose, falling hair and scaly skin, eye symptoms varying in severity from an inflamed condition of the cornea to its complete opacity in cataract (Fig. 10–8), digestive disturbances, nerve lesions (severe cases show paralysis of hind legs), poor utilization of food, increasing weakness, and death.

Riboflavin is needed in the diet of all monogastric animals tested, including the mouse, guinea pig, monkey, cat, fowl, pig, dog, fox, horse, fish, and even the young calf before the rumen starts to function. Many deficiency signs similar to those seen in the rat are seen in these animals. Riboflavin is added routinely as a supplement to commercial animal feeds.

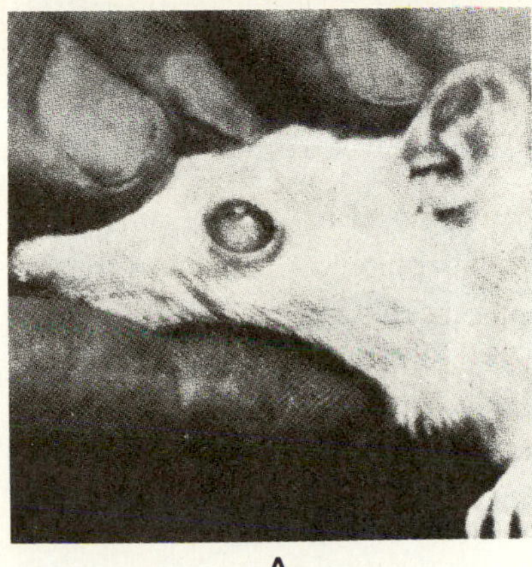

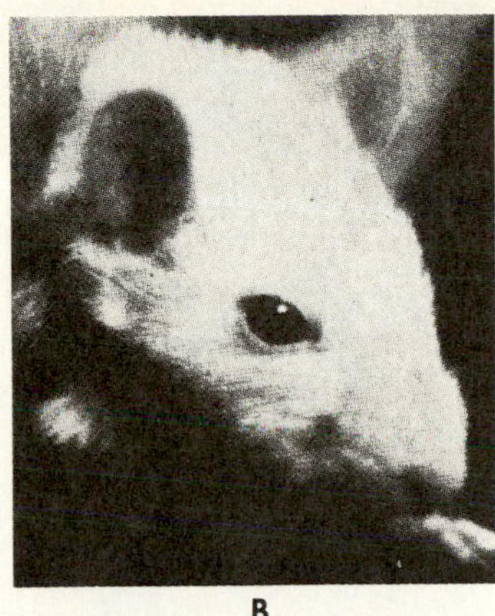

A B

Figure 10–8 Two views of the same rat. A, After cataract developed in the left eye as a result of riboflavin deficiency. B, Several weeks after administration of riboflavin, the right eye thus being saved. Also note the marked improvement of the rat's general condition as the result of riboflavin administration. (Courtesy of Paul L. Day and the *American Journal of Public Health.*)

In humans, symptoms of riboflavin deficiency are similar to those seen in animals, but they are less specific and less severe. W. H. Sebrell and R. E. Butler, who first studied experimental deficiency of riboflavin in human beings, reported as characteristic symptoms reddening of the mouth, a sore red tongue (glossitis), and *cheilosis,* a condition of cracks on the lips, mainly in the corners of the mouth (20). These symptoms were cured when riboflavin was given.

Other investigators have reported eye disorders in riboflavin-deficient persons such as dimness of vision and burning of the eyes. Cataracts, seen in riboflavin-deficient animals, are not seen in humans with a mild degree of riboflavin deficiency (21). Skin abnormalities, including a greasy scaly dermatitis on the face (see Fig. 10–9) and on the scrotum in the male, are common signs of severe riboflavin deficiency (22). Symptoms of general debility and behavioral changes, similar to those seen in pellagra, may also be associated with a deficient intake of riboflavin.

Ordinarily it takes several months for symptoms of riboflavin deficiency to appear, but M. Lane and co-workers developed an acute deficiency in humans within ten to twenty-five days by using a riboflavin *antagonist*[2] in a semisynthetic riboflavin-free diet (23). The resulting symptoms seen in the six test subjects were first, sore throat or mouth; followed by the typical reddening and swelling of the mucous membrane of the mouth and throat; cheilosis; glossitis; dermatitis of the face, ears, and other parts of the body; and anemia. Anemia was a "new" symptom, so it appears that riboflavin deficiency interferes with the production of red blood cells in humans, as has been reported in animals. All these symptoms were rapidly and completely reversed after administration of riboflavin.

[2]A nutritional antagonist is a compound whose structure is so similar to a specific nutrient that it can substitute for the nutrient in certain enzyme systems for which the specific nutrient is necessary, thus leading to at least partial inactivity of these systems. Hence, an effect similar to a deficiency is produced in a short time. True nutritional antagonism, or *competitive inhibition,* can always be overcome by high enough levels of the nutrient in question. The riboflavin antagonist used by Lane et al. (21) was *galactoflavin,* in which galactitol has been substituted for ribitol in the vitamin. Antagonists of this type exist for many of the other vitamins.

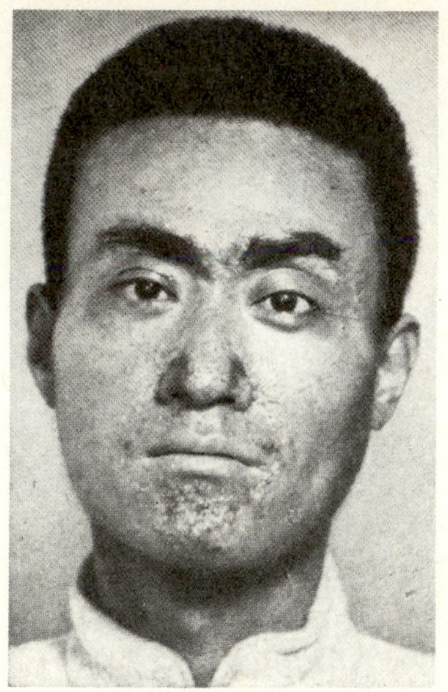

A

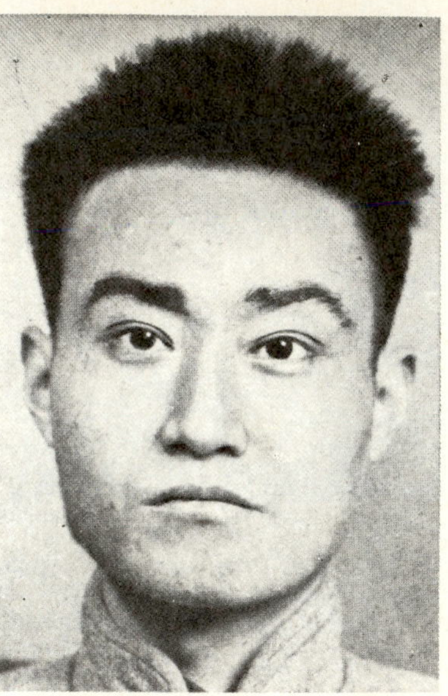

B

Figure 10–9 Patient before and after treatment for riboflavin deficiency. A, Scales and sores on the forehead, eyes, nose, cheeks, lips, and chin, and in the folds around nose and mouth. B, After treatment with riboflavin, 15 mg the first two days, 10 mg for the next two days, and 5 mg daily for one week. (Courtesy of Bernard Read and H.C. Hou, Shanghai, Wm. Heinemann, Ltd., London, and the *Chinese Medical Journal*.)

Recommended Allowances of Riboflavin

The daily riboflavin allowances recommended by the Food and Nutrition Board have been based for practical purposes on a value of 0.6 mg of riboflavin for every 1000 kcal consumed for people of all ages (1). This is about 20 percent over the apparent minimum requirement of about 0.5 mg per 1000 kcal, a rather small margin of safety in comparison with the safety margins for many of the other vitamins. This figure does not allow too great a leeway for "dietary indiscretions" of individuals, at least not over long periods.

The recommended dietary allowance (RDA) for college-age men is 1.7 mg per day, and for college-age women it is 1.3 mg per day. The need for riboflavin increases during pregnancy and lactation, as is true with all B vitamins.

Some evidence exists from recent studies in Gambia that the requirement of pregnant and lactating women is about 2.5 mg of riboflavin per day, somewhat higher than the U.S.RDA (24). The conclusions were based on biochemical status tests but need further study.

See Table 10–3 and inside front cover for more details on allowances. A minimum of about 1.2 mg of riboflavin per day in adults is necessary to maintain adequate body stores and normal urinary output even if the caloric intake is below 2000 kcal.

Riboflavin Intakes

Low riboflavin intakes are still seen in segments of the population in North America and in many other areas of the world.

Intake in the United States and Canada. Severe riboflavin deficiency once was fairly common, especially in the South, and wher-

Table 10–3 RECOMMENDED ALLOWANCES FOR RIBOFLAVIN*

	Age	*Allowance, mg/day*
Males	11–14 years	1.6
	15–22 years	1.7
	23–50 years	1.6
	51 years and over	1.4
Females	11–14 years	1.3
	15–22 years	1.3
	23–50 years	1.2
	51 years or over	1.2
	Pregnant	+0.3
	Lactating	+0.5

*From the Food and Nutrition Board, 1980.

See Appendix Table 1 for recommendations of FAO/WHO and of other countries. The Canadian allowance is set at 0.5 mg per 1000 kcal of food rather than at any specific set figure.

ever milk, the best dietary source, was not consumed regularly. After 1941, the start of the food-enrichment program (see Chap. 18), cases of clinically apparent deficiency of riboflavin in humans became very rare. Concentrates of riboflavin, from synthetic or fermentation sources, used in current food-enrichment programs in the United States, contribute an average of about 0.33 mg of riboflavin per person per day. This is about one-fourth of the requirement, a very significant amount.[3] Not all states, however, require food-enrichment programs, and the riboflavin intake of many persons, up to 30 percent in some subgroups, in these and other states is still well below recommended allowances (4,5,25–29).

Chronic borderline or low-riboflavin intakes are most likely to occur in persons with inadequate intake of basic or enriched foods, especially milk or milk products. In the United States and Canada low intakes have been recently reported in various vulnerable groups such as adolescents (25), children (26), low socioeconomic groups of adults (27), women of child-bearing years (28), and the aged, especially those in nursing homes and/or other institutions (21,29). In many of these studies biochemical measurements were made that correlated with the low-intake values. The most commonly used test for riboflavin intake is measurement of the red blood cell enzyme *erythrocyte glutathione reductase,* which requires a riboflavin coenzyme for its activity. Other clinical signs of low-riboflavin intake were seen in some of these studies.

Women taking oral contraceptives were found by several research groups to be less apt to have increased riboflavin requirements than was formerly believed. Persons with high-alcohol intakes are more likely to have low-riboflavin intakes.

Many studies can be cited, on the other hand, showing few, if any, low-riboflavin intakes in great numbers of healthy, well-fed population groups in the United States (4,5,30,31). Many people—30 to 40 percent—take some sort of nutrient supplement, most of which contain riboflavin (25,31,32).

Because infants generally consume a large amount of breast milk or cow's milk, their average consumption of riboflavin is well above the recommended allowance. Only when milk is not consumed is it necessary to be concerned about an infant's riboflavin intake, and most commercial milk substitutes supply liberal amounts (see Chap. 23).

Intake in Other Countries. Riboflavin deficiencies, often with typical and more severe clinical symptoms, exist in India, China, Africa (24), Europe, Ireland, the United Kingdom, and elsewhere (see supplementary readings in the Appendix). Low intakes are of epidemic proportions in developing countries. It is important, therefore, that many

[3]The wholesale cost of riboflavin from such sources is only about 15 cents per 1000 mg (1 gm)—more than a year's requirement for one person.

more efforts be devoted in all countries to increasing intakes of riboflavin and other key nutrients as well, such as vitamin D, folacin, vitamin A, calcium, and iron. To accomplish this, new programs in nutrition education, distribution of free and low cost foods to the poor, and enrichment of foods will be needed.

One of the major reasons for the low consumption of riboflavin is that many persons in all countries do not use milk in any form or they use it very sparingly (25,28). It is clear that people not consuming milk products must eat liberal quantities of other good sources of riboflavin to maintain an adequate intake (see Fig. 10–10).

Riboflavin in Foods

Sources. Riboflavin (most often in combined forms) is widely, but not abundantly, distributed in both plant and animal tissues. It is made by all higher plants, chiefly in the green leaves. Younger parts of the plant contain more than older parts. Fruit, nonleafy vegetables, beans, nonenriched grains, potatoes, and other roots and tubers rank from poor to very poor sources (see Table 10–4).

Liver, kidney, heart, and yeast are the

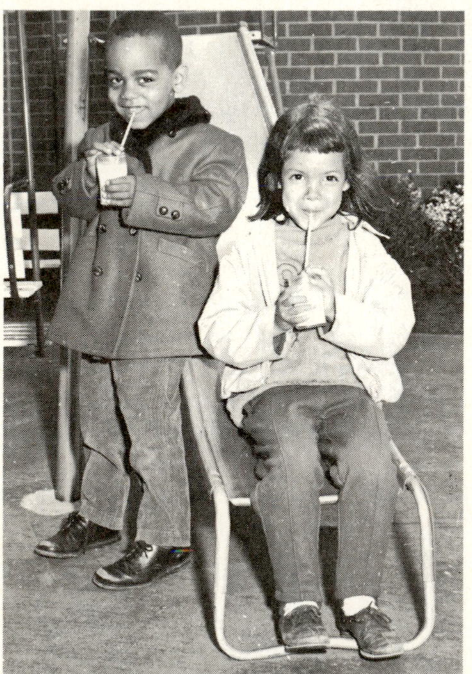

Figure 10–10 Milk supplies about 35 percent of all the riboflavin in the food supply of the United States. (Courtesy of U.S. Department of Agriculture.)

Table 10–4 EXAMPLES OF FOOD SOURCES OF RIBOFLAVIN[a] (BASED ON AVERAGE SERVING SIZES)

Rich sources[b]—1 to 6 mg per serving
Liver, kidney, and heart.
Excellent sources—0.4 to 1.0 mg per serving
Breakfast cereals (wheat)—enriched, burrito (beef), hamburger (large, with bun), milk (whole, low-fat, or skim), and yogurt.
Good sources—0.2 to 0.4 mg per serving
Breakfast cereals (non-wheat)—enriched, cheese (blue or cottage), chili (with meat), eggs (two), enchilada, ice cream, meat (beef, lamb, pork), mushrooms, pancakes, poultry (light-without skin, or dark meat), salmon, spaghetti—enriched, sprouts, tostada (with cheese), turnip greens, wheat germ, and white flour—enriched (1 cup).
Fair sources—0.1 to 0.2 mg per serving
Asparagus, almonds, banana, beet greens, bread (2 slices—enriched), brussel sprouts, cake—enriched flour, candy (with milk or nuts), cheese (1 oz), cornmeal—enriched, fish, macaroni—enriched, peas (fresh or frozen), pizza (cheese), poultry (light meat), spinach, squash, strawberries, taco (beef), wheat (bran or whole grain), and wheat farina—enriched.
Poor Sources—0.05 to 0.1 mg per serving
Beans, beer (1 glass), broccoli, citrus and citrus fruit, corn (fresh or frozen), cornmeal—not enriched (maize), cow peas, granola, lettuce, melons, oatmeal, peas (canned), peppers, potatoes (baked or boiled), soups (without meat or milk), soybeans, sweet potatoes, Swiss chard, shredded wheat cereal, and tomatoes.

Table 10–4 continued

Very poor sources—less than 0.05 mg per serving
Apples, apricots, beets, bread (white)—not enriched, cabbage, candy, carrots, cauliflower, celery, chick peas, cookies, cornmeal—not enriched (maize), fats and oils, mustard greens, peaches, peanuts, pears, potatoes (chips or french fries), rice, sugar, tofu.

[a]See Table 2 in Appendix for detailed figures on riboflavin content of foods. For additional values not listed there see sources in the footnotes to Appendix, Table 2, and also Dong, M. H., et al.(13) (for 81 foods and dishes as served), Ensminger, A. H., et al.(33), and Gordon, D. T., et al.(34).

[b]Other rich sources (supplements) of riboflavin are available but are not served with meals. These are yeast, with about 0.3 to 0.7 mg per tablespoon depending on the yeast, and pure riboflavin, which is available in many different concentrations.

richest sources of riboflavin, though consumption of these is low. Milk, milk products, enriched cereals, lean meats, poultry, and eggs are good to very good sources, and as a group contribute over 80 percent of the riboflavin in American diets. Milk and milk products, alone, provide 36 percent of U.S. riboflavin intake. Whole-grain cereals have only a moderate content of riboflavin. When enriched with riboflavin to the level of whole grains, however, bread and cereals contribute one-fourth of the riboflavin to the average American diet—a reflection of the large amount consumed of these foods. Green vegetables and tomatoes are only poor to fair sources of riboflavin, although they provide most other vitamins and minerals.

Effects of Processing, Light, and Cooking. It is fortunate that riboflavin is stable enough on heating that little of it is destroyed in ordinary cooking processes, although some may be lost by solution in water in which foods are cooked or canned. Losses also can occur from exposure to light if the cooking is done in open vessels. In fact, riboflavin is so sensitive to light than when someone is using a dilute solution of it in a laboratory—such as when assaying it in foods—it is routine practice to turn off the lights and pull down the shades to darken the room as much as is practical.

Riboflavin is stable to heating in neutral or acid solutions, but it may be destroyed by heating in alkaline solution. For instance, the use of sodium bicarbonate in the cooking of vegetables to keep them green can also destroy riboflavin. Average losses of riboflavin in processing and cooking are 10 to 20 percent depending on the food, the amount of heat, light, and on other processing conditions (35).

Because of the importance of milk as a dietary source of riboflavin, the possible destruction of this vitamin on exposure of milk to light needs to be emphasized. Before the 1960s clear glass bottles of milk were delivered on the doorsteps of homes—a practice still very common in many countries. It is now rare in North America, at least, partly because a glass bottle left standing on the doorstep in direct sunlight may lose 50 to 70 percent of its riboflavin potency in two hours (36). The use of opaque cartons cuts down losses from exposure to sunlight or from display lighting in foodstores. Even so, it is best to keep milk as much as possible in a cool, dark place, such as the refrigerator. Only minor losses of riboflavin occur in pasteurization of milk.

Because of the destructive effect of light on riboflavin, low levels of the vitamin have been observed in newborn infants receiving phototherapy in the treatment of jaundice (37). This is of interest, but one should not conclude that persons spending long hours in the sun need extra riboflavin.

Discovery and Properties

In 1933, chemists in Germany found that rats grew faster when given a dietary source of a yellow compound called ovoflavin, which they isolated from egg white (*flavus* means "yellow"). It was soon shown that the flavin pigment that had been isolated and that was essential for rats was the same as the pigment associated with the classic "yellow enzyme," isolated by O. Warburg in Germany in 1931, and similar to the yellow pigment isolated from heart muscle by A. Szent-Györgyi and co-workers in 1932, which was later shown to be an important coenzyme. This proved to be the first demonstration of a vitamin-coenzyme relationship and opened the door to modern nutritional biochemistry. The name riboflavin was given by P. Karrer of Switzerland to the yellow pigment in the coenzyme in 1935.[4]

One of the most important chemical properties of riboflavin is its change to a colorless form *on reduction* (addition of hydrogen molecules), and its *reoxidation* (removal of hydrogen) to its orange-yellow color by exposure to oxidizing agents. This forms the basis of its metabolic role in the body.

Metabolism of Riboflavin

Free riboflavin, such as is found in milk, eggs, and enriched foods, is absorbed in the small intestine directly into the blood stream. Bound forms must first be split in the intestine, although riboflavin is quite readily available (38). Once it enters the blood, it is carried by certain proteins and distributed to all cells of the body.

Riboflavin's metabolic role revolves chiefly around the two important coenzymes vital to every cell and in which most of the riboflavin in the body exists—*flavin mononucleotide* (or riboflavin monophosphate) and the more common *flavin adenine dinucleotide* (FAD), composed of riboflavin monophosphate with additional phosphate and sugar groups plus adenine, a purine. These coenzymes are attached with various degrees of tenacity to a number of highly important enzymes in the body, the *flavoproteins,* which catalyze oxidation-reduction reactions. Most of these enzymes act as hydrogen carriers, passing this element along from one substance to another until its atoms are finally united with oxygen atoms, by special enzymes, to form molecules of water (see Fig. 10–11). Riboflavin-containing compounds, therefore, are essential for the metabolism of carbohydrates, of amino acids, and of fats. During this process, energy is released gradually and made available to the cell. It is of interest that several of these enzymes contain a metal—for example, molybdenum or iron—demonstrating again the important interrelationships between vitamins and minerals.

Among the various riboflavin-containing enzymes in the body are *glutathione reductase* of the red blood cell, used in studies of intake, and various *dehydrogenases, oxidases, and transferases* (38). These enzymes are essential not only for energy formation but for a wide variety of functions, including thiamin and vitamin B-6 metabolism, nerve formation, hemoglobin formation and iron metabolism, lipid metabolism, niacin formation from tryptophan, adrenal gland function, collagen formation, and immune mechanisms.

Because riboflavin is essential for so many cellular reactions in the body, it is clear why its lack causes damage to many different types of tissues and that sufficient intake of it is necessary to promote the welfare of the body as a whole.

There does not appear to be any specialized mechanism for storage of riboflavin, although muscle tissues may retain considerable amounts even in riboflavin deficiency. Unused riboflavin is excreted in the urine. Reports of toxicity are very rare (39).

PANTOTHENIC ACID

Pantothenic acid is a dietary essential for humans and animals and plays an unusually

[4]Karrer and the German R. Kuhn, working independently, first synthesized riboflavin in 1935. Karrer was also the first to synthesize carotene and made other important discoveries in nutrition. He was awarded the Nobel Prize in 1937.

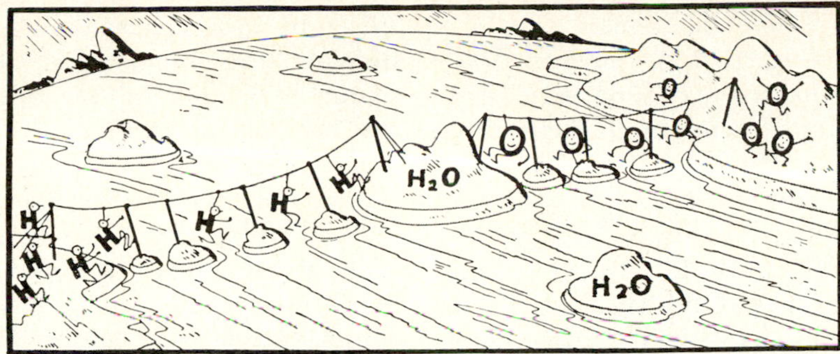

Figure 10–11 Diagram to illustrate how enzymes or coenzymes, which contain vitamins, may act as stepping stones for oxygen or hydrogen atoms in bringing about oxidation-reduction in living tissues. Thiamin, riboflavin, and niacin form part of enzymes and coenzymes that function in this manner. The hydrogen and oxygen atoms, separated by an otherwise formidable barrier, are enabled by the use of stepping stones (enzymes) and the handrails (coenzymes) to move toward each other and ultimately unite to form molecules of water (H_2O). (Adapted from W.O. Kermack and P. Eggleton: *The Stuff We're Made Of,* Edward Arnold & Co., London.)

important role in the body. It is so widely distributed in most foods, however, that a deficiency has not been seen in populations consuming ordinary foods in the United States or in any other country.

Discovery

The name pantothenic acid, derived from the Greek, meaning, "from everywhere," was given in 1933 by R. J. Williams, then of Oregon State, to an unknown factor in various biological materials necessary for the growth of yeast. (Williams, still working, in retirement, at the University of Texas, is a brother of the late R. R. Williams, who first synthesized thiamin.) Later, pantothenic acid was found to be the third member of the vitamin B complex needed by higher organisms. Therefore, it is discussed in this order, after riboflavin.[5]

After much painstaking research, primarily using young chicks as test animals, workers at the Universities of California and Wisconsin, in 1939, announced that a highly active preparation of the "chick-antidermatitis factor" and Williams's pantothenic acid had identical growth activity (40). In 1940, its structure was determined and it was synthesized by Williams (see formula in the Appendix) (41). Stable crystalline salts of pantothenic acid are readily available, such as synthetic sodium or calcium pantothenate.[6]

Deficiency Symptoms

Humans. Deficiency symptoms in humans, produced experimentally in volunteers by use of a purified diet and a specific antagonist, include fatigue, headache, sleep disturbances, personality changes, nausea, abdominal distress, numbness and tingling of hands and feet, muscle cramps, impaired coordination, and loss of antibody production (42). All symptoms are cured by the administration of pantothenic acid. A well-defined deficiency of pantothenic acid has not been observed in humans under natural conditions.

Experimental Animals. Pantothenic acid

[5]Pantothenic acid, before its structure was known, was called by several other names, now obsolete, including filtrate factor, chick antidermatitis factor, factor 2, vitamin B-x, and vitamin B-3. Note that the term vitamin B-3, often used today in current health food literature for niacin, has no historic significance and is incorrect. (See N. Engl. J. Med., *291*:263, 1974.)

[6]The D isomer of synthetic salts of pantothenate is the natural active form.

deficiency in experimental animals is readily obtained by feeding them on purified diets or natural diets heated over long periods to destroy this vitamin. Deficient chickens have a characteristic dermatitis of the beak, eyes, and feet. They grow poorly, and if not given pantothenic acid, death results in three or four weeks (see Fig. 10–12). In other animals, a deficiency of pantothenic acid affects many tissues, and, in general, causes poor growth and faulty reproduction. It is of interest that graying of the hair is produced in pantothenic acid-deficient rats, monkeys, dogs, and foxes; color usually can be restored by added pantothenate in the diet. In humans, this relationship between pantothenic acid intake and graying of hair has not been seen. (Adding extra amounts of pantothenic acid to human diets does not change the color of gray hair.)

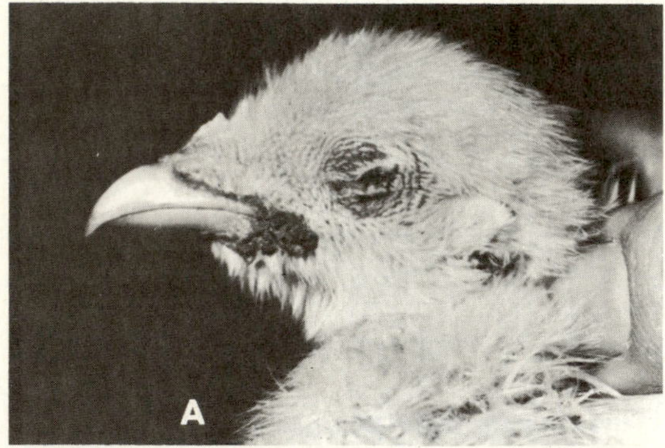

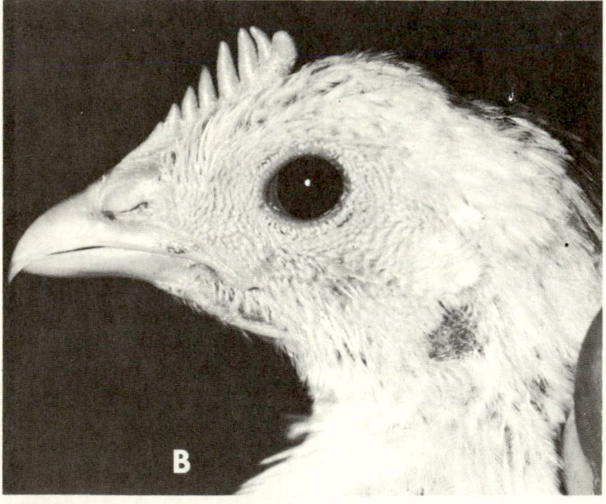

Figure 10–12 A, Chick after being fed a diet deficient in pantothenic acid. The eyelids, corners of the mouth, and adjacent skin are inflamed. The growth of feathers is retarded, and the feathers are rough. B, The same chick after three weeks on a diet containing pantothenic acid. The lesions are completely cured. (Courtesy of the Upjohn Company.)

In many species deficient in pantothenic acid, degenerative changes are found in nerve tissues and especially in the adrenal glands, which may become enlarged, reddened, and hemorrhagic. The role of pantothenic acid in the activity of the adrenals was found when it was shown to be part of a coenzyme, coenzyme A, needed for making certain hormones (cortisone and two related hormones) formed in the outer portion or cortex of these ductless glands. These hormones have important regulatory influences on metabolism and indeed are essential for life.

The Role of Pantothenic Acid in the Body

The physiological role of pantothenic acid is involved primarily with coenzyme A,[7] one of the most important substances in body metabolism. As part of coenzyme A, pantothenic acid is essential for the intermediary metabolism of carbohydrates, fats, and proteins, for their synthesis, breakdown, and release of energy. It functions primarily by effecting the removal or acceptance of important chemical groups with 2, 3, 4, or more carbon atoms at a time. Acetyl-coenzyme A is the most abundant form. Coenzyme A is needed for the formation of such important sterols as cholesterol and the adrenocortical hormones. It is also essential for the synthesis of acetylcholine, an important regulator of nerve tissue, and for making

[7]Coenzyme A, discovered in the 1940s, consists of a complicated molecule, *phosphopantetheine* (composed of pantothenic acid, a phosphate group, and reduced sulfur) plus two additional phosphate groups, a pentose, and adenine (a purine).

many other important compounds in the body (43).

Coenzyme A is essential for so many chemical reactions in the body, such as those necessary for energy release and for building many essential complicated compounds out of simpler ones, that pantothenic acid has been said to "sit at the crossroads of metabolism."

Pantothenic acid functions also as a component of the enzyme *fatty acid synthetase* involved in fatty acid synthesis in the body. It has many other functions including maintenance of blood-sugar levels, of hemoglobin structure, of nerve and brain tissue, of muscle tissue, and of a defense system against infection.

In many of these reactions of pantothenic acid, the coenzymes of riboflavin, thiamin, biotin, niacin, and pyridoxal are also involved, as well as the minerals phosphorus, sulfur, magnesium, and manganese, showing again how vitamins and minerals are interrelated.

Requirement and Nutritional Status

A formal recommended dietary allowance for pantothenic acid has not been set by the Food and Nutrition Board on the basis that "isolated dietary deficiencies are unlikely." Since marginal deficiencies may exist, however, a "safe and adequate daily dietary intake" has recently been set (1). A range of 4 to 7 mg a day is suggested for all adults until better information is available (see Table 10–5 for more details).

An average level in "adequate" diets is probably about 7 mg per day and ranges normally between 4 and 20 mg (1,44,45). Instances of intakes as low as 1.1 mg a day have been seen in two small samples of teenage girls, a level that would be expected eventually to result in a deficiency if continued.

Recent studies have found intakes of pantothenic acid of 3.75 mg a day in a Utah nursing home (not including beverages) (46), 6.1 mg in a composite Canadian diet (47), 5.1 mg in a British diet (48), and 11.5 mg in an "average American diet" (49). These figures are within the earlier estimates and are within the range suggested as safe and adequate. No specific deficiency signs accountable to pantothenic acid were obvious in any of the persons surveyed in these studies, but more such studies are needed.

Human milk has about 2.2 mg of pantothenic acid per liter, so the daily infant requirement would be expected to be less than this. Cow's milk has about 3.4 mg per liter.

Since processing of food can, in some instances, result in appreciable losses of pantothenic acid, it is possible that unrecognized borderline deficiencies may exist in human populations, such as in multiple nutritional deficiencies associated with lack of good food for any reason, and with alcoholism. Such deficiencies, if they exist, would occur only in connection with other deficiencies in humans and would likely escape detection because of emphasis on other nutrients.

Deficiencies of pantothenic acid have been seen, though rarely, in farm animals (swine) fed "natural rations." As a result, synthetic

Table 10–5 ESTIMATED SAFE AND ADEQUATE DAILY INTAKES OF PANTOTHENIC ACID[a]

Group	*Age (years)*	*Range in mg*
Infants	0–0.5	2
	0.5–1	3
Children	1–3	3
	4–6	3–4
	7–10	4–5
Adolescents	11–16	4–7
Adults	17 and on	4–7

[a]From Food and Nutrition Board, 1980(1). No Canadian recommendations have been offered, nor estimations for pregnancy and lactation.

pantothenic acid is often added to commercial swine rations. How a deficiency could develop under such conditions is not clear, but this points out the need for many more studies with this vitamin in human nutrition. Availability of pantothenic acid from foods may be low under certain conditions. A recent study in humans indicated only about half of the pantothenic acid in an "average American diet" was bioavailable from natural food (5.8 mg available out of 11.5 mg in the diet) (49).

Pantothenic Acid in Foods

Sources. Pantothenic acid exists in all cells of living tissues and therefore is present in all natural foods, usually in combined forms. All foods in the four food groups contain pantothenic acid, but foods especially rich in it are yeast, liver, eggs, wheat and rice germ or bran, peanuts, and peas. Moderate to good amounts are contained in such foods as meat, milk, poultry, whole grains, broccoli, mushrooms, and sweet potatoes. Most vegetables and fruits and refined foods contain lesser amounts. White flour, precooked rice, corn flakes, and many processed foods (50) are poor sources of the vitamin. None is present, of course, in salad oils, shortening, sugar, and similar products. See detailed values in Table 2 of the Appendix or in other tables (3,33,50).

Effects of Processing. Processing and refinement of foods as well as milling of grains can result in considerable losses of pantothenic acid. Losses of up to 50 percent and even more may occur in processing and storage of frozen vegetables and meats. Similar losses occur in many canned food products. Persons on low-energy diets may well choose diets below 4 mg of pantothenic acid per day if care is not taken (50).

Synthetic calcium pantothenate is quite widely used today in vitamin supplements and to fortify a few breakfast foods, though usually only in trivial amounts. It is not a toxic substance, but there is no reason to consume more than what is found in a good basic diet (39).

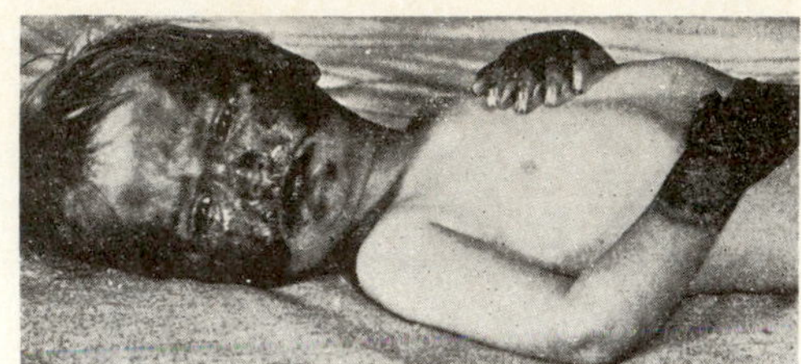

Figure 10–13 Pellagra in a child, showing typical red rash on face and hands on parts of body exposed to sunlight. (Courtesy of Dr. John A. McIntosh.)

NIACIN

Niacin is a collective term including two natural forms of the vitamin (vitamers)[8] *nicotinic acid* and *nicotinamide*. Either compound, alone or in combination with the other, will prevent or treat *pellagra,* a fatal skin disease (see Fig. 10–13).

Deficiency Symptoms

The tissues that show damage as a result of niacin deficiency are chiefly the skin, the gastrointestinal tract, and the nerves.

Pellagra existed in some parts of Europe for more than 200 years, especially in areas where corn (maize) formed a large part of the diet before a cure was found. Its most striking and characteristic symptoms include a reddish skin rash, especially on the face, hands, and feet when they are exposed to sunlight, which later makes the skin dark and rough (see Figs. 10–13 and 10–14)(22). This condition gave rise to the name pellagra in 1771 from the Italian *pelle agra,* meaning "painful, or rough skin." The skin

[8]Vitamers are any of two or more compounds that relieve a deficiency of a specific vitamin.

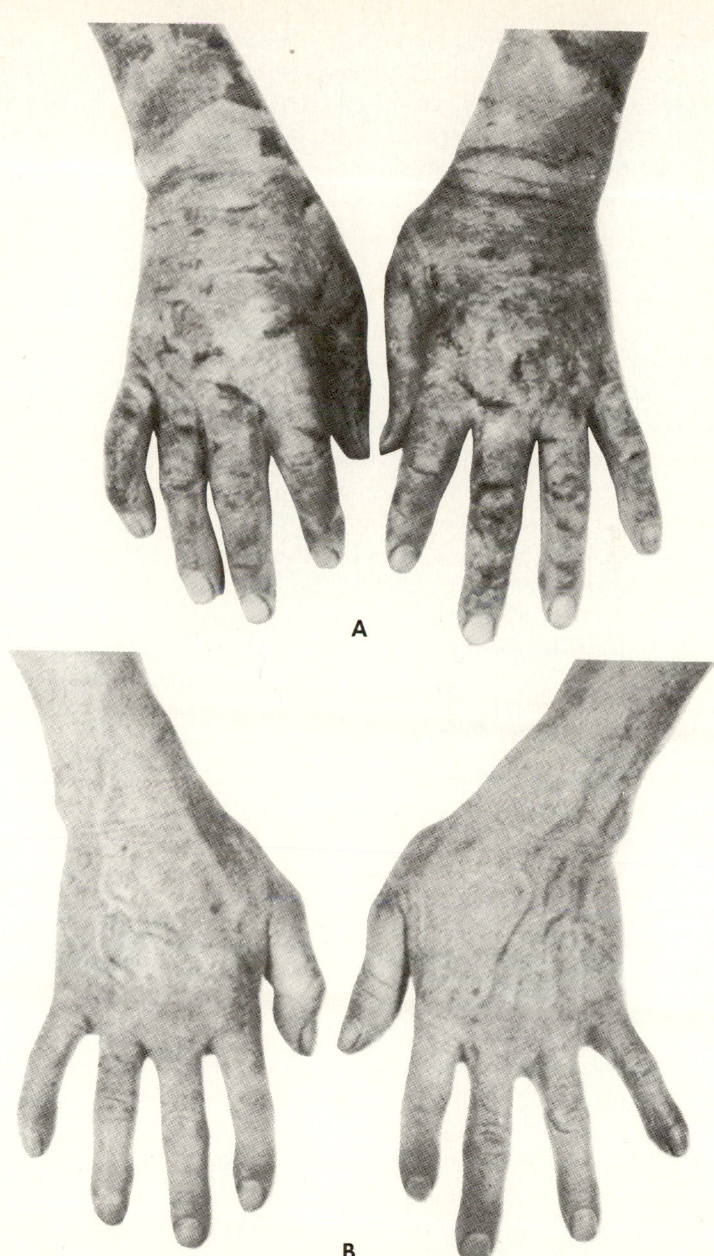

Figure 10–14 Cure of pellagrous lesions on hands on an adult by a diet rich in B vitamins, especially niacin. A, Hands of pellagra patient. B, Same patient after 2 weeks of corrective diet. (From Spies: *Rehabilitation through Better Nutrition.* Philadelphia, W.B. Saunders, 1947.)

rash always appears on both the left and right sides of the body at the same time—that is, it is bilaterally symmetrical.

Other symptoms include a sore mouth and tongue, and inflamed membranes in the digestive tract, with bloody diarrhea in the later stages. There may also be distressing nervous and mental disturbances, such as irritability, anxiety, depression, and in advanced cases, delirium, hallucinations, confusion, disorientation, and stupor. Many mental institutions in the United States had large numbers of such persons before the cure was discovered. Physicians sometimes referred to pellagra symptoms as "the three Ds—dermatitis, diarrhea, and dementia." Still other symptoms are loss of weight, anemia (which may be associated with deficiencies of other B vitamins), and dehydration, from diarrhea.

Less acute symptoms of niacin deficiency may be difficult to recognize. Changes in the tongue are among the earliest signs of niacin lack and may be used to detect it. Mild pellagra may occur in infants and children in whom the usual pellagra symptoms are lacking. Weakness and failure to grow properly, however, respond favorably to treatment with niacin. Hence, we see that this vitamin is necessary for growth and for health of tissues, and it also promotes appetite, proper functioning of the digestive tract, and good utilization of foodstuffs in the body.

Discovery and Properties

The history of the discovery of the pellagra-preventing factor is as interesting as a detective story (6,7,51).

Though a few early physicians were convinced that pellagra was caused by dietary deficiencies, it was commonly thought in the early 1900s that it might be due to an infectious agent or to some toxic substance present in corn (maize) or developed in corn (maize) that had spoiled. About 1907, pellagra became prevalent in the southern part of the United States, and cases increased in number so rapidly, mainly in adult females, that in 1915 more than 10,000 persons died of it. In 1917–1918 there were 200,000 cases of pellagra in the United States, not limited to the South, but found throughout the whole country.

This situation was of great concern to the United States Public Health Service, which instituted special studies of the disease under the direction of Joseph Goldberger. By then, opinion was divided as to whether pellagra was due to poor sanitation or diet. Later, when Goldberger had induced the disease solely by feeding a "poor" diet to volunteer convicts and had prevented its incidence in various institutions by improvement of the diet, it was established as a disease of dietary deficiency.[9] Goldberger proved that the disease could be prevented by giving people liver, yeast, lean meats, milk, or other foods rich in B-complex vitamins (52).

The exact nature of the pellagra-preventing substance in Goldberger's diets remained a mystery until C. A. Elvehjem and co-workers, of the University of Wisconsin, showed in 1937 that blacktongue—an analogous disease in dogs—could be cured by giving *nicotinic acid* or the closely related *nicotinic acid amide* (nicotinamide), which they isolated from liver (53). Administration of one or both of these was soon shown by several investigators to cure the most striking and characteristic symptoms of pellagra in humans. Even before these discoveries, preventive dietary measures had been instituted in the southern states that resulted in marked decrease in pellagra incidence until, by 1945, acute cases were seldom seen.

Another chapter in the story of pellagra prevention was completed in 1945–1950 when it was discovered that the amino acid tryptophan was converted, in part, to nicotinic acid in the body of humans and animals and that sufficient amounts of tryptophan alone could overcome pellagra in the absence of dietary niacin. The *niacin activity* of any food, then, is derived from the amount of available niacin *and* tryptophan present (see later sections).

Properties of Niacin. Nicotinic acid had been originally discovered and named in

[9]Goldberger proved in 1916 that pellagra was not an infectious disease when he and a group of fifteen volunteers, in a heroic and crucial experiment, inoculated themselves with blood, swabbed their throats with saliva, and swallowed the excreta of patients severely ill with pellagra. Although some of the volunteers felt a bit squeamish, none became ill with pellagra afterward (6).

1867 by the German chemist C. Huber. He made it by chemical treatment of nicotine—of the tobacco plant, from which it derived its name.[10] It sat on laboratory shelves untested for many years while thousands of persons were dying from pellagra. No one knew then that there was a relationship.

Nicotinic acid and the related compound—nicotinamide—are white compounds, soluble in water and stable to both heating and oxidation, as well as to acids and alkalis. They are more resistant to destruction than any of the B-complex vitamins.

Chemically, these nitrogen-containing compounds are among the simplest of the vitamins (see formulas in the Appendix); one contains an organic acid group (—COOH) and the other has an amino group (—NH_2) substituted in the acid group.

The name niacin was adopted in 1971 by the American Institute of Nutrition and international agencies for all forms of the vitamin, and the term *niacin activity* for combined activity of nicotinic acid and its derivatives (2).[11] The word niacin was originally coined in 1942 to be used as the popularized name instead of nicotinic acid. This was to avoid any possible implication that these normal nutrients are related in activity to nicotine, the alkaloid in tobacco. The word niacin, however, now refers to the two forms of the vitamin. Niacin is present in foods or tissues in either free or combined forms, sometimes bound so tightly that it is not always available to the body.

Tryptophan Relationship. For many years before the discovery of niacin it had been known that eating diets high in corn (maize) increased the incidence of pellagra, as has been noted. The reason for this was a puzzle to early nutrition workers. Also they were puzzled by the fact that some foods, such as milk and eggs, were found to have greater pellagra-preventing potency than could be explained on what little was known about the nature of the protective factor. Goldberger at first suspected protein had something to do with pellagra and even cured a few patients by feeding them tryptophan, but this work was not followed up when it was found that yeast and liver extracts very low in protein were even more effective.

It was not until 1945 that W. A. Krehl and coworkers at the University of Wisconsin opened the door that led to the explanation of the causal relation of corn (maize) and pellagra. They found that either niacin or tryptophan overcame a niacin deficiency in rats on a high-corn diet (54). Some of the tryptophan, it turned out, was being converted in the body to niacin. Corn is known to be especially imbalanced in regard to tryptophan (it has a low amount in relationship to the other amino acids).

It was soon discovered by means of other animal studies that the simultaneous presence of three conditions was responsible for the pellagra-producing effect of corn: (1) the low amount of available niacin, (2) the low amount of tryptophan, and (3) a dietary imbalance caused by the presence of relatively large amounts of other amino acids in proportion to tryptophan in corn (55). Other foods low and unbalanced in respect to tryptophan, such as gelatin, give about the same effect as corn when fed to experimental animals, as do various mixtures of amino acids devoid of tryptophan. *All three conditions must be present at once to produce pellagra.* The relatively low content of both tryptophan and niacin in corn as compared to that in rice and wheat is shown in Table 10–6.

The above studies explained why some foods, such as milk and eggs, have far greater pellagra-preventing potency than

[10]Nicotine itself has no vitamin activity.

[11]Recently this vitamin has been called, wrongly, "vitamin B-3" in certain health food literature. There is no historic basis for this terminolgy, and its use is to be deplored. A few researchers called nicotinic acid vitamin B-5 in the early days before it was identified, but not vitamin B-3.

Table 10–6 RELATIVE AMOUNT OF TRYPTOPHAN AND NIACIN IN RICE, WHEAT, AND CORN (MAIZE)[a]

	Total Protein	*Tryptophan*	*Niacin*
Rice, white, per 100 gm	7.5 gm	115 mg	2.0 mg
Whole wheat, per 100 gm	13.0 gm	168 mg	4.3 mg
Whole corn, per 100 gm	9.0 gm	55 mg	2.0 mg

[a]In relationship to protein level.

would be expected from their actual content of niacin. Such foods are low in niacin but carry proteins that are high in the amino acid tryptophan, thus furnishing the body with protection from pellagra by enabling it to build niacin within the tissues.

Tryptophan has a sparing action on the amount of niacin necessary because during its breakdown in the body part of it is metabolized to a precursor substance *(quinolinic acid)* from which niacin can be formed in the body. A number of steps are involved.

Soon after this discovery, it was shown that humans could substitute tryptophan for niacin at a ratio of about 60 parts of tryptophan to one part of niacin—about the same ratio as had been found in animals (43). If sufficient tryptophan is eaten (amounts generally higher than in average diets), niacin itself is no longer essential in the diet—all the niacin required would then be made within the body.

Niacin Equivalents. It should be evident from the foregoing discussion that the actual requirement for niacin varies with the nature of the diet—mainly whether the protein furnishes much or little tryptophan. To adjust for this, recommended allowances are now given in terms of *niacin equivalents* (NE)—dietary sources of niacin plus the amount that can be made in the body from food sources of its precursor, tryptophan. For practical purposes, then, one niacin equivalent is defined as 1 mg of niacin or 60 mg of tryptophan (or combinations thereof) (1,43).

A food that provides a large amount of tryptophan may be an excellent source of niacin equivalents even though its niacin content is not high. A quart of milk daily, for instance, suffices to prevent pellagra, although its content of niacin is relatively low. Its high content of tryptophan can be counted on to furnish additional niacin in the body, which must be added in calculating its "niacin equivalence," as shown in Figure 10–15.

Niacin equivalents of foods can be calculated from food composition tables that give both the niacin and the tryptophan content of foods. In the absence of information on the tryptophan content, one can estimate that the protein of meats contains 1.1 percent tryptophan, eggs 1.5 percent, milk products 1.3 percent, fruits and vegetables 1.0 percent, and corn (maize) products 0.6 percent of tryptophan (56).

Recommended Allowances of Niacin

Recommended allowances for niacin equivalents (NE) have been established by the United States Food and Nutrition Board. These replace the former allowances for niacin alone. A college-age woman has an allowance of *14 mg per day of niacin equivalents,* and a college-age man *19 mg per day* because

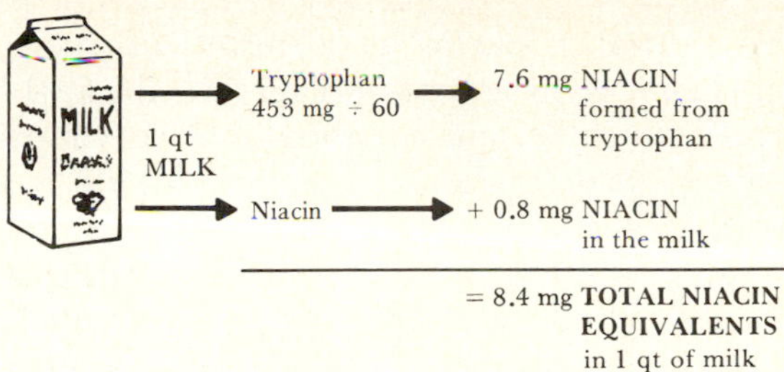

Figure 10–15 Calculating the niacin equivalents in a quart of milk. To the niacin that is carried as such in the milk (0.8 mg per quart) is added the amount that may be expected to be formed in the body from its tryptophan content (453 mg per quart). Assuming that approximately 1 mg of niacin is formed for each 60 mg of tryptophan, 453 ÷ 60 = 7.6 mg of niacin might be expected to arise from the tryptophan content of the milk, bringing the *total niacin equivalents* of a quart of milk up to 8.4 mg.

of average size differences. The allowances decrease somewhat with age because of decreased energy needs. See Table 10–7 for more details on allowances.

The amounts shown in Table 10–7 are approximately 20 to 40 percent greater than the minimum requirement, which is about 10 to 12 mg of niacin equivalents per day. They are based primarily on the energy requirement of an average individual, as are the requirements for thiamin and riboflavin, because of the essential role of these vitamins in energy formation from carbohydrates and fats. The Food and Nutrition Board has recommended a value of 6.6 mg of niacin equivalent per 1000 kcal (4200 kJ). Even if less than 2000 kcal is consumed per day, the board states that adults should not eat less than 13 mg per day.

Table 10–7 RECOMMENDED ALLOWANCES FOR NIACIN EQUIVALENTS(NE)*

	Age	*Allowance, mg NE/day*
Males	11–18 years	18
	19–22 years	19
	23–50 years	18
	51 years and over	16
Females	11–14 years	15
	15–22 years	14
	23 years and over	13
	Pregnant	+2
	Lactating	+5

*From the Food and Nutrition Board, 1980.

See Appendix Table 1 for recommendations of other countries and U.N. agencies. These are similar to the 1983 Canadian allowance of 6.6 NEs per 1000 kcal.

Intake of Populations

Most diets consumed in the United States supply from 500 to 1000 mg or more of tryptophan daily and 8 to 17 mg of niacin for a total of 16 to 31 mg of niacin equivalents per day, according to the Food and Nutrition Board (1). The *average* intake, therefore is higher than the recommended allowance, even though individual diets might be borderline in their content of niacin equivalents.

Clinical signs and biochemical and dietary evidence of low-niacin intakes are seldom reported in North America today. Low intakes might be expected to occur, however, in alcoholics, those taking drugs that increase the need for niacin, persons on high-corn diets (unenriched or not treated with lime), certain groups of the elderly, and persons with very poor eating habits.

Most of the dietary surveys being reported today only give intakes of niacin itself—figures that are quite meaningless without knowing tryptophan intakes and without clinical and biochemical measurements of status. Also to be considered in determining the extent of niacin deficiency are the recent studies that demonstrate that much of the niacin in many foods, especially grain products, appears to be only 20 to 40 percent available to the body (57). Niacin is bound in foods to various compounds, thought to be glycoproteins, primarily.

Pellagra itself is seldom seen in the United

States today partly as a result of food-enrichment programs. Pellagra is still fairly common in certain countries such as China where corn (maize) is a major part of the diet. In those parts of Latin America where large amounts of corn (maize) are a principal source of energy, however, pellagra is seldom seen. This is because it is common practice to soak the corn in lime, a practice that makes the niacin in corn more available to the body.

Corn (maize) and sorghum are rich in the amino acid *leucine.* It has been proposed that the high content is a major reason for the pellagragenic (pellagra-producing) action of these grains in India where much is consumed. This is an active research area, although it is evident the overall effect of leucine by itself cannot be as important as first reported (58).

Niacin Equivalents in Foods

Values for the content of niacin itself in foods have limited use unless the amount of tryptophan in the food is also considered. Most food composition tables, including Appendix Table 2 and the new USDA tables, give values for niacin only since good information on the tryptophan content of foods is not available. Niacin values for food are, of course, useful when NE values are not available. The NE values can be roughly calculated by the method previously mentioned (page 262).

Table 10–8 gives estimates of a few niacin equivalents for some representative raw foods, taking into account both niacin and tryptophan. In examining this table, one can see that it should not be difficult to secure the recommended amounts of niacin equivalents from normal diets such as are advised for meeting other nutritive requirements.

As for sources of the two vitamin forms (vitamers) themselves, in general animal products contain the vitamin as nicotinamide, while in plant products most of it is present as nicotinic acid. Both have about the same niacin activity for humans.

Both forms of niacin are among the most stable of all the B vitamins in processing and cooking. Niacin is lost, of course, in milling of foods, in blanching of vegetables in preparation for freezing, and in cooking in water if the water is discarded (59).

As with most other vitamins, the most inexpensive source of niacin is the synthetic form, many tons of which are used for food enrichment and for vitamin supplements each year. As previously pointed out, however, people should depend on traditional foods for their source of nutrients and not on pure compounds, at least for routine purposes. Nicotinic acid is available in wholesale quantities at a price of only about 1 cent per gm, sufficient to supply 25 percent of the daily allowance for one person for 100 days. Obviously, the cost of enrichment of foods with niacin, an important practice, is negligible. The once dreaded pellagra, as a worldwide disease wherever corn (maize) is a basic food, should be a disease of the past.

The Role of Niacin in the Body

The chief function of niacin in the body is to form the active portion of coenzymes that play an essential role in tissue oxidations (hydrogen transport), and it thus is necessary for the health of all tissue cells. Nicotinamide, in both free and combined form, is carried in the blood and found in all tissues, but most richly in liver, kidney, heart, brain, and muscles.

Niacin's metabolic role revolves around its presence in two important coenzymes essential to all life. These two coenzymes are *nicotinamide adenine dinucleotide* (NAD), which contains nicotinamide, two ribose groups, two phosphate groups, and adenine (a purine), and *nicotinamide adenine dinucleotide*

Table 10–8 NIACIN EQUIVALENTS OF SOME REPRESENTATIVE FOODS[a] (TOTAL NIACIN ACTIVITY PLUS MG TRYPTOPHAN ÷ 60)

Food	*Niacin Equivalent mg/100 gm*	*Food*	*Niacin Equivalent mg/100 gm*
Almond	6.4	Lamb	8.2
Apple	0.2	Milk, cow's, pasteurized	0.9
Asparagus	1.9	Milk, human	0.5
Banana	0.9	Parsley	2.4
Bean, lima	4.7	Pork	5.4
Beef	7.3	Rice, brown, dry	6.3
Beet root	0.7	Rice, milled, dry	4.9
Brussels sprouts	1.9	Sesame seed, dry	10.2
Carrot	0.7	Soybean, dry	11.1
Cashew nut	8.1	Spinach	1.2
Cauliflower	1.3	Sunflower seed	8.8
Chicken	10.9	Sweet potato	1.0
Chickpea	4.9	Wheat germ	8.6
Cornmeal, dry	2.9	Wheat, whole, dry	7.1
Egg, whole	3.2	Yeast, brewer's	45.0
Fish, trout	11.5		

[a]Calculated from niacin values in USDA Handbook 8 and from tryptophan values in FAO: *Amino-Acid Content of Foods and Biological Data on Proteins,* Rome, 1970, and Orr, M. L., and Watt, B. K.: *Amino-Acid Content of Foods,* Washington, D. C., U.S. Department of Agriculture, 1957. Based on fresh, raw, edible portion. Availability differences have not been considered.

phosphate (NADP), which is similar to NAD but contains an extra phosphate. (These two coenzymes are called NADH and NADPH when they are in the reduced form.) They play several different roles in cellular metabolism. Their most important function is to help bring about the action of enzymes known as dehydrogenases, which are essential in the course of oxidation-reduction reactions. For instance, the enzyme lactic dehydrogenase in tissues oxidizes lactic acid to pyruvic acid only in the presence of NAD. A second function of the niacin coenzymes, when in the reduced form, concerns the reduction of riboflavin-containing coenzymes and enzymes. In these reactions, hydrogen is passed along the reduced niacin coenzymes to a riboflavin-containing coenzyme and then to the cytochromes and eventually to oxygen, with the formation of water. Lack of niacin to form these coenzymes in sufficient quantities handicaps vital chemical processes and may result in injury to tissues throughout the body.

Toxicity and Use as a Drug

One could eat up to 30 times or so of the RDA of niacin without the appearance of toxic symptoms. Nicotinic acid, though not the amide form, acts as a drug when taken in large amounts—2 to 3 gm per day—resulting in vascular dilation or "flushing" of the skin or even a red rash. The compound is often prescribed by physicians for cardiovascular diseases and for treatment of other clinical symptoms, though its value for these purposes is in doubt. Especially dubious is the current use of high levels of niacin for the treatment of allergies, for increased athletic performance, and for schizophrenia and other mental diseases. These practices are widely promoted, mainly by those who are most apt to benefit financially by the practice. Niacin, along with other vitamins, is available in health food stores at most any concentration desired, which tends to support these seemingly useless practices. High doses of niacin or any vitamin should not be used without the advice of competent physicians (39).

This is not to say that niacin is not necessary for optimal performance and for the formation and maintenance of brain tissues—evidence shows that it is. These functions are fully satisfied, however, by amounts of niacin within the recommended allowances.

QUESTIONS

1. For thiamin, riboflavin, and niacin give the chief use, or uses, of each in the body, its RDA, and the symptoms resulting from deficiency.

2. What relationships, if any, do the diseases beriberi, cheilosis, and pellagra have to your usual diet? Explain.

3. Many persons consume pantothenic acid in vitamin supplements. Is this practice of any use? Are pantothenic acid deficiencies likely to be occurring? Explain and support your answer.

4. Is pellagra a clear-cut deficiency disease resulting from lack of niacin alone? If not, enumerate what other nutrition deficiencies are likely to occur as a result of a diet consisting mainly of corn meal and grits, white flour and rice, and fatty salt pork. What foods would you introduce to improve the diets?

5. Estimate the niacin equivalents in serving sizes of five different foods of different types not listed in Table 10–8. Use information given in the section describing niacin equivalents in this chapter and in Table 2 of the Appendix. Show your calculations.

Note: For additional questions on the B vitamins (covering both Chapters 10 and 11) see end of Chapter 11.

References

General

1. Food and Nutrition Board: *Recommended Dietary Allowances.* 9th Ed. Washington, D.C., National Research Council, National Academy of Sciences, 1980.
2. Nomenclature policy: Generic descriptors and trivial names for vitamins and related compounds, J. Nutr., *113*:7, 1983; I.U.N.S. Recommendations, Nutr. Abst. Rev., *48*:831, 1978.
3. U.S. Department of Agriculture: *Composition of Foods: Raw, Processed, Prepared.* Agriculture Handbook, No. 8, 1963 (partially republished—Sections 1–9, 1976 to 1983).
4. Pao, E. M., and Mickle, S. J.: Food Tech., *35* (Sept.):58, 1981.
5. U.S. Department of Agriculture: *Food and Nutrient Intakes of Individuals in One Day in the U.S., Spring 1977.* USDA Consumer Nutrition Center, Hyattsville, Maryland, Prelim. Rept. No. 2, 1980. (Also see other reports in this series.)

Thiamin

6. McCollum, E. V.: *A History of Nutrition.* Boston, Houghton Mifflin Co., 1957.
7. Guggenheim, K. Y.: *Nutrition and Nutritional Diseases, The Evolution of Concepts.* Lexington, Mass., D. C. Heath and Co., 1981.
8. Zuidema, P. J.: Trop. Geogr. Med., *32*:195, 1980.
9. Melnick, D., et al.: J. Nutr., *18*:593, 1939; Jolliffe, N., et al.: Amer. J. Med. Sci., *198*:198, 1939; Williams, R. D., et al.: Arch. Intern. Med., *69*:721, 1942; Williams, R. D., et al.: Arch. Intern. Med., *71*:38, 1943; Hulse, M. C., et al.: Ann. Intern. Med., *21*:440, 1944.
10. Bonjour, J. P.: Internat. J. Vit. Nutr. Res., *50*:321, 1980; Somogyi, J. C., et al.: J. Nutr. Sci. Vitaminol., *26*:221, 1980; Hoyumpa, A. M., Jr.: Amer. J. Clin. Nutr., *33*:2750, 1980; Shaw, S., Gorkin, B. D., and Lieber, C. S.: Amer. J. Clin. Nutr., *34*:856, 1981; Inokuchi, T., et al.: J. Nutr. Sci. Vitaminol., *27*:263, 1981; Nutr. Rev., *40*:50, 1982. (All on alcohol and thiamin.)
11. Rizek, R. L., and Jackson, E. M.: *Current Food Consumption Practices and Nutrient Sources in the American Diet.* Consumer Nutrition Center, Human Nutr. Sci. Educ. Admin., USDA, Hyattsville, Maryland, June, 1980.
12. Yearick, E. S., Wang, M. L., and Pisias, S. J.: J. Gerontology, *35*:663, 1980; Owen, G. M., et al.: Amer. J. Clin. Nutr., *34*:266, 1981. O'Hanlon, P., et al.: J. Amer. Dietet. Assoc., *82*:646, 1983. (Each on thiamin intakes. Also see ref. 26 in Chap. 8 and Supplementary Readings for Chap. 1, 8, and 10.)
13. Dong, M. H., et al.: J. Amer. Dietet. Assoc., *76*:156, 1980.
14. (On thiamin stability in foods) Luh, B. S., Karbass, M., and Schweigert, B. S.: J. Food Sci., *43*:431, 1978

(beans); Ang. C. Y. W., et al.: J. Food Sci., *43*:1024, 1978 (beef-soy patties, chicken); Keagy, P. M., Conner, M. A., and Schatzki, T. F.: Cereal Chem., *56*:567, 1979 (enriched cookies); Augustin, J., et al.: J. Food Sci., *44*:216, 1979 (potato products); *46*:1697, 1981 (home-prepared potato products); Hall, K. N., and Lin, C. S.: J. Food Sci., *46*:1292, 1981 (microwave, chicken); Kamman, J. F., Labuza, T. P., and Warthesen, J. J.: J. Food Sci., *46*:1457, 1981 (pasta); Lee, F. V., Khan, M. A., and Klein, B. P.: J. Food Sci., *46*:1560, 1981 (chicken); Dahl-Sawyer, C. A., Jen, J. J., and Huang, P. D.: J. Food Sci., *47*:1089, 1982 (microwave); Dexter, J. E., Matsuo, R. R., and Morgan, B. C.: Cereal Chem., *59*:328, 1982 (enriched spaghetti). (Also see Supplementary Readings, Chap. 8.)

15. Vimokesant, S., et al.: J. Nutr. Sci. Vitaminol., *22*(Suppl.):1, 1976; Rungruangsak, K., et al.: Amer. J. Clin. Nutr., *30*:1680 and 1686, 1977; Wills, R. B. H., and McBrein, K. J.: Food Chem., *6*:111, 1980–81; Ruenwongsa, P., and Pattanavibag, S.: Nutr. Rept. Internat., *27*:713, 1983.
16. Williams, R. R., and Cline, J. K.: J. Amer. Chem. Soc., *58*:1504, 1936.
17. Grijns, G.: Geneesk. Tijdschr. v. Ned. Ind. 1, 1901 (as seen in McCollum, ref. 4).
18. Jansen, B. C. P.: Nutr. Abstr. Rev., *26*:1, 1956.
19. Rindi, G.: Acta Vitaminol. Enzymol., *4*:59, 1982.

Riboflavin

20. Sebrell, W. H., and Butler, R. E.: U.S. Public Health Rept., *53*:2282, 1938; *54*:2121, 1939.
21. Skalka, H. W., and Prchal, J. T.: Cataracts and riboflavin deficiency. Amer. J. Clin. Nutr., *34*:861, 1981; Metab. Pediatr. Ophth., *5*:17, 1981.
22. For highly illustrative colored photographs of most nutritional deficiencies in man, including thiamin, riboflavin, and niacin deficiencies, see the recent book by D. S. McClaren: *Color Atlas of Nutritional Disorders.* Chicago, Year Book Medical Publishers, 1981.
23. Lane, M., et al.: J. Clin. Invest., *43*:357, 1964.
24. (Riboflavin needs in pregnancy and lactation) Bates, C. J., et al.: Amer. J. Clin. Nutr., *34*:928, 1981; and *35*:701, 1982; Int. J. Vit. Res., *52*:14, 1982; Riboflavin requirement of rural women and children. Nutr. Rev., *40*:300, 1982.
25. (Adolescents) Lopez, R., et al.: Amer. J. Clin. Nutr., *33*:1283, 1980 (in New York City—low socioeconomic status, of mixed ethnic groups).
26. (Children) Blumenthal, D. S., et al.: Nutr. Rept. Internat., *23*:327 and 377, 1981 (Blackfeet Indians, Montana); Owen, G. M., et al.: Amer. J. Clin. Nutr., *34*:266, 1981 (Apache Indians, New Mexico).
27. (Adults—mixed ethnic background) Koh, E., and Chi, M. S.: Amer. J. Clin. Nutr., *34*:1562, 1981 (men and women in Mississippi); Ziegler, R. G., et al.: J. Nat. Cancer Inst., *67*:1199, 1981 (black men in Washington, D.C.).
28. (Women) Clarke, H. C.: Int. J. Vit. Nutr. Res., *51*:293, 1981 (women during childbirth, Toronto); Foss, S. B., and Keith, R. E.: Nutr. Rept. Internat., *26*:613, 1982 (professional women in Alabama); Roe, D. A., et al.: J. Amer. Dietet. Assoc., *81*:682, 1982 (in family planning clinics); Belko, A. Z., et al.: Amer. J. Clin. Nutr., *37*:509, 1983 (effect of exercise).
29. (Aged) Chen, L. H., and Fan-Chiang, W. L.: Int. J. Vit. Res., *51*:232, 1981 (in central Kentucky); Harill, I., Kunz, M., and Kylen, A.: J. Nutr. Elderly, *1* (No. 3/4):3, 1981 (nursing-home women in Colorado); Garry, P. J., et al.: Amer. J. Clin. Nutr., *36*:902, 1982 (in New Mexico); O'Hanlon, P. et al.: J. Amer. Dietet. Assoc., *82*:642, 1983 (in Missouri).
30. (Riboflavin intakes close to or above RDA levels) Kerr, G. R., et al.: Amer. J. Clin. Nutr., *35*:294, 1982 (Hanes I data); Harrill, I., et al.: Nutr. Rept. Internat., *25*:189, 1982 (Western USA); Sempos, C. T., et al.: J. Amer. Dietet. Assoc., *81*:35, 1982 (Wisconsin nursing homes).
31. Garry, P. J., et al.: Amer. J. Clin. Nutr., *36*:902, 1982 (elderly in New Mexico, with and without supplements).
32. See all of citations given in ref. 27, Chap. 8.
33. Ensminger, A. H., et al.: *Foods and Nutrition Encyclopedia.* Clovis, Calif., Pergus Press, 1983.
34. Gordon, D. T., et al.: J. Agric. Food Chem., *27*:483, 1979 (thiamin, riboflavin, and niacin in Pacific seafoods).
35. (On stability in foods) Augustin, J., et al.: J. Food Sci., *47*:274, 1982 (potato products); Woodcock, E. A., et al.: J. Food Sci., *47*:545, 1982 (pasta). Also see the studies of Luh (1978), Ang (1978), Kamman (1981), and Dexter (1982) and their co-workers cited in ref. 14; also see Supplementary Readings, Chap. 8.
36. Williams, R. R., and Cheldelin, V. H.: Science, *96*:22, 1942; Peterson, W. J., et al.: J. Amer. Chem. Soc., *66*:662, 1944; Ziegler, J. A.: J. Amer. Chem. Soc., *66*:1039, 1944; Stamberg, O. E., and Theophilus, D. R.: J. Dairy Sci., *28*:269, 1944; Allen, C., and Parks, O. W.: J. Dairy Sci., *62*:1377, 1979 (fluorescent light effects).
37. Anon.: Riboflavin under the lights (editorial). Lancet *1*:1191, 1978; Gromisch, D. S., et al.: J. Pediatr., *90*:118, 1977.
38. Rivlin, R. S. (ed.): *Riboflavin.* New York, Plenum Press, 1975; Merrill, A. H., Jr., et al.: Formation and mode of action of flavoproteins. Ann. Rev. Nutr., *1*:281, 1981.
39. Rosenberg, I. H., et. al.: Report of FDA panel on Vitamin and Mineral Drug Products for Over-the-Counter Human Use. Federal Register, *44*(No. 53):16126, March 16, 1979.

Pantothenic Acid

40. Jukes, T. H.: J. Amer. Chem. Soc., *61*:975, 1939; Woolley, D. W., Waisman, H. A., and Elvehjem, C. A.: J. Amer. Chem. Soc., *61*:977, 1939.
41. Williams, R. J., and Major, R. T.: Science, *91*:246,

1940; Stiller, E. T., et al.: J. Amer. Chem. Soc., *62*:1785, 1940.

42. Bean, W. B., and Hodges, R. E.: Proc. Soc. Exp. Biol. Med., *86*:693, 1954; Hodges, R. E., et al.: J. Clin. Invest., *37*:1642, 1958; *38*:1421, 1959; Amer. J. Clin. Nutr., *11*:85, 1962; *11*:187, 1962.
43. Goodhart, R. S., and Shils, M. E. (eds.): *Modern Nutrition in Health and Disease.* 6th Ed. Philadelphia, Penn., Lea and Febiger, 1980 (see chapter by H. E. Sauberlich on pantothenic acid, p. 209; and M. K. Horwitt on niacin, p. 204).
44. Cohenour, S. H., and Calloway, D. C.: Amer. J. Clin. Nutr., *25*:512, 1972; Fry, P. C., Fox, H. M., and Tao, H. G.: J. Nutr. Sci. Vitaminol., *22*:339, 1976; Fox, H. M., and Linkswiler, H.: J. Nutr., *75*:451, 1961.
45. Chung, A. S. M., et al.: Amer. J. Clin. Nutr., *9*:573, 1961 (intakes given for pantothenic acid, vitamin B-6, folacin, and vitamin B-12); Hoppner, K., Lampi, B., and Smith, D. C.: Can. Inst. Food Sci. Tech. J., *11*:71, 1978 (pantothenic acid, vitamin B-12, and biotin).
46. Walsh, J. H., Wyse, B. W., and Hansen, R. G.: Ann. Nutr. Metab., *25*:178, 1981; also see Song, W. O., et al.: Fed. Proc.(abst.)., *42*:831, 1983 (in pregnant and lactating Utah women).
47. Hoppner, K., Lampi, B., and Smith, D. C.: Can. Inst. Food Sci. Tech. J., *11*:71, 1978.
48. Bull, N. L., and Buss, D. H.: Human Nutr.: Appl. Nutr., *36A*:190, 1982.
49. Tarr, J. B., Tamura, T., and Stokstad, E. L. R.: Amer. J. Clin. Nutr., *34*:1328, 1981.
50. Walsh, J. H., Wyse, B. W., and Hansen, R. G.: J. Amer. Dietet. Assoc., *78*:140, 1981 (content of 75 processed and cooked foods).

Niacin

51. Carpenter, K. J.: *Pellagra.* Benchmark papers in biochemistry, Vol. 2. Stroudsburg, Penn., Hutchinson Ross Publishing Co., 1981; Sebrell, W. H., Jr. (Chairman): Conquest of pellagra (a symposium). Fed. Proc., *40*:1519, 1981.
52. Goldberger, J., et al.: U.S. Pub. Health Rept., *30*:3117, 1915; *31*:3159 and 3336, 1916; *33*:2038, 1918; and four reports in *35*:1920. Goldberger was aided considerably by the early work of C. Voegdin (J. Amer. Med. Assoc., *63*:1094, 1914).
53. Elvehjem, C. A., et al.: J. Amer. Chem. Soc., *59*:1767, 1937; J. Biol. Chem., *123*:137, 1938.
54. Krehl, W. A., Sarma, P. S., Teply, L. S., and Elvehjem, C. A.: Science, *101*:489, 1945; J. Nutr., *31*:85, 1946.
55. Briggs, G. M., et al.: J. Biol. Chem., *161*:749, 1945; *165*:739, 1946; J. Nutr., *32*:659, 1946; *45*:345, 1951; Krehl, W. A., et al.: J. Biol. Chem., *162*:403, 1946; *166*:531, 1946.
56. Except for the factor for milk products, these estimates are proposed by M. K. Horwitt, A. E. Harper, and L. M. Henderson in their article, Niacin-tryptophan relationships for evaluating niacin equivalents (Amer. J. Clin. Nutr., *34*:423, 1981). (These authors rightly make a plea for the U.S. government to change the food labeling requirements so that niacin equivalents can be used instead of just the niacin value, which can be misleading. Under the present regulations, eggs and milk have to show less niacin activity than corn products.)
57. (On bioavailability.) Carter, E. G. A., and Carpenter, K. J.: Nutr. Res., *1*:571, 1981 (in sorghum); Amer. J. Clin. Nutr., *36*:855, 1982 (in wheat bran); J. Nutr., *112*:2091, 1982 (12 foods, using a rat assay).
58. Patterson, J. I., et al.: Amer. J. Clin. Nutr., *33*:2157, 1980 (human niacin studies with leucine and vitamin B-6) (see this paper for earlier references on this topic); Ohguri, S.: J. Nutr. Sci. Vitaminol., *26*:141, 1980.
59. (On losses in food) Lee, C. Y., Massey, L. M., Jr., and Van Buren, J. P.: J. Food Sci., *47*:961, 1982 (losses of vitamins in processing of peas). Also see studies of Luh (1978), Augustin (1981), and Dexter (1982) and their co-workers in ref. 14; and Augustin, et al. (1982) in Ref. 35.

11 Vitamin B Complex II: Vitamin B-6, Biotin, Folacin, Vitamin B-12, Vitamin-like Substances

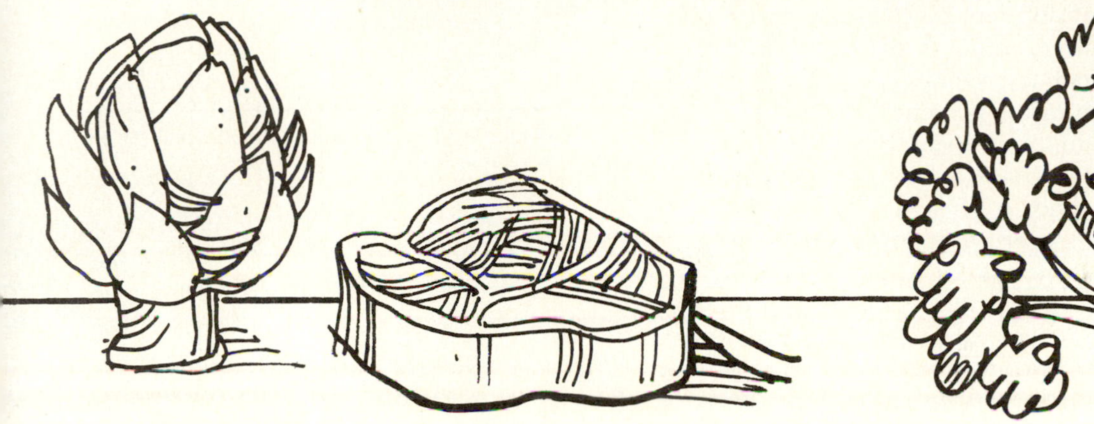

The vitamins discussed in Chapter 10 (thiamin, riboflavin, pantothenic acid, and niacin) were the first four of the B-complex to be discovered. Newer members of the B-complex vitamins, identified since 1938, are examined here. They are vitamin B-6, biotin, folacin, and vitamin B-12 plus various vitamin-like substances. Their chemical structures are given in the Appendix.

Since they are newer, they are receiving a large share of attention from nutritionists, biochemists, and clinicians. Also, these newer B vitamins tend to be more limited in usual American diets because they are not used as often in fortification programs as are most of the more established, older B vitamins. These newer B-complex vitamins are therefore especially popular among those who follow the controversial "health food" movement.

VITAMIN B-6

Vitamin B-6, first isolated in 1938 by S. Lepkovsky at the University of California, Berkeley, is the group name for three compounds: pyridoxine, pyridoxal, and pyridoxamine. These *vitamers*[1] are widely distributed in foods, usually as the phosphate esters, with about equal vitamin B-6 activity. They are white solids of rather simple chemical structure (see Appendix). Pyridoxine is the compound we hear about the most and is often called, by itself, vitamin B-6. This is an inaccurate use of the word since pyridoxine is just one of three compounds that all together are vitamin B-6.

[1]Defined in Chapter 10, page 258.

Deficiency Symptoms

Symptoms of severe vitamin B-6 deficiency in humans are similar in some respects to those seen in niacin and riboflavin deficiency (1,2,3). A common symptom is a greasy (seborrheic) *dermatitis* around the eyes, in the eyebrows, and at the angles of the mouth, along with soreness of the mouth and a smooth, red tongue. An early metabolic symptom of deficiency is the excretion in the urine of large amounts of *xanthurenic acid,* an abnormal tryptophan derivative, which turns green in the presence of iron salts.

Later symptoms include dizziness, other skin disorders, nausea, vomiting, weight loss, irritability and confusion, anemia, kidney stones, and severe nervous disturbances including convulsions. Deficient monkeys show also symptoms of atherosclerosis. Most of these symptoms, except kidney stones, can be corrected within several days, even within a few minutes for some symptoms, by administering vitamin B-6. Persons with intakes of vitamin B-6 just slightly below their individual requirements ("borderline" intake) may show none of these clinical symptoms but would show biochemical changes in their tissues, as will be discussed later.

Recommended Allowances for Vitamin B-6

One of the main functions of vitamin B-6 in the body is to assist in the metabolism of protein and amino acids. The more protein we eat the greater are our requirements for vitamin B-6. Americans normally consume about twice as much protein as they actually need. Therefore, U.S. recommended allowances for vitamin B-6 are somewhat higher than those of countries where protein intakes are normally lower.

The most recent recommended dietary allowances (RDA) of vitamin B-6, for persons over eleven years of age, are given in Table 11-1 (for values for infants and children see complete recommended dietary allowance [RDA] table inside the front cover). These allowances are based, primarily, on customary high U.S. protein intakes. They also reflect the range of requirements observed in various research studies and on the uncertainty of the availability of the vitamin in ordinary foods (1,3). Thus, if one is routinely consuming 50 grams (gm) of protein a day, for example, his or her vitamin B-6 allowance is likely to be considerably less than the value shown in Table 11–1. Persons eating very high quantities of protein will have larger requirements than shown in the table.

Table 11–1 RECOMMENDED ALLOWANCES FOR VITAMIN B-6[a]

	Age	*Allowance, mg/day*
Males	11–14 years	1.8
	15–18 years	2.0
	19 years and over	2.2
Females	11–14 years	1.8
	15 years and over	2.0
	Pregnant	+0.6
	Lactating	+0.5

[a]From the Food and Nutrition Board, 1980 (1). For additional values see inside front cover.

The new Canadian standards for vitamin B-6 are based directly upon a ratio of 15 micrograms (μg) of vitamin B-6 per gram of protein (equal to 1.5 milligrams [mg] per 100 gm). This is an easy way to express requirements, but there are other factors besides protein that affect the requirement of vitamin B-6.

Measuring Nutritional Status and Intake

There is no one approved method of measuring the degree of vitamin B-6 deficiency of an individual or a population. Studies of dietary intake and the occurrence of symptoms, alone, are not reliable. Current biochemical methods being studied include measurements of pyridoxal phosphate levels in blood and red blood cell transaminase (which contains vitamin B-6). Urinary levels of vitamin B-6 and of levels of metabolites of vitamin B-6 or tryptophan are also used in measuring vitamin B-6 status.

There is a great concern as well as ever-increasing evidence that, in rather large segments of the population of the United States, normal diets may be borderline or low in this vitamin (1,3,4). In fact, there is more evidence of low intakes of vitamin B-6 today than of any other vitamin. Overall, there is good information showing lower body stores and generally increased needs for this vitamin in persons with poor eating habits, in persons on low-calorie diets, in pregnancy and lactation, in the elderly, and in alcoholics. This situation also exists in various pathologic and genetic disturbances and in persons receiving high-protein diets or certain common drugs such as isoniazid, penicillamine, and oral contraceptives and other steroids. When there is an increased need, it must be met by a source of vitamin B-6 in some form—often more than the amounts readily available in usual diets—unless more foods are to be enriched with this vitamin or unless they are selected with considerable care.

Diets of foods commonly available in the United States can be devised with as little as 0.4 to 0.5 mg per day, well below the requirement. For instance, K. E. Cheslock and M. T. McCully (5) saw symptoms of vitamin B-6 deficiency in humans fed specially selected common cereal products, fruits, milk, vegetables, and other foods low in vitamin B-6 (many of which had been highly processed).

The actual intake of vitamin B-6 by adults in the United States varies considerably; it ranges somewhere between 0.5 mg to 1.5 mg in poor diets and up to 2 or 3 mg or more in many diets (3,4,6). Recent government surveys (three-day intakes) in the United States show that only 20 percent of the large population studied consumed more than the RDA values, and 51 percent of the population ate less than 70 percent of the RDA (7).

Many studies show large numbers of persons of all ages with low intakes of vitamin B-6 and with biochemical signs of deficiency, not only in the United States but in other countries as well (3,8).

Vitamin B-6 in Foods

Sources. The distribution of vitamin B-6 in foods follows the general pattern of that of most of the other B vitamins. Good sources are whole-grain cereals, potatoes and some other vegetables, turnip greens, salmon and most other fish, poultry, lean red meats, beans, and seeds, as well as most of the basic foods in lesser amounts. (See Table 11–2 and Table 2 of the Appendix for more details. Values are given in terms of total vitamin B-6 activity, combining the three naturally occurring forms of the vitamin.)

In the milling of white flour, more than 75 percent of the vitamin B-6 content of wheat is lost; it is not added in white-flour enrichment programs. There are many good arguments that this should be done since synthetic pyridoxine is quite inexpensive—about 20 cents per 1000 mg.

Pure sugar and fat, of course, are devoid of vitamin B-6, as they are of other vitamins. Processed or refined foods are generally much lower in vitamin B-6 than the natural food, often less than half. Flour, white bread, precooked rice, noodles, macaroni, and spaghetti are quite low in vitamin B-6. A diet composed solely of these foods low in vitamin B-6, or similar ones, would eventually cause a vitamin B-6 deficiency (along,

Table 11–2 EXAMPLES OF AMOUNTS OF VITAMIN B-6 IN VARIOUS FOOD SOURCES (BASED ON AVERAGE SERVING SIZES)[ab]

Excellent sources - 0.6 mg to 1.0 mg per serving (or more if totally enriched)
Bananas; Beef, dried and creamed; Breakfast cereals (if totally enriched); Chicken, fried or roasted; Enchiladas, beef; Fish (salmon, tuna, etc.); Liver (poultry, beef, calf); Turnip greens, boiled
Good sources - 0.3 mg to 0.59 mg per serving
Avocado; Beans, navy, canned (with pork and tomato sauce); Beef, roast, hamburger, rib, steak, stew; Breakfast cereals, 25% enriched; Fish, most varieties; Lamb, broiled; Pork, lean, broiled, roasted; Potatoes, baked, boiled; Sweet potatoes, boiled in skin; Tomato juice (¾ cup); Turkey
Fair sources - 0.15 mg to 0.29 mg per serving
Brussel sprouts; Hamburger, with a bun; Lamb, roasted; Melon, cantaloupe; Milk (2 cups); Peppers, green, raw; Potatoes, french fried; Prunes, cooked; Rice, brown; Sausage, pork; Spinach
Poor to fair sources - 0.06 mg to 0.14 mg per serving
Apples; Asparagus; Beans, lima; Beef, corned (canned); Broccoli; Cabbage; Cauliflower; Bread, whole wheat (2 slices); Breakfast cereals, granola, corn (maize) meal, wheat meal, cooked; Cottage cheese; Corn, sweet; Eggs (two); Egg plant; Frankfurter; Grapes; Milk (1 cup), all types; Mustard greens; Onions; Oranges; Peanuts, roasted; Peas, green, frozen; Pizza, cheese and sausage; Raisins; Strawberries; Tomatoes; Yogurt (1 cup)
Very poor sources - less than 0.06 mg per serving
Bacon; Beans, green; Beets, sliced; Bread (2 slices), cracked wheat, French, raisin, white (enriched); Breakfast cereals, corn flakes, puffed rice, wheat flakes, oatmeal; Cake, all types; Candy, all types; Carrots, raw; Celery; Cheese, cheddar, Swiss processed; Cookies, all types; Fats and oils, all types; Fruit, most all types (apples, apricots, cherries, grapefruit, peaches, pears, plums, etc.); Ice cream; Lettuce; Nuts (almonds, pecans); Peanut butter; Peas, canned; Pies, most types; Potato chips; Rice, white; Sausage and bologna; Spaghetti, Sugar

[a]The serving sizes are those used in Table 2 of the appendix on which this table is based. For details of vitamin B-6 levels in these foods see that table. For additional values see the footnotes to the appendix Table 2 and also see: Dong, M. H., et al.: J. Amer. Dietet. Assoc. *76*:156, 1980 (for foods as served in dining halls); Vanderslice, J. T., et al.: J. Food Sci., *46*: 943, 1981 (in breakfast cereals); Guilarte, T. R., et al.: J. Nutr., *111*:1869, 1981 (breakfast cereals); Augustin, J., et al.: Cereal Foods World, *27*:159, 1982 (cereals and baked goods); Bupurao, S., and Tulpule, P. G.: Indian J. Nutr. Dietet., *18*:3, 1981 (foods of India).

[b]Of major interest, this table demonstrates, well, the large number of common, well-liked foods that are very poor sources of vitamin B-6.

probably, with deficiencies of many other nutrients).

It should be obvious that vitamin B-6 is not one of the "lesser vitamins" in terms of its food distribution and its importance to good health. One must choose one's food with at least some degree of nutritional knowledge in order to have a sufficient amount. Well-planned food-enrichment programs with vitamin B-6 will, no doubt, also prove to be useful.

Effects of Processing. Considerable vitamin B-6 has already been processed out, or wasted, by the time consumers purchase foods in the market place. Still, the total amount available per person in "market basket" foods averages about 2.3 mg per day. It comes mainly from meat, poultry, and fish, which supply about 41 percent of our intake (see Fig. 11–1). About 52 percent comes about equally from potatoes, other vegetables, flour and cereals, fruits, and dairy products. The other 7 percent comes chiefly from legumes and eggs.

One often sees the above "2.3 mg a day" figure, for available vitamin B-6, quoted by various persons as evidence that we have sufficient vitamin B-6 available in our food supply. It should be kept in mind, however, that this is only an average figure and does not include further processing or cooking losses in the home or in restaurants or other places where food is consumed outside the home. This loss amounts to 15 to 30 percent average reduction of vitamin B-6 intake. Two of the natural forms of vitamin B-6 (pyridoxamine and pyridoxal) are especially sensitive to exposure to air, light, and heat. As a result the cooking or processing of foods,

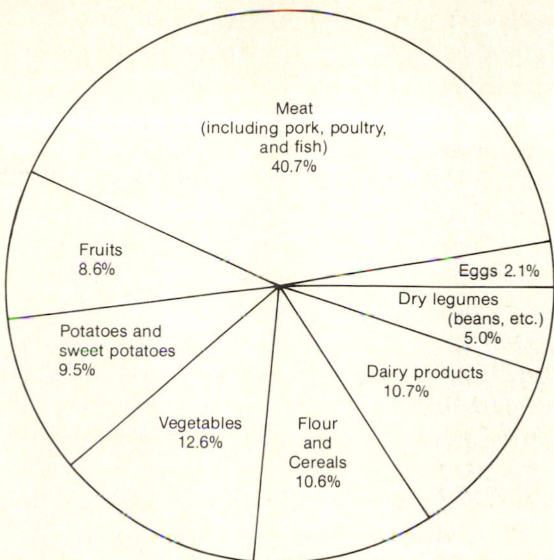

Figure 11–1 Contributions of major food groups to vitamin B-6 supplies. (United States figures for 1980.) This includes the amounts supplied by enriched cereals. It does not include 0.2 percent from miscellaneous sources. The total amount available is 2.3 mg per capita per day, before processing and cooking.

especially from animal sources, may destroy up to 50 percent of the vitamin B-6 activity. Considerable research is still being done on factors affecting vitamin B-6 retention in various foods (9).

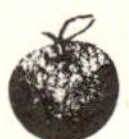

health considerations

Instability in Infant Formulas

People responsible for our food supplies, and people who cook at home and in institutions, should keep in mind the instability of vitamin B-6. The following account is a dramatic example of what happens when they forget.

In 1951, over 300 babies six weeks to six months old in various parts of the United States, fed solely on a well-known brand of a commercial infant food, began to develop irritability, muscular twitchings, and convulsions. Those babies who were fed the company's canned liquid product became seriously ill, while others fed a similar formula, of the same brand sold in dry, powdered form were not ill. Lee Kline, then of the United States Food and Drug Administration, recognizing the similarity of these convulsive seizures to those seen in young rats deprived of vitamin B-6, suggested the infants might be ill because of lack of this vitamin. When vitamin B-6 was given to them, they promptly recovered. The heat used to sterilize the liquid product in cans had been high enough to destroy (or make unavailable) most of the vitamin B-6, a fact no one had noticed or would have thought important if they had noticed. Today, because of the proved need for this vitamin in infants' diets, this company and other manufacturers of infant foods take special precautions to make sure that it is present.

The previous sentence also appeared in the last edition of this textbook in 1979. The authors' professed faith in manufacturers of infant foods was shaken in March, 1982, however, when the Food and Drug Administration announced the third urgent recall in a week's time of 3 million cans of a well-known brand of infant foods suspected of being very low in vitamin B-6. In the most serious cases reported of infants said to have consumed the products, investigators found permanent brain damage and symptoms like those of cerebral palsy.[2]

This example is a rather isolated instance, considering the vast sales of infant formulas in the United States, but it is nevertheless serious. The authors recall that several years before this incident, another company withdrew its infant formulas because a number of infants developed serious chloride defi-

[2]Reported in the CNI Weekly Report, March 18, 1982, of the Community Nutrition Institute, Washington, D.C.

ciencies (see Chap. 14). Chloride had been known for many decades to be required but apparently it was forgotten by those responsible both for the federal standards and for the contents of the company's formula.

The authors refrain from predicting the safety of infant formulas, at least until the government sets the final form of long-awaited guidelines. Interestingly, these guidelines were tentatively and hurriedly approved just a few days after the recall in March 1982. Those companies that pretest the safety of their formulas and new products with experimental animals are most likely to have the safest products.

The Metabolism of Vitamin B-6

Functions. Once absorbed, all three forms of vitamin B-6 are converted to *pyridoxal phosphate*—the coenzyme form—which has many important roles in metabolism, particularly in that of protein and amino acids. Interestingly, one of the many specific functions of pyridoxal phosphate is as a catalyst in the formation in the body of niacin from tryptophan. Animals deficient in vitamin B-6 are unable to do this, which may partially explain why symptoms of vitamin B-6 deficiency in humans are similar to those seen in pellagra.

Pyridoxal phosphate is essential for several highly important reactions in the body concerned with amino acid metabolism. The most important of these reactions involving pyridoxal phosphate (and, to some extent, pyridoxamine phosphate) are known as transamination and decarboxylation.

Transamination is the shifting of an amino group (-NH_2) from a donor amino acid to an acceptor acid to form another amino acid. By this type of reaction, the building of certain amino acids from nonnitrogen-carrying acids formed in metabolism is made possible. *Decarboxylation* is the removal of carbon dioxide (CO_2) from an amino acid.

Vitamin B-6 is necessary for the formation in the body of at least three vital physiological regulators (hormones or similar compounds) from the amino acids histidine, tryptophan, and tyrosine. It is also essential for the oxidation of amino acids for energy. Pyridoxal phosphate also catalyzes the removal of SH groups from sulfur-containing amino acids.

As many as fifty specific reactions of amino acids requiring pyridoxal phosphate as a coenzyme have been discovered. In addition to the functions listed above, vitamin B-6 (along with many other B vitamins) is essential in the body for the breakdown of glycogen to glucose for the production of energy.

Absorption. Free pyridoxine hydrochloride, the form of vitamin B-6 in vitamin supplements, is nearly 100 percent absorbed from the intestine. The forms of vitamin B-6 in foods, however, are bound to proteins, which need to be broken down in the intestine. This process is accomplished with varying degrees of efficiency so that amounts of vitamin B-6 activity in foods ranging from about 60 to 90 percent are absorbed and enter the blood stream. Dietary fiber appears to have little or no effect on such absorption, although the vitamin B-6 in whole-wheat bread is absorbed about 5 to 10 percent better than from white bread. The type of food consumed, the possible presence of binding agents, and a person's use of drugs and alcohol affect the absorption of vitamin B-6 (3,10). This is another good reason for people to make certain that they consume at least the RDA level on a regular basis.

Vitamin B-6 is necessary in the metabolism of polyunsaturated fatty acids and for conversion of linoleic acid to arachidonic acid. It is involved in red cell regeneration and normal functioning of nervous tissues. Vitamin B-6 is also known to perform many vital functions in the brain, where the concentration is much higher than in blood—up to 25 to 50 times higher (3,11). Mammals deficient in vitamin B-6 show impaired antibody responses, more so than with deficiencies of any other B vitamins (3,12). It has been proven that this remarkable vitamin plays a major role in the protection against many infections and diseases.

Toxicity, and Use as a Drug

Vitamin B-6 is not very toxic. Toxicity signs have been observed in humans, though rarely, with levels of 100 to 200 mg of vitamin B-6 per day (13). Most individuals appear to be able to tolerate still higher levels (2,3,13). It is metabolized rapidly, much of it being excreted as *pyridoxic acid,* a normal metabolic derivative of vitamin B-6.

Because of vitamin B-6's low toxicity and because of its well-known nutrient functions, it has been widely tested by physicians for possible use in treating certain clinical disorders (or it has been used as a placebo). Its pharmaceutical use has had various degrees of apparent success. A list of examples is given in the references (also see supplementary readings in the Appendix) (2,3,13,14). It would be unwise for anyone to use megadoses of vitamins such as vitamin B-6 for these or any other purposes without the close supervision of a reliable physician. Any kind of disease that might require unusually high levels of vitamin B-6 is likely to have more than one cause, and one should not try to diagnose such diseases for one's self.

BIOTIN

Biotin was first shown to be a vitamin in 1940 by Paul György, who named it vitamin H, a term no longer used. It was synthesized and its structure determined in 1942 (see Appendix for its formula). It is a white substance and contains sulfur in the molecule, as does thiamin. It is quite resistant to heat in cooking, processing, and storage.

Biotin is just as vital as any other vitamin to body tissues because they cannot synthesize it. Since the last edition of this text there have been a number of important developments in clinical areas concerning biotin. For practical purposes, however, there is still no need to be concerned about eating greater amounts of biotin than are found in normal diets. (A major reason for this is that intestinal microorganisms make large amounts.) Therefore, only the basic facts about this interesting B vitamin will be discussed.

Deficiency Symptoms of Biotin

Symptoms of biotin deficiency are seldom seen in humans, although they can exist. Such a deficiency in adults results in pathologic changes in the skin and tongue, loss of appetite, nausea and a low-grade anemia, lassitude, intense depression, sleeplessness, and muscle pain. Injections of biotin give marked improvement of symptoms in three to four days.

Recently, clear examples of biotin deficiency have been produced in children and adults receiving nutrients by intravenous feeding (parenteral nutrition), but without biotin, a vitamin for which physicians in the past have had little concern (15). The above symptoms were seen plus a severe rash, depression, lethargy, and loss of hair. The symptoms were arrested and eventually disappeared by administering biotin (15).[3]

Even more dramatic are the reports of the lifesaving use of biotin in infants with inherited absence of several enzymes essential for biotin absorption—all biotin-containing *carboxylases.* Injection of biotin brought about improvement, in just a matter of hours (16). Thereafter, large amounts of biotin given orally were effective. The biotin-deficient infants showed a variety of metabolic disorders, including acidosis, ketosis, and rash, all

[3]The treatment of hair loss with biotin prompted the appearance in the marketplace of biotin-containing lotions and tonics for "regenerating hair." These products are quite worthless since biotin deficiency does not exist in normal populations.

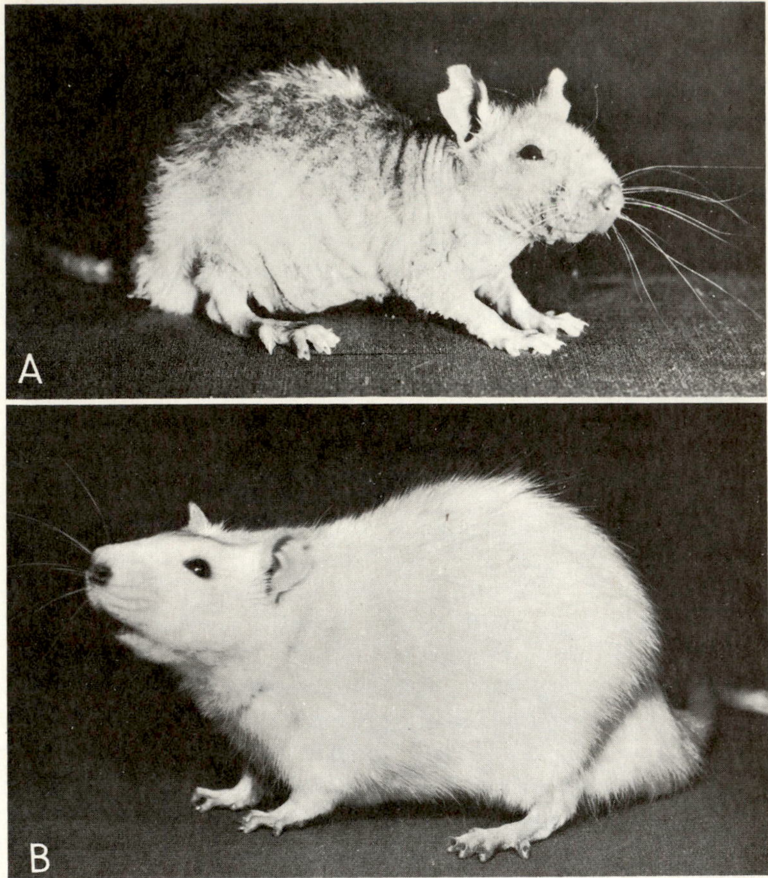

Figure 11–2 A, Rat after being fed a diet deficient in biotin, to which raw egg white was added. Growth has been retarded, and there is a generalized inflammation of the skin. B, The same rat after three months on a diet containing adequate amounts of biotin. Growth is normal, and the skin lesions are completely healed. (Courtesy of the Upjohn Company.)

indicating the importance of biotin to the body.

More recent studies have shown that giving pregnant women with a family history of this inherited condition high levels of biotin during the fifth month prevents all symptoms of biotin deficiency in their infants at birth (17). This finding represents another important clinical advance with the use of one of the B vitamins.

It has been known since the 1920s that the feeding of raw egg white to animals or to humans will produce a disorder later shown to be due to a biotin deficiency (see Fig. 11–2). In humans, this illness would affect only those persons who consumed large amounts of raw egg whites—eight to ten per day—without extra biotin sources. The occasional eating of a few raw eggs, as in eggnog, does not, however, produce a biotin deficiency.

Biotin deficiency from raw egg white is due to the presence in the white of a special protein called *avidin,* which combines with biotin in the intestinal tract, thus rendering the biotin unabsorbable. This so-called egg white injury can be overcome by ingesting sufficient biotin, though it takes more than that present in an equivalent number of egg yolks. Cooking egg white, even briefly, destroys the biotin-binding action of avidin, so normally there is no need to be concerned about this danger, although examples keep showing up in the medical literature.

Requirement for Biotin

For the first time, based on the recognition of a clinical role for biotin, the U.S. Food and Nutrition Board recently set a tentative "safe and adequate daily dietary intake" of biotin—100 to 200 μg per day for adults. (See inside back cover for levels suggested for lower age groups.) It is believed that conventional mixed American diets supply approximately this amount per day. There is some evidence, however, that the amount of biotin in normal diets might be lower than this figure—30 to 70 μg per day (18). If that is true, probably the provisional minimum "adequate" level set by the Board will be lowered in the future.

This discussion of requirements is a moot point, since the amount of biotin excreted in the urine and feces of normal adults is greater than the known intake. Synthesis of biotin from microorganisms in the intestinal tract accounts for this difference, though little is known about the availability to the tissues of biotin produced in the lower tract. Biotin deficiency in human populations is not likely to occur because of intestinal synthesis, a situation similar to that of vitamin K.

It is of interest that monogastric farm animals, such as poultry and swine, readily develop biotin deficiency if it is left out of their experimental diets. Intestinal synthesis is insufficient to take care of their needs. Considerable evidence exists that for breeding swine, natural-grain diets need supplementation with biotin. In other words, biotin should not be totally ignored, especially if animals or humans are given antibiotics or other antibacterial drugs for long periods.

Biotin in Foods

Biotin is widely distributed in those foods known to be good sources of other B vitamins. Liver, kidney, yeast, and egg yolks are especially good sources. Whole grains, breads, fish, peanut butter, nuts, beans, meat, and dairy products are also good sources. Vegetables, fruits, and potatoes are rather poor sources, as is white bread (19). Much needs to be learned yet about the availability of biotin from these food sources. What little evidence there is indicates that the biotin in some cereals, for example, may be very poorly absorbed, at least in experimental animals. The subject is still relatively new.

The Role of Biotin in the Body

Metabolic reactions requiring biotin are very important in the synthesis of fatty acids, in the production of energy from glucose, and in the formation of nucleic acid, glycogen, several amino acids, and protein.

Most biotin in the body is combined in various enzymes by means of chemical union with the amino acid lysine. When thus bound to an enzyme, biotin plays an important role in essential *carboxylation reactions,* in which carbon dioxide is transferred from the enzyme complex to other compounds. These reactions are reversible and are closely involved with those of pantothenic acid (coenzyme A). Biotin at high levels has not been found to be toxic (13).

FOLACIN

Folacin[4] (folic acid and related vitamers), the next to last of the B vitamins to be discovered, is essential for all vertebrates, including humans, for normal growth and reproduction, the prevention of blood disorders,

[4]According to international rules of nomenclature, the term folacin is used here as the generic description for folic acid and related compounds exhibiting the biological activity of folic acid. There is no single compound with the name folacin. The word folate is used often in biochemical literature for salts of folic acid but is not properly used in nutrition literature for lack of specificity.

important biochemical mechanisms within each cell, and the prevention of a variety of symptoms in different species.

The name folic acid, the forerunner of the term folacin, was suggested in 1941 by H. K. Mitchell, E. E. Snell, and R. J. Williams of the University of Texas for a highly purified growth factor for bacteria. It is derived from the latin *folium* ("foliage" or "leaf"), because it was first isolated from spinach leaves and was known to be widely distributed in green, leafy plants.

Identification and Properties

Folacin exists in several different forms in nature making up the folacin group of compounds. These different forms have similar activity when fed to higher animals. The first of the folacin group to be obtained in crystalline form was *folic acid,* known chemically as *pteroylmonoglutamic acid,* isolated from natural materials in 1943. It is a bright yellow powder quite soluble in slightly alkaline or acid solutions, readily destroyed by heat when in an acid solution, but reasonably stable when in neutral or alkaline solutions, especially in the absence of air. (The structural formula may be seen in the Appendix.) This parent compound is the most common form of the vitamin, used in laboratory diets, for enrichment purposes, and for vitamin tablets. It is usually called just folic acid.

Folic acid, which probably does not exist free in nature—is formed by the linkage of three compounds: *pteridine,* a yellow phosphorescent pigment related to the yellow pigment in butterfly wings (the Greek word for wing is pteron); *para-aminobenzoic acid* (a growth factor for bacteria); and the amino acid *glutamic* acid.

Para-aminobenzoic acid has considerable folacin activity when fed to deficient animals in which intestinal synthesis of folacin takes place; in fact, in the rat and mouse dietary para-aminobenzoic acid can completely replace the need for a dietary source of folacin in this manner. This explains why para-aminobenzoic acid was once considered to be a vitamin in its own right. Obviously, since it does exist in the free form in some foods, it can be considered a dietary precursor of folacin, but it is not a vitamin itself, though often listed as one.

In addition to the parent folic acid with only one glutamic acid group in the molecule, a number of *conjugated forms* of folacin exist in foods. Two common ones have either three or seven glutamic acid groups per molecule (20). These conjugated forms serve as the major precursors of the vitamin in the diet. The coenzyme form, *tetrahydrofolic acid,* the most common form in the body, is also widely distributed in foods. Another form of folacin which is active metabolically and which occurs in food is *10-formyltetrahydrofolic acid,* a reduced form of folic acid. Methyl derivatives of folic acid are also found in nature.

Various synthetic derivatives of folic acid, not present in foods, are antagonists of folic acid and are widely used in the treatment of leukemia and certain other types of cancer.

Deficiency Symptoms of Folacin

Folacin deficiency in humans results in a smooth, red tongue, gastrointestinal disturbances, and diarrhea; but the primary symptom is a blood disturbance called macrocytic anemia. In this anemia, the mature red blood cells are fewer in number, larger in size, and contain less hemoglobin than normal. The young red blood cells in the bone marrow (megaloblasts) fail to mature in a person deficient in folacin. Administration of folacin by mouth or injection results in prompt formation and development to maturity of a very large number of new red blood cells.

Certain anemias that develop during pregnancy, infancy, and childhood respond well to treatment with folacin, as do those seen in sprue or pellagra as a result of poor intestinal absorption. Anemias resulting primarily from dietary lack of iron and certain other causes are not relieved by it. In pernicious anemia (see vitamin B-12) there is some initial response to folacin with increased level of red cells, but it is not as marked as it is after the person has been given much smaller amounts of vitamin B-12. The nervous symptoms often seen in pernicious anemia cannot be cured by treatment with folacin.

Recommended Allowances

Folacin is now recognized as being one of the "problem nutrients" in the United States. A deficiency in humans is known to occur under "normal" conditions, especially during the later stages of pregnancy and lactation when the incidence of deficiency may be quite marked (1,21,22).

A total of 400 μg (0.4 mg) per day of folacin activity is recommended for adult men and women, as seen in Table 11–3. This figure takes into account possible losses from cooking, from poor absorption, and from the varying activity of the several forms of folacin in foods.

The recommended allowance provides an especially wide margin of safety since an intake of about 100 to 200 μg per day is sufficient to maintain body stores. Many persons in the United States and other countries obtain less than the RDA and, if the intakes are not too low, appear to be healthy (21,22,23,24). The Canadian recommended allowance provides a smaller safety margin.

Table 11–3 RECOMMENDED ALLOWANCES FOR FOLACIN AND VITAMIN B-12[a]

	Age	*Folacin Activity, μg/day*	*Vitamin B-12 Activity, μg/day*
Males	11 years and over	400	3
Females	11 years and over	400	3
	Pregnant	800	4
	Lactating	500	4

[a]From the Food and Nutrition Board, 1980 (1). Also see inside front cover for other age groups and Table 1 in Appendix for recommendations of FAO and certain other countries.

Intakes of Populations and Nutritional Status

Average American intakes are generally over the RDA for folacin, but certainly not always (21–24). Especially low intakes or low tissue levels are often seen in persons suffering from sprue, in infants of low birth weight or on unsupplemented milk diets, in persons who made very poor food choices (or on strict, low-caloric, reducing diets), in the aged (4,25), in alcoholics (26), and in pregnant women (2,22). There is no normal need for larger intakes of folacin than the RDA or than the levels in a well-balanced diet (although well-balanced diets are not always possible for a number of reasons).

Methods of measuring the degree of folacin deficiency in humans, and the various factors affecting it, have been reviewed in detail recently by V. Herbert and co-workers (21) and by M. S. Rodriguez (23).

Folacin in Foods

Sources. Information about the folacin activity of foods for humans is incomplete because of the difficulty of assaying the many different forms of folacin in terms of animal activity. The richest sources, however, are liver, yeast, and leafy vegetables, as seen in Table 11–4 and Table 2 of the Appendix. Good sources are dried legumes; green vegetables such as asparagus, lettuce, and broccoli; fresh oranges; and whole-wheat products.

Poor sources include most meats, eggs, root vegetables, most fruits, white flour and products made with highly milled cereals, most desserts, and processed milks—espe-

Table 11–4 EXAMPLES OF FOOD SOURCES OF FOLACIN*

Food Source *(in terms of 100 gm)*	Per Serving: Approximate Measure	Weight	Free Folacin	Total Folacin
		gm	μg	μg
Almonds	1 c	142	47	136
Bananas, raw	1 medium	119	26	33
Bread				
White	1 slice	25	3	10
Whole-wheat	1 slice	28	8	16
Cantaloupe	1 c	145	3	9
Cheddar cheese	1 c, shredded	113	1	20
Collard greens, raw	1 c	55	—	56
Cottage cheese	1 c, packed	245	—	29
Eggs, hard-cooked	1 medium	44	—	22
Garbanzo beans	1 c	200	64	398
Ground beef, cooked	3 oz	85	—	3
Lasagna	10 oz portion	280	—	62
Milk, cow, fluid, whole, pasteurized	1 c	244	12	12
Milk, human	1 fl. oz	31	1	2
Oatmeal, dry	1 c	80	13	42
Orange juice	1 c	248	84	136
Peanuts, roasted	1 c	144	35	153
Pinto beans, cooked	1 c	190	—	112
Pizza, cheese, frozen	1/8 pie	67	—	24
Pork, cooked, lean	3 oz	85	—	4
Potatoes, cooked				
French-fried	10 pieces	50	4	11
Mashed	1 c	210	10	21
Poultry				
Chicken and turkey, dark meat, cooked	3 oz	85	—	6
Rice, brown	1 c	185	22	30
Soybeans, dry	1 c	210	158	359
Spinach, cooked	1 c	180	108	164
Tuna, canned	3 oz	85	7	13
Wheat germ, toasted	1 oz	28	35	118
Yeast				
Baker's dry, active	1 pkg.	7	10	286
Brewer's, debittered	1 tbsp	8	14	313
Yogurt	1 c	245	—	27

*From Perloff, B. P., and Butrum, R. R.: J. Amer. Dietet. Assoc., *70*:161, 1977. These values are being used in the revision of Handbook 8 of U.S.D.A. Values are also given for "free folacin" in this reference, representing the amount that is available to the assay microorganism (*Lactobacillus casei* generally) before treatment of the food with conjugase enzymes. "Total folacin" shown here represents values more similar to conditions in the intestine of humans and are better values to use in calculating dietary intakes. Also see Butterfield, S., and Calloway, D. C.: J. Amer. Dietet. Assoc., *60*:310, 1972, new Handbook 8 values, and values listed in Appendix, Table 2.

cially dried milks. Sugar and table fats and oils supply no folacin. Diets made up entirely of natural foods low in folacin have produced folacin deficiencies in animals and humans.

Folacin compounds differ in their ability to cross intestinal barriers, depending on the degree of conjugation with glutamic acid or the nature of other types of binding—generally with protein. Hence, tables of folacin composition in foods, especially foods in the raw state, should be looked at with a degree of caution.

Effect of Heat and Processing. The folacin content of foods is partially destroyed by heating or processing at high temperatures. Normal cooking temperatures of 110° to 120° for ten minutes can cause losses up to 65 percent. Fresh leafy vegetables stored at room temperature for three days may lose up to 70 percent of their folacin activity. Generally, less folic acid is lost by microwave cooking than by conventional cooking methods.

As a general guide to ensure ample folacin in a daily diet, the best advice, as with all the nutrients, is to choose one's daily diet from the traditional foods in the four food groups, according to energy needs. Obviously the choice of at least one serving of green, leafy vegetables per day contributes significantly to meeting the daily requirement of folacin.

For recent references on folacin distribution in foods and its stability in cooking and processing, see supplementary readings in the Appendix.

The Role of Folacin in the Body

After absorption, whichever form of folacin is eaten is converted by the body to several active coenzyme forms, the parent form being tetrahydrofolic acid. These coenzyme forms are distributed throughout the body but are most abundant in the liver. Probably their primary function is to serve as carriers for single-carbon groups (specifically, the formyl and hydroxymethyl groups), which are essential for the building of purines and pyrimidines. These compounds are, in turn, needed for synthesis of nucleic acids, which are vital to all cell nuclei. This explains the important role of folacin in cell division and in animal reproduction.

Folacin coenzymes also are responsible for synthesis of certain amino acids, especially glycine and serine, used in the formation of body proteins. These reactions require ascorbic acid for maintaining folic acid in its reduced form, and they also require coenzymes of vitamins B-6 and B-12, again demonstrating the interdependence of various vitamins.

The folacin coenzymes are also necessary for the breakdown of many, if not all, amino acids. For instance, in folacin deficiency in humans and animals, the amino acid histidine is imperfectly utilized, resulting in increased amounts of an abnormal derivative in the urine.[5]

Coenzymes derived from folacin also serve as a source of carbon and hydrogen atoms in the synthesis of methyl groups and thus function with choline, betaine, and methionine in supplying *labile methyl groups* to the body (see also section on choline). In most animals, folacin cannot be depended on to supply the entire requirement of methyl groups.

There is good recent evidence that certain folacin-binding proteins exist in liver cells and elsewhere that also play a specific role in metabolism (27).

Toxicity and Use as a Drug

Folacin is quite free of toxic responses (13,21). Individuals have taken more than 15 mg a day over long periods without detrimental effects. Nevertheless, no one should try to diagnose his or her condition and take high levels of folacin or any other nutrient without close supervision by a physician. Even for a relatively nontoxic vitamin the danger is mainly that the person in seeking to cure one disease might easily miss the presence of a more serious one.

In some instances physicians use larger

[5]Formiminoglutamic acid (FIGLU). This is the basis for one of the laboratory tests for folacin deficiency.

than usual amounts of folacin when working with patients, such as those in mental depression, those already receiving drugs antagonistic to folacin (such as estrogens and oral contraceptives, anticonvulsant drugs, certain anticancer drugs, and sulfa drugs), and those with certain inborn errors of metabolism (21,28). It is known that immune functions are related to folacin intake (12).

There is no evidence that intakes of folacin suppress any cancers in humans (29). Various cancers in animals, however, especially experimental leukemias, are greatly affected by folacin levels of the diet. The several folacin antagonists are among the best of the antileukemia drugs available in humans. They are also widely used for certain other forms of cancer.

VITAMIN B-12

Vitamin B-12 was the last vitamin to be discovered (1948), thus completing the B-complex vitamin jigsaw. Distinguishing characteristics are its red color, the presence in its molecule of cobalt and phosphorus, and unlike any other vitamin, the inability of higher plants to synthesize it. Its most important deficiency state is *Addisonian pernicious anemia* (21).

Identification and Properties

Pernicious anemia has long been known and was given its name because it arose from some factor inherent in the body, did not respond to any known treatment, and eventually culminated in death. In 1849 T. Addison, an English physician, gave a detailed description of its symptoms. No treatment could be found, however, until, in 1926, G. R. Minot and W. P. Murphy of Boston announced that feeding large amounts of liver (¼ to ½ pound, or 113 to 227 gm per day) restored a normal level of red blood cells in cases of this disease (30). This indicated that the disease might well be related to nutritional factors. For this discovery they shared the Nobel Prize. Later, concentrates of liver were made available, obviating the necessity of eating large amounts of this food. Biochemists began a long series of attempts to isolate the active component present in liver concentrates, which was then called the *antipernicious anemia factor.*

In 1948 F. L. Rickes and coworkers, of Merck and Co., New Jersey, announced the isolation from a liver concentrate of a crystalline, red pigment, which they called vitamin B-12 (31). In the same month, E. L. Smith, of England, isolated two similar red, noncrystalline pigments from liver concentrate (31). In New York, R. West showed that injections of vitamin B-12 induced a dramatic beneficial response in patients with pernicious anemia (31). The vitamin was isolated by the Merck group with the use of a convenient test developed at the University of Maryland by M.S. Shorb and G. M. Briggs (32). This test, which used *Lactobacillus lactis* Dorner (a bacterium), saved much work when compared with the former tests, which had to be made with humans with pernicious anemia or with experimental animals.

Vitamin B-12 is the group name for several *corrinoids,* named because of their *porphyrin*-like structure.[6] They are nitrogenous basic substances with very large, complicated molecules. (See formula in Appendix.) Its cobalt constituent occupies the center of the molecule and may be attached to various chemical groups including a cyanide (CN) group—in which case the compound is called *cyanocobalamin.* This is rarely found in nature but is a stable form used commercially as a drug. If the cobalt is bound to a

[6]Porphyrin-like structures are found also in the "heme" part of the hemoglobin in blood and in chlorophyll in plants. They consist basically of four nitrogen-containing rings bound together with a mineral element in the center.

hydroxyl group (OH), it is called *hydroxocobalamin,* probably the most common form in the body.

One coenzyme form of vitamin B-12 contains an *adenosine*[7] molecule in place of the cyanide or hydroxyl group and is thought to be the most common form of vitamin B-12 in foods. *Methylcobalamin* is another form of the vitamin with a coenzyme role. All these forms of vitamin B-12 have about equal vitamin B-12 activity when in the diet.

The structure of cyanocobalamin was first determined in 1955 by Dorothy Hodgkins and co-workers (33). She later received the Nobel Prize.

Vitamin B-12 is the most complicated of all the vitamins. It has been synthesized—by Woodward's group at Harvard using a very complicated and expensive procedure. Fortunately, highly active vitamin B-12 concentrates can be produced inexpensively by the vitamin industry from cultures of certain bacteria and fungi grown in large tanks containing special media. These concentrates are universally used as the source of vitamin B-12 in vitamin supplements and in commercial rations for animals.

Neither humans nor animals can synthesize vitamin B-12 in their tissues, and, unlike any other vitamin, higher plants are unable to synthesize it. Thus, all the vitamin B-12 available to humans and animals comes originally from that produced by bacteria and fungi, either directly or indirectly. It is present in milk and red meats because of microbial synthesis in the rumen, which provides more than an ample amount. Considerable vitamin B-12 can be made in the intestines of humans as well. Rich soils and cloudy water from farm ponds are often good sources of vitamin B-12 for monogastric farm animals also because of microbial production. It is not readily destroyed by cooking.

[7]Adenosine is a nucleoside and consists of a purine (adenine) combined with a pentose sugar, ribose.

Vitamin B-12 Deficiency Symptoms

Humans. Vitamin B-12 deficiency in humans may occur in several ways: as a result of a simple dietary lack, possible only in vegetarians, or as a result of insufficient absorption from the intestine no matter how much is eaten. When the latter is due to lack of vitamin B-12-binding proteins in the intestine, the *intrinsic factor,* classic pernicious anemia results. Vitamin B-12 deficiency is occasionally seen also in persons with total or partial removal of the stomach by surgery, those infested with parasites such as the fish tapeworm (not uncommon in some countries), or persons with tropical anemias, sprue, and other conditions in which intestinal absorption is insufficient.

In an uncomplicated dietary deficiency of vitamin B-12, symptoms such as sore tongue, weakness, loss of weight, back pains, tingling of the extremities, apathy, and mental and other nervous abnormalities may develop. Anemia is rarely seen. On the other hand, in pernicious anemia, anemia and degeneration of the spinal cord are the major signs—though without treatment the other symptoms may appear and eventually will result in death.

Absorption of vitamin B-12 depends on the intrinsic factor, which has been identified as a mucoprotein that binds tightly to the vitamin and facilitates its absorption. In many cases of pernicious anemia its normal action is prevented by the presence of an antibody. In cases resulting from a metabolic defect, thought to be inherited, the body is unable to secrete the intrinsic factor and usually certain other gastric juices. This failure results in inability to absorb vitamin B-12 from the intestinal tract. Hence, there is a low level of vitamin B-12 in the blood and an inability of new red blood cells to develop normally, resulting in *megaloblastic anemia.* Various neurological symptoms may also precede or follow the anemia.

As little as 1.5 μg of vitamin B-12, injected intramuscularly each day[8] in a pernicious anemia patient, will result in restoration of a normal red cell count and gradual disappearance of all the other symptoms. Because the inherent defect of faulty absorption persists, pernicious anemia patients must continue to receive vitamin B-12 in some manner which by-passes the intestinal tract. The intrinsic factor, in purified form and bound to vitamin B-12, is now commonly used in the oral treatment of the disease. Because these treatments are successful, severe symptoms are seldom seen now in persons with pernicious anemia.

The oral administration of massive amounts of vitamin B-12 alone is not always successful, so is used very little in the treatment of pernicious anemia.

Animals. Cattle and sheep, grazing on plants grown on cobalt-poor soil develop symptoms of cobalt deficiency, which include loss of weight, weakness, and anemia. The injection of vitamin B-12, but not of cobalt, relieves all these symptoms, proving that the cobalt lack resulted in inability of the microorganisms in the rumen to synthesize the vitamin. Because cobalt is one of the constituents of the vitamin B-12 molecule, it is obvious that it is required by all animals that are chiefly dependent on microbial synthesis in the intestine for their supply of this vitamin.

Deficiencies in rats, fowl, young calves, monkeys, pigs, and many other species are readily obtained merely by leaving the vitamin out of the diet and at the same time preventing the animal from eating litter, soil, its feces, or extra sources of cobalt. Deficient animals show poor growth and reproductive disorders, and in severe cases they die. Pigs may show nervous irritability.

If true vegetarians lived in a cobalt-free environment, they would show more evidences of vitamin B-12 deficiency for the same reasons.

[8]Usually injections are spaced a month or so apart, so that much larger amounts are routinely given.

Recommended Allowances and Intake of Populations

Allowances. The recommended dietary allowance for vitamin B-12 in the United States is 3 μg per day for adolescents and adults of all ages, assuming that at least 50 percent is absorbed (1). This is an extremely small amount to keep a whole body in good health! No other nutrient is needed in such small levels. A whole year's requirement is only about 1 mg—an amount just barely visible.

Allowances for women during pregnancy and lactation are slightly higher, as shown in Table 11-2 and inside the front cover. Of course, persons with pernicious anemia, who do not absorb the vitamin, will respond to 3 μg of vitamin B-12 only if it is injected. As little as 0.1 μg per day can give a small response when injected in deficient persons, making vitamin B-12 one of the most potent compounds known. Our basic minimum requirement is about 1 μg, with no margin of safety.

The vitamin B-12 content of diets in those developing countries where foods of plant origin are more common may be low or borderline, and straightforward vitamin B-12 deficiencies are not unknown. For instance, vitamin B-12 deficiency in infants can occur frequently in certain areas of the world where intakes of animal products by mothers are low. In studies of pregnant mothers in southern India, S. J. Baker and coworkers reported that "babies born and suckled by vitamin B-12-deficient mothers may have lower body vitamin B-12 stores, may receive less vitamin B-12 in breast-milk feeds, and may be in danger of developing frank vitamin B-12 deficiency" (34).

Likewise, children who live exclusively on plant foods ("vegans") may show symptoms of vitamin B-12 deficiency after extended periods (see Health Considerations section on vegetarianism). Deficiency signs, or low serum vitamin B-12 levels, have also been seen in adults, especially child-bearing women, after eating vegetable and grain diets for several years—even in the absence of pernicious anemia (35).

All such examples are due to a straightforward deficiency. Normally, the total body stores of vitamin B-12 in wellfed adults are as much as 5 to 10 mg. These reserves are sufficient to last as long as two to three years, or much longer, even in the absence of a vitamin B-12 supply—but eventually a deficiency will occur if vitamin B-12 is not obtained.

Nutritional Status. On an average, most people in North America receive considerably more vitamin B-12 than their requirement because of the abundant supplies of inexpensive foods of animal origin that they eat by choice. A daily intake of one or two glasses of milk plus an egg or two and a serving of meat, fish, or poultry—easily obtainable in most diets—satisfies our basic needs for vitamin B-12.

The recent large government survey on nutrient intakes of the United States population indicated that considerable numbers of people eat relatively few animal products, either by choice, or because of higher costs (7). About 35 percent of the U.S. population ate less than the RDA levels of vitamin B-12; nearly half of those fell below 70 percent of the RDA. Since the minimal requirement is probably around 1 μg per day and intestinal microbes synthesize the vitamin, there is no cause for concern about these figures.

Most Seventh Day Adventists, who are lacto-ovo vegetarians, regularly drink several glasses of milk per day and consume eggs, which satisfies their vitamin B-12 needs. The controversial question of nutrition for those persons who prefer to eat no animal products at all is discussed in the section "Health Considerations."

Vitamin B-12 in Foods

There is no vitamin B-12 in plant products, such as grains, vegetables, and fruits, except trace amounts that might be absorbed from the soil while the plant is growing. Soil is one of the better sources of vitamin B-12 because of its high bacterial content. There is no vitamin B-12 present in normal yeast,[9] the traditional source of other B-complex vitamins. The richest sources are liver and organ meats. Muscle meats, fish, eggs, shellfish, milk, and most milk products, except butter, are good sources, while evaporated milk and yogurt are fair sources. (See Table 11–5 for examples of good sources and Table 2 of the Appendix for more values in foods.) The coenzyme form of the vitamin, which accounts for a major protion of vitamin B-12 in food, is not very resistant to the heat used in processing procedures or to light. Up to 10 percent is lost in milk during pasteurization, and 40 to 90 percent in evaporated milk.

Meat, including poultry and fish, contributes about 72 percent of the approximately 5 μg or so of vitamin B-12 consumed in the typical United States daily diet; eggs contribute 8 percent, and dairy products 18 percent. A small amount is provided in fortified cereals. Canadian intakes are higher, since Canadians consume a higher percentage of animal foods (18).

The most inexpensive sources of vitamin B-12 are microbial growth concentrates. One year's supply for one normal person costs about 3 cents! These concentrates have not been used much to enrich food, for there has as yet been no demonstrated means of suitably doing so in vegetarian societies.

[9]However, some special yeasts containing vitamin B-12 are available. They have been grown on media very rich in the vitamin, which is then absorbed in the yeast cell.

Table 11–5 EXAMPLES OF FOOD SOURCES OF VITAMIN B-12*

Food Source	*Vitamin B-12, μg/100 gm*
Beef	1.4
Cheese	
Cheddar	1.0
Cottage	1.0
Chicken meat	0.4
Clams, raw, meat only	98
Cod, dehydrated, slightly salted	10
Crab, cooked or canned	10
Eggs, whole	2.0
Herring, Atlantic	
Raw	10
Canned	8
Kidney, raw	
Beef	31
Calf	25
Lamb	63
Liver, raw	
Beef	80
Lamb	104
Mackerel, Atlantic raw	9
Milk,	
Human	0.02
Whole fresh	0.4
Yogurt	0.1
Oysters, Eastern, raw	18
Sardines, Atlantic, canned	10
Liverwurst	14

*Adapted from Orr, M. L.: USDA Home Econ. Res. Rept. *36,* 1969. Also see Appendix, Table 2.

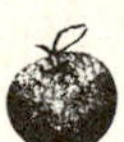

health considerations

Vegetarianism: Nutritional Aspects

There are many kinds of vegetarians, including those who eat no foods of animal origin (true vegetarians, or "vegans"), those who eat no animal flesh but consume milk and/or eggs (lacto-ovo vegetarians), and those who eat some marine foods and possibly poultry but no red meats. Then there are vegetarians who "hardly ever" eat meat. These last two kinds may have no difficulty obtaining enough vitamin B-12 and other borderline nutrients depending on how often they deviate from the vegetarian path.

Some of the special nutritional problems that vegetarians face are outlined in this section and in the supplementary reading in the Appendix. The student who is considering being a vegetarian should look at all the facts before making a choice. No specific attempt is made here to make that choice. It can be an important decision since it involves many other issues, and more nutrients, than vitamin B-12.

Vitamin B-12 need not be of as great concern for adult, nonpregnant vegetarians as it is for pregnant women, infants, and children. Traditional vegetarian cultures appear to adapt to low intakes of vitamin B-12, perhaps by consuming diets that favor intestinal microbial production. For example, in India, where there are many vegetarians, the normal average intakes of 0.5 to 1.0 μg of vitamin B-12, along with its intestinal synthesis, appear to cover dietary needs and to leave a small margin of safety (36). In rural areas of certain Third World countries unintentional microbial and soil contamination of water supplies is fairly common, which provides an appreciable though unsafe source of vitamin B-12. This may help to explain why vitamin B-12 deficiency is not more widespread among vegetarians in those countries. In developed countries more reliable vitamin B-12 sources are available for vegetarians (see preceding sections on intake and food).

Since true vegetarians obtain their needed nutrients entirely from cereals, fruits, legumes, nuts, and vegetables, they need to give special attention to obtaining adequate intakes of good-quality protein, calcium, zinc and iron (and certain other trace elements), riboflavin, vitamin D, vitamin B-6, and niacin-active substances. Plant foods are not consistently good sources of these nutrients. In the United States more than 50 percent of each of these important nutrients comes from red meat, poultry, dairy products, fish, and sea foods. Yet, only about 40 percent of the calories consumed come from animal foods. (This is not counting the nutrients added to fortified foods or from vitamin-mineral supplements.)

Plant foods, if carefully chosen, can provide adequate amounts of all the above nutrients, other than vitamin B-12. The point is, however, that it is not easy to obtain nutrients this way and that true vegetarians must take more than the usual care to insure such intake and also that of vitamin B-12.

Persons considering vegetarianism should also examine the various health indicators of true vegetarians in various countries of the developing world. They should consider, for comparison purposes, only those areas where ample foods of plant origin are readily available rather than areas where food in general is in short supply. What about mortality rates? Overall physical fitness? Are people in these areas healthier or less healthy than nonvegetarians? Why?[10]

Seventh Day Adventists in the United States have excellent health statistics, considerably better than those of the average American. Is it because they eat smaller amounts of flesh foods, or none at all, or is it primarily because of other factors such as their greatly reduced intake of alcohol, coffee, and tobacco smoke? What is the effect of their special physical fitness and antistress programs? These health records should be compared with the records of members of the Church of Jesus Christ of Latter-day Saints ("Mormons"), whose life-style is similar to that of the Adventists but who consume foods of animal origin in about the same amounts as do nonvegetarians. The health statistics of the Mormons are about equal to those of the Seventh Day Adventists and far better than those of the average American. Why? Why do the health records of "average Americans" vary from one end of the scale to the other, many being as healthy as members of the two religious groups mentioned.

More important, prospective vegetarians who plan to be parents should read about the severe nutritional problems of infants and children of strict vegetarians described in the selected references in this text (37).

[10]If there is difficulty in finding a country that consists almost entirely of pure vegetarians and where ample amounts of foods of plant origin are readily available to all, it is worth inquiring into the reasons for this also. Are people in such countries vegetarian by choice or by necessity?

The Role of Vitamin B-12 in the Body

Vitamin B-12 is absorbed only to the extent of 30 to 70 percent in normal persons, and none is absorbed in persons with pernicious anemia. Once in the body it is converted to one of the coenzyme forms, if it is not already in that form. The coenzymes circulate in the blood combined with one of several proteins, including *transcobalamin* and *cobalophilin* (R-proteins) (38). Vitamin B-12 is stored in the liver and kidney. It is essential for the normal functioning of all body cells, particularly those of the bone marrow, the nervous system, and the gastrointestinal tract.

A major role of vitamin B-12 in metabolism is in the formation of nucleic acids by aiding in the synthesis of various purine and pyrimidine intermediates, similar to the function of folacin. Coenzyme B-12 also participates, often with pantothenic acid, in the unique but essential *isomerism reactions,* in which several carbon units are rearranged within a molecule, such as in the formation of an amino acid, aspartic acid. Coenzyme B-12 also is involved, along with choline, folacin, and methionine, in the synthesis and transfer of labile methyl groups. Methyl groups have many functions in the body including the synthesis and metabolism of nerve and spinal cord tissue (see the section on choline).

Use as a Drug

Because it is not toxic (13,21), vitamin B-12 is used quite widely in treating various other diseases than pernicious anemia. These include certain neurological diseases, mental disorders, and certain inherited metabolic errors. Success is obtained only when the condition is due to vitamin B-12 deficiency (21,39). Otherwise, taking extra vitamin B-12 serves no function, with or without the supervision of a physician. One questionable aspect of this practice is that the vitamin B-12 in most vitamin supplements on the market contains about 10 to 30 percent of inactive vitamin B-12 analogues whose safety has been neither proved nor disproved (40).

Vitamin B-12 promises to be one of the most important vitamins for humans. Understanding its functions makes it possible to use vegetable, legume, and cereal foods much more wisely in the human diet in the event of future population pressures, famine, and shortage of foods of animal origin. Also, vitamin B-12 is one of the major reasons foods of animal origin remain relatively inexpensive in developed countries. Rations for these animals can now be made without expensive animal products, which were necessary in the feed before the advent of vitamin B-12.

VITAMIN-LIKE AND OTHER RELATED SUBSTANCES

The eight B vitamins needed by humans have been discussed in Chapters 10 and 11 (see Fig. 11-3). In addition, foods contain certain other substances that have many characteristics similar to those of vitamins (see Chap. 8). These are choline, inositol, carnitine, taurine, and still others. Considerable research has been done, lately, on these substances resulting, in the case of carnitine, for example, in the saving of lives of many children with genetically induced vitamin-like deficiencies. A much better understanding of their role is now possible through the use of parenteral nutrition and modern analytical methods.

The health-conscious student and other consumers are asking many questions about these vitamin-like substances since they are favorite topics of certain vitamin supplement suppliers and are often described in health-food literature.

What are the facts?

Choline

Choline is not accepted as a vitamin for humans, though it is a vitamin for many animal species (1,41). In the form of *acetylcholine* in the body of all species, animal and human, choline is vital for nerve functioning as a *neurotransmission* agent. It is also an essential component of several phospholipids vital in lipid metabolism—notably lecithin and sphingomyelin, which together make up 70 to 80 percent of the phospholipids in the animal body. The human body is able to synthesize what choline it needs except, possibly, in infancy.

Identification and Properties. Choline (from *chole* the Greek word for "bile") was isolated from bile in 1862 by a German chemist. Its vitamin nature, for animals, was not appreciated fully until the early 1940s when it was shown that it is essential for growth of rats.

Before that, in 1930, *lecithin,* a phospholipid that contains choline, was shown to prevent the accumulation of excessive fat in the liver (fatty livers) of dogs. By feeding dogs components of lecithin, C. H. Best[11] and his coworkers at the University of Toronto, be-

[11]Best was one of the discoverers of insulin.

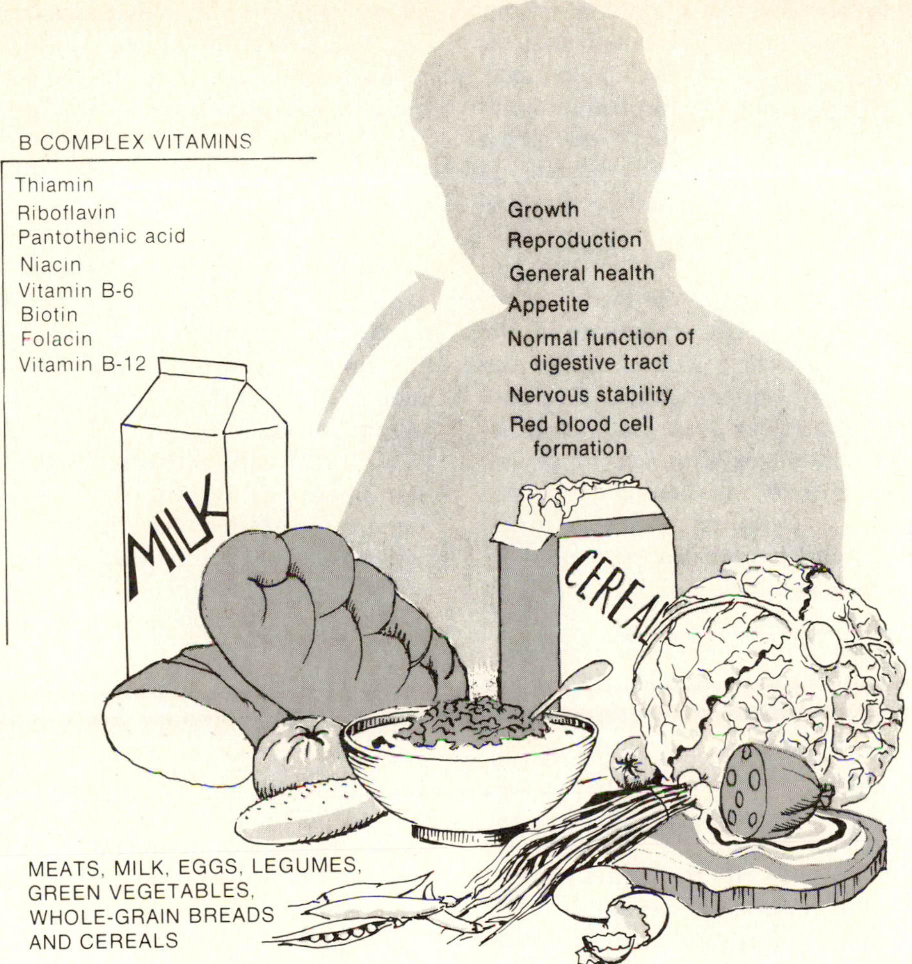

Figure 11–3

tween 1932 and 1935, showed that choline was the part of the lecithin[12] molecule that prevented the occurrence of fatty livers in rats fed diets low in protein and high in fat, cholesterol, or sucrose. *Betaine,* a closely related substance in certain foods, acted less efficiently than choline. Best's work was done before any other B-complex vitamin was available in pure form, and he considered choline as only an accessory food factor. By 1942, the vitamin nature of choline was fully confirmed by many other workers, who used experimental animals.

Choline, a relatively simple molecule, contains three methyl groups (—CH_3) and is strongly alkaline in its free form (see formula in Appendix). It is a water-soluble white syrup that takes up water rapidly on

[12]Lecithin is often added to dietary supplements sold in health-food stores and is said to aid in the utilization of cholesterol, among other claims. There is no evidence that lecithin is a dietary necessity. Of course, it does provide choline and, thus, can overcome a choline deficiency in animals.

exposure to air (hygroscopic) and readily forms more stable crystalline salts with acids such as choline chloride or choline bitartrate. In foods, it exists primarily in phospholipids or as the water-soluble sulfate or phosphate salts. It is heat-resistant and remains at nearly a constant level in dried foods when stored over long periods.

The Role of Choline in the Body. Choline has many important functions in the body. As a constituent of the phospholipids it is essential for cell membrane structure and for the transport and metabolism of fats; as a constituent of *acetylcholine* it plays a role in the normal functioning of nerves; and it serves as a source of labile methyl groups, which are essential in metabolism.

The methyl group ($—CH_3$) is found in many organic substances, but in most of them it is fixed and not detachable. When a methyl group is present in such a form that it can be transferred from one compound to another, it is called a labile methyl group and the process is called *transmethylation.* The body has a pool of labile methyl groups contributed from various sources, which it uses for such purposes as the formation of creatine (important in muscle metabolism) and for methylating certain substances for excretion in the urine. These methyl groups are also used in the synthesis of several hormones, such as adrenalin, and have other essential roles. Among the dietary sources of labile methyl are choline (or related substances), the amino acid methionine, and, in addition, folacin and vitamin B-12.

Deficiency Symptoms. Feeding insufficient choline to rats, mice, guinea pigs, rabbits, pigs, monkeys, calves, and dogs results in fatty livers in four to six weeks. In addition, depending on the type of diet and the length of time the deficient diet is fed to them, symptoms such as poor growth, edema, and an impaired cardiovascular system are seen, the last of which results in hemorrhagic lesions in the kidneys, heart muscles, and adrenal glands.

Requirement and Intake of Populations. The U. S. Food and Nutrition Board does not suggest a recommended allowance for choline because there is little or no evidence that it is required in the diet of humans. It is estimated that an average mixed diet for adults in the United States contains about 300 to 700 mg per day of choline and betaine, or about 0.06 to 0.14 percent of the diet. Human milk contains about 145 mg per liter, nearly 0.1 percent of total solids. These amounts, if needed, are adequate when compared with known requirements of laboratory animals. Additional intake of choline, as in special food supplements, is unnecessary and unwise.

Recently, fifteen patients receiving parenteral nutrition solutions low in choline and methionine developed very low levels of choline in the blood (42). Whether this condition reflects a true choline deficiency remains to be seen because of the lack of evidence for human need for choline (42). If it is needed, one would expect infants and young children especially to show a need, since, generally, it is the young of experimental animals fed deficient diets that are primarily affected. It would not be wise, based on our knowledge of choline, to give infants and children a choline-free diet for any extended time. In fact, a committee of the American Academy of Pediatrics has recommended that choline be added to infant formula diets in amounts similar to those in breast milk as a precaution until more is known about it. Parenteral nutrition solutions with no choline but *ample methionine* have been given to adults for long periods with apparent success.

Fatty infiltration of the liver is commonly

seen, especially in chronic alcoholics or in persons on very low-protein diets (for, example, in children with kwashiorkor). Choline and other lipotropic agents have been used by physicians in attempts to cure these disorders, but the results have been inconsistent and disappointing. Other clinical responses to dietary choline or lecithin, or both, indicate that these substances have potential use as pharmacological agents for certain mental and nerve disturbances in humans. There is considerable interest in the use of oral choline (generally fed as lecithin) as a therapeutic agent in protecting against loss of memory in conditions resembling senility (see supplementary readings in the Appendix). In general, success, if any, has been very limited.

Choline in Foods. Choline is present in all foods in which phospholipids occur liberally, as in egg yolk, whole grains, legumes, meats of all types, and wheat germ (19,43). Fresh egg yolk contains about 1.5 percent choline—probably the richest natural source—and beef liver contains about 0.6 percent. Legumes, such as soybeans, peas, and beans, contain from 0.2 to 0.35 percent; vegetables and milk have moderate choline activity. Most other foods, including fruits, have little or no choline activity.

Inositol

Another vitamin-like substance is inositol. It is required in the diet of certain species of fish and, under certain conditions, of the rat and the male gerbil (44).

Inositol[13] is often listed among the B-complex vitamins on labels of health products, in textbooks, catalogs, magazines, and diets. Inositol is the basic constituent of *phytic acid* in cereals, and, like choline, is an important component of certain phospholipids in the body. Most of the higher animals and humans, however, appear capable of synthesizing all the inositol needed (44,45). Nevertheless, it still remains at the least as an essential growth factor for certain yeasts (as one of the "bios" group), for many bacteria, and for several lower organisms up to and including several species of fish.

Recently, there has been renewed interest in inositol. More and more studies are indicating a dietary need for inositol in certain experimental situations in animals. Deficiencies can be readily produced in rats when the ratio of polyunsaturated fatty acids to saturated fatty acids is changed. (See supplementary readings in the Appendix for more information.)

Inositol is widely distributed in nature; there is roughly about the same amount as choline in a day's diet—225 to 1500 mg a day (46). In 1982 the U.S. Food and Drug Administration set a minimum level of 4.0 mg of inositol per 100 kcal for infant formulas. This is the level recommended by the American Academy of Pediatrics as a safe minimum until more information is obtained.

Inositol is closely related to simple sugars in structure, with the formula $C_6H_{12}O_6$. Since it contains no nitrogen, if it were ever found to be a vitamin it probably would not be a member of the B-complex.

Carnitine

Another vitamin-like substance receiving much attention recently is *carnitine.* It has been known for many years to be an essential growth factor for certain insects and was once called vitamin B_T.

Similar in some respects to choline and inositol, carnitine is a vital coenzyme in animal tissues and is involved in fat and muscle metabolism within the cells. It is similar to a

[13]Inositol is a group name for several closely related substances. The major one in foods, and the most biologically active, is *myoinositol.*

vitamin with the exception that in normal conditions higher animals synthesize their total needs within the body from lysine and methionine. Carnitine has three active methyl groups in the molecule and is very similar to choline in structure. However, it cannot replace choline in preventing a choline deficiency.

The current nutritional interest in carnitine stems from examples in the clinical literature of patients of all ages becoming at least partially "deficient" in carnitine. This condition has occurred, for example, after parenteral feeding in small infants of a carnitine-low formula (for newborn babies a dietary source appears to be essential), and in certain types of metabolic errors. A number of good reviews on carnitine and its physiological role are available for the reader who wants detailed information (47). (Also see supplementary readings in the Appendix.)

Normal persons synthesize all the carnitone they need so there is no reason to take supplements. Besides, large amounts are widely distributed in foods of animal origin.

Taurine

Taurine is a very simple organic compound containing sulfur. Tissues of cats and, it appears, of human infants cannot manufacture taurine in sufficient rate to take care of their needs. A dietary need for it in cats has been clearly established but not yet in human infants.

Taurine has the formula $NH_2CH_2CH_2SO_3H$. Obviously sulfur amino acids are involved in its biosynthesis under ordinary conditions.

Taurine is a precursor, with sterols, of the bile acid *taurocholic acid*. Its exact function is not known, and at this point there is no evidence that we need it. It is synthesized in ample amounts in adult tissues, it appears. Large amounts are widely distributed in animal tissues and thus taurine is readily available in foods of animal origin. Excellent recent reviews on taurine are available (48).

Growth Factors for Lower Organisms or for Cell Culture

A number of other compounds in foods, popular in the health-food industry, are essential for certain lower forms of life but not for higher animals (1). None of these are vitamins for humans, and we have no need to consume extra amounts of these under any condition.

Para-aminobenzoic Acid. One of these constitutents of foods is *para-aminobenzoic acid,* often incorrectly listed with the B vitamins. It is an important growth factor for lower animals, but in the diet of higher animals it serves only as a sparing factor for folacin. It has no vitamin activity in animals receiving ample folacin and can no longer be considered a vitamin, contrary to its listing in many vitamin preparations on the market.

Other Growth Factors. There are many other natural, organic growth factors, other than the vitamins, necessary for cell culture and for lower forms of life. They include lipoic acid (also called thioctic acid), nucleotides, nucleic acids, purines and pyrimidines, biopterin, peptides, sterols, hematin, coenzyme Q (ubiquinone), asparagine, certain proteins, nerve-growth factors, orotic acid, lecithin, natural chelating agents, pimelic acid, various polyamines, and pteridines. None of these are needed by humans, but they are all present in foods. None fit the definition of a vitamin (1,2).

Unidentified Growth Factors. There may well be other biologically active substances in foods essential for human health under conditions not recognized now. Some of the compounds listed above as growth factors may someday prove to be more important, just as choline, carnitine, inositol, and taurine, formerly on this list, proved to be vitamin-like substances.

Other compounds that promote growth in animals, or have some other beneficial effect, probably exist in natural foods or may be synthesized by intestinal bacteria. These compounds are being studied in various laboratories and are conveniently termed unidentified factors (49). Whether any of these "unidentified factors" for animals turn out to be B vitamins or whether they will be needed by humans remains to be seen. In any event, if such unidentified vitamins actually do exist, they are no cause for concern as long as one eats a variety of foods that supply ample amounts of all the B vitamins.

Nonnutrient Substances

It is of historical interest that over the years during which the B vitamins were developed, other numbers were temporarily used to name biologically active fractions of active materials in well-conducted laboratory tests. In this way the names vitamin B-4, B-7, B-8, B-10, B-11, B-13, and B-14 have all been used in the literature. Likewise, there has been use of the terms vitamin F, G, H, I, J, L, M, N, P, Q, R, S, T, U, and V in the nutrition literature. None of these are recognized today, for good reasons, by official nomenclature bodies.

Pangamic acid and *laetrile,* popular fads, are in no way to be considered vitamins. They are not nutrients in any sense, nor do they serve any known function (50).

QUESTIONS

(Note: These questions cover both chapters 10 and 11.)

1. Either make out a day's menus for what you would consider an attractive diet, or write down your actual food intake for an average day. Specify the amounts of each food consumed. Consult the tables in this chapter and in the Appendix for the amounts of riboflavin, vitamin B-6, folacin, and vitamin B-12 in foods. Add up the total quantities of each which would be provided in the day's diet that you have planned or consumed.

2. What is the recommended allowance for the above four B vitamins for a person of your sex, size, and degree of activity. If you are not receiving sufficient amounts, what foods fairly rich in these four vitamins might you add to your diet to increase your intake?

3. Give the chief nutritional functions for each of the following vitamins: folacin, vitamin B-12, vitamin B-6, and pantothenic acid. Can you give any examples of interrelations between different B-complex vitamins?

4. What types of foods, used freely in the diet, ensure a sufficient intake of the whole group of B vitamins?

5. Name three B-complex vitamins that are most likely to lose activity by commercial processing, and home preparation and cooking. What can be done to reduce these losses?

6. List eight B-complex vitamins needed by humans. Discuss why choline is not necessary for humans. Are there other B vitamins needed by humans than the eight listed here? Explain your answer.

References

Vitamin B-6

1. Food and Nutrition Board: *Recommended Dietary Allowances.* 9th Ed. Washington D.C., National Research Council, National Academy of Science, 1980.
2. Goodhart, R. S., and Shils, M. E. (eds.): *Modern Nutrition in Health and Disease.* 6th Ed. Philadelphia, Penn., Lea and Febiger, 1980, p. 216.
3. Munro, H. N. (Chairman): *Human Vitamin B-6 Requirements.* Committee on Dietary Allowances, Food and Nutrition Board, National Research Council, National Academy of Sciences, Washington, D.C., 1978.
4. See general surveys of vitamin intakes in the U.S. given in refs. 12–14, Chap. 1, and refs. 24–26, Chap. 8.
5. Cheslock, K. E., and McCully, M. T.: J. Nutr., *70*:507, 1960.
6. (On vitamin B–6 intakes) Singleton, N., Overstreet,

M. H., and Schilling, P. E.: J. Nutr. Elder., *1*:77, 1980 (in elderly); Windham, C. T., et al.: J. Amer. Dietet. Assoc., *78*:587, 1981 (nutrient consumption patterns, U.S.); Allington, J. K., Matthews, M. E., and Johnson, N. E.: J. Amer. Dietet. Assoc., *82*:377, 1983 (in 14 nursing homes).

7. Pao, E. M., and Mickle, S. J.: Food Tech., *35* (Sept.): 58, 1981.
8. (On vitamin B–6 status) Fries, M. E., Chrisley, B. M., and Driskell, J. A.: Amer. J. Clin. Nutr., *34*:2706, 1981 (Virginia preschoolers); McCoy, J. H.: Nutr. Rept. Internat., *23*:713, 1981 (immune relation, young girls in Kentucky); Shizukuishi, S., Nishii, S., and Folkers, K.: J. Nutr. Sci. Vitaminol., *27*:193, 1981 (University of Texas students); Chen, L. H., and Fan-Chiang, W. L.: Internat. J. Vit. Nutr. Res., *51*:232, 1981 (elderly in Kentucky); Bamji, M. S., and Premp, K.: Nutr. Rept. Internat., *24*:649, 1981; and *23*:785, 1981 (in India); Bapurao, S., and Tulpule, P. G.: Ind. J. Nutr. Dietet., *18*:7, 1981 (various regions in India); Russ, C. S., et al.: Nutr. Rept. Internat., *27*:867, 1983 (in depressed patients); Bailey, L. B., et al.: Fed. Proc. (abst.), *42*:831, 1983 (low-income adolescents in Florida).
9. (On vitamin B–6 stability in foods) Evans, S. R., Gregory, J. F., III, and Kirk, J. R.: J. Food Sci., *46*:555, 1981 (dehydrated food); Ang, C. Y. W.: J. Food Sci., *47*:336, 1982 (poultry meat); Soetrisno, U., Holmes, Z. A., and Miller, L. T.: J. Food Sci., *47*:530, 1982 (heated soybeans); Navankasattusas, S., and Lund, D. B.: J. Food Sci., *47*:1512, 1982 (thermal systems). (Also see ref. 3, this chapter, and Supplementary Readings, Chap. 8, 10, and 11, for additional references on this topic.)
10. (On bioavailability) Leklem, J. E., et al.: J. Nutr., *110*:1819, 1980; Gregory, J. F., III, and Kirk, J. R.: Nutr. Rev., *39*:1, 1981; Tarr, J. B., Tamura, T., and Stokstad, E. L. R.: Amer. J. Clin. Nutr., *34*:1328, 1981; Middleton, H. M., III: J. Nutr., *112*:269, 1982.
11. Dakshinamurti, K.: Neurobiology of pyridoxine. Adv. Nutr. Res., *4*:143, 1982.
12. Beisel, W. R.: Single nutrients and immunity. Amer. J. Clin. Nutr., *35* (Suppl. 2, Feb.):417, 1982.
13. Report of FDA Panel on Vitamin and Mineral Drug Products for Over-the-Counter Human Use, U.S. Federal Register, *44* (No. 53): 16126, March 16, 1979.
14. Harrison, A. R., et al.: Brit. Med. J., *282*:2097, 1981 (in bladder stones); Ellis, J., et al.: Res. Comm. Chem. Path. Pharm., *33*:331, 1981 (in carpal tunnel syndrome); Acta Vitaminol. Enzymol., *4*:27, 1982 (in autistic children); Mattes, J. A., and Martin, D.: Human Nutr.: Appl. Nutr., *36A*:131, 1982 (in premenstrual depression); Dorsey, J. L., et al.: Fed. Proc., *42*:556 (abst.), 1983 (no effect in premenstrual acne and tension); Schuster, K., et al.: Fed. Proc., *42*:553 (abst.), 1983 (lack of effect in morning sickness).

Biotin

15. (Parenteral nutrition deficiencies) Nutr. Rev.: *39*:274, 1981; Mock, D. M., et al.: New Eng. J. Med., *304*:820, 1981; McClain, C. J., Baker, H., and Onstad, G. R.: J. Amer. Med. Assoc., *247*:3116, 1982; Innis, S. M., and Allardyce, D. B.: Amer. J. Clin. Nutr., *37*:185, 1983; Levenson, J. L.: J. Parenter. Enter. Nutr., 7, 181, 1983.
16. (Inherited biotin-responsive disorders—some examples) Thoene, J., et al.: New Eng. J. Med., *304*:817, 1981; Packman, S., et al.: J. Pediatr., *99*:418 and 421, 1981; Roth, K. S., et al.: Clin. Chim. Acta, *109*:337, 1981; Narisawa, K., et al.: J. Inher. Metab. Dis., *5*:67, 1982; Wolf, B. et al.: New Eng. J. Med., *308*:161 (letter), 1983.
17. Packman, S., et al.: Lancet, *1*:1435, 1982; Roth, K. S., et al.: Pediatr. Res., *16*:126, 1982.
18. (On the biotin content of diets) Hoppner, K., et al.: Canad. Inst. Food Sci. Technol. J., *11*:71, 1978 (in a composite Canadian diet—60 μg/day); Bull, N. L., and Buss, D. H.: Human Nutr: Appl. Nutr., *36A*:190, 1982 (in a British food supply—33 μg/day).
19. Ensminger, A. H., et al.: *Foods and Nutrition Encyclopedia,* Clovis, Calif. Pergus Press, 1983 (this book has extensive food composition tables, including many biotin values); Wilson J., and Lorenz, K.: Food Chem., *4*:115, 1979 (with biotin and choline values, and many references to previous tables).

Note: for additional recent information about other aspects of biotin not covered here, see ref. 1; p. 274 of ref. 2 (J. M. Appel and G. M. Briggs); p. 16143 of ref. 13; and p. 210 of ref. 19; and supplementary readings in Appendix.

Folacin

20. (Reviews about pteroylglutamate metabolism) Covey, J. M.: Life Sci., *26*:665, 1980; Kisliuk, R.L.: Mol. Cell. Biochem., *39*:331, 1981; McGuire, J. J., and Bertino, J. R.: Mol. Cell. Biochem., *38*:19, 1981. Matthews, R. G. (chm.): Fed. Proc., *41*:2599, 1982.
21. Herbert, V., Colman, N., and Jacob, E.: Folic acid and vitamin B-12. In Goodhart and Shils (eds.): *Modern Nutrition in Health and Disease* (see ref. 2), p. 229 (a detailed review on function, nutrition status measurements, relationship to diseases, etc.). Also see Nutr. Rev., *40*:246, 1982 for a reprint of a classic folacin deficiency study which Dr. Herbert performed on himself.
22. Bailey, L. B., et al.: Amer. J. Clin. Nutr., *33*:1997, 1980 (low-income women, Florida); Letsky, E. A.: Human Nutr.: Appl. Nutr., *36A*:245, 1982 (a review); Nutr. Rev., *40*:235, 1982; Bates, C. J., et al.: Human Nutr.: Appl. Nutr., *36A*:422, 1982 (on normal folacin intakes and RDA levels).
23. (Examples of folacin status and intakes, general) Rodríguez M. S.: A conspectus of research on folacin requirements of man. J. Nutr., *108*:1983, 1978

(a review); Martinez, O. B.: Canad. J. Public Health, *73*:109, 1982 (school children in Canada); Areekul, S.: J. Med. Assoc. Thailand, *65*:1, 1982 (in Thailand); Johnson, A. A., Latham, M.C., and Roe, D. A.,: Amer. J. Public Health, *72*:285, 1982 (in English-speaking Caribbean); Milne, D. B., et al.: Amer. J. Clin. Nutr. (abst.), *37*:701, 1983.

24. (Examples of folacin states and intakes, U.S.A.) Butte, N. F., Calloway, D. H., and Van Duzen, J. L.: Amer. J. Clin. Nutr., *34*:2216, 1981 (Navajo pregnant and lactating women); Bailey, L. B., et al.: Amer. J. Clin. Nutr., *35*:1023, 1982 (black and Spanish-American adolescents in low-income urban areas, Florida); Bailey, L. B., et al.: Nutr. Res., *2*:397, 1982 (adolescents from rural areas, Florida).
25. (Examples of folacin status in the aged) Baker, H., et al.: J. Amer. Geriat. Soc., *26*:218, 1978 (in New Jersey); Bailey, L. B., et al.: Amer. J. Clin. Nutr., *32*:2346, 1979 (low-income black elderly in Florida); Rosenberg, I. H., et al.: Amer. J. Clin. Nutr. *36*:1060, 1982 (free-living elderly, a review).
26. (Folacin and alcohol) Halsted, C. H.: Amer. J. Clin. Nutr., *33*:2736, 1980 (a review); Hillman, R. S., and Steinberg, S. E.: The effects of alcohol on folate metabolism. Ann. Rev. Med., *33*:345, 1982.
27. Wagner, C.: Cellular folate binding proteins: function and significance. Ann. Rev. Nutr., *2*:229, 1982.
28. Folate-responsive homocystinurea and "schizophrenia." Nutr. Rev., *40*:242, 1982.
29. Committee on Diet, Nutrition, and Cancer report, National Academy of Sciences, Washington D.C., 1982.

Vitamin B-12

30. Minot, G. R., and Murphy, W. P.: J. Amer. Med. Assoc. *87*:470, 1926.
31. Rickes, E. L., et al.: Science, *107*:396, 1948; *108*:135, 1948; Smith, E. L.: Nature, *161*:638, 1948; *162*:144, 1948; West, R.: Science, *107*:398, 1948.
32. Shorb, M. S.: J. Biol. Chem., *169*:455, 1947; Science, *107*:397, 1948; Shorb, M. S., and Briggs, G. M.: J. Biol. Chem., *176*:1463, Shorb, M. S., and Briggs, G. M.: Univ. Maryland Agric. Exp. Station Bull. A-66, June, 1952.
33. Hodgkin, D. C., et al.: Nature, *176*:325, 1955; *179*:64, 1956.
34. Baker, S. J., et al.: Brit. Med. J., *5293*:1658, 1962.
35. Saraya, A. K., et al.: Amer. J. Clin. Nutr., *23*:1378; 1970; *24*:622, 1971; Dong, A., and Scott, S. C.: Ann. Nutr. Metab., *26*:209, 1982.
36. Baker, S. J., and Mathan, V. I.: Amer. J. Clin. Nutr., *34*:2423, 1981.
37. (On infants and children of strict vegetarians) Wighton, M. C., et al.: Med. J. Austral. *2*:1, 1979 (a case of brain damage); Dwyer, J. T., et al.: Amer. J. Dis. Children, *133*:134, 1979 (rickets); Dwyer, J. T., et al.: J. Amer. Dietet. Assoc., *77*:434, 1980 (depressed anthropometric measurements); Davis, J.R., Jr., Goldenring, J., and Lubin, B. H.: Amer. J. Dis. Children *135*:566, 1981 (vitamin B–12 deficiency); Lacroix, J., et al.: Arch. Fr. Pediatr., *38*:233, 1981 (breast-fed infant of a vegetarian mother); Dwyer, J. T., et al.: Amer. J. Clin. Nutr., *35*:204, 1982 (preschool children of "macrobiotic" parents); Dwyer, J.: Compreh. Ther., *9*:23 (April), 1983; Sanders, T. A. B., and Purves, R.: J. Human Nutr., *35*:349, 1981 (vegan preschool children); Shinwell, E. O., and Gorodischer, R.: Pediatrics, *70*:582, 1982 (multiple deficiency in infants in a vegan community in Israel); Curtis, J. A., et al.: Canad. Med. Assoc. J., *128*:150, 1983 (rickets). (Most of these studies were made in the United States. These are selected papers; similar studies could probably be found pertaining to nonvegetarian families, but the incidence of deficiency among vegetarians is higher.)
38. Jacob, E., Baker, S. J., and Herbert, V.: Vitamin B–12 binding proteins. Physiol. Rev., *60*:918, 1980; Seetharam, B., and Alpers, D. H.: Absorption and transport of cobalamin (vitamin B–12). Ann. Rev. Nutr., *2*:343, 1982.
39. Roach, E. S., and McLean, W. T.: Neurological disorders of vitamin B–12 deficiency. Amer. Family Physician, *25*:111, 1982; Evans, D. L., et al.: Amer. J. Psych., *140*:218, 1983.
40. Herbert, V., et al., New Eng. J. Med., *307*:255, 1982.

Vitamin-like Substances (Choline, Inositol, Carnitine, Taurine)

41. Appel, J., and Briggs, G. M.: Choline (a review). In Goodhart and Shils (eds.): *Modern Nutrition in Health and Disease* (see ref. 2), p. 282; Zeizel, S. H.: Dietary choline: biochemistry, physiology, and pharmacology. Ann. Rev. Nutr., *1*:95, 1981; Ensminger, A. H ., et al.: *Foods and Nutrition Encyclopedia* (see ref. 19), p. 413.
42. Burt, M. E., Hanin, I., and Brennan, M. F.: Lancet, *2*:638, 1980 (choline "deficiency" in parenteral nutrition).
43. Ensminger, M. E., and Olentine, C. G., Jr.: *Feeds and Nutrition—Complete*. Clovis, Calif., Ensminger Publishing Co., 1978 (extensive tables of choline content of feeds and many foods).
44. (Inositol reviews) Appel, J., and Briggs, G. M.: Inositol (a review). In Goodhart and Shils (eds.): *Modern Nutrition in Health and Disease* (see ref. 2), p. 286; Holub, B. J.: The nutritional significance, metabolism, and function of myo-inositol and phosphatidylinositol in health and disease. Adv. Nutr. Res., *4*:107, 1982.
45. Clements, R. S., Jr., and Diethelm, A. G.: J. Lab. Clin. Med., *93*:210, 1979 (reports that the kidney may synthesize up to 4 gm. of inositol a day).
46. Clements, R. S., Jr., and Darnell, B.: Amer. J. Clin. Nutr., *33*:1954, 1980 (provides an extensive table on the inositol content of foods).
47. (Reviews on carnitine) Frenkel, R. A., and McGarry, J. D. (eds.): *Carnitine Biosynthesis, Metabolism, and Functions*. New York, Academic Press, 1980; Tao, R. C., and Yoyshimura, N. N.: J. Parenter. Ent.

Nutr., *4*:469, 1980; Bray, D. L., and Briggs, G. M., in Goodhart and Shils (eds.): *Modern Nutrition in Health and Disease* (see ref. 2), p. 291; Nutr. Rev., *38*:25, 310, 338, 1980; and *39*:24, 385, 400, 406, 1981; Broquist, H. P., and Borum, P. R.: Carnitine biosynthesis, nutritional consequences. Adv. Nutr. Res. *4*:181, 1982; Lancet, *2*:1027, 1982; Broquist, H. P. (Chairman): Carnitine biosynthesis and function. Fed. Proc., *41*:2840–2862 (5 papers), 1982; Borum, P.: Carnitine. Ann. Rev. Nutr., *3*, in press, 1983.

48. (Taurine reviews) Huxtable, R. J.: Fed. Proc., *39*:2678, 1980; Huxtable, R. J., and Pasantes-Morales, H.: Taurine in nutrition and neurology. Adv. Expt. Med. Biol. *139*:567, 1981; Hayes, K. C.: Taurine in metabolism. Ann. Rev. Nutr., *1*:401, 1981.

49. Lofgren, P. A., et al.: Proc. Soc. Exp. Biol. Med., *147*:331, 1974; Blair, R., Scott, M. L., and Young, R. J.: J. Nutr., *102*:1529, 1972; Smith, J. L., et al.: New Eng. J. Med., *306*:1013, 1982 (also see editorial by W. G. M. Hardison on unidentified essentials, Gastroenterology, *83*(Oct.):935, 1982).

50. Herbert, V.: *Nutrition Cultism, Facts and Fictions.* Philadelphia, Penn., George F. Stickley Co., 1980 (on laetrile and pangamic acid); Herbert, V., Legal aspects of specious dietary claims. Bull N.Y. Acad. Med., *58*:242, 1982 (reprinted in J. Canad. Dietet. Assoc. *44*:12, 1983).

Note: For additional resources on the B–complex vitamins, see supplementary readings in the Appendix for Chap. 1, 8, 10, and 11. Also see journals and review series listed at the end of Chap. 1 for current information being published on these topics.

12 Vitamin C: Ascorbic Acid and Dehydroascorbic Acid

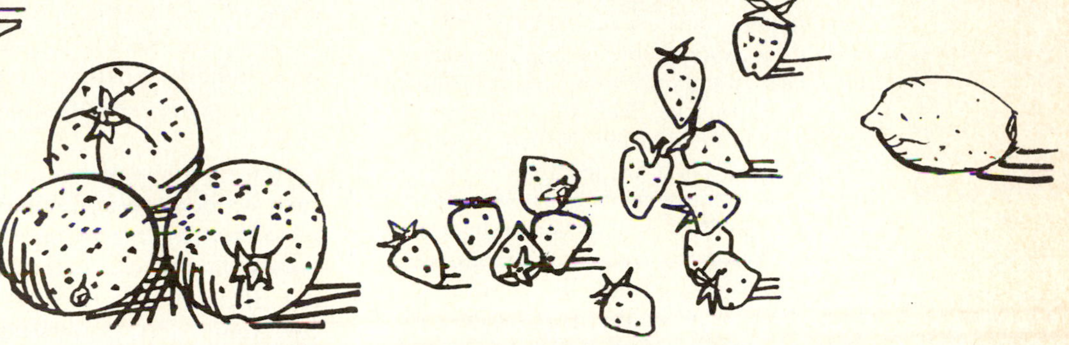

One of the most important of the vitamins is vitamin C, which prevents scurvy. *Scurvy,* a disease that affects connective tissue, has been recognized for more than thirty-five centuries. In the eighteenth century probably more sailors died of it than were killed in battle or lost at sea. Scurvy results from a deficiency of vitamin C and can therefore be prevented or treated with either *ascorbic acid* or *dehydroascorbic acid.* Both these closely related compounds are present in food and have similar vitamin C activity. Thus, the term vitamin C is not synonymous with ascorbic acid, as is commonly thought, but is a group name for the two compounds.

In scurvy, connective tissues cannot be properly built or maintained. This results in the breaking open of small blood vessels; in reddening and bleeding of sensitive tissues (especially evident in the skin all over the body and in the gums of the mouth); loose teeth; general weakness; and death. Except in extreme cases these conditions can be reversed when adequate vitamin C is given—with no permanent damage resulting.

When the vitamins were identified in the first half of the twentieth century, vitamin C was arbitrarily given third place in the vitamin alphabet. The reason is that Elmer V. McCollum used rats instead of guinea pigs in his classic studies on "fat-soluble A" and "water-soluble B." Rats do not get scurvy in the dietary absence of vitamin C because they make their own vitamin C; guinea pigs do get scurvy because they, like humans, cannot make their own.

DESCRIPTION OF VITAMIN C

Vitamin C is set apart from the other vitamins by a number of distinguishing characteristics.

1. The vitamin C-active compounds are relatively simple organic acids with a structure similar to the 6 carbon sugars (see formula in the Appendix). They are composed only of carbon, hydrogen, and oxygen and, unlike the B-complex vitamins, have no nitrogen.
2. Only a few animal species require vitamin C. They lack an enzyme (to be described) that, if present, allows the liver, or kidney in some species, to make ascorbic acid from glucose. It has therefore been argued that vitamin C is not a vitamin but a hormone, which a few species are genetically unable to manufacture. In humans, however, vitamin C fulfills all the requirements of a vitamin.
3. Vitamin C is one of the most unstable of all vitamins, readily destroyed in processing, cooking, drying, or overheating.
4. There are only a few good dietary sources of vitamin C,—certain fruits and green vegetables. Grains, nuts, beans, and most foods of animal origin, except for liver and fresh milk, are devoid of vitamin C.
5. Humans need more vitamin C than any other vitamin. The requirement is about 20,000 times the requirement for vitamin B-12, for example. This difference has little or no nutritional significance and the recommended intake, 60 milligrams (mg) a day is still a very small amount, relative to the total amount of foods we eat.

Deficiency Symptoms

Lack of vitamin C can result in acute or latent scurvy.

Acute Scurvy. The effects of an acute lack of vitamin C have been thoroughly studied by R. E. Hodges, E. M. Baker, H. Sauberlich, and others (1). Five male prisoners volunteered to be placed on a vitamin C–deficient diet for eighty-four to ninety-seven days. The first symptoms of deficiency seen were fatigue, rough skin (hyperkeratosis), pink or hemorrhagic skin follicles (see Fig. 12–1), hemorrhages in the eye, coiled hairs, and gum changes. They were followed by pains in the joints, changes in the salivary and tear glands, loss of dental fillings, dental caries, tender mouth, dryness and itching of skin, and excessive loss of hair. The skin changes were noted as early as twenty-nine days, several weeks before the occurrence of swollen and bleeding gums, contrary to common beliefs. Giving vitamin C overcame all the symptoms eventually (after three to ten weeks).

Acute scurvy presents such a dramatic picture of degeneration in many body tissues (skin, teeth and gums, blood vessel walls, bones, cartilage and muscle tissues) that it is not difficult to recognize. Because these severe symptoms are prevented by taking even moderate amounts of fresh or cooked fruits and vegetables, full-blown scurvy is very seldom encountered.

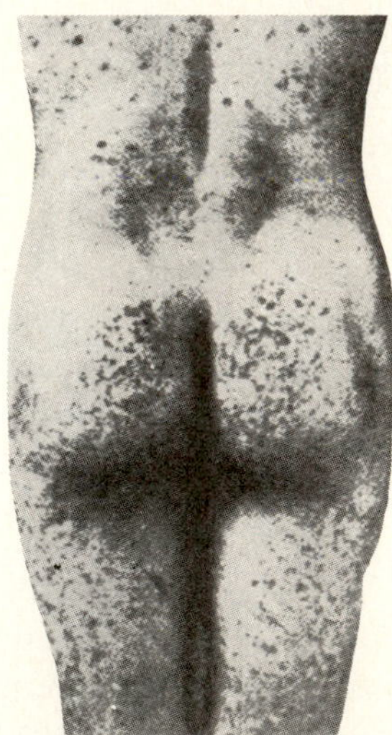

Figure 12–1 A typical case of adult scurvy, showing the numerous petechiae—spots where blood has effused to the skin. (From L. J. Harris: *Vitamins in Theory and Practice.* New York, Macmillan Co., 1955.)

Latent Scurvy. A condition with less severe symptoms, known as subacute or latent scurvy, still occurs (though infrequently) among infants fed almost exclusively on heat-treated milk or gruels, when sources of vitamin C are not used or are unobtainable. A deficiency shows up in persons whose intake is just below the borderline of sufficiency, when there is greater need of the vitamin (as in growth), or when there are conditions of physiological stress or infection (2,3).

In young children, symptoms of latent scurvy are failure to grow properly, weakness, restlessness, irritability, swollen joints, and tenderness of the lower extremities (Fig. 12–2). Signs of vitamin C deficiency in older children and adults are usually listlessness, lack of endurance, fleeting pains in the legs and joints (often mistaken for rheumatism), small hemorrhages under the skin, and gums that bleed easily.

Scurvy in Certain Animals. Humans, monkeys, guinea pigs, certain fish and marine animals, and certain species of bats, birds, and fowl (for example, the ptarmigan) are the only common species of higher animals dependent on the vitamin C contained in their food for the prevention of scurvy.

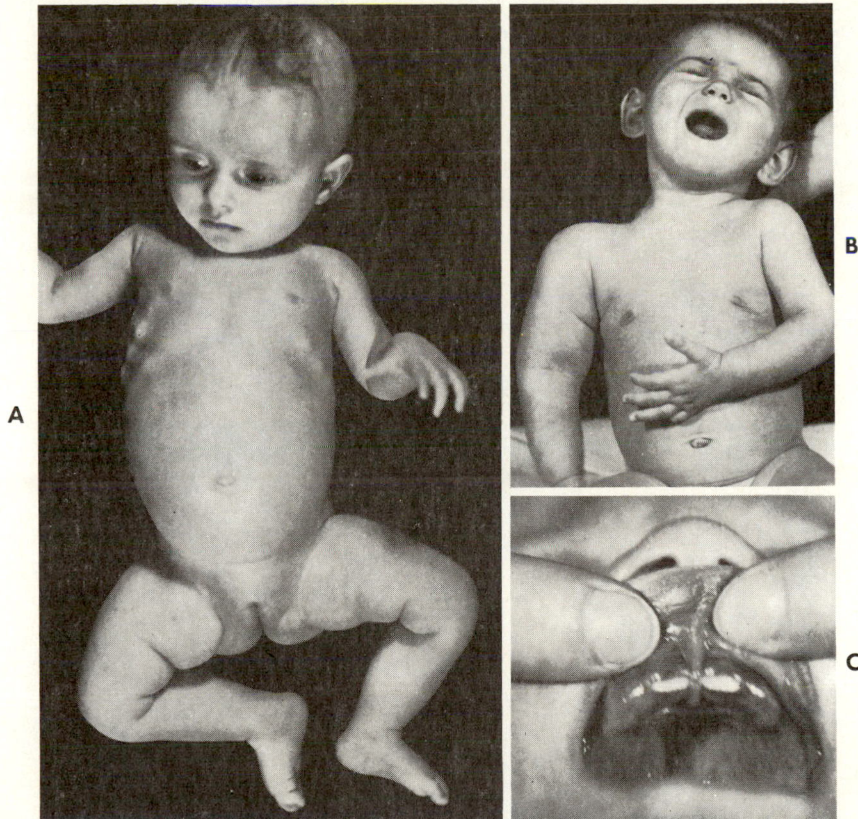

Figure 12–2 Infant scurvy. A, Characteristic postion, with legs flexed at hips and knees, and thighs externally rotated. B, The infant becomes irritable when handled. C, Gums are swollen and boggy. (From Cecil-Conn: *The Specialities in General Practice.* 2nd ed. Philadelphia, W.B. Saunders Co.)

All other common higher animals (including dogs, cats, rabbits, rats, poultry and most birds, cows, and horses) can synthesize the vitamin C they need in their bodies from glucose and galactose. This *biosynthesis* requires a specific enzyme, *L-gulonolactone oxidase,* which is not present in the species that develop scurvy (4).

Scorbutic symptoms in guinea pigs, for classroom demonstration purposes, can be readily obtained merely by feeding a commercial rabbit feed (containing no added vitamin C) to young guinea pigs. The symptoms are readily cured by giving sources of vitamin C (Fig. 12–3), with no permanent harm to the animal.

Biosynthesis in Certain Species. The activity of the enzyme necessary for vitamin C biosynthesis from glucose is known to be affected by a variety of factors including genetic, seasonal, and sexual differences, and differences among species (5). M. Cummings considers vitamin C deficiency to be an "inborn error of metabolism" and speculates that there may be humans who by fortunate genetics synthesize sufficient vitamin C in their bodies (6). This remains to be seen. In a recent experiment the missing enzyme necessary for biosynthesis of vitamin C was ingeniously implanted or injected into guinea pigs given a vitamin C-deficient diet (7). A "pronounced" increase in vitamin C in the plasma was obtained and deficiency symptoms were reversed.

From these demonstrations, one might speculate that in the distant future people may not need a dietary source of this vitamin. Until then, however, we definitely need a dietary source. Natural foods containing vitamin C are inexpensive, easy to obtain, tasty, and a good source of other nutrients.

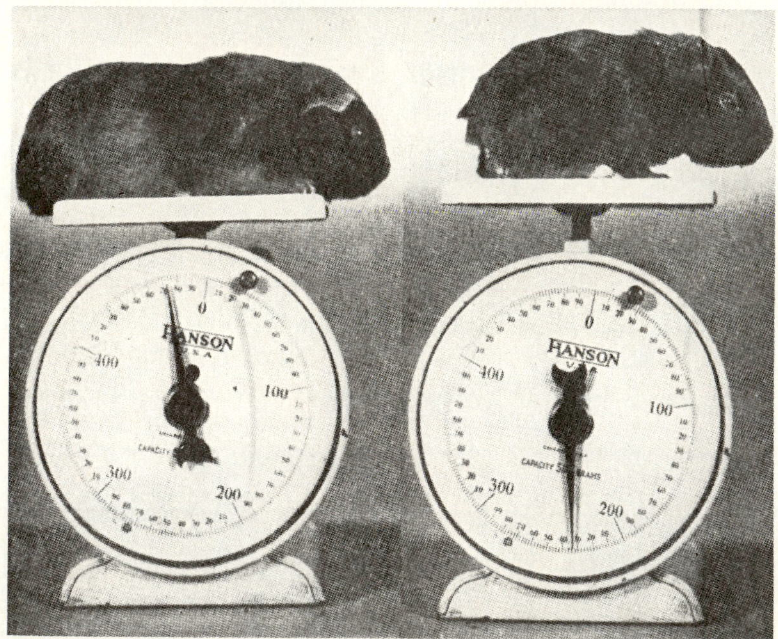

Figure 12–3 Stunting of growth due to lack of vitamin C. The guinea pig at the right, which had a vitamin C-deficient diet, was in poor condition and weighed only 234 gm. The guinea pig at the left, on the same diet plus tomato juice, weighed 473 gm. (Courtesy of Dr. F. F. Tisdall, Toronto.)

Recommended Allowances

The absolute minimum requirement of vitamin C per day to prevent scurvy appears to be only about 10 mg. This amount, however, provides no reserve for building and maintaining tissue. The Food and Nutrition Board of the United States set in 1980 a recommended daily allowance at 60 mg per day for adult males and females (8). This figure is higher than the previous recommendation; it was changed in order to provide a generous increment for individual variability, adequate stores in tissue, and a surplus to compensate for potential losses in food. The Food and Nutrition Board recognizes that the allowances are still not necessarily adequate to meet the additional requirement of persons depleted by disease, traumatic stress, or prior dietary inadequacies. For values showing the current dietary recommendations for pregnancy and lactation and for other details, see Table 12–1 and table inside front cover.

Table 12–1 RECOMMENDED DIETARY ALLOWANCES FOR VITAMIN C*

	Age	*Allowance, mg/day*
Males	infants	35
	1–10 years	45
	11–14 years	50
	15 years and over	60
Females	infants	35
	1–10 years	45
	11–14 years	50
	15 years and over	60
	pregnant	+20
	lactating	+40

*From Food and Nutrition Board, 1980 (8).

The amount of vitamin C recommended daily varies from country to country because different criteria are used and because further research is still needed. This is a controversial area in which many views are presented in the scientific literature (8,9) and by interested, but not always bias-free, writers. Under normal conditions, 60 mg a day appears to the authors to be more than adequate for satisfying the requirement and maintaining ample stores in the body.

Adequacy of Intake

Unless a survey of vitamin C is recent, it should be regarded with some degree of caution because of changing food habits and new practices of fortifying foods. In surveys made in the United States and Canada, clinical signs of scurvy are rarely seen (10). In fact, since knowledge of the protective action of citrus fruits and other fresh fruits and vegetables has become widespread, actual epidemics of scurvy, as were seen centuries ago, have completely disappeared. Since rice is very low in vitamin C, persons eating extremely simple diets based on rice (such as the "macrobiotic" diet) have been known to develop severe scurvy. Such instances are very rare in the Americas.

In spite of the almost total absence of clinical symptoms, there is much evidence, made by biochemical measurements and by reliable surveys, that many persons in the United States do not receive sufficient vitamin C by recommended dietary allowance (RDA) standards. For example, the study of E. M. Pao and S. J. Mickle of the U.S. Department of Agriculture (USDA) shows that 26 percent of 37,785 individuals in the country reported intakes of less than 70 percent of the RDA for vitamin C (11). Only 59 percent had intakes of 100 percent of the RDA or over. G. M. Owen and co-workers studied the nutrition of Apache Indian preschool children in New Mexico and found that almost 40 percent of those between two and five years old had daily vitamin C intakes of 30 mg or less (well below the recommended allowances) (12). Other recent surveys show low intakes of vitamin C in a significant proportion of women during reproductive years, at least by RDA standards (13).

Still other recent studies show that elderly persons may have low intakes of vitamin C (14). Also it is known that the utilization of vitamin C in those who drink alcoholic beverages in excess may be impaired (15).

The amount of vitamin C *available* in the food supply to the average person is considerably higher than average *intake* because of waste of food and destruction during storage, processing, and cooking.

Vitamin C in Foods

Sources. For vitamin C we are dependent almost entirely on certain *fruits* and *vegetables*. They contain the most vitamin C when eaten fresh, uncooked, or previously frozen. Fresh milk contains small amounts of vitamin C and pasteurized milk only negligible amounts. Breast milk provides adequate amounts for infants as long as the mother's intake of vitamin C meets recommended allowances. What little vitamin C might be in meat, poultry, and fish is destroyed in cooking. Eggs, cereal, sugar, and fats, nuts, dried legumes, and dried fruits contain either very little or none at all.

Certain kinds of fruits and vegetables are unusually rich in vitamin C (see Table 12–2). Citrus fruits, strawberries, and cantaloupe lead the fruits in vitamin C content, with the exception of two very rich sources rather uncommon in the United States except in health-food stores. These are a West Indian Cherry *(acerola)* and a Peruvian jungle fruit *(camu-camu)* (16). Rose hips are another concentrated, though variable, source of vitamin C, but they too are not widely available. These exotic fruits are unnecessarily expensive and have no special value other than their vitamin C content.

Green leafy vegetables, green peppers, broccoli, brussels sprouts, and cauliflower have a high content of vitamin C and are very good sources even after cooking. Raw cabbage, turnips, salad greens, and tomatoes are also good sources. Potatoes contribute considerable amounts of vitamin C when cooked at moderate temperatures. In large quantities they are still a principal source of vitamin C in areas of the world where other sources are not easily available. Dehydrated potatoes are an undependable source, unless fortified with vitamin C (see Table 12–3). Much of the vitamin C is retained in the normal processing of French fries and potato chips. Most cooked and canned vegetables and fruits provide some vitamin C but in smaller and more variable amounts than the corresponding fresh foods. Freezing, however, preserves most of the vitamin C activity. Frozen orange juice is one of our best sources, and is widely used in countries where refrigerators are available.

Pure ascorbic acid is available in stores wherever vitamins are sold, in very inexpensive form—for as little as 0.5 cent or less per 100 mg (which is more than a day's supply).[1] This costs less than an equivalent amount in natural foods, but such foods (except for the acerola and camu-camu berries) also supply a variety of minerals and other vitamins and are to be preferred whenever possible. For this reason, the authors do not recommend the various high-vitamin C, imitation fruit drinks on the market as routine sources of vitamin C for children or adults, except when no other source is available.

It should be understood that there is considerable variability in the vitamin C content of fruits and vegetables and that the figures given in Table 12–2 represent only approximate mean values. The vitamin C content of plant foods varies greatly with different varieties of the same plant, with soil and climate, and especially with the amount of exposure to sunlight and the degree of ripeness of the fruit. In general, the more

[1]The cost per unit may vary considerably. The natural active form of ascorbic acid is the L-isomer, and this is equal in every way to the synthetic L-isomer, the usual commercial form.

Table 12–2 FRUITS AND VEGETABLES AS SOURCES OF VITAMIN C*

Food	*Vitamin C (mg/100 gm, Edible Portion)*	*Food*	*Vitamin C (mg/100 gm, Edible Portion)*
Fruits, fresh		Vegetables (cont.)	
Strawberries	59	Cauliflower	78
Oranges (or juice)	50	Spinach	51
Frozen orange juice	45	Cabbage	47
Lemons (or juice)	46	Rutabagas	43
Grapefruit (or juice)	38	Dandelion greens	35
Frozen orange-grapefruit juice	41	Asparagus	33
Cantaloupe	33	Chard	32
Honeydew melon	23	Okra	31
Berries (except strawberries		Beet greens	30
and blueberries)	21	Beans, lima, green	29
Pineapple, fresh	17	string, green	19
Avocados	14	Peas, green	27
Blueberries	14	Radishes	26
Bananas	10	Onions, young, green	25
Cherries	10	mature	10
Apricots	10	Tomatoes	23
Peaches	8	juice, canned	16
Apples		Squash, summer	22
Grapes		winter	13
Pears	7	Sweet potatoes	21
Plums		Potatoes	20
Watermelon		Lettuce, green	18
Vegetables		Parsnips	16
Kale, leaves only	186	Corn, sweet	12
Turnip greens	139	Cucumbers	11
Peppers, green	128	Beets	10
Broccoli	113	Celery	9
Brussels sprouts	102	Lettuce, head	6
Mustard greens	97	Eggplant	5
Collards	92	Carrots	8

*Figures are from U.S. Department of Agriculture Handbook No. 8, *Composition of Foods—Raw, Processed, Prepared*, 1963. See Appendix for further details. All values are computed on a raw basis before cooking, unless indicated otherwise.

mature a plant becomes, the less vitamin C it contains; the more sunlight a plant receives, the more vitamin C it contains. Different varieties of apples and oranges have been found to vary considerably in vitamin C content. Even allowing for such variations, certain fruits and vegetables are much richer in this vitamin than others.

An undetermined amount of vitamin C activity is reaching the American public by way of a common and safe food additive closely related to ascorbic acid, *isoascorbic acid* (or *erythorbic acid*), with antioxidant activity similar to that of vitamin C. Isoascorbic acid, however, has only about 5 percent of the vitamin activity of ascorbic acid (17).

Losses in Processing. Further variations in the vitamin C content of foods must be expected because of losses of this vitamin during storage, processing (canning or drying), and cooking.[2] Vitamin C is very susceptible to destruction under these conditions because it is so water-soluble, is easily

[2]See supplementary reading for Chapter 8 and this chapter in Appendix for more information on vitamin C stability in foods.

Table 12–3 RETENTION OF VITAMIN C DURING PROCESSING OF POTATOES*

State of Processing	*Mean Total Vitamin C (Fresh Weight Basis) mg/100 gm*
Raw potatoes	26.5
Fresh mashed	13.6
Reconstituted, dehydrated granules	6.7

*From Bring, S. V., and Raab, F. P.: J. Amer. Dietet. Assoc., 45:149, 1964.

oxidized, and is destroyed by certain enzymes. Leafy vegetables (with large surface areas) lose more vitamin C in storage than do root vegetables or tubers. Refrigeration during storage reduces losses, and in markets, more of the vitamin is retained if vegetables are kept in crushed ice.

In preparation of raw foods for canning, quick freezing, or drying, a brief blanching with steam favors retention of vitamin C because the steam destroys the enzymes present that hasten destruction of the vitamin. There is least loss of vitamin C when foods are preserved by quick freezing, as with frozen orange juice. Most losses occur when foods are preserved by drying, especially if they are exposed to sunlight in the process. Commercially canned foods may compare favorably in vitamin C content with home-cooked products if the fruits or vegetables reach the cannery fresh from nearby fields and are heated quickly in vacuum-sealed cans. The vitamin C content of canned fruit juices will vary considerably unless fortified with vitamin C or unless it is specially protected in canning.

Because vitamin C is water-soluble, considerable amounts of it may be lost in the liquid in which the food is canned if the liquid is discarded. In drying fruits, sulfuring before drying and rapid drying (away from sunlight) favor retention of the vitamin content, but dried fruits cannot be counted on as a source of much vitamin C.

The amount of vitamin C lost in home cooking varies greatly. If short boiling times and small amounts of water are used, however, and if the water is consumed there is little loss. It has been observed that ascorbic acid in vegetables can be protected somewhat by boiling the cooking water for a minute before adding the food. Boiling removes the oxygen dissolved in water, thus preventing oxidative destruction of some of the ascorbic acid.[3] For example, loss of ascorbic acid from cabbage boiled fifteen minutes starting in cold water is 25.5 percent compared with a 1.8 percent loss when cooked in water that has been boiled one minute (18).

The loss in vitamin C content in home cooking also depends on numerous factors including the nature of the food; whether it is acid or alkaline; the period and degree of heating; and, especially, the extent to which the food is exposed to water and to air in the cooking process. The oxidation of ascorbic acid in foods is hastened by the enzyme *ascorbic acid oxidase*, which is present but inactive in raw fruits and vegetables and which becomes active when leaves or fruits are damaged by drying, bruising, or cutting. Retention of the vitamin is favored by cooking with peel left on or in large pieces and cooking with as much exclusion of air as possible (tightly covered vessel or pressure cooker). Increased losses of the vitamin result from contact with copper or iron in preparing or cooking the food, or from mashing the food

[3]Probably practical only where vitamin C is scarce and expensive and the value of one's time in the kitchen is not in question. The monetary value of the vitamin C gained by such a procedure (and which can easily be replaced by some other food or supplementary source) is less than the value of one moment's time in many countries. Of course, the flavor of the food may also be changed by these procedures, which also needs to be considered. (This points out again the necessity of nutrition education for all people who prepare food so that one can weigh these factors for oneself).

and leaving it in a hot place or exposed to the air. The practice of holding cooked foods warm for prolonged periods of time, such as on steam tables in cafeterias, may result in significant losses of vitamin C (50 to 75 percent).

Conserving Vitamin C in Home Cooking. It is foolish to allow vitamin C, which is essential for health, to be lost before foods are served. Because it is the most easily destroyed of the vitamins, its conservation presents a special problem. Reasons for the following special precautions in handling fresh fruits and vegetables should be self-evident if one keeps in mind, as stated before, that vitamin C is water-soluble and that heat, alkaline reaction, and, above all, exposure to air hasten its destruction. The following practical suggestions are also useful in preserving most other water-soluble vitamins in foods in home cooking.

1. Buy fresh fruits and vegetables in small enough quantities so that they will be used without long periods of storage at room temperature. Keep them at low temperatures (in a refrigerator, if possible).
2. Prepare them (paring and cutting up) immediately before they are to be cooked or served raw; do not let them stand in water or exposed to air before cooking; serve promptly; do not keep hot for long (or reheat) before serving.
3. Cook in as small a quantity of water and for as short a time as feasible; cook by steaming or broiling (instead of boiling) and with "skins" left on when possible; keep cooking vessels tightly covered.
4. Never add soda in cooking vegetables and do not use copper cooking vessels if you want to preserve vitamin C (the presence of either alkali or copper hastens vitamin destruction).
5. Do not allow frozen foods to thaw out for long periods before cooking; keep them in the refrigerator and start cooking in a frozen state in small amounts of boiling water.
6. Juices of fresh fruits are best prepared just before serving. Acid juices (orange, grapefruit) may, however, be left in a covered glass or plastic container in the refrigerator several weeks with little loss in vitamin C value. The liquid should nearly fill the container, leaving a minimum of air above the surface.

The above suggestions are helpful but need not be slavishly followed.

Obtaining Vitamin C in a Day's Menu. Table 12–4 illustrates various fruit and vegetable combinations that will furnish at least 75 percent of a person's daily RDA. Combinations I and II represent a more expensive way to obtain vitamin C (that is, fresh fruits, especially out of season), while combinations III and IV are examples of more economical sources of vitamin C (available throughout the year).

Of interest are the latest USDA figures on food sources of vitamin C consumed by the American public in a year—a reflection of average food habits. The largest contributors

Table 12–4 EXAMPLES OF FOOD COMBINATIONS THAT FURNISH A GENEROUS DAY'S SUPPLY OF VITAMIN C

Food	*Vitamin C (mg)*
I	
Strawberries, 2/3 cup	60
Cooked summer squash, 1/2 cup	10
	70 mg
II	
Cantaloupe, 1/2 melon, 6 in. diameter	50
Asparagus, 4 stalks	18
	68 mg
III	
Tomato, 1 medium, fresh	35
Sweet potato, 1 medium, baked or boiled with skin	20
	55 mg
IV	
Grapefruit juice, 1/2 cup, canned	41
Lima beans, 1/2 cup cooked	14
Potato, 1 medium, baked or boiled with skin	16
	71 mg

are vegetables, which contribute 51 percent of our vitamin C. Citrus fruits supply 29 percent, and all other fruits, including those fortified with synthetic vitamin C, supply 12 percent for a total of 41 percent from fruit. (Of the 51 percent from vegetables, potatoes make up 14 percent; dark green and deep yellow vegetables, 9 percent; and tomatoes and all other vegetables, 28 percent.) Thus, fruits and vegetables supply 92 percent of our vitamin C intake in foods, demonstrating the importance of this food group.

Figures on the percentage of vitamin C intake from synthetic sources (used in fortified foods or taken as vitamin supplements) are not readily available but probably range between 20 and 30 percent of the total intake on a per capita basis. This figure varies considerably with each individual. Recent studies have verified that vitamin C is the most popular vitamin supplement. It is regularly used by 15 to 40 percent of the population, depending on the study (see ref. 25 and 27 in Chap. 8 for more details). Large numbers of people are taking 2 or more grams a day (11 percent of the users in the study by M. H. Read and co-workers)—a level the authors of this book consider potentially toxic and unnecessary. (See section on toxicity and supplementary readings in the Appendix.)

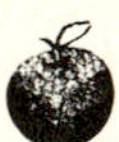

health considerations

Toxicity of Vitamin C

Many millions of Americans, as has just been said, consume high levels of supplements of vitamin C in the belief that this practice will improve their health. Sometimes they do so under the care of a physician, but more often they diagnose their own condition. It is possible that more people take more vitamin C at high levels and, hence, as a drug than any other drug (except aspirin). (See the discussion on megavitamins in the section on health considerations in Chap. 8.)

The practice of taking high levels of ascorbic acid without the advice of an expert is not without its problems. First, although ascorbic acid is generally nontoxic, it is a chemical, as is any drug. At excessively high levels, say more than 1000 mg per day, toxicity signs have been seen, including absorption of excessive iron, excretion of high levels of uric acid in the urine, and gastrointestinal symptoms such as diarrhea (8). Second, if the body takes in more than 250 to 300 mg of ascorbic acid per day, it becomes saturated within a few days and either does not absorb extra amounts or absorbs and excretes them.

The Food and Nutrition Board recognizes that extra amounts of vitamin C, up to 200 to 250 mg a day (the amount in several glasses of orange juice along with other fresh fruit) may be needed "under acute emotional or environmental stress, such as exposure to elevated temperatures" (8). The term elevated temperatures would include not only fever but also high environmental temperatures over extended periods, as experienced by, say, mine workers or foundry workers.

If extra vitamin C is desired for any reason the authors are of the opinion that there is never a need to consume more than 200 to 250 mg a day. (See supplementary readings.)

THE HISTORY OF VITAMIN C

Attempts to treat the ancient disease of scurvy led to the discovery that a disease could be caused by lack of some intangible component of the diet and to the eventual isolation of the lacking substance as a vitamin. This is one of the most fascinating stories of achievement in the development of nutrition as a science.[4]

Treatment of Scurvy

Scurvy is one of the oldest diseases; early descriptions date from as far back as about 1500 B.C. Symptoms of gangrene of the gums, loss of teeth, and painful legs in soldiers were described by Hippocrates about 450 B.C. From records of the crusaders in the Middle Ages, it is evident that they, too, suffered from scurvy. In the fifteenth and sixteenth centuries, it was a scourge throughout Europe, so much so that philosophers wondered if all disease might be outgrowths of scurvy. It was particularly prevalent and severe on long voyages of sailing ships, in besieged cities, and in times of crop failures—in short, wherever fresh foods were unavailable. When Vasco de Gama made his long voyage around the Cape of Good Hope, nearly two-thirds of his crew perished from scurvy. The lives of many of the men with the explorer G. E Cartier, when obliged to spend the winter of 1535 in Canada, were saved because they learned from the Indians that a "brew" made from the growing tips of the spruce and other trees was a cure for this malady. (It is obvious now that the "brew" contained vitamin C.)

In 1753, James Lind, a Scottish naval surgeon, published what became a famous report of experiments made on ships of the British navy, proving that oranges and lemons prevented or cured the disease (19). His classic studies generally are considered the first experiments to show that an essential food element can prevent a deficiency disease.

[4]Persons interested in more detail on this subject will find a list of general references on the history of vitamin C in the supplementary readings in the Appendix.

The experiences of Lind, Cartier, and others gradually became well known, so that by the time of the historic voyage of Captain James Cook (1772–1775), enough was known about the prevention of scurvy to cause Cook to stock the ship with fresh fruits and vegetables at every port visited, thereby keeping the men well throughout the long trip. Cook also recognized that sauerkraut was "antiscorbutic" (prevented scurvy) and supplied the ship with large quantities of it, stating that it was "not only a wholesome vegetable food, but, in my judgment, highly antiscorbutic, and spoils not by keeping it" (20). Not until 1795, however, were citrus fruits (lime juice) required on ships of the British navy, a practice that provided British sailors with the nickname "limeys."

The explorers of the New World introduced the potato to Europe. Consequently, as potatoes (a good source of vitamin C) became a food staple there, scurvy disappeared. Epidemics of scurvy reappeared on several occasions after disastrous failures of the potato crop in certain regions, as in Norway and in Ireland. While it became generally recognized that citrus fruits and fresh vegetables were preventives against scurvy, nearly 150 years elapsed before the potency of these foods was explained as due to the presence in them of a specific substance known as a vitamin.

Identification

In the first decades of the twentieth century it became clear that there were at least three distinct nutritional deficiencies in humans and animals—scurvy, pellagra, and rickets (see Chap. 8).

In 1912, the terms "scurvy vitamine" and "antiscorbutin" were first used in the literature for the scurvy-preventing substance (21). The letter C for the antiscorbutic factor (or "water-soluble C") was first used by British scientists in 1918 and 1919 (22). This practice led directly to the use in 1921 of the term vitamin C for the substance by F. O. Santos and others (23), following J. C. Drummond's suggestion of combining the word vitamin with the letters then in use (24).

In 1928, the Hungarian-born scientist A. Szent-Györgyi, first isolated what is now known as ascorbic acid (he called it "hexuronic acid") from oranges, cabbages, and adrenal glands, although he did not recognize it as vitamin C and did not try it in the treatment of scurvy (25). In 1932, C. G. King and W. A. Waugh isolated from lemon juice a crystalline material that possessed antiscorbutic activity in guinea pigs (26). They found that their compound was identical with the substance isolated by Szent-Györgyi (who, as a result, in 1933 called it ascorbic acid, a shortened form of the "*a*nti*scorb*u*ic* factor" (27). Shortly afterward, the structure of L-ascorbic acid was announced, and it was synthesized in the laboratory, starting with the sugar galactose and later with glucose (Fig. 12–4).

Both the ascorbic acid and the dehydroascorbic acid in foods contribute to the vitamin C activity in the body. In living plant and animal tissues, this oxidation-reduction between the two substances is *reversible*. When dehydroascorbic acid is further oxidized, however, it loses its vitamin C activity, and the reaction is not reversible—that is, it cannot be reduced to form dehydroascorbic acid again.

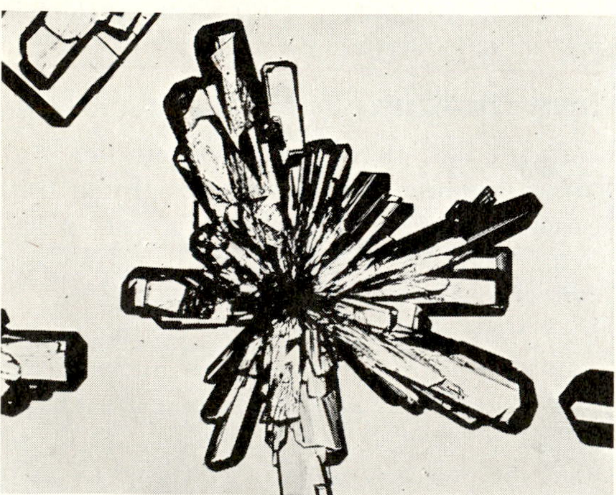

Figure 12–4 Photomicrograph showing crystalline structure of pure ascorbic acid. (Courtesy of Merck & Company.)

METABOLISM OF VITAMIN C

Once vitamin C is absorbed in the body it helps to maintain strength of connective tissue and blood vessels, aids in metabolism, and protects against infections.

Absorption

Vitamin C taken in food is absorbed into the blood stream chiefly from the ilium of the small intestine by an active transport system within a few hours after it is ingested. It can also be absorbed directly through the tissues of the mouth, in part (28). The level of vitamin C in the blood plasma is increased only temporarily, because the vitamin is taken up by the tissues and any excess is excreted promptly. Intravenously injected ascorbic acid is excreted within one to three hours. Although the body has limited ability to store vitamin C, it is present in higher concentrations in glandular tissues, especially in the adrenal glands. The amount of vitamin C in the body tissues depends on the quantity in the food and the rate at which it is utilized in and excreted from the body. About 10 to 30 mg of vitamin C appears to be the amount utilized in the body per day in normal adults. This amount does not, however, allow for adequate body stores of the vitamin. An intake of 60 mg per day will maintain a normal body pool of about 1500 mg, enough to maintain body stores for three or four weeks even if no vitamin C is consumed at all. There is no evidence that saturation of the tissues with vitamin C is essential to optimal health.

Metabolic Role of Vitamin C

Although the exact manner in which vitamin C functions in metabolism is yet to be explained, it is assumed that because of its instability—its property of being reversibly oxidized and reduced—it plays some part vital to the welfare of cells and tissues throughout the body. Just as hemoglobin and other iron-containing pigments in the body are capable of alternately taking on and giving up oxygen (reversible oxidation-reduction), so ascorbic acid is able alternately to lose and take on hydrogen. It thus can act as a "hydrogen carrier," and as such it may have an essential role in the metabolism of carbohydrates or proteins, or both. Whatever the explanation, the widespread tissue damage seen in scurvy makes it apparent that this vitamin is needed by many kinds of tissues, and hence its role would seem to be a fundamental one.

Clues to the functions of vitamin C come chiefly from the symptoms seen in scurvy. So many apparently unrelated tissues show damage that only some of its functions can be discussed here.

Formation of Collagen. The main type of tissue showing marked damage in scorbutic animals is *connective tissue.* The reason is primarily that *collagen,* a protein important in the formation of skin, tendon, and bone, as well as supportive tissue, is not properly formed when there is vitamin C deficiency. Normally collagen contains the amino acid *hydroxyproline,* which is obtained by conversion from the amino acid *proline.* In vitamin C deficiency, this conversion does not take place. Consequently, this results in the many characteristic signs of scurvy, including disorganization of bone and tooth calcification and delayed healing of tissue in burns and wounds. Both animal and human studies indicate that a sufficiently low dietary intake of this vitamin results in delayed healing and less strength of the healed wound, whereas administration of vitamin C under such conditions promotes sound healing of wounds.

Other Metabolic Functions. Vitamin C appears to help maintain strength in blood vessels, a function unrelated to maintaining collagen in connective tissue. Small blood vessels under the skin tend to hemorrhage, especially when suction or pressure is applied. This tendency has been used as a rough test for the lack of vitamin C (the *capillary fragility test*). Examination of the rate of blood flow in scorbutic guinea pigs has revealed a marked sluggishness of the blood flow in vessels that are greatly dilated.

Vitamin C also takes part in a number of reactions involving other amino acids, such as tyrosine and tryptophan, and the vitamin folacin. In addition, it influences the formation of hemoglobin and deposition of iron in liver tissue. One of the most interesting aspects of vitamin C's influence on iron metabolism is its ability to increase the amount of iron absorbed from the intestine. Thus, vitamin C, when taken with iron supplements or iron-containing foods, will allow more of the iron to be absorbed and therefore be available for use by the body. This action, in turn, causes some destruction of vitamin C as a result of oxidation, a fact considered in setting the RDA at 60 mg per day.

Because the adrenal glands contain more vitamin C than most other tissues, it is believed that vitamin C is involved in some way with the secretion of hormones of the adrenal cortex.

As yet no evidence has been found that the vitamin functions as a coenzyme or as a specific component of any particular enzyme system, as do many of the other vitamins. Rather, its participation appears to be general, and it is required in the metabolism of many substances in the body. Just how or why vitamin C is concerned in so many and such varied chemical changes that are parts of normal metabolism in the tissues is not yet known, but enough is known to establish it as a very important substance for our physical well-being.

Proposed Clinical Uses

Vitamin C is also useful in protecting the body against infections and bacterial toxins. In infants with scurvy their lowered resistance to infections is notable.

Infections apparently decrease the amount of ascorbic acid in tissues and body fluids; normal recommended intakes of vitamin C are thought to be helpful in enabling the body to combat infections. There is as yet little evidence that amounts greatly in excess of normal recommended intake confer extra benefits, except after deprivation or during periods of unusual physical stress.

The apparent role of vitamin C in maintaining normal immunological and other body defenses may well explain its reported effects in certain clinical situations, including cancer (see the section on health considerations). Quite convincing evidence of an immunological or bactericidal function for vitamin C has been observed in recent experiments with a variety of levels of intake of vitamin C under a wide range of conditions (29).

Because vitamin C is inexpensive and not likely to be toxic and has the magic name of a vitamin, physicians occasionally prescribe it for their patients rather than provide no treatment at all. In such instances, it is usually given beyond RDA amounts. Because it is popular and widely available in stores, many people prescribe it for themselves without the guidance of a physician, as has been noted. Vitamin C is widely misused.

Vitamin C has been claimed to be helpful in reducing blood lipids, atherosclerosis, and heart disease. Although it does, in fact, lower blood lipids in experimental animals, what little evidence there is for such an effect in humans is not convincing (30). Evidence that a deficiency of vitamin C causes abnormal lipoprotein patterns is much more believable, although further work is needed before definite conclusions can be made (31).

Ascorbic acid, at 200 mg per day, seems to have legitimate use in treating a rare inherited metabolic disease of childhood known as the Chediak-Higashi syndrome (32). Limited other uses exist when a vitamin C deficiency occurs for any reason. In spite of claims to the contrary, however, there is no satisfactory evidence that high levels of vitamin C help in treating diabetes, arthritis, stress, bladder stones, allergies, and the like. These claims are often seen in health-food magazines and similar media that advertise vitamin C supplements.

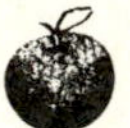

health considerations

Colds, Cancer, and Smoking

Vitamin C has been linked with three areas of health that concern large numbers of people—the common cold, cancer, and smoking.

Colds. The possibility suggested by Linus Pauling in 1970 (33) that very large intakes of vitamin C are necessary to protect against the common cold is without good scientific foundation. There is little acceptable evidence that a high intake of vitamin C will prevent colds any better than RDA levels. Nevertheless, it would be wise to make sure that one's intake of vitamin C is up to the RDA at all times, especially during the winter.

In any event, the large amounts of vitamin C often suggested for treatment of colds are usually far higher than the RDA, and higher than would be normally supplied by natural foods. Any beneficial effect that might be obtained by high amounts of ascorbic acid, therefore, would be a pharmaceutical rather than a nutritional effect. Results of most of the well-controlled studies on the use of large amounts of vitamin C for colds have been negative (34). On the other hand, T. N. Anderson and other scientists found some positive effects in the treatment of colds with vitamin C at levels above the RDA (35). Anderson suggested about 250 mg per day, which seems a more reasonable amount for the treatment of colds than higher levels —if extra vitamin C is useful at all. More evidence is needed before extra vitamin C is accepted as an effective way to treat a cold.

Cancer. Much interest and controversy exist today over the role of vitamin C, at normal or pharmacological levels, in the prevention and treatment of certain types of cancer. In the past several years it has become increasingly evident that certain nutrients, including vitamin C, do indeed help to prevent the occurrence of various cancers (see ref. 24, Chap. 9). For instance, the National Academy of Science's 1982 report "Diet, Nutrition, and Cancer" concluded that "the limited evidence suggests that vitamin C can inhibit the formation of some carcinogens and that the consumption of vitamin-C-containing foods is associated with a lower risk of cancers of the stomach and esophogus." A number of references are cited in the Academy report and at the end of this chapter, that give further information on this important topic (36).

As with news such as this about any nutrient, one should not jump to a conclusion too fast. Cancer is a very complicated disease. The important point is that one should consume at least the recommended allowance for vitamin C. There is no acceptable evidence that "mega" amounts are more effective. The allowances set by the Food and Nutrition Board take into account the amount necessary for cancer prevention.

Smoking. Claims have been made over the years that smoking greatly increases the body's need for vitamin C. Recent research shows there is some truth to this claim. The quantitative relationships are not clear, nor is it clear whether the relationship is due to actual destruction, or reduced availability, of ascorbic acid. Heavy smokers do have lowered blood levels of vitamin C, but the biochemical reason for that condition has not yet been established (37). In any event there is evidence that heavy smokers need more vitamin C than that supplied by the recommended dietary allowances, but this subject needs more research also. The Food and Nutrition Board considered the effect of smoking in setting the RDA at 60 mg per day for adults.

FLAVONOIDS AND RELATED SUBSTANCES

Various pigments and related compounds in citrus fruits and other plants are advertised widely in health-food literature as sources of "vitamin P." Chief among them are certain *flavonoids* (called "bioflavonoids by the health-food industry), including *hesperidin,* and *rutin.* These have been reported to have limited vitamin C-sparing activity in experimental animals. There is no evidence today that these compounds in otherwise nutritionally complete diets have activity similar to that of a vitamin (38). They may well serve, however, as pharmaceuticals. They can protect against capillary fragility, for instance, under special experimental conditions in animals, but this has not been demonstrated to take place in humans. Nutritionists in most countries (except, primarily, the Soviet Union) have not accepted "vitamin P" as either a separate entity or as a significant vitamin C-sparing factor. The term vitamin P, therefore, must be considered obsolete.

QUESTIONS

1. From what materials was ascorbic acid first isolated as a pure substance? What type of chemical compound is it? Why was the name ascorbic acid given to it? Where does it occur in nature? In the human body? How stable is the substance when kept in dry, solid form? In water solution with alkaline reaction? In acid solution? What other conditions affect its stability, and why?

2. Why was scurvy a prevalent disease among crews on long sea voyages and early explorations? Why is it possible for modern astronauts to remain in space for long periods without fear of their succumbing to scurvy? What foods or other substances were known to prevent or cure scurvy long before it was recognized that their efficacy was due to the presence in all of them of a definite compound that might be classed as a vitamin? Give the symptoms of acute scurvy and explain the widespread tissue damages in the light of one of the chief functions of vitamin C in the body—that is, the formation and maintenance of intercellular and connective tissue substances.

3. Why do humans and guinea pigs develop scurvy when the diet is lacking in vitamin C, while dogs, rats, and other animals do not? Do plants need vitamin C, and if so, how do they obtain it? Give three characteristic symptoms of subacute or latent scurvy in infants and three symptoms in adults that indicate the diet has furnished too little vitamin C. From consideration of the results of lack of this vitamin, what would you conclude are its main uses in the body?

4. What classes of foods contribute little or no vitamin C in the diet, at least in the condition in which they are eaten? What classes of foods furnish the major part of the vitamin C intake? Consult Table 12–2 and list the five fruits and five vegetables richest in vitamin C in the raw state. List the ten that have the next highest vitamin C content per 100 gm, either fruits or vegetables, in order of their relative vitamin C content when raw. Rearrange these twenty fruits and vegetables in the order of the vitamin C contribution that is made by average serving of each, with average allowance for loss of vitamin C in cooking, as given in Table 2 of the Appendix.

5. What is the recommended daily allowance of vitamin C for a normal woman? For a teenage boy? For a pregnant woman? If 10 mg of vitamin C per day protects an adult against scurvy, what is the use of consuming the recommended allowance? Is there any point in taking about twice the recommended allowance daily? Is a high level of vitamin C intake practical, or even possible, in some parts of the world? Name three countries in which the available foods and dietary customs make it probable that the average intake of vitamin C is low.

6. List five foods that provide vitamin C at low or moderate cost. Plan a day's diet, at low or moderate cost, that would furnish the RDA of vitamin C for an adult.

7. Plan a day's meals for yourself with some food that is a good source of vitamin C in each meal. Compute how many milligrams of vitamin C this diet would provide and compare with the standard allowance.

8. Give methods of conserving vitamin C in foods during storage and preparation for the table.

References

1. Hodges, R. E., et al.: Amer. J. Clin. Nutr., *22*:535, 1969; *24*:432, 1971; Baker, E. M., et al.: Amer. J. Clin. Nutr., *19*:371, 1966; *22*:549, 1969; *24*:444, 1971.
2. Hodges, R. E.: Ascorbic acid (Chapter 6K). In Goodhart, E. S., and Shils, M. E. (eds.): *Modern Nutrition in Health and Disease.* 6th ed. Philadelphia, Penn., Lea and Febiger, 1980, p. 259 (also see p. 690).
3. Ginter, E.: World Rev. Nutr. Dietet. *33*:104, 1979.
4. Chaudhuri, C. R., and Chatterjee, I. B.: Science, *164*:435, 1969; Chatterjee, I. B., et al.: Nature, *192*:163, 1961; Chatterjee, I. B.: World Rev. Nutr. Diet., *30*:69, 1978.
5. Jenness, R., Birney, E. C., and Ayaz, L.: Comp. Biochem. Physiol., *67B*:195, 1980. Also see Rucker, R. B., et al.: Amer. J. Clin. Nutr., *33*:961, 1980.
6. Cummings, M.: Amer. J. Clin. Nutr., *34*:297, 1981.
7. Sato, P. H.: Molecular Pharm., *18*:326, 1980; Sato, P. H., and Grahn, I. V.: Arch. Biochem. Biophy., *210*:609, 1981.

8. Food and Nutrition Board: *Recommended Dietary Allowances.* 9th Ed. Washington D.C., National Research Council, National Academy of Sciences, 1980.
9. (Vitamin C requirement) Irwin, I. M., Hutchins, B. K.: J. Nutr., *106*:823, 1976; Kallner, A. B., Harmann, D., and Hornig, D. H.: Amer. J. Clin. Nutr., *34*:1347, 1981: Garry, P. J., et al.: Amer. J. Clin. Nutr., *36*:332, 1982; Hornig, D.: Trends Pharm. Sci., *3*:294, 1982.
10. Koh, E. T., and Chi, M. S.: Amer. J. Clin. Nutr., *34*:1562, 1981.
11. Pao, E. M., and Mickle, S. J.: Food Tech., *35* (Sept.):58, 1981.
12. Owen, G. M., et al.: Amer. J. Clin. Nutr., *34*:266, 1981.
13. Wassertheil-Smoller, S., et al.: Amer. J. Epidem., *114*:714, 1981 (in women during reproductive years); Bowering, J., Lowenberg, R. L., and Morrison, M. A.: Amer. J. Clin. Nutr., *33*:1987, 1980 (in pregnant women in East Harlem).
14. (On vitamin C needs of elderly) Baker, H., et al.: J. Amer. Geriat. Soc., *27*:444, 1979; Bates, C. J., et al.: Brit. J. Nutr., *42*:43, 1977; Schorah, C. J., et al.: Amer. J. Clin. Nutr., *34*:871, 1981; Garry, P. J., et al.: Amer. J. Clin. Nutr., *36*:332, 1982; Lewis, J. S.: Amer. J. Clin. Nutr., *37*:331, 1983; Goodwin, J. S., et al.: J. Amer. Med. Assoc., *249*:2917 (1983) (also see editorial by M. Raskin on p. 2939).
15. (On vitamin C and alcohol) Bonjour, J. P.: Int. J. Vit. Nutr. Res., *49*:436, 1979; Majumdar, S. K., et al.: Int. J. Vit. Nutr. Res., *51*:274, 1981; Fazio, V., et al.: Amer. J. Clin. Nutr., *34*:2394, 1981.
16. Derse, P. H., and Elvehjem, C. A.: J. Amer. Med. Assoc., *156*:1501, 1954; Bradfield, R. B., and Roca, A.: J. Amer. Dietet. Assoc., *44*:28, 1964.
17. Wang, M. M., Fisher, K. H., and Dodds, M. L.: J. Nutr., *77*:443, 1962; Goldman, H. M., Gould, B. S., and Munro, H. N.: Amer. J. Clin. Nutr., *34*:24, 1981.
18. Roy, J. J., and Biswas, S. K.: Ind. J. Med. Res., *50*:259, 1962.
19. Lind, J.: Treatise on Scurvy (first published in 1753). Reprinted, and edited by C. P. Stewart and Douglas Guthrie. Edinburgh University Press, 1953.
20. Editorial: Captain James Cook (1728–1779). J. Amer. Med. Assoc., *209*:1217, 1969.
21. Funk, C.: J. State Med., *20*:341, 1912 (as reprinted in Goldblith, S. A., and Joslyn, M. A.: *Milestones in Nutrition.* Westport, Conn., Avi Publishing Co., Inc., 1964, pp. 145–171); Holst, A., and Frölich, J.: Z. Hyg., *72*:1, 1912.
22. Hardin, A., and Zilva, S. S.: Biochem J., *12*:408, 1918; Drummond, J. C.: Biochem. J., *13*:77, 1919.
23. Santos, F. O.: Proc. Soc. Exp. Biol. Med., *19*:2, 1921; McClendon, J. F.: J. Biol. Chem., *47*:411, 1921.
24. Drummond, J. C.: Biochem J., *14*:660, 1920.
25. Szent-Györgyi, A.: Biochem. J., *22*:1387, 1928.
26. King, C. G., and Waugh, W. A.,: Science, *75*:357, 1932; Waugh, W. A., and King, C. G.: J. Biol. Chem., *97*:325, 1932; and King, C. G.: Physiol. Rev., *16*:238, 1936.
27. Szent-Györgyi, A., and Haworth, W. N.: Nature, *131*:24, 1933.
28. Sadoogh-Abasian, F., and Evered, D. F.: Brit. J. Nutr., *42*:15, 1979.
29. (On immune systems) Leibovitz, B., and Siegel, B. V.: Internat. J. Vit. Nutr. Res., *48*:159, 1978; Nutr. Rev., *36*:183, 1978; Lancet, *1*:308, 1979; Anthony, L. E., et al.: Amer. J. Clin. Nutr., *32*:1691, 1979; Anderson, R., et al.: Amer. J. Clin. Nutr., *33*:71, 1980; Ramirez, I., et al.: J. Nutr., *110*:2207, 1980; Delafuente, J. C., and Panush, R. S.: Internat. J. Vit. Nutr. Res., *50*:44, 1980; Prinz, W., et al.: Internat. J. Vit. Nutr. Res., *50*:294, 1980; Sakamoto, M., et al.: J. Nutr. Sci. Vitaminol., *27*:367, 1981; Kay, N. E., et al.: Amer. J. Clin. Nutr., *36*:127, 1982; Patrone, F., et al.: Acta Vitaminol. Enzymol., *4*:163, 1982.
30. (On vitamin C and blood lipids) Khan, A. R., and Seedarnee, F. A.: Atherosclerosis, *39*:89, 1981; Johnson, G. E., and Obenshain, S. S.: Amer. J. Clin. Nutr., *34*:2088, 1981; Wahlberg, G., and Walldius, G.: Atherosclerosis, *43*:283, 1982; Burr, M. L., et al.: Human Nutr.: Clin. Nutr., *36C*:135 and 399, 1982.
31. Horsey, J., et al.: J. Human Nutr., *35*:53, 1981.
32. Nutr. Rev., *35*:170, 1977; Boxer, L. A., et al.: Brit. J. Haematol., *43*:207, 1979.
33. Pauling, L.: *Vitamin C and the Common Cold.* San Francisco, W. H. Freeman and Co., 1970; Pauling, L.: *Vitamin C, the Common Cold, and the Flu.* San Francisco, W. H. Freeman and Co., 1977.
34. (On vitamin C and colds): Miller, J. Z., et al.: J. Amer. Med. Assoc., *237*:248, 1977; Kent, S.: Geriatrics, *33*(Oct.):91, 1978; Pitt, H. A., and Costrini, A. M.: J. Amer. Med. Assoc., *241*:908, 1979; Coulehan, J. L.: Postgrad. Med., *65*:153, 1979; Baird, I. M.: Amer. J. Clin. Nutr., *32*:1686, 1979.
35. (On "treatment" of colds) Anderson, T. W.: Acta Vitaminol. Enzymol., *31*:43, 1977; Contemp. Nutr. (General Mills), *3* (Oct.):1, 1978; Davies, J. E. W., et al.: Biochem. Med., *21*:78, 1979; Wilson, C. W. M.: Acta Vitaminol. Enzymol., *2*:120 (abst.), 1980; Carr, A. B., et al.: Med. J. Aust., *2*:411, 1981.
36. (On vitamin C and cancer) Weisburger, J. H., et al.: Prevent. Med., *9*:352, 1980 (stomach); Graham, S., et al.: Amer. J. Epidem., *113*:675, 1981 (larynx); Kolonel, L. N., et al.: Amer. J. Clin. Nutr., *34*:2478, 1981 (stomach); Wassertheil-Smoller, S., et al.: Amer. J. Epidem., *114*:714, 1981 (cervix); Ziegler, R. G., et al.: J. Nat. Cancer Inst., *67*:1199, 1981 (esophagus in black men); Morigake, T., and Ito, Y.: Cancer Letters, *15*:255, 1982 (cell culture); Greco, A. M., et al.: Acta Vitaminol. Enzymol., *4*:155, 1982 (lung and bladder cancer); Consumer Reports, *48*(May):243, 1983.
37. (On vitamin C and smoking) Keith, R. E., and Driskell, J. A.: Nutr. Rept. Internat., *21*:907, 1980; Kallner, A. B., Hartmann, D., and Hornig, D. H.: Amer. J. Clin. Nutr., *34*:1347, 1981; Ginter, E.:

Amer. J. Clin. Nutr., *35*:1043, 1982 (letters to editor); Keith, R. E., and Driskell, J. A.: Amer. J. Clin. Nutr., *36*:840, 1982; Mossholder, S. B., and Keith, R. E.: Fed. Proc. (abst.), *42*:1065, 1983.

38. (On flavonoids) Baird, I. M., et al.: Amer. J. Clin. Nutr., *32*:1686, 1979.

Also see supplementary readings in the Appendix.

13 Water and Minerals

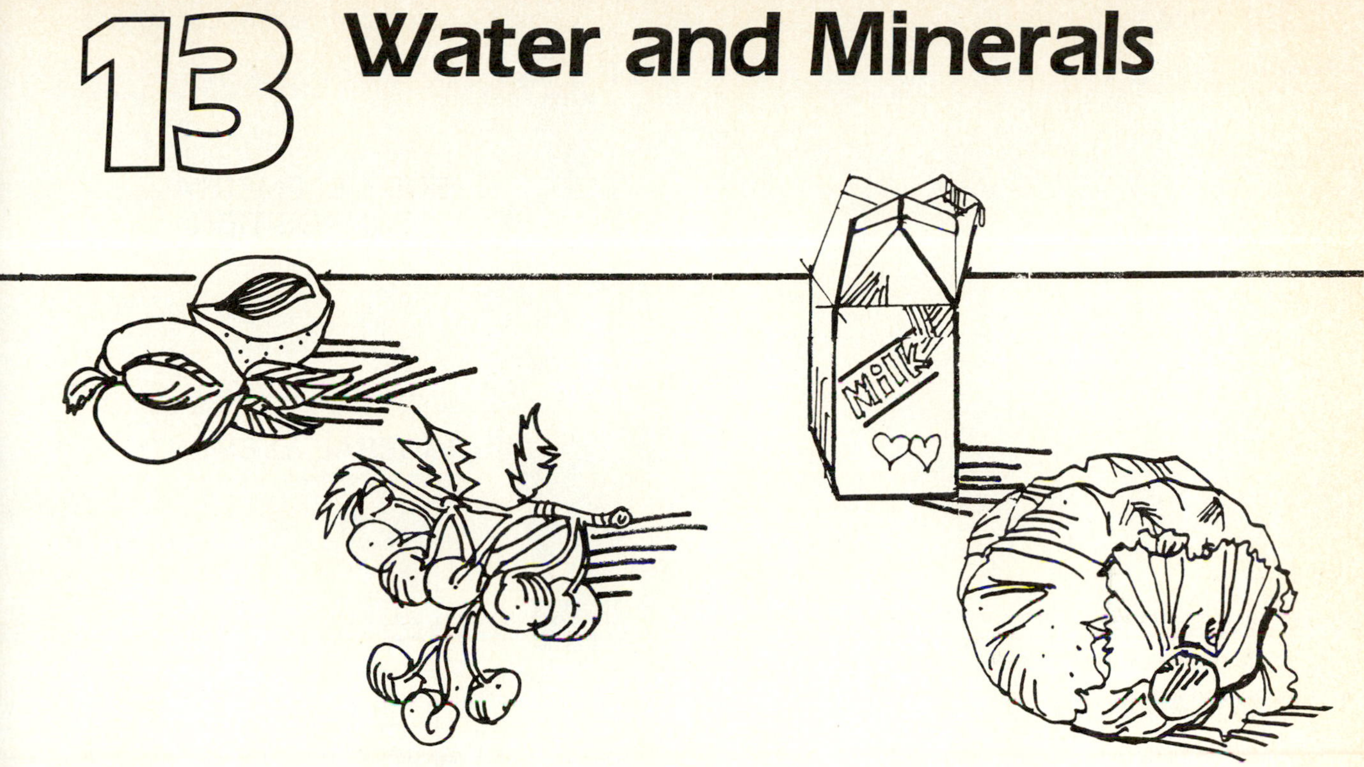

The chemical elements, in many different combinations, are the building blocks of the human body (see Fig. 13–1). This chapter will discuss water, made up of the elements oxygen (O) and hydrogen (H), and introduce the elements, or minerals, of nutritional importance.

WATER

Water (H_2O) is essential to all living organisms, plant and animal. It is the major constituent of body fluids, making up about half of body weight. Water is a simple compound of 2 atoms of hydrogen with 1 of oxygen, and it is thought to have a tetrahedral (four-sided) structure, as shown in Figure 13–2 (1).

Water occurs in nature in solid, liquid, and gaseous states as ice or snow, water, and steam respectively. It is a unique chemical that has properties different from those of any other liquid. For example, water has its maximum density at 4°C, just above the freezing point; that is, it expands upon freezing rather than contracting as do most substances. This property allows lakes and rivers to freeze from the surface down, since ice formed on top insulates the underlying water. Water also has an unusually high melting point, boiling point, and heat capacity as compared with other molecules of similar atomic structure and molecular weight.

Water is, also, an important biological solvent in which a multitude of chemical substances essential for life are dissolved. A relatively large amount of heat is needed to vaporize it, which makes perspiring a very effective means of dissipating body heat.

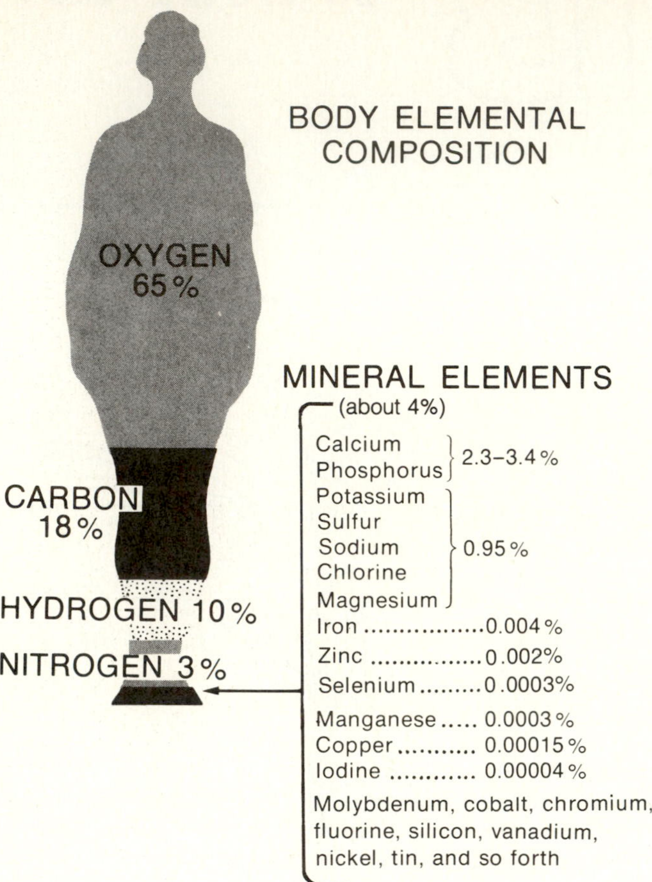

Figure 13–1 The nonmetallic elements oxygen carbon, hydrogen, and nitrogen together make up 96 percent of the body weight, leaving only 4 percent for all the various mineral elements. Calcium and phosphorus are the mineral elements present in largest amounts, but these amounts vary considerably, depending on the reserves of these two elements stored in the bones. Substantial quantities of potassium, sulfur, chlorine, sodium, and magnesium also are present in the body. These seven elements are referred to as macrominerals, whereas iron, manganese, copper, zinc, cobalt, iodine, and many other elements present in the body in trace amounts are called trace minerals or trace elements.

Water is second only to oxygen (which with hydrogen makes up three-fourths of body weight) in importance to the body. A healthy adult may live for weeks without food but only for a few days without water. A person can lose all reserve carbohydrate (glycogen) and fat and about half the body protein without real danger, but a loss of 10 percent of total body weight as water is serious, while a loss of 20 to 22 percent is fatal.

Body Content and Regulation

Body Water. Water makes up about 60 percent of total body weight in average adult males and 50 percent in average adult females. This percentage varies inversely with the fat content of the body; that is, when less fat is present, water is a greater percentage of body weight and vice versa. Water makes up a higher proportion of body weight in infants than in older children and adults; in the newborn it is approximately 77 percent of body weight. With advancing age, the percentage of body water declines to about 45 to 50 percent.

Fluid Compartments. Total body water is distributed between two major fluid compartments: Approximately 60 to 75 percent is located in the *intracellular fluid compartment,* or all of the water within cells. The remaining 25–40 percent is present in the

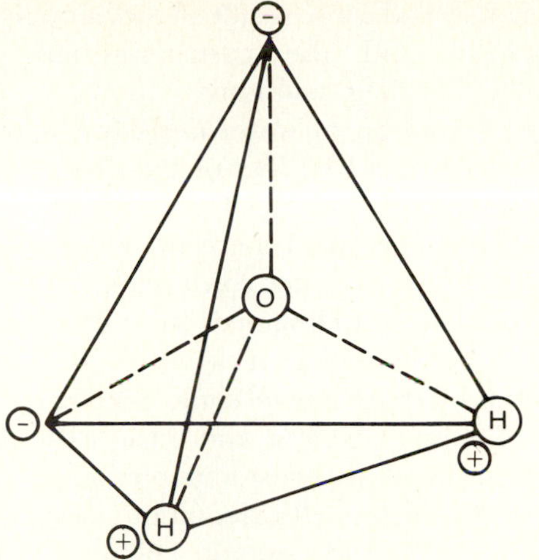

Figure 13–2 Tetrahedral character of the water molecule (H = hydrogen, O = oxygen, − = electron) (1).

extracellular fluid compartment, all the fluids not present in cells. (See Fig. 13–3.)

The extracellular fluid compartment is further divided into an *interstitial fluid compartment* (water between cells) and the *intravascular fluid compartment* (plasma, the noncellular portion of blood in the blood vessels).

The composition of the fluid within the cells is different from that of the fluid outside the cells, The extracellular fluid contains a relatively large amount of sodium and chlorine and is equivalent to a 0.9 percent solution of common salt (sodium chloride). Small amounts of potassium, calcium, magnesium, phosphorus, and sulfur also are present. This composition is about the same as is thought to have been present in the ancient seas where simple life forms first began. Besides the inorganic salts, extracellular fluid contains dissolved carbon dioxide, protein, a small amount of organic acids, and, of course, other organic compounds.

The intracellular fluid is quite different from the extracellular fluid in composition. The former is particularly high in potassium and phosphorus. It contains more magnesium, sulfur, and protein than does the extracellular fluid but less carbon dioxide and much less sodium and chlorine.

Regulation. It is surprising that the concentration of a substance as freely moving as water is different in these separate compartments. One reason is the nature of the membranes that surround the cells. These membranes are semipermeable: That is, they are freely permeable to water. Small molecules like the mineral salts diffuse through them; but other substances with larger molecules (such as proteins) are held back. The distribution of water inside and outside the cells depends on adequate protein and balanced mineral intakes. Sodium and potassium are the principal minerals responsible for water balance. (See Chap. 14.)

If there is a loss of water in the fluid outside the cell, or if the concentration of dissolved substances in this outside fluid increases, water will flow from the cell through the cell membrane into the outside fluid until a balance is achieved. The reverse process also occurs, with water flowing into the cell if the concentration of dissolved substances is higher within the cell than in the outside fluid.

The concentration of dissolved substances, or solute particles, is measured in units of *osmolality,* and the passage of water across

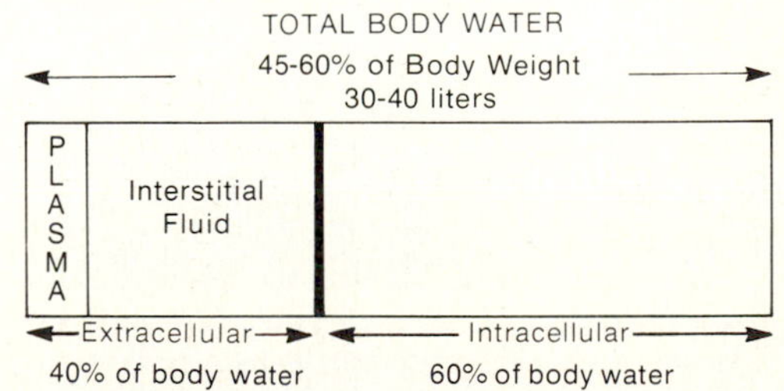

Figure 13–3 The extracellular fluid and intracellular fluid of the body are quite different in composition. Each compartment is maintained in homeostasis by active, energy-requiring body processes.

a semipermeable membrane as described above is called *osmosis*. Ionized *electrolytes* are important factors in osmolality and will be discussed in the next chapter. Basically, the interchange of water among the cells, circulatory system, and extracellular spaces depends on their concentrations of proteins and electrolytes.

Water Deficiency Symptoms

An adequate fluid intake is even more important than an adequate supply of calories. (See Fig. 13–4.) Water deficits can arise from inadequate water intake and from excessive losses of water from the body. Water in sufficient quantities to replace normal body losses, such as from evaporation from the skin, must be taken in each day or water depletion results. Increased losses, requiring increased intake or a consequent deficiency, may occur in conditions affecting the skin (burns), heavy sweat losses, the kidney (water not conserved as a result of hormonal dysfunction), and the gastrointestinal tract (watery diarrhea, vomiting).

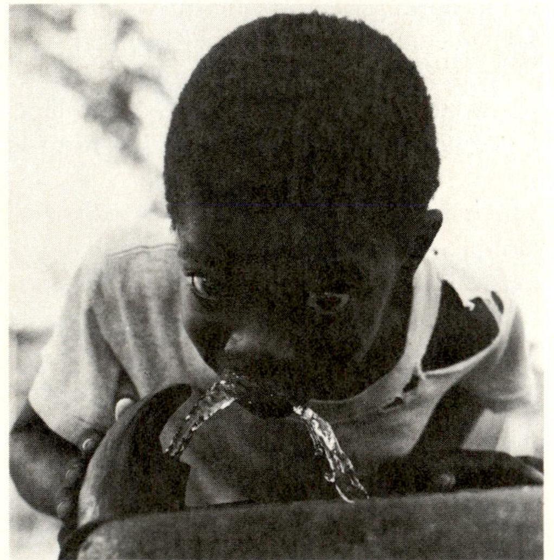

Figure 13–4 The need for water ranks second only to the need for air. Provision of safe public water supplies is an important indirect nutritional measure, by reducing the spread of disease and its concomitant nutritional costs and by freeing women and children from the burden of carrying water. Water can provide some essential minerals, including fluorine, and must be protected from environmental pollutants. (Courtesy of Laurel Stradford, Chicago.)

The first sign of water depletion is thirst. Thirst occurs when loss of total body water amounts to 1 or 2 percent or when loss amounts to about 1 percent of total body weight. If water is not consumed, *dehydration* progresses as delineated in Figure 13–5. With a water depletion of up to 10 percent, a person can perform some physical work, but efficiency is low and heat exhaustion takes place. With greater depletion of body water, weakness, disorientation, circulatory insufficiency, and loss of kidney function result.

The ability to function physically is greatly affected by continuing water depletion, even if the condition does not progress to acute life-threatening stages. Generalized symptoms of abnormal function, such as headaches, nervousness, loss of appetite, digestive disturbances, and inability to concentrate, have been correlated with chronic water depletion. Water is given partial credit for the first successful climb of Mount Everest. The successful team drank 3 to 4 liters (3.2 to 4.2 quarts) of water a day to make up for losses resulting from hyperventilation (increased breathing rates). This occurred in the high mountain air, while at least one unsuccessful team had previously attempted the climb with water rations of one liter or less.

An inadequate water intake for meeting needs for optimal digestive functioning may also be signaled by constipation. Initial treatment prescribed usually includes increased intake of water and other fluids.

Water Balance

To maintain *homeostasis,* or the normal balance, in the body's water supply, daily intake must equal daily output (see Fig. 13–6). The average daily turnover of water in normal persons ranges from 2 to 3 liters (about 2.1 to 3.2 quarts).

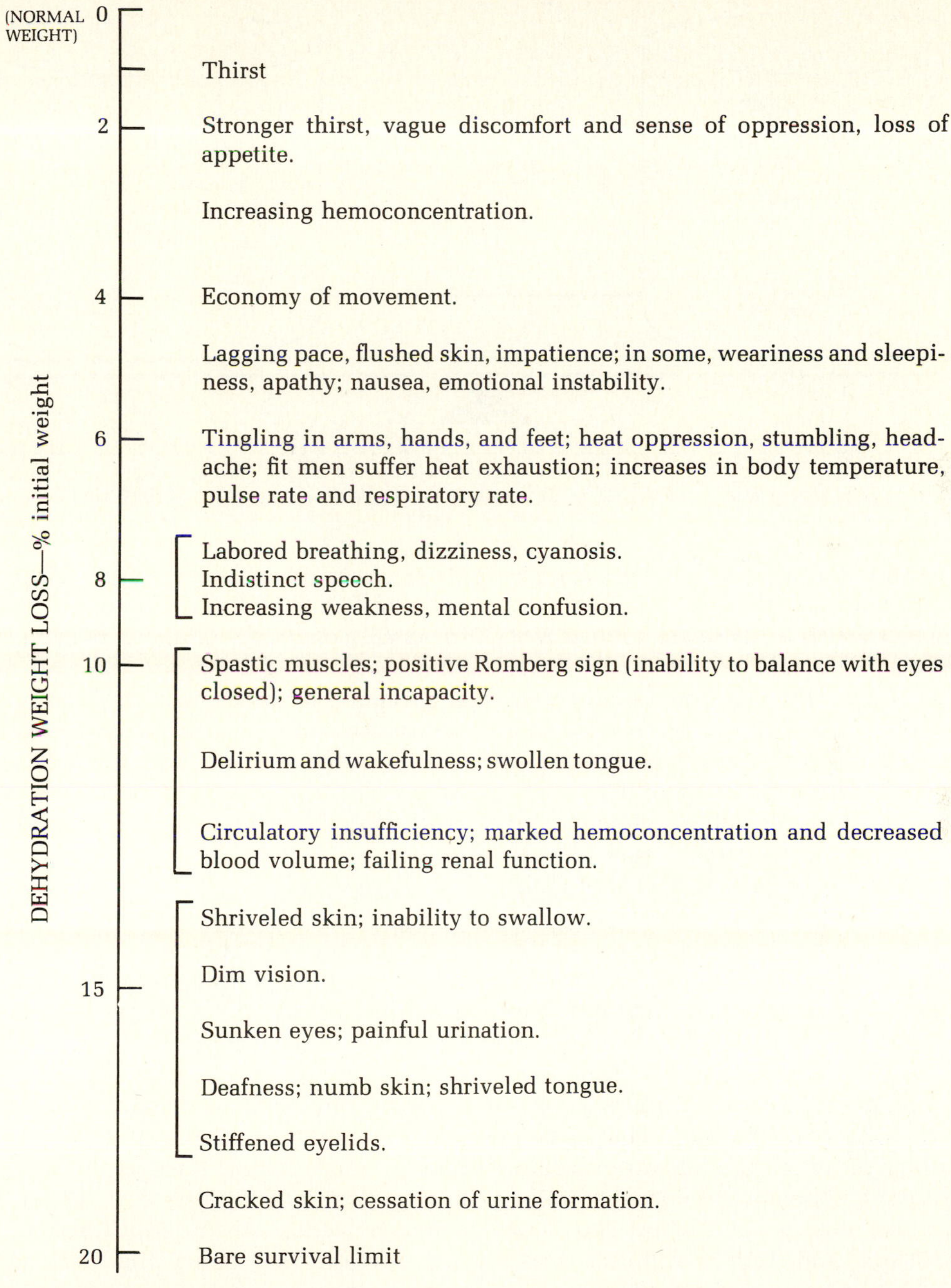
SPECTRUM OF DEHYDRATION
(NORMAL WEIGHT) 0
Thirst
2
Stronger thirst, vague discomfort and sense of oppression, loss of appetite.
Increasing hemoconcentration.
4
Economy of movement.
Lagging pace, flushed skin, impatience; in some, weariness and sleepiness, apathy; nausea, emotional instability.
6
Tingling in arms, hands, and feet; heat oppression, stumbling, headache; fit men suffer heat exhaustion; increases in body temperature, pulse rate and respiratory rate.
Labored breathing, dizziness, cyanosis.
8
Indistinct speech.
Increasing weakness, mental confusion.
10
Spastic muscles; positive Romberg sign (inability to balance with eyes closed); general incapacity.
Delirium and wakefulness; swollen tongue.
Circulatory insufficiency; marked hemoconcentration and decreased blood volume; failing renal function.
Shriveled skin; inability to swallow.
15
Dim vision.
Sunken eyes; painful urination.
Deafness; numb skin; shriveled tongue.
Stiffened eyelids.
Cracked skin; cessation of urine formation.
20
Bare survival limit
Death
DEHYDRATION WEIGHT LOSS—% initial weight

Figure 13–5 Spectrum of dehydration. (After Roth, E. M. (ed.): *Compendium for Development of Human Standards in Space System Design,* Vol. 3 NASA, 1967.)

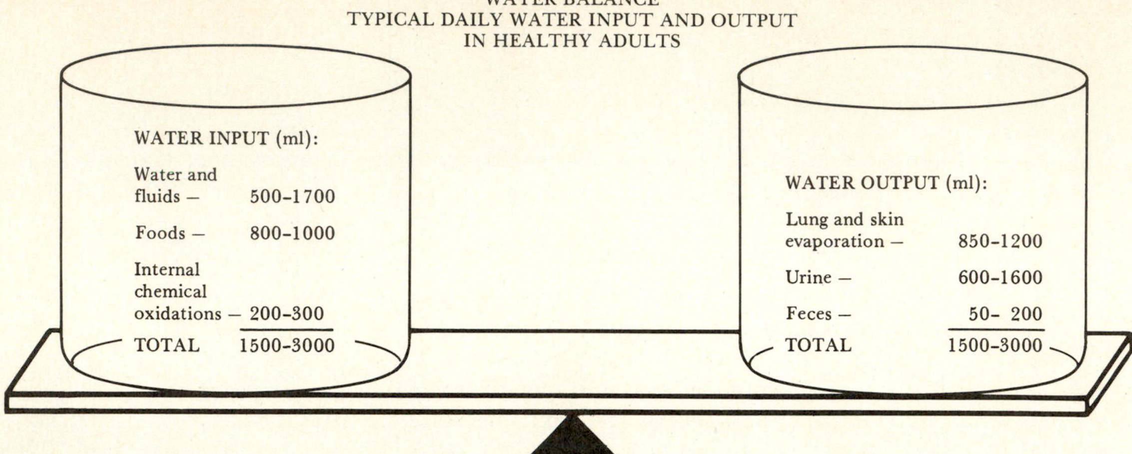

Figure 13–6 A *negative water balance* exists when the output (right side) exceeds the input (left side), and a *positive water balance* exists when the input is at least sufficient to balance the output of water. A negative balance, or a water deficit, stimulates drinking and kidney water conservation. Water excess stimulates water excretion and inhibits thirst.

Intake and Losses. Water intake includes the fluid consumed and the water contained in foods eaten, such as fresh fruit and vegetables. Water is also formed in the body by the oxidation of fats, amino acids, and sugars. Complete oxidation of 100 grams (gm) of fat yields 107 gm water; 100 gm carbohydrate yields 55 gm water; and 100 gm protein yields 41 gm water. The volume of this *water of oxidation,* or *metabolic water,* makes up about 10 to 20 percent of the total daily water requirement.

Total water intake from foods and fluids for an adult ranges from about 1.5 liters to nearly 3 liters. A recent survey showed that the beverages most frequently consumed by children and teenagers are milk and milk drinks, at an average of 500 milliliters (ml), or 17.5 ounces (oz), per day. The second most popular beverage groups were carbonated and noncarbonated sweetened drinks and tea, at an average of 350 ml (11.7 oz) per day. Fruit and vegetable juices were third at 215 ml (7.5 oz) per day (2).

Water losses occur daily in normal people in the urine, gastrointestinal tract, skin, and lungs. Water evaporates from the skin and is exhaled from the lungs. These *insensible water losses* account for a major portion of the daily water loss. Urinary losses vary widely and depend on fluid intake and the action of the *antidiuretic hormone* (ADH), which decreases excretion of water by the kidneys. Normally only a small fraction (3 to 7 percent) of daily water loss occurs through the feces.

Regulation. Many variables influence water balance in the body, including the amount of fluid consumed, protein and mineral content of the diet, physical activity, metabolic and respiratory rates, and body temperature.

Thirst, the urge to drink, is very important in regulating intake of fluid. For persons in good health, thirst is the best guide to the amount of fluid needed. Thirst is regulated by centers in the *hypothalamus,* which is the area at the base of the brain adjacent to the pituitary gland. If the hypothalamic thirst centers do not function properly, the thirst mechanism may not function correctly, and severe dehydration may occur. The thirst mechanism is inhibited when total body water is replenished.

Loss of water, as well as intake, can be regulated to maintain water balance. Net water loss increases secretion of ADH, whose name means "against water loss." ADH is formed in the hypothalamus and is stored and released in the posterior lobe of the pituitary gland. One major stimulus to the release of this hormone is an increase in the salt concentration of the blood supply to the hypothalamus. This increase occurs when water has decreased in relation to the salts in the blood. Another stimulus comes from receptors in the circulatory system itself and is communicated to the hypothalamus through the nervous system. Once released, the hormone exists in the blood stream for only about sixty to ninety minutes; and during this time it exerts an antidiuretic effect on the kidney, which results in reabsorption of water that was on its way to being excreted. This method of control of water lost from the body by the kidneys is an extremely important regulatory mechanism. (See also the section on excretion.)

Toxicity

Going without water can have serious, even fatal, consequences, as noted, but most people are surprised to learn that too much water can also threaten life. Water excess, also referred to as *water intoxication,* or *overhydration,* occurs because water intake far exceeds water output.

Generally, excessive water intake alone is not the cause of water intoxication, although that relation has been documented in extreme cases. Deliberately induced water intoxication is always dangerous, and fatalities have been reported. Basically, water is taken in faster than the kidneys can excrete it. The cause is usually psychogenic although a neurologic condition must be considered. Headache and vomiting are the first symptoms. There are also abdominal cramps, and in later stages, edema, convulsions, circulatory failure, and death.

Factors that may contribute to water excess, in addition to drinking, are administration of excess intravenous fluid, diminished capacity of the kidney to excrete water as a result of various renal disorders, and inappropriate or excessive secretion of the ADH. Inappropriate ADH secretion has been observed in several clinical conditions including head injuries and meningitis. Early identification of this condition is important so that fluid intake may be restricted.

A few cases of water intoxication in infants have been reported (3). The cause appears to be giving excessive amounts of water between feedings or giving an excessively diluted formula, either deliberately or inadvertantly.

Requirements

Water requirements of infants and children are proportionately higher than those of adults. Both body surface area and metabolic rate per unit of body weight are higher in infants and children than in adults, and water loss under sedentary conditions in a comfortable environment is roughly proportional to the metabolic rate. Children are also more active than many adults and so need additional water to cover the loss of sweat. To quantify this difference in terms of body weight, the daily need for fluid by adults is equivalent to about 4 percent of their body weight, while in infants, fluid need per day equals a full 10 to 15 percent of body weight.

Water requirements are related to, and can be expressed in terms of, energy consumption. Under conditions of moderate temperature and exercise, the minimal adult water requirement according to the Food and Nutrition Board is about 1 ml per kcal of energy expenditure, or about 2.5 liters (2.6 qt) a day. Infants require about 1.5 ml per kcal. The requirements are increased in hot environments and with strenuous activity and increased body temperature. If the urine volume is low, it is an indication that fluid intake should be increased.

The requirement for water can also be expressed as one cup of water for each 200 kcal in the diet. One way for us to be sure we are meeting the water requirement is to drink about three more cups of water a day than our thirst tells us that we need. If any of this water is excessive, the kidneys will excrete it very easily. Water needs also increase with high intake of protein and salt, characteristic of the "typical" American diet. Pregnant women and nursing mothers have higher water needs and requirements which relate to their increased energy needs and the need for maintenance of lactation in the nursing mother.

Sources

Water in the body is derived from three different sources:

1. solid foods consumed
2. fluids consumed (water, soup, coffee, tea, fruit juice, and other beverages)
3. metabolic processes

Solid foods contain a great deal of water—ranging from about 5 percent in very dry foods such as crackers to more than 90 percent in juicy fruits and vegetables such as tomatoes, eggplant, cauliflower, lettuce, strawberries, and watermelon. Even such a solid food as bread contains about 30 to 35 percent water (see Table 13–1); the majority of foods we eat are more than one-half water. Our daily intake of solid food contains about 1 liter (slightly over 1 qt) of water.

Roughly half of the water in the body comes from the fluids consumed. As has been discussed, the amount of fluid we need to drink is variable, depending on the magnitude of water loss and on the type of foods eaten; usually about 6 cups of water from fluids is sufficient. There is no objection to a person's drinking fluids on an empty stomach or drinking water with meals. Large quantities of an iced beverage, however, may cause some mild, temporary gastric distress.

Water of oxidation has been described previously. Its volume is about 300 ml a day (well over a cup).

Supplies of Drinking Water

Drinking water is usually not "pure" water; it nearly always contains some minerals. The amount of minerals present depends almost entirely on the source of the drinking water. Rain is a relatively pure source of natural water, although it contains dissolved gases from the air as well as traces of chlorides, sulfates, nitrates, and ammonia. Water from streams and lakes in mountainous dis-

Table 13–1 WATER CONTENT OF FOODS*

Food	*Percent water by weight*
Fresh vegetables and juices	90–95
Watermelon	93
Soft drinks, beer, soups	88–92
Fresh fruits and juices	85–90
Milk, cow's, whole	87
Potatoes	80
Avocados, bananas, sweet potatoes	75
Eggs	74
Cooked dry beans, cereals	70
Veal, 12% fat (thin)	71
Beef, 24% fat (utility)	62
34% fat (good)	55
46% fat (prime)	45
Tuna fish, canned, drained	60
Bread	30–35
Iced cake	20
Honey	17
Wheat flour	12
Dry beans	10
Crackers, ready-to-eat cereals	2–4
Nuts	2–4

*Data from U.S. Department of Agriculture Handbook No. 8. Washington, D.C. Values are approximate.

tricts is relatively free from organic impurities but may contain some dissolved minerals; water from nonmountainous lakes and rivers runs a risk of being contaminated. Water from springs and wells has filtered through the ground and thus has been more or less purified of organic contaminants, but it still may contain minerals. Bottled water, sold commercially for use in homes and offices, either is bottled from some natural source or is distilled water to which standard amounts of minerals have been added. (See also the section on health considerations.) Distilled water is produced by converting water (sea water or tap water for example) to steam and cooling the steam in a clean collecting system. Dissolved materials remain behind, so that distilled water contains only the substances taken up from the storage containers and pipe systems. Deionized water, with ions removed by absorption, is used in some homes, often unnecessarily.

Minerals, or inorganic salts, in small amounts are not objectionable in drinking water; in fact drinking is one way of consuming small quantities of some of the essential minerals. Organic matter in drinking water is not desirable because it encourages bacterial growth. Also specific organic compounds may have a toxic potential if they are present in high enough amounts.

Hard water is water containing the soluble salts of calcium and magnesium, primarily as bicarbonates, chlorides, and sulfates. These salts tend to prevent the detergent action of soaps with water. Iron compounds may also be present. *Soft water* is water in which the calcium and magnesium levels are low. Hard water can be changed to soft water by special softening processes, which often substitute sodium for the calcium and magnesium. Persons watching their sodium intake should be aware of the sodium content of their drinking water, particularly if it is soft water.

Contaminants. Contaminants in water can be divided into five groups: (1) microorganisms (bacteria, viruses, parasites), (2) particulate matter, (3) inorganic solutes, or minerals, (4) organic solutes, and (5) radionucleotides. Historically, the first group was the greatest concern because of the diseases they cause. These diseases include typhoid fever, cholera, bacillary dysentery, and amebic dysentery. Today microorganisms are controlled by methods of *water treatment* such as chlorination, sedimentation, and filtration.

Public drinking water is usually made safe by the use of *chlorine.* This substance has been used to purify water supplies since Jersey City began to chlorinate its water in 1907. Other substances used for control of microorganisms are ozone and chlorine dioxide.

The federal safe drinking water amendments of 1977 direct the Environmental Protection Agency (EPA) to review periodically, with the National Academy of Sciences, information on the safety of drinking water. In the 1979 review, the use of chlorination, and the other two methods listed above, were upheld as the best currently available methods of disinfecting water (4).

The EPA also has the task of evaluating possible water contaminants. It is responsible for the development of guidelines for the removal of substances in water such as pesticides and toxic metals.

It should be noted that the essential minerals in small quantities are not generally considered to be water contaminants but instead may contribute to meeting daily needs of these required nutrient elements (5).

Quality. Water should be safe to drink; attractive in appearance, taste, and odor; and usable for a multitude of household and industrial purposes. The impurities in water include the disease-producing organisms and other specific contaminants mentioned earlier. They can also include extremely fine particles from the erosion of clay deposits into water, and algae, which can produce colors and tastes. Organic materials can also produce odors and tastes. Some impurities may arise from the water supply system itself, such as corrosion products of zinc, copper, iron, and lead from old pipes. Iron and manganese are known to give a metallic taste to drinking water.

The quality of water from some surface and ground sources is usually satisfactory for ordinary uses, but water may be chlorinated as a precaution against chance contamination by microorganisms.

Chlorination itself has recently been reported to be linked in some studies to increased cancer rates in some communities. However, the studies do not establish a causal relationship (6).

The World Health Organization and the U.S. Public Health Service have established a standard of biological quality for drinking water. This standard is that there should be not more than one disease-producing bacteria (coliform organism) per 100 ml of water. There are still so many parts of the world without safe and sanitary drinking water that the United Nations has declared 1981-1990 as the International Drinking-Water Supply and Sanitation Decade (7).

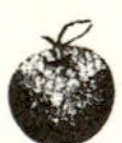

health considerations

Bottled Water

Is water worth 25 cents a glass? The advertisers for imported and domestic bottled water hope to convince consumers that it is, even though tap water is nearly free. Bottled-water consumption has become a trend in some areas of the United States. To the extent that it replaces overuse of alcoholic beverages there is no question that it benefits health.

As for taste, the winner of a recent Consumer Reports test of tap water and three dozen unmarked varieties of bottled water was tap water from New York City. All but one of the tested sparkling waters, which contain bubbles of carbon dioxide that can exaggerate unwanted flavors, were perceived to have at least some bitter taste (8).

Technically, all water except distilled water is mineral water. California recently instituted regulations that define a mineral water as having 500 parts per million or more of "total dissolved solids," a figure that acts as a general standard. The U.S. Department of Agriculture (USDA) has not yet officially defined mineral water. So-called mineral waters may have as much as 200 to 400 milligrams (mg) of sodium per 8-oz glass. People watching their intake of sodium should be aware of this fact.

The decision to substitute bottled water for tap water sometimes follows publicity about constituents of tap water. Because water is a natural solvent, and even "pure" rain water contains many other substances such as dissolved gases, it is not surprising that there are minerals in tap water. There has been no evidence of harmful effects of normal constituents of most all tap water in the United States.

Water Activity of Foods

Food has been preserved by drying, so that it resists microbial and chemical deterioration, since antiquity. The physical-chemical basis of this process was not described until the 1950s when the concept of water activity (a_w) was introduced.

The *water activity* of a food is defined as the ratio of the vapor pressure of water in the food divided by the vapor pressure of pure water at the same temperature (9). Water activity is an important factor influencing the growth of microorganisms. Maximum water activity standards have been established for various food products so that spoilage and growth of food-poisoning microorganisms may be prevented.

It is now generally accepted that water activity is more closely related to the physical, chemical, and biological properties of foods than is total moisture content, the previous measure used. For example, water activity, as well as water temperature, may have direct effects on certain chemical reactions, enzyme reactions, and the growth rate of organisms. Specific aspects of food such as aroma, flavor, texture, and stability have all been shown to be related to specific narrow ranges of water activity. The concept of water activity is of particular interest and importance to food scientists and food technologists, since it relates to the effects of water on changes that occur during storage. Thus it is an influence on food processing and storage practices, such as the processing and preservation of leafy vegetables, cheese, and dried fish.

Metabolism and Function

As a major constituent of the cells of all animal and vegetable tissue, water is present in every chemical reaction that takes place in every cell in the body. In many reactions, such as hydration, when the water molecule is added to a substance, water actually enters into the reactions.

Water is the main component and medium of all body fluids, secretions, and excretions: blood plasma, lymph, bile, digestive juices, urine, and perspiration. In it are dissolved or suspended the vital chemicals of the body. (See Table 13-2 for a summary of water's important functions in the body.)

Ingested Water. Most of the water consumed is reabsorbed throughout the length of the intestinal tract. Only about 100 to 200 ml of water are lost daily in the stool. Depending on the rate of growth, about 0.5 to 3 percent of the fluid intake is actually retained by the body. The rest is lost through normal physiological processes. (See the section on water balance and the following section on excretion.)

Although not much water is absorbed in the stomach, water is necessary throughout the gastrointestinal tract for digestion. The products of digestion are made soluble in water and pass through the intestinal cell walls to enter the blood stream. There, the water of the blood carries the nutrients to all cells of the body and carries away the waste products: carbon dioxide to the lungs and excess salts and nitrogen compounds to the kidneys.

During a twenty-four-hour period, more than 7.6 liters (8 qt) of water are secreted into the digestive tract in the form of digestive juices. This water is also reabsorbed with the products of digestion. Thus, the body recycles its water content over and over for different purposes before excreting it.

Excreted Water. As noted in the section on water balance, water is excreted primarily through the kidneys as urine, the skin as perspiration, and the lungs as water vapor in expired air.

The waste products along with large volumes of water leave the blood stream and

Table 13–2 THE FUNCTIONS OF WATER IN THE BODY

- Major component of cell structure and body fluids
- Medium for cellular reactions
- Transport of nutrients, ions, and oxygen
- Part of chemical digestion process
- Transport and excretion of waste products
- Regulation of body temperature
- Cushion for body tissues
- Lubrication for body joints
- Moisture for respiratory system function
- Necessary for proper muscle structure and function

are collected in the collecting tubules of the nephron, the basic structural unit of the kidney. Much of the water and certain useful nutrients are reabsorbed during their passage through these tubules. The kidneys actively secrete other substances to form the final product—urine. Urine is secreted continuously (although more rapidly under certain stimuli) and is collected in the urinary bladder.

The kidneys of an average healthy adult filter a total quantity of about 200 liters (about 50 gallons) of water a day. Most of this (about 99 percent) is recycled water and is again reabsorbed into the blood for reuse. The final amount of water excreted as urine is highly variable and is dependent upon the amount lost through other channels and on the amount of water intake. Urine is about 96 percent water.

The amount of water lost through the skin is influenced by body area, body temperature, environmental temperature, and the level of physical activity. Under usual conditions this water evaporates as fast as it is excreted through the skin through the process of *insensible perspiration.* The amount lost is about 800 ml daily with no loss of salt unless there is a high activity level and/or a high environmental temperature. In these conditions water loss from the skin can go much higher (up to 2500 ml per hour has been reported) and visible perspiration results. It contains salt, other electrolytes, and other substances found in blood plasma.

The loss of water through the lungs is about 400 ml a day and is increased by strenuous activity, high altitudes, and low humidity (such as those encountered by the climbers of Everest).

Regulation of Excretion through the Kidneys. Water loss in the urine is under the control of a pituitary-renal mechanism. The pituitary gland secretes the antidiuretic hormone discussed previously, which causes the kidneys to conserve water. This is accomplished through the effect of the ADH on increasing water reabsorption by the renal tubules, and the result is a low-urine output and a high-urine osmolality (high concentration of dissolved solutes). In contrast, the absence of the ADH results in an increased urinary water loss, since the tubules no longer have the ADH stimulus to increase water reabsorption. Urine volume is increased and osmolality is decreased. Specialized *osmoreceptors,* which are located in the hypothalamus, monitor the osmolality of body fluid and influence the rate of secretion of the ADH, which will in turn regulate the osmolality to its relatively constant level.[1] This is an example of *feedback control,* such as is found in many other important systems of the body.

For a summary of factors influencing the release of ADH from the posterior pituitary gland, see Table 13-3.

Dietary factors can also be important in renal excretion. For example, coffee and tea act as *diuretics* by increasing urine flow, as a result of their content of caffeine and related substances. These increase the rate of blood flow through the kidneys and alter the transport of salts and water by tubule cells. Another diuretic, alcohol, brings about increased urine flow by depressing the production of ADH. There is a limit to the extent of concentration that the kidneys can achieve, and if substances to be excreted are present in excessive quantities additional water is required to dilute them. Normally, drinking more water can supply this need, but if the water supply is limited, the extra water needed is drawn from body fluids or tissues. This is why drinking sea water, which has a high content of salts, takes water

[1]In the healthy person, plasma osmolality remains at 285-295 milliosmoles (units of measure for osmolality) per kilogram (kg) regardless of day-to-day changes in water and solute intake.

Table 13–3 FACTORS THAT AFFECT ANTIDIURETIC HORMONE SECRETION

INCREASED ANTIDIURETIC HORMONE SECRETION (and subsequent renal conservation of water):

- Increased osmolality of extracellular fluid
- Decreased vascular or extracellular fluid volume (body water deficiency)
- Certain drugs (e.g., nicotine)
- Pain, anxiety

DECREASED ANTIDIURETIC HORMONE SECRETION (and subsequent increased urinary water loss):

- Decreased osmolality of extracellular fluid
- Increased volume of extracellular fluid (body water excess)
- Certain drugs (e.g., alcohol)

away from the body and thus is damaging to water-deprived castaways. Excretion of the large amounts of urea formed as a result of a very high protein intake may also require extra water.

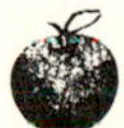

health considerations

Water and the Athlete

Mistaken beliefs and well-meaning but potentially harmful practices concerning the water intake of athletes abound (see also Chap. 21). One such false belief is that water should not be consumed during strenuous activity; some coaches feel that drinking water during exercise will lead to muscle weakness and cramps. Thus, they may limit the water intake of players before a game, not realizing that fatigue and body dysfunction may be caused by excessive dehydration.

The fact is that water in sufficient quantities seems to improve physical effort, as has been previously pointed out. In experiments with dogs, giving them additional water has been shown to produce an increase in endurance and working ability up to 80 percent. The dogs performed longer on a treadmill test, expending only 1,191 kcal without extra water and 2,141 kcal with an average of 1.5 liters (about 1.5 qt) of extra water (10).

Since it is now more thoroughly understood that water restriction impairs performance, and dehydration limits the capacity to perform physical tasks, athletes and coaches need to be aware of the signs of a negative water balance so that the hazards of water deprivation may be avoided (11). One sign is diminished volume of urine; volume should be maintained at no less than about 900 ml (almost 1 qt) a day.

An athlete may lose large amounts of water, even 3 to 4 liters (about 3 to 4 qt), during strenuous exercise. Unless this loss is replaced at frequent intervals during the physical activity, heat exhaustion can develop. During a prolonged period of training and competition in hot weather, athletes should drink about 500 ml or so (about 2 cups) of water fifteen minutes before the competition. Lost fluids should continue to be replaced during and/or after the event. Athletes should not depend only on thirst to tell them when water is needed. Both athletes and coaches should be aware of the hazards of water deprivation so that it can be avoided (11).

The salt lost in sweat can be readily replenished with food intake, and should normally not be taken with the water. (See also Chap. 14.)

Another practice seen in some sports is attempt at rapid body weight reduction by severe water restriction. Dehydration can result from forced deprivation of water and can reduce cardiac function, possibly resulting in heart rate abnormalities. Such a practice should not be followed before a sports event or at any other time.

Air Travel. Water loss during air travel is a commonly overlooked problem. The extremely dry air inside the cabin, in combination with rapid air circulation of the plane's ventilation system, can result in very large losses of water by evaporation through the skin. During a three and one-half hour flight in a standard commercial jet, as much as 1 liter, or 1 quart, of water can be lost by one person.

Rehydration Therapy. One advance in nutrition as it relates to water is *oral rehydration* applied to children suffering from dehydration and diarrhea. This recently accepted method, in which liquids are given by mouth rather than through the veins as was previously thought necessary, has been shown to be life saving in many circumstances (12). This method is especially useful in developing countries where the problems of infections are numerous and health workers are few.

Heart Disease. Interest in, and research on, the relationship of the composition of drinking water to heart disease has recently increased (13). Most of the studies have dealt with the calcium and magnesium found in hard water or with the possibility that soft water (low in calcium and magnesium) may dissolve toxic metals from water pipes. Relationships for several drinking-water constituents have been reported, but no single factor has been found to be strongly and consistently associated with heart disease. For example, there is some evidence of an association between several inorganic substances in water—sodium, lead, nitrates, calcium, and magnesium—and blood pressure, but the evidence is insufficient to prove any direct relationship. Some studies, first reported in 1957 in Japan, point to an association of soft drinking water and higher rates of death from coronary heart disease.

Three hypothetical reasons for these associations are as follows. (1) The elemental constituents of hard water exhibit a protective effect, possibly by lowering intestinal absorption of toxic metals. (2) Trace elements normally associated with hard water could provide a protective effect. (3) Trace constituents present in soft water (such as cadmium and lead) could have a harmful effect on health. These hypotheses are being actively studied. It is also as yet unclear whether the reported adverse effect of soft water on the incidence of heart disease in some studies may be due to increased hardening of the arteries, increased high blood pressure, or possibly increased heart rate abnormalities.

Since not all of these studies have been confirmed, the association of soft water to heart disease remains just that, an association and not a proven fact. Based on current knowledge, individuals should not hesitate to drink soft water.

MINERALS—GENERAL

About ninety chemical elements occur in nature. (See the Periodic Table of the elements in the Appendix.) The five elements that make up 94 percent of the earth, from the most to the least common, are iron, oxygen, silicon, magnesium, and nickel. Several of the ninety elements have qualities such as radioactivity, inert gaseous form, or high toxicity that make them clearly unsatisfactory for incorporation in living organisms. At the present time, about twenty-four of the ninety are thought to be essential to life. They include the elements hydrogen and oxygen, combined in water, which, together with carbon and nitrogen, make up 96 percent of body weight and 99 percent of the body's atoms. They also include inorganic elements, most of which are minerals, which will be discussed generally here and in particular in succeeding chapters.

A *mineral* is defined as a naturally occurring inorganic substance with a characteristic set of physical properties. The *nutrient minerals* are themselves elements and thus are chemically simpler substances than the vitamins, which are organic compounds composed of elements such as carbon, hydrogen, and oxygen.

It is interesting to note that only two of the twenty-four or so elements known to be essential for human and animal life have an atomic number over 34. Both of them (molybdenum and iodine) are needed in only trace amounts. The four most abundant elements in living organisms listed previously all have atomic numbers under 10. The seven next most abundant (calcium, phosphorus, potassium, sulfur, sodium, magnesium, and chlorine), all minerals, have atomic weights under 21. These eleven elements together make up more than 99.9 percent of the atoms in the human body.

Functions

Minerals, like vitamins, are not formed in the body but must be supplied from an external source. Their presence or absence means the difference between normal and abnormal functioning of the body. As a group, the nutritionally essential minerals are vital for optimal health and well-being; they are needed for the normal structure and function of body cells, tissues, and systems. Typical physiological functions include bone formation, enzyme activation, maintenance of water balance, and hormonal function. Individual minerals have special functions, which will be discussed separately.

Discovery

Knowledge about the character of the elements has developed relatively recently. Ancient peoples were aware of the existence of gold, silver, copper, tin, lead, iron, tin, and mercury since these elements occur free in nature, but they did not understand their role as chemical elements. The early Greeks thought that all material was made of certain basic elements, but they proposed only four—earth, water, air, and fire. The Swiss-born alchemist Paracelsus, in the early 1500s, attempted to explain substances by three alchemical building blocks: sulfur, "the principle of combustion"; salt, "the fixed part left after burning"; and mercury, "the essential part of all metals." The alchemists were interested in making precious metal, and Paracelsus proposed that gold and silver were combinations of sulfur and mercury.

The British scientist Robert Boyle, in the *Skeptical Chemist* (1661), first defined the word element, in the sense that it retained until the discovery of radioactivity in 1896, as a form of matter that could not be split into simpler forms. One of the first true elements to be isolated was phosphorus by a German alchemist, Hennig Brand, in 1669. The first scientific list of the then-recognized elements was made by the "Father of Chemistry," Antoine Lavoisier of France, in 1789. There were thirty-three substances on the list, twenty-three of which were actual elements and ten of which eventually proved to be compounds.

The development of a new scientific technique occasionally led to several elements being discovered in succession. In 1807, for example, Sir Humphrey Davy had used electrical current to break compounds down into elements and soon discovered potassium, sodium, aluminum, barium, calcium, magnesium, and strontium. By the end of the nineteenth century, a total of eighty-two elements had been identified.

Element 43, which had not been previously identified, was discovered by Emilio Segré in the 1930s by bombarding molybdenum with charged particles in a cyclotron. He called the newly discovered element technetium since it was the first element actually produced by humans using artificial technical methods. It is unstable and does not exist long in nature. Nearly all recently identified elements have been discovered in this general manner. All elements with a nuclear charge number of 85 or over are unstable; weighable quantities do not exist in nature and they depend on modern nuclear techniques for their formation.

Macrominerals and Trace Elements

Seven minerals that are present in the body in amounts greater than 0.01 percent of body weight are the *macrominerals,* or major minerals. They are required in the human diet in amounts larger than 100 mg per day. Minerals that are present in the body in extremely small amounts and are required in amounts less than 100 mg per day are *microminerals,* or *trace elements.* (See Chap. 16 and 17.) Both are necessary for the biochemical and physiological well-being of the human organism. They are listed in Table 13-4.

The macrominerals are the electrolytes sodium, potassium, and chloride (see Chap. 14) and calcium, phosphorus, and magnesium (see Chap. 15). Inorganic forms of these six macrominerals take care of all their dietary needs. Sulfur is also considered a macromineral and is unique as a mineral nutrient in being required almost exclusively in the form of sulfur-containing amino acids; limited use can be made of sulfur salts.

The trace elements include nickel, vanadium, silicon, and arsenic, microminerals that are thought to be probably essential in very small quantities but for which no specific requirements have been set. Tin, boron, tungsten, cadmium, and lead are trace elements for which human requirements are unknown; some animal studies suggest that they may have essential functions, but the evidence is not yet conclusive nor convincing (see Chap. 17).

Table 13–4 ESSENTIAL DIETARY MINERALS AND ELEMENTS

Macrominerals	*Trace Elements or Microminerals*
Sodium	Iron
Potassium	Iodine
Chlorine	Copper
Calcium	Manganese
Phosphorus	Zinc
Magnesium	Fluorine
Sulfur[a]	Cobalt[a]
	Molybdenum
	Selenium
	Chromium
	Nickel
	Vanadium
	Silicon
	Arsenic (?)

[a]Needed in organic form.

Minerals as Salts and in Organic Compounds

An element is "in the free state" when it is not chemically combined with another element. About thirty elements (including gold, zinc, platinum, and copper) may be found in the free state in nature. Body tissues generally do not use minerals in the free state but only when they are combined with another element in the form of *inorganic salts.*

The general definition of a *salt* is the combination of any negatively charged element or group (except hydroxyl, OH^-) with any positively charged element or group (except hydrogen, H^+). The exceptions exist because of the formation of *acids* with the H^+ addition, and *bases* with the OH^- addition. Table salt, the combination of Na^+ with Cl^-, is the best known example of a salt.

Minerals may be present as salts in foods, but they return to their *ionic* (positively or negatively charged element) state during digestion. The important electropositive elements (cations) for the body's functions are Ca^{++} for calcium; Mg^{++} for magnesium; K^+ for potassium; and Na^+ for sodium. The important electronegative elements (anions) are P^{---} for phosphorus (also with 5 negative charges); S^{--} for sulfur (also with 4 and 6 negative charges), and Cl^- for chloride.

These mineral ions are water-soluble, and the small amounts necessary are important throughout the body for such functions as activation of enzymes and maintenance of water and acid-base balance (see also Chap. 14).

While some minerals exist in foods and tissues as inorganic salts, several others are found in organic complexes, bound to or part of an organic compound. Examples include iron in the hemoglobin molecule, which we ingest in meat, cobalt in the structure of vitamin B-12, iodine in the hormone thyroxine, and sulfur in amino acids. Most of the essential trace elements are constituents of enzymes. Utilization of the mineral in organic form depends on such factors as solubility, strength of chemical bonds, and absorbability. Since minerals are basic elements, they are not broken down or digested into any other substances but maintain their original chemical form.

Dietary Essential Elements

In the latest edition of the Food and Nutrition Board's recommended dietary allowances (RDA), specific dietary allowances are included for calcium, phosphorus, magnesium, iron, zinc, and iodine; estimated safe and adequate daily dietary intake ranges are set for copper, manganese, fluoride, chromium, selenium, molybdenum, sodium, potassium, and chlorine. Nickel, vanadium, and silicon are listed as elements that may prove to be essential for humans. Cadmium, lead, and mercury are toxic elements, probably not essential, which can be present in foods at levels high enough to be of concern. There are also many elements ubiquitous in nature and commonly found in animal tissues for which no metabolic role has yet been identified. Some appear to be harmless, some toxic. (See Chap. 17.)

The recommended dietary allowances for the essential macro- and microminerals are summarized inside the front and back covers and are also presented in the appropriate chapter. The range of recommended dietary allowances is from 150 micrograms (μg) a day for iodine to 1200 mg a day for calcium and phosphorus.

Deficiencies

Research in recent years has increased knowledge and appreciation of the nutritional importance of adequate supplies of the essential minerals in our diet. Deficiency states in humans involving zinc, copper, chromium, selenium, and molybdenum have been described within the past two decades. Electrolyte deficiencies and imbalances can be life threatening. Calcium, iron, and iodine deficiencies (and others) have been clinically described for some time.

Toxicity

Above a defined level, all the elements are toxic to humans; good health is achieved when the balance of elements is correct in terms of body requirements. Specific toxic effects in humans have been described for each of the elements.

The mineral elements have been divided into four categories with respect to pollution hazard: low, moderate, high, and very high. Those mineral elements classified as "very high" are silver, gold, cadmium, chromium, copper, mercury, lead, antimony, tin, thallium, and zinc (14). Although the majority of these elements have relatively high molecular weights and are not essential nutrients, one will recognize three nutrient minerals in the list. Their listing simply confirms that nearly everything is toxic if present in high enough quantities.

Metabolism of Minerals

Minerals vary in the amounts absorbed, in their form of transport in the body, in the exact function they perform, and in their routes of excretion. The location of absorption, the same for all minerals, is throughout the small intestine. Some are absorbed in the free ion form, and others require carrier molecules. Retention of elements in tissues usually depends on associations with organic compounds. It is estimated that for every gram of protein retained by the body, such as during growth, 0.3 gm of mineral matter is deposited.

Interactions between and among mineral elements must be recognized in considering their nutritional effect on the body. While some interactions, such as that of calcium and zinc, are well defined, others are as yet poorly understood.

Minerals ingested together in a meal may compete in the process of absorption. Also, high intakes of one mineral can influence the handling of a second mineral not ingested at the same time. For example, if one mineral is constantly ingested in high quantities, such as with routine mineral supplementation, a blocking protein may be formed in the intestine. This blocking protein may act to block another, chemically similar mineral as well as the first mineral (it should be remembered that some essential minerals differ by only one or two protons in the nucleus). The result can be that an unwanted and unforeseen deficiency of the second mineral is produced.

Distribution in Food

In planning a diet that will furnish enough of any mineral element, one must consider three questions. (1) How much of the mineral element is present in different foods? (2) What foods furnish it in easily utilizable form? (3) Which of the foods are rich enough in the mineral to contribute substantially to the daily quota?

The answers to these questions are discussed in the chapters on the individual minerals. The first and third questions can also be approached by looking up foods in the Table of the Nutritive Value of Foods in the Appendix for those minerals listed there (calcium, phosphorus, magnesium, sodium, potassium, zinc, copper, and iron).

Authorities agree that, in general, a daily diet made up of a wide variety of foods chosen with some degree of care from each of the basic four food groups, and consumed in quantities sufficient to meet total energy needs, almost certainly will provide the nutrient minerals in required quantities. (See "Health Considerations.")

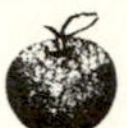

health considerations

Mineral Supplements

With increasing knowledge about the importance of the essential minerals to health, many adults are concerned about taking mineral supplements in the form of pills and capsules. In most instances, the authors do not recommend supplements unless prescribed by a responsible physician. A well-balanced, varied diet supplying the recommended number of calories is sufficient to meet the basic mineral needs. In addition, detrimental mineral interactions may occur if high quantities of minerals are regularly consumed, resulting possibly in decreased utilization of some of the essential minerals. The net effect of mineral supplements may be more harmful than beneficial, and adverse effects from nutrient imbalance may outweigh the supposed benefits of the additional minerals.

Therefore, if one is on a low-calorie diet and there is a question about mineral adequacy, it is best to supplement with foods rich in the minerals in question. Many mineral-rich foods are also low in calories and make good, protective foods for those on diets. (A few examples include vegetables such as brussel sprouts and broccoli; green leafy vegetables and beans; whole-grain products; seafood, fish, poultry, eggs, and lean meat; and skim milk and lowfat yogurt or cottage cheese.) Food sources of iron, calcium, magnesium, and zinc are especially important.

In instances of extreme diets or health-related questions, the physician should make the final decision as to the need for specific mineral supplements.

For a discussion of supplements in the diets of infants and children, see Chapter 23; also see Chapter 20.

For exceptions to the general advice on mineral supplements given in this section, see the discussions of each individual mineral in the appropriate chapters.

QUESTIONS

1. How much water is present in the body? How does water content change with age? Into what compartments is water divided?

2. By what routes is water lost from the body? What is the first sign of water depletion? What is the average range of daily water loss from the body?

3. Keep a record of your total intake of water for one day—that is, the amount taken as water, soup, tea, coffee, milk, and other beverages. How does your intake compare with the amount that most persons should take either in beverages or as drinking water? What is meant by "metabolic water"?

4. How much additional water intake is needed to compensate for the amount lost as sweat produced from playing tennis for one hour indoors? (Use the data on energy cost of activities given in Chap. 6.)

5. What is the ADH and what are two factors that increase its secretion? Decrease its secretion?

6. List five physiological functions of water in the body.

7. Which elements are most abundant in the body? What substances are classed as mineral, or ash? Why? How much mineral is found in the body?

8. What differentiates a macromineral from a trace element? Explain the difference between a vitamin and an essential mineral.

9. Describe the general functions of the essential minerals and why they are needed by the body.

10. Identify some common foods that are relatively low in calories but good sources of minerals. Choose one of these foods and calculate, for one macromineral and one trace element, the percentage of the RDA that would be supplied by one average serving of this food. (Use the Recommended Dietary Allowances table inside front cover and the Nutritive Value of Foods in the Appendix.)

References

1. Leung, H. K.: Structure and properties of water. Cereal Foods World, *26*:350, 1981.
2. Stults, V. J., Morgan, K. J., and Zabik, M. E.: Children's and teenagers' beverage consumption patterns. School Food Service Research Rev., *6*:20, 1982.
3. Partidge, J. C., et al.: Water intoxication secondary to feeding mismanagement. Amer. J. Dis. Children, *135*:38, 1981.
4. Safe Drinking Water Committee, National Research Council: *The Disinfection of Drinking Water.* Board on Toxicology and Environmental Health Hazards, Assembly of Life Sciences, National Research Council, 1979.
5. Masironi, R.: Trace elements in water. Nutr. Food Sci., No. *56*:15, 1979, Masironi, R.: How trace elements in water contribute to health. WHO Chronicle, *32*:382, 1978.
6. Maugh, T. H.: New study links chlorination and cancer. Science, *211*:694, 1981.
7. A challenge to developing countries: the International Drinking-Water Supply and Sanitation Decade, 1981–1990. WHO Chronicle, *34*:327, 1980.
8. The selling of H_2O. Consumer Reports, *45*:531, 1980.
9. Labuza, T. P.: The effect of water activity on reaction kinetics of food deterioration. Food Tech., *34*:36, 1980; Rockland, L. B., and Nishi, S. K.: In-

fluence of water activity on food product quality and stability. Food Tech., *34*:42, 1980; Franks, F.: Cereal Foods World, *27*:403, 1982.
10. Young, D. R., et al.: Effect of time after feeding and carbohydrate or water supplement on work in dogs. J. Appl. Physiol., *14*:1013, 1959.
11. Committee on Nutritional Misinformation, National Research Council: Water deprivation and performance of athletes. Food and Nutrition Board Statement, National Academy of Sciences, 1974.
12. Hirschhorn, N.: Oral rehydration therapy for diarrhea in children—A basic primer. Nutr. Rev., *40*:97, 1982.
13. (Water hardness and cardiovascular disease) Comstock, G.: J. Env. Pathol. and Toxicol., *4*:9, 1980; Folsom, A. R., and Prineas, R. J.: Amer. J. Epidem., *115*:818, 1982; Joyce, M.: J. Environ. Health, *43*:134, 1980.
14. Bowen, H. J. M.: *Trace Elements in Biochemistry.* New York, Academic Press, 1966.

14 The Electrolytes (Sodium, Potassium, and Chlorine) and Acid-Base Balance

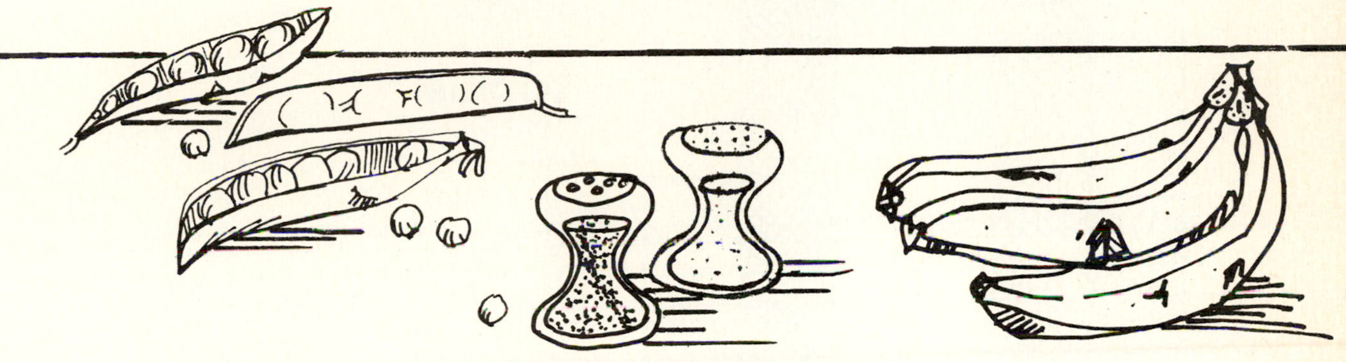

The preceding chapter discussed the importance of water to the body. One vital role of water is to serve as a medium for the dissolved salts necessary for proper functioning of the body. Salts dissolved in water and in body fluids and cells are considered to be completely separated into their electrically charged *ions.*[1] For example, the salt sodium chloride (NaCl), becomes Na^+ and Cl^- in solution. Chemicals such as the salts that separate into oppositely charged ions are also called *electrolytes;* nonelectrolytes are substances that do not separate into ions. Glucose and urea are two examples of nonelectrolytes. Electrolytes in solution, because of the charged ionic particles, will conduct an electric current. (A battery works on this principle.)

The sum of the positive ions (*cations*) in an electrolyte solution must equal the sum of the negative ions (*anions*), according to *the law of electric neutrality.* This law also holds true in the body; in Figure 14–1 the two columns representing anions and cations in either fluid compartment must be equal to each other. This figure also represents the relative differences in the major cations (Na^+ and K^+), and the major anions (Cl^- and phosphate [$HPO_4^{=}$]) in extracellular versus intracellular fluids.

The electrolyte ions, since they are particles, are largely responsible for normal conditions of *osmotic pressure,* which is directly proportional to the number of particles in a solution.

[1]A positively charged ion is electron-deficient (it has lost one or more electrons when dissolved in water); a negatively charged ion has surplus electrons (it has gained electrons when dissolved).

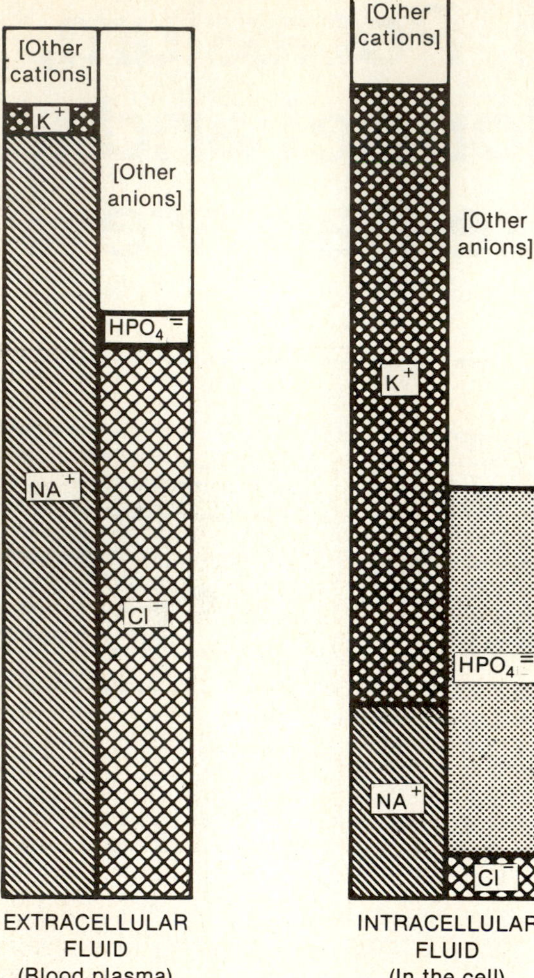

Figure 14–1 Relative differences of sodium, potassium, chloride, and phosphate in the electrolyte content of intracellular and extracellular fluid. Other electrolytes which have important roles in body fluids include the cations calcium and magnesium and the anions sulfate and carbonate. Much of the energy produced in the body's metabolic processes is used to establish and maintain the high concentration of K^+ and the low concentration of Na^+ within the cells, the opposite of the relative concentrations of these electrolytes in the fluids outside the cell. (See also Chap. 13.) This electrolyte relationship is necessary for normal functions of living cells and body systems.

Electrolyte imbalances, along with water balance disturbances, can cause a multitude of physiological problems. Thus, an intricate knowledge of the functions and balance of electrolytes is very important to those in health fields, particularly to those caring for persons with kidney, metabolic, and nutritional problems and those on diuretics.

The electrolytes that are also nutrient elements are sodium, potassium, and chloride, to be discussed in this chapter, and calcium and magnesium (and phosphorus as phosphate), which will be discussed in the following chapter.

SODIUM

Sodium, the sixth most abundant element on earth, is a soft, white, silvery metal. Sodium's symbol, Na, is from the Latin *natrium,* which means "soda." It is a very active element chemically, combining easily with other elements to form many different compounds, of which NaCl, or table salt, is the most familiar. Pure sodium is not found in nature; it was first isolated by Sir Humphry Davy in 1807. When the atom of sodium loses its outer-shell electron, it becomes a positively charged ion, which is relatively stable and is important to normal body functioning.

The terms sodium and salt are sometimes used interchangeably, but their meanings need to be clearly differentiated. One recent survey indicated that these two terms had equal meaning for two-thirds of the respondents (1). *Sodium* is the elemental nutrient while *salt* commonly means sodium chloride, which contains about 40 percent of sodium. Salt is also a general term for any compound with a positive and a negative ion. One should keep the differences firmly in mind, whether reading through this chapter or reading labels on foods.

Salt in History

A significant portion of the sodium in the human diet has long been derived from sodium chloride. Salt was probably the first food additive ever used, as soon as people discovered its ability to flavor food and to preserve meat and fish. There are many written references to salt throughout history. In Job 6:6 we find the following, "Can that which is unsavory be eaten without salt? Is there any taste in the white of an egg?"

The importance of salt as an item of commerce also dates back to ancient times. Salt trading was an active enterprise in antiquity and the Middle Ages as inland peoples traded with coastal peoples for the salt they needed. The word salary comes from the use of salt as a form of payment to Roman soldiers. Close association of salt with money was also noted by the Venetian merchant Marco Polo during his travels in China in the 13th century; he found that salt, in the form of salt cakes stamped with the khan's sign, was used as payment for gold.

The most abundant and widespread source of salt is the ocean. For centuries people have evaporated sea water in the sun or boiled it over fires to obtain the salt. There are also natural salt deposits, which have been mined. (See Fig. 14–2.)

Sodium Deficiency Symptoms

In a classic experiment with a dairy herd, S. M. Babcock of the University of Wisconsin investigated the need of animals for salt. One-half of the herd were given their usual feed, which included salt; the other half were given unsalted feed. The effect of salt deprivation did not show up immediately, although the salt-deprived cows soon showed by their actions, such as licking the soil, that they craved salt. Gradually they lost appetite, became emaciated, gave less milk, and produced very weak calves, which frequently did not live. In similar experiments, when salt was re-fed to cows, they experienced a dramatic return to their former state of good health. In later animal experiments, it was proven that sodium itself, not only as sodium chloride, is an essential nutrient.

In humans the signs of sodium deficiency or depletion include loss of appetite, loss of thirst, severe muscle cramps and weakness,

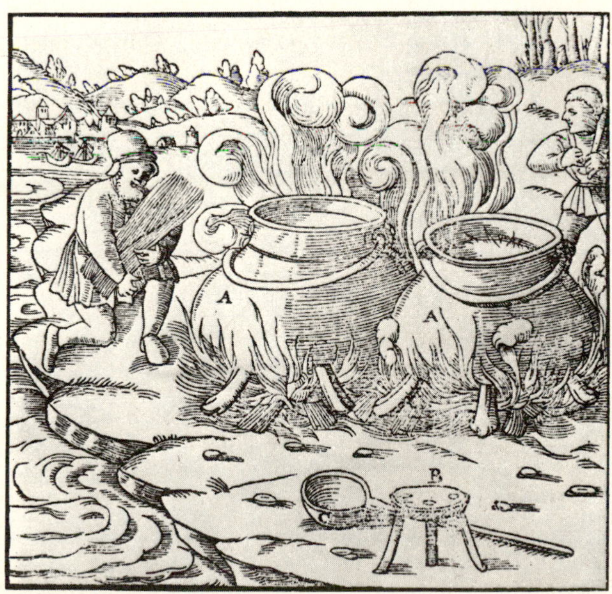

Figure 14–2 Salt has always been a desired commodity for food flavoring and preservation. Here the boiling of sea water or brine for extraction of salt is depicted (from a 16th century drawing) (2).

vomiting, irritability, low serum sodium (hyponatremia), and ultimately confusion, circulatory collapse, coma, and death.

Sodium deficiency or depletion is unusual in healthy persons because normal diets easily contain the minimal sodium requirements. Sodium deficiency is possible in areas where meat and fish are scarce and where vegetables are the primary food.

Acute sodium depletion may occur, however, in conditions of ill health, such as diarrhea and kidney disease, or of excessive sweating caused by heavy physical activity in hot climates. In the tropics, workmen may lose 10 or 15 liters of sweat a day, an amount that contains 10 grams (gm) or so of sodium chloride. Although the normal kidney can compensate for most of this salt loss, ongoing losses that are not matched by increased intakes may lead to sodium depletion.

Chapter 13 has discussed the importance of replacing the water losses from heavy sweating, such as may occur in athletic events, with frequent intakes of water. If more than 3 liters of water are drunk to replace sweat loss, then extra salt may be needed, and it can usually be taken either with snacks or a meal (3). If a liquid replacement solution is used, about 2 gm of salt per liter, or 2 teaspoons of salt per gallon, is sufficient and safe. Use of salt tablets is *not* recommended.

Sodium Requirements and Intakes

Sodium is an essential nutrient; we would not be able to survive on a sodium-free diet. Like other electrolytes, it cannot be stored or manufactured in the body but must be taken in food. The precise minimum daily requirement of sodium for adults has not been definitely established, since the body conserves this element so effectively. The absolute minimal requirement may be approximately 200 milligrams (mg), an amount that would replace the minimal amount of sodium lost from the body.

For infants and children, the minimal requirement is somewhat less; one liter of breast milk contains 160 mg per liter, which is sufficient to keep infants in sodium balance. In pregnancy, the sodium requirements increase by about 70 mg a day more than for nonpregnant females; this amount is easily provided by the diet.

The Food and Nutrition Board has published "safe and adequate daily dietary intake ranges" for sodium and other electrolytes, which are presented in Table 14–1. In the United States today, sodium chloride is second only to sugar in the total amount

Table 14–1 ESTIMATED SAFE AND ADEQUATE DAILY DIETARY INTAKES OF THE MINERAL ELECTROLYTES[a]

	Age (years)	*Sodium (mg)*	*Potassium (mg)*	*Chloride (mg)*
Infants	0–0.5	115–350	350–925	275–700
	0.5–1	250–750	425–1275	400–1200
Children and Adolescents	1–3	325–975	550–1650	500–1500
	4–6	450–1350	775–2325	700–2100
	7–10	600–1800	1000–3000	925–2775
	11+	900–2700	1525–4575	1400–4200
Adults		1100–3300	1875–5625	1700–5100

[a]Because there is less information on which to base allowances, these figures are not given in the main table of RDA and are provided in the form of ranges of recommended intakes. Source: Food and Nutrition Board, National Academy of Sciences, 1980.

added to food each year. When adults have free access to salt, their intake of sodium ranges between 2300 mg and 6900 mg (4). (This is equivalent to about 6 to 17 gm of sodium chloride). The 1978 Food and Drug Administration (FDA) diet studies lead to an estimate that an adult consumes an average of about 5000 mg of sodium a day. This is equivalent to about 12 gm of sodium chloride. The average daily intake of sodium, in sodium chloride equivalents, amounts to more than 9 pounds (4 kg) of salt consumed by each person per year.

The salt intake of infants increases three- to four-fold when the infant begins to consume the family's table foods and ceases its diet of no-added-salt, prepared infant foods (5).

Recent concern and publicity about a possible link between high blood pressure and a high sodium intake (see section on this topic) has helped to spur consumer interest in levels of salt consumption. According to a recent survey, about three of four consumers interviewed said that they try to avoid serving foods high in salt content (6).

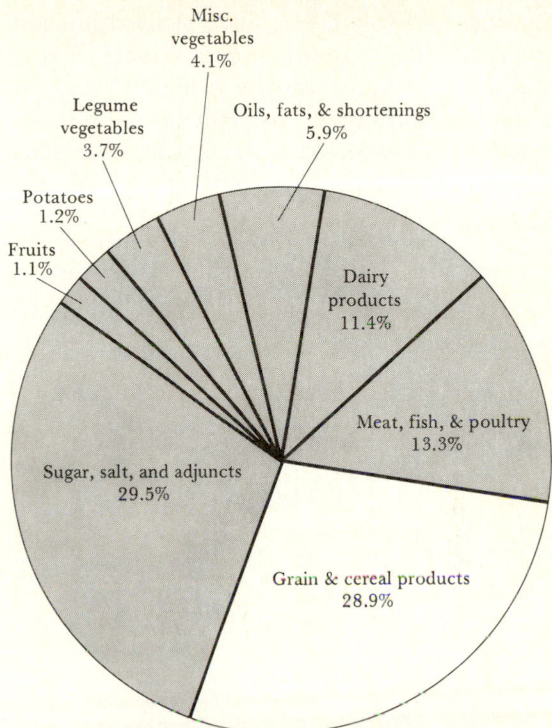

Figure 14–3 Average sodium content by commodity groups in adult market baskets (collections of retail food from four U.S. geographic regions). (Adapted from the FDA 1978 Total Diet Studies data, as published in "Sodium and Potassium in Foods and Drugs," American Medical Association.) (7) It can be seen that cereals and grains make up the largest source of sodium after table salt, then meat, fish and poultry, and the third food group as sodium source is milk-dairy products. Soups are not differentiated on this graph, but dietary recall surveys have indicated that soups may contribute up to 10 percent of a typical day's sodium intake from foods (8).

Food Sources of Sodium

Sodium chloride and other sodium compounds accumulate in foods in three ways: (1) as a natural food ingredient, (2) as an addition during processing for flavoring and/or preserving, and (3) added by the consumer, usually as table salt, in preparing and eating foods at home. Only about 25 to 30 percent of the average daily intake is found naturally in foods. Groups of foods and how much they contribute to average sodium intake are shown in Figure 14–3.

Nearly all foods contain at least small quantities of sodium. Cheese and shellfish are rich sources of sodium; and milk, meat, fish, poultry, and eggs make significant contributions. Fresh fruits and vegetables are very low in this nutrient, but commercially processed vegetables routinely have additional salt for flavor. Cereals, bread, and baked goods contain moderate amounts. Water supplies and boiled water are quite variable in sodium content but may add to the daily total intake. Commercial fruit-flavored drinks and soft drinks, including diet drinks, can also be not insignificant sources of sodium. In addition, salted snack foods add significant amounts of sodium if eaten frequently and in large quantities. Other possible sources of sodium in the diet are monosodium glutamate (MSG), soy sauce, and baking powder.

Processed foods, including frozen dinners, canned and dry soups, tomato juice, cheese, and canned tuna, can be especially high in sodium content because salt and other sodium compounds have been added to them. For example, just one 8-ounce (oz) serving of canned tomato soup contributes about 75 percent of the lower level and 25 percent of the upper level range of sodium intake suggested by the Food and Nutrition Board.

Since there is much current interest in lower intakes of salt, it should be pointed out that sources of sodium are very often good sources of other important nutrients such as vitamins and other minerals. Because of this relationship, sharply decreasing or eliminating meats, dairy foods, and whole grain foods from one's diet simply to control sodium intake is not recommended for the average healthy person.

The sodium content of some representative foods is presented in Table 14–2, and of various beverages in Table 14–3.

Nonfood products may also be a source of sodium in the diet; for example, antacid medications sometimes contain significant amounts of sodium. There are also about 70 sodium-containing compounds that may be added to foods; a recent FDA study found that more than 75 percent of the food brands surveyed listed one or more sodium-containing substances in their ingredient lists(10). It should be remembered that on a

Table 14–2 SODIUM AND POTASSIUM CONTENT OF SOME REPRESENTATIVE FOODS*
(For Values of Other Common Foods, see Table 2 of Appendix)

Food, 100 gm	*Sodium, mg*	*Potassium, mg*
Apple	1	110
Banana	1	370
Bread, salted	536	273
Bread, unsalted†	38	120
Broccoli, cooked	10	267
Butter, salted	987	23
Butter, unsalted	10	10
Carrot, raw	47	341
Cheese, cheddar	700	82
Chicken, broiled	66	274
Corn, canned, with salt	236	97
Corn, salt-free pack	2	97
Dates, dry	1	648
Egg, cooked in shell	122	129
Hamburger, cooked	47	450
Liver, calf's, fried	118	453
Milk, whole, fluid	50	144
Orange	1	200
Pickle, dill	1428	200
Popcorn, plain	3	660
Popcorn, with oil and salt	1940	512
Potato, French fried	6	853
Potato, French fried, with salt	236	853
Potato chips, salted	up to 1000	1130
Rice, cooked, salted	358	43
Spinach, cooked, no salt	50	324
Tomato, raw	3	244
Tomato juice, canned, with salt	200	227
Wheat, puffed, without salt	4	340
Wheat, puffed, with salt and sugar	161	99

*From Watt, B.K., and Merrill, A.L.: *Composition of Foods: Raw, Processed, Prepared.* Washington, D.C., U.S. Department of Agriculture Handbook No. 8, 1963, except where noted. Where unspecified, values refer to foods cooked without salt.

†Sodium value is for yeast-leavened bread without added salt or sodium propionate (preservative), made with 3 to 4 percent nonfat dry milk solids.

Table 14–3 SODIUM CONTENT OF VARIOUS BEVERAGES[a]

Beverage, 8 oz	*Sodium, mg*
Milk (whole, lowfat, or skim)	120–145
Chocolate milk	150
Tomato juice (6 oz) salt added	555
Apple juice	3
Bottled water:	
Perrier	3
Vichy	330
Coffee, Tea	2
Coca-Cola	18
Seven-Up	60
Diet Pepsi	42
Diet Squirt	2
Diet Rite Cola	62

[a]Values are from manufacturers' data, the USDA, and published reports (9).

food label, the higher on the list an ingredient is placed the larger the quantity of that substance there is in the product. A partial list of these sodium-containing substances is found in Table 14–4.

Sea salt is consumed by many persons throughout the world, some by necessity and some by choice. See Table 14–5 for typical sea salt, sea water, and table salt composition.

The Role of Sodium in the Body

The availability and absorption of sodium in the diet is excellent; virtually all the sodium that is ingested is absorbed in the intestinal tract, mainly in the small intestine. The amount of sodium contained in the body of the average adult male is about 65 gm. Of this total amount 38 gm is found outside cells, 21 gm is in the skeleton, and 6 gm is present inside the body's cells.

Functions. Sodium is the predominant positive ion (cation) in the fluid outside the cells and in the circulating fluids of the body. Potassium is the predominant cation inside the cell. (Refer to Fig. 14–1.) The mechanism that maintains this difference, which is very important for water balance and for normal cellular structure and function, is the *sodium pump.* This action of the cell membrane transports sodium out of the cell and potassium into the cell. Energy is required for this process. If the sodium pump were not present, the cell interior would draw in water from the fluids outside of the cell and would eventually rupture.

Sodium is also important in the transmission of nerve impulses, maintenance of osmotic equilibrium and extracellular fluid volume, heart function, acid-base balance, and the metabolism of protein and carbohydrate.

Table 14–4 SOME SODIUM-CONTAINING SUBSTANCES COMMONLY USED IN THE PREPARATION AND PROCESSING OF FOOD

Sodium Terms To Look for on Labels	
Sodium ascorbate	Disodium inosinate
Sodium citrate	Disodium guanylate
Baking soda	Sodium ferrocyanide
Sodium chloride	Sodium triosulfate
Sodium caseinate	Celery salt
Sodium acid pyrophosphate	Sea salt
Sodium phosphate	Disodium dihydrogen pyrophosphate
Sodium bisulfite	Sodium hexametaphosphate
Disodium phosphate	Sodium gluconate
Sodium iron pyrophosphate	Sodium nitrite
Sodium benzoate	Sodium erythorbate
Garlic salt	Sodium nitrite
Calcium disodium EDTA	Baking powder
Sodium carboxymethyl cellulose	Anhydrous disodium phosphate
Monosodium glutamate	Sodium biphosphate
Sodium preservatives	Salt pork
Trisodium citrate	Brine
Sodium aluminosilicate	Dioctyl sodium sulfosuccinate
Sodium stearoyl-2-lactylate	Onion salt
Sodium propionate	Sodium hydroxide
Sodium saccharin	Sodium metaphosphate
Sodium tripolyphosphate	Sodium thiosulfate
Sodium alginate	Flour (self-rising)

Table 14–5 COMPOSITION OF SEAWATER, SEA SALT, AND TABLE SALT

	*Sea Water** *(per kg)*	*Sea Salt†* *(per kg)*	*Table Salt* *(per kg)*
Sodium, gm	10.6	275	400
Calcium, gm	0.4	8.6	
Magnesium, gm	1.27	34	
Potassium, gm	0.38	1.13	
Silicon, gm	.02-4.0	- ‡	
Iron, μg	2-20	100	
Zinc, μg	5	0.15	
Selenium, μg	4	-	
Lead, μg	4	-	
Tin, μg	3	-	
Cobalt, μg	0.1	0.1-1.0	
Manganese, μg	1-10	0.03-0.3	
Molybdenum, μg	0.5	0.013	
Nickel, μg	0.1	-	
Vanadium, μg	0.3	-	
Copper, μg	3.6	20	
Chloride, gm	19.0	505	600
Bicarbonate, gm	0.14	-	
Nitrate, mg	.001-0.7	-	
Sulfate, gm	2.65	18.3(S)	
Bromine, mg	65	-	
Iodine, μg	50	1.5	
Phosphorus, μg	1-100	0.3	
Fluorine, mg	1.4	.033	

*From Altman, P. L., and Dittmer, D. S.: *Environmental Biology,* Washington, D.C., FASEB, 1966.

†From Kaufman, D. W.: *Sodium Chloride. The Production and Properties of Salt and Brine.* ACS Monograph Series. New York, Reinhold, 1960.

‡(-) indicates no information.

Regulation. The control of the whole body content of sodium (as well as of potassium and water) is regulated by the kidney. Malnutrition can damage the kidney's ability to handle heavy loads of salt, resulting in higher than normal salt levels in the body. (Malnutrition can also impair the normal functioning of the sodium pump.)

The vast majority of ingested sodium is excreted in the urine. During periods of sodium deprivation, the kidney conserves sodium very efficiently.

The hormone *aldosterone* plays a major role in the maintenance of sodium homeostasis, or balance. This hormone comes from the adrenal gland and acts on the tubules of the kidney *nephron* (the structural unit of the kidney) to increase the retention or reabsorption of sodium by the body. If aldosterone levels are low, most of the sodium will not be retained but will be excreted in the urine. See Figure 14–4 for summary of this basic regulatory mechanism. With this knowledge, it is easy to see why a disorder of the adrenal gland, if it resulted in an absence of aldosterone, would seriously jeopardize normal sodium balance in the body by causing increased and constant sodium loss in the urine.

Conversely, if there is improper or diseased kidney function, there is a risk that salt will not be excreted in sufficient quantities, causing a sodium excess in body tissues. This excess in turn draws more water to the tissues so that the normal concentration of body salt can be maintained, thus causing

Situation	*Aldosterone Level*	*Action of Aldosterone on Kidney Tubule*	*Result*
Sodium in diet decreased	Rises	Increased sodium reabsorption (sodium retained in body)	Sodium in urine decreases to very low levels
Sodium in diet increased	Falls	Decreased sodium reabsorption (more sodium excreted in urine)	Sodium in urine at relatively high levels

Figure 14–4 Regulation of sodium excretion by the hormone aldosterone, secreted by the adrenal gland.

edema (excess fluid in body tissues), a frequent symptom of kidney disease.

Another influence on sodium excretion seems to be one of the relatively recently discovered *prostaglandins* (hormone-like chemicals formed from a fatty acid precursor). It has been found to affect the regulation of sodium reabsorption in the kidney tubules (11).

In addition to urinary excretion, sodium can be lost from the body in a variety of body fluids, such as gastrointestinal secretions and perspiration.

Toxicity of Sodium

There is no doubt that sodium can be dangerous and even fatal when consumed in very large amounts. Salt poisoning, although rare, is difficult to treat. The increased sodium in the plasma and the body impairs the kidney's ability to excrete excess solute, and kidney damage may occur.

Humans are well equipped to cope with low sodium intakes, since the kidney can conserve sodium very well when necessary. The kidney has no efficient mechanisms, however, to eliminate a large excess of sodium.

The results of chronic, less dramatic, sodium excess, which may be considered to exist in the American diet, is a controversial subject, which usually centers on the relationship of sodium intakes to blood pressure.

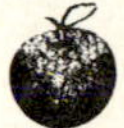

health considerations

Blood Pressure

The possible relationship of sodium intake to high blood pressure[2] is an issue of concern to many. High blood pressure (*hypertension*), generally defined as a blood pressure over 140 (systolic) and/or 90 (diastolic),[3] is a major contributing factor to heart disease and stroke, and it affects about 40 million people in the United States today. The cause of most cases of high blood pressure is unknown.

It is known that significant restriction of sodium intake seems to help lower blood pressure in people already affected by hypertension. Thus, low-sodium diets are usually advised for those under medical care for hypertension. Nevertheless, it does not necessarily follow that consuming less sodium will prevent high blood pressure in people whose blood pressure is normal.

In fact, only about 20 percent of the population is at genetic risk of developing

[2]Blood pressure is defined as the force that flowing blood exerts against artery walls. Systolic pressure occurs when the heart contracts; diastolic pressure, when the heart relaxes between contractions.

[3]Blood pressure is measured in millimeters of mercury (mmHg). The upper level (as usually written) is the systolic pressure, and the lower level, the diastolic pressure. An average healthy blood pressure is 120/80.

hypertension. The other 80 percent of the population are not likely to develop this disease, so any sodium-hypertension relation is not likely to affect them. For those who are at risk, sodium consumption at present levels may help increase their chances of developing high blood pressure.

The evidence for a sodium-blood pressure link is mainly drawn from studies of large populations in which areas of high levels of sodium consumption also tend to have more cases of high blood pressure. Studies such as these are not able to prove a cause-and-effect relationship because, for example, there may be other unidentified reasons for the elevated blood pressure.

A sodium-blood pressure link in animals has been proven: a high sodium intake causes high blood pressure to develop in rats that are susceptible. To date, however, there is no evidence of an actual cause-and-effect relation between salt and high blood pressure in humans.

Recent recommendations have asserted that, even though the majority of the population are not at particular risk from hypertension, most people should moderately decrease their sodium intake. There is certainly no foreseeable harm to be derived from this recommendation. The suggested intake level is about 5 to 6 gm of sodium chloride, or about half of the present level of salt intake. Individuals may, of course, receive advice from their physician to restrict salt to even lower levels. Some suggestions for reducing salt are presented in Figure 14–5.

With the promulgation of these recommendations regarding sodium, consumer interest in the sodium content of foods has increased (12), food experts are reminding us that low-sodium diets do not have to be "bland and tasteless" (13) and the Food and Drug Administration is planning a five-point program that includes the monitoring of the sodium content of the national food supply and new requirements for the sodium content of foods (14).

TO AVOID TOO MUCH SODIUM

Learn to enjoy the unsalted flavors of foods.

Cook with only small amounts of added salt.

Add little or no salt to food at the table.

Limit your intake of salty foods, such as potato chips, pretzels, salted nuts and popcorn, condiments (soy sauce, steak sauce, garlic salt), cheese, pickled foods, cured meats.

Read food labels carefully to determine the amounts of sodium in processed foods and snack items.

Figure 14–5 Suggestions for moderately reducing sodium intake. Source: "Nutrition and Your Health—Dietary Guidelines for Americans," USDA and USDHHS, 1980.

Potassium may also have a significant role in the blood-pressure puzzle. When it is added to the diet of experimental animals, high blood pressure is reduced. It is interesting that, in general, diets high in sodium are often low in potassium. These relationships lead some to reflect that recommendations for less sodium might include encouragement for adequate intake of potassium.

POTASSIUM

Potassium, like sodium, is a soft, whitish, silvery metal, which is chemically very active. Its symbol, K, comes from the Latin *kalium,* meaning "potash," from which its name in English derives. Potash is the alkaline ash of vegetable substances, which is used as a plant fertilizer. Potassium is not found in a free state in nature but is widely distributed in compounds (potassium salts). It was discovered by Davy in 1807.

Potassium is one of the most abundant elements in the body. The total potassium content of the adult body is about 150 to 250 gm. There is some evidence that this total may decrease with age (15). Unlike sodium in the body, potassium is located almost entirely within the cells. It is the primary ion in the intracellular fluid, with a concentration 20 to 30 times that found outside the cell.

Only about 2 percent of body potassium is located in extracellular fluids and bone.

Body potassium is located chiefly in muscle cells; it is also found in skin and other tissues. Potassium is so nearly a constant component of normal lean body tissues that one method of estimating the amount of lean tissue in a living person is by measuring the amount of potassium present.

The body does not store potassium; it must be constantly replenished in the diet. Determinations of the level of potassium in the blood are not necessarily an accurate reflection of total potassium in the body, but these levels are still the major way clinically to detect serious potassium imbalances.

Potassium Deficiency Symptoms

Since potassium is widely found in foods, a pure dietary deficiency is unlikely. Deficiencies are primarily seen in conditions of ill health, such as diarrhea and vomiting, when potassium losses increase, and when medications are given that may cause increased potassium excretion. Diuretics given to increase water excretion and as part of therapy for high blood pressure are a prime example of such medication.

Potassium deficiency affects the kidney, the heart, and the muscles. With severe deficiencies, the kidney shows decreased ability to concentrate the urine as it should, the muscles show degeneration and scarring, and the heart may show an irregular beat. Signs of deficiency in the affected person include loss of appetite, constipation, muscle weakness, fatigue, apathy, confusion, and a depressed mood. Potassium levels in the blood are lowered *(hypokalemia)*. If the potassium deficiency is not recognized and corrected, muscle paralysis and life-threatening heart problems may ensue.

Although healthy people on normal diets as a rule easily receive sufficient potassium, those on very low-calorie reducing diets run a risk of inadequate intake of this nutrient as well as others. This risk is one important reason why a health professional should be involved when people need significantly to reduce calories.

Another special group who should be aware of potential potassium depletion are athletes. Athletes and others who do hard physical work in hot climates may be at risk for a potassium deficiency because of increased losses in sweat. It has been suggested that feelings of weakness and tiredness over a long period of time in an otherwise healthy athlete may be related to this condition, and that athletes in hot climates should be aware of the importance of replenishing potassium by eating potassium-rich foods (16). Short-term exercise, however, apparently does not cause significant potassium depletion (17).

Potassium deficiency is also seen in malnourished children; both low intake of potassium and increased loss in diarrhea are contributing causes. Another probable cause is an impairment of the sodium pump, a defect that compounds problems of sodium and potassium balance.

Another condition that may be associated with hypokalemia is hospitalization. It has been documented that hospitalized patients are more likely than others to have low potassium levels. Of course these patients often already have a medical problem, which may be intensified by inadequate nourishment in the hospital.

Potassium Requirements and Intakes

Potassium is an essential nutrient; without it an organism would die. The Food and Nutrition Board has estimated the minimal requirement for infants and children, based on natural losses, to be about 90 mg a day, and it is thought that adults are able to maintain potassium balance at levels only slightly higher. A specific minimal requirement for adults has not been established. The "safe and adequate" intake levels for adults are set at approximately 1900 to 5600 mg a day. (Refer to Table 14–1.)

The average dietary intake of potassium is about 2500 to 3000 mg a day for an adult, about 1775 mg a day for an average toddler, and about 1550 mg a day for infants (18). The adult values are well within the safe and adequate ranges; the toddler and infant values are somewhat elevated.

As discussed in the previous section, potassium losses in perspiration increase when people do hard physical work in hot climates. Therefore, the potassium requirement for such workers (or athletes) increases, and their intakes should be at the upper levels of the safe and adequate range. The amount of potassium that can be lost in perspiration under the above conditions is approximately 300 mg per hour, thus the specific potassium replacement need can be estimated.

Potassium in Foods

Most foods, except fats and sugar, contain at least some potassium; therefore, a diet sufficient in energy and protein usually contains enough potassium as well. Foods particularly rich in potassium include citrus fruits, prunes, dates, figs, apricots, bananas, tomatoes, potatoes, and green vegetables such as brussels sprouts. Both preservation and cooking tend to deplete the potassium in foods; fruits and vegetables contain more potassium when raw than when cooked, canned, or frozen.

Foods relatively low in potassium include cereals, cheese (the potassium in milk is largely lost in the whey), and eggs. It is interesting to note that a selection of foods that provides a favorable balance of potassium also provides a fairly low level of dietary sodium. Table 14–2 lists several foods with their contents of sodium and potassium, and Figure 14–6 shows the contribution of typical foods to potassium intake.

When discussing possible dietary sources of potassium, one must include commercial potassium chloride (KCl) supplements, for medicinal use when prescribed by a physician. Chloride is the anion generally desirable in a potassium replacement preparation, since a chloride depletion usually accompanies hypokalemia, the condition for which the supplement is given. Potassium chloride may also be a partial or complete substitute for sodium chloride, but this type of *salt substitute* should be used only upon medical advice because of the risk of potassium excess.

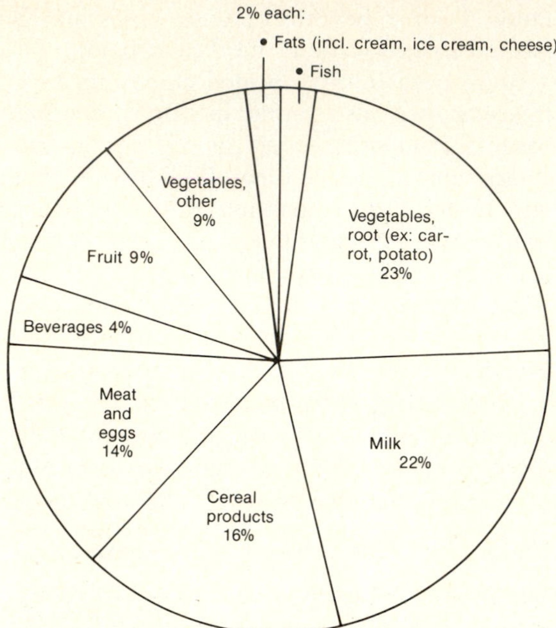

Figure 14–6 Contributions of various foods to total potassium intake. These figures are based on the British diet (19).

In addition, many vitamin-mineral-supplements contain potassium, and labels should be carefully read, especially if one must watch potassium levels in the diet (20).

The Role of Potassium in the Body

Potassium is very well absorbed through the intestinal tract; only about 10 percent of the amount ingested is not absorbed. Once absorbed, it is present in plasma and cells in the free ionic form, K^+. There is also a small amount of potassium within cells that is bound to protein.

Regulation. Any potassium in excess of body needs is usually excreted in the urine. Potassium losses can also occur in perspiration and in feces, but the kidney is the primary organ of excretion. Fairly large differences in intake can be tolerated without changing the all-important potassium concentration in the plasma (see section on toxicity) because of the kidney's fine ability to regulate the amount of potassium excreted.

This regulation of body potassium depends on the same system that regulates sodium balance—reabsorption into the body or secretion into the urine, whichever is needed, of the ion in question by specialized kidney tubules. Also, an increase of aldosterone causes decreased excretion of potassium, as it does of sodium. Basically, however, humans are better equipped to cope with a relatively high intake of potassium than with a chronically low intake. The kidney is not able to conserve potassium as effectively as it does sodium. Although low intakes of potassium are compensated for by decreasing potassium excretion somewhat, there is still an average potassium loss in urine that amounts to about 600 mg a day or more.

Regulation on the cellular level is based on transport processes that move the potassium ion across the membranes of the kidney cells. Intestinal cells have a similar capability, since potassium can also be secreted into the intestinal tract.

If there is a sudden large intake of potassium, the cells of the body assist the kidney in its attempt to lower potassium concentrations in the plasma by temporarily taking in more potassium than usual. The hormone *insulin* is known to affect this potassium uptake by cells, and potassium levels in the plasma may serve to increase insulin release from the pancreas (21).

Functions. Potassium plays its major role in living cells as a co-factor for enzymes that are needed to synthesize protein and starch and for other metabolic processes. Two other important functions of potassium, as of sodium, are regulation of water in the body and participation in buffering systems, and thus in the acid-base balance, of the body. Control of exchangeable K^+ is the physiological means of controlling intracellular volume. Potassium is also necessary for proper functioning of the muscles. For example, optimal levels of potassium (and magnesium) ions in the tissues are essential to the structure and function of the heart muscle. In addition, the relative concentrations of sodium and potassium across the cell wall determine the electric potential of the cell membrane and thus are responsible for the normal conduction of nerve impulses.

Toxicity of Potassium

If potassium is injected quickly into the bloodstream, it is extremely toxic; its major target is the heart. Relatively small increases (threefold or so) in potassium levels in the blood can cause abnormalities in the heart beat or even heart stoppage; potassium toxicity can cause sudden death.

Excess potassium may cause muscle weakness, mental confusion, numbness and tingling of the extremities, cold and pale skin, and abnormalities of heart rhythm that are detectable on electrocardiograph tests. Most cases of *hyperkalemia* (high levels of potassium in the blood) are seen in patients with diminished renal excretion mechanisms. In addition, decreased aldosterone levels may contribute to a high potassium level.

It is clear from a knowledge of the risks of potassium toxicity that taking extra potassium in pills, liquids, or salt substitutes without medical advice is not recommended. At least one adult fatality from excess, indiscriminate use of a prescribed KCl medication has been reported and an infant died when its mother gave it KCl for "colic" on the advice of a "health" book (22).

Like all nutrients, potassium in recommended amounts is necessary and safe; taken in excess, it may be very dangerous.

CHLORINE

Chlorine (Cl), a common water purifier and bleach, is also an essential element for all higher animals and humans. It was first chemically prepared in 1774 by Scheele. In 1810, Davy recognized it as an element, and named it chlorine, from the Greek *chloros*, meaning "greenish-yellow," after its color. In nature it always exists in a combined form, most commonly in soluble chlorides. It is in this *chloride* (Cl^-), or electrolyte, form that it is an essential nutrient, not its gaseous state.

The body contains about 1.17 gm chloride per kilogram (kg) of fat-free body weight, or about 0.15 percent of total body composition. The chloride, as well as sodium, content may be slightly decreased in the elderly. Chloride is normally a major constituent of extracellular fluids, but small quantities are also found within cells. Chloride is abundant in gastric secretions and in cerebro-spinal fluid. Relatively low concentrations are seen in muscle and nerve tissue.

Deficiency Symptoms

Chloride deficiency is rare because chloride is widely available in foods and in table salt, or sodium chloride.

More than usual losses of chloride may occur in repeated vomiting, as well as in diarrhea and heavy perspiration. Equal loss of both sodium and chloride leads to a decrease in body water. Decreased intake may occur on severe sodium-reduced diets. A general sign of low chloride is a metabolic alkalosis, (a high base to acid ratio in body tissues) and a low level of chloride in the blood.

The need for chloride was dramatically demonstrated in 1979 when a type of infant formula was inadvertantly made with insufficient chloride to meet minimal infant requirements. Infants fed this formula as their primary food became ill, they failed to gain weight, and suffered from constipation and alkalosis, as well as low levels of chloride in the blood and other electrolyte abnormalities. When chloride was added, the infants promptly improved. Consequently, the chloride-deficient formula was identified and recalled. These events showed that a low intake of chloride can induce a state of severe deficiency, and they reaffirmed the essential role of chloride, independent of sodium, in nutrition (23).

Chloride Requirements and Intakes

The Food and Nutrition Board's safe and adequate daily dietary intakes for chloride (see Table 14–1) are calculated from the suggested sodium intakes, since intake and losses of chloride are closely tied to those of sodium. The suggested range of intake of chloride for adults is 1700 to 5100 mg a day. A precise minimal requirement is not set. Average intakes range from about 3500 to 9000 mg a day in adults, about 600 mg in infants, and about 1800 mg in children.

If sodium intake is severely restricted, as in heart or kidney disease, chloride intake is also decreased and it may be necessary to provide alternative chloride sources. Alternatives include other chloride-containing salt substitutes to be taken on medical advice.

Food Sources

Chloride in our diet is provided almost entirely by sodium chloride. Chloride presence in a few foods is presented in Table 14–6.

Human milk provides between 280 and 420 mg of chloride per liter. In later infancy, chloride is supplied primarily as sodium chloride, with chloride intake parallel to that of sodium as in adults.

Table 14–6 CHLORIDE IN DIFFERENT FOOD SAMPLES, IN PARTS PER MILLION[a]

Sample	*Cl^- Found, Parts Per Million (ppm)*
Fish tissue	2840
Plant tissue	873
Beef extract	4890
Orange juice	735
Tomato juice	1093
Grapefruit juice	450
Milk	1050

[a]From Sekerka and Lechner (24) (ppm is mg/kg).

The Role of Chloride in the Body

Chloride is absorbed readily in the intestinal tract; it is actively absorbed by the lining cells of the large intestine.

Functions. The chloride ion plays an important role in the fluid and electrolyte balance, as well as in the acid-base equilibrium. It is an essential component of gastric juice as part of the *hydrochloric acid* (HCl) necessary for digestion. In nerve cells, the chloride ion tends to stabilize the electrical potential of the membranes and may also be involved in activating nerve impulses. Research interest in chloride transport across epithelial (lining) cell membranes has recently increased. Recognition is growing that active chloride transport may be the primary ionic movement responsible for a number of the body's secretory processes.

Chloride also crosses the red blood cell membrane readily, an ability termed the *chloride shift.* The chloride shift is of particular physiological importance because it allows the blood to carry more carbon dioxide to the lungs.

Regulation. Chloride regulation is associated with the regulation of the major positive ions because of the need to maintain electrical neutrality in the cells.

Excretion of chloride from the body is chiefly through the urine, usually about 4200 mg a day. It can also be lost in perspiration and gastrointestinal secretion. Aldosterone's action on chloride parallels its effect on sodium, that is, it enhances renal tubular reabsorption of this ion. Thus, when aldosterone release is stimulated by low sodium levels, chloride as well as sodium is conserved. Active reabsorption of chloride occurs in specialized cells in the ascending tubule of the nephron. A defect of this process of chloride reabsorption could lead to excess loss of chloride in the urine.

Toxicity of Chloride

Elemental chlorine gas is a poison and has been used for chemical warfare. A specific toxicity syndrome for chloride has not been reported in humans.

ACID-BASE BALANCE

Acid-base balance is a term used to describe the regulation of the hydrogen ion (H^+) concentration in the body fluids. The *pH measurement*[4] refers to the hydrogen ion concentration of a solution; a solution with a pH of 7 is *neutral* (acids and bases are balanced), one with a pH of 0 to 6.9 is *acidic,* and one with a pH of 7.1 to 14 is *alkaline* (or *basic*). An *acid solution* has more hydrogen ions than a neutral solution, an *alkaline solution* contains fewer hydrogen ions than a neutral solution, and in a *neutral solution,* the hydrogen ions equal the alkaline (basic) ions (ions which will accept acids). A simple chemical definition of an *acid* is a hydrogen ion donor, and a *base* is a hydrogen ion acceptor.

[4]The symbol pH technically stands for the negative logarithm of the H^+ concentration. This explains why a higher H^+ concentration results in a low pH, or acid concentration.

The cells of the body function best in a slightly alkaline medium and will be unable to function if the level of hydrogen ions within the cells or in fluids surrounding the cells differs too widely from the optimum. There are complex protective mechanisms for keeping the blood and tissue fluids within a narrow pH range (7.35 to 7.45). A pH level below 7.1 or above 7.6 is usually incompatible with life since at these degrees of acidity or alkalinity the cellular processes and enzyme systems cannot function properly.

Acid is produced constantly as a result of the metabolic process of the body, yet in the healthy person, an excess of the H^+ ions produced does not accumulate.

Regulation of Hydrogen Ions Formed During Metabolism

Ultimately the excretion of hydrogen ions exactly balances their production. The body accomplishes this "balancing act" by three main mechanisms:

1. *Buffering systems of the blood stream.* A *buffer* is a substance that can combine with H^+ when the solution is too acidic and release H^+ when conditions change. See Figure 14–7 for a description of the major buffering system in the body, the *carbonic acid-bicarbonate buffer system.* Another important buffer is the hemoglobin molecule in the red blood cells.
2. *Kidney (renal) mechanisms.* One important function of the kidney is to regulate the concentration of the bicarbonate ion that is needed in the body's key buffer system. It does this by restoration and resorption of bicarbonate when needed. It also can excrete acid as $H_2PO_4^-$ and excrete ammonia, NH_4^+.
3. *Lung (respiratory) mechanisms.* The respiratory mechanism for regulation of acid-base balance is closely related to the bicarbonate buffer system. When carbonic acid is produced, it forms CO_2, which is then "blown off," or exhaled from the lungs. (Water is also produced in the reaction.) Rapid breathing blows off more CO_2 and thus more acid is excreted. If the body has an acid excess, such as occurs in uncontrolled diabetes, rapid deep breathing usually results. On the other hand, shallow or inefficient breathing, such as may be present in some lung disorders, causes less acid to be excreted, and thus more accumulates in the blood stream.

Figure 14–7 ACID-BASE BALANCE: ACTION OF A PHYSIOLOGIC BUFFERING SYSTEM (The Carbonic Acid-Bicarbonate System)

A. *Situation:* A strong acid (with many free H^+ ions) enters the blood plasma. Unchecked, these would cause a rapid decrease in blood pH.
Buffer Action: The bicarbonate ions in the plasma rapidly combine with the hydrogen ions to form carbonic acid, a weak acid. A weak acid "holds on" to H^+ ions, allowing the pH to drop only minimally.
Chemical Notation of Action:

$$H^+ + HCO_3^- \leftrightharpoons H_2CO_3$$

(Bicarbonate Carbonic Acid)

(Note: the carbonic acid then is able to be converted into water (H_2O and carbon dioxide (CO_2); the latter can then be excreted through the lungs.)

B. *Situation:* A strong base (with many free OH^- ions) enters the blood stream. Unchecked, these would cause a rapid increase in blood pH.
Buffer Action: One of the free OH^- *(hydroxyl)* groups attracts a hydrogen ion from carbonic acid, forming water and a bicarbonate salt.
Chemical Notation of Action:

$$NaOH + H_2CO_3 \rightarrow HOH + NaHCO_3$$

(Base) (Carbonic Acid) (H_2O) (Water) (Bicarbonate Salt)

Figure 14–7 It can be seen from Example A that *bicarbonate ions* have a vital role in the control of excess acid in the blood stream. A decline in these buffer ions can lead to acidosis. Other buffer systems include the buffering action of hemoglobin and other proteins carried in the blood stream, as well as other chemical buffer systems such as phosphate.

The renal response to acid-base imbalances takes longer (over a day) than the buffer-system responses (within minutes and hours). The kidney's role in acid excretion is nevertheless very important, and impaired kidney function can lead to body *acidosis* (an increase of H^+ ions that outstrips the buffer capacity). If acidosis from any cause persists, the dangerous condition of *acidemia* (pH in the blood below 7.35) may result. (*Alkalosis* is the condition of too much base in the body and can lead to undesirable *alkalemia,* pH in the blood over 7.45.)

The electrolytes also have roles in maintaining acid-base balance, for example, sodium participates in the kidney's H^+ ion excretion mechanisms. Potassium concentrations in the blood are influenced by pH levels in the blood, if acidosis exists, K^+ in the blood is also usually high.

Acid Formers and Base Formers

Nutrient elements and foods are said to be acid formers or base formers depending on how they change the pH of the urine. (See also Table 14–7.) The elements phosphorus, sulfur, and chloride form acids upon oxidation (that is, form a compound that can donate a hydrogen ion); sodium, potassium, calcium, and magnesium form bases (that is, form compounds that can then accept a hydrogen ion).

The nineteenth-century French scientist Claude Bernard, one of the founders of modern physiology, was the first to record the correlation between foods consumed and acid production in the body when he noted that rabbits who were given a meat diet began producing an acid, rather than their usual alkaline, urine. Most protein foods contribute to an acid urine because of sulfur-containing amino acids (methionine and cysteine), which release sulfate, an acid former, on oxidation. The exception is milk, which, although protein-rich, also contains calcium, a base former, and this base-forming effect predominates.

Most fruits and vegetables contribute to an alkaline urine. Their residue after oxidation is richer in the alkaline-forming ions (such as Na^+ and K^+) than in acid-forming ions, and they also can contain organic anions that yield the bicarbonate ion when metabolized. A few fruits (for example, plums, prunes, and cranberries) contain high quantities of organic acids, which are also eliminated in the urine as a type of acid, and thus are acid formers.[5]

Table 14–7 THE CHIEF ACID- AND BASE-FORMING COMPONENTS OF THE DIET

Acid-Forming on Oxidation	*Base-Forming on Oxidation*
ELEMENTS	
Phosphorus	Sodium
Sulfur	Potassium
Chloride	Calcium
	Magnesium
FOODS	
Meat, poultry, fish	Most fruits
Eggs	Vegetables
Cereal products	Milk[b]
Bread	Nuts
Corn	
Cranberries, plums[a]	

[a]These are acidic owing to their content of organic acids which yield acidic end-products in metabolism. Most other organic acids are converted to carbon dioxide and water.

[b]Milk is a base-former mainly because of the calcium it contains.

In general, then, diet determines whether the urine is acidic or not. In practice, however, unless one is a strict vegan (that is, eliminates all meat and eggs from the diet), the urine pH is not generally on the alkaline side (26).

The typical American diet usually has a balanced content of acid- and base-forming foods, and the urine's alkalinity or acidity does not affect the status of one's health under normal conditions.

[5]Although most fruits are base forming, many fruit juices are high in acid content and do in fact have acid pH levels as consumed. (Most foods contain little if any preformed acids.) For example, the approximate pH's are grapefruit juice 3.5, orange juice 3.8, apple juice 3.6, cranberry juice 2.7, and tomato juice 4.3(25). All these fruit juices still lead to the formation of alkaline end products when oxidized and thus are still termed base-formers.

Likewise, eating an excess of acid-forming or base-forming foods does not have any significant effect upon pH level in the blood in the healthy person because of the body's fine-tuned regulatory processes for acid-base balance. In infants, however, specially acidified formulas have been shown to produce acidosis. Acidified formulas are no longer recommended for use, and modifications of protein in newer formulas make the acidified preparations unnecessary.

Individual adults need not be concerned about the acidity or alkalinity of their body chemistry. The body's physiologic processes keep it in excellent acid-base balance. Special remedies for "acid blood" are just not necessary for healthy people; our own acid-base buffering and regulating systems function better than anything money can buy.

QUESTIONS

1. What is the difference between an electrolyte and a nonelectrolyte? Give an example of each. What is the major positive ion of the extracellular fluid? The intracellular fluid? What is the sodium pump?

2. Is the body able to store sodium or potassium? What is the estimate of the minimal safe allowance for sodium? How does this compare with average adult intakes of sodium? Explain the difference between someone's *salt* intake and his or her *sodium* intake.

3. What foods are high in sodium content? Which are low? Recall the foods you ate yesterday and estimate how much sodium was included in that meal (using Table 2 in the Appendix). Is the total amount within the range of the "safe and adequate daily intake"? (Remember, if you added salt to foods, you will be underestimating your intake.)

4. What is the name of the hormone that is critical to normal sodium balance in the body? What is the action of this hormone if the sodium level of the diet becomes too low?

5. What foods are high in potassium content? Which are low? How does potassium deficiency occur? What are the symptoms? What are the risks of high levels of potassium in the blood? About how much potassium should be taken daily?

6. What is the other element in table salt in addition to sodium? Is it considered an essential nutrient? Why or why not? Are deficiency states of this element known?

7. What is meant by acid-base balance? What does "pH" measure? What is a simple definition of an acid?

8. What are the body's protective mechanisms against becoming too acidic or too basic? Describe one of these mechanisms.

9. Name two base-forming elements and two base-forming foods. Why are they called base formers? Do they cause any major changes in the body's acid-base balance?

References

1. Wyatt, C. J.: Adequacy of food labeling for consumers on limited sodium diets. J. Food Sci., *45*:259, 1980.
2. Bloch, M. R.: Salt in human history. Interdisc. Sci. Rev., *1*:336, 1976.
3. Food and Nutrition Board: *Recommended Dietary Allowances.* 9th Ed. Washington, D.C., National Research Council, National Academy of Sciences, 1980.
4. Dahl, L. K.: Salt and hypertension. Amer. J. Clin. Nutr., *25*:231, 1972.
5. Committee on Nutrition, American Academy of Pediatrics: Sodium intake of infants in the United States. Pediatrics, *68*:444, 1981.
6. Sloan, A. E.: Sodium: a potential problem for the cereal industry. Cereal Foods World, *26*:57, 1981; Miller, R. W.: The public knows and cares about sodium. FDA Consumer, *17*(April):10, 1983.
7. Vetter, J. L.: Technology of sodium in bakery products. Cereal Foods World, *26*:64, 1981; White, P. L., and Crocco, S. C. (eds.): *Sodium and Potassium in Foods and Drugs.* Chicago, American Medical Assoc., 1980: Council on Scientific Affairs: Sodium in processed foods, J. Amer. Med. Assoc., *249:* 784, 1983.
8. Abraham, S., and Carroll, M. D.: Fat, cholesterol and sodium intake in the diet of persons 1–74 years: United States. Advance Data, National Center for Health Statistics, No. 54, February 27, 1981.

9. Iannaccone, S., Potter, J. D., and Robertson, S. P.: Sodium content of bottled sparkling water (letter). J. Amer. Med. Assoc., *244*:437, 1980; Hewitt, M. I.: Sodium content of diet drinks (letter). Obesity/Bariatric Med., *4*:3, 1975.
10. Lecos, C.: A touch of salt for food labels. FDA Consumer, *16*:8, 1982.
11. Levin, M. L.: Renal control of sodium homeostasis. Ann. Clin. Lab. Sci., *11*:322, 1981.
12. The Gallup Organization, Inc. : *The Gallup Study of Changing Food Preparation and Eating Habits.* Princeton, N.J., The Gallup Organization, June 1980.
13. Kris-Etherton, P. M., et al.: Teaching principles and cost of sodium-restricted diets. J. Amer. Dietet. Assoc., *80*:55, 1982.
14. Shank, F. R., et al.: Perspective of Food and Drug Administration on dietary sodium. J. Amer. Dietet. Assoc., *80*:29, 1982; Shank, F.R. et al.: FDA perspective on sodium. Food Tech., *37*(No. 7):73, 1983; Forbes, A. L., and Miller, R. W.: The case for moderating sodium consumption. FDA Consumer, *15*:9, 1981; Hayes, A.H. Jr.: FDA's dietary sodium initiative—in the war against hypertension, a new weapon. Public Health Rept., *98*:207, 1983.
15. Cox, J. R., and Shalaby, W. A.: Potassium changes with age. Gerontology, *27*:340, 1981; Lye, M.: Distribution of body potassium in healthy elderly subjects. Gerontology, *27*:286, 1981.
16. Mirkin, G., and Hoffman, M.: *The Sportsmedicine Book.* Boston, Little Brown and Co., 1978.
17. Costill, D. L., Cote, R., and Fink, W. J.: Dietary potassium and heavy exercise: effects on muscle water and electrolytes. Amer. J. Clin. Nutr., *36*:266, 1982.
18. Potassium, sodium intake high in adult, infant, toddler diets. Food Chem. News, *21*:25, 1979; Walker, M. A., and Page, L.: Nutritive content of college meals. J. Amer. Dietet. Assoc., *70*: 260, 1977.
19. Bull, N. L., and Buss, D. H.: Contributions of foods to potassium intakes. Proc. Nutr. Soc., *39*:31A, 1980.
20. Schneiweiss, F.: Potassium: is it a necessary component of vitamin-mineral dietary supplements? Contemp. Pharm. Prac., *4*:78, 1981.
21. Cox, M., Sterns, R. H., and Singer, I.: The defense against hyperkalemia: the roles of insulin and aldosterone. New Eng. J. Med., *299*:525, 1978.
22. FDA proposes GRAS affirmation for potassium chloride. Food Chem. News, *24*:32, 1982.
23. Grossman, H., et al.: The dietary chloride deficiency syndrome. Pediatrics, *66*:336, 1980; Hill, F.D., and Bowie, M.D.: Chloride deficiency syndrome due to chloride-deficient breast milk. Arch. Dis. Childhood, *58*:224, 1983.
24. Sekerka, I., and Lechner, J. F.: Ion selective electrode for determination of chloride ion in biological materials, food products, soils, and waste water. J. Assoc. Off. Anal. Chem., *61*:1493, 1978.
25. Flick, A. L.: Acid content of common beverages. Digest. Dis., *15*:317, 1970.
26. Chan., J. C.: Nutrition and acid-base metabolism. Fed. Proc., *40*:2423, 1981.

15 Calcium, Phosphorus, and Magnesium

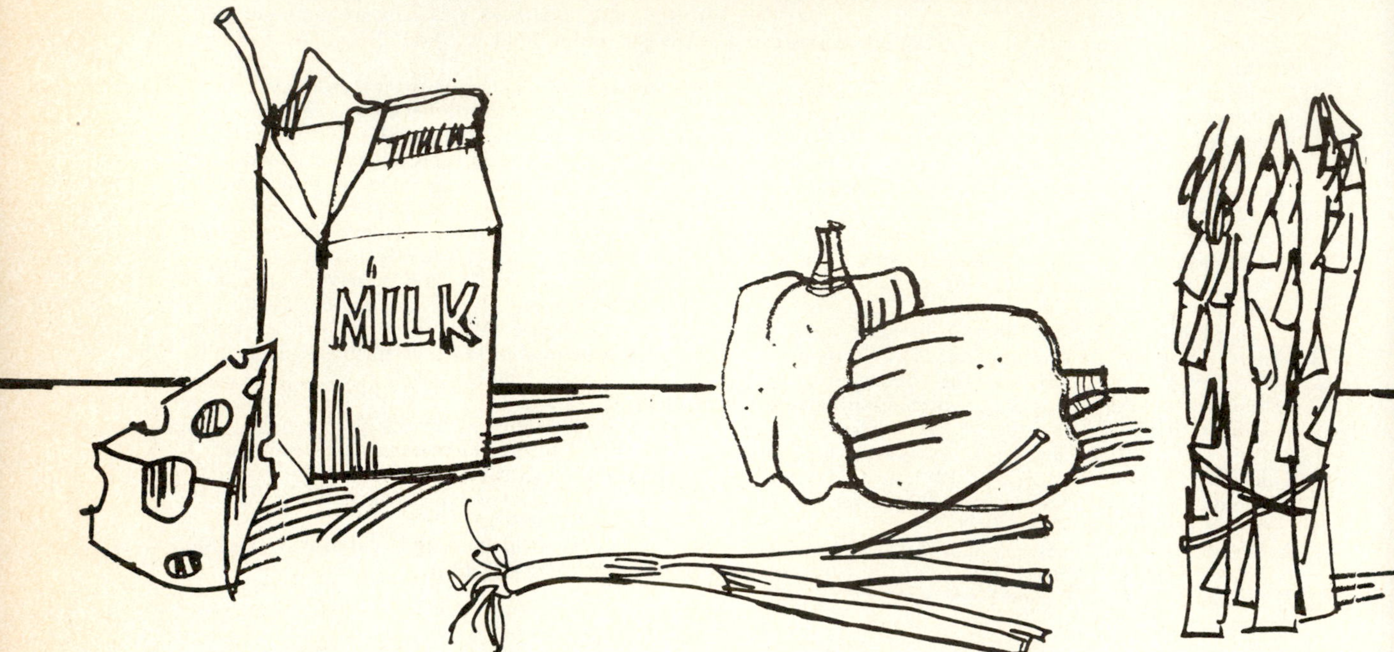

The previous two chapters discussed the body's need for water and the electrolytes (sodium, potassium, and chlorine). These three elements plus calcium, phosphorus, and magnesium make up the six *macrominerals* essential in our diets. They are present in the body in relatively large amounts and are required in the diet in considerably larger quantities than the trace elements (Chap. 16 and 17).

CALCIUM

Calcium (Ca) is the fifth most abundant element on the earth's crust. It is a silvery white metallic element that tarnishes on exposure to air and burns in oxygen. The name is derived from the Latin *calx,* meaning "lime," which is also the origin of the word chalk. Calcium does not exist in nature in the free state; it was isolated by Sir Humphrey Davy in 1808. Calcium compounds, however, are widely distributed. They exist often as a phosphate or carbonate in such common substances as chalk, granite, eggshell, seashells, "hard" water, bone, and limestone. Nearly all calcium compounds can serve as a source of calcium in the diet.

Calcium makes up from 1.5 to 2.2 percent of the human body; the amount present in a 70-kilogram (kg) adult is about 1200 grams (gm) (nearly 3 pounds).

Deficiency Symptoms

A deficiency of calcium is most apparent in the young of any species because of the great demand for calcium to form bone and teeth. The effects of such a deficiency dur-

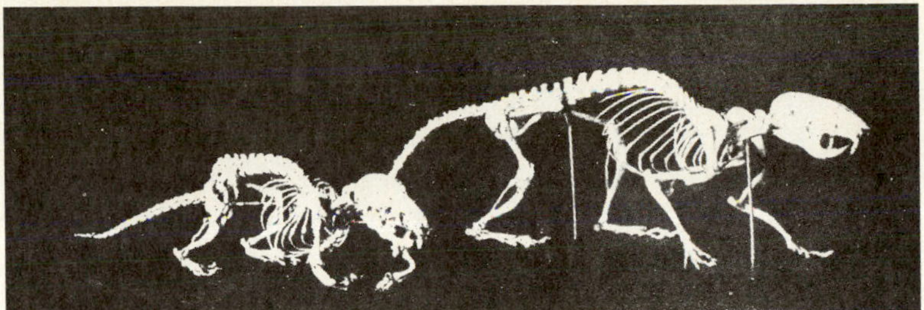

Figure 15–1 Skeletons of twin albino rats, showing influence of calcium content of the diet on the growth and character of the bones. Right, this rat, fed a diet adequate in calcium, attained full growth and had strong bones. Left, this rat received a diet deficient in calcium. Its growth was stunted, and its bones were soft and fragile, and more or less deformed. (Courtesy of Sherman and MacLeod and the *Journal of Biological Chemistry.*)

ing the growth period are manifested in one or more of the following ways:

1. stunted growth
2. poor quality of bones and teeth
3. malformation of bones (rickets)

When the lack of calcium has not been too severe, no effect may be noted in the size of the body, but the bones may either be delicate and brittle or remain soft and pliable because too little mineral salts are deposited in them. The skeleton of the smaller rat in Figure 15–1 shows both stunting in size of bones and their poor quality as exemplified in brittleness and certain deformities. The child suffering from rickets shown in Figure 15–2 evidences the bone deformities peculiar to that disease—narrow chest, enlargement of bones at their ends (seen at knees), and bowlegs resulting from inability of soft bones to bear the body weight. This disease can be caused by lack of either calcium, phosphorus, or vitamin D, or combinations of all three nutrients. The bone deformities of rickets may persist in later life, the narrow pelvic cavity being a complicating factor in pregnancy.

The teeth are largely formed during the latter part of fetal life and during infancy. Any lack of calcium during this period is likely to result in malformed teeth and jaws or in poor-quality teeth that are more subject to decay in later life.

In parts of the world where food supplies and living conditions are poor, conditions that indicate calcium deficiency may be found frequently, in both children and adults. When milk and meats are scarce or unavailable, a large proportion of the diet must come from vegetable sources, especially cereals. Such diets are usually low in calcium, as well as deficient in the quantity and biological value of the proteins supplied. Populations do adapt to low-calcium diets (see section on absorption), their children grow, and acute bone disease does not appear as a major problem. Children in such countries,

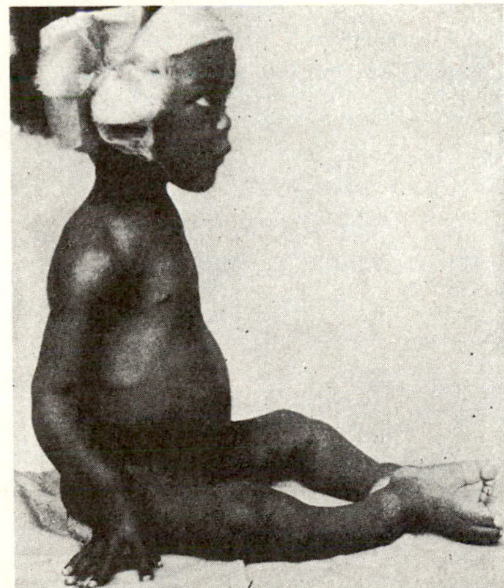

Figure 15–2 Rachitic child—note bowlegs with enlargement of bones about joints, deformity of chest, and enlargement of abdomen. (From Morse: *Clinical Pediatrics.*)

however, are often as much as three years behind in growth rate, as compared with well-nourished children, and the shorter stature attained by many of the adults suggests strongly that the low level of calcium intake (probably accompanied by other dietary lacks) may have prevented them from growing to the full height of which they were genetically capable. Children of such parents, when given a more nutritionally adequate diet, respond with increased growth rate and by adulthood are considerably taller than their parents.

A lifetime of a low-calcium intake may be a contributing factor to a state of gradual demineralization of bony tissues known as *osteoporosis* ("porous bones"). (See the section on health considerations.) A disease with somewhat similar symptoms, *nutritional osteomalacia,* occurs fairly commonly in parts of the world but is largely due to lack of vitamin D, although calcium or phosphorus, or both, also may be lacking.

States of low levels of calcium in the blood, which can be caused by disturbances in normal body regulatory functions, are termed *hypocalcemia* and can have serious effects. Symptoms include muscle pains and cramps, numbness, stiffness and tingling of hands and feet, and muscle spasms that may progress to convulsions. This range of symptoms caused by low-calcium levels is called *tetany.*[1]

Recently, it has been noted that persons with high blood pressure may have associated abnormalities in calcium levels in the blood (1). The reason for this relationship has yet to be clarified.

Calcium's protective action against rickets (antirachitic properties), as well as the general health benefits of calcium-containing compounds, has been recognized since ancient times. Calcium was one of the first nutrients shown to be essential in the diet. In 1842 the French scientist M. Chossat showed experimentally that pigeons required calcium salts. Before 1920 many other experiments proved the need of all animals for both calcium (2) and phosphorus (3). Well-controlled experiments with humans are more recent.

Requirement and Allowances

Requirement. Calcium is continuously being lost from the body through excretion in the urine and feces and, to a small extent, through the skin. The minimum requirement in the case of adults is the amount needed to balance these losses.

Attempts to fix a minimum requirement were at first based on balance experiments similar to those described for nitrogen balance (Chap. 4), but for calcium this method proved to have some drawbacks. Since the absorptive adaptations to changed levels of intake are slow, a person may take a certain amount of time to adapt to a lower calcium intake. Yet in time adaptation does occur, and thus investigators have been unable to give an exact figure for the minimum calcium requirements for adults. Estimates range from about 400 to 650 mg per day for an adult of average weight with ideal absorption and other ideal conditions.

Several well-known earlier studies have claimed that humans can adapt, with time, to lower calcium intakes and maintain calcium balance on intakes as low as 200 to 400 mg daily (4). Although it is true that a higher proportion of calcium is utilized on a low intake than when it is liberally supplied, most of the national populations that maintain calcium equilibrium on low calcium intakes live in either tropical or semi-tropical areas (where abundant sunlight favors calcium utilization by forming vitamin D in the body), or they may have hitherto unrecognized sources of calcium in the diet. Such sources include white clay quite commonly con-

[1]Not to be confused with the term *tetanus,* which is an infectious disease caused by bacteria and is preventable by immunization.

sumed in some cultures (a practice known as *pica*); the lime-steeped corn used for making tortillas in Mexico; and the "stone powder," which is essentially calcium carbonate, added to rice during its milling in Formosa.

In a review of the extensive literature on calcium balance experiments, M. A. Ohlson has stated, "Few adults eating diets characteristic of our society are in equilibrium on intakes of less than 500 mg (0.5 gm) per day (5). The Food and Nutrition Board's opinion on this subject is that "no advantage accrues from such [200–400 mg] low intakes, and for a variety of reasons it seems unwise to recommend such a low calcium intake."

Recommended Allowance for Adults. The Food and Nutrition Board in 1980 kept its recommended allowance for calcium at 800 mg per day for adults. The Board, in discussing the allowance, states: "Collectively, the possible effects of high dietary intakes of protein and phosphate on [increasing] urinary calcium and enhanced bone resorption, respectively, along with the possibility of reduced calcium absorption with advancing age, argue for recommending an ample intake of calcium" (6).

The recommended amount is based on estimates of daily calcium losses in adults of about 175 mg in the urine and 125 mg in the feces, for a total of at least 300 mg. Minor amounts of calcium may be lost in perspiration (at least 20 mg per day), but they need be taken into account only in instances of excessive perspiring as a result of physical activity at high environmental temperatures. Assuming that 40 percent of ingested calcium is absorbed, 800 mg per day are needed in the diet. This allowance provides a factor of safety above the bare maintenance requirement and covers individual differences of need and of the ability to utilize calcium from the diet. Despite the usually lesser weight and lighter skeletal structure of women, the same amount is recommended for women as for men in order to cover menstrual losses and to provide a reserve store in the body to meet needs of pregnancy and lactation. Table 15-1 gives the recommended dietary allowance (RDA) for young people and adults for both calcium and phosphorus (see RDA table inside front cover for allowances for younger children). The recommended allowances of calcium vary from country to country (see Appendix, Table 1C), ranging from as low as 400 mg a day up to 1000 mg. These differences are to be expected until more research is done on the subject. At this time, the authors advise students to use for themselves that figure recommended by the highest nutrition authority in their own country (in the United States it is the Food and Nutrition Board) because of different national dietary and environmental conditions.

A Food and Agriculture Organization (FAO) and World Health Organization (WHO) FAO/WHO committee has proposed intakes of calcium between 400 and 500 mg per day as "suggested practical allowances" for adults, especially for countries where calcium-rich foods such as dairy products are

Table 15–1 RECOMMENDED DIETARY ALLOWANCES PER DAY FOR CALCIUM AND PHOSPHORUS*

	Age (yrs)	*Calcium (mg)*	*Phosphorus (mg)*
Males	11–14	1200	1200
	15–18	1200	1200
	19–22	800	800
	23–50	800	800
	51+	800	800
Females	11–14	1200	1200
	15–18	1200	1200
	19–22	800	800
	23–50	800	800
	51+	800	800
	Pregnant	+400	+400
	Lactating	+400	+400

*From Food and Nutrition Board, 1980 (6).

either not plentiful or unavailable (7). More recent studies suggest that this figure may be inadequate (8).

Allowances during Childhood, Pregnancy, and Lactation. Adults need calcium and phosphorus only for maintenance of a body already built, but children need also a "growth quota." Extra amounts of these elements are required not only for the growth of bones but also for their strengthening by further deposits of calcium phosphate. The bones of a newborn infant are more flexible and of lower mineral content than those of an adult, a provision of nature that makes birth easier. As the child grows, the relative proportion of calcium phosphate in the bones must be increased so that they will become stronger and more rigid, in order to bear the weight of the body and to be less easily broken. The teeth are formed and partially calcified in the latter months of fetal life, and their calcification is practically completed by the time the child is two to three years old. For children from one to ten years of age, the calcium and phosphorus allowances are the same as adults, 800 mg. Per unit of weight, growing children may need 2 to 4 times as much calcium as does an adult.

Children will continue to grow on diets that supply less than desirable amounts of calcium or phosphorus, but the bones and teeth will not be of as good a quality, or growth may not be so rapid as with a more liberal allowance of these elements. If the quantity of either element is too limited, growth may be stunted. During the rapid growth in the period of preadolescence and puberty (eleven to eighteen years), a higher intake is recommended—1200 mg. At levels of 1000 to 1500 mg daily of each of these elements in the diet, children have shown "maximum retention"—that is, as much calcium and phosphorus is provided as the body can store (9). Greater amounts would normally be excreted by the body.

Women in the latter half of pregnancy and those who are nursing their babies have considerably higher calcium and phosphorus needs than do normal adults, since the mineral needs of the growing fetus or infant must be met through the mother's body. For mothers, as well as for growing children there should also be a plentiful supply of vitamin D so that optimal calcium absorption and utilization can occur. (See Chap. 9.) A liberal intake of calcium is especially important during lactation, in order to provide for the secretion of calcium-rich milk without undue drain on the reserve stores of calcium in the mother's own body (Fig. 15–3). The recommended allowance for pregnancy in a woman nineteen or over is 1200 mg of calcium. (See Table 15–1.)

Intakes of Population Groups

How adequate are freely chosen diets in the United States as to the amount of calcium they supply? The answer depends upon which index, or standard, is used and which age and sex group are considered. Then, too, a survey of an *average* population does not mean too much, since adequate calcium intakes are so dependent upon the consumption of milk or milk products by individuals, which varies widely. Whenever milk intake is low, calcium intakes are very likely to be low unless other calcium sources are substituted. Fifteen to 25 percent of the American population consume very little, or no, milk, which is directly indicative of the extent of inadequate calcium intakes.

Within a family, fathers and adolescent boys are most likely to eat food that meets the recommended allowances of calcium, while mothers, pregnant and lactating women, and adolescent girls are least likely to do so. Statistics in the United States show that females twelve and over, on the average, consume below 80 percent of the RDA for calcium (10). Since this is an average figure, it means that there is no question that calcium intakes are significantly low in many

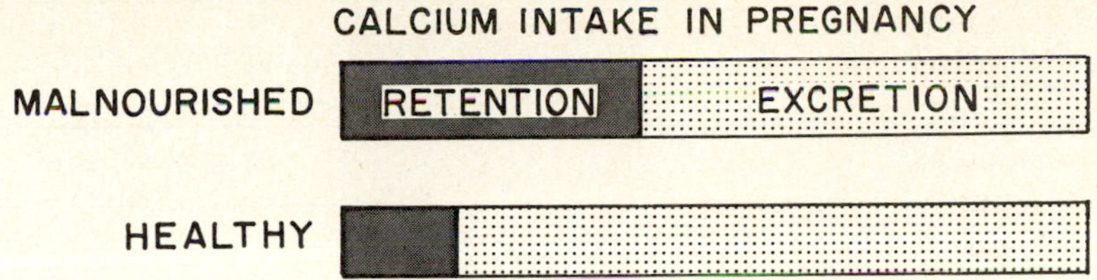

Figure 15–3 Some women enter into pregnancy with too low reserves of those nutrients that can be stored in the body because of previous inadequate diets. Calcium is one of the nutrients most likely to be furnished in less than optimum amounts in American diets. This diagram shows that, when given a relatively rich supply of calcium during pregnancy, the previously malnourished woman retained a good percentage of it, thereby building up her body reserves of this element. The woman whose diet before pregnancy had been adequate and whose stores of calcium were therefore higher had less need to store it and hence retained a smaller percentage of the calcium furnished by the diet than the other woman. (Adapted from Macy and Williams: *Hidden Hunger.* Lancaster, Pa., Jacques Cattell Press, 1945.)

individual females. Males tend to consume more calcium than females at all age periods, no doubt because their total intake of food is greater.

Overall, it appears that perhaps 10 percent of the American population is consuming less than one-half of the recommended allowance of calcium (11), an inadequate amount. About 20 to 40 percent of men in the population appear to consume less than two-thirds of the RDA; 50 to 60 percent of adolescent girls and about 60 percent of women aged thirty-five to seventy-four also fall into this category of calcium intake (12). Other groups consume intakes closer to the RDA.

Records of growth of children and of osteoporosis in older individuals are as useful indicators of calcium (and phosphorus) deficiencies as any available. The extensive *Ten-State Nutrition Survey in the United States* showed that 10 to 50 percent of children (six years or less) from low-income families in different states were "one or more standard deviations below Iowa growth standards (13). Also, the incidence of osteoporosis in older females is known to be very high. (See health considerations section on osteoporosis, p. 367.)

Calcium in Foods

Sources. Table 15–2 gives examples of foods containing calcium and phosphorus. The first column of figures under each mineral element gives the amount furnished in an average serving of each food in the condition in which it is eaten (cooked or raw). The second column shows the number of milligrams present in 100 gm of the food substance. Thus, cheddar cheese ranks high in calcium (750 mg) on a 100 gm basis, but an average serving, or 1-oz portion, would contribute only 225 mg, which is slightly less than the amount furnished by an 8-oz glass of milk. On a weight basis, milk (which is 87 percent water) is not so high in calcium and phosphorus as dried beans or dried figs, but it is at or near the top of the list for both elements in the amount furnished in an average serving. Dried fruits and dried beans do not usually contribute large amounts of calcium to the diet, because dried fruits ordinarily are eaten in small quantities and dried beans increase in water content on cooking.

To generalize, foods may be grouped according to their contributions of calcium in the ordinary diet as follows:

excellent sources—hard cheeses, milk, most dark green, leafy vegetables, and soft fish bones
good sources—softer cheeses, ice cream, broccoli, baked beans, dried legumes, and dried figs
fair sources—cottage cheese, light cream, oranges, dates, salad greens, nuts, lima beans, parsnips, and eggs
poor sources—most other fruits and vegetables, grains, and meats

Table 15–2 REPRESENTATIVE FOODS, WITH CALCIUM AND/OR PHOSPHORUS CONTENT

Calcium (mg)

Food	Per Average Serving	Per 100 gm
Sesame seeds, whole, ¼ c	348	1160
Milk, 8 oz glass, ½ pt	285	118
Salmon, red, canned with bones, ⅖ c	259	259
Sardines, canned in oil, 2 fish, drained	174	435
Cheese, American cheddar, 1 oz	225	750
*Leafy vegetables, avg. ½ c cooked	140	167
Ice cream, plain, avg. ¾ c	123	123
†Molasses, medium, 2 tbsp	116	290
Artichokes	102	51
Broccoli, ⅔ c	88	88
Baked beans, canned with		
molasses, ½ c	82	56
tomato sauce ½ c	70	49
Cream, light, 7 tbsp	74	97
Orange, 1 medium	62	40
‡Cottage cheese, 2 round tbsp	52	96
String beans, ⅔ c, cooked	50	50
Parsnips, ½ c, cooked	44	57
Lima beans, ½ c, cooked	38	47
Salad greens, raw, avg. 2 large or 4–5 small leaves	34	68
Sesame seeds, hulled, ¼ c	33	110
Egg, 1 large	26	54
Figs, dried, 1 large	25	125
canned, 3, with juice	13	13
Bread, whole-wheat, 1 slice	23	96
white, 1 slice (4% milk solids)	19	79
Peanut butter, 2 scant tbsp	22	74
Peas, canned, ½ c	20	25
Apricots, dried, cooked, 4 halves	20	22
Orange juice, 6 oz	20	25
Dates, 3–4 pitted, 1 oz	22	72
Prunes, 4–5 medium, cooked	17	25
Grapefruit, ½ medium	16	16
Cereal, whole-grain, avg. ⅔–¾ c, cooked	8–15	9

Phosphorus (mg)

Food	Per Average Serving	Per 100 gm
Liver, fried, 2 slices, 75 gm	311	358
Milk, 8 oz glass, ½ pt	227	93
Cod steak or sole, 100 gm	220	220
Lamb, leg, roast, 2 slices, 100 gm	208	208
Beef, rib roast, 1 slice, 100 gm	186	186
hamburger, ¼ lb, 85 gm	165	194
Baked beans, canned, ½ c	120	92
Cheese, American cheddar, 1 oz	140	478
Peanut butter, 2 scant tbsp	118	393
Shredded wheat, 1 biscuit	102	360
Whole-wheat cereal, ½ c, cooked	113	83
Oatmeal, ⅔–¾ c, cooked	105	57
Cottage cheese, 2 round tbsp	108	189
Egg, 1 large	101	210
Ice cream, plain, avg., ¾ c	99	99
Cream, light, 7 tbsp	77	77
Broccoli, ⅔ c	76	76
Nuts, mixed, 1–12 nuts, ½ oz	67	446
Parsnips, ½ c, cooked	62	80
Lima beans, ½ c, cooked	97	121
Peas, canned, ½ c	62	77
Corn, canned, ½ c	43	52
Cauliflower, ¾ c, cooked	42	72
Leafy vegetables, ½ c, cooked, avg.	45	45
Bread, whole-wheat, 1 slice	60	263
white, 1 slice (4% milk solids)	21	92
Apricots, dried, cooked, 3 halves	34	34
Figs, dried, 1 large	33	111
canned, 3, with juice	21	35
Prunes, 4–5 medium, cooked	27	40
Dates, 3–4 pitted, 1 oz	18	60
Orange, 1 small	37	37
String beans, ⅔ c, cooked	19	23
Grapefruit, ½ medium	16	16

*Including dandelion, mustard, turnip greens, collards, and kale, but excluding spinach, beet greens, and chard, in which calcium is in a poorly utilizable form.

†The calcium in molasses is due to addition of lime to neutralize acid in refining sugar; it is in lowest concentration in light molasses and highest in the blackstrap variety.

‡Calcium content of cottage cheese varies according to whether it is made from sour milk or by addition of rennin to sweet milk.

Eggs and nuts (which are high in phosphorus) are of only moderate calcium content, while meat, poultry, and fish are calcium-poor. Most fruits and vegetables, bread, and breakfast cereals contain relatively minor quantities, but if eaten in considerable quantities, they may add appreciably to the calcium intake.

As shown in Table 15–3 and Figure 15–4, about 75 percent of all the calcium in the American food supply comes from dairy products (other than butter). The rest is about equally distributed among meat, eggs, vegetables, beans, and cereals. Enrichment of foods with calcium is not common. Certain food processing techniques do add calcium to some convenience foods, a practice that underscores the importance of food labeling.

Obtaining the Calcium Allowance in the Diet. Calcium is one of those nutrients most likely to be provided by the diet in less than recommended or optimal quantities. It is not difficult, however, to obtain the recommended allowance of 800 mg daily if one includes 2 cups (1 pint, or about 480 ml) of milk or its calcium equivalent in milk products other than butter. In Table 15–4, four groups of foods are given, each of which furnishes the recommended calcium allowance for a day, with the amount of milk decreasing in each group from left to right (from 1½ pints, which furnishes more than the day's allowance, to none). It should be noted that diets that contain lesser amounts of milk (or none in group 4), depend on cheese or ice cream, as well as green leafy vegetables and broccoli, as major sources of calcium.

Other foods in an average diet—some of which are classed as fair, moderate, or even poor sources of calcium—may together contribute significant amounts toward the day's total intake. Two servings each of fruit and vegetables (other than green, leafy ones or

Table 15–3 SOURCES OF CALCIUM AND PHOSPHORUS BY FOOD GROUPS, SELECTED YEARS*

	Calcium (Percent)					*Phosphorus (Percent)*				
Food Group	1909–1913	1947–1949	1957–1959	1967	1980†	1909–1913	1947–1949	1957–1959	1967	1980†
Dairy products, excluding butter	67.7	74.2	76.5	76.1	**71.6**	27.5	37.1	38.3	36.3	**32.6**
Meat, poultry, fish, including fat pork cuts	4.2	3.5	3.3	3.7	**4.2**	20.0	21.0	23.0	26.5	**28.6**
Dry beans, peas, nuts, and soybean products	3.2	2.5	2.6	2.6	**3.1**	5.4	5.6	5.7	5.7	**6.4**
Potatoes, sweet potatoes	2.5	1.2	1.0	0.9	**1.0**	6.9	4.2	3.8	3.7	**3.6**
Vegetables (excluding potatoes, sweet potatoes)	7.1	7.0	6.2	6.1	**6.7**	4.5	5.7	5.3	5.4	**5.7**
Fruit	2.1	2.4	2.1	2.1	**2.5**	1.7	2.0	1.9	1.8	**2.2**
Flour and cereal products	7.4	3.3	3.3	3.4	**3.8**	26.6	15.1	12.9	12.4	**13.4**
Other foods‡	5.7	5.5	5.0	5.0	5.1	6.8	9.2	9.0	8.3	**7.6**
Total§	100.0	100.0	100.0	100.0	**100.0**	100.0	100.0	100.0	100.0	**100.0**
Quantity per capita per day (mg)	817	996	979	946	**N/A**	1561	1554	1530	1544	**N/A**

*From Marston, R., and Friend, B., *National Food Situation,* 1977.
†Source: USDA.
‡Includes eggs.
§Components may not add to total because of rounding off to closest figure.
N/A = Not available.

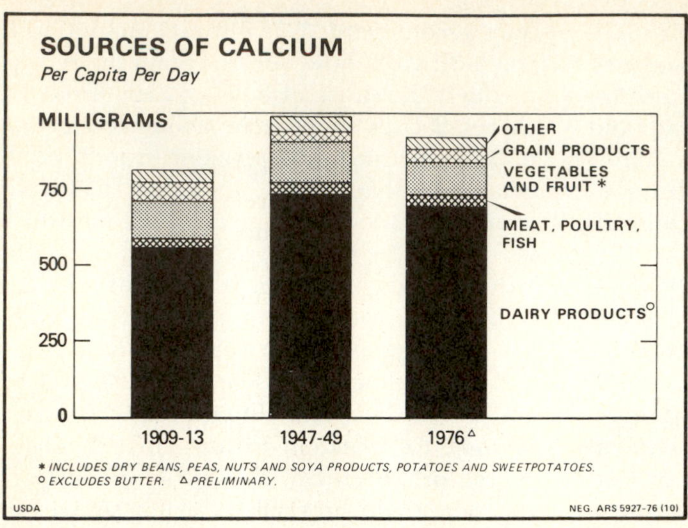

Figure 15–4 Food sources and average *per capita* intake of calcium from 1909 to 1976. (From Marston, R., and Friend, B.: Nutritional review, reprinted from *The National Food Situation.* Hyattsville, Md., U.S. Department of Agriculture Agric. Res. Serv., Consumer and Food Economics Institute Report CFE (Adm.)-299-11, Jan. 1977.)

broccoli) contribute about 100 to 150 mg calcium, while four to six slices of bread or a serving of cereal might contribute 75 to 150 mg, especially if whole-grain cereals or bread made with added milk solids are used. The typical American dietary pattern of bread and butter, meat and potatoes, other vegetable, salad or fruit, and dessert can be expected to supply only about 300 mg of calcium daily. Two cups of milk in the daily diet would bring the total intake up to the recommended allowance, yet only a relatively small portion of American women have this amount of milk in their diet.

It is also important to consider which foods carry calcium in forms that are readily absorbed from the intestine and hence available for use in the body. The calcium in milk

Table 15–4 FOODS THAT FURNISH THE ADULT RECOMMENDED CALCIUM ALLOWANCE (800 mg daily)

Group 1	*Calcium, mg*	*Group 2*	*Calcium, mg*	*Group 3*	*Calcium, mg*	*Group 4*	*Calcium, mg*
Milk, 1½ pts	855	Milk, 1 pt	570	Milk, ½ pt	285	Cheese, American cheddar, 1½ oz	337
		Cottage cheese, 2 round tbsp	52	Cheese, American cheddar, 1 oz	225	Ice cream, plain, ⅙ qt	123
		Bread, whole-wheat, 4 slices	92	Bread, whole-wheat, 5 slices	95	Bread, whole-wheat, 4 slices	92
		Orange, 1 medium	62	Orange juice, 8 oz	24	Turnip greens, ¾ c, cooked	138
		Green beans, ¾ c, cooked	45	Broccoli, ⅔ c	88	Beans, baked, with molasses, ½ c	82
			821	Carrots, diced, ⅔ c	33	Egg, 1 medium	27
				Cream, light, 4 tbsp	61	Hamburger, lean, 85 gm	10
					811		809

is highly utilized by the body, and its availability is not altered by pasteurization. Broccoli, cauliflower, and kale rank almost with milk in availability of their calcium content, while that in carrots, lettuce, string beans, and almonds has been shown to be only slightly less well assimilated. Leafy vegetables whose calcium is fairly well utilized include kale, cabbage, collards, turnip greens, and probably also mustard and dandelion greens. Spinach, chard, and beet greens have much of their calcium in insoluble combination with oxalic acid, and hence in a form unavailable to the body, but this condition is not detrimental if there is plenty of absorbable calcium in the diet; furthermore, these greens are valuable sources of iron and vitamin A.

The inclusion of at least *2 cups of milk* daily in the diet of adults is urged as the chief means for obtaining the calcium quota, as well as for the high-quality proteins and vitamins that milk provides. Children should generally receive *3 cups of milk* or its equivalent each day. Those who do not drink milk should have it incorporated in cooked foods wherever possible, and they might eat more cheese. Hard cheeses have much higher calcium content than soft cheeses with higher water content; cottage cheese has only about one-seventh as much calcium as a hard cheese like cheddar (American), but one-cup of it can take the place of one-half cup of milk in calcium value. The wider use of green, leafy vegetables, including salad greens, would help to reinforce the diet in calcium, as well as in other minerals and vitamins.

If calcium is taken in pills (by doctors's advice), it should be in the form of some soluble salt, such as calcium lactate. Unless there is some excellent reason (as, for example, an allergy to milk or intolerance to appreciable amounts of lactose), it is far better to revise the diet to include more calcium-rich foods, which furnish, along with calcium, other minerals, vitamins, and amino acids essential for body welfare.

The Role of Calcium in the Body

After calcium is absorbed in the body, its level in the blood is carefully regulated. The ratio of calcium to phosphorus affects the amount absorbed. Calcium functions chiefly to build the skeletal structure.

Absorption and Retention. The absorption of calcium from the intestinal tract varies with different individuals and under different conditions, but it is not as complete as for some other nutrients. Generally, only 20 to 40 percent of the calcium intake is absorbed. In the first place, any calcium that is in organic combination must be set free in soluble form before it can be absorbed; in the second place, various substances or conditions in the intestinal tract may contribute to the formation of insoluble (and hence unabsorbable) compounds.

Recent evidence has clarified that calcium absorption occurs by two processes: active transport and diffusion (14). Vitamin D apparently affects both processes.

The relative absorption may vary under special conditions or with individual foods. Some of the factors that either favor or hinder the absorption of calcium and the closely related mineral phosphorus from the intestinal contents are listed briefly in Table 15–5.

The fact that *oxalic acid* in certain foods (for example, rhubarb, cocoa, and spinach) forms an insoluble salt with calcium (calcium oxalate) and that *phytic acid* in the outer coats of cereals can tie up much of the calcium and phosphorus in insoluble compounds, is not considered of major practical importance, provided the supply of these elements in the diet is liberal enough that sufficient absorbable calcium and phosphorus remain to meet body needs.

Table 15–5 ABSORPTION OF CALCIUM AND PHOSPHORUS FROM THE INTESTINAL TRACT

Factors Favoring Absorption	*Factors Hindering Absorption*
Acid reaction in upper intestinal tract.	Alkaline reaction in lower intestinal tract.
Normal digestive activity and normal motility of intestinal tract.	Large amounts of fiber in diet.
Calcium and phosphorus in diet in about equal amounts.	Laxatives or any circumstances that induce diarrhea or hypermotility of the intestine.
The fat-soluble vitamin D.	Large excess of either element in comparison with the other (Ca:P ratio unbalanced).
Need for higher amounts of these mineral elements by the body.	With excess calcium present, insoluble Ca salts may be formed with phytin (complex P compound in cereals), oxalic acid (in certain leafy vegetables), and unabsorbed fatty acids.
Vitamin D.	Excess of iron, magnesium, or aluminum forms insoluble phosphates.
Calcium or phosphorus deficiency.	Vitamin D deficiency.
Low calcium intake.	Menopause.
Parathyroid hormone.	Old age.
Pregnancy, lactation.	

Excessive amounts of fatty acids in the intestine can also tie up calcium by forming insoluble "soaps," but this fact, too, appears to have little practical significance when persons are eating normal diets. The amount of vitamin D available in the body, however, does play an important role in both the absorption and utilization of calcium.

Possibly even more critical factors influencing the relative amounts of calcium and phosphorus that are absorbed and retained in the body are the body's need for these elements, especially calcium, and the level of intake to which the body has become adapted. If a person regularly takes in large amounts of calcium, the body adjusts by absorbing less calcium. On the other hand, people may adjust to a lower level of calcium intake by more efficient absorption and decreased excretion of this element, thus conserving sufficient calcium for upkeep of body tissues. But in the case of calcium the readjustment process may take many weeks, or months. In an infant or young child, or in an adult during healing of bone fractures, absorption of calcium is relatively more efficient, so that a larger percentage of the intake is available for the building or strengthening of bone tissues. Absorption efficiency also increases in pregnancy or in an adult after a fairly long period on a low-calcium intake. Thus, the relative amounts of calcium retained in the body vary, depending on the age of the person, previous dietary habits, and the level of the current supply.

Regulation. Calcium in the blood is maintained at the optimal level mainly through the action of two hormones with opposing actions. When the level rises above normal, *calcitonin,* from the thyroid gland, stimulates bone formation, and calcium is removed from blood and deposited in bone. When the level drops below normal, *parathyroid hormone* (PTH), from the parathyroid glands, stimulates bone demineralization, resulting in a movement of calcium from bone to blood. It also stimulates absorption of calcium from the intestines and inhibits loss in the urine. Thus, in addition to its other functions, bone serves as a store of calcium that can be drawn upon for the regulation of the level of this important mineral in blood. This type of balance, with the calcium ion freely exchanging between bone and the blood stream yet maintaining a relatively constant level in the blood, is known as a *dynamic equilibrium* (see Fig. 15–5).

Regulation of absorption by gastrointestinal mechanisms according to body need has already been discussed. Basically, if there is a shortage of calcium in the body, absorption increases. The increased uptake is directly stimulated by the active form of vitamin D in the body (see Chap. 9). Other influences have been listed in Table 15–5.

Factors that influence sodium reabsorption in the kidney also influence calcium retention (except in the distal tubule of the nephron where sodium is actively absorbed). A high-protein intake increases kidney excretion of calcium, as does decreased physical activity. Parathyroid hormone increases calcium reabsorption from the urine being formed. All in all, kidney mechanisms play a relatively small role in maintaining calcium balance. Calcium can also be secreted into the intestinal tract by intestinal lining cells as another form of excretion.

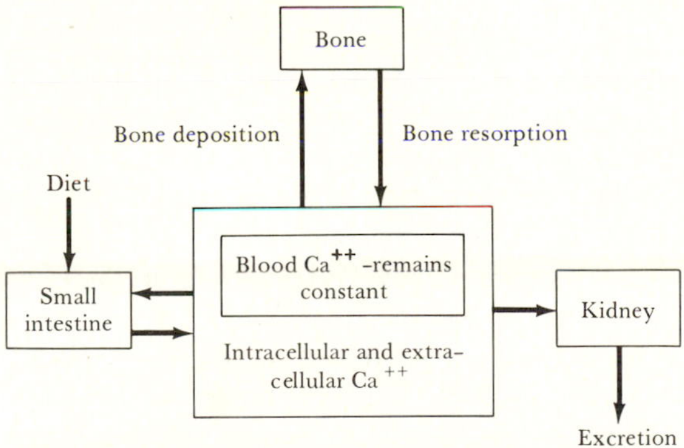

Figure 15–5 *Dynamic Equilibrium of Calcium in the body.* As a result of the body's homeostatic (balancing) mechanisms, the calcium in blood and in tissue fluids remain at a very constant level. The above diagram is a simplified representation of this complete regulatory system and of the role of the ongoing turnover of bone calcium. The level of calcium in the blood depends on a balance between calcium from intestinal absorption and bone resorption on the one hand, and calcium lost from the blood by bone formation and by excretion through the kidney on the other. Several factors which affect this equilibrium are discussed in the text, but a full understanding of all the cellular and hormonal mechanisms involved still awaits further research.

The Calcium-to-Phosphorus Ratio. The ratio of calcium to phosphorus (Ca:P) in the diet is known to affect the amount of calcium absorbed in experimental animals. In the animals studied (usually rats), a Ca:P ratio of about 2:1 results in optimal calcium absorption, and a relationship of calcium intake to phosphorus intake of 1:1 or 2:1 appears to avoid excess calcium loss from bone storage areas (see also the health considerations section on osteoporosis). The exact influence of Ca:P ratio changes in humans, however, is not completely understood, since some studies have shown that the above animal results may not apply to primates or humans.

The RDA figures for calcium and phosphorus are based on a 1:1 relationship, although the Food and Nutrition Board acknowledges that humans can probably tolerate a wider range, from 2:1 to 1:2 proportions of calcium to phosphorus. It is generally recognized, however, that excess intakes of phosphorus (more than double those of calcium) can lead to calcium loss from bones and from the body.

In the 1970s, the Food and Drug Administration (FDA) estimated the average Ca:P ratio in American diets to be about 1:1.5 or so for adults, and 1:1 for infants and toddlers. Others have estimated the ratio in adults to be even closer to the 1:2 range. For a comparison, New Zealand figures have indicated the ratio in an average diet of about 1:1.8, so it is not just the American diet but more likely all Western diets that seem to be in excess of the theoretical 1:1 ratio.

For individuals, the Ca:P ratio can vary significantly depending, for example, on how much milk is consumed. A 1:4 ratio can occur if only 400 mg a day is taken in, as could happen easily if one had no milk, and a ratio much closer to 1:1 would result when milk intake reached 3 or 4 cups a day. Milk, cheeses, and green leafy vegetables are among the relatively few foods that provide lesser amounts of phosphorus than calcium. Meats, poultry, and fish furnish 15 to 20 times as much phosphorus as calcium.

Most authorities agree that more studies are needed to clarify the optimal Ca:P ratio for humans.

Functions. Calcium and phosphorus together make up three-fourths of the mineral content of the body, and the calcium present is twice that of phosphorus. Ninety-nine percent of this calcium plays a major role in the structure of bones and teeth. A strong, well-developed skeletal system fulfills a number of functions. It gives form to the body, affords protection to the brain and the visceral organs, serves as an anchor for muscles that allow body movement, and is the site of blood formation.

Bone is a connective tissue of which about 30 percent is organic matter (cells and fibers) that is embedded in mineral matter (70 percent). The mineral part is composed mostly of tiny crystals of calcium phosphate[2] but includes smaller amounts of magnesium, sodium, and carbonate. The metabolism of bone is so slow that formerly this tissue was thought of chiefly as inert material drawn on only in instances of great need. It is now recognized, however, that bone is a living tissue that undergoes remodeling throughout adult life.

The microscopic structure of bone is such that none of the mineral crystals is far from a blood vessel, an arrangement that favors exchange of minerals and nutrients between bone tissues and body fluids. The most readily available supply of calcium and phosphorus in bones is found in the *trabeculae*—columns of crystalline calcium compounds that grow from the inner surface of the cavity at the bone's end and that project toward the center in such a way as to act as braces in strengthening the end of the bone (see Fig.15–6). The more abundant the supply of calcium in the food, the greater is the development of bone trabeculae; when dietary calcium is inadequate over a considerable period, these structures may be practically absent. Within the cavity, blood vessels and intercellular fluid come into intimate contact with the mineral material in the trabeculae, so that it may be readily taken up by the blood stream to meet minor fluctuations in blood calcium.

[2]Hydroxyapatite, $Ca_{10}(PO_4)_6(OH)_2$ is the complex bone salt.

Although only 1 percent of the body's calcium is found in the blood, the extracellular fluid, and within the cells of body tissues, this small amount is of vital physiological importance. Calcium is one of the essential factors for blood clotting, affects muscle tone and irritability, is required for normal nerve transmission, and is involved in the secretion of hormones. The proper balance between calcium ions on the one hand and sodium, potassium, and magnesium ions on the other is necessary for normal rhythmical contraction and relaxation of the heart muscles. Calcium also activates several enzymes important in metabolism. When the level of blood calcium is subnormal, these functions cannot be fulfilled; the heartbeat becomes erratic, muscles contract spontaneously (tetany), and death may result.

The essential roles of calcium in skeletal structure and cellular functions have been known for years. More recently it has been recognized that most calcium effects are mediated by way of *calcium-binding proteins.* One of these proteins, *calmodulin,* appears to be the major intracellular receptor for calcium and thus be an important regulator of calcium's cellular functions (15).

Toxicity of Calcium

Hypercalcemia is the term used to designate elevated levels of calcium in the blood. The causes of hypercalcemia are numerous and are often related to clinical conditions. One

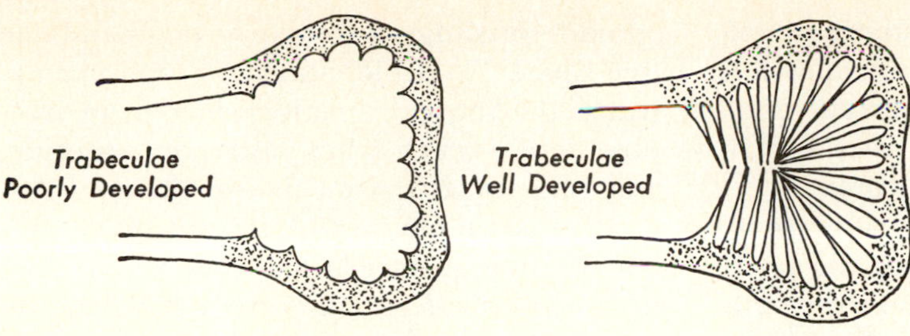

Figure 15–6 Diagrammatic representations of bone trabeculae showing poor or good development according to whether the food calcium intake is low or liberal. (From Sherman, H. C.: *Chemistry of Food and Nutrition.* New York, Macmillan Co., 1952.)

fairly common cause is prolonged immobilization, for example as a result of a fractured limb or illness, since increased bone resorption can take place under these conditions. If kidney functions are normal, the calcium excess in the blood can be excreted. Another cause is increased production of the parathyroid hormone and vitamin D intoxication.

Signs of high levels of calcium in the blood may include muscle weakness, loss of appetite, nausea and vomiting, constipation, loss of weight, and fever. Increased calcium levels also lead to less sodium reabsorption by the kidney, causing increased urination and thirst resulting from excess sodium and water loss.

Toxicity directly resulting from ingested excesses of calcium is essentially unknown in healthy individuals because of the body's ability to control the amount of calcium absorbed through the intestinal walls.

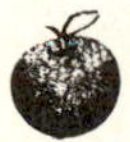

health considerations

Osteoporosis

Can osteoporosis be prevented and treated by sufficient or increased calcium (16)? Studies of the nutritional intake of older Americans show that osteoporosis, a loss of the internal mineral mass of bone, also called *osteopenia* (meaning "too little bone"), is the most frequently found disorder. As many as nine out of ten older, white females have some evidence of this condition, and one in five will suffer a hip fracture or vertebral fracture as a result. These fractures, when the result of osteoporosis, need not be caused by an accidental injury but can occur from an internal crushing of the weakened bone as it finally gives way to the stress of weight-bearing. The seriousness of hip fractures in the elderly is underscored by the fact that 15 to 30 percent of those who experience them will eventually die from resulting complications. Associated medical costs amount to about a billion dollars a year.

Women are at significantly greater risk for osteoporosis than men, since they have a less dense bone structure from youth onward. Apparently as a result of heredity, blacks have an increased bone density throughout their life span; thus black women are less likely than white women to develop osteoporosis. A few women already show a reduction in bone mass by as early as age twenty-five, and most show some decrease by thirty-five to forty. Most acceleration in loss, however, occurs after menopause, which is why estrogen replacement therapy (to compensate for a drop in estrogen production during menopause) has had much success. Without any type of preventive measures, a woman's total bone mass at age eighty may be only a half of what it was at age forty.

A major influence on the degree of bone loss at every age is thought to be a woman's calcium intake: The calcium demands of pregnancy and lactation and inadequate calcium intakes in lower-energy diets are thought to "drain" the body stores of calcium, located in bone. On any one day, it is estimated that as many as 75 percent of all women are not consuming the recommended intake of 800 mg of calcium.

In osteoporosis, the minerals that make up the bone structure are lost from the bone, released into the circulation, and eventually excreted without a corresponding bone build-up, as would occur if normal homeostatic mechanisms were working. Signs of osteoporosis can include back pain and bone deformity ("dowager's hump"), as well as fractures. Symptoms may lead to decreased activity, which in turn worsens the condition by accelerating bone loss itself. There may also be no obvious symptoms at all.

Osteoporosis no doubt has a number of nutritional and other causes working together. The exact underlying mechanisms are still not understood. Nevertheless, the influence of calcium and/or the Ca:P ratio on the development and treatment of the condition is thought to be significant. In fact, the strongest evidence for the role of dietary calcium deficiency is that experimental treatment of osteoporosis with oral calcium supplements decreases age-related bone loss. Thus, bone loss can be prevented or slowed both by estrogen replacement therapy and also by supplementation of the diet with calcium (1 gm daily is the amount often used). Estrogen therapy has been shown to increase calcium absorption in most postmenopausal women.

The total daily calcium intake required to maintain bone mass and proper calcium balance in a postmenopausal woman is now thought to be approximately 1.2 to 1.5 gm daily. This figure is higher than the present RDA, and significantly higher than most intakes in this age group. Thus, some bone disease experts are recommending calcium supplementation of the diet of all postmenopausal women if dietary intake does not reach 1.5 gm. *Fluoride* has also been used as an additional agent to help strengthen bone (see Chap. 17). In identified osteoporotic patients, the most dramatic reduction in fracture rate occurs when estrogen, fluoride, and calcium are given in combination. Another potentially useful suggestion is frequent walking, since lack of exercise can lead to increased calcium loss from bone. It also makes sense for younger people, especially women, to give some special attention to their daily calcium intake so that they are sure that they are meeting at least the recommended allowance.

In conclusion, although much research is still in progress, most authorities agree that calcium has a definite role in the prevention and treatment of osteoporosis.

PHOSPHORUS

Phosphorus (P), a nonmetallic element, was first isolated in elemental form in 1669 by the German alchemist Hennig Brand. It created much interest, since this element, in the unnatural free form, glows in the dark, and breaks into fire spontaneously upon exposure to air. It exists in nature only in the combined forms (usually with calcium) in such sources as bone and rock phosphates. Phosphorus is widely used in matches, detergents, and fertilizers. A frequent ingredient in food additives, it helps cure and retain moisture in food, as well as preserving color, flavor, and tenderness in meat.

Phosphorus is present in the human body at a level of about 1 percent. It accounts for about one-fourth of the body's total mineral content.

Deficiency Symptoms

Phosphorus deficiency is well recognized in animals, where it is characterized by poor bone mineralization and the occurrence of bone fractures. It sometimes occurs in cattle grazing on soil that has been depleted of phosphates (by crops or leaching, for example), for the grass grown on such soil is of low phosphorus content. Such a deficiency is evidenced by decrease or distortion of the appetite (desire to eat bones and wood), emaciation, weakness, and eventually death.

Phosphorus deficiency seldom develops in normal humans because of its wide distribution in food. Deficiencies are present, however, in several clinical conditions, such as in some persons who frequently take antacids, since aluminum-containing antacids can block the intestinal absorption of phosphorus. Lowered phosphorus levels may also accompany persistent vomiting, disorders of vitamin D metabolism, kidney or liver disorders, alcoholism, malabsorption, or the administration of nonphosphate-containing intravenous fluids. Up to about 20 percent of all hospitalized patients have been identified as having low levels of phosphorus in the blood (17).

Persons with symptomatic deficiencies show loss of appetite, weakness, muscle tremors, bone pain, demineralization of bone, and loss of calcium. A low phosphorus level in the blood can result in abnormalities of oxygen delivery in the body and disorders of platelets and red blood cells. Extremely low levels can result in seizures and coma. Chronically low levels cause *osteomalacia,* bone softening as a result of reduced mineral content. All of these symptoms can be reversed by the administration of phosphorus.

Allowances and Intakes

The Food and Nutrition Board has given specific recommended dietary allowances for phosphorus since 1968 (8). Prior to that time, it was simply noted that "diets sufficient in calcium and protein are probably adequate in phosphorus." Without other evidence available, the allowances for phosphorus were made the same as for calcium (except for infants). See Table 15–1 and the RDA table inside front cover. The allowance for a normal adult is 800 mg a day and for teenagers 1200 mg a day. About twice as much calcium as phosphorus is present in bones and teeth, but because of the much higher amounts of phosphorus in soft body tissues and in our food supply, it is estimated that the requirement is similar to that for calcium. These figures should be considered only preliminary, since much more research needs to be done before more specific recommendations can be made.

The level of phosphorus in the average American diet, based on studies done during the 1970s, is about 45 to 62 mg phosphorus per 100 kcal. Thus, if a person consumed 2000 kcal a day, the phosphorus intake would be around 900 to 1200 mg, and if he or she consumed 2700 kcal/day, the intake would probably be from 1200 to 1700 mg. These approximate intake figures are also commonly expressed as 15 mg phosphorus per gram of protein, or 1.5 to 1.6 mg phosphorus to 1 mg calcium. Children's intakes tend to be proportionally greater (mg per kcal ingested) than those of adolescents and adults (18).

Phosphorus in Foods

Phosphorus is associated chiefly with protein-rich foods and cereal products. It is found in many foods that contribute little calcium, as well as along with calcium in milk and its products. Rich sources of phosphorus in the diet are meats (especially organs), fish, and poultry; eggs; cheese and milk; nuts; legumes; and all foods made from grains, especially whole grains. Fruits (especially dried ones) and vegetables contribute lesser amounts of phosphorus to the diet. In general, edible roots, stems, and flowerets of plants contain similar amounts of both calcium and phosphorus, but plants concentrate calcium in the green leaves and phosphorus in the seeds (grains). The darker green leaves have higher calcium content than light green ones (for example, the inner leaves of head lettuce). Phosphorus is carried in foods more liberally than is calcium, and many foods that provide little calcium, such as meats, are excellent sources of phosphorus. (Refer to Table 15–2 for some examples of phosphorus content in foods.) Since its distribution follows that of protein, a diet that supplies adequate amounts of protein is usually adequate for phosphorus.

Table 15–3 and Figure 15–7 show that in the American food supply, more than half of the phosphorus usually comes from two major sources: milk products and meat and fish products. Flour and cereal products contribute 12 percent of the supply. The rest comes largely from eggs, potatoes, beans, and other vegetables. Sugar and fats provide only trace amounts of calcium and phosphorus.

Since vegetables generally are not rich sources of phosphorus, persons consuming typical vegetarian diets, especially those low in milk products, might easily be deficient in this element as well as in other nutrients. It is well known that farm animals fed diets composed only of grains, legumes, and green, leafy feeds must have supplementary phosphorus (as well as calcium) in order to have adequate growth and bone structure.

Phosphorus is also found in some food additives. If a person consumes daily large amounts of convenience and snack foods, the additives in them may account for as much as 20 to 30 percent of the phosphorus in the diet. A high phosphorus intake from additives may have some effect on iron and calcium absorption, at least in animals. That is another reason why people should avoid over-dependence on convenience foods by eating a variety of foods every day. The FDA has stated that "there is no reason to believe that the phosphates used in food processing at present are hazardous when used at current levels" (19).

The Role of Phosphorus in the Body

Absorption and Regulation. Seventy percent of the dietary intake of phosphorus is absorbed, as free phosphate, from the intestine. Some of the absorption occurs in proportion to water movement across the intestinal wall; another portion of the total appears to be independent of the water absorption.

Factors that influence the absorption of phosphorus include an excess of dietary

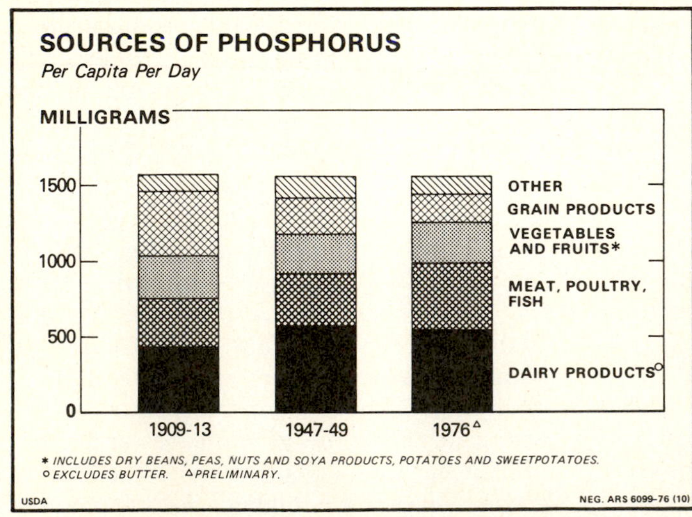

Figure 15–7 Food sources and average *per capita* intake of phosphorus from 1909 to 1976. It can be seen that over 50 percent of our current phosphorus intake (1980 figures are similar to 1976) comes from meat and dairy products, whereas a larger proportion used to be from grains. The total amount of phosphorus *per capita* per day has stayed quite constant. (Note: an exception to the figures on this chart is in infants; two thirds to all of their phosphorus intake comes from milk alone.) (From Marston, R., and Friend, B.: Nutritional review, reprinted from *The National Food Situation.* Hyattsville, Md., U.S. Department of Agriculture Agric. Res. Serv., Consumer and Food Economics Institute Report CFE (Adm.)-299-11, Jan. 1977.)

zinc, which results in decreased phosphorus (as well as calcium and magnesium) absorption in rats. The amount of fiber ingested has not been shown significantly to affect phosphorus absorption.

Vitamin D is an important regulator of phosphorus in the body. It stimulates intestinal absorption of phosphorus, increases its mobilization from bone, and increases its retention in the kidneys. Parathyroid hormone decreases retention (reabsorption) of this element by the kidney. The inorganic phosphorus level of the blood is kept quite constant by means of the above processes.

Phosphorus is excreted in the urine and feces. Its principal site of reabsorption in the kidney is the proximal tubule of the nephron.

Functions. Phosphorus is one of the most important nutrients known. It takes part in almost every metabolic reaction in the body and also has an important structural function in combining with calcium in the formation and strengthening of bone tissues. In fact, about 80 percent of the phosphorus in the body is in the bones and teeth. The remaining 20 percent, found in the blood and tissues, performs a number of other critical functions.

Inorganic phosphates (PO_4^{-3} ions, or radicals) in the blood act as buffer substances that assist in maintaining blood neutrality and the acid-base balance of the blood. Phosphorus, as phosphate, is an essential constituent of nucleic acids and nucleoproteins in cell nuclei and cytoplasm, which play a key role in reproduction, transmission of hereditary traits, cell division, and protein synthesis within the cells. Phosphates are also a component of phospholipids, which promote the emulsification and transport of fats and fatty acids, as well as the permeability of cell membranes. For this reason, phosphorus is important in normal transmission of nerve impulses. Also, phosphorus is indispensable to the oxidation of carbohydrates, by which much of the energy for body processes is obtained; it links with glycogen and glucose to activate them for oxidation, and it is a part of several enzymes or coenzymes that are essential to this oxidation. Adenosine mono-, di-, and triphosphates are among the most vital of all body substances for regulating hormone activity and for providing quick release of energy in muscular contraction.

Phosphorus is highly reactive and imparts this property to substances with which it is combined. Phosphorus is present in or combines readily with proteins, lipids, or carbohydrates. Chemically inert substances such as glucose and fats become highly reactive in tissue metabolism and more readily transported in body fluids by combination with phosphate radicals. From one-half to two-thirds the phosphorus in blood is contained within the red cells.

Toxicity of Phosphorus

An excess of phosphorus has been shown to result in a decrease of the calcium level in the blood and to inhibit bone mineralization. A decreased calcium level can lead to tetany, a condition that has occurred in infants given formulas too high in phosphorus in relation to calcium. The adverse effects of excessive dietary phosphorus on bone development are most apparent in animals such as the chick, in which bone formation and remodeling occur rapidly. (See section on the calcium-to-phosphorus ratio for more information on the relationship between these two elements in the diet.) Because laxatives and enemas may contain phosphates, their excessive use may lead to phosphate toxicity, with a life-threatening decreased calcium level in the blood as a possible result (20). The main problem so far recognized with high phosphate levels in the blood is the fact that calcium levels decline as phosphate levels rise.

MAGNESIUM

Magnesium (Mg) is a silvery white metallic element related closely to calcium and zinc. The eighth most plentiful element in the earth's crust (2.5 percent), it is the lightest structural metal and is found widely distributed in a variety of compounds. Magnesium alloys (usually containing over 75 percent of this mineral) are used in airplanes, parts of cars (up to 90 lb [41 kg] in a Volkswagen), ladders, portable tools, luggage, vacuum cleaners and as the silverlike material that provides the light in flares, flash bulbs, and fireworks. Magnesium is also the major mineral in asbestos, talcum powder, and dolomite limestone (a fertilizer).

Even more important than these industrial uses is magnesium's centrality to the energy cycle required for all life. It is the central component of *chlorophyll,* the well-known green pigment of all higher plants. One of the most important biological processes, photosynthesis, is dependent on the magnesium-containing chlorophyll molecule; this process harnesses the sun's energy, with water and carbon dioxide, to produce glucose and oxygen. A plant without adequate magnesium will become stunted and will have pale yellowish leaves as a result of the lack of chlorophyll. When magnesium is restored to the soil, the plant will again grow and its leaves will return to their normal green color.

Magnesium is a major mineral component of sea water (0.13 percent), from which life and chlorophyll originally evolved. It is estimated that each cubic mile of sea water contains 6 million tons of magnesium, so it appears that we will have enough in the future to take care of our needs!

Magnesium is the fourth most abundant cation in the human body, after calcium, potassium, and sodium. The body contains about 20 to 28 gm of magnesium, more than half of which is found in the complex salts that make up bone. The remainder is found chiefly within the cells of tissues and organs such as the skeletal muscles and the heart, kidney, and liver. Only about 1 percent of body magnesium is extracellular, existing in the body fluids and taking part in the transfer by osmosis of water into and out of the cells. Most magnesium circulates in body fluids in ionic form, but about 35 percent of magnesium in blood serum is bound to protein. Bone magnesium and blood magnesium are exchangeable as needed for balance in the body.

Deficiency Symptoms

Symptoms of magnesium deficiency are slow to develop in humans because of reserve stores in the body. Symptoms of deficiency in animals are first, failure to grow, followed by pallor, weakness, low level of magnesium in the blood, excessive irritability of nerves and muscles, irregular heartbeats, heart and kidney damage, and convulsions or seizures, especially when the animal is suddenly disturbed. Death can result in a few weeks' time in small animals fed magnesium-deficient diets.

In humans, clinical magnesium deficiency is usually a result of excessive losses of magnesium from the kidney or digestive tract. The conditions that cause such loss include malnutrition, diabetes, malabsorption, prolonged diarrhea, and alcoholism. Low magnesium levels can also be seen in persons receiving diuretics for long periods and in some surgery patients who are on restricted diets. Deficiencies have also been noted in some people on a liquid protein diet, as well as in hospital patients receiving intravenous fluids without magnesium over a long period.

Deficiency signs in humans are similar to those first identified in experimental animals. Symptoms include weakness, muscle pain and cramps, vertigo, twitching and tremors, muscle spasms, and convulsions, all indications of neuromuscular over-excitability. (Tetany, a specific type of muscle rigidity, has been described in relation to magnesium depletion, but it is usually related to the low calcium levels that may coexist with some instances of low magnesium.) Behavioral disturbances, including apathy, delirium, and depression, are another sign. Dangerous changes in heart rhythm may also be seen (see also the health considerations section on heart disease on p. 376).

The body's protective action against a state of magnesium depletion rests primarily with the kidney, which retains the element when losses begin to exceed input. Levels of magnesium in the blood usually remain within the normal range until the deficiency is fairly severe.

On the other hand, even though body stores of magnesium are normal, levels in the blood may decline after periods of extreme stress. This apparent breakdown of the normal regulation processes (although possibly serving a physiological purpose of which we are not presently aware) has been shown to occur in animals after the stress of severe cold and in humans after serious injury or extensive surgery. These lowered levels alone may result in some of the signs of magnesium deficiency just described.

Magnesium deficiency is clearly an important concern for professional nutritionists and clinicians (21). The reader need remember chiefly that a deficiency of magnesium is extremely unlikely in normal persons eating a variety of wholesome foods.

Discovery

Most Americans are familiar with "milk of magnesia" (magnesium hydroxide) and Epsom salts[3] (magnesium sulfate). Salts of magnesium have been known through the ages for their healing properties. An unknown Roman claimed many centuries ago that "magnesia alba" (white magnesium salts from the district of Magnesia in Greece, for which the element was eventually named) cured many ailments. The Scottish chemist Joseph Black, working with this substance (now known to be magnesium carbonate), discovered in 1755 that magnesium was an element. Like many other elements, it was first isolated by Sir Humphry Davy, in 1808.

Magnesium was found to be present in the human body in the 1850s and to be essential for plant life in 1860. Not until 1926 did the French chemist J. Leroy, working with mice, prove that magnesium is an essential nutrient for the animal body. Later, in the United States, E. V. McCollum and co-workers described the wide range of deficiency signs in rats and dogs, including what they termed *magnesium tetany,* a form of convulsions in which the nerves and muscles are affected (22). Indications that magnesium was required by humans were published within the next decade (1933–1944). More complete proof of human need for magnesium has since been shown by a number of scientists (6), and deficiency states in humans have now been clearly defined (21). This is a very active research area.

Allowances and Intakes

The magnesium requirement depends upon body size and composition of the diet. A great amount of calcium in the diet, for instance, is known to compete with the absorption of magnesium. Protein, phosphorus, and vitamin D levels also influence the requirement. Requirements are higher during pregnancy and lactation.

The latest RDAs for magnesium are summarized in Table 15–6 and are given in detail inside the front cover. For magnesium, the allowances are from 25 to 50 percent higher than minimal requirements (which

[3]Named after Epsom, a village south of London, found in 1618 to have a water supply with wound-healing properties and a laxative effect. "Epsom salts" were the substance formed after evaporation of the water.

Table 15–6 RECOMMENDED DIETARY ALLOWANCES FOR MAGNESIUM*

	Age (yrs)	*Magnesium (mg/day)*
Males	11–14	350
	15–18	400
	19–22	350
	23–50	350
	51+	350
Females	11–14	300
	15–18	300
	19–22	300
	23–50	300
	51+	300
	Pregnant	450
	Lactating	450

*From Food and Nutrition Board, 1980 (6).

range between 200 and 300 mg per day for adults) to allow for individual differences, normal stresses, and variations in diet. An additional allowance of 150 mg per day is recommended for pregnant and lactating women.

The average American diet contains an estimated content of about 120 mg of magnesium per 1000 kcal (6). Thus, a person taking in 2000 kcal would receive approximately 240 mg of magnesium, and a 2800 kcal diet would contain about 340 mg. These figures are close to the allowances.

Some concern has been voiced, however, that magnesium intakes may not actually be at optimal levels, especially for those on diets containing relatively large amounts of starches, potatoes, fatty meats, and dairy products (foods that are not rich in magnesium). Recent studies provide the following information about actual intakes and food magnesium content:

1. Analyses of student meals at a university cafeteria showed that their magnesium content was lower than the RDA.
2. At least some adolescent females may lose more magnesium than they take in(23).
3. In another group of adolescent females, the calculated magnesium intake was only two-thirds of the RDA. Blood values for magnesium were within normal limits.
4. From 13 to 35 percent of preteen females were found to consume less than 67 percent of the RDA (24).
5. A group of economically privileged American mothers had a mean intake of 60 percent of the RDA.
6. Athletes have moderately decreased magnesium levels in the blood.
7. A 1977 U.S. Department of Agriculture dietary survey showed that average daily magnesium intakes of women were slightly more than 200 mg, and for men, close to 300 mg. Females age twelve and over averaged 69 to 79 percent of the RDA; boys and men, 80 to 89 percent (10).

It can be seen that there is room for improvement in reaching 100 percent of the recommended allowances for magnesium in most of the groups studied.

Magnesium in Foods

Distribution of magnesium in foods tends to follow that of protein and phosphorus. Whole grains, nuts, beans, legumes, and green, leafy vegetables are good sources. Animal products, including meat and milk, are only poor to fair sources. Processing of foods can result in great losses. Thus, there is little left in rice and white flour (about 20 percent of that in the whole grain) and practically none in sugar, alcohol, or fats and oils. Boiling of vegetables can cause losses if the water is discarded. Table 15–7 gives figures for magnesium distribution in some common foods.

In an average American diet, most of the magnesium comes from fruits and vegetables (22 percent), cereal products and flour (21 percent), meat, poultry, fish, and eggs (20 percent), milk and milk products (17 percent), nonalcoholic beverages (12 percent), legumes (5 percent), and other foods, including desserts and chocolate (3 percent) (USDA figures from 1977) (10).

Table 15–7 EXAMPLES OF MAGNESIUM DISTRIBUTION IN COMMON FOOD

Food	*Magnesium in Edible Portion, mg/100 gm**	*Magnesium in Average Serving, mg*	*Food*	*Magnesium in Edible Portion, mg/100 gm**	*Magnesium in Average Serving, mg***
Apples, raw, unpared	8	10	Lettuce	11	10
Bananas, raw	33	55	Liver, beef	13	15
Beans, raw, canned, baked	37	35	Macaroni, cooked	20	25
Beans, snap, frozen	21	15	Milk, whole	13	30
Beef, hamburger, broiled	25	20	Oatmeal, cooked	21	30
Beet greens	106	80	Orange juice, frozen	10	20
Bread, white	22	5	Peaches, raw	10	12
Bread, whole-wheat	78	10	Peanuts, roasted	173	50
Cabbage, raw	13	10	Peas	35	15
Cake, (Angel Food)	—	10	Potatoes, unpeeled, baked	34	45
Carrots, raw	23	15	Rice, brown, cooked	29	40
Chard, Swiss	65	45	Rice, white, cooked	8	10
Cheese, cheddar	45	8	Soybeans, cooked	265	80
Chicken, white meat	19	10	Spinach	88	60
Chocolate, sweet	107	35	Sweet potatoes	31	40
Cocoa, dry powder	420	20	Tomatoes, raw	14	20
Coffee, instant, dry powder	456	10	Turnip greens	58	20
Corn flakes	16	4	Walnuts, black	190	20
Eggs, whole	11	6	Wheat, shredded (cereal)	130	65
Flour, whole-wheat	133	—	Wheat germ	336	90
Flour, all-purpose	25	—	Yeast, brewer's	231	10

*Watt, B. K., and Merrill, A. L.: *Composition of Foods: Raw, Processed, Prepared.* Washington, D.C., U.S. Department of Agriculture Handbook No. 8, 1963.

**Source: Table 2, Appendix.

The Role of Magnesium in the Body

Absorption and Regulation. Magnesium salts (like those of calcium) are usually rather insoluble, so that their absorption, which occurs when magnesium is in its ionic, dissolved form, is relatively inefficient. The use of high levels of salts such as magnesium sulfate as laxatives depends on the fact that they draw much water into the intestinal tract by osmosis because they are so poorly absorbed.

About 30 to 40 percent of ingested magnesium is normally absorbed, nearly all in the small intestine. This amount will vary depending on the amount of magnesium in the diet, For example, if magnesium intake is low, up to 75 percent may be absorbed. In active transport across the intestinal membrane, magnesium salts seem to use the same route as calcium salts, so that a high intake of either interferes with the absorption of the other. (Unlike calcium, there is little excretion of magnesium through the intestine, except that which is unabsorbed from the food.) Vitamin D increases the absorption of magnesium as well as of calcium. Substances that may decrease the amount of magnesium absorbed include excess fiber and phytate.

The body's balance of magnesium is primarily regulated by the kidney. The normal kidney is able to conserve magnesium efficiently when necessary, thus, low levels of magnesium in the urine are an early sign of magnesium deficiency. Levels in the blood are kept within a narrow range by the kidney, the parathyroid hormone, and other regulatory mechanisms.

Sixty or 70 percent of intake is lost (without being absorbed) in the feces. Of that absorbed, the urine is the primary route of eventual excretion. Small amounts are lost in perspiration. Urinary excretion usually amounts to about one-third of intake. Factors that increase excretion of magnesium are increased calcium in the body, diuretics, and an increase in extracellular fluid; factors that inhibit excretion include a low level of magnesium in the blood (this stimulates parathyroid hormone, which decreases urinary losses of both calcium and magnesium).

A continuing obligatory loss of magnesium occurs even with very low magnesium intake. Thus, a magnesium deficiency can possibly result from long-term inadequate dietary intake, especially with the added stress of serious illness or conditions causing excess magnesium losses.

Functions. Magnesium is essential to the activities of all the body's cells. Aside from its role as part of bone structure, its main function is to activate numerous enzyme systems that control carbohydrate, fat, and electrolyte metabolism and active transport across cell membranes. Magnesium is necessary for the important chemical reaction oxidative phosphorylation, which converts adenosine diphosphate (ADP) to adenosine triphosphate, with a high energy bond (ATP). It is a co-factor for all of the important actions of ATP in the processes of metabolism, that is, it activates the enzymes that transfer the high-energy phosphate groups. Magnesium is also necessary for the maintenance of the normal structure of ribosomes and thus for protein synthesis.

With this understanding of the importance of magnesium to vital enzyme functioning, it becomes clear why it is considered essential for the transmission of nerve impulses, for normal contraction of muscles in the heart and throughout the body, and for normal metabolism and growth of body cells and tissues. Other roles of magnesium include an ability to act as a metabolic antagonist to some of the actions of calcium and to stimulate the normal release and the activity of parathyroid hormone.

Toxicity of Magnesium

Too much magnesium has toxic effects, including loss of reflexes, drowsiness, respiratory and central nervous system depression, coma, and, ultimately, death. Toxicity may occur with over-administration of magnesium salts in clinical situations (for example, when magnesium is used for an anti-convulsant action). It can also occur in persons with kidney failure, since the healthy kidney is an all-important regulator of normal magnesium balance.

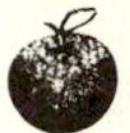

health considerations

Magnesium and Heart Disease

A deficiency of magnesium has been suggested as a cause of coronary artery disease of the heart and associated sudden death. Various evidence supports this hypothesis (25).

One known effect of low magnesium levels is heart rhythm abnormalities (arrhythmias); magnesium therapy has improved arrhythmias as well as heart muscle performance after damage resulting from lack of oxygen. Studies of animal muscle function seem to substantiate the clinical impressions of the benefit of magnesium in these conditions. For example, magnesium-deficient diets have been shown to predispose experimental animals to metabolic alterations in heart muscle fibers.

In addition, chronic magnesium deficiency in animals (dogs) have been shown to result in microscopic changes in the coronary arteries, as well as fibrotic (scarlike) changes within the heart muscle itself, which were followed by calcium deposition. Other possible alterations affecting heart function when magnesium is deficient include secondary changes in other important electrolytes with known heart effects, such as potassium and calcium. Additional potential deleterious effects of low magnesium levels on the heart's blood vessels (important since the heart muscle depends on blood brought through a limited number of coronary arteries) appear to include interference with (1) normal tone and tension in the muscles of the artery walls and (2) normal calcium functions and distribution in the cells of these muscles. The influence on tension properties can lead to spasm of the small arteries of the heart, with resultant decreased blood supply to the affected heart areas, possibly leading to symptoms of a heart attack.

Also reported have been associations between sudden death from heart disease and low magnesium content of drinking water in certain geographic areas. (See also Chap. 13.) Lower than normal levels of magnesium have been found in heart muscle of victims of sudden cardiac death (although it is possible that this is an association rather than a causal relationship). Other studies have pointed to a relation between diseases that result in high blood pressure and decreased levels of magnesium; this relationship has also been shown in experimental animals.

Thus, evidence is accumulating to indicate that magnesium may be more important in heart and blood vessel health than previously recognized. From a practical standpoint, this evidence can be viewed as another reason to aim for a wide variety of healthful foods to assure consistent, fully adequate magnesium intakes.

QUESTIONS

1. Where in the body is most of the calcium and phosphorus found? What function to they serve in this tissue? In what other tissues do these mineral elements occur, and what are their functions there?

2. List three possible signs of an inadequate calcium intake in a child. What special advantages are there in a liberal intake of both calcium and phosphorus for young children? Why are the needs for these two elements greater in pregnant women and nursing mothers than in other adults?

3. Can the body build up reserve stores of calcium and phosphorus, provided the diet supplies more than enough to meet current body needs? Where are these elements stored? What are the bone trabeculae, and what is the advantage of having them well developed?

4. What are two hormones that help to regulate the calcium level in the blood? Which one increases calcium levels and how does it accomplish this?

5. Look up the minimum requirement and recommended allowance for calcium and phosphorus in your age group. Then multiply the number of full glasses of milk that you drink in a typical day by 290 mg (the amount of calcium in 8 oz of milk). Does the result approach your calcium allowance? If not, look up some other foods in Table 2 of the Appendix that would allow you to reach the recommended amount of calcium.

6. Name three factors that have a favorable influence and three that have an unfavorable influence on absorption of calcium from the intestinal contents. What vitamin exerts an important influence on the utilization of calcium and phosphorus? Explain how the body may adapt to varying levels of calcium intake.

7. Name four specific foods that are comparatively rich in calcium and four rich in phosphorus. What is the Ca:P ratio for each of these foods? (Look up the Ca and P content for each.) Which are closest to a 1:1 ratio? Which classes of food contribute phosphorus liberally but carry little calcium? Why is the average diet less likely to be high in calcium than in phosphorus?

8. Why are some authorities recommending a calcium intake of more than 800 mg a day for older women?

9. Does phosphorus in the "average" American diet tend to be lower or higher than the RDA? What is a common source of phosphorus in convenience and processed foods? Is there a danger in high phosphorus levels in the blood?

10. What is the mineral essential for photosynthesis, and why? List two minerals essential to the body's oxidative processes. Which minerals discussed in this chapter affect the rhythm of the heart?

11. The first patient to receive an artificial heart experienced muscle convulsions, or seizures, a few days after the surgery. His physicians said these were due to a "chemical imbalance," which they soon corrected, with the help of some supplemental feeding. Which mineral or minerals discussed in this chapter do you think could have been responsible?

References

1. Kesteloot, H., and Geboers, J.: Calcium and blood pressure. Lancet, *1*:813, 1982; McCarron, D. A.: Low serum concentrations of ionized calcium in patients with hypertension. New Eng. J. Med., *307*:226, 1982; McCarron, D. A., Morris, C. D., and Cole, C.: Dietary calcium in human hypertension. Science, *217*:267, 1982. (Also see Science, *219*:112, 1983.)
2. Osborne, T. B., and Mendel, L. B.: J. Biol. Chem., *34*:131, 1918.
3. McCollum, E. V.: Amer. J. Physiol., *25*:120, 1909; Hart, E. B., McCollum, E. V., and Fuller J. G.: Univ. Wis. Agric. Exp. Stat. Res. Bull. No. 1, 1909; Plimmer, R. H. A.: Biochem. J., *7*:34, 1913; Forbes, E. B., and Keith, M. H.: Ohio Agric. Exp. Stat. Tech. Ser. Bull. No. 5, 1914.
4. Hegsted, D. M., Moscoso, J., and Collazos, C.: J. Nutr., *46*:181, 1952; Nicolaysen, R., et al.: Physiol. Rev., *33*:424, 1953.
5. Ohlsen, M. A.: J. Amer. Dietet. Assoc., *31*:333, 1955.
6. Food and Nutrition Board: *Recommended Dietary Allowances.* 9th Ed. Washington, D.C., National Research Council, National Academy of Sciences, 1980.
7. FAO Nutrition Meetings Report: *Calcium Requirements.* Series No. 30. Rome, 1962.
8. Heaney, R. P., Recker, R. R., and Saville, P. D.: Calcium balance and calcium requirements in middle-aged women. Amer. J. Clin. Nutr., *30*:1603, 1978; Matkovic, V., et al.: Bone status and fracture rates in two regions of Yugoslavia. Amer. J. Clin. Nutr., *32*:953, 1979.
9. Sherman H. C., and Hawley, E.: J. Biol. Chem., *55*:375, 1922; Daniels, A. L., et al.: J. Nutr., *10*:373, 1935; Stearns, G., and Jeans, P. C.: Proc. Soc. Exp. Biol. Med., *32*:428, 1934; Stearns, G.: J. Amer. Med. Assoc., *142*:478, 1950.
10. Consumer Nutrition Center: *Food and Nutrient Intakes of Individuals in One Day in the United States, Spring 1977. Nationwide Food Consumption Survey 1977–1978,* Preliminary Rep. No. 2, USDA, Science and Education Administration, September, 1980.
11. Abraham, S., et al.: *Dietary Intake Findings, U.S. 1971–1974,* HANES Rept., Pub. No. (HRA)*17*-1647, 1977, Hyattsville, Maryland, U.S. Dept. of Health, Education, and Welfare (National Center for Health Statistics); Lowenstein, F. W.: Amer. J. Clin. Nutr., *29*:918, 1976.
12. Pao, E. M., and Mickle, S. J.: Problem nutrients in the United States. Food Tech., *35* (Sept.):58, 1981.
13. Center for Disease Control: *Ten-State Nutrition Survey in the United States, 1968–1970*(preliminary report). Washington, D.C., U.S. Department of Health, Education, and Welfare, 1971.
14. Wasserman, R. H.: Intestinal absorption of calcium and phosphorus. Fed. Proc., *40*:68, 1981.
15. West, W. L., et al.: Calmodulin-regulated enzymes: modifications by drugs and disease (a symposium). Fed. Proc., *41*:2251, 1982; Stinson, S.: Calmodulin structure and function clarified. Chem. and Eng. News, June 2, 1980, p. 18; Cheung, W. Y.: Calmodulin. Sci. Amer., *246*:62, 1982.
16. (Osteoporosis and calcium-related dysfunctions) Albanese, A. A., et al.: Nutr. Rep. Internat., *24*:403, 1981; Lancet, *2*:423, 1982; Draper, H. H., et al.: (symposium): Fed. Proc., *40*:2417, 1981; Gordan, G. S.: West. J. Med., *133*:331, 1980; Heaney, R. P.: J. Amer. Med. Assoc., *245*:1362, 1981; Lee, C. J., Lawler, M. S., and Johnson, G. H.: Amer. J. Clin. Nutr., *34*:819, 1981; Marcus, R.: Metabolism, *31*:93, 1982; Whedon, G. D.: New Eng. J. Med., *305*:397, 1981; Recker, R. R.: Contemp. Nutr. (General Mills), *8*(No. 5): 1, 1983.
17. Juan, D., and Elrazak, M. A.: Hypophosphatemia in hospitalized patients. J. Amer. Med. Assoc., *242*:163, 1979.
18. Greger, J. L., and Krystofiak, M.: Phosphorus intake of Americans. Food Tech., *36*:78, 1982.
19. GRAS affirmations proposed for phosphates. Food Chem. News, Dec. 24, 1979, p. 58.
20. McConnell, T. H.: J. Amer. Med. Assoc., *216*:147, 1971; Rao, K. J.: N.Y. State J. Med., *76*:968, 1976; Sotos, J. F. : Pediatrics, *60*:305, 1977.
21. (Magnesium deficiency) Abdulla, M.: Nutr. Rev., *38*:99, 1980; Lancet, *1*:523, 1976; Nutr. Rev., *37*:6, 1979; Flink, E. B.: Acta Medica Scand., suppl. 647, 1981; Gitelman, H. J., and Welt, L. G.: Ann. Rev. Med., *20*:233, 1969; Wacker, W. E. C., and Parisi, A. F.: New Eng. J. Med., *278*:658, 1968.

22. Kruse, H. D., Orent, E. R., and McCollum, E. V.: J. Biol. Chem., *96*:519, 1932; *100*:603, 1933; Orent, E. R., Kruse, H. D., and McCollum, E. V.: Amer. J. Physiol., *101*:454, 1932; J. Biol. Chem., *106*:573, 1934.
23. Greger, J. L., et al.: Calcium, magnesium phosphorus, copper, and manganese balance in adolescent females. Amer. J. Clin. Nutr., *31*:117, 1978.
24. Huber, H. G., Disney, G. W., and Mason, R. L.: Urinary excretion and dietary intake of magnesium in girls. Nutr. Rept. Internat., *23*:127, 1981.
25. (Magnesium and heart disease) Altura, B. M., and Altura, B. T.: Fed. Proc., *40*:2672, 1981; Altura, B. M., et al.: Artery, *9*:212, 1981; Karppanen, H.: Artery, *9*:190, 1981; Manthey, J., et al.: Circulation, *64*:722, 1981; Shine, K. I.: Amer. J. Physiol., *237*:H413, 1979; Turlapaty, P. D. M. V., and Altura, B. M.: Science, *208*:198, 1980; Ebel, H. and Gunther, T.: J. Clin. Chem. Clin. Biochem., *21*: 249 (a review), 1983.

16 The Trace Elements Iron, Iodine, Copper, and Manganese

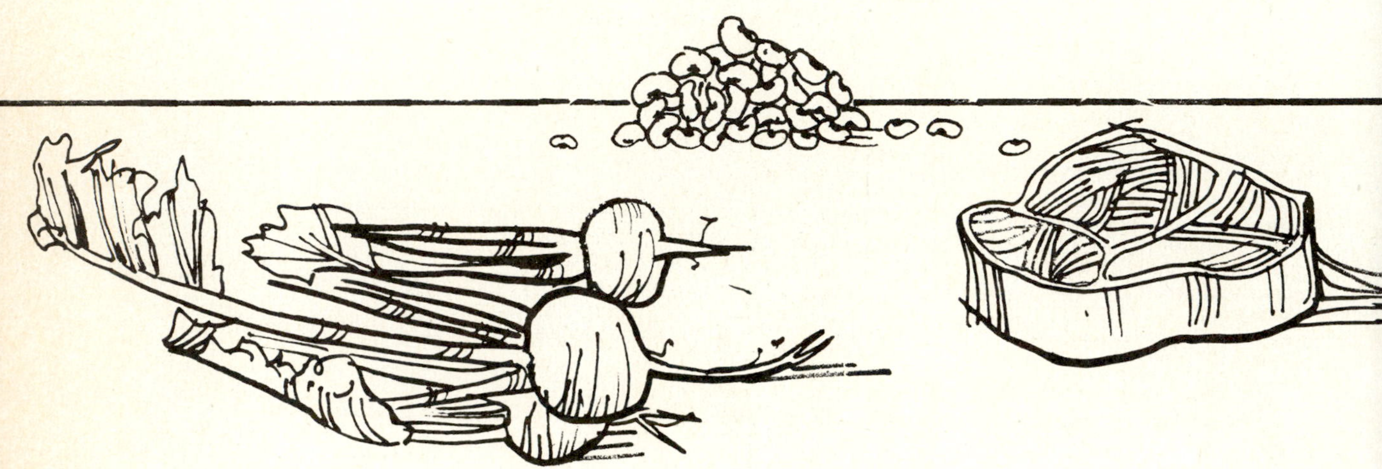

The six macrominerals discussed so far (plus organic sulfur) make up 99 percent of the mineral content of the body. The trace elements, which represent the other 1 percent, make up in importance what they lack in size. They are just as vital to our health as are water, oxygen, energy sources, amino acids, the essential fatty acids, and the macrominerals, which we have already considered.

This chapter introduces the trace elements and discusses iron, iodine, copper, and manganese—the first of the trace elements found to be required. The other, "newer," trace elements will be discussed in the next chapter. Much interesting experimental work is being conducted worldwide on all the trace elements.

TRACE ELEMENTS

The *essential trace elements* can be defined simply as those elements necessary in the diet of humans or animals in trace amounts—less than 100 milligrams (mg) per day for humans. This is an arbitrary dividing line, of use chiefly to students and teachers.

The word trace was given to these elements by early nutritionists before modern methods of analyzing food and tissues were available. The levels present were just barely discernible in a qualitative way only and, therefore, were said to be present in trace amounts—hence "trace elements."

Measuring Trace Elements

The requirements for the trace elements range from milligram quantities for iron, zinc, and manganese down to microgram quantities for some of the newly discovered elements such as selenium, chromium, and vanadium. They are measured in foods and tissues in concentrations of parts per million (ppm) or sometimes in amounts as low as parts per billion (ppb). One ppm equals 1 mg per kilogram (kg), and one ppb equals 1 microgram (μg) per kg. A combined total of only about 25 to 30 grams (gm) of all trace elements, about 1 ounce (oz), exists in the human body as compared with over 1000 gm of calcium alone.

The Essential Trace Elements

There is no one convenient way to classify trace elements in nutrition because they vary so much in function, distribution, level at which they are needed, and chemical properties. To call them the minor elements is very misleading. Table 16-1 lists the fourteen essential trace elements in about the order of discovery of their nutritional importance, the order in which they will be discussed. Ten of these have been proven to be required by humans, either by their known role in essential body functions or by direct experimental evidence. Four more can be assumed to be needed by humans since they are required by experimental animals.

Since the last edition of this textbook in 1979, two trace elements, molybdenum and selenium, formerly in the "needed by animals" category, have been proven to be

Table 16–1 TRACE ELEMENTS, ESSENTIAL AND NONESSENTIAL

Essential Trace Elements	*Examples of Trace Elements Present in Food for Which No Essential Role Is Proven, or Considered, for Higher Animals*	
Essential for humans:	Possibly essential in animals (claims have been made in the literature):	
1. Iron	Boron	
2. Iodine	Lead	
3. Copper	Tin	
4. Manganese	Tungsten	
5. Zinc	Cadmium	
6. Fluorine	Element known to have a biological role in plants:[c]	
7. Cobalt[a]	Boron	
8. Molybdenum	No essential role known in plants or animals (examples):	
9. Selenium	Aluminum	Lithium
10. Chromium	Antimony	Mercury
Essential for animals:[b]	Barium	Platinum
11. Nickel	Beryllium	Rubidium
12. Vanadium	Bismuth	Silver
13. Silicon	Bromine	Strontium
14. Arsenic	Cadmium	Titanium
Total: 14 essential trace elements	Gallium	Zirconium
	Germanium	Others
	Gold	

[a]Needed by man in the organic form, as vitamin B-12 (but can be utilized by many animal species in inorganic form for vitamin B-12 synthesis).

[b]The need by man has not yet been proved for these but can be assumed from their role in animals. (See Chap. 17.)

[c]In addition to boron, certain other trace elements are required by plants in common with animals (see text). Bromine can substitute for chlorine requirements in most plants. Higher plants *do not require* iodine, fluorine, chromium, nickel, arsenic, or vanadium as far as is known, and do not generally require selenium, cobalt, silicon, or sodium.

required by humans. Understandably, studies with humans, when feasible, are much more expensive and difficult to conduct than studies with animals.

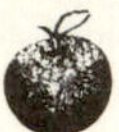

health considerations

"Organic" Foods

Because we hear so much today about "organic" foods (meaning "organically grown" foods), it is important to look briefly at the role of trace elements in the nourishment of plants used as food sources. Sellers of "organic" foods state that food labeled organic is produced with the use of humus and organic fertilizers, and without the use of chemical pesticides, herbicides, hormones, antibiotics, or food additives. There is no easy way to corroborate most of these claims, and except for the possibility that certain trace elements might be present in higher levels, there is no basis for claiming significant nutritional superiority of such foods.

"Organic" foods are not likely to be any less free of contamination with filth, mold or bacterial growth, natural toxins, or heavy metals (such as mercury or lead) than the same natural foods sold at regular food stores usually at much lower prices.

Of the essential trace elements listed in Table 16–1, only iron, copper, manganese, zinc, molybdenum, and boron are essential for the growth of most plants. From these elements in inorganic form, plus nitrogen, sulfur, calcium, phosphorus, chlorine, potassium, magnesium, water, carbon dioxide, and sunlight (energy), the plant is able to grow normally and make within its own tissues all the carbohydrates, fiber, protein, fat, vitamins, pigments, flavors, and other substances that make up plant foods as we know them.

None of the substances known to be required in the soil for plant growth are needed in the organic form—in fact, organic sources of the elements must first be broken down to inorganic forms before they can be absorbed by the plant root tips. (Certain organic plant hormones in soil can be exceptions.) This explains why the term organic food is a misnomer. All foods of plant or animal origin are basically organic in the chemical sense regardless of how they are grown.

Plants have the ability to absorb into their tissues trace elements from the soil whether or not they are required. This fact is usually fortunate because foods derived from these plants can later serve as sources of these trace elements for humans and animals (unless, of course, excessive amounts of toxic elements are absorbed by the plant). The level of all trace elements in plant tissues, and to a small extent the level of certain other minerals, protein, and vitamins, is influenced by the level of these trace elements in the soil (1,2). In some situations, such as the levels in plant food of iodine, copper, zinc, chromium, and selenium, the influence of soil elements can be considerable. Climate, temperature, chemical composition of the soil, and other environmental conditions can also affect plant composition.

Thus, theoretically, plant foods raised on soils with "natural," or organic, fertilizers containing many trace elements, such as compost and farm manures, could be nutritionally superior to plant foods raised on soil deficient in trace elements. But they would be superior only if they made up a major part of a person's diet over a long period of time and if other sources of these trace elements were not available.

In terms of an individual's nutritional needs, he or she should keep in mind that those trace minerals that occur in different amounts in the soil: (1) are not usually in short supply in farm soils but, if they are, could be added as inorganic fertilizers; (2) are generally present in adequate amounts in a mixed diet consisting of a variety of foodstuffs and iodized salt; and (3) can be added to foods by other means such as enrichment programs (although that is not done generally except for iron and iodine).

The foregoing discussion is not meant to underrate the value of compost, farm manures, and other organic fertilizers. They are very useful, though not necessary, for plant growth and soil texture. It needs to be made clear, however, that, nutritionally speaking, "organically grown" foods serve no essential nutritional needs and have no special magic (see Fig. 16–1). Furthermore, there are insufficient supplies of organic fertilizer available to raise all the crops necessary to feed the American population—or any other large population. Inorganic fertilizers and approved food additives serve an essential function in providing an abundant amount of relatively inexpensive, nutritionally valuable foods. (See also supplementary readings in the Appendix.)

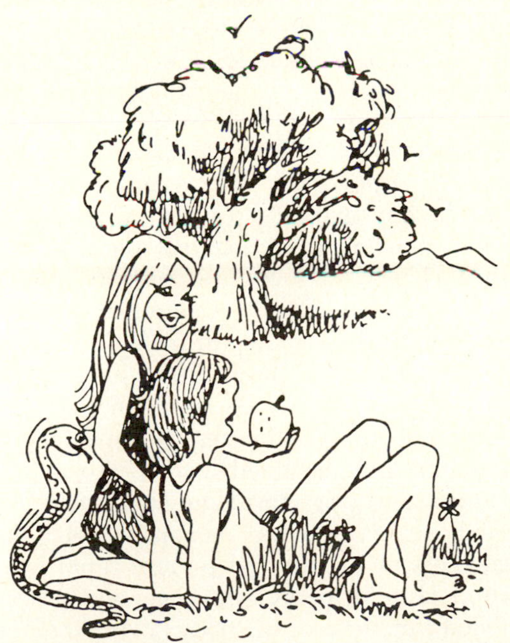

"Is it organic or inorganic?"

Figure 16–1 "Is it organic or inorganic?" (Courtesy, USDA.) See Ensminger et al., 1983 (3).

Trace Elements in Foods

As explained, the amount of many trace elements, especially the micronutrients, in plants depends to some extent on the soil in which the plant is raised. For that reason no attempt is made here to provide tables of distribution in plant foods of many of the trace elements discussed in these two chapters. Such information would be quite meaningless. As a general rule, however, since plant cells require certain trace elements for their growth, a diet consisting of a variety of plant foods from various geographical areas would almost always provide reasonably good sources of trace elements. Foods of animal origin, though, such as eggs, red meat, fish, milk, poultry, and sea foods, are more likely to contain fairly constant and adequate amounts of essential trace elements because animals will not grow or reproduce if the trace elements are absent from their diet or their tissues. This is one of the major reasons nutritionists generally recommend some animal foods as part of a normal diet.

The processing of foods, if severe and if anything is discarded, can be just as detrimental to trace minerals as to vitamins. Boiling or blanching of foods (and discarding the water) or removal of the endosperm of grains are examples of processes that can remove trace elements. Few trace elements are present in highly processed foods such as starch, sugar, gelatin, fats, and oils, or in foods made from these products, such as soft drinks, desserts, or hard candies.

Trace Element Metabolism in the Body

Absorption. As a general rule, all the trace elements, except cobalt, are absorbed (or can be) in the inorganic form before being utilized by the body. Some minerals present in organic forms in the food must be split off to the free inorganic form before absorption. Others, such as iron in meat and chromium, are better absorbed in organic forms, though inorganic forms are quite well utilized. It is also a general rule that trace elements in food may not be readily available from the intestine and, in such instances, are only partially absorbed. Because such small amounts of trace elements are present in the intestine, their availability to the body can be affected by the level of other minerals as well as by the presence of various organic compounds such as *oxalates, phytates,*[1] or other organic *chelating*[2] compounds (natural or synthetic compounds that can chelate, or "tie up" an element, thus preventing its absorption). Specific exceptions and examples will be discussed individually.

Function. The trace elements have no common biological role other than that they usually function in the body at the cellular level, often as constituents of enzymes or as enzyme activators. Their function is not unlike that of vitamins in some ways. Some of the trace elements function in the body as constituents of important organic compounds, such as iron in *hemoglobin* and iodine in the hormone *thyroxine.*

The specific role of each element, if known, will be discussed individually. The function of some of the newly discovered essential elements is unknown. (See Chap. 17.)

IRON

Iron and its alloys such as steel are very familiar substances to everyone. Iron is the major element of the earth (35 percent—greater than oxygen at 30 percent and silicon at 15 percent), making up the major part of the earth's interior. Its chemical symbol is Fe, from the Latin *ferrum.*

Deficiency Symptoms

Iron deficiency (primarily anemia) is the most common nutritional deficiency in North America; it affects about 15 to 25 percent of the overall population, depending partially on the standard of measurement. These figures apply in all affluent societies and in developing nations, illustrating the importance of trace elements. Deficiencies in iron are most widespread in certain subgroups such as infants and children since rapid growth imposes great need for iron. Deficiencies are common in women during child-bearing years, but they are present in persons of all ages and in all socioeconomic levels.

Anemia. The most common sign of iron deficiency in humans is *iron-deficiency anemia,* in which the level of hemoglobin in the red cells is reduced and the red cells themselves are smaller (a condition called, technically, a *microcytic hypochromic anemia,* meaning that the cells are smaller and paler).

Iron-deficiency anemia, like anemias from other causes, reduces the oxygen-carrying capacity of the blood, resulting in lowered muscular and tissue performance in all of its aspects. If severe, it produces such symptoms as paleness of the skin, the lips and other mucous membranes; chronic fatigue, weakness, and lessened work performance; coldness and tingling of the hands and feet; inability to exercise normally including shortness of breath and a more rapid heart rate; lack of appetite; and a general slowing of vital functions of the body (2–4). Note that these symptoms are common to all anemias and are effectively treated with iron only if they result from an iron deficiency.

[1]The phytates are especially abundant in whole wheat but also occur in other grains. They are salts or esters of phytic acid containing inositol and phosphates as the base.

[2]From the Greek, meaning "claw of a crab."

Iron-deficiency anemia may be precipitated in young women whose diets are on the borderline of adequacy for iron when the onset of menstruation results in increased losses of iron from the body. More common than outright anemia in very young women are the low stores of body iron with which they come into the age of possible pregnancy. Pregnancy may precipitate iron-deficiency anemias because of the increased need for iron both for blood in the unborn child and for building up a store of iron in the placenta and in the infant's liver. The child may be born with a good store of iron in its own liver but at the cost of depletion of the mother's store. Repeated pregnancies are especially costly to iron stores in the mother's body (see Chap. 22).

Anemia most frequently results from low stores of iron, which can be caused by inadequate dietary intake, blood loss, or malabsorption of iron. There are many other possible causes of anemia, however, such as deficiency of another nutrient or inability to mobilize stored iron.

Other Deficiency Symptoms. Iron is a vital component of *myoglobin,* a red protein in muscle, and of numerous *cytochrome and other enzymes* essential for oxygen and electron transport throughout all the cells of the body. It is no wonder, then, that iron-deficiency signs can be seen even if a person has neither low hemoglobin levels nor anemia. These signs include, also, poor growth and reproduction, reduced physical fitness and work performance, lowered scholastic performance, and apparently, increased behavioral problems (4). Important changes in resistance to disease, including reduced immune functions, are also seen in conditions of iron deficiency, especially in infants and children (5).

Without having anemia, iron-deficient persons may also have such specific symptoms as thin, brittle, flattened, or spoon-shaped fingernails. Other symptoms are digestive disturbances, and changes in the mouth, esophagus, and intestinal tissues and function (4). Data are not sufficient to conclude that stomach, esophageal, or other types of human cancer are related to iron deficiency, though this is an active area of research (6).

As with all essential nutrients, severe iron deficiency over long periods will result in morbidity and eventually death.

Allowances and Intake of Populations

Allowances. It is difficult to fix any exact figure regarding the minimal requirements for iron, because of the many variables. Chiefly because of the very limited absorption in the intestine of iron, the recommended intake has to be much higher (about 10 times) than the actual tissue requirements.

Taking all these variables into consideration, the Food and Nutrition Board recommends a 10-mg per day allowance for men and postmenopausal women and an 18-mg per day allowance for other women (7). The recommendation, based on an assumed average availability of 10 percent of the iron in food, provides for retention in the body of 1 mg per day for men and postmenopausal women and 1.8 mg per day for other women. The recommended iron allowances for both sexes and for different periods of life are given in Table 16–2.

Any period in which growth takes place calls for an additional allowance of iron; such periods include pregnancy, lactation, and childhood from infancy through adolescence. With infants, requirements for iron to support rapid growth are relatively high per unit of body weight because of the small weight, but they are not high quantitatively (see Chap. 23). The iron requirements for small growing children are relatively high, as is the requirement for older boys and girls

TABLE 16–2 RECOMMENDED DAILY IRON ALLOWANCES[a]

	Age (yrs)	Iron (mg)
Infants and children	0–½	10
	½–3	15
	4–10	10
Males	11–18	18
	19 on	10
Females	11–50	18
Pregnant		>18[b]
Lactating (first 2–3 mo.)		18[c]
Lactating (beyond 2–3 mo.)		18
	51 on	10

[a]From Food and Nutrition Board, 1980 (7). See Appendix Table 1A to 1D for recommendations of other countries and WHO/FAO.

[b]The Food and Nutrition Board states "The increased requirement during pregnancy cannot be met by the iron content of *habitual diets* in the United States, nor by the existing iron stores of *many women;* therefore, daily supplements of iron are recommended. These *usually range from 30 to 60 mg/day;* the amount should be determined by the physician administering prenatal care" (p. 138, italics added) (7). These high levels are within the range of a usual therapeutic dose but beyond what could be obtained from foods.

A more logical and conservative allowance value of 20 to 40 mg/day for pregnancy can be derived from the statement in this same report, page 137–138 (7), that "Pregnancy increases the requirement to approximately 3.5 mg of iron per day, with a range from 2 to 4 mg." An allowance, therefore, of 35 mg per day, with a range from 20 to 40 mg during pregnancy could then be chosen on the same basis as the other iron allowance values were chosen—from consideration of an average of 10 percent absorption of dietary iron. This range of allowances is much closer to Canadian and international (FAO/WHO) allowances. This can be derived from food supplies with special care, though with typical American diets it would be easier to obtain this amount from iron supplements taken with the advice of a physician (see Chap. 22).

[c]The Food and Nutrition Board further states (7), "Iron needs during lactation are not substantially different from those of nonpregnant women, but continued supplementation of the mother for 2–3 months after parturition is advisable in order to replenish stores depleted by pregnancy."

during the growth spurt that occurs in the teenage period (eleven to eighteen years).

The U.S. recommended dietary allowance (RDA) of 18 mg per day for teenagers is designed to permit optimum storage of iron against possible drains on iron reserves, especially in young women because of menstruation, pregnancy, and lactation. The standardization of recommendations for iron intake among different countries is difficult because of the influence of so many factors on the iron requirement, including levels of intake of animal foods (which increase iron availability) and the level of vitamin C in the diet.

The Food and Agriculture Organization (FAO) and World Health Organization (WHO) recommendations for women of childbearing age, in countries where intakes of animal foods are less than 10 percent, is 28 mg per day, and 14 mg when animal foods supply 25 percent or more of calories. (See footnote to Table 16–2.)

Intakes. Inadequacy of iron in the diet to meet body needs, as evidenced by the frequent occurrence of nutritional anemia, is common in the United States and most other countries. Iron intakes continue to be low despite programs of moderate food enrichment and increased, although limited, programs in nutrition education. Refining and processing of foods, the great decrease in use of cast-iron cooking equipment in food manufacturing and in kitchens, decreased needs for energy (food), and lack of nutrition knowledge have been major reasons for low iron intakes.

To meet the RDA, a diet requires at least an average of 8 mg, or so, of iron for every 1000 kcals (8). Unfortunately, intakes in the United States average less—about 6 to 7 mg per 1000 kcals, and still less in various subgroups (9). This means that persons with requirements of 18 mg per day who are restricting themselves to 1500 to 2000 kcals per day are likely to receive too little iron.

Indeed, current studies of Americans continue to show large numbers of persons with intakes of iron well below the RDA levels. The recent U.S. Department of Agriculture (USDA) dietary survey of 37,700 Americans indicates that iron is one of the major "problem nutrients," with 32 percent of the population receiving less than 70 percent of the RDA (10).

Many recent studies, mostly in North America but applicable everywhere, show similar examples of widespread low-iron intakes in various subgroups of society, including infants and children (11), pregnant women (12), the elderly (13), ethnic groups (11–14), handicapped children (15), and still other groups (8–10,16). In many of these studies, dietary surveys were combined with various biochemical measurements to prove that deficiency symptoms were due to inadequate iron intakes.

Determining Iron Status

Various methods or combinations of methods are used to determine if someone, or a group of people, is receiving sufficient iron (4,10–17). Dietary intake values, along with determinations of hemoglobin, hematocrit (a method of measuring the amount of blood cells), and serum iron and/or ferritin levels are most commonly chosen for tests on populations. Many more specific clinical procedures are available. The iron content of hair is not a sensitive measure of iron status. Regardless of the method, one should not attempt to diagnose one's iron status or the extent of any nutritional deficiency unless under the supervision of clinically trained experts. One should be very wary especially of impressive-looking computerized printouts of the results of hair analysis and inadequate diet histories. (See Chap. 17.)

Iron in Foods

Amounts of iron in an average serving of some typical basic foods, not taking into account differences in availability, are given in Table 16–3 (see Table 2 of the Appendix for more information on these and other foods). In many instances, the distribution of iron follows that of other mineral elements, as it is relatively high in foods of low moisture content and low in fresh fruits and vegetables, which contain large amounts of water and fiber. Milk, which is one of the best sources of many other nutrients, is poor in iron. Organ meats, such as liver and the blood-forming organs (spleen and bone marrow, seldom consumed in the United States), are unusually rich in iron.

Good sources of iron are lean meats, legumes, nuts, dried fruits, poultry, fish, whole grains or enriched cereal foods, and most green, leafy vegetables.

Some wines are fair to good sources of iron. Such foods as dark molasses, raisins, and nuts (often presented as rich sources of iron) are used infrequently or in small servings, so that they do not constitute as important sources of this element as some staple foods of lower iron content—such as whole-grain or enriched breads and cereals. Unenriched, highly milled cereals or bread, sugar, and fats are either very low or lacking in iron. Some water supplies are high in iron, but water is not a dependable source.

The iron content of plant foods is not affected much by soil content, nor is the composition of milk, including human milk, influenced appreciably by the iron content of the diet. The lower iron content of veal is an exception.

Effect of Enrichment with Iron. The addition of iron salts to bread, breakfast cereals, flour, and other cereal products in conjunction with the food-enrichment program has been a considerable help in raising the available iron content of the American diet. Approximately 25 percent of total iron intake comes from enrichment sources.

Effective July 1983, the U.S. government has issued a final rule on enrichment standards for bread, rolls, and buns at 12.5 mg

Table 16–3 TYPICAL SOURCES OF IRON, ABOUT IN DECREASING ORDER OF CONTENT (not considering availability)[a]

Food	*Size of Serving*	*Mg per Average Serving*
Liver:		
Pork, fried	1 slice (85 gm)	24.7
Lamb, broiled	2 slices (90 gm)	16.2
Calf, fried	1 slice (85 gm)	12.1
Beef, fried	1 slice (85 gm)	7.5
Chicken, cooked	3 livers (75 gm)	6.3
Baked beans, canned:		
pork and molasses	½ cup (130 gm)	3.0
alone	½ cup (130 gm)	2.6
Meats (lean or medium fat):		
Beef, round, cooked	1 large hamburger (85 gm)	3.0
rib roast, cooked	3 slices (100 gm)	2.6
Pork, chop, cooked	1 medium large chop (85 gm)	2.7
Lamb, shoulder, cooked	3 pieces (85 gm)	1.6
Chicken, fried	1 medium piece (100 gm)	1.3
Fish, cooked (cod, tuna, salmon, sardines, etc.):	1 medium filet (100 gm) or 3½ oz	1.0–2.4
Grains, whole, not cooked:		
Corn flour	1 cup (117 gm)	2.1
Rice, white, dry	½ cup (100 gm)	1.5
Wheat, whole, flour	1 cup (120 gm)	4.0
Fruits, dried (uncooked):		
Apricots	4 halves (30 gm)	1.6
Prunes	4–5 medium (30 gm)	1.3
Raisins	3 Tbsp (30 gm)	1.0
Legumes:		
Soy beans	½ cup, cooked (90 gm)	2.5
Peanut butter	2 Tbsp (30 gm)	0.6
Lima beans, fresh	½ cup, cooked (85 gm)	2.2
Peas, fresh, green	½ cup, cooked (80 gm)	1.4
Molasses:		
Medium color	1 Tbsp (20 gm)	1.2
Blackstrap	1 Tbsp (20 gm)	3.2
Eggs, whole:	2 medium (100 gm)	2.2
Leafy vegetables:		
Spinach	½ cup, cooked (90 gm)	2.0
Beet greens	½ cup, cooked (100 gm)	1.9
Chard	½ cup, cooked (100 gm)	1.8
Kale (leaves only)	1 cup, cooked (110 gm)	1.8
Turnip greens	½ cup, cooked (90 gm)	1.0
Vegetables, cooked:		
Potatoes, sweet	1 medium (150 gm)	1.0
white	1 medium (150 gm)	0.8
Broccoli	⅔ cup (100 gm)	0.8
Brussels sprouts	5–6 medium (100 gm)	1.1
Cauliflower	¾ cup (100 gm)	0.7
Carrots	⅔ c, diced (100 gm)	0.6
String beans	¾ cup (100 gm)	0.6
Beets	2, 2-in diameter (100 gm)	0.5
Bread:		
White, enriched	2 slices (50 gm)	1.4
Whole-wheat	2 slices (50 gm)	1.6
White, unenriched	2 slices (50 gm)	0.3

continued

Table 16–3, continued

Food	*Size of Serving*	*Mg per Average Serving*
Breakfast cereals, whole grain (oats, corn, wheat, rice):	See label on package—range from 0.2 to 0.7 mg unenriched, up to 10 mg enriched, per serving	(see label)
Fresh fruits and fresh vegetables:	100 gm serving, mostly	0.3–0.6
Milk, whole, fluid, cow's:	½ pt, or 8 oz glass (246 gm)	0.12
Human	½ pt, or 8 oz (246 gm)	0.07

[a]Values are from Adams, C.: "Nutritive Value of American Foods in Common Units," USDA Handbook No. 456, 1975, unless noted otherwise. Figures for milk, eggs, and poultry products are from the new Handbook 8 (Nos. 1 and 5), 1976–1978. Bread values are from Table 2 in the Appendix. For recent total non-heme iron values for certain muscles of beef, pork, and lamb see Schricker, B. R., et al.: J. Food Sci., *47*:740, 1982.

per pound (lb) and for enriched flour at 20 mg per lb. Over 2 million lbs of iron sources are used per year in U.S. food-enrichment programs. The most widely used source of iron is "elemental iron" made up of extremely fine metallic iron particles, which are generally as available to the body as the natural, non-heme iron (from non-meat sources) in foods. Ferric phosphate and ferrous sulfate are used to a somewhat lesser extent to enrich foods, as are still smaller amounts of other approved iron compounds.

Recent limited use of iron-fortified milk in Mexico and of iron-fortified table salt in rural and urban areas in India has met with considerable success in combating iron deficiency (17).

Effect of Processing and Cooking. The amount of iron in processed and manufactured foods can be quite variable, a fact to keep in mind when using food composition tables. The use of iron (in contrast to steel) cooking utensils in food manufacture and in the kitchen is a useful source of iron, but it can make the iron content too high (18). The iron in canned applesauce, tomato sauce, and crushed pineapple is known to increase at least twenty fold if the cans are stored at room temperature for four months and then left opened in a refrigerator for one week (Greger) (18).

The iron content of foods is related to a number of other conditions, not the least of which is the acidity of the food in the can. Iron toxicity is known to exist, for example, in certain members of the Bantu tribe in South Africa who have used iron utensils in cooking and in the brewing of alcoholic beverages. In the United States, toxicity from the normal iron in foods is unknown except in a rare genetic disease in which iron accumulates *(hemochromatosis).*

The iron content of foods can also be raised by contamination from other sources, such as the grinding together of metal plates during milling of cereals, and from grinding of foods with traditional metal kitchen ware (19).

The milling of cereals can remove up to 75 percent of the iron depending on the degree of milling. Blanching, freezing, cooking, and canning of foods have only modest effects on iron levels. Baking, long heating, and storage, however, can quite markedly reduce the availability of various forms of iron present in foods, especially of added iron compounds (20).

The consumer should learn to read food labels and, if in doubt about the iron content of a particular manufactured food, write to the manufacturer.

Availability and Absorption

It may now be seen that various tables of iron composition of foods are of only limited use because they do not reflect the increased availability of *heme iron* for absorption compared with that of *non-heme iron.* (Heme iron is an organic form of iron found primarily in hemoglobin and, to a smaller extent, in myoglobin of muscle and in certain enzymes.) Neither do they reflect the fact that absorption of iron depends greatly on the body's need for iron and also on the presence of ascorbic acid, and other dietary factors. Iron absorption from various foods can range from 1 to 3 percent up to 50 or 60 percent or more, depending on these different circumstances (2,3,7,21).

Differences in the terms availability and absorption are slight when used with trace elements, and they are often used interchangeably. *Availability,* as used here, is a nutritional term that applies to the amount of a substance in food that can be absorbed. *Bioavailability* is a shortened term used popularly for "biological availability," which for nutrients is synonomous with "availability." *Absorption* is a physiological process involving the passage of substances through the intestinal wall.

In the small intestine, the epithelial cell lining the intestinal wall (the *mucosal cell*) is the key to the mechanism of iron absorption. This cell takes in either heme or free iron by regulating procedures not fully understood—possibly hormonal regulation. Absorption takes place mainly in the upper part of the small intestine.

Under average conditions with mixed diets, generally only about one-tenth of the iron in the diet is absorbed—about 1 to 1.5 mg a day. This is the actual body requirement for iron. For practical purposes, this means that the amount of iron that should be eaten is about 8 to 12 times this level. The rest is unabsorbed and excreted in the feces. Factors affecting these generalities are described below.

Heme and Non-heme Iron. When iron is consumed as meat (heme iron) proteins, it is normally 15 to 35 percent available, about 3 to 6 times more than iron from non-heme sources. It has been shown that the heme molecule itself, especially when eaten with meat, fish, or poultry, may be absorbed directly into the intestinal mucosa cells before iron is released. It is affected minimally by other dietary factors. Meat contains about 40 percent of heme iron and about 60 percent of non-heme iron, though this percentage varies considerably. (See references in footnote to Table 16–3.) In Western countries heme iron accounts for only 10 to 15 percent of all the dietary iron.

The iron in other non-heme food sources, such as grains, vegetables, fruit, eggs, milk, and cheese, is only about 2 to 5 percent available under normal conditions. Thus, the total heme and non-heme iron of meat, fish, and poultry is 2 to 3 times as available as the iron from non-heme sources alone. Obviously one's dietary requirement for iron is based in part on the type of food eaten.

Effect of Diet on Availability of Nonheme Iron. Numerous dietary factors affect the availability of non-heme iron in the intestine. The intestinal contents form a "pool" of enhancing and inhibitory substances including ascorbic acid, phytates, tannins, fiber, proteins, chelating agents, and others. The amount of iron absorbed from this pool can vary quite remarkably (21). Iron is more readily absorbed in the less oxidized form—as ferrous rather than ferric iron. Ferrous sulfate is generally used as a standard in absorption studies and is usually absorbed at nearly the maximum rate of 20 to 40 percent (not more because of the control mechanisms). Factors favorable for absorption of non-heme iron are as follows:

1. normal acidity of the gastric juice secreted in the stomach
2. the presence of reducing substances (such as ascorbic acid) that can change ferric iron to the more readily absorbable ferrous forms. (Considerably more nonheme iron is absorbed, for

example, when 25 mg or more of vitamin C is present in a meal.)

3. a well-balanced diet in which a fair proportion of the iron is provided in meat, poultry, or fish and there are not too many foods in which the iron is not very available as a result of the presence of inhibitory factors

Surprisingly, eggs[3] and green, leafy vegetables, such as spinach, formerly famous for their iron content, are relatively poor sources of available iron (only 2 to 5 percent of their iron is absorbed). *Phytic acid,* found especially in grains, reduces absorption by forming insoluble compounds with iron, as it does with calcium. This accounts for the poor absorption of iron from whole wheat (also about 2 to 5 percent), explaining the high incidence of anemia in countries whose population depends on whole wheat as its major carbohydrate source.

The iron in rice, corn, and beans is likewise poorly absorbed. When these plant foods are eaten with ascorbic acid or meat, their iron availability is approximately doubled.

Among the foods that increase absorption are those that contribute ascorbic acid, citric acid, amino acids, certain chelates, and meat protein. For instance, a glass of orange juice increases non-heme iron absorption threefold. The iron in human breast milk is nonheme iron but is more available than heme iron in an infant. About 50 percent of such iron is absorbed.

Among the foods that lower iron absorption are egg yolk,[3] soybean proteins, and foods containing tannins (such as millet, sorghum cereals, and tea). Foods that contribute oxalates, carbonates, phosphates, and extra zinc salts, along with certain fiber components of corn and wheat, may also inhibit absorption. The lack of normal acid secretion by the stomach may be an inhibitory factor. These inhibitory effects may be partially overcome by eating meat, extra ascorbic acid, or, of course, extra iron supplements.

[3]The phosphoprotein, phosvitin, of egg yolk is claimed to bind the iron of egg in the digestive tract. The practical significance of this, considering the overall "pool" of iron in the digestive contents, has been recently questioned. This remains a current controversial area. (See Miller, J., and Nnanna, I.: J. Nutr. *113*:1169, 1983.)

Effect of Body Needs and Blood Losses on Absorption of Iron. The extent of the *body's* need for iron is the major factor that controls the relative amount of iron absorbed; this makes differences in degree of utilization of iron from different types of food of less importance. If the margin between the total amounts needed and those furnished by the food intake is small, the relative utilization from all types of food will be "stepped up." If only small amounts of iron are needed for body maintenance, less will be absorbed and much of the food iron will remain unabsorbed to be discarded in the feces—that is, the degree of availability will be lower for all types of food.

The body guards its iron stores very carefully and reuses any that is broken down in the body over and over again. The body recycles about 35 to 40 mg of iron a day. Only the small amounts of iron lost in the bile, urine, sweat, hair, sloughed-off skin, nails, and menses need to be replaced—normally about 1 or 1.5 mg a day. Normal menstrual losses of iron average about 15 to 20 mg per period (representing a total of about 35 to 45 milliliters [ml] of blood). There is considerable variation among women, however (4). In one large study more than 10 percent of women lost 40 mg or more of iron per menstrual period. This represents a need for an extra 14 mg of iron per day in the diet, or a total daily need of 24 mg by U.S. standards. The choice of contraception methods may also affect the extent of blood losses in women.

Because considerable iron is needed when large amounts of blood are lost, as in blood donations (450 ml, or about 200 mg of iron) or in bleeding from wounds, the body uses its unique, built-in control mechanism, which allows the intestine to absorb more iron when the need is greatest. The body can also inhibit absorption, in part, when there is an excess. Unusually high iron needs also may be precipitated by hemorrhages (either sudden loss of much blood or long-continued pathological bleeding such as with hemorrhoids, ulcers, or malignancies). Such losses may occur in both men and women.

The body tends to replace a major loss of iron for hemoglobin building at a rate far in excess of that supplied in the diet and for this it mobilizes stored iron, especially the more labile types. The need for extra iron under these circumstances is far in excess of the amounts supplied by normal absorption of dietary iron from the intestine. This in turn promotes more efficient absorption of food iron.

A diet that offers a plentiful supply of all substances needed for rebuilding blood (especially protein and including some rich sources of iron, such as liver and meats) often is adequate to rebuild blood supplies, provided there are normal reserves of iron in the body. If the previous diet has been too low in iron to provide such reserve stores, or if the current diet is low in iron, extra iron supplements are needed to promote rapid blood regeneration.

The presence or absence of anemia and the amount of body stores of iron greatly affect body needs. Adult men with stores of 500 mg of iron will absorb more iron than those with 1000 mg of iron, both within normal ranges. In adult women the stores are lower, generally not exceeding 500 to 700 mg. Many women in both industrialized and developing countries have little or no iron stores. Persons with no stores of iron and who are anemic will absorb it at the highest rate possible—up to 35 percent.

The Metabolism of Iron in the Body

Once iron is inside the mucosal cell it can be either transferred (and later released) to the tissues with the aid of a protein known as *transferrin* or stored in the mucosal cell or other cells in the form of the unique proteins *ferritin* and *hemosiderin* (see Fig. 16–2).

Iron Compounds in the Body. Iron, being a component of essential metabolic enzymes in every cell, is in every part of the body (see Table 16–4). The adult human body contains a total of about 3 to 5 gm of iron.

Most of the iron (60 to 70 percent) is present in the blood as hemoglobin in red blood cells. *Hemoglobin* is a red compound consisting of two tightly connected parts: *globin,* a protein, and *heme,* a nonprotein substance that contains iron in the ferrous state. Each molecule of hemoglobin can carry four molecules of oxygen and is essential for oxygen transfer in the blood. A total of about 800 to 900 gm (2 lb) of hemoglobin is present in an adult man, representing the major chemical component of blood other than water. Normally hemoglobin is present in blood at a level of about 12 to 15 gm per 100 ml (except in anemic persons, in whom the amount in rare instances is as low as 5 to 8 gm per 100 ml). Hemoglobin contains about 0.33 percent iron.

The next largest concentration of iron (about 20 to 30 percent) is that stored in combination with proteins, such as ferritin and hemosiderin, primarily in the liver, spleen, and bone marrow.

The minor quantities of iron (about 10 percent) found in other tissues are nevertheless vitally important, as is evidenced by their locations:

1. in the chromatin network in cell nuclei
2. in *cytochrome* (an iron-containing pigment) in protoplasm of cells, and in numerous enzymes

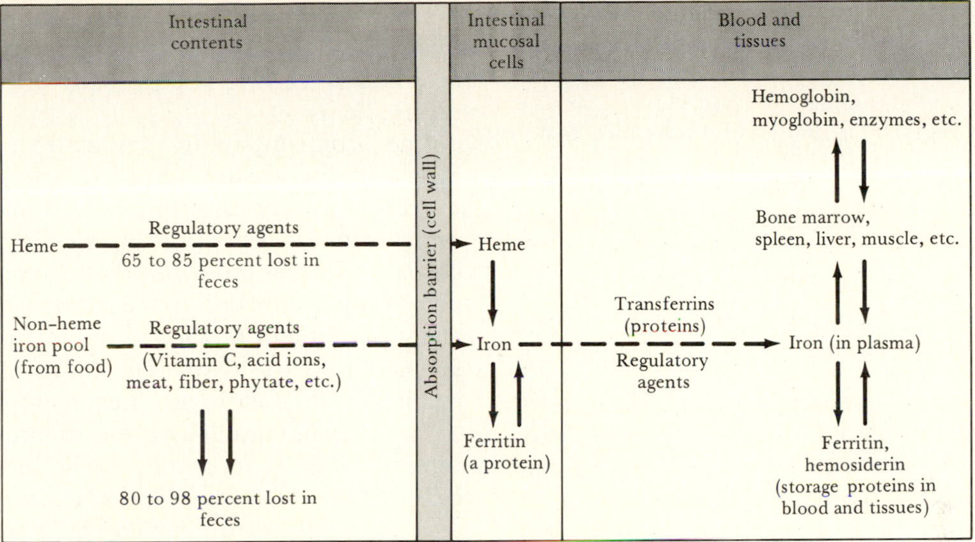

Figure 16–2 Diagram of absorption of iron from the intestine into the blood and tissues.

Table 16–4 TYPICAL AMOUNTS OF IRON COMPOUNDS IN THE BODY[a]

Form of Iron in Body	*Iron Containing Compound*	*55 kg (121 lb) Female*	*70 kg (154 lb) Male*
		mg	mg
Active functional compounds	Hemoglobin	1750	2220
	Myoglobin	170	250
	Heme enzymes	50	75
	Non-heme enzymes	62	91
	Transferrin-iron	3	4
	Subtotal	2035	2620
Storage compounds	Ferritin	200	650
	Hemosiderin	65	275
	Subtotal	265	925
Other body iron (in hair, skin, nails bones, and other tissues)	Miscellaneous iron compounds	200	455
	Total body iron	2500 mg	4000 mg

[a]Adapted from Bothwell, T. H., et al.: *Iron Metabolism in Man.* Oxford, Blackwell Scientific Publications, 1979; Hallberg, L.: 1982 (cited in ref. 21); and other sources.

(cytochrome oxidases, catalase, and *phenylalanine hydroxylase)* that help catalyze oxidation-reduction and hydroxylation processes in body tissues

3. in myoglobin in muscles, a substance that is closely related in chemistry and function to hemoglobin but is fixed in muscle tissue (and that constitutes about 7 percent of the total body iron)

In all these sites, the iron-containing compounds are involved in the vital life processes of all cells and tissues (see Fig. 16–3).

Function. Iron owes its usefulness in the body to its special ability to be reversibly oxygenated—that is, to take on oxygen and later give this oxygen up to other substances. By means of this property, the iron-containing hemoglobin in red blood cells can take on extra oxygen when blood circulates through the lungs, can then carry oxygen to the tissues, and there can pass it on to the tissue cells for oxidative processes necessary to their life. Venous blood, which owes its bluish color to the presence of reduced hemoglobin, takes on excess carbon dioxide (a waste product of tissues) and is returned to the lungs, where it loses carbon dioxide and takes on another load of oxygen, becoming bright red again when *oxyhemoglobin* is formed. When insufficient iron is available

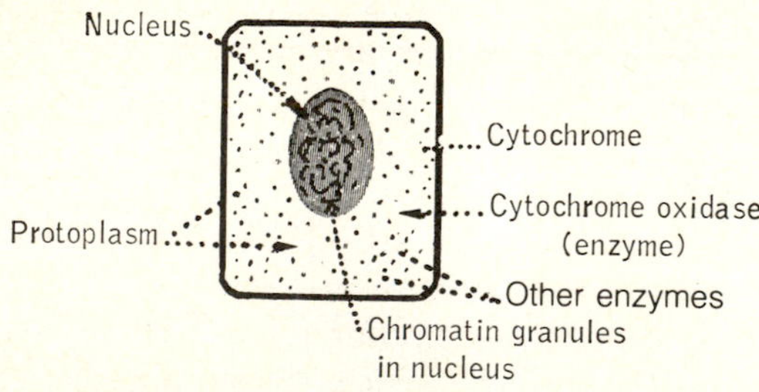

Figure 16–3 Small amounts of iron are found in every tissue cell—in chromatin granules in the cell nucleus and in the protoplasm as the pigment cytochrome, the enzyme cytochrome oxidase, and in other enzymes. These iron-containing substances are largely responsible for the uptake of oxygen by the cells and for the use of oxygen in their life processes.

to the body, less hemoglobin is formed (anemia), and these oxygen-carrying mechanisms are reduced, giving rise to many physiological problems.

The iron-containing pigments and enzymes in the tissues serve to bring about transfers of oxygen within cells in much the same manner. The cytochromes and cytochrome oxidases (enzymes that contain iron) have been estimated to be responsible for about 90 percent of the energy transfers associated with the oxidative phases of tissue respiration. Catalase, another example of a heme-iron-containing enzyme, is present in relatively high concentrations in red blood cells and in other tissue cells. Catalase protects the cell from damage by peroxides. Iron-containing enzymes are also necessary for connective tissue biosynthesis.

Among the billions of red blood cells (about 4.5 to 5 million per cubic millimeter of blood), there are continual casualties and calls for replacements; the lifetime of such cells has been determined by use of isotopes to be about four months. Red blood cells are formed in the bone marrow and destroyed chiefly in the spleen. Not only is iron needed for their formation, but also protein (for the protein part of hemoglobin) and other materials for the *stroma,* the body of the red blood cell in which hemoglobin is embedded. When the cells disintegrate, the main nonprotein portion of hemoglobin is split into oxidized heme, an iron-containing dark brown substance *(hematin),* and a pigment *(bilirubin).* Almost all the iron and much of the bilirubin are saved to be used over again in new red corpuscles. The excess is secreted in bile and contributes to the normal color of feces.

The body has a store of readily available iron, a "labile pool of iron," made up of recently absorbed iron plus that recently released by the breaking down of red blood cells. This iron is used by preference for hemoglobin in building new red cells. Other stores of iron (as in the liver) may be somewhat less readily available, and the fixed iron in tissue cells cannot be generally drawn upon even in times of great need.

Toxicity of Iron

As with all trace elements, the toxic level of iron is easily reached by taking in sources outside a normal food supply. The safe range with most of the trace elements for chronic intakes is within about 10 to 50 times the requirement. With iron, the safe range is about 10 to 30 times the allowance, though "iron overload" can occur with less intake over long periods (4,7,22).

In the United States, toxicity from the normal iron in foods is unknown except in a rare genetic disease in which iron accumulates *(hemochromatosis)*.

Some people find they have very limited tolerance for single doses of highly ionizable forms of iron (such as ferrous sulfate) if eaten in a supplement in amounts much over 200 to 250 mg a day. A greater health problem in America is the accidental intake by small children of large amounts of iron pills. Single intakes of only 200 to 400 mg of iron (equivalent to only a dozen or so iron pills) have caused severe symptoms of iron poisoning in young children. Fewer deaths have been reported with the advent of safety caps.

IODINE

Iodine (I) is a nonmetallic, blackish gray element essential in the diet for the formation in the thyoid gland of two hormones, *thyroxine* and *triiodothyronine*, both containing iodine in their structure (see Fig. 16–4). These important hormones are required in the body for growth, reproduction, nerve formation and mental health, bone formation, protein synthesis, and cellular oxidative processes, including serving as the major regulators of energy metabolism in all its aspects. Without iodine in the diet none of these things can occur.

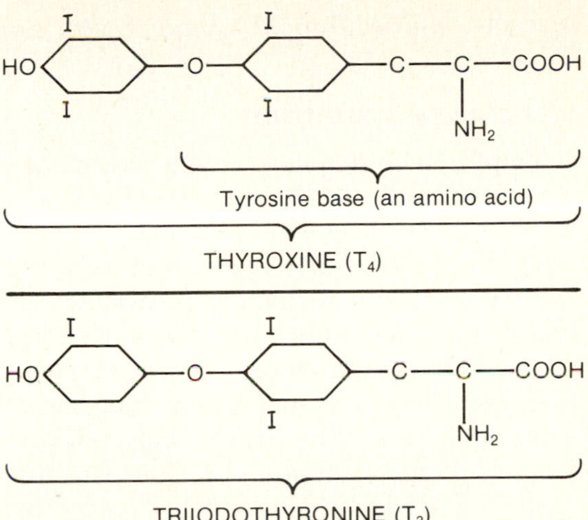

Figure 16–4 Formulas for the two thyroid hormones, thyroxine (T_4—with 4 iodine molecules) and triiodothyronine (T_3—with 3 iodine molecules). These are shown in simplified form not showing all the C and H atoms. There is about 20 times as much T_4 hormone in the body as T_3, though T_3 is about 3 times more active.

Iodine is a *halogen* along with chlorine, fluorine, and bromine—all are gases when in the free form. Iodine has the highest molecular weight (127) of any of the essential elements. It is not required for the growth of plants so its presence in plant foods depends on the concentration of soil, water, and the environment. Iodine is present in animal tissues and in seawater and sea weeds. Crude sea salt prepared by drying seawater is not likely, however, to be a good source of iodine.

Though there has been considerable unplanned improvement in America iodine intake in recent years (almost to the point of too much), iodine deficiency is unfortunately widespread in many other parts of the world. The result is high incidences of goiter, an enlargement of the thyroid gland. Also *cretinism* (reduced stature and mentality) may result in children born from iodine-deficient (hypothyroid) mothers or from mothers whose thyroid gland could not function properly.

Deficiency Symptoms

Simple, or endemic, goiter is an enlargement of the thyroid gland in the neck as a result of insufficient iodine. The gland enlarges in an attempt to compensate for the shortage of iodine, which is an essential ingredient for making its hormones (see Fig. 16–5). Females are more subject to goiter than males, and it is most likely to appear at adolescence and pregnancy. This disorder was prevalent for centuries before its cause was recognized.

Goiter was known in China as early as 3000 B.C. and was treated effectively by feeding seaweed or burnt sponge to those affected. In 1820 the Swiss physician J. R. Coindet provided evidence that the then newly discovered iodine was the curative agent in seaweed and burnt sponge. Though the idea was not universally accepted then, in retrospect it is clear that iodine was one of the first nutrients to be recognized as essential for humans or animals. Vitamins, amino acids, and the concept of essential elements were not known at the time. It took nearly a century before the finding was put to widespread use.

Studies on Goiter in the United States. Several sets of events around 1917 and 1918 directed the attention of the public and of

Figure 16–5 Goiter, the result of chronic iodine shortage in diet and drinking water, affects entire communities. Schoolchildren with the typical swollen necks in an East African village. (Photo WHO/FAO, 1982.)

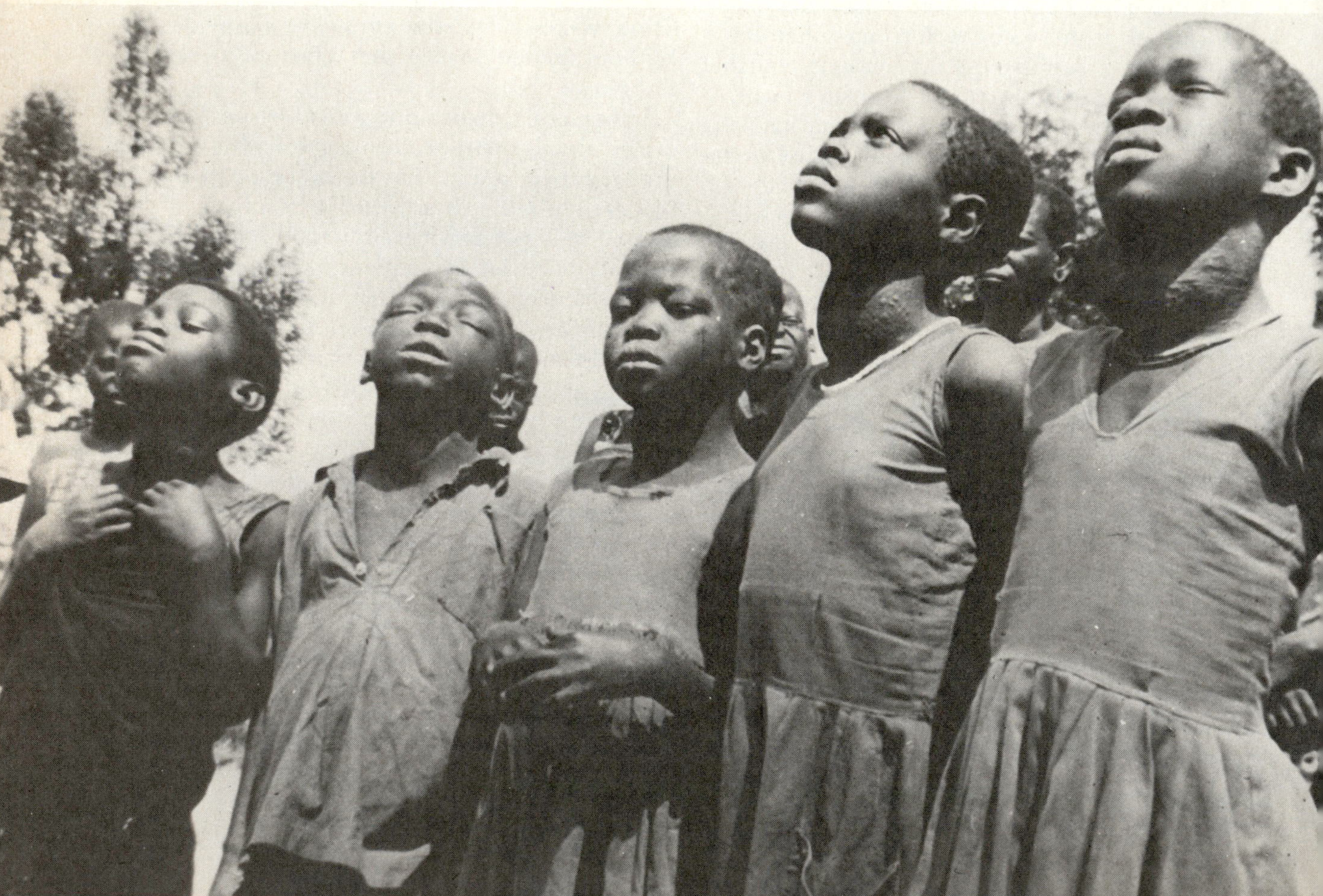

scientists to the distribution of simple goiter in different parts of the United States (Fig. 16–6). One was the publication of figures on the incidence of goiter among men drafted during World War I, which showed that this disorder was most prevalent in the basin of the Great Lakes and in the Pacific Northwest in the United States and Canada. In areas adjacent to the ocean, where both soil and foods grown on it were relatively iodine-rich and where seafoods were commonly eaten, goiter proved to be almost nonexistent.

Another event was that farm animals in goitrous regions showed the same evidence of iodine deficiency as humans, and their tendency to produce stillborn or weak and sickly young was a source of concern and a financial loss to farmers.

A third event was the work of D. Marine and O. P. Kimball, who, on the basis of evidence accumulated over a period of six years, administered small doses of iodine to school children in Akron, Ohio, where mild goiter was common among adolescent girls. Small doses of potassium iodide were given during two ten-day periods each year to about 800 girls, while about 1,800 untreated girls of the same age group served as controls. No goiter developed in the treated group, while 26 percent of the control group developed enlarged thyroids in the same period (23, 24).

Then in 1918, E. B. Hart and H. Steenbock published results of a study of the "hairless pig malady," a condition in which apparently normal sows gave birth to still-

Figure 16–6 A "goiter map" of the then 48 states in 1917–1918 showing (in black) the regions where goiter among draftees was most prevalent. Goiter also occurred fairly commonly in the shaded and dotted states, but was almost totally absent in the states in white. The use of preventive measures (iodine in drinking water and iodized salt) greatly reduced the incidence of simple goiter, even in the states where it was most prevalent. (From Love and Davenport: *Geographic Distribution of Simple Goiter among Drafted Men, 1917–18.* U.S. Department of Public Health.)

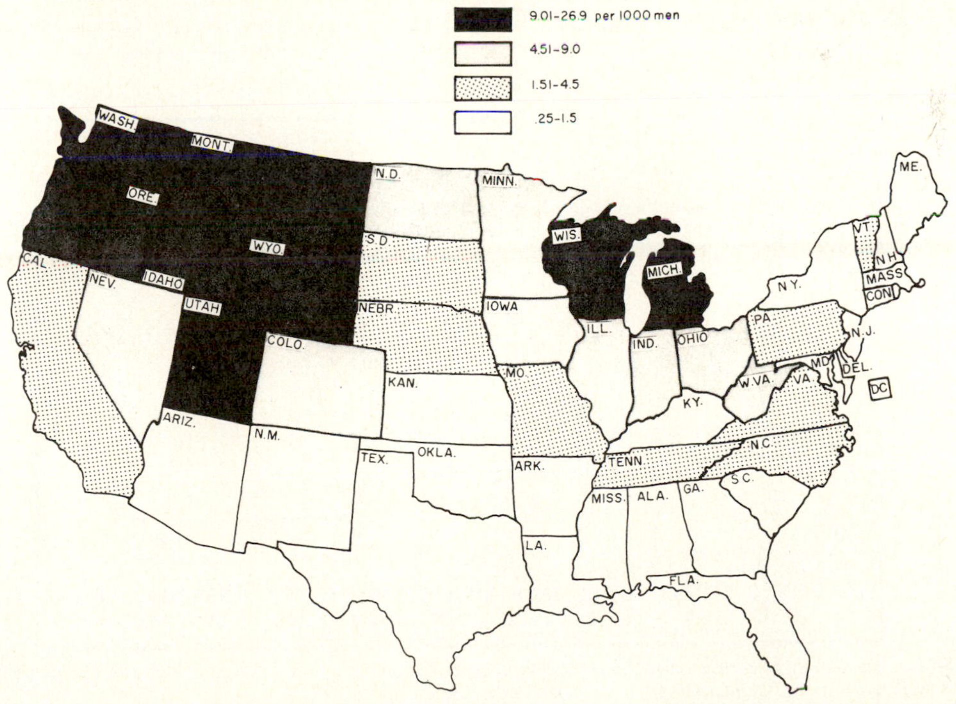

born young that were nearly hairless and had thick, goitrous necks (25). This condition was found to be the result of iodine deficiency, and the addition of iodide to the feed enabled the sows to produce normal young. The hairless pig malady is similar to endemic cretinism in severely handicapped and dwarfed children born with underdeveloped thyroids as a result of a deficiency of iodine in their mothers during the first three months of pregnancy or before conception. Cretinous children, in addition to being undersized and mentally slow, are often partly or almost entirely deaf. They generally have short lifespans.

These studies and others established without question the practicability of prevention of simple goiter by administration of small quantities of some iodine compound (Fig. 16–7).

Control of Goiter. The use of iodized salt (or some other carrier) is now recommended in all localities where simple goiter is endemic. Iodization of salt is required by law in Switzerland, Canada, Colombia, Guatemala, and many other countries. In the United States, the iodization of salt is not legally mandatory but is very common. Educational campaigns have wisely encouraged its widespread use. Under the current Food and Drug Administration regulation, iodized table salt must be labeled, "This salt supplies iodide, a necessary nutrient." Uniodized salt is labeled, "This salt does not supply iodide, a necessary nutrient." In the United States and Canada, iodized salt contains 0.1 percent of potassium iodide, or its equivalent, supplying 76 μg of iodine per gm of salt.

The foregoing account illustrates how the need for trace elements was established and reminds us that some health problems that were once considered a natural part of life no longer need to exist. Nevertheless, despite the easy remedy for iodine deficiency, goiter is still one of the most common nutrition-related diseases in the world, affecting 200 million people. It is rife in both developed and developing countries, such as Austria, China, northern India, South and

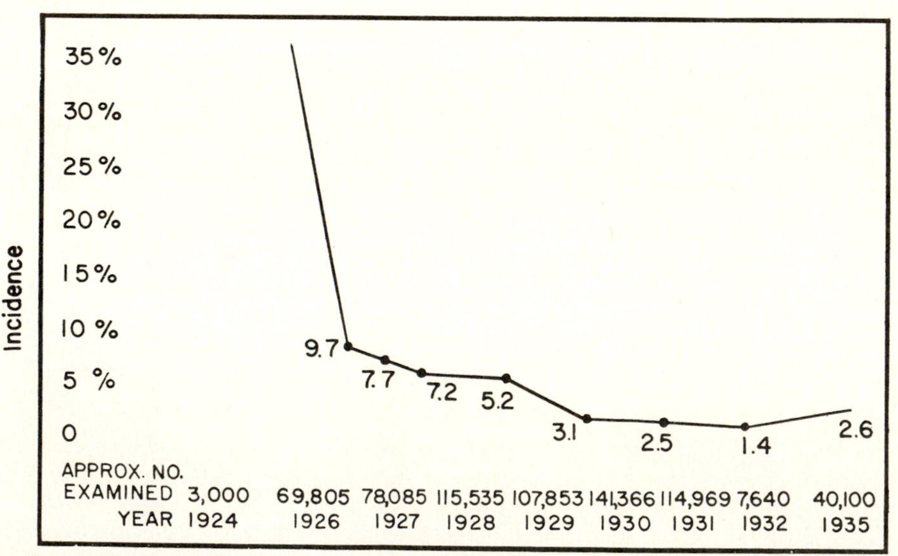

Figure 16–7 The marked decrease in simple goiter among Detroit school children between 1924 and 1935, due to the use of iodized salt. (From Kimball, O. P.: *Journal of American Medical Association,* 1937.)

Central America, Greece, and Yugoslavia. Educational, medical, and public-health agencies have much work to do before goiter is finally eradicated. Injections of iodized oil can serve as a suitable iodine source in areas lacking in iodine and in countries where the use of iodized salt is not possible. It should be stressed, however, that once a goiter has developed in adult life, taking supplementary iodine will not decrease its size.

Other Causes of Goiter. Enlarged thyroid gland can also be caused by eating large amounts of foods such as turnips, cabbage, cassava, and rutabagas over long periods of time. Such foods contain natural antithyroid compounds called *goitrogens,* which inhibit the formation of thyroid hormones. The thyroid glands enlarge in their attempt to make as much thyroid hormone as possible. Normal consumption of these foods, as in the United States, is in no way harmful.

Certain drugs such as thiouracil and several sulfa drugs also have a goitrogenic effect, and there are known inherited defects that can cause goiter.

Iodine Allowances and Intake

Allowances. Recommended allowances for iodine have been set in the United States at about 2 times the minimal amount essential to maintain a normal balance in order to ensure a margin of safety. The current recommendation for the iodine allowance for all persons—men and women—from age eleven on is 150 μg (0.15 mg) a day (7). The needs are increased during pregnancy (by 25 μg more) and lactation (50 μg more). See RDA tables (inside front cover) for the details of needs of other age groups. Iodine intakes at this level have no harmful effects and serve to build up a reserve store in the thyroid gland for use in emergencies. Possibly the smallness of the quantities of iodine required may best be appreciated by considering that the standard allowance of iron for an adult woman for only three days (54 mg) would weigh about the same as a whole year's allowance (55 mg) of iodine. It is truly a "trace" element.

Intake. According to studies by the Food and Drug Administration (FDA), a dramatic change in iodine intake has occurred in the United States in recent years. The iodine content of the American food supply has changed markedly (see Fig. 16–8). Since the 1960s it has increased from 3 to 13 times the recommended levels (9,26). It has reached such high levels that there are concerns about possible toxicity. Recent extensive surveys showed "market basket" food supplies averaged about 490 μg of iodine per 2000 kcal with wide variations. The inclusion of iodized table salt in the surveys would have contributed still more iodine, as would extra oral supplements of iodine, especially kelp (seaweed) products (26). A typical meal at a fast-food store (a Big Mac hamburger, french fries, and a milkshake) contributed about 450 μg of iodine. In a study of frozen fried chicken dinners, an average of 970 μg of iodine—and up to 4700 μg—was found per dinner.

Iodine in Food

Among the sources of iodine in the current American food supply, other than iodized salt, are dairy products, which now contribute the largest share of our intake of iodine (56 percent). This iodine comes partly from cleansing agents containing iodine (*iodates* and *iodophors*), used in processing milk on the farm and in dairies, and partly from cattle producing the milk, many of which are being fed more iodine than necessary to protect against iodine deficiency (27).

Iodates and iodophors are also used as cleaning agents in bread and cereal processing plants, which may account for the high contribution of iodine from this food group (16 percent). Neither grain nor milk is

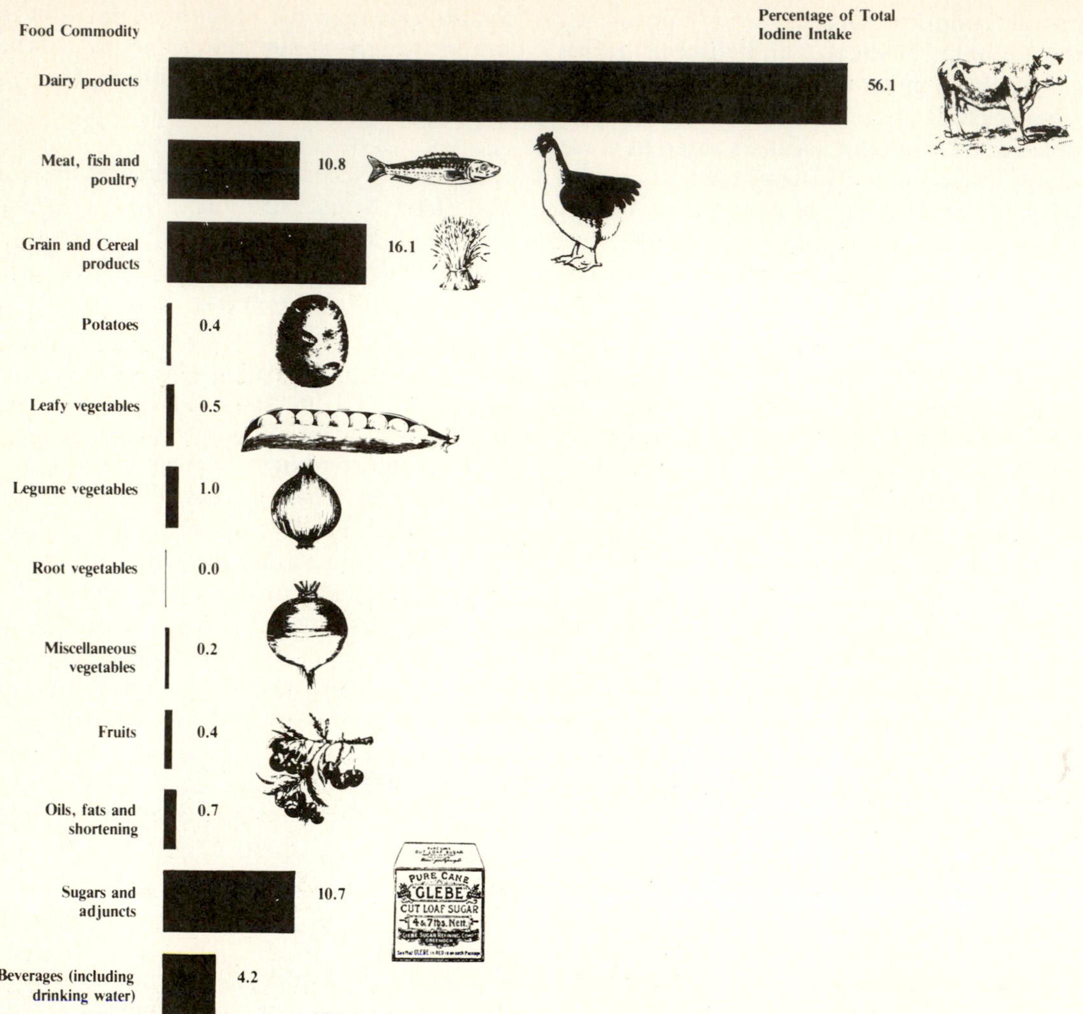

Figure 16–8 Sources of iodine in an adult diet, giving percent of total iodine intake. Source: U.S. Food and Drug Administration, FDA Consumer, *15* (April): 15, 1981. *The contribution of table salt was not considered in these studies.* These percentages were based on studies showing iodine in average diets at a level of 488 mcg per 2000 kcal. The values reflect contamination of food supplies with iodine sources. Studies are in progress on the bioavailability of these new sources of iodine and on means to reduce their content in American diets. (Source: FDA Consumer, 1981.)

generally considered a rich source of iodine under ordinary circumstances. A number of bread companies formerly used iodine compounds in dough conditioners. Their use for that purpose has dropped considerably since the concern about extra sources of iodine in our food supply.

About 10 percent of the iodine comes from candy, sugared breakfast cereals, cake mixes, and other confectionary products. These foods often contain the common food color FD&C Red No. 3, which contains more than 50 percent iodine. It is not known yet how much of the iodine in these products is available to the body, but there is little evidence that it is not available (26).

Still other sources of iodine are kelp often used in seasoning mixes, and food additives derived from algae such as *carrageenan.* Dietary supplements often are also sources of extra iodine.

In many areas of the world, foods do not have extraneous sources of iodine. Foods raised in high-iodine areas then become the best sources of iodine; they include sea food, meat, milk, poultry, eggs, vegetables, fruit, and whole grains (also dried seaweed in countries where it is customarily eaten). On the other hand, all plant foods in low-iodine areas are low in iodine. Therefore, to put iodine values in food composition tables would be most misleading.

Persons living in nongoitrous areas are practically certain to obtain enough iodine to meet their requirement from water supplies, and from any well-balanced diet—one not too high in cereals and highly refined foods. Those living in goitrous regions may supplement their diet with seafoods and vegetables or other foods shipped in from regions where there is more iodine in the soil. However, by using iodized salt, or other fortified food, people in almost any area may be assured of getting their quota of this element without considering the small and variable amounts provided by the diet.

The Metabolism of Iodine

Iodine is readily absorbed in the upper part of the intestine as iodide ions. It may also be absorbed through the skin, if applied. Estimates of the total amount in the body range from 15 to 30 mg, about the size of a matchhead. Of this small amount, about three-fifths is concentrated in the thyroid gland, and the rest is mostly in the circulating blood.

Iodine serves but one purpose in the body—namely, to form an integral part of the thyroid hormones thyroxine and triiodothyronine. When carried to the tissues, these hormones are quantitatively the most important single factor in determining the rate of basal metabolism. The thyroid hormones also have other vital roles in health and reproduction, which, from a nutritional viewpoint, are likewise essential roles of dietary iodine (see Chap. 6). The level of the thryoid hormones in the blood is controlled by release or suppression of the thyroid-stimulating hormone from the pituitary gland.

Approximately 30 percent of the iodine in the body is normally removed by the thyroid gland, where most of it is stored as the complex protein *thyroglobulin.* The salivary glands, certain vital parts of the brain, the gastric lining, and the lactating mammary glands absorb more than other tissues, but only the thyroid can make the hormones. The remainder is excreted in the urine, with minor amounts in the feces.

Iodine appears to be less involved in protection from infectious disease or cancer than certain other trace elements (4–6).

Toxicity of Iodine

Intakes of iodine in the United States, though high and of concern, are below toxic levels (7,26,27). Levels of iodine up to 2 to 3 mg per day have been taken over long periods by persons with normal thyroids without apparent health problems (2,7,22,26,27). Current high intake should be watched, however, especially by thyroid-sensitive persons. Very high levels of iodine intake can act as a goitrogen. Treating oneself with compounds of iodide or concentrates of iodine in dried seaweed over long periods is a hazardous procedure.

COPPER

Copper (Cu) was the third trace element found to be a dietary essential, as a result of studies by University of Wisconsin biochemists in 1928 (28).

Shortly thereafter, in the early 1930s, the Canadian E. S. Mills and the American

H. W. Josephs provided evidence that copper was more effective than iron alone in overcoming the anemia of milk-fed infants (29,30). Although their findings were not accepted at first, there is now proof that copper deficiency exists in humans receiving low-copper diets (2,4,7,31).

Copper deficiencies in adults are unknown except under experimental conditions. However, because the copper content of refined foods is not a certain entity and because of the recognition of copper deficiency in infants fed natural diets, it is important to have an understanding of its distribution in food and its role in the body.

Deficiency Symptoms

Symptoms of copper deficiency in infants and in the few adults studied include anemia, a low level of a type of white blood cells (neutropenia), pallor, bone and connective tissue disorders, and disorders of blood lipid metabolism.

These symptoms are seen in infants with a rare genetic disturbance called *Minkes steely-hair syndrome,* which involves impaired copper absorption. Additional symptoms are growth retardation, convulsions, scurvy-like conditions, problems with temperature regulation, hair like steel wool (sparce and brittle), and an early death. They can be treated with high doses of copper (2,4,31).

In copper-deficient animals a variety of these and other symptoms occur, including skeletal defects, bone fractures, lung disorders, gray or depigmented hair (see Fig. 16–9), faulty wool or hair structure, degeneration of the nervous system, cardiovascular lesions, internal hemorrhages, and a variety of reproductive disorders (2). Under natural conditions, copper deficiencies occur in animals in areas where the copper content of the soil and the environment is very low, or when there are excessive zinc or molybdenum levels. Otherwise they are rarely seen.

Requirements and Intake

Recognizing the clinical importance of copper, the Food and Nutrition Board has recently recommended 2 to 3 mg of copper for persons over eleven years of age as an "estimated safe and adequate" daily intake. Evidence is accumulating, however, that symptoms of copper deficiency do not appear with intakes of 1.3 mg to 1.5 mg a day. Since this lower level is closer to average intake values, it is likely that the estimated adequate level may be lowered in the future. Recent studies show that not more than 25 percent of daily diets contain 2 mg or more of copper (32). Copper deficiencies have occurred in patients fed parenteral nutrition solutions with low copper levels.

L. M. Klevay and co-workers of the USDA have shown incidence of blood lipid and cholesterol disturbances in humans when they are fed higher than desirable zinc-copper ratios. High zinc levels are known to cause reduced copper absorption. A desirable ratio would be about 7 parts of zinc to 1 of copper. According to Klevay and his colleagues, most American diets have larger ratios than this and inadequate copper levels (less than 2 mg a day). This is still a controversial area (32).

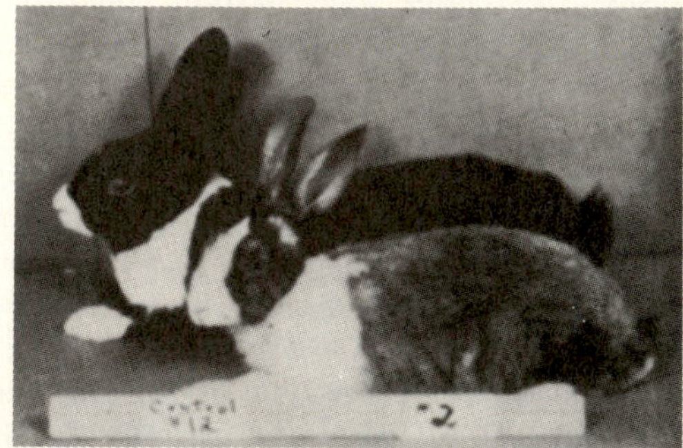

Figure 16–9 The rabbit in the back received sufficient copper in his diet. The rabbit in the foreground, after 6 weeks on a copper deficient diet, displayed smaller size and hair depigmentation. (From Hunt, C.E., and Carlton, W.W.: J. Nutr., *87*:385, 1965.)

Klevay and others, in a study of thirteen men in a metabolic ward for thirty days, suggest that the requirement for copper is about 1.55 mg per day. They further show that this value "substantially exceeds the amount of copper found in many conventional diets (33).

A recent study from Israel reports that a normal, healthy, six-month-old infant on a diet of cow's milk and corn (maize) meal developed a copper deficiency anemia (34). He responded to copper treatment but not to iron, folacin, or vitamin C. This and the Klevay studies, obviously, may show copper to be far more important than it is considered at present.

A recent Canadian study of 100 women averaging about thirty years of age showed an average intake of 1.9 mg a day of copper, exceeding the Canadian allowance (35).

Copper in Foods

Copper occurs along with other mineral elements in all natural foods. The richest sources are organ meats, shellfish, nuts, dried legumes, and cocoa. Cow's milk is a very poor source of this element, as are many other foods. Human milk contains an adequate amount. The amount of copper in the diet depends on both the choice of foods and the locality in which they are produced.

Copper may be inadvertently added to foods in processing, as occurs during the pasteurization of milk by passing it over copper rollers, or from cooking in copper utensils. Copper levels may be reduced, on the other hand, by the refinement of food. It would be extremely difficult, though, to obtain an insufficient supply of copper in one's diet when eating a variety of foodstuffs. Natural drinking water often supplies the entire requirement, for example—especially in homes with copper plumbing (36).

New data on the copper content of foods are available in the recent literature (37). Also see Appendix Table 2 and the new USDA Handbook 8.

Metabolism of Copper in the Body

Availability and Absorption. Normally about 20 to 50 percent of the copper eaten is absorbed. In addition to the inhibition of absorption by high zinc levels, absorption may also be hindered by the consumption of large amounts of antacid tablets. Such amounts were recently reported to have caused a copper deficiency in a thirty-six-year-old woman who was eating an otherwise normal diet (38).

High-protein diets are known to increase copper absorption in humans. In addition to high intakes of zinc and antacids, excessive molybdenum is known to make copper unavailable to experimental animals. Fiber and phytates appear to have only a minor effect on copper availability.

Distribution and Function. A total of 75 to 150 mg of copper is present in the entire human adult body, most of it bound to various essential proteins. Most of the body copper is in blood and muscle, though the brain, heart, liver, eye, hair, and kidney have higher concentrations, suggestive of important functions in these tissues.

In the blood serum most of the copper is present in the protein *ceruloplasmin,* which is essential for iron utilization. Copper is a constituent of a number of important enzymes including *cytochrome oxidases, phenylalanine hydroxylase, tyrosinase, superoxide dismutase,* and *monoamine oxidase.*

Thus, it plays a role in many essential reactions in the body, including the synthesis of hemoglobin (or release of iron for this purpose), the metabolism of glucose and release of energy, the formation of phospholipids in the nerve wall, and the formation of connective tissue.

Clinical Aspects of Copper

Wilson's disease is a rather rare chronic metabolic disease in humans, in which the body has great difficulty in disposing of excess copper; the copper is stored in the liver and other tissues (such as the eyes), finally resulting in toxic concentrations. The level of ceruloplasmin in blood serum is usually very low. Copper-low diets of "normal foods" have been developed and are used as part of the clinical management of the disease.

The copper in hair is claimed by various commercial laboratories to indicate the level of copper in individuals. It is not a reliable indicator, however. (See discussion on hair minerals in Chap. 17.)

The apparent success of various organic compounds in treating certain inflammatory diseases has aroused considerable interest (39). Copper deficiency is known to impair various immune functions, such as the prevention of tumors, in experimental animals. The human aspects of these studies, if any, are not known at this time (5,6).

MANGANESE

Manganese (Mn) is easily confused with magnesium (Mg) because the names are similar, both names being derived centuries ago from the white magnesium salts "magnesia alba." Both are essential nutrients, but most of the similarity stops there.

Inorganic manganese has been known to be a dietary essential for all higher animals ever since the original discovery in 1931 in several laboratories (by Hart, McCollum, and their associates) that it was essential for growth of rats (40). Later it was shown to be essential for poultry (a deficiency resulted in a tendon and bone disorder), swine, guinea pigs, cattle, and other animals (2).

Undoubtedly manganese is an essential nutrient for humans, even though what signs would identify a deficiency of it have never been determined with certainty. Impaired blood clotting, lowered cholesterol in blood serum, color changes in the hair, and dermatitis have been seen in very limited clinical studies that require confirmation (41). In any event, the dietary requirement is so low in comparison with the abundant amounts in our environment and in most foods that a deficiency in populations would be quite unlikely.

Deficiency Signs

Manganese deficiency occurs chiefly under experimental conditions. It may be caused either by simply feeding fowl natural grain and legume diets or by feeding manganese-low diets to several species of animals.

The resulting symptoms of deficiency include failure to grow, interference with sexual processes, and inability to produce normal young (42). In rabbits, there are deformations of bone. In fowls, a manganese-deficient ration is the chief cause of a disorder called "slipped tendon," resulting in deformed legs, which could be a source of economic loss to poultry producers. The routine addition today of small amounts of manganese to the ration prevents development of this disease (55 mg per kg of diet is needed by fowl, a relatively high level compared with the normal need of mammals). The brain and nervous system of laboratory animals are particularly susceptible to both manganese deficiency and manganese toxicity.

Requirement, Intake, and Food Sources

The "safe and adequate" recommended requirement for manganese was established in 1980 by the Food and Nutrition Board at 2.5 to 5.0 mg per day for adults (see inside front cover for other age groups). The minimal requirement is not yet known. The few studies made show dietary intakes well above

2.5 mg a day, which are fully adequate to take care of the body's needs.

Manganese is widely distributed in foods of plant and animal origin, especially nuts, vegetables, and fruits, though it is partially lost along with other trace elements in food refining. It is relatively nontoxic.

The Role of Manganese in the Body

Absorption of manganese ranges from only 1 to 20 percent of intake. Like iron absorption, it depends on dietary intake and need. High intakes of iron and of calcium decrease manganese absorption. The human body apparently contains only about 20 mg of manganese so there is little storage.

Manganese has many essential functions in each cell of the body. The highest concentrations in the body are in the pituitary gland, lactating mammary glands, liver, pancreas, kidney, intestinal wall, and bone.

Manganese is an important catalyst and is a co-factor or component of many enzymes in the body.[4] Because of its relationship to these enzymes, manganese functions in: synthesis of complex carbohydrates (mucopolysaccharides) in cells, utilization of glucose, lipid synthesis and metabolism, nerve cell metabolism, cholesterol synthesis, normal pancreas development, muscle contraction, prevention of skeletal defects, prevention of sterility, and other vital functions. Few trace elements have as many metabolic functions.

QUESTIONS

1. In what special tissue is most of the iron in the body found, and in what special substance in this tissue? What function does it fulfill in this tissue, and what chemical property enables it to carry out this function? How do the smaller amounts of iron located in tissue cells help in oxidation-reduction processes vital to the life of cells?

2. What is the recommended dietary allowance for iron daily for a man? A woman? At what periods of life is the need for this element increased, and why? Explain how iron is conserved by the body and how a liberal supply of it in the diet can build up reserve stores that protect the body in times of extra need.

3. Record all the foods you ate on a typical day, with quantities of each, and calculate the amount of iron they furnished. Use either Table 16–3 for iron content of foods or the table in the Appendix or both. Does the amount of iron in this day's diet come up to your RDA? If not, what changes could be made to furnish more iron? (Changes, if any, should be palatable, economical, and provide food you would eat routinely.) Do not use iron supplements for these calculations.

4. Does your state (or province, territory, district) have standards or requirements for iron enrichment? If so, how do they differ from national standards? If not, discuss whether you think the difference is important.

5. What are the symptoms of iron-deficiency anemia, and under what conditions may it be caused? Does the existence of anemia necessarily mean that the diet furnished less than normal amounts of iron? Give reasons for your answer. What other nutritional factors besides iron are important in preventing anemia?

6. Can the body utilize inorganic and organic iron equally well? In what form or forms is iron most readily absorbed from the intestine? Mention three conditions that are favorable and three that are unfavorable to iron absorption. To what extent may the degree of availability and absorption of iron be influenced by the relative need of the body for iron?

7. How many liters of blood are present in a typical female body? A male body? How many pints is this? (A pint is the usual amount given in

[4]Manganese is present in such enzymes as pyruvate carboxylase, and superoxide dismutase (which also contains copper), and is a co-factor in the metabolism of liver arginase, phosphoglucomutase, polymerase (for mucopolysaccharide formation), galactotransferase, acetyl-CoA carboxylase, and others.

a blood transfusion.) How much extra iron per day should a person consume who is donating blood every three months?

8. Why is iodine essential in small amounts for body welfare? In what tissue is it concentrated, and what is its function there? Can iodine be stored in the body and, if so, where? What is a ductless gland? A hormone? The names of the two iodine-containing hormones of the thyroid gland? The influence of these hormones on body metabolism (tissue oxidations)?

9. Simple goiter is a deficiency disease caused by lack of what element? In what regions is it most prevalent, and why? At what periods of life is it most likely to develop, and why? What public health measure has been used successfully in preventing simple goiter?

10. Is copper an essential element? If so, for what major purpose is it necessary? Why does a rat become anemic if kept a long time on a diet consisting only of cow's milk? Why can such an anemia not be cured by giving either iron alone or copper alone? Explain why most people are sure of getting enough copper in their food to meet their requirement.

11. Why is manganese essential for humans? How much manganese, roughly, do you eat each day (no calculation necessary)? Compare this with your allowance for magnesium.

References

1. (On trace element content of foods and soil relationships) Reid, R. L., and Horvath, D. J.: Soil chemistry and mineral problems in farm livestock (a review—300 references). Anim. Feed Sci. Tech., *5*:95, 1980; Furr, A. K., et al.: J. Agric. Food Chem., *29*:156, 1981 (minerals in vegetables raised on different soils); Watkinson, J. H.: Amer. J. Clin. Nutr., *34*:936, 1981 (selenium levels in humans and soil); Chang, A. C., et al.: Effects of sludge application on the Cd, Pb, and Zn levels of selected vegetable plants, Hilgardia (U. Calif. Exp. Stat.), *50*(Nov.):1, 1982; Gupta, U. C., et al.: Canad. J. Soil Sci., *62*:145, 1982 (selenium levels on barley vs. soil levels). Also see current issues of the Journal of Plant Nutrition, Soil Science, and related journals.
2. Underwood, E. J.: *Trace Elements in Human and Animal Nutrition.* 4th Ed. New York, Academic Press, 1977; Underwood, E. J.: J. Human Nutr., *32*:253, 1978 and *35*:37, 1981.
3. Ensminger, A. H., et al.: *Foods and Nutrition Encyclopedia,* Clovis, Calif., Pergus Press, 1983 (iron, p. 1246; iodine, p. 1242; copper, p. 476; manganese, p. 1370; organic foods, p. 1693; minerals, p. 1508; anemia, p. 76; goiter, p. 1083).

Iron

4. Goodhart, R. S., and Shils, M. E. (eds.): *Modern Nutrition in Health and Disease.* 6th Ed. Philadelphia, Penn., Lea and Febiger, 1980 (see E. Beutler, p. 324, on iron; R. R. Cavalieri, p. 395, on iodine; and T. Li and B. L. Vallee, p. 408, on copper, manganese, and other trace elements).
5. Gross, R. L., and Newberne, P. M.: Physiol. Rev., *60*:188, 1980; Beisel, W. R.: Single nutrients and immunity. Amer. J. Clin. Nutr., *35* (Suppl. No. 2, Feb.): 417–458, 1982.
6. Committee on Diet, Nutrition, and Cancer: Washington, D.C., National Academy of Sciences, 1982.
7. Food and Nutrition Board: *Recommended Dietary Allowances.* 9th Ed. Washington D.C., National Research Council, National Academy of Sciences, 1980.
8. Windham, C. T., et al.: J. Amer. Dietet. Assoc., *78*:587, 1981.
9. Harland, B. F., et al.: J. Amer. Dietet. Assoc., *47*:16, 1980 (a study on "market basket" diets); Lynch, S. R., et al.: Amer. J. Clin. Nutr., *36*:1032, 1982 (iron status of elderly Americans).
10. Pao, E. M., and Mickle, S. J.: Food Tech., *35* (Sept): 58, 1981. (This study is based on a three-day dietary survey, which has been recently criticized for not "catching" all food intake—by a factor of up to 25 percent. Even with an adjustment by this percentage, the study still shows millions of persons in the U.S. with low iron intakes. Also see following references, 11–16.)
11. (Children) Bailey, L. B., et al.: Nutr. Rev., *2*:397, 1982 (adolescents in low-income rural households, black and white, in Florida); Bailey, L. B., et al.: Amer. J. Clin. Nutr., *35*:1023, 1982 (urban low-income adolescents, black and Spanish-American, in Florida); Martinez, O. B.: Canad. J. Public Health, *73*:109, 1982 (young school children in Canada).
12. (Pregnant women) Bowering, J., et al.: Amer. J. Clin. Nutr., *33*:1978, 1980 (low-income Puerto Rican and black women in New York); Letsky, E. A.: Human Nutr.: Appl. Nutr., *36A*:245, 1982 (a review); Jackson, R. T., and Latham, M. C.: Amer. J. Clin. Nutr. *35*:710, 1982 (in Liberia).
13. (Elderly) Harrill, I., et al.: J. Nutr. Elderly, *1* (No. 3/4):3, 1981 (nursing home residents); Kerr, G. R., et al.: Amer. J. Clin. Nutr., *35*:294, 1982 (white and black subjects); Harrill, I., et al.: Nutr. Rept. Internat., *25*:189, 1982 (5 ethnic groups); Sempos, C. T., et al.: J. Amer. Dietet. Assoc., *81*:35, 1982 (14 Wisconsin nursing homes); Lynch, S. R., et al.: Amer. J. Clin. Nutr., *36*:1032, 1982 (a review); Nordstrom,

J. W.: Nutr. Rept. Internat., *25*:97, 1982; O'Hanlon, P., et al.: J. Amer. Dietet. Assoc., *82*:646, 1983 (elderly Missourians); Johnson, A. A. et al.: Fed. Proc., *42*:1181(abst.), 1983 (low income, aged blacks).

14. (Ethnic groups) Haider, S. Q., and Wheeler, M.: J. Amer. Dietet. Assoc., *77*:677, 1980 (black and hispanic teenage girls in Brooklyn); Margolis, H. S., et al.: Amer. J. Clin. Nutr., *34*:2158, 1981 (Eskimo children, Alaska); Johnson, A. A., Latham, M. C., and Roe, D. A.: Amer. J. Public Health, *72*:285, 1982 (English-speaking Carribbean—a review).
15. Caliendo, M. A., Booth, G., and Moser, P.: J. Amer. Dietet. Assoc., *81*:401, 1982 (in developmentally delayed children in Washington D.C. area).
16. Cook, R. A., et al.: Nutr. Rept. Internat., *19*:179, 1979 (Maine adults); Schafer, R. B., et al.: Home Econ. Res. J., *8*:190, 1980 (470 women in 7 states); Foss, S. B., and Keith, R. E.: Nutr. Rept. Internat., *26*:613, 1982 (single, professional Alabama women).
17. Rivera, R., et al.: Amer. J. Clin. Nutr., *36*:1162, 1982 (milk fortification in Mexico); Working Group on Fortification of Salt with Iron: Amer. J. Clin. Nutr., *35*:1442, 1982 (India).
18. (On containers and cooking utensils as a source of iron in foods) White, H. S.: J. Home Econ., *60*:724, 1968 (cast-iron cookware); Franz, K. B., and Kennedy, B. M.: New Eng. J. Med., *293*:1265, 1975; Mertz, W.: J. Amer. Dietet. Assoc., *77*:258, 1980 (see p. 260 on cookware effects); Greger, J. L., and Baier, M.: J. Food Sci., *46*:1751, 1981 (19 types of canned and bottled foods); Rosanoff, A., and Kennedy, B. M.: J. Food Sci., *47*:609, 1982 (apples).
19. Cunningham, H. M., and O'Brien, R.: J. Food Sci., *37*:572, 1972 (metal particles in commercially ground cereals); Kuhnlein, H. V., and Calloway, D. H.: J. Food Sci. *44*:282, 1979 (Hopi Indian diets); Greenhouse, R.: Ecol. Food Nutr., *10*:221, 1981 (Pima Indian foods).
20. (On stability of iron in processed foods) Lee, K., and Clydesdale, F. M.: J. Food Sci., *45*:1500, 1980 (effect of baking); Weaver, C. M., et al.: Cereal Chem., *58*:120, 1981 (effect of milling on trace elements in oats and barley); Lee, K., Clydesdale, F. M.: J. Food Sci., *46*:1064, 1981 (heat effects in canned spinach); Clemens, R. A.: J. Food Sci., *47*:228, 1982 (effect of storage and heat on a liquid milk-based product).
21. (Selected references on iron availability and absorption) Bowering, J., Sanchez, A. M., and Irwin, M. I.: J. Nutr., *106*:985, 1976 (a review with 752 references); Hallberg, L.: Bioavailability of dietary iron in man. Ann. Rev. Nutr., *1*:123, 1981 (a review with 90 references); Rao, B. S. N.: Brit. Med. Bull., *37*:25, 1981 (a review); Hallberg, L.: Human Nutr.: Clin. Nutr., *36C*:259, 1982 (a review for the general reader); Monsen, E. R., and Balintfy, J. L.: J. Amer. Dietet. Assoc., *80*:307, 1982; Sabry, J. H., and Grief, H.: J. Canad. Dietet. Assoc., *43*:132, 1982; Turnland, J. R., et al.: Amer. J. Clin. Nutr., *35*:1033, 1982 (in elderly men); Charlton, R. W., and Bothwell, T. H.: Ann. Rev. Med., *34*:55, 1983 (a review); Bjorn-Rasmussen, E.: Lancet, *1*:914, 1983 (present knowledge and controversies—a review). Also see supplementary readings for additional information on this topic.
22. Rosenberg, I. H., et al.: Report of FDA panel on vitamin and mineral drug products for over-the-counter human use. Federal Register, *44* (No. 53): 16126, March 16, 1979 (see iron, p. 16182; iodine, p. 16181; copper, p. 16175; manganese, p. 16189); Fenner, L.: FDA Consumer, *16* (Feb.):27, 1982 (on accidental toxicity in children).

Iodine

23. Marine, D., and Kimball, O. P.: Arch. Intern. Med., *25*:661, 1920; J. Amer. Med. Assoc., *77*:1068, 1921.
24. Marine, D., and Kimball, O. P.: J. Lab. Clin. Med., *3*:40, 1917 (reprinted in Nutr. Rev., *33*:272, 1975).
25. Hart, E. B., and Steenbock, H.: J. Biol. Chem., *33*:313, 1918.
26. Taylor, F.: Iodine—going from hypo to hyper. FDA Consumer, *15* (April, No. 3):15, 1981; Park, Y. K., et al.: Estimation of dietary iodine intake of Americans in recent years. J. Amer. Dietet. Assoc., *79*:17, 1981.
27. Hemkin, R. W., Fox, J. D., and Hicks, C. L.: J. Food Protect., *44*:476, 1981; Bruhns, J. C., et al.: J. Food Protect., *46*:41, 1983.

Copper

28. Hart, E. B., Steenbock, H., Waddell, J., and Elvehjem, C. A.: J. Biol. Chem., *77*:797, 1928.
29. Mills, E. S.: Canad. Med. Assoc. J., *22*:175, 1930, and Amer. J. Med. Sci., *182*:554, 1931.
30. Josephs, H. W.: Bull. Johns Hopkins Hosp., *49*:246, 1931 (also see Lewis, M. S.: J. Amer. Med. Assoc., *96*:1135, 1931; Usher, S. J., MacDermott, P. N., and Lozinski, E.: Amer. J. Dis. Children, *18*:642, 1935).
31. (Reviews on copper in human nutrition) Mason, K. E.: A conspectus of research on copper metabolism and requirements of man. (879 references) J. Nutr., *109*:1979, 1979; Kay, R. G.: Zinc and copper in human nutrition. J. Human Nutr., *35*:25, 1981; Sandstead, H. H.: Copper bioavailability and requirements. Amer. J. Clin. Nutr., *35*:809, 1982.
32. (On zinc-copper ratios.) Klevay, L. M.: personal communication. Also see Klevay, L. M., et al.: J. Amer. Med. Assoc., *241*:1916, 1979; Klevay, L. M.: Interactions of copper and zinc in cardiovascular disease. Ann. N. Y. Acad. Sci., *355*:140, 1980; Also see Sandstead, H. H.: J. Amer. Med. Assoc., *245*:1528, 1981; and Amer. J. Clin. Nutr., *35*:809, 1982.
33. Klevay, L. M., et al.: Amer. J. Clin. Nutr., *33*:45, 1980; Klevay, L. M., Amer. J. Clin. Nutr., *37*:717 (abstract), 1983.
34. Naveh, Y., et al.: Pediatrics, *68*:397, 1981.
35. Gibson, R. S., and Scythes, C. A.: Trace element intakes of women. Brit. J. Nutr., *48*:241, 1982.
36. Sharrett, A. R., et al.: Environ. Res., *28*:456, 1982.

37. (On copper content of foods) Allen, K. G. D., and Klevay, L. M.: Nutr. Rept. Internat., *22*:389, 1980 (breakfast cereals); Freeland-Graves, J. H., et al.: J. Amer. Dietet. Assoc. *77*:648, 1980 (vegetarian foods); Leung, C., Koehler, H. H., and Hard, M. M.: J. Amer. Dietet. Assoc., *80*:530, 1982 (Fe, Cu, and Mn in prepared hospital food); Mbofung, C. M. F., and Atinmo, T.: Nutr. Rept. Internat. *26*:767, 1982. (Nigerian foods and diets); Kenny, M. A., and Thimaya, S.: J, Amer. Dietet. Assoc., *82*:509, 1983 (various teas).
38. Van Kalmthout, P. M., et al.: Dig. Dis. Sci., *27*:859, 1982.
39. Sorenson, J. R. J. (ed.): *Inflammatory Diseases and Copper*. Clifton, N.J., Humana Press, 1982.

Manganese

40. Kemmerer, A. R., Elvehjem, C. A., and Hart, E. B.: J. Biol. Chem., *92*:623, 1931; Orent, E. R., and McCollum, E. V.: J. Biol. Chem., *92*:651, 1931 (also see McCarrison, R.: Ind. J. Med. Res., *14*:641, 1927).
41. Leach, R. M., and Lilburn, M. S.: Manganese metabolism and its function. World Rev. Nutr. Dietet., *32*:123, 1978 (see their ref. 15.)
42. Hurley, L. S.: Teratogenic aspects of manganese, zinc, and copper nutrition. Physiol. Rev., *61*:249, 1981.

17 The Newer Trace Elements

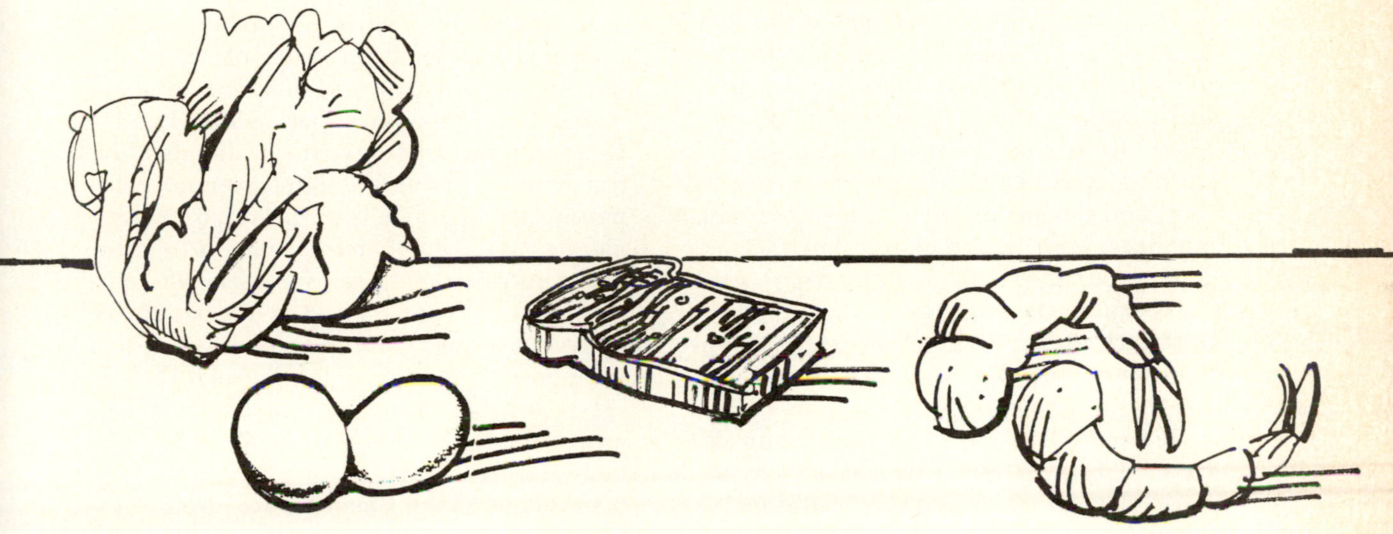

Chapter 16 presented the "older" trace elements, those accepted before the 1960s as being needed by humans and animals. This chapter examines relatively "new" trace elements found in the last twenty-five years to be essential and still being studied. The newer essential trace elements are zinc, fluorine, cobalt, molybdenum, selenium, chromium, nickel, vanadium, silicon, and possibly arsenic. It would be difficult to pinpoint any one essential trace element as the most important. Each is vital.

Overview

The introductory section to the older trace elements in Chapter 16 discussed, briefly, the distribution of trace elements in food, the effects of processing, absorption and bioavailability, and the variety of functions in the body. These topics will be discussed in this chapter only when specifically relevant to understanding a particular element.

This chapter will, however, be concerned with areas of particular research interest or controversy. One of the most investigated questions in nutrition today is, "Which of the newer trace elements are essential for humans—and which are not?" This question will be considered in the course of discussing vanadium, arsenic, tin, lead, nickel, silicon, boron and other elements that have been proposed as essential for certain species.

Another controversial area is the widespread use of analysis of minerals in the hair to provide an indication of the level of intake of trace elements. Still another controversial topic is the possible role of certain trace elements in preventing cancer.

Nonessential Elements and Minerals. In addition to the essential trace elements, this chapter will consider the more important of the dozens of *nonessential elements,* for which there is no known nutritional need. Examples are aluminum, bromine, barium, rubidium, cadmium, strontium, lithium, and mercury. These nonessential elements, along with the essential elements, make up the total of the ninety-one or so stable natural elements listed in the periodic table in the Appendix. Many are widely distributed in soils, water supplies, and plants. Hence, they are in our food and our bodies, generally in very small amounts. Over all, roughly 0.05 to 0.2 percent of our diet is likely to be composed of nonessential elements. Because a number of them are very toxic it is important to have knowledge about them. (See also Table 16–1.)

Determination of Essentiality of Elements. How is the essential nature of a trace element determined? The trace elements discussed in this chapter are especially difficult to study in humans and in experimental animals because of the difficulty in obtaining dietary ingredients, drinking water, and environment completely free of these elements. Investigators have to be meticulous in order to avoid possible contaminating sources of the element being studied. Dietary ingredients have to be specially purified. It is not uncommon to use special plastic isolators in which to maintain the animals and to remove dust particles, carriers of trace elements, from the air by special filters (see Fig. 17–1).

Deficiencies of trace elements may also be obtained by raising plants on soils deficient in a specific element that the plant does not require or requires in very small amounts such as iodine, selenium, molybdenum, and chromium. Then, diets made from these plants can be fed to animals in experimental situations to study a lack of a specific element.

In studies with humans, deficiencies of selenium, zinc, chromium, and other elements have been unexpectedly obtained by the long-time, routine clinical use of highly complex sterile solutions of nutrients containing, supposedly, all known trace elements. These mixtures are widely used in hospitals and in home care when a person is unable to eat in a normal manner (as a result of a digestive disease or surgery of digestive organs). These liquid mixes are given either by tube bypassing the upper part of the digestive tract *(enteral nutrition),* or intravenously, bypassing the digestive tract entirely *(parenteral nutrition).* (For further information on these liquid nutrition mixtures, see, especially, current issues of the *Journal of Parenteral and Enteral Nutrition.*) It should be obvious that without the recent advances in such life-saving techniques major progress in medicine would not be possible (1).

Levels of Trace Elements Required. Estimations of the amount required of a trace element may be determined by *mineral balance studies,* which measure intakes against outputs in urine, perspiration, and feces. Balance studies have been conducted for all the minerals and for nitrogen but are not feasible with organic compounds, which metabolize. Less is known about the amounts required by humans for the elements described in this chapter than for any other class of nutrients, with the possible exception of the electrolytes. This is because their nutrient nature has been discovered only relatively recently. Studies with humans are especially difficult to undertake, but a number of such studies are now in progress. Zinc is the only mineral discussed in this chapter with an established recommended dietary allowance. In the United States "safe and adequate daily dietary intakes" were suggested in 1980 by the Food and Nutrition Board for several other elements—fluorine, molybdenum, selenium, and chromium (2).

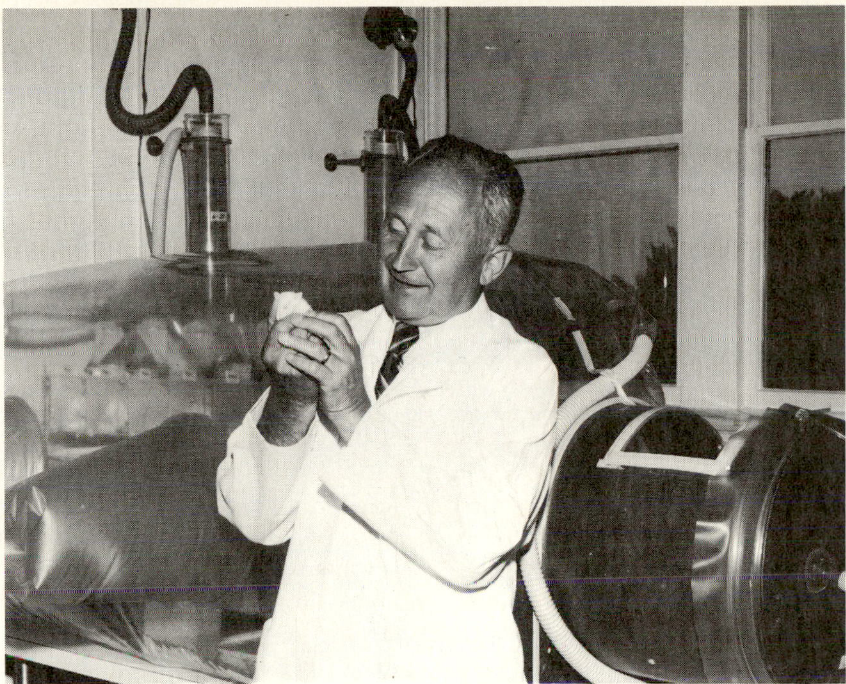

Figure 17–1 The late Dr. Klaus Schwarz, in whose laboratories the growth effects of selenium, chromium, and vanadium were demonstrated. Mineral contamination from the environment was eliminated by use of the isolator and air filters shown here.

The need by humans for nickel, vanadium, and silicon, known to be essential for experimental animals, has not yet been confirmed by scientific study. The need by experimental animals for arsenic and possibly other elements is a current area of research.

For more specific information about these newer trace elements see the references at the end of the chapter, the supplementary readings in the Appendix, and current copies of journals listed at the end of Chapter 1.

ZINC

Zinc is a silver-blue mineral. It has been known for centuries as an important mineral in commerce. Zinc is a constituent, with copper, of brass. We commonly encounter zinc in such forms as the coating of galvanized iron and as a component of flashlight batteries. About 2 grams (gm) are present in the adult human body.

The first clear-cut proof that zinc is needed by mammals was shown by nutritionists at the University of Wisconsin working with rats in 1934 (3). Zinc is known to be very important in the diet of all animal species studied, including rats, cattle, sheep, dogs, pigs, mice, and poultry (4,5). (See Fig. 17–2.) It is necessary for growth, reproduction, and the health of all tissues. Not until the 1960s was it proven to be required by humans as well as farm animals (6). Zinc deficiency can occur in both when certain combinations of natural foods are consumed. In other words, contrary to former opinion, it is now known that one can not take for granted that his or her intake of zinc will be

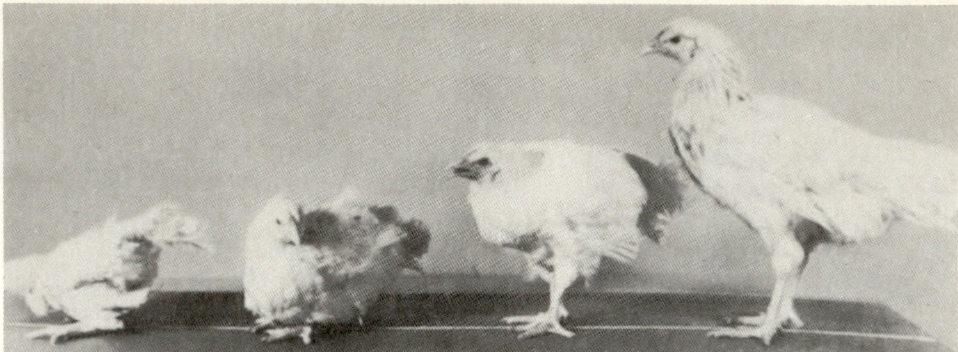

Figure 17–2 These four chickens are all 10 weeks old. From left to right, they were fed increasing amounts of zinc. Note the retarded growth, poor feathering, and difficulty in standing up in the deficient animals. (Courtesy of the American Zinc Institute.)

satisfactory no matter what foods are eaten.

Zinc is a constituent of dozens of different body enzymes, each of which is vital for the growth and metabolism of body cells and tissues. No other nutrient functions as a part of so many different enzymes.

Zinc has become one of the most studied of all trace elements, rivaling iron in popularity not only with nutritional scientists but also with health-food advocates. In 1982 about 400 scientific papers on zinc nutrition were published.

Zinc Deficiency Symptoms

Deficiency in Animals. Symptoms of zinc deficiency in animals include retarded growth, loss of appetite, skin disorders, dental decay, many reproduction problems, and abnormal bone metabolism (4). In zinc-deficient pigs, an increase in zinc intake prevents or cures *parakeratosis,* a disease characterized by roughening of the skin and loss of hair. This formerly caused economic losses to pig farmers. Zinc-deficient dogs develop similar skin disorders, including hair loss and open sores and crusts (7). Zinc is now routinely added to commercial animal feed as an insurance against deficiency.

Deficiency in Humans. In humans, zinc is essential for normal growth, tissue and wound repair, skin structure, prevention of infection, reproduction, growth of all tissues, taste perception, and prevention of "dwarfism," or greatly reduced stature (2,6). Some areas of the Middle East, where zinc deficiency in humans was first found, have a high incidence of dwarfism combined with sexual immaturity. In classic nutrition studies, a group of young men aged eighteen to nineteen, thought to be "dwarfs," increased in stature and developed normal secondary sexual characteristics after being given supplemental doses of zinc (6,8).

Studies in the United States have shown that some segments of the population have marginal zinc deficiency. The first and now classic of these studies was on school children in the Denver area. They were found to have low levels of zinc in their hair, impaired taste acuity, poor appetite, and retarded growth. These symptoms were corrected by giving them more zinc (9). Since then, numerous studies have confirmed and extended these early observations, as discussed in the following pages. (See also the supplementary readings in the Appendix.)

Effect on Pregnancy and Reproduction. The role of zinc in the prevention of abnormalities in the fetus has been clearly demonstrated in a number of important studies with animals (4,10). Consequently, a number of researchers have recently suggested that in human pregnancy a deficiency of zinc would be likely to lead to smaller babies and, in severe instances, to cleft palates, nerve and brain disorders, and other congenital malformations (10,11).

Reproductive disorders such as reduction of testes size, failure of sperm production, and reduced male hormone (testosterone) have been known to occur in zinc-deficient male animals (4) and humans (12,13). These deficiencies are correctable by giving the subjects proper supplements of zinc.

Effect on Nerves, Learning, and Behavior. In recent studies, zinc deficiency has been shown to affect adversely nerve and brain function, learning, and behavior (14). A. S. Prasad and his colleagues reported apathy, lethargy, amnesia, and mental retardation (often associated with irritability, depression, and paranoia) in zinc-deficient humans (15).

Effect on Immunological Functions. Zinc is one of the most important of the many nutrients necessary for proper immunological functioning of the body, including the activity of the *thymus gland* (16–18). Bacterial and viral infections and all other immune disorders are likely to be more severe and life-threatening to populations of all ages with a low intake of zinc. Zinc deficiency may be seen early in life and may occur at anytime through adulthood (19) and old age (20). A recent study at the University of California at Davis showed that offspring of pregnant mice that were moderately deficient in zinc had depressed immunological functioning for six months. Depression persisted to a lesser extent for three generations of mice, even though the offspring were fed a normal diet (21).

It needs to be noted that there is no evidence that humans who consume larger amounts of zinc than the recommended allowance will improve their immunity, prevent disease, or prevent or cure any of the deficiency symptoms mentioned in these paragraphs.

Effect on Taste and Smell. The relation of zinc to the ability to taste and smell is a controversial area of research. In the early 1970s R. I. Henkin reported that giving zinc to patients increased their senses of taste and smell (cited in [2]). Since then some researchers have confirmed this finding (14,22), but others have been unable to do so (23).

Evaluation of the research indicates that when persons are actually deficient in zinc, their ability to taste and smell can be reduced. This condition is likely to exist especially in an unknown percentage of persons who have some disease or may be genetically susceptible. Impaired senses of taste and smell, however, can result from a number of other causes. Unless zinc deficiency is the cause, no amount of extra zinc will cure the symptoms.

Zinc in Acne and Congenital Skin Disorders. Since skin disorders are a common sign of severe zinc deficiency, it is logical to ask if acne can be corrected by eating extra amounts of zinc-rich foods. The acne common among teenagers is not due to a zinc deficiency and so cannot be effectively treated with zinc (see ref. 23, Chap. 9). Acnelike skin disorders, however, although not common, can occur in persons deficient in zinc (24). Skin rashes may also occur on other parts of the body even if the face remains clear. Such zinc-related disorders can be prevented by the person's eating the recommended allowance of zinc per day. It is that easy and simple, but zinc will not prevent more common kinds of acne (see Fig. 17–3).

An acne-like condition, *acrodermatitis enteropathica,* is a rare but serious congenital disease in infants. It responds dramatically to zinc therapy, indicating that a genetic defect in zinc absorption or metabolism is respon-

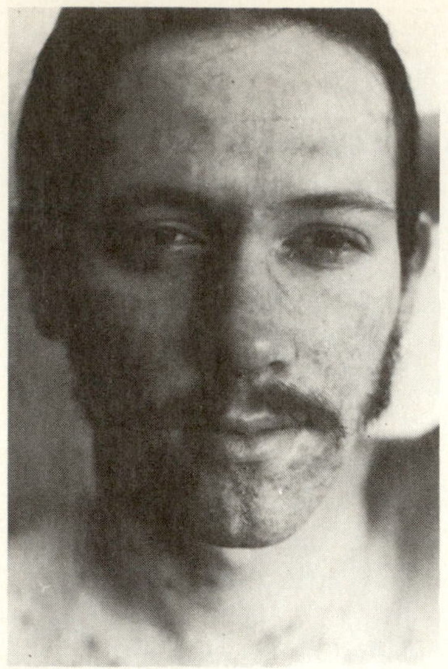

A. Zinc deficient

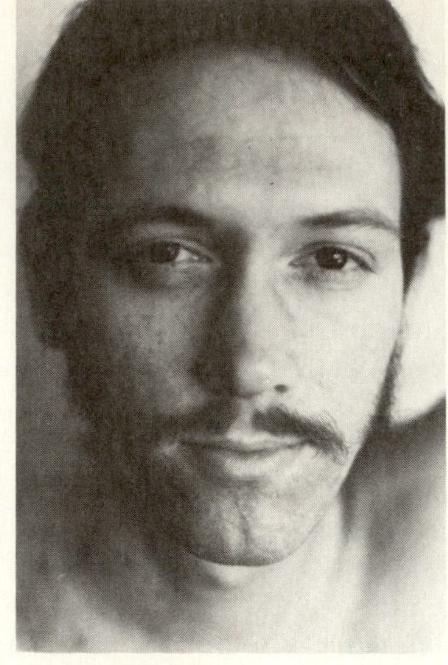

B. After 4 days of zinc treatment

Figure 17–3 A. An acne-like condition in a young male volunteer after eating a zinc-deficient diet for four weeks. B. After 4 days of zinc administration. Note nearly complete disappearance of symptoms. Courtesy of Dr. Janet King, University of California, Berkeley.

sible (13,16,25). Children with this disorder may also lose hair, have diarrhea, be psychologically disturbed, and fail to thrive—all symptoms of the lack of zinc. One cause, at least, is lack of available zinc in breast milk of certain mothers, a condition thought to be inherited but possibly the result of inadequate intake of zinc during pregnancy. The loss of immunological functions from zinc deficiency may be related (25).

Zinc in Parenteral Nutrition and Other Clinical Situations. Examples of people with classic symptoms of zinc deficiency continue to be described in nutrition literature because zinc has been often unintentionally left out of parenteral solutions fed to infants (26) and adult patients (1,27).

The relation of zinc deficiency to the incidence of cancer is an active research area. According to the National Academy of Sciences, not enough information is available yet to enable us to draw any conclusions (28). Under different experimental conditions zinc can either encourage or retard certain cancers. It would be foolish to take extra amounts of zinc, beyond that in a well-balanced diet, to prevent cancer without the close supervision of a physician.

Zinc is being prescribed by physicians, or studied experimentally, for use in a variety of conditions. They include certain chronic liver diseases (especially as related to alcoholism), malabsorption syndromes (as in cystic fibrosis), sickle-cell disease, parasitic infestations, surgery, burns, and chronic fevers (13,18,29). It might be expected that when zinc is deficient for any reason a supplemental intake of zinc would be beneficial. In fact, the chances that only zinc is deficient in such situations is slim; other nutrients are likely to be low as well. The effectiveness of zinc therapy alone in these conditions remains to be proven.

Other Deficiency Symptoms in Humans. When a nutrient is involved in as many enzyme systems in the body as zinc is, it is to be expected that many other specific signs of deficiency will be discovered. Among those recently reported but in need of further study are interference with metabolism of alcohol and with vitamin A metabolism (resulting in night blindness), eye defects at birth, a nonmotile small intestine, bone-growth deformities, reduced protein and carbohydrate metabolism, high levels of lipids in the blood, reduced growth-hormone levels, loss of appetite (anorexia), and diarrhea (4,13,16).

When one reads about all the dire things that can happen when zinc is low in the diet, one is tempted immediately "to go" and buy a zinc supplement. This course is not advised. If a person is low in zinc, other nutrients are likely to be missing from the diet as well. Correcting one's diet so that it contains recommended levels of zinc and other nutrients is the proper course to take. The way to achieve such a balanced diet is explained in later sections and in Chapter 20. Nevertheless, people who cannot obtain sufficient zinc in their diet for any reason should take extra supplements of zinc. This course is advised until various governmental agencies require that white flour and other processed cereals be enriched with zinc up to, at least, the original level found in the natural grains.

Recommended Allowances for Zinc

The recommended dietary allowances (RDA) for zinc in the United States are given in Table 17–1. They are set at 15 milligrams (mg) a day for both men and women for reasons outlined by the Food and Nutrition Board (2). It is interesting that the U.S. allowances are about 50 percent greater than the Canadian "recommended intakes," which average around 8 mg per day for females and 9 mg per day for males (see Appendix, Table 1). A person's basic requirement does not differ whether he or she lives north or south of the border. The differences reflect in part differences in the interpretation of "allowance" and "recommended intake." The authors think the Board's figure is justified by the reasons given in the report. These differences will no doubt diminish as more research is done and as the diets of the two populations become more similar.

Table 17–1 RECOMMENDED ALLOWANCES FOR ZINC[a]

	Age	*Allowance mg/day*
Children	1–10 years	10
Males	11–51 years and older	15
Females	11–51 years and older	15
	Pregnant	20
	Lactating	25

[a]From the Food and Nutrition Board, 1980 (2).

Intakes and Their Measurement

The typical American diet supplies an average of about 10 to 15 mg of zinc per day (2,30). The amount absorbed varies with the kind of diet (see the next section). Intake in many instances is less than the RDA, indicating that: (1) there are many people with borderline intake, (2) we should take extra care in planning our meals to obtain sufficient zinc, or (3) the allowance is set too high. The authors think the first and second conclusions are correct.

The degree of zinc deficiency in the body is not easy to measure in the absence of symptoms. Common practice is to measure levels of zinc in blood serum, although these can be affected by non-nutritional factors such as oral contraceptives, circadian rhythms, short-term fasting, and infection (31). Levels of zinc in the hair (see later discussion), levels in the blood serum containing the enzyme *alkaline phosphatase,* and "salivary sediment zinc" have all been suggested as measures of the degree of zinc deficiency in the body, but there are problems with each of these methods (31). Normal zinc levels in blood serum average about 100 to 120 micrograms (μg) per 100 milliliters (ml). Levels below 80 μg would be considered low.

Effect of Increased Age. Older persons require no more zinc than younger persons do (2,32). In fact there is some recent evidence that older people may require somewhat less than 15 mg per day (33,34). H. H. Sandstead and his colleagues suggest that in elderly persons reduced consumption of protein and phosphorus, as well as other factors, may reduce the zinc requirement (34). Nevertheless, it is becoming increasingly clear from biochemical tests and/or dietary surveys that intakes of zinc by the elderly often are low—at least less than ideal (34,35). (See also the discussion on copper-zinc ratios in Chap. 16.)

Pregnancy and Infancy. The increased allowance for zinc in pregnancy is based on increased physiological needs (2). (See also Chap. 22.) Recent studies in four different countries have demonstrated a gradual decrease in zinc levels in blood serum during the course of pregnancy (36). No specific zinc-deficiency signs in the mothers or their infants were correlated in any of these studies with the reduced levels in the blood. These studies indicate, however, that the normal zinc intake in pregnancy is generally low. These indications are confirmed by recent studies of pregnant women in India and of low-income women of Mexican descent in Los Angeles (37). Intakes averaging only about 8 to 10 mg per day were found.

Nutrition workers in Turkey, in 1980, noted that the amount of zinc in more than 100 pregnant women studied varied with their socioeconomic background. Women of low socioeconomic status had low levels of zinc in their blood plasma. Better nourished women of middle and high socioeconomic status had normal zinc levels (38).

Additional evidence for the greater need for dietary zinc in pregnancy was obtained in recent studies of 270 pregnant New Orleans adolescents of low socioeconomic status (39). Those with the lowest levels of zinc had the highest incidence of hypertension and toxemia.

Low, but not necessarily inadequate, zinc intakes and/or zinc levels in blood were found in infants in Canadian studies (40). (See also Chap. 23.)

Effect of Alcohol. Experiments with animals have shown that alcohol intake can provoke zinc-deficiency disturbances in growth and in pregnancy (41). A number of earlier studies with humans have shown similar relationships. Recently, for example, researchers at the Nassau County Alcoholism Treatment Services in New York found that twenty children of alcoholics had "depressed zinc levels" and the boys in the group were found to be "below the controls in mental ability" (42). Though a direct cause and effect relation is not proved by these preliminary studies, their implications are important. There are indications, also, that low levels of zinc are partially responsible for the well-known *fetal alcohol syndrome* (43).

Further evidence of the association between alcohol toxicity and the degree of zinc deficiency in the body is the 1982 case report of a thirty-three-year-old alcoholic woman who developed zinc-deficiency symptoms including a severe rash on her face (an acrodermatitislike condition) and on other parts of her body. Treating her with extra zinc completely healed her rash in five days (she later died from liver cirrhosis) (44). Although this is just one case, the conclusions we can draw from all of these studies with alcohol and zinc are obvious.

Other Studies of Intake. Many other factors affect zinc intake and the degree of zinc deficiency in an individual. One of the most important is the extent and rate at which dietary zinc is absorbed into the blood stream, in other words the bioavailability of zinc as affected by conditions in the intestine including fiber and other dietary components (see next section).

The use of vitamin and mineral supplements, practiced by large segments of the American population, also affects zinc intake, depending on the level of zinc in the supplement (see Chap. 8). For example, in a recent study of several hundred persons in Colorado, 8 percent of young women (age eighteen to thirty) and 10 percent of young men took zinc supplements that were not part of a vitamin-mineral supplement. About twice that percentage of people over sixty were found to be taking special zinc supplements (45).

According to other studies, the amount of dietary zinc necessary to maintain a zinc balance ranges from 8.5 mg a day in adults in India to 20 mg in pregnant American women (46). Most of the zinc lost from the body is in the feces, and most of the rest is excreted in the urine. Very little, less than 0.5 mg, is lost in menstrual fluid. Generally about 1 mg a day of zinc is lost in sweat, a fact that may explain the low levels of zinc in the blood of a group of 160 male and female athletes training in West Germany studied in 1981 (47).

Hair Zinc Analysis. Within the past several years at least thirty to forty scientific papers, generally from reliable laboratories, have described experiments using hair analysis as one of several methods to measure zinc status. This is a justifiable use of the procedure. The method seems most sensitive when applied to infants and children with mild deficiencies. Several authors, however, have not been able to find a relationship of hair values to zinc intake (48–51).

A number of laboratories have tested, in some cases successfully, zinc in hair as the sole biochemical measure of zinc levels (48). Values of zinc tend to run around 100 to 200 μg per gm of hair. Though the procedure has obvious value in certain situations, continued research on the method and interpretation of the results is needed (49).

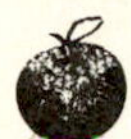

health considerations

Hair Analysis for Trace Minerals

Background. In recent years the number of nutritionists using scalp hair as a convenient tissue as a legitimate measure of the mineral status in populations (as distinct from individuals) has greatly increased. Hair is easier and more convenient to handle than blood, urine, or feces. Hair is relatively easily transported to central laboratories, where it is washed, stored, and analyzed by modern instruments.

A sample consists of only about 0.5 to 1 gm of hair, about the weight of one or two paper clips, usually from several sites just above the nape of the neck. The first several centimeters (an inch or so) of hair, fairly close to the skin, are considered the least contaminated and represent about two months of recent growth.

There are a number of problems in using mineral analysis of hair to diagnose health conditions. These include contamination by trace elements in shampoos and soaps, bleaches, dyes, hair lotions, and other environmental sources. Hair color makes a difference, as does age and sex, hormone levels, disease, and many other factors. Also it is not yet clear what levels of specific trace elements mean in terms of the physiology and pathology of the body in the absence of other analytical data.

Theoretically, for groups of people, levels of a trace element in hair should reflect levels of body stores. Also, theoretically, the presence of toxic elements, such as cadmium, lead, and mercury, in the hair of such groups should reflect recent contamination of the body by these elements. In practice, however, these conditions do not usually apply.

Misuse and Misinterpretation of Hair Analysis

A number of opportunistic health professionals in the United States and other countries have hastened to persuade a health-minded but confused public of the value of hair analysis. For a substantial fee anyone can have a complete mineral analysis of his or her hair as a primary means of detecting "nutritional problems." The individual obtains a referral from a health-food store, physician, chiropractor, or other health professional or by responding to a magazine advertisement or some other source. Generally the individual is asked to submit a dietary history, also. Literally hundreds of thousands of people, including many students, have participated in these schemes. For their money they receive computerized advice in an attractive form from doctors who, in most instances, have never examined or met them.

The authors have no major quarrel with the analytical procedures themselves, though the values obtained can vary considerably as results of tests of the same person's hair from different laboratories reveal. Proper washing procedures are not always used, and not all trace elements can be measured with accuracy. The authors maintain, however, that the interpretation of the analytical results can be clearly fraudulent. Generally, very comprehensive computerized evaluations are returned to the customer along with some dire warning about "abnormal patterns" of minerals in the hair and suspected "dangerous" body contamination by cadmium, lead, mercury, or some toxic minerals. In order to rid the body of these toxic minerals the computer prints out an "individualized" list of vitamins and minerals or suggests other types of supplements, such as a garlic mixture, which the "patient" is advised to take. Generally the levels of vitamins suggested are in "meganutrition" doses (see Chap. 8), many times larger than the recommended allowances.

The companies supplying this information may suggest specific generic formulas rather than specific products. Fraud is evident, however, when the customer discovers that the only conveniently available commercial products that can fulfill the suggested formula are obtained only from cooperating health-food stores or from the health professionals directly connected with the laboratory making the report. Consequently, the customer pays much more money than necessary for useless products of questionable safety.

The authors fully support the warnings made by established scientists about these offers of computerized information (50). They deplore the use of vitamins and minerals in megadoses without properly qualified medical advice. They urge the student to read the scientific literature evaluating mineral analysis of hair before spending money on a commercially sponsored test (48–51).

Zinc in Foods

As an essential trace element for all plant and animal cells and tissues, zinc is present in all foods. Foods from animal sources and whole grains contain more zinc per serving, in general, than fruits, vegetables, white flour, and refined foods. Zinc is not used as yet in food-enrichment programs.

Table 17–2 lists the approximate zinc content of representative types of food based on individual servings. For details of the approximate zinc servings of common foods see Appendix (and refs. 52,53). Red meats, liver, oysters, beans, whole grains, chick

Table 17–2 APPROXIMATE ZINC CONTENT OF REPRESENTATIVE FOODS BY SERVING SIZE[a]

Class of Food and Serving Size	*Mg/Serving*
Beans and Legumes	
Canned, ½ cup	1.0
Lima, ½ cup	0.4
Beverages	
Beer, 1½ cup	0.2
Carbonated, ¾ cup	0.01
Coffee, 1 cup	0.03
Bread (1 slice)	
White	0.2
Whole wheat	0.2
Cakes and Cookies 50 gm	0.2 to 0.5
Candy 30 gm	0.1
Cereals, breakfast (30 gm)	
Corn flakes	0.1
Cream of wheat	0.3
Granola	1.0
Shredded wheat	0.9
Bran flakes	3.7
Cheese, 30 gm (1 oz)	0.8 to 1.1
Chickpeas, ½ cup	2.7
Eggs, 2 scrambled	1.4
Fish, 110 gm	1.0 to 2.0
Fruit, per avg. fruit	0.05 to 0.3
Grains, 100 gm, dry (whole)	
Corn (maize)	1.8
Oats	3.7
Rice	1.3
Wheat	4.5
Meat, red, 90 gm	
Beef	3.7 to 5.0
Lamb	3.0 to 3.6
Liver, calf	5.2
Pork	2.7
Milk, 1 cup	
Whole, 2%, skim	1.0 to 1.1
Milkshake	1.0
Yogurt, fruit	1.5
Nuts, 30 gm	
Almond	0.4
Cashew	1.3
Peanuts	0.9
Walnut	0.8
Pasta, avg. serving	0.6 to 1.4
Potatoes	
White, 1 large	0.4
Chips, French fries	0.2
Sweet potato, 1 large	1.0
Poultry, 60 gm	
Dark meat	1.7
Light meat	1.5
Seafood, 100 gm	
Clams, canned	1.2
Lobster	2.2
Oysters, Pacific[b]	9.0
Soups, 1 cup	0.2 to 1.5
Vegetables	
Avg. serving	0.1 to 0.8
Beets, ½ cup	0.5
Cabbage, 1 cup	0.3
Peas, ½ cup	0.6

[a]Adapted from references to Table 2, Appendix.

[b]Eastern oysters are reported to have 75 mg per 100 gm by Murphy, E. W., et al.: J. Amer. Dietet. Assoc., *66*:345, 1975, the original source of some of these data. That figure is in doubt, though oysters raised in high zinc waters could probably contain that much.

peas, and poultry are the richest sources of zinc. Milk products, eggs, fish, nuts, some breakfast cereals, other seafoods, and sweet potatoes are among the good sources. There are many fair or poor sources especially among the fabricated and imitation foods. As discussed in the next section, the zinc in foods of plant origin is not always absorbed as well from the intestine as zinc from animal foods. Not considering differences in availability, meat, poultry, and fish supply almost half of the zinc intake of the American population. Dairy products supply about 20 percent and grain products about 13 percent. (For more details of zinc in our food see Fig. 17–4.) Animal foods contribute about 70 percent of our zinc supply. Vegetarians may need to be careful to consume

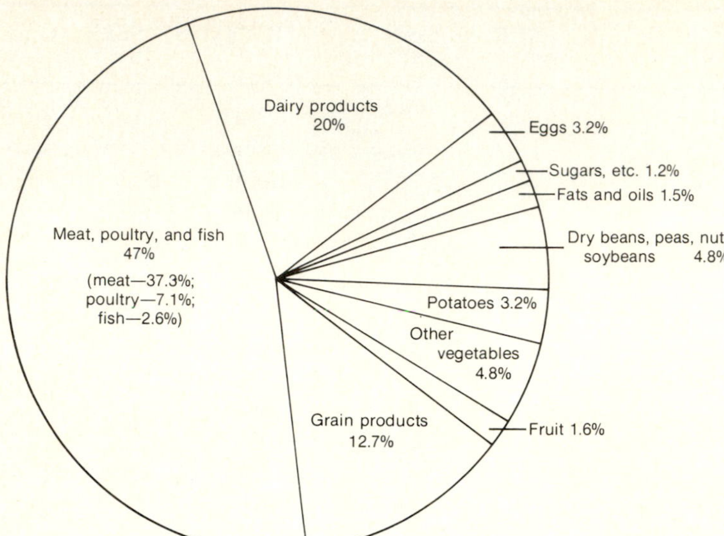

Figure 17–4 Contributions of major food groups to zinc supplies in the United States for 1980. (Source: Welsh, S.O., and Marston, R.: Zinc levels in the U.S. food supply, 1909-1980, Food Technol., *36* (Jan.): 70, 1982.)

ample zinc, as well as vitamin B-12, since many authorities (but not all) think the zinc in vegetable foods is less available (54).

Because of the way zinc is distributed in food, zinc-rich meals are among the most expensive in America. H. H. Sandstead has calculated that on the basis of average eating patterns it costs at least $1.59 a day to prepare meals containing sufficient zinc (34). People with less money than this to spend on food would be likely to have insufficient zinc.

A major reduction of zinc in the American food supply is caused by milling white flour from whole wheat, a process in which nearly 80 percent of the zinc content is lost (and eventually fed to farm animals). Unfortunately, manufacturers do not enrich white flour with zinc, as they do with iron and certain vitamins. When zinc is added to foods it is generally as the sulfate or oxide salts.

Only modest amounts of zinc are lost in cooking, since zinc, like all minerals, is not destroyed by heat. In the cooking of pasta products, for example, there is little or no loss of zinc (55).

Zinc Metabolism

Absorption. Zinc absorption is influenced by many factors including food, hormonal levels, various drugs, and gastrointestinal diseases. It also varies widely depending on the level of zinc in the diet and the presence in the intestine of interfering substances such as phytate, fiber, protein, and phosphorus and other minerals. Zinc occurring in animal products is absorbed about twice as well as zinc in plants. Therefore, unless one is a vegetarian, one should consume a balanced diet containing sufficient animal foods to ensure an adequate intake of zinc.

The body needs to absorb into the blood stream about 2.5 to 4.0 mg of zinc per day, our basic needs. Since only 10 to 40 percent of the zinc consumed is absorbed, the requirements have been adjusted to allow for the zinc not absorbed (2). It is believed that zinc combines in the intestine with a low-molecular-weight ligand (a co-binding agent) to ease its absorption. Other chelating agents may also assist in absorption, though they may also hinder (thus the chelated zinc supplements on the market serve little known purpose). The ligand, believed to be *picolinic acid* and/or *citric acid,* serves a useful purpose in breast-fed infants by aiding the absorption of the limited supplies of zinc in breast milk. Zinc absorption is an active and important area of current research (56). Excellent reviews are available (34,57). (See also supplementary readings.)

Distribution. Once zinc enters the cells of the intenstinal wall it may combine with one of many proteins, it may be stored temporarily, or it may pass into the blood stream. There it is generally combined with a protein and travels throughout the body, where it is active, and necessary, in every cell. About 60 percent of the body's zinc is located in the muscle, 20 percent in bones and skin, and 20 percent in other tissues.

Concentrations of zinc in the human body are highest in the liver, bones, epidermal tissues, prostate gland, testes, sperm cells, hair, nails, eyes, and blood. It metabolizes rapidly in the pancreas, kidneys, and pituitary gland. In the blood, 75 percent of the zinc is in the red cells.

Zinc circulates back into the intestine indirectly by way of bile and pancreatic secretions and directly through the intestinal wall. About 95 percent of what the body takes in is excreted in the feces and most of the rest in the urine.

Function. Zinc enzymes, all *metalloproteins,* are necessary for the metabolism of every cell in the body. One of them, for example, is *thymidine kinase,* essential for the formation of all nucleic acids and cellular proteins (13,58).

Zinc is important as an active component of the enzyme *carbonic anhydrase,* which functions in maintaining equilibrium between carbon dioxide and carbonic acid ($CO_2 + H_2O \leftrightarrows H_2CO_3$) in tissues. It also catalyzes the reaction in which hydrogen may be split off from carbonic acid. In addition, zinc activates enzymes that aid the digestion of proteins by hydrolyzing specific peptide linkages. It is part of alkaline phosphatase, an enzyme essential in bone metabolism and a constituent or activator of a number of other enzymes. Collagen, vital for bone and skin formation cannot be made without zinc. Zinc is believed to be necessary for the action of the hormone insulin and the follicle-stimulating and luteinizing hormones secreted by the anterior pituitary gland. Zinc is also essential for vitamin A metabolism. In light of these functions it is no wonder that zinc-deficiency symptoms develop so readily and so severely.

Toxicity of Zinc

Zinc has been considered one of the least toxic trace elements. The older literature reported that levels of oral zinc sulphate, supplying 150 to 200 mg of zinc per day over periods of several months, did not show obvious side effects (59). That is about 10 to 15 times the amount found naturally in diets. On the other hand, in a 1980 study of twelve healthy men, a level of 160 mg of zinc per day, as zinc sulfate, for five weeks reduced levels of desirable blood lipids (the high-density lipoproteins) (60).

In more recent studies, women fed 50 and 100 mg of zinc per day for eight weeks did not show the changes in lipids in the blood as clearly, but they reported some nausea, bloating, and cramps (61). These symptoms, along with diarrhea and fever, are the usual indications of zinc toxicity. Such symptoms were seen in patients in Brazil given, in error, 100 mg of zinc a day intravenously for a short period. The patients returned to normal when the levels were lowered to normal (59a).

Increasing evidence indicates that any level above 15 to 25 mg of zinc per day may depress copper absorption and utilization. Higher levels, when copper intakes are low, increase the chances of copper deficiencies (2,4,34). (See also the section on copper in Chap. 16.)

In 1982 an international committee of the Food and Agriculture Organization (FAO) and the World Health Organization (WHO) established the "Provisional minimum tolerable daily intake" of zinc as 15 to 50 mg per 50 kilograms (kg) of body weight.

Zinc salts are quite poisonous if taken in large amounts (several grams) at one time. For instance, poisoning has been known to occur from drinking acid fruit drinks stored in galvanized (zinc-lined) containers.

FLUORINE

Fluorine (F), generally accepted as an essential nutrient for humans, is a lively topic. It promotes strong reactions both in the laboratory and among citizens considering the fluoridation of public water supplies. The name fluorine was suggested in 1811 by the French scientist André Marie Ampère. It was first isolated in 1886 by another French scientist, Henri Moissan. The terms fluorine and fluoride will be used interchangeably in this discussion.

Fluorine is a very reactive gas, closely related to the other halogen gases—chlorine, iodine, and bromine. It is widely distributed in soil, water, plants, food, and bones in its ion form, fluoride. It is present in natural ores such as fluorspar and in rock phosphate, a fertilizer that contains 3 to 4 percent fluorine. An adult body contains an average of 2 to 3 gm of fluoride (62), at least 100 times as much as the rest of the trace elements to be discussed in this chapter (except silicon). As with many other elements, there is not much difference between the required amount and a chronic level of toxicity.

Fluorine Deficiency Symptoms

A deficiency of fluorine causes an increased incidence of dental caries (decay) and possibly osteoporosis. No specific metabolic role is known yet for fluorine. Proof of its essentiality for teeth and bones has not been obtained beyond doubt. Its importance for teeth, however, is sufficient reason for national and international agencies to consider it essential for all practical purposes and to recommend it for everyone (2,4,63). Its use in dental care in recent years has saved billions of dollars in the United States alone—not to mention reducing the number of toothaches!

Interest in fluorine at first centered on the harmful effects of abnormally high concentrations of it in drinking water in certain areas of the world. Consumption of such waters was shown to be the cause of mottled tooth enamel (chalky spots that later stain dark brown). Mottling may appear in the teeth of children and persist into adult life. In the United States, this tooth disorder was endemic before the 1930s in certain areas in Arizona, Colorado, the Texas panhandle, and elsewhere. Although disfiguring, mottling of teeth seemed to do no harm. Later studies indicated that the teeth of children living in these areas were more resistant to decay than the teeth of children in areas where the fluorine content of drinking water was lower (64).

The effect of raising the fluorine level in low-fluorine water supplies to a point where it might protect teeth against caries without being harmful was then tested. It was found that if the fluorine concentration was over about 2 parts per million (2 mg per liter of water), some very small degree of mottling of the enamel of teeth was seen; if it was about 1 part per million, no harmful effects were observed and the incidence of decay in children's teeth was reduced by 50 percent or more. This discovery led to the practice of fluoridating in the 1940s.

It is now clear that regulation of the fluorine content of water, either by adding fluorides in localities where there is a deficiency or by removing excesses beyond a range of 0.7 to 1.2 parts per million (ppm), is now a scientifically accepted, safe, economical, and efficient public health measure (2,63,65). See Chapter 24 for further discussion of the dental aspects of fluoridation.

Recommended Intakes of Fluorine

The latest Food and Nutrition Board's report on recommended allowances sets an "estimated safe and adequate" daily range of recommended intakes for fluorine at 1.5 to 4.0 mg per day for adults (2). (See Table 17–3 for values for other age groups.) These suggested ranges are obtained readily in areas with fluoridated water levels in the 0.7 to 1.2 ppm range. In such areas no extra amounts are needed or desirable.

There is no established level of recommended intake of fluorine for adults for aid in the possible prevention of bone disorders. The amounts prescribed, usually drug levels (20 to 60 mg a day), are much higher than caries-preventing levels. They are generally close to toxic levels and require the supervision of a physician. Fluorine is often consumed in conjunction with high-calcium sources (and with other forms of treatment) to prevent osteoporosis, or demineralization of the bones (see calcium, Chap. 15) (63).

In Pregnancy. University of Miami researchers have recently reported the unexpected finding that fluorine supplementation of the diet of pregnant women almost completely eliminated dental caries in their offspring (66). The women, living in fluoridated-water areas, consumed tablets with 1 mg of fluorine daily between the third and ninth month of pregnancy. Best results were said to be obtained when the tablets were taken between meals without other foods or drugs that might reduce absorption. The researchers reported no medical or dental defects such as mottling of teeth. They did find slightly larger weights at birth. These studies need further confirmation, but they appear interesting, especially since an infant's teeth start to form at the tenth to the twelfth week of pregnancy. The researchers attributed the results to the development of an "immunity," which is not proved.

Table 17–3 SAFE AND ADEQUATE RECOMMENDED INTAKES FOR FLUORIDE[a]

Ages	*Years*	*Range in mg*
Infants	0–0.5	0.1–0.5
	0.5–1.0	0.2–1.0
Children	1–3	0.5–1.5
	4–6	1.0–2.5
	7–10	1.5–2.5
Adolescents	11+	1.5–2.5
Adults		1.5–4.0

[a]From the Food and Nutrition Board, 1980 (2).

Workers in Finland recently found that breast milk of women in fluoridated-water areas had almost twice as much fluoride as the breast milk of women living in nonfluoridated-water areas (67). This fact is of interest because breast milk has been considered to be very low in fluoride and not affected by the mother's diet. The amounts found in the group drinking fluoridated water were still only 0.01 ppm, much lower than those in cow's milk.

People in Nonfluoridated Water Areas. Persons of all ages in areas where water is nonfluoridated should consume fluorine within the range of recommended intakes. These amounts are especially important for all infants and children during tooth-forming years. Tablets and toothpastes containing fluoride are reliable sources of this element.

Animal Requirement. The indications in the early 1970s of the possible necessity of fluorine for maximum growth rates of rats and for reproduction in mice have not yet been confirmed (4). Also, no other animal species has demonstrated deficiency signs in the absence of fluorine in the diet. That does not prove that fluorine is not essential—it means only that more research is needed before a final decision should be made.

Fluorine in Food

No specific fluorine values for food are given here or in government food-composition tables because the amount of fluorine in plant foods or animal products is dependent largely upon the level in the environment (such as soil, water, and air) or the amount in the feed. Fluorine is not an essential element for plants, so it is not always present in significant amounts in foods from plants.

Very few foods contain more than 1 to 2 ppm of fluorine (unless such foods are raised in a high-fluorine environment), and most contain less. Generally, meats, poultry, and ocean fish (especially when eaten with bones) are dependable sources; whole grains and fruit and fruit juices when produced in areas with higher fluoride levels in the soil and water are good sources. Soft drinks and other beverages made in fluoridated-water areas are also good sources. Mechanically separated meat (with undetectable bone particles) and tea (about 0.2 to 0.3 mg per cup) are among the highest sources. Bone meal, sometimes used as a mineral supplement, is very rich in fluorine (normally 300 to 600 ppm). A normal day's diet in the United States contains about 0.3 to 0.6 mg of fluorine (as fluorides), not including the amount in drinking water. Including drinking water, a normal intake would be about 1 to 2.5 mg per day in adults.

The fluorine content of infant formulas and foods varies somewhat depending on whether they are processed in fluoridated-water areas or not. Daily levels of intake of fluorine by two- to six-month-old, nonbreast-fed infants are known to vary from 0.05 mg to 0.76 mg per day (68). The amount of fluoride supplied by breast milk is about 0.01 mg per day or less.

A comprehensive study made in 1980 showed that typical daily diets of two-year-old children ("market basket" diets) in four regions of the United States varied from 0.18 mg to 0.31 mg of fluoride, not counting the drinking water (69). Children in the Los Angeles area, where the water was not fluoridated, had less fluorine available to them per day than the estimated recommended intake. Pediatricians have established new standards for fluoride supplements for infants and children in nonfluoridated-water areas because of inadequate intakes otherwise (70). The suggested intakes are within the ranges of those shown in Table 17–3. Unfortunately, some parents, through carelessness, indifference, or ignorance, may not provide such supplements regularly.

The most reliable source of fluorine, therefore, is fluoridated water. In some countries where fluoridation of water supplies is not possible, other means of providing fluorine may be used. Fluoridated salt is used in some parts of the world, and fluoridated sugar is being tested in others. Some sugars, especially brown sugar, are fairly rich sources even without extra fluoride. Fluoridated milk is common in Britain, especially in schools. Sea salt is not a reliable source of fluorine.

Metabolism of Fluorine

Fluorine is readily absorbed from the intestine and is distributed widely in the body, with highest concentration (up to 0.5 percent on a dry basis) in the teeth and bones. The urine is the main route of excretion. About 80 percent of ingested fluorine is excreted in children and up to 98 percent in adults. Aluminum, found in antacids, markedly decreases intestinal absorption of fluorine.

As previously mentioned, there is no known specific metabolic role for fluorine. It is known to activate certain enzymes and to inhibit others. All that can be said with certainty is that fluorine is necessary for maximal resistance to dental caries as a structural component of normal teeth.[1] Recent studies incidate that fluoride increases the calcium-to-phosphorus ratio of the specific mineral salts of the teeth, thus increasing resistance to action of plaque acids (62,71). The preventative and metabolic roles of fluorine are a controversial but active area of research (72). The high therapeutic doses of fluorine prescribed indicate that its action may not be physiologically normal.

Toxicity of Fluorine

Fluorine has a small safety range—as small as just about any element. The range is wide enough, however, for safe accommodation of normal fluctuations in the fluoride content of foods without risk of toxicity. Several million Americans live in communities with water levels of natural fluorine from 1.2 to 4 ppm without any handicap other than slight mottling of the teeth. Their general health is otherwise satisfactory.

When animals or humans are exposed to intakes of fluorine higher than about 20 mg per day over long periods of time, or when there is environmental contamination, *fluorosis* can result. It is manifested by deformed teeth and bones and other toxic symptoms (4,73). It has been fully demonstrated, however, that fluorine in drinking water, when present at a level of about 1 ppm, is not harmful to humans or animals, regardless of the amount of water consumed.

The effect of adding fluorine to water over a long period of time needs continually to be reassessed, as pointed out recently by D. H. Leverett of the Eastman Dental Center in Rochester, New York (74). It has long been known that animals eating plants very high in fluoride in contaminated industrial areas (around aluminum factories, for example) can show symptoms of fluorosis. Recent studies have demonstrated that this is a continuing problem (75). In some areas of the southwestern desert from Texas to Nevada, plants and water naturally have high fluoride levels, often bordering on toxic levels. Cattle grazing on such lands have developed fluorosis, reminding us of the high incidence of mottled teeth in humans known to occur in those areas.

[1]The form of fluorine in teeth and bones has been postulated to be chiefly *fluorapatite* ($CaF_2 \cdot 3\ Ca_3(PO_4)_2$), but this is not proven.

COBALT

Cobalt (Co), known since 1742, was the seventh trace element to be recognized, in 1935, as a dietary essential, in studies with cows and sheep (ruminants). It is required by humans and monogastric animals only in the organic form—as a constituent of vitamin B-12. Hence, whether one considers it an essential trace element for humans is a matter of semantics. There can be no question that all plant-eating animals require inorganic cobalt unless they obtain vitamin B-12 from some other source.

Sheep and cattle grown on pastures in cobalt-deficient areas of Australia, Canada, New York, Florida, and elsewhere develop symptoms of progressive anemia, muscular atrophy, listlessness, extreme emaciation, and eventually death (sometimes called wasting disease) (4). About 2 mg of cobalt added per kg of feed is all that is needed to overcome the deficiency.

The major role of cobalt in the body (if not the only role) is to serve as part of vitamin B-12. This fact can be proven by injecting vitamin B-12 into cobalt-deficient cows and sheep. This measure overcomes all symptoms, whereas injecting equivalent amounts of cobalt has no effect. Cobalt had been effective in ruminants because microorganisms in the rumen synthesize vitamin B-12. Without cobalt there is no synthesis and all the symptoms are, in effect, due to the lack of vitamin B-12.

To some extent, humans also have this ability to synthesize vitamin B-12 from cobalt by microorganisms, a fact that probably explains, in part, why true vegetarians can live many years without vitamin B-12 itself in the diet. Synthesis in the intestine is not assured in humans at all, so we regard the human need of cobalt in terms of the intact vitamin B-12 molecule and not in terms of inorganic cobalt itself.

The question of whether cobalt is an essential trace element or not is somewhat similar to the situation with the mineral sulfur. Sulfur, as studied in Chapter 4, is a constituent of the amino acids methionine and cystine. Inorganic sulfur in the diet serves little, if any, practical purpose except in ruminants, which can make their own methionine and cystine from free sulfur in the rumen.

There is no evidence that humans need ever be concerned about their intake of inorganic cobalt. In other words, a cobalt deficiency has never been described for humans and would be difficult to obtain. The normal day's intake of 150 to 600 μg of inorganic cobalt is far greater than any possible requirement. Cobalt ions are distributed throughout the body, especially in the liver and heart. The entire human adult body has only about 1.5 mg of cobalt, a smaller amount than that of any other essential mineral.

Cobalt is present in almost all foods in small and varying amounts. Since we really do not have to worry about it, and there is no recommended intake (2), to present figures would serve no purpose. There appears to be no shortage, and our concern, actually, in human nutrition is about vitamin B-12 and not cobalt.

Large amounts of cobalt in the diet of humans and animal species other than ruminants cause stimulation of bone marrow, with excessive production of red corpuscles (polycythemia) and higher than normal hemoglobin. Toxic reactions from unusually large levels in food have been known.

MOLYBDENUM

With the discovery in 1953 that *molybdenum* (Mo) is a component of the essential enzyme *xanthine dehydrogenase* (and later other enzymes), a new era of essential microelement research was ushered in (4,13).

Deficiency Symptoms

The first molybdenum deficiency in humans was found in 1981 in a surgery patient given a much purified parenteral nutrition solution high in sulfur amino acids. After several months the patient developed rapid rates of heartbeat and breathing, headache, night blindness, mental disturbances, irritability, nausea, and vomiting. After several days these symptoms developed into edema, lethargy, disorientation, and coma. The patient had biochemical signs of deficiencies of two of the three major enzymes involved in sulfur and purine metabolism, *sulfite oxidase* and *xanthine oxidase*. Since these enzymes were known to contain *molybdenum*, it was given intravenously, resulting in an improved clinical condition and reversal of the biochemical defects (76). Molybdenum is now added to all parenteral nutrition solutions, needless to say.

The situation just cited was very unusual, and a person with any of these symptoms should not conclude that he or she has a molybdenum deficiency. Besides, no human deficiencies of molybdenum have ever been reported in normal people eating a varied diet because molybdenum is so widely distributed in foods, in amounts well within the requirements.

A few examples of a rare genetic disturbance with symptoms similar to those just described have been reported. Such persons have very low amounts of the molybdenum-containing enzymes, since they cannot make the recently discovered "molybdenum cofactor" (77). This is a derivative of *biopterin,* a small molecule similar to the pterin part of the folic-acid molecule. It is required for the activity of these molybdenum-containing enzymes.

Certain animals (rats, poultry, and sheep) have been made artificially deficient by giving them low levels of molybdenum, often accompanied by the antagonistic action of other trace elements such as copper or tungsten. Such animals produce weak and malformed young. Sulfate intake in animals has a marked effect on molybdenum amounts. High dietary sulfate inhibits absorption and increases urinary excretion of molybdenum.

Though a few tables of food composition giving the molybdenum content of foods are available (78,79), the authors do not give values here and the new U.S. Department of Agriculture (USDA) food-composition tables do not list molybdenum, either. The reasons are that data are very limited, molybdenum content varies greatly depending on the soil where the food was grown, and there is little evidence that molybdenum deficiency can ever occur in humans. There is no need to worry about molybdenum intake on the basis of present knowledge.

Metabolism of Molybdenum

Molybdenum is rapidly absorbed in both organic and inorganic forms. The main route of excretion is the urine. It is not stored in the body—the entire adult body contains only about 10 mg (62).

In addition to the two important enzymes previously mentioned, another molybdenum-containing enzyme is *aldehyde oxidase,* vital in liver metabolism.

Toxicity of Molybdenum

Severe molybdenum toxicity, molybdenosis, in animals, particularly cattle, has been seen in many parts of the world where the soil has a high molybdenum content. Symptoms include weight loss, growth retardation, and changes in connective tissue (4,80).

SELENIUM

The element selenium (Se) is closely related chemically to sulfur but is much less abundant. It was discovered and named by the Swedish chemist Baron Jöns Jakob Berzelius in 1817. It is now clear that selenium is just as important a nutrient for humans as better known trace elements such as zinc, iron, and copper. Since it is widely distributed, we are not likely to be consuming too little of it. Deficiencies in humans have been described in the past several years for the first time, giving rise to an explosion of research.

Deficiency Symptoms

Animal scientists first became interested in selenium when it was determined in the 1930s that soils and certain plants in parts of western North America and in other parts of the world contained levels of selenium that were toxic to farm animals. Grazing animals in such seleniferous areas developed symptoms of *alkali disease,* or *blind staggers,* characterized by stiffness and lameness, loss of hair, deformed hoofs, blindness, paralysis, and eventually death (4).

It was with considerable surprise, then, that an element this toxic was found to be nutritionally essential. In the 1950s K. Schwarz and C. M. Foltz produced dietary liver necrosis (death of liver tissue as a result of a deficiency), poor growth, and death in rats fed special diets containing torula yeast (which is very low in selenium and vitamin E). Less than 0.5 ppm of selenium, when it was identified as the missing component, was found to be as effective as 50 ppm of vitamin E, which it replaced. Later work has shown that selenium has specific functions in addition to its vitamin E-sparing effect. It now appears that much of the need for vitamin E is to spare the selenium requirement.

In Animals. Besides poor growth and liver necrosis in rats, a wide variety of deficiency signs were found in animals deficient in both selenium and vitamin E. Extensive striated muscular degeneration, known widely as *white muscle disease,* or *nutritional muscular dystrophy,* occurs in young sheep, cattle, horses, and rabbits under farm conditions. It occurs in many areas of the United States (mainly west of the Rocky Mountains and east of the Mississippi River (see Fig. 17–5) and other parts of the world, such as New Zealand, where soils are deficient in selenium. As many as 20 to 30 percent of all lambs in some flocks may be affected, for example.

Selenium-deficient chicks develop large greenish blue spots under the skin because of blood leakage from capillaries and soon die. Selenium-deficient mice develop damaged hearts. Pigs deficient in selenium and vitamin E develop diseased livers and die without warning.

Selenium, in the absence of much higher amounts of vitamin E (the requirement of which is greatly reduced by selenium), is essential for reproduction in all animals studied. It is commonly added to the diet of livestock in selenium-deficient areas a practice recently approved by the U.S. government.

In Humans. New Zealand, one of the many countries with a low level of selenium in soils and water supplies, has become a leading center for selenium research. A. M. van Rij, M. F. Robinson, and colleagues demonstrated in 1979, and since, clear-cut deficiencies of selenium in humans given parenteral nutrition solutions (81). One of their patients, a thirty-seven-year-old woman, developed severe muscle pain and eventually an inability to walk. Levels of

Figure 17–5 Selenium-deficient and selenium-excess areas in the lower United States (approximate). (Adapted from U.S. government figures. See Muth and Allaway: J. Amer. Vet. Med. Assoc., *142*:1379, 1963; and Kubota, et al.: J. Agric. Food Chem., *15*:448, 1967.) Values for Hawaii and Alaska not available.

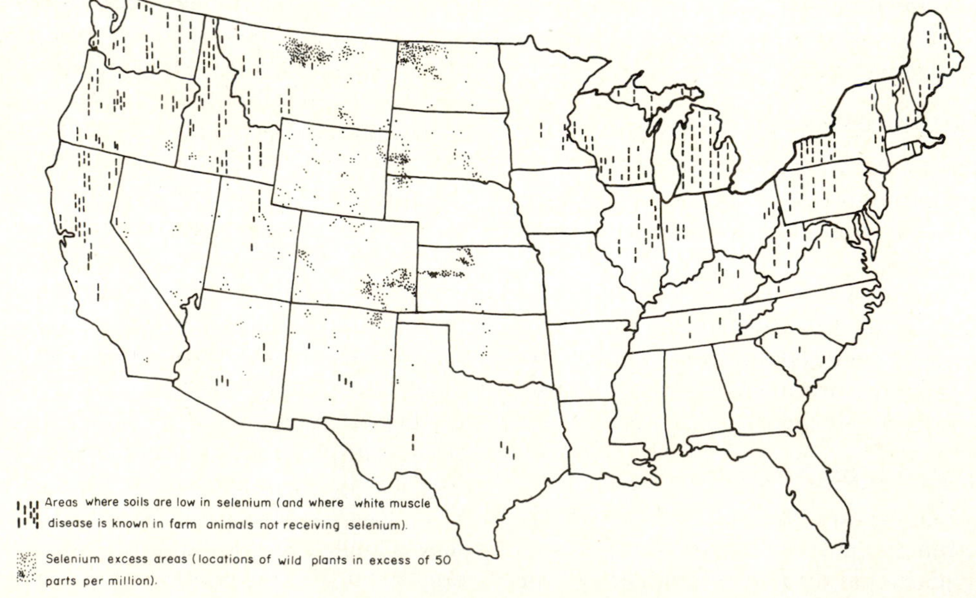
Areas where soils are low in selenium (and where white muscle disease is known in farm animals not receiving selenium).
Selenium excess areas (locations of wild plants in excess of 50 parts per million).

selenium in her blood were lower than had ever previously been reported. After she was injected with 100 μg of selenium a day, in the form of *selenomethionine* (one of the common organic forms in food and the body), her symptoms disappeared in a week.

About the same time, in 1979, Chinese researchers reported an epidemic of heart-muscle disorders, primarily in children and child-bearing women living in a large area from the northeastern part of China to the south west (82). The disease, known as *Keshan disease,* or *cardiomyopathy*, a disorder of the heart muscles, is characterized by heart enlargement, a fast rhythm, abnormal electrocardiograms, and in severe cases, heart failure and death. (Disorders of the heart muscles had been known to occur in certain selenium-deficient animals.) The Chinese researchers already knew that soils in that area were low in selenium. As a result of the epidemic, they further discovered that foods grown in the area and the body tissues of the population were also low in selenium. For a four-year period they fed 36,000 children selenium orally, with the result that most of the symptoms cleared up and the death rate was considerably reduced. The researchers stated that other trace elements such as molybdenum, might be involved as well.

More recently, reports are available elsewhere of several cases of selenium deficiency in patients, both young and old, who were receiving parenteral nutrition (83). Cardiomyopathy was the major clinical symptom (see later section). It should now be clear to all physicians that parenteral nutrition solutions are not nutritionally complete unless selenium is present. Several other researchers have urged these selenium additions to parenteral nutrition solutions and have made studies to find levels which are adequate (83,84).

According to a letter to the editor of the *New England Journal of Medicine,* a "selenium deficiency," including low selenium levels in the blood, heart muscle damage, and an enlarged liver, was recently seen in a two-year-old girl in Nassau County, New York (85). Her diet had consisted of "grits, sausage, and beans for breakfast, a frankfurter and beans at lunch, and pork and beans with rice for supper." Her only beverage was water or Kool-Aid. She was said to have "improved steadily" at home after receiving selenium supplements in the hospital. Her heart problem, however, did not disappear, indicating that she could well have had other problems or other nutritional deficiencies.

One should not make final conclusions from such information, even if it appears in the best of medical journals, until more evidence is available. The authors of this book, along with other researchers (86), consider single case histories with poor experimental control insufficient evidence of selenium deficiency. The selenium levels in the blood and some of the biochemical characteristics of any person will rise if given extra selenium, even if he or she is not selenium deficient.

Selenium Requirements

Since selenium deficiency in humans has been recognized, the Food and Nutrition Board has tentatively recommended "estimated safe and adequate daily dietary intakes" of 0.05 to 0.2 mg (50 to 200 μg) of selenium for college-age persons. (See Table 17–4 and inside the back cover.)

These recommendations suggest several new areas for future research on selenium. One is to refine further the requirement for any particular age and sex group. Another is to study the effect of disease on selenium requirements. Two further areas of research are to determine how to ensure adequate intakes and to find the best clinical and biochemical measurements for the determination of the adequacy of selenium intakes. (These steps for selenium are an example of the procedure for every other known nu-

Table 17–4 SAFE AND ADEQUATE RECOMMENDED INTAKES FOR SELENIUM AND CHROMIUM[a]

Ages	*Years*	*Range in mg*
Infants	0–0.5	0.01–0.04
	0.5–1.0	0.02–0.06
Children	1–3	0.02–0.08
	4–6	0.03–0.12
	7–10	0.05–0.2
Adolescents	11+	0.05–0.2
Adults		0.05–0.2

[a]From the Food and Nutrition Board, 1980 (2).

trient after its essential nature was first established.) Progress is now being made (84,87), but there are indications that the minimum requirement for adults should be at least 40 percent higher than the minimum proposed by the Food and Nutrition Board to maintain usual body stores. Several researchers have proposed still higher minimums to prevent certain types of cancer and other diseases (see later sections).

Selenium Intakes and Status Measurement

A person in North America whose diet consisted of mixed foods of different origins would most likely have an intake of 75 to 200 μg of selenium a day. Ranges will vary from one part of the continent to another and from country to country depending largely on cultural habits and selenium levels in soils and water. A number of studies are available showing a wide variety of figures (88). People eating very poor diets in selenium-deficient areas may well have low levels of this element, but it is too early yet to define a "low level." Long-term daily intakes of 28 to 32 μg of selenium have not been associated with any adverse health effects in New Zealand. Requirements in the United States should not be any different.

There is no one best way to determine if a person or a community is receiving ample selenium. Many factors must be studied including dietary intakes, clinical signs, and biochemical status. Among biochemical measurements are levels of selenium in blood serum along with levels of glutathione peroxidase of the red blood cell (81,83,87,89). Other measurements used, experimentally and less successfully, involve hair, nails, and urine.

Selenium in Food

Selenium, probably bound to protein, occurs naturally in all seafood, meat, and those grains raised on selenium-containing soils. Dairy products and eggs are generally fair sources. Fruits and vegetables are very low in it. Levels in most plants depend entirely on the level of selenium in the soil. Variations of more than 100-fold are known to occur, so tables of the selenium content of food are quite useless. The few wild plants[2] that accumulate the element in selenium-rich soils contain toxic levels (from 0.1 to 1 percent of selenium) for any grazing animals that might consume them.

Considerable losses of selenium can occur in food processing and cooking. (See Fig. 17-6.)

Metabolism of Selenium

More than half of dietary selenium is absorbed, depending on many factors. It is excreted in both urine and feces. The total body stores average only about 20 mg, about the size of a match head (62). Selenium is bound to proteins in animal tissues. Its most important function is as part of the enzyme *glutathione peroxidase,* essential along with other enzymes and vitamin E for protecting the cells against damage from peroxides and free radicals. Each molecule of glutathione

[2]Gray's vetch and woody aster.

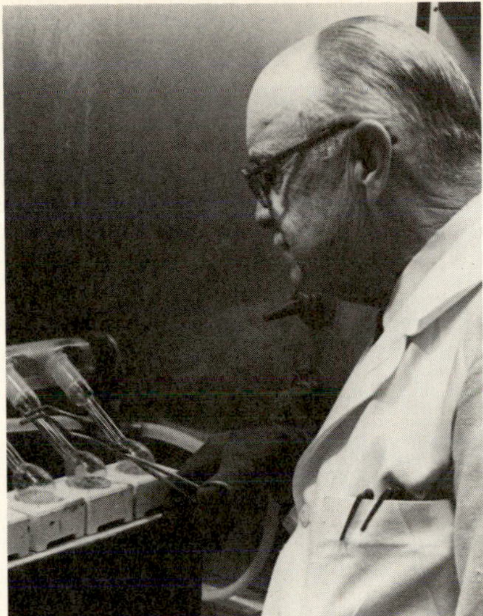

Figure 17–6 A. L. Moxon tests selenium content of foodstuffs grown in Ohio or purchased from local grocers or supermarkets.

peroxidase contains 4 molecules of selenium. The enzyme is a strong antioxidant, which protects cellular membranes. Liver has the highest glutathione peroxidase activity; and erythrocytes, heart muscle, lungs, and kidneys have moderately high activity. Recent evidence indicates the enzyme is contained in blood platelets in rather large amounts and functions in the metabolism of arachidonic acid and the hormone prostaglandin. Several selenium-containing proteins have been found in mammalian tissues which are distinct from glutathione peroxidase (90). Other functions of selenium in the body appear to include the formation of connective tissue and the conversion of the amino acid cysteine to methionine.

Selenium and Chronic Diseases

The discovery of various abnormalities in selenium-deficient humans and animals has opened a floodgate of speculation on the relationship of selenium to chronic diseases. A group of influential studies showed decreased immunological function in selenium-deficient animals (18). Papers have been published on the possible linkage of selenium deficiency in humans with atherosclerosis, cardiovascular disease, cancer (see the following section), muscular dystrophy, cystic fibrosis, alcoholic cirrhosis, hypertension, and the treatment of inborn errors of metabolism. Much more work must be done before any conclusions can be drawn about selenium's preventative effect on any of these diseases.

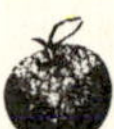

health considerations

Cancer: Selenium and Other Trace Elements

A number of experiments with animals has demonstrated that certain cancers can be reduced or alleviated by doses of oral selenium. The amounts range from slightly above the requirement to levels approaching toxicity. Based on these animal studies, epidemiologists have compared selenium levels with the incidence of certain cancers. Although epidemiological studies are fraught with difficulties, there are some encouraging indications that normal selenium levels can be helpful against certain cancers.

The Committee on Diet, Nutrition, and Cancer of the National Research Council, in their recent report, reviewed a large number of epidemiological reports dealing with selenium and a variety of cancers (28). They concluded, "both the epidemiological and laboratory studies suggest that selenium may offer some protection against the risk of cancer. However, firm conclusions cannot be drawn on the basis of the present limited evidence. Increasing the selenium intake to more than 200 micrograms/day (the upper limit of the range of Safe and Adequate Daily Dietary Intakes . . . by the use of supplements has not been shown to confer health benefits exceeding those derived from the consumption of a balanced diet." They further state, "Although these studies generally demonstrated an inverse relationship between the level of selenium and the risk of cancer, it is not clear whether this relationship applies to all cancer sites or only to specific cancer sites, such as those in the gastrointestinal tract. There are as yet no data from case-control or cohort studies."

The Committee further examined the epidemiological and experimental literature on the other trace elements in the treatment of cancer (28). In no instance were they as encouraging as their statement about selenium. With most other elements, except for the possibility of thyroid cancer and iodine intakes, they found no positive evidence. The authors of this book consider the conclusions of the Committee about trace elements and cancer to be positive, reasonable, and properly conservative, indeed representative of the best scientific opinion on the subject.

Often the public is faced with claims that supplements of one nutrient or another are necessary to prevent cancer. These supplements may be very expensive and in some instances contain close to toxic levels of one or more nutrients. The correct response is obviously to examine with skepticism the source and the motives of any statements different from the conclusions of the committee.

Toxicity of Selenium

Selenium is a very toxic element, as described earlier. This fact was established by years of study with farm animals raised in areas with high levels of selenium in the soil (4). Levels in animals' diets or herbage of above 5 to 10 ppm are considered to be toxic. This is equivalent to about 2.5 to 5 mg a day in humans, or about only 13 to 20 times the highest recommended "safe" level. These high levels are not possible for persons living on a diet of mixed foods. Unlimited amounts of selenium supplements, however, are sold widely on the open market. Over-zealous persons might easily consume too much. It is of interest that one sign of the intake of excessive selenium in humans is a garlic-like odor on the breath from selenium metabolites (91). The toxicity of selenium is affected, experimentally, by the levels of copper, cadmium, mercury, arsenic, and other minerals.

CHROMIUM

Very few persons would have guessed before 1959 that chromium, the mineral most of us know as that which makes the shiny "chrome"-plated bumpers and strips on automobiles, is essential in the diet of mammals, including humans (4,91).

Chromium (Cr) was originally discovered in 1797 by the French chemist Louis Nicolas Vauquelin (who also isolated the first amino acid). It was named from the Greek word *chroma,* meaning "color." It has been known for many years to be present in food and animal tissues. In 1959, K. Schwarz and W. Mertz, then of the U.S. National Institutes of Health, made the important discovery that very small amounts of chromium (only when in the stable trivalent state as Cr^{3+}) were necessary in the diet for normal metabolism of blood glucose in the rat (92). They tested more than forty-seven different elements before they announced the specificity of chromium as the *glucose tolerance factor* (GTF).

Deficiency Symptoms

In studies made in the late 1960s, poorly nourished children in Turkey and Lebanon showed signs of poor glucose utilization. These signs disappeared in a number of instances when small amounts of chromium (250 μg) were added to the diet (93). In these countries chromium levels of some soils and water supplies are low. The effects

were thought to be due to a role of chromium in insulin metabolism. Similar insulin-like effects have been seen in a few diabetic adults elsewhere who apparently were deficient in chromium.

Two reports of specific deficiencies of chromium, in patients receiving parenteral nutrition solutions, have been recently published. In the first, in 1977 studies in Toronto, a patient developed weight loss, diabetes-like symptoms, nerve degeneration, and other signs. In the second, a similar case developed in Boston. In both cases all symptoms were reversed by the addition of chromium (94).

In rats, mice, and monkeys, a chromium deficiency results in decreased growth and increased mortality, as well as a decreased rate of glucose removal from the blood. In other studies, an organic form of chromium, the GTF, has been isolated from brewer's yeast. It contains chromium, nicotinic acid, glycine, glutamic acid, and cysteine (95). Its exact chemical nature is still unknown, but it appears to have greater potency when fed than equivalent amounts of inorganic chromium.

Requirement and Measurement

The new safe and adequate ranges of recommended daily intake for chromium are the same as for selenium, 0.05 to 0.2 mg per day (50 to 200 μg) for adults. These levels for all age groups are given in Table 17–4. A typical daily intake in the United States usually ranges between 50 and 120 μg.

Work is in progress to determine better methods of measuring the degree of deficiency of chromium in an individual or a population. Hair samples are used quite widely (96), often in connection with other tissues. The interpretation of the results, however, has the same problems as for zinc in hair (50,51). Chromium in the blood, considered by itself, is not a reliable indicator of status.

Recent studies have confirmed earlier indications that chromium intakes reduce levels of undesirable blood lipids (97). This fact further strengthens the argument that chromium helps protect against atherosclerosis. More work is needed in this area.

Chromium in Foods

Good food sources of chromium are meats and fats such as corn oil, in which it exists as an impurity. Fruits, vegetables, seafood, and drinking water are generally poor sources. The amount of chromium in plant foods depends to a large extent on the amount in the soil. Tables of chromium content of representative foods are available—but are not to be trusted.

Processing and refining reduce the chromium content of foods considerably. For instance, white sugar contains very little, and white flour has much less than whole wheat.

Of significance in considering food sources of chromium are the early studies of Mertz and Schwarz, who produced a chromium deficiency in rats by feeding them on commercial stock diets of natural foodstuffs. They found that brewer's yeast is a particularly rich source of chromium—hence beer is also a good source.

Chromium is not toxic in the forms and levels found in foods, and excesses are rapidly excreted.

Metabolism of Chromium

Absorption from the intestine varies considerably, depending on the form of chromium. Inorganic chromium compounds are 1 to 3 percent absorbed, while the chromium in the GTF is 10 to 25 percent absorbed. The human body contains only a small amount of chromium—about 6 mg—which decreases with age.

Chromium has a variety of functions, including: (1) stimulation of enzymes involved in glucose and energy metabolism and (2) stimulation of synthesis of fatty acids and

cholesterol in the liver. Other functions are (3) involvement in insulin metabolism and (4) a role as a part of several other enzymes, including one of the protein-digesting enzymes in the intestine.

NICKEL

Nickel (Ni), the metal of which the U.S. five-cent piece is made, was discovered by the German scientist A. F. Cronstedt in 1751. It is included among the essential trace elements because deficiencies have been obtained in experimental animals and it is present in *nickeloplasmin,* a serum protein in rabbits and humans. There are no known deficiency symptoms in humans.

Nickel-deficient chickens were found in 1970 by F. H. Nielsen of the USDA to have slightly enlarged hocks, thickened legs, bright orange leg color (instead of pale yellow-brown), dermatitis, and a "less friable liver" (4,5,98). Feeding them nickel at a level of 3 to 5 mg per kg of diet corrected these minor abnormalities. Deficiencies have also been obtained by other scientists in the United States and Germany in rats, pigs, sheep, and goats. Nickel is known to activate several enzyme systems, although whether this is a specific function is not known. It is present in high levels in ribonucleic acids for reasons that are not yet clear. Its need is most clearly seen in diets low in iron and/or protein. Copper is also closely related to nickel.

Nickel is widely distributed in foods. The deficiency in chickens was produced after careful removal of all sources of nickel, although corn (maize) was one of the ingredients of the diet. A deficiency in humans has never been seen and would be unlikely to occur except under unusual conditions, such as after long periods of parenterally feeding a low-nickel solution. Nickel concentration in blood serum is elevated in humans following myocardial infarction, stroke, and severe burns, but the cause of this increase is not known (4). A normal diet would supply about 0.1 to 0.5 mg per day, and any requirement for the element must be less than this. No provisional RDA has been given for nickel as yet. Dietary nickel is 1 to 10 percent absorbed. Most of the absorbed nickel is excreted in the feces along with unabsorbed nickel. Only about 10 mg is said to exist in an entire adult body (62).

VANADIUM

The twelfth essential trace element is vanadium (V). It was identified in 1831 by the Swedish scientist N. G. Sefström, who named it after Freya Vanadis, the Norse goddess of beauty. It was long known to be present throughout the plant and animal kingdoms and to be required by several lower organisms. Preliminary studies in 1970 with chickens (showing reduced growth of feathers), by USDA scientists L. L. Hopkins and H. E. Mohr, and with rats, by Purdue University scientists, indicated that vanadium was an essential trace element (99).

Its need by higher animals was amply proven by Schwarz (100). (See Fig. 17–1.) The growth of rats raised on special deficient diets in "ultraclean" conditions was increased over 40 percent in a twenty-one to twenty-eight day period by the addition of 0.25 to 0.5 mg of vanadium (as sodium orthovanadate) per kg of diet. (See Fig. 17–7.) Other effects observed were loss of hair, a seborrhea-like condition (oily skin), and loss of muscle tone.

New interest in vanadium is due to the discovery by L. C. Cantley and colleagues that very small, normal physiological amounts are a powerful regulator of intercellular sodium (98,101). Vanadium does this by inhibiting the action of an enzyme in red blood cells called *erythrocyte* (Na^+, K^+)*—ATP-ase.* This

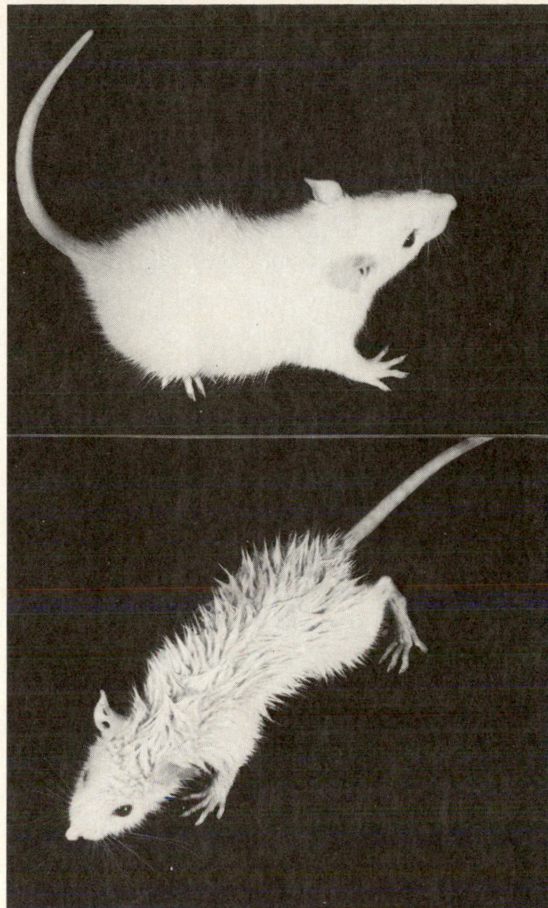

Figure 17–7 Vanadium deficiency. Upper animal: outside control, kept under conventional conditions on vanadium deficient purified diet. Lower animal: maintained for 28 days on the same diet in the trace element sterile environment system. (Courtesy of Dr. K. Schwarz.)

knowledge may have considerable clinical application in the control of edema, hypertension, and other disorders. (See supplementary readings in the Appendix.) Deficiency symptoms have not yet been described in humans.

No figure can be given for the vanadium requirement for humans, but it would be in the range of only 0.1 and 0.3 mg per day. Normal diets contain about 10 times this amount, so deficiencies would be very rare under usual conditions. The amount of vanadium in our foods and in the environment appears to be considerably lower than the toxic level. Toxic levels in animals (25 ppm) produce growth depression and increased mortality (4).

SILICON

One of the newer trace elements shown to be essential for animals (chickens and rats) is silicon (Si). This element, named from the Latin word *silex,* meaning "flint," is the most abundant mineral element on the earth's surface. Its most common form is silicon dioxide (SiO_2), also called silica (in such forms as sand and quartz). It was originally discovered as an element by Berzelius in 1823.

Silicon had long been known to be required by certain lower forms of life and by some plants (such as rice), but its need by animals was unexpected and constitutes a major nutrition discovery. E. M. Carlisle reported in 1972 that silicon is needed in microgram amounts for normal growth and bone development in the chick (102). Silicon deficiency, as shown in later but independent studies, produced growth retardation and bone changes in the skull of rats raised in an environment free of trace mineral contamination (103).

Silicon is present in bone in highest concentrations in regions of active growth, which suggests that it has a role in bone mineralization and connective-tissue synthesis. High-silicon content of connective tissue is thought to be due to its presence in mucopolysaccharides, important in connective-tissue formation. Silicon is present at the highest level in lymph nodes. High concentrations also occur in the skin, the aorta, the trachea, and the tendons. More recent studies prove its importance in the formation and metabolism of the skeleton, especially the skull (5,104).

Silicon is widely distributed in foods. Therefore, common over-the-counter silicon for strengthening bones is useless. No observation of a deficiency in humans has yet been made.

Silicon in the diet occurs as monosilicic acid, as solid silica, and as a form bound to organic compounds. Human intake has been estimated to be as much as 1 gm a day, which places it in the category of a macromineral. The adult human body has a total of about 18 gm, about the same as magnesium (62).

Little is known about requirements, which are probably well under 1 gm a day. No provisional allowance can be set for silicon because of lack of information. It does not appear to be toxic in the levels usually found in foods, although silicosis of the lungs from inhalation of excessive amounts of silicon-containing particles is a common symptom among workers in certain industries.

ARSENIC

The trace mineral most recently shown to have an apparent essential role, at least in experimental animals, is arsenic (5,105). Evidence is not yet totally conclusive. Rats maintained in a special trace-mineral-free environment on arsenic-free diets demonstrated slower growth, a rough coat, and an enlarged spleen. Chickens and pigs also appear to benefit from added arsenic (105,106). The severity of deficiency symptoms is related to the level of zinc and perhaps other minerals in the diet.

Most foods contain less than 0.5 ppm arsenic. Fish and seafoods contain 2 to 10 ppm. A deficiency has never been seen in humans. It would seem unlikely because of the widespread distribution of arsenic in foods.

Arsenic is well known for its toxicity. Acute oral poisoning causes nausea, vomiting, diarrhea, and severe abdominal pains. Chronic exposure to smaller toxic levels produces headache, confusion, convulsions, weakness, and muscular aches.

THREE ELEMENTS OF POTENTIAL INTEREST

Three trace elements—lead, boron, and tin—may at some time prove important to human nutrition.

Lead

Interesting reports on the obtaining of a lead deficiency in rats have appeared in German publications since 1981. Rats fed diets with as little as 0.045 ppm of lead showed growth reduction, enzyme changes, and blood disturbances after a second generation (107). Control rats were fed 1.0 ppm of lead and had none of these symptoms. A close relationship of iron and copper levels of the diet was found, which may be crucial to the results.

It will take several years to confirm and extend these findings. Meanwhile, nutritionists in the United States and elsewhere are showing proper restraint in not accepting the essentiality of lead until more data are available (5). This skepticism about new trace minerals is sensible, especially when there is no known metabolic role.

Lead is known primarily for its toxic effects in children and adults. Children who have chewed on window sills, toys, or other surfaces painted with lead-containing paints have suffered ill effects. Lead glazes on ceramic dishes can also be damaging. Acid fruit juices should not be kept more than a few hours in any suspected container; in fact, lead-glazed dishes should not be used for food. A small but significant source of extra lead in our food supply is from the lead solder in cans. By the year 1988 it is expected that this source of lead will be completely eliminated in the United States.

Lead has been found in high concentrations in plants and soils near highways owing to discharges of lead from automobile engines.

Boron

Boron is probably the only trace element required by most all plants that does not appear to be required by animals (4). Many nutritionists have tested it, however, under a variety of conditions without providing evidence for its essential nature.

Therefore, a recent report from USDA mineral researchers indicating a growth response to boron in the absence of vitamin D is of interest (108). Calcium metabolism may be affected. Further work will be necessary to confirm this finding.

Boron in some form or another is found in about every home medicine cabinet. Many reports exist of toxicity in children who have innocently consumed these medicines in large amounts.

Tin

In 1970 Schwarz and colleagues observed a growth effect of tin in specially isolated rats. Unfortunately, this observation has never been able to be repeated in other laboratories. Hence there is not enough evidence to consider tin to be essential.

Tin is not very toxic, and if acid fruit juices or similar products dissolve appreciable amounts of tin from a tin-plated can it is not well absorbed by humans (though the iron might be). A normal tin intake is probably in the range of 1.5 to 5 mg a day, depending on the amount of canned food eaten.

NONESSENTIAL TRACE ELEMENTS

As stated in the introduction, there are many other trace elements present in plants and animals. Some of these could theoretically be shown to be essential in the diet of higher animals at some time in the future. If the trend over the past twenty years continues, other essential trace elements will be found.

There are small pieces of evidence, such as a requirement by plants or lower organisms, or a catalytic role demonstrated in isolated systems, for a possible future role in nutrition for certain elements. For instance, *cadmium* is found associated with zinc in at least one natural protein. Also *tungsten* is part of an essential enzyme for at least one microbe.

Many elements are widely distributed in nature in most plant and animal foods in minute amounts, for example, aluminum, antimony, barium, bromine, gallium, germanium, niobium, rubidium, silver, strontium, titanium, and zirconium. In spite of their widespread occurrence, there is no evidence as yet that any of these elements plays an essential role in higher animals, and they must be considered as nonessential elements at this time. Likewise, such elements as gold, cesium, lithium, and mercury are widely distributed in nature, but this does not prove, or even indicate, any essential function. It is well to remember, however, that nickel, selenium, chromium, silicon, and vanadium were listed with these nonessential elements just a few years ago.

It is both interesting and important to call attention to the fact that, although small amounts of trace elements may be required for body welfare, any of them, whether essential or not, are toxic when too large amounts are taken into the body. Sometimes the margin between optimal intake and toxic amounts is not very wide. For example, too large a dose of iodine may overstimulate or inhibit the function of the thyroid gland, or too small an intake may result in enlargement of this gland in simple goiter. With fluorine, about 3 to 10 times the amount that provides protection against dental caries will cause some degree of mottling of teeth. All the metallic elements are stored in the liver, so that the amount in the body may accumulate to toxic levels. Hence, it is unwise to supplement the diet with high levels of any trace mineral, because all are toxic in sufficient amounts.

Especially of interest today are mercury, aluminum, lead, and cadmium because of their presence in toxic amounts in certain segments in the environment. Mercury, though naturally occurring in small amounts, has increased in concentration in the environment because of industrial wastes. It has been found to be close to toxic levels in some samples of seafoods. Toxic levels have been reached in isolated instances in Japan and the United States. The highest permissible level in American foods is 0.5 ppm.

Aluminum toxicity is seen in patients with renal failure who are treated with aluminum compounds to decrease phosphorus levels in plasma. In addition, the concentration of aluminum is increased in a disease of early senility (Alzheimer's disease). Aluminum cooking utensils yield only traces of aluminum, far below levels that might be toxic.

The practice of *pica* (109), an unnatural but common craving to eat laundry starch, clay, ashes, dirt, ice, or similar material, is seen most often in women and young children in times of stress such as in pregnancy or lactation. It may be due, partially, to a natural craving for trace minerals, especially iron. Pica sometimes involves toxic elements such as lead and should be avoided as much as possible. It will cease only as a result of nutrition education and good eating habits.

One cannot avoid eating traces of toxic elements no matter how carefully one tries not to do so. The authors recommend being aware of public health and government agencies whose job it is to monitor and control levels of toxins in our food and environment. They have a good record of success.

No attempt is made in this text to cover the toxicity or pharmaceutical use of the nonessential minerals or other compounds found in food. Interested readers will find the listing of some reviews on this topic in the supplementary readings in the Appendix. (Also see Chap. 18.)

QUESTIONS

1. Prepare in detail two daily menu plans that will supply 15 mg, or more, of zinc per day. Use the food-composition table in the Appendix. Where values are unavailable you may estimate them based on Table 17–2. How would you add 5 mg a day more for pregnancy? Do you think the RDA allowance for zinc is too high—or too low? Why?
2. Is fluorine an essential nutrient? In what body tissues is it concentrated? What is the effect of too high an intake, and at what level of fluorine in drinking water do such effects occur? What level in water supplies is safe and yet provides protection against tooth decay? (See Chap. 24.) Why has fluoridation of public water supplies met opposition in some communities, and is such opposition warranted? Is your own drinking water fluoridated?
3. Name four trace elements discussed in this chapter (other than zinc and fluorine) that are accepted as essential nutrients for humans. On what types of evidence is their acceptance based? Can you name two enzymes that contain and presumably are activated by one or more of these elements?
4. How many of the trace elements listed in this chapter are beneficial and essential in small quantities but toxic at higher levels of intake? Why may it be unsafe to take tablets or capsules as vitamin-mineral supplements if the kinds and amounts of minerals they contain are considerably above the allowance? Describe a situation, if any, of a reasonable use for a vitamin-mineral supplement with RDA levels of nutrients present. Give detailed reasons for your choice.
5. Working with the text and available references, what is the minimum and maximum level of selenium you should consume each day? Dis-

cuss in detail whether the selenium content of your present diet is within this range and why? If not should you be concerned? Why?

6. Is some form of cobalt essential for humans? For what animals is it essential? What are the symptoms of cobalt deficiency, and how may it be caused? In what vitamin is cobalt found and why is anemia a prominent symptom of cobalt deficiency in ruminants such as sheep or cattle?

7. Discuss the pros and cons of mineral analysis of hair.

References

1. (On parenteral nutrition) Expert Panel, Amer. Med. Assoc.: J. Parenter. Ent. Nutr., *3*:263, 1979; Alemdaroglu, T., and Berthon, G.: Inorg. Chim. Acta, *56*:115, 1981; Nutr. Rev., *40*:19, 1982; Ferrara, J., Fabri, P. J., and Carey, L. C.: J. Parenter. Ent. Nutr., *6*:140, 1982; Greig, P. D., Baker, J. P., and Jeejeebhoy, K. N.: Ann. Rev. Nutr., *2*:179, 1982; Miratallo, S. M.: Drug Intell. Clin. Pharm., *17*:189, 1983.
2. Food and Nutrition Board: *Recommended Dietary Allowances.* 9th Ed. Washington, D.C., National Research Council, National Academy of Sciences, 1980; Mertz, W.: J. Amer. Dietet. Assoc., *76*:128, 1980.

Zinc

3. Todd, W. R., Elvehjem, C. A., and Hart, E. B.: Amer. J. Physiol., *107*:146, 1934; Stirn, F. E., Elvehjem, C. A., and Hart, E. B.: J. Biol. Chem., *109*:347, 1935; (also see J. Nutr., *6*:289, 1933).
4. Underwood, E. J.: *Trace Elements in Human and Animal Nutrition.* 4th Ed. New York, Academic Press, 1977; Underwood, E. J.: J. Human Nutr., *35*:37, 1981.
5. Mertz, W.: Science, *213*:1332, 1981.
6. Prasad, A. S., et al.: J. Lab. Clin. Med., *61*:537, 1963; Prasad, A. S., et al.: Amer. J. Clin. Nutr., *12*:437, 1963; Sandstead, H. H., et al.: Amer. J. Clin. Nutr., *20*:422, 1967; Prasad, A. S.: Amer. J. Clin. Nutr., *20*:648, 1967; Carter, J. P., et al.: Amer. J. Clin. Nutr., *22*:59, 1969.
7. (On zinc deficient dogs) Sanecki, R. K., Corbin, J. E., and Forbes, R. M.: Amer. J. Vet. Res., *43*:1642, 1982.
8. Prasad, A. S., et al.: Arch. Intern. Med., *111*:407, 1963; Brewer, G. J., and Prasad, A. S.: *Zinc Metabolism: Current Aspects in Health and Disease.* New York, Alan R. Liss, Inc., 1977 (see Chapter 1 by J. A. Halsted); Halsted, J. A., et al.: Amer. J. Med., *53*:277, 1972; Mahloudji, M., et al.: Amer. J. Clin. Nutr., *28*:721, 1975.
9. Hambidge, K. M., et al.: Pediatr. Res., *6*:868, 1972.
10. (On fetal abnormalities in animals from zinc deficiency) Blamberg, D. L., et al.: Proc. Soc. Exp. Biol. Med., *104*:207, 1960; Kleinholz, E. W., et al.: J. Nutr., *75*:211, 1961; Hurley, L., and Swenerton, H.: Proc. Soc. Exp. Biol. Med., *123*:692, 1966; Apgar, J.: J. Nutr. *100*:470, 1970; Hurley, L. S., Gowan, J., and Swenerton, H.: Teratology, *4*:199, 1971; Hurley, L. S.: *Developmental Nutrition,* Englewood Cliffs, N.J., Prentice Hall, 1980; Hurley, L. S.: Physiol. Rev., *61*:249, 1981; Cerklewski, R. L.: J. Nutr., *111*:1780, 1981.
11. (On fetal abnormalities in humans from zinc deficiency) Jameson, S.: Effects of zinc deficiency in human reproduction. Acta Med. Scand., Supplement 593, 1976; Crosby, W. H., et al.: Amer. J. Obst. Gyn., *128*:22, 1977; Cavdar, A. O., et al.: Amer. J. Clin. Nutr., *33*:542, 1980; Cherry, F. F., et al.: Amer. J. Clin. Nutr., *34*:2367, 1981; Hurley, L. S.: Teratology, *25*:123, 1982; Soltan, M. H., and Jenkins, D. M.: Brit. J. Obst. Gyn., *89*:56, 1982.
12. (On male reproductive disorders in humans) Abbasi, A. I., et al.: J. Lab. Clin. Med., *96*:544, 1980; Castro-Magana, M., et al.: Amer. J. Dis. Children, *135*:322, 1981; Netter, A., Hartoma, R., and Nahoul, K.: Arch. Androl., 7:69, 1981.
13. Li, T., and Vallee, B. L.: The biochemical and nutritional roles of other trace elements (Chapter 9B). In Goodhart, R. S., and Shils, M. E. (eds.): *Modern Nutrition in Health and Disease.* 6th ed. Philadelphia, Penn., Lea and Febiger, 1980.
14. (On nerve changes in zinc deficiency) Dreosti, I. E., et al.: Life Sci., *28*:2133, 1981; Hesketh, J. E.: Int. J. Biochem., *13*:921, 1981; Hughes, R. N., and Horsburgh, R. J.: Nutr. Res., *2*:513, 1982; Massaro, T. J., Mohs, M., and Fosmire, G.: Physiol. Behav., *25*:117, 1982; Pfeiffer, C. C., and Braverman, E. R.: Zinc, the brain and behavior (a review). Biol. Psych., *17*:513, 1982 (with 125 references some from non-peer-reviewed sources).
15. Prasad, A. S., Rabbani, P., and Abbash, A.: Ann. Int. Med., *89*:483, 1978.
16. Hansen, M. A., Fernandes, G., and Good, R. A.: Ann. Rev. Nutr., *2*:151, 1982 (a review on nutrition, especially zinc, in immunity—248 references). For papers not cited in this review see next four references.
17. (On immune function and zinc in animals) Nutr. Rev. *38*:288, 1980; Beach, R. S., et al.: J. Nutr. Rev., *110*:805, 1980; Frost, P., et al.: Proc. Soc. Exp. Biol. Med., *167*:333, 1981; Fraker, P. J., et al.: J. Nutr., *112*:1224, 1981; Golub, M. S., et al.: Fed. Proc., *42*:820 (abst.), 1983.
18. Beisel, W. R.: Single nutrients and immunity. Amer. J. Clin. Nutr., *35* (Suppl., Feb.):417–439, 1982.
19. (On immune function in adults) Allen, J. I., Kay, N. E., and McClain, C. J.: Ann. Int. Med., *95*:154, 1981; Nutr. Rev., *40*:72, 1982; Briggs, W. A., et al.: Kidney Internat., *21*:827, 1982.
20. (On immune function in elderly) Steidemann, M.,

and Harrill, I.: Nutr. Rept. Internat., *21*:931, 1980; Duchateau, J., et al.: Amer. J. Med., *70*:1001, 1981; Wagner, P. A., et al.: Internat. J. Vit. Nutr. Res., *53*:94, 1983.

21. Beach, R. S., Gershwin, M. E., and Hurley, L. S.: Science, *218*:471, 1982.
22. (On taste and smell—positive findings) Mahajan, S. K., et al.: Amer. J. Clin. Nutr., *33*:1517, 1980; Buzina, R., et al.: Amer. J. Clin. Nutr., *33*:2262, 1980; Wright, A. L., et al.: Amer. J. Clin. Nutr., *34*:848, 1981; Sandstead, H. H., et al.: Amer. J. Clin. Nutr., *36*:1046, 1982.
23. (On taste and smell—negative findings) Greger J. L., and Geissler, A. H.: Amer. J. Clin. Nutr., *31*:633, 1978; Nutr. Rev. *37*:283, 1979 (see response by R. I. Henkin, in *38*:228, 1980); Vreeman, H. J., et al.: Nephron, *26*:163, 1980.
24. (On zinc-related acne) Baer, M. T., et al.: Arch. Derm., *114*:1093, 1978; Michaëlsson, G.: Oral zinc in acne. Acta Derm., Supplement 89, 1980.
25. (On congenital skin disorders and zinc) Krieger, I., and Evans, G. W.: J. Pediatr., *96*:32, 1980; Nutr. Rev., *39*:168, 1981; *40*:78, 1982; *40*:84, 1982; Zimmerman, A. W., et al.: Pediatrics, *69*:176, 1982; Krieger, I., Evans, G. W., and Zelkowitz, P. S.: Pediatrics, *69*:773, 1982.
26. (On zinc deficiency and parenteral nutrition in infants) Latimer, J. S., McClain, C. J., and Sharp, H. L.: J. Pediatr., *97*:434, 1980; Thorp, J. W., et al.: Amer. J. Clin. Nutr., *34*:1056, 1981; Vileisis, R. A., et al.: Amer. J. Clin. Nutr., *34*:2653, 1981; Weber, T. R., et al.: J. Pediatr. Surg., *16*:236, 1981; Nutr. Rev., *40*:81, 1982.
27. (On zinc deficiency and parenteral nutrition in adults) Phillips, G. D., and Garnys, V. P.: J. Parenter. Ent. Nutr., *5*:11, 1981; McClain, C. J.: J. Parenter. Ent. Nutr., *5*:424, 1981; Tasman-Jones, C.: J. New Zeal. Dietet. Assoc., *35* (April):27, 1981; Ize-Lamache, L., et al.: Arch. Invest. Méd. (Mexico), *12*:241, 1981; Mozzillo, N., et al.: Lancet *1*:744, 1982.
28. Committee on Diet, Nutrition, and Cancer: *Diet, Nutrition and Cancer,* Washington D.C., National Academy Press, 1982 (Chapter 10).
29. (Zinc in clinical trials) Nutr. Rev., *38*:365, 1980 (Down's syndrome); Brewer, G.: Amer. J. Hemat., *10*:195, 1981 (sickle cell); Prasad, A. S., et al.: Amer. J. Hemat., *10*:119, 1981 (sickle cell); Solomons, N. W., et al.: Nutr. Rev., *1*:13, 1981 (cystic fibrosis); Olsson, R.: J. Roy. Soc. Med., *212*:191, 1982 (biliary cirrhosis); Tiber, A. M., and Mukherjee, M. D.: Amer. Family Phys. *26*:167, 1982 (on clinical deficiencies in general); Nutr. Rev., *40*:175, 1982 (nightblindness in sickle cell); *40*:109, 1982 (Crohn's disease).
30. (Zinc intakes of adults) Hunt, I. F., et al.: Amer. J. Clin. Nutr., *32*:1511, 1979 (low-income pregnant women of Mexican descent); Klevay, L. M., Reck, S. J., and Barcome, D. F.: J. Amer. Med. Assoc., *241*:1916, 1979 (in hospital diets); Freeland-Graves, J. H., Bodzy, P. W., and Eppright, M. A.: J. Amer. Dietet. Assoc., *77*:655, 1980 (vegetarian students); Harland, B. F., et al.: J. Amer. Dietet. Assoc., *47*:16, 1980 (U.S. "market basket"); Srivastava, U., et al.: Nutr. Rept. Internat., *24*:1139, 1981 (student meals in Montreal, Canada); Anderson, B. M., Gibson, R. S., and Sabry, J. H.: Amer. J. Clin. Nutr., *34*:1042, 1981 (vegetarian women in Ontario); Gibson, R. S., and Scythes, C. A.: Brit. J. Nutr., *48*:241, 1982 (women in Ontario); Welsh, S. O., and Marston, R. M.: Food Tech., *36* (Jan.):70, 1982 (a review of zinc intakes in U.S.).
31. (On measuring zinc status) Kasarskis, E. J., and Schuna, A.: Amer. J. Clin. Nutr., *33*:2609, 1980; Freeland-Graves, J. H., et al.: Amer. J. Clin. Nutr., *34*:312, 1981; Danks, D. M.: Amer. J. Clin. Nutr., *34*:278, 1981; Wada, L. L., and King, J. C.: Compr. Therapy, *9* (4):45, 1983.
32. Hsu, J. M.: Current knowledge on zinc, copper and chromium in aging. World Rev. Nutr. Dietet., *33*:42, 1979.
33. Bunker, V. W., et al.: Human Nutr.: Clin. Nutr., *36C*:213, 1982 (balance studies).
34. Sandstead, H. H., et al.: Amer. J. Clin. Nutr., *36*:1046, 1982 (a good review, 115 references).
35. Wagner, P. A., et al.: Amer. J. Clin. Nutr., *33*:1771, 1980 (low-income black Americans); Wagner, P. A., et al.: Nutr. Res., *1*:565, 1981 (elderly women); Sempos, C. T., et al.: J. Amer. Dietet. Assoc., *81*:35, 1982 (14 nursing homes); Allington, J. K., et al.: J. Amer. Dietet. Assoc., *82*:377, 1983 (14 nursing homes).
36. (On low serum zinc in pregnancy) Prema, K., et al.: Ind. J. Med. Res., *71*:547, 1980 (in India); King, J. C., Stein, T., and Doyle, M.: Amer. J. Clin. Nutr., *34*:1049, 1981 (Berkeley); Vir, S. C., Love, A. H. G., and Thompson, W.: Amer. J. Clin. Nutr., *34*:2800, 1981 (Ireland); Dreosti, I. E., et al.: Nutr. Rev., *2*:591, 1982 (Australia); Swanson, C. A., and King, J. C.: J. Nutr., *112*:697, 1982 (Berkeley).
37. Mittal, R., et al.: Ind. J. Nutr. Dietet., *19*:117, 1982; Hunt, I. F., et al.: Amer. J. Clin. Nutr., *32*:1511, 1979; *37*:572, 1983.
38. Cavdar, A. O., et al.: Amer. J. Clin. Nutr., *33*:542, 1980.
39. Cherry, F. F., et al.: Amer. J. Clin. Nutr., *34*:2367, 1981.
40. Gibson, R. S., and DeWolfe, M. S.: J. Canad. Dietet. Assoc., *41*:206, 1980 (intakes); Acta Paediatr. Scand., *70*:497, 1981 (serum levels).
41. Ruth, R. E., and Goldsmith, S. K.: J. Nutr., *111*:2034, 1981; Silverman, B., and Rivlin, R. S.: J. Nutr., *112*:744, 1982; Ghishan, F. K., et al.: J. Lab. Clin. Med., *100*:45, 1982.
42. Kern, J. C., et al.: J. Psych. Treat. Eval., *3*:169, 1981.
43. Nutr. Rev., *40*:43, 1982.
44. Ilchyshyn, A., and Mendelsohn, S.: Brit. Med. J., *284*:1676, 1982.
45. Harrill, I., and Bowski, M. M.: J. Nutr. Elderly, *1*:51, 1981.

46. Spencer, H., et al.: Amer. J. Clin. Nutr., *32*:1867, 1979; Swanson, C. A., and King, J. C.: J. Nutr., *112*:697, 1982; Rao, B. S. N.: Nutr. Rept. Internat., *26*:915, 1982.
47. Haralambie, G.: Internat. J. Sports Med., *2*:135, 1981.
48. (Examples of the sole use of hair zinc in zinc status studies) O'Leary, M. J., Mata, L. J., and Hegarty, P. V. J.: Amer. J. Clin. Nutr., *33*:2194, 1980 (Costa Rican infants and preschoolers); Moser, P. B., Krebs, N. K., and Blyler, E.: Nutr. Res., *2*:585, 1982 (small-for-age-children in Washington, D.C. area); MacDonald, L. D., Gibson, R. S., and Miles, J. E.: Acta Paediatr. Scand., *71*:785, 1982 (breast-fed versus bottle-fed infants); Dorea, J. G., et al.: Ecol. Food Nutr., *12*:1, 1982 (children of poor families in Brazil); Dorea, J. G., et al.: Human Nutr.: Appl. Nutr., *36A*:63, 1982 (urban children in Brazil); Dorea, J. G., et al.: J. Trop. Pediatr., *29*:58, 1983 (malnourished infants).
49. (Evaluation of hair-zinc analysis. Also see refs. 36, 48, 50, and 51.) Gentile, P. S., et al.: Pediatr. Res., *15*:123, 1981; Nutr. Rev., *40*:74, 1982.
50. Herbert, V., and Barrett, S.: *Vitamins and "Health" Foods: the Great American Hustle.* Philadelphia, Penn., George F. Stickley Co., 1981; Hambidge, K. M.: Amer. J. Clin. Nutr., *36*:943, 1982; Meister, K. A.: ACSH News Views (Amer. Council Sci. Health), *3*(No. 2):11, 1982; Fenner, L.: FDA Consumer, *17*(April):16, 1983.
51. (On hair trace-element analysis) Chittleborough, G., and Steel, B. J.: Sci. Total Environ., *15*:25, 1980; Gibson, R. S.: J. Human Nutr., *34*:405, 1980; Toribara, T. Y., et al.: Anal. Chem., *54*:1844, 1982; Laker, M.: Lancet *2*:260, 1982 (also see pp. 554 and 608); Holzbecher, J., and Ryan, D. E.: Clin. Biochem., *15*:80, 1982; Gibson, R. S.: Amer. J. Clin. Nutr., *37*:37, 1983.
52. (On zinc content of foods) Haeflein, K. A., and Rasmussen, A. I.: J. Amer. Dietet. Assoc., *70*:610, 1977; Banerjee, S., and Pal, B.: Ind. J. Nutr. Dietet., *16*:320, 1979 (foods of India); Freeland-Graves, J. H., et al.: J. Amer. Dietet. Assoc., 77:648, 1980 (74 vegetarian foods); Allen, K. G. D., and Klevay, L. M.: Nutr. Rept. Internat., *22*:389, 1980 (breakfast cereals); English, R.: J. Food Nutr., *38*:63, 1981 (Australian foods); Leung, C., et al.: J. Amer. Dietet. Assoc., *80*:530, 1982 (hospital foods). Also see references in Appendix, Table 2.
53. Kirkpatrick, D. C., et al.: Canad. Inst. Food Sci. Tech. J., *13*:154, 1980 (on baby foods and intake of zinc by infants).
54. (Vegetarian diets) Freeland-Graves, J. H., Bodzy, P. W., and Eppright, M. A.: J. Amer. Dietet. Assoc., 77:655, 1980 (also see Amer. J. Clin. Nutr., *33*:1757, 1980); Anderson, B. M., Gibson, R. S., and Sabry, J. H.: Amer. J. Clin. Nutr., *34*:1042, 1981; King, J. C., Stein, T., and Doyle, M.: Amer. J. Clin. Nutr., *34*:1049, 1981; Ellis, R., et al.: J. Amer. Dietet. Assoc., *81*:26, 1982; Abu-Assal, M., and Craig, W. J.: Fed. Proc., *42*:552 (abst.), 1983.
55. Ranhotra, G. S., et al.: Nutr. Rept. Internat., *26*:821, 1982.
56. (Current studies on zinc availability in humans) Greger, J. L., and Snedeker, S. M.: J. Nutr. *110*:2243, 1980 (effect of protein and phosphorus); Sandström, B., et al.: Amer. J. Clin. Nutr., *33*:739 and 1778, 1980; Aamodt, R. L., et al.: Amer. J. Clin. Nutr., *34*:2648, 1981 (procedures); Solomons, N. W., and Jacob, R. A.: Amer. J. Clin. Nutr., *34*:475, 1981 (effect of heme and nonheme iron); Casey C. E., et al.: Pediatrics, *68*:394, 1981 (human milk vs. cow's milk); Saleh, A., et al.: Nutr. Rev., *1*:327, 1981 (effect of yeast); Janghorbani, M., et al.: Amer. J. Clin. Nutr., *36*:537, 1982 (protein sources); Solomons, N. W., et al.: J. Nutr., *112*:1809, 1982 (soybean protein effect); Nutr. Rev., *40*:76, 1982 (iron effect); Turnlund, J. R., et al.: Amer. J. Clin. Nutr., *35*:1033, 1982 (procedures); Payton, P., et al.: Gastroenterology, *83*: 1264, 1982 (procedures); Bodwell, C. E.; Cereal Foods World, *28*:342, 1983 (effect of soybean protein); Solomons, N. W., et al.: Amer. J. Clin. Nutr., *37*:566, 1983 (effect of tin); Anderson, H. L., et al.: Fed. Proc., *42*:1183 (abst.), 1983 (beef vs. soy-meat analog).
57. (Reviews) Solomons, N. W.: Amer. J. Clin. Nutr., *35*:1048, 1982; Solomons, N. W.: J. Amer. Dietet. Assoc., *80*:101, 1982; Kelsay, J. L.: Cereal Chem., *58*:2, 1981.
58. Roth, H. P., and Kirchgessner, M.: Zinc metalloenzyme activities. World Rev. Nutr. Dietet., *34*:144, 1980.
59. a) Faintuch, J.: J. Parenter. Ent. Nutr., *2*:640, 1978; b) Nutr. Rev., *40*:72, 1982.
60. Hooper, P. L., et al.: J. Amer. Med. Assoc., *244*:1960, 1980.
61. Freeland-Graves, J. H., et al.: Amer. J. Clin. Nutr., *35*:988, 1982.

Fluorine

62. Masironi, R.: WHO Chronicle, *32*:382, 1978.
63. Schamschula, R. G., and Barmes, D. E.: Fluoride and health: dental caries, osteoporosis, and cardiovascular disease. Ann. Rev. Nutr., *1*:427, 1981.
64. Dean, H. T., et al.: Public Health Rept., *56*:761, 1941.
65. Shaw, J. H., and Sweeney, E. A.: Nutrition in relation to dental medicine (Chapter 30). In Goodhart, R. S., and Shils, M. E. (eds.): *Modern Nutrition in Health and Disease.* 6th Ed. Philadelphia, Penn., Lea and Febiger, 1980.
66. Glenn, F. B., Glenn, W. D., and Duncan, R. C.: Amer. J. Obst. Gyn., *143*:560, 1982; also see Teuscher, G. W.: J. Dent. Children, *48*:2, 1981.
67. Esela, S., et al.: Brit. J. Nutr., *48*:201, 1982.
68. Singer, L., and Ophaug, R. H.: Pediatrics, *63*:460, 1979.
69. Ophaug, R. H., Singer, L., and Harland, B. F.: J. Dent. Res., *59*:777, 1980.

70. Driscoll, W. S., and Horowitz, H. S.: Amer. J. Dis. Children, *133*:683, 1979; AAP Committee on Nutrition: Pediatrics, *63*:150, 1979; Barness, L. A.: Pediatrics, *67*:582, 1981.
71. Ingram, G. S., and Nash, P. F.: Caries Res., *14*:298, 1980.
72. (Fluoride and bone relationships) Riggs, B. L., et al.: J. Amer. Med. Assoc., *243*:446, 1980 (see editorial on p. 463); Stein, I. D., and Granik, G.: Calcif. Tissue Internat., *32*:189, 1980; Ream, L. J.: Cell Tissue Res., *221*:421, 1981; Briancon, D., and Meunier, P. J.: Orthop. Clin. North Amer., *12*:629, 1981; Mohamedally, S. M., Phil, M., and Wix, P.: Fluoride, *15*:137, 1982; Riggs, B. L., et al.: New Eng. J. Med., *306*:446, 1982; Williams, C. C.: Clin. Invest. Med., *5*:195, 1982; Bikle, D. D.: Ann. Int. Med., *98*:1013 (editorial), 1983.
73. Brit. Med. J., *282*:253, 1981.
74. Leverett, D. H.: Science, *217*:26, 1982.
75. Crissman, J. M., Maylin, G. A., and Krook, L.: Cornell Vet., *70*:183, 1980 (on inadequate New York and Federal standards for fluoride pollution); Ammerman, C. B. (Chairman): J. Dairy Sci., *51*:744–774 (5 papers), 1980 (on fluoride toxicosis in cattle); Kubota, J., Naphan, E. A., and Oberly, G. H.: J. Range Manag., *35*:188, 1982 (on high plant levels of fluorine around thermal springs in Nevada); Andrews, S. M., et al.: Fluoride, *15*:56, 1982 (on contaminated grasslands and potential food sources).

Molybdenum

76. Abumrad, N. N., et al.: Amer. J. Clin. Nutr., *34*:2551, 1981.
77. van der Heiden, C.: Clin. Biochem., *12*:206, 1979; Johnson, J. L., et al.: Proc. Nat. Acad. Sci., *77*:3715, 1980; Rajagopalan, K. V., et al.: Fed. Proc., *41*:2608, 1982 (a review).
78. Tsongas, T. A., et al.: Amer. J. Clin. Nutr. *33*:1103, 1980.
79. Schlettwein-Gsell, D., and Mommsen-Straub, S.: Int. J. Vit. Nutr. Res., *43*:110, 1973 (a review of molybdenum distribution); Deosthale, Y. G.: Ind. J. Nutr. Dietet., *18*:15, 1981 (common Indian foods).
80. Mills, C. F. (Chairman): *Symposium on metal toxicities.* Proc. Nutr. Soc. (U.K.), *38*:235, 1979.

Selenium

81. van Rij, A. M., et al.: Amer. J. Clin. Nutr. *32*:2076, 1979; van Rij, A. M., et al.: J. Parenter. Ent. Nutr., *3*:235, 1979; Thomson, C. D., and Robinson, M. F.: Amer. J. Clin. Nutr., *33*:303, 1980; van Rij, A. M., et al.: J. Parenter. Ent. Nutr., *5*:120, 1981; Robinson, M. F., et al.: New Zeal. Med. J., *93*:289, 1981; Thomson, C. D., et al.: Amer. J. Clin. Nutr., *36*:24, 1982.
82. Keshan Disease Research Group: Chinese Med. J., *92*:471 and 477, 1979; Lancet, *2*:889, 1979; Nutr. Rev., *38*:278, 1980. (Also see the entire Aug. 1982 issue of Acta Nutrimenta Sinica, V. 4, No. 3, on this topic.)
83. (On selenium deficiency in parenteral nutrition) Johnson, R. A., et al.: New Eng. J. Med., *304*:1210, 1981; King, W. W. K., et al.: New Eng. J. Med., *304*:1305, 1981; Young, V. R.: New Eng. J. Med., *304*:1228, 1981 (an editorial); Fleming, C. R., et al.: Gastroenterology, *83*:689, 1982; Shils, M. E., Levander, O. A., and Alcock, N. W.: Amer. J. Clin. Nutr., *35*:838, 1982 (abst.); Kien, C. L., and Ganther, H. E.: Amer. J. Clin. Nutr., *37*:319, 1983.
84. (On adequacy of selenium levels in PN solutions) Smith, J. L., and Goos, S. M.: J. Parenter. Ent. Nutr., *4*:23, 1980; also see ref. 27 (Phillips; McClain).
85. Collipp, P. J., and Chen, S. Y.: New Eng. J. Med., *304*:1304, 1981.
86. Sartiano, G. P., et al.: New Eng. J. Med., *307*:558, 1982.
87. (On estimation of requirements) Perona, G., et al.: Brit. J. Haemat., *42*:567, 1979 (in pregnancy and newborns); Amin, S., et al.: Nutr. Metab., *24*:331, 1980 (in prematures); Levander, O. A., et al.: Amer. J. Clin. Nutr., *34*:2662 (Se balance in young men); Butler, J. A., Whanger, P. D., and Tripp, M. J.: Amer. J. Clin. Nutr., *36*:15, 1982 (in pregnant women and animal models).
88. (On selenium intakes) Gibson, R. S., and DeWolfe, M. S.: J. Canad. Dietet. Assoc., *41*:206, 1980 (infants in Nova Scotia); Thomson, C. D., and Robinson, M. F.: Amer. J. Clin. Nutr., *33*:303, 1980 (New Zealand); Levander, O. A.: Contemp. Nutr. (General Mills), *5* (No. 11):1, 1980; McConnell, K. P., et al.: Nutr. Rev., *1*:235, 1981 (hospital diets in Washington, D.C.); Welsh, S. O., et al.: J. Amer. Dietet. Assoc., *79*:277, 1981 (Maryland residents); Smith, A. M., Picciano, M. F., and Milner, J. A.: Amer. J. Clin. Nutr., *35*:521, 1982 (infants in Illinois); Gibson, R. S., and Scythes, C. A.: Brit. J. Nutr., *48*:241, 1982, and Fed. Proc. (abst.), *42*:816, 1983 (women in Ontario).
89. (On selenium status measurement) Valentine, J. L., Kang, H. K., and Spivey, G. H.: Environ. Res., *17*:347, 1978 (blood, urine, hair); Lane, H. W., Dudrick, S., and Warren, D. C.: Proc. Soc. Exp. Biol. Med., *167*:383, 1981 (red blood cells and plasma); Thamaya, S., and Ganapathy, S. N.: Sci. Total Environ. *24*:41, 1982 (serum and hair); Hojo, Y.: Bull. Environ. Cont. Tox., *29*:37, 1982 (urine creatinine level); Steiner, G., et al.: Europ. J. Pediatr. *138*:138, 1982 (plasma glutathione oxidase); Kasperek, K., et al.: Biol. Tr. Elem. Res., *4*:29, 1982 (platelet selenium); Feldman, E. B., et al.: Amer. J. Clin. Nutr. (abst.), *37*:714, 1983; Levander, O. A., et al.: Amer. J. Clin. Nutr. *37*:887, 1983 (use of blood parameters to measure availability); Lane, H. W., et al.: Proc. Soc. Exp. Biol. Med., *173*:87, 1983 (of elderly subjects in Texas); Verlinden, M., et al.: Biol. Tr. Elem. Res., *5*:91 and 103, 1983 (of Belgian population).

90. Burk, R. F., and Gregory, P. E.: Arch. Biochem. Biophy., *213*:73, 1982.
91. Ensminger, A. H., et al.: *Foods and Nutrition Encyclopedia,* Clovis, Calif., Pergus Press, 1983, p. 1985.

Chromium

92. Schwarz, K., and Mertz, W.: Arch. Biochem. Biophys., *85*:292, 1959; Fed. Proc., *20*:111, 1961; Mertz, W.: Fed. Proc., *26*:186, 1967; Physiol. Rev., *49*:163, 1969.
93. Hopkins, L. L., Jr., Ransome-Kuti, O., and Majaj, A. S.: Amer. J. Clin. Nutr., *21*:203, 1968; Gürson, C. T., and Saner, G.: Amer. J. Clin. Nutr., *24*:1313, 1971.
94. Jeejeebhoy, K. N., et al.: Amer. J. Clin. Nutr., *30*:531, 1977 (Toronto); Freund, H., et al.: J. Amer. Med. Assoc., *241*:496, 1979 (Boston).
95. Mertz, W.: Nutr. Rev., *33*:129, 1975; Toepfer, E. W., et al.: J. Agric. Food Chem., *25*:162, 1977; Haylock, S. J., et al.: J. Inorg. Biochem., *18*:195, 1983.
96. (Examples of hair chromium studies) Shapcott, D., et al.: Clin. Biochem., *13*:129, 1980 (pregnant women); Gibson, R. S.: J. Human Nutr., *34*:405, 1980 (a review); Rabinowitz, M. B., et al.: Metabolism, *29*:355, 1980 (diabetic men); Vobecky, J., et al.: Nutr. Rept. Internat., *22*:49, 1980 (mental patients); Saner, G.: Amer. J. Clin. Nutr. *34*:853, 1981 (also see *35*:776, 1982) (pregnant women in Turkey); Kasperek, K., et al.: Sci. Total Environ., *22*:149, 1982 (Egyptian population).
97. Offenbacher, E. G., Pi-Sunyer, F. X.: Diabetes, *29*:919, 1980 (elderly subjects); Riales, R., and Albrink, M. J.: Amer. J. Clin. Nutr., *34*:2670, 1981 (adult men); Abraham, A. S., et al.: Atherosclerosis, *41*:371, 1982 and *42*:185, 1982 (atherosclerosis in rabbits).

Nickel and Vanadium

98. Nielsen, F. H., et al.: J. Nutr., *109*:1623, 1979; Nielsen, F. H.: Evidence of the essentiality of arsenic, nickel, and vanadium and their possible nutritional significance. Adv. Nutr. Res., *3*:157, 1980; Nielsen, F. H., Hunt, C. D., and Uthus, E. O.: Ann. N. Y. Acad. Sci., *355*:152, 1980.
99. Hopkins, L. L., Jr., and Mohr, H. E., in Mertz, W., and Cornatzer, W. E. (eds.): *Newer Trace Elements in Nutrition.* New York, Marcel Dekker, Inc., 1971; Fed. Proc., *30*:462, 1971; Strasia, C. A., and Smith, W. H.: J. Animal Sci., *31*:1027, 1970 (abst.).
100. Schwarz, K., and Milne, D. B.: Science, *174*:426, 1971.
101. Cantley, L. C., Jr.: J. Biol. Chem., *252*:7421, 1977.

Silicon

102. Carlisle, E. M.: Science, *167*:179, 1970; Carlisle, E. M.: Science, *178*:619, 1972 (reprinted in Nutr. Rev., *40*:210, 1982).
103. Schwarz, K., and Milne, D. B.: Nature, *239*:333, 1972.
104. (On silicon metabolism) Carlisle, E. M.: J. Nutr., *106*:478, 1976; *110*:352, 1980; *110*:1046, 1980: Calcif. Tissue Res., *33*:27, 1981; Carlisle, E. M., and Suchil, C.: Fed. Proc., *42*:398 (abst.), 1983.

Arsenic

105. Neilsen, F. H., Givand, S. H., and Myran, D. R.: Fed. Proc., *34*:923, 1975; Uthus, E. O., and Nielsen, F. H.: Interaction between arsenic and zinc in the chick. Fed. Proc., *39*:904, 1980; Neilsen, F. H.: Adv. Nutr. Res., *3*:157 (see ref. 98), 1980.
106. Anka, M., et al.: Arsenic—a new essential trace element (tr.). Arch. Tierenahr., *26*:742, 1976.

Lead

107. Reichlmayr-Lais, A. M., and Kirchgessner, M.: Z. Tierphy., Tierern. Futter., *46*:1, 1981; also, Ann. Nutr. Metab., *25*:281, 1981 (anemia, etc.); Arch. Tierern., *31*:731, 1981 (depletion studies); Kirchgessner, M., and Reichlmayr-Lais, A. M.: Int. J. Vit. Nutr. Res., *51*:421, 1981; also, Biol. Trace Elem. Res., *3*:279, 1981 (both on iron relationship).

Boron

108. Hunt, C. D., and Nielsen, F. H., in Howe, J. M., et al. (eds.): *Trace Element Metabolism in Man and Animals.* Canberra, Australian Academy of Sciences, 1982, p. 597. Hunt, C. D., and Nielsen, F. H.: Fed. Proc. (abst.). *42*:398, 1983.

Pica

109. Danford, D. E.: Pica and Nutrition. Ann. Rev. Nutr., *2*:303, 1982 (a review, 224 references).

(See also references and supplementary readings for Chap. 13 [Introduction to Minerals] and Chap. 16 [Trace Elements I].)

18 Food: Our Source of Nutrients and Nonnutrients

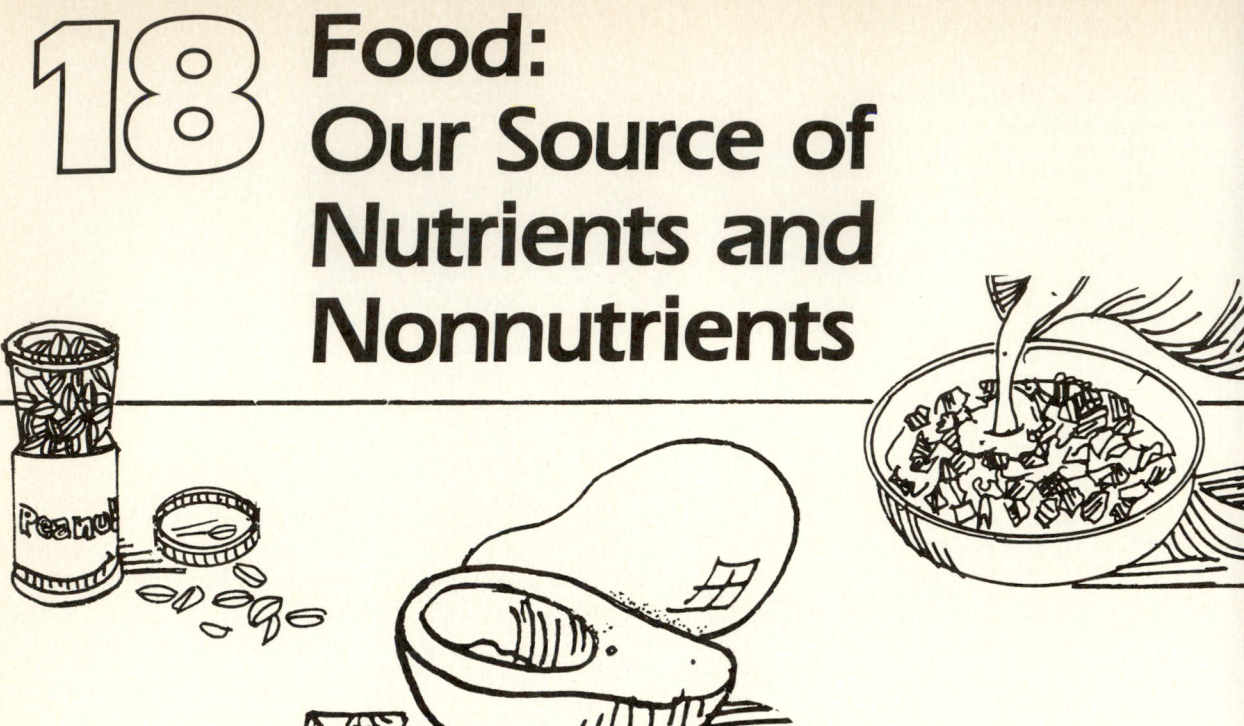

So far this book has emphasized the forty-five or so individual nutrients, including water and fiber, making up 98 percent or more of nearly all our foods. Small amounts of thousands of nonnutrient compounds that have barely been mentioned complete its composition. Most of these are naturally present in foodstuffs—a few are food additives. These nonnutrients make up as much as 1 or 2 percent or more of the composition of some foods. They greatly influence food's nature, taste, appearance, safety, and acceptability. Some may be removed or destroyed by preservation and processing methods, while still others are formed during processing.

It would not be wise or practical, except for medical reasons, to attempt to live solely on mixtures of synthetic or purified nutrients. Commonly available foodstuffs are preferred. Not only are they economical and practical for essential nourishment, but they also offer variety and sensory pleasure, satisfy the appetite, and serve social and religious needs.

DEFINITION AND TYPES

Nutrition was defined in Chapter 1 as "the science of *food* as it relates to optimal health and performance." Now that the major structural components of all food, the nutrients, have been described, food can be defined. A definition must include both traditional, basic foods and new, twentieth-century manufactured products.

Definition

The word food has its origin in the old Anglo-Saxon word *foda*, from which the English word fodder is also derived. Food means different things to different people depending on their occupation, geographical location, culture, religion, economic and social situation, scientific training, and other circumstances. From the viewpoint of nutrition, *food* is defined as those substances that are consumed in solid or liquid form that provide energy and nutrients necessary for optimal health and performance.[1] This definition is broad and includes everything consumed, alone or in combination, that provides energy or one or more of the nutrients (water, carbohydrate, fat, protein or amino acids, vitamins, and/or minerals). Ideally, foods are consumed in balanced amounts over a day's period primarily as meals made from basic foodstuffs, or their equivalent. Not everyone agrees, however, that "food" must serve a nutritional function or that everything that serves a nutritional function is food (2).

Foods That Provide Only One or Two Nutrients. In addition to substances that provide many nutrients, those that provide only one or two, even in small amounts, must be considered foods. They include water, sugar, oils and fats, alcoholic beverages, vinegar, monosodium glutamate, salt, honey, soft drinks, pancake syrup, most candies, or a vitamin C tablet. A "calorie-free" soft drink or a cup of tea or coffee provide water, a nutrient, so they count as foods. Diets consisting only of such foods would be exceedingly poor, but when mixed with adequate amounts of basic foods these substances can become part of a good diet.

Nonnutrients in Food. As has been noted, food also includes nonnutrients naturally present. These include literally hundreds of nitrogen-containing compounds as well as flavors, volatile substances, pigments, flavonoids, naturally occurring toxins and drugs (such as caffeine), steroids, nonessential minerals and other elements, and still other substances that serve no nutritional function. If these were isolated and eaten by themselves for any reason they would not be considered food because they would serve no nutrient function. Some would then serve as drugs.

Other nonnutrients forming an integral, and often a necessary, part of foods are the many food additives present intentionally or unintentionally (to be discussed later in this chapter). A few of these, such as phosphates, spices, and herbs, supply minerals or vitamins so are foods in their own right.

Nonfood Substances. About the only substances taken into the body that are not considered food by this broad definition are drugs and medicines. When they are not a natural part of commonly available foodstuffs—and few are today—they are not foods. The dividing line often becomes a political and a legal question, such as whether alcohol sources such as beer and liquor are foods, and whether megadoses of vitamins sold over the counter in a drug store are foods.

Traditional and New Types

The most basic of the traditional types of food for humans are rice, wheat, and lesser amounts of other grains, which make up 70 to 80 percent of the world's food supply. Legumes provide another 10 to 15 percent, followed by vegetables, fruit, fish and meat, milk, poultry, eggs, nuts, and sweeteners. In the United States, Canada, and other developed countries, relatively larger amounts of animal products, sugars, and isolated fats and oils are consumed. For example, the major foods in the United States are dairy products, vegetables, meat (including poul-

[1] Food could not be defined in the past from a chemical or nutritional viewpoint until most of the nutrients and other ingredients were known (1). The legal definition of food by the Food and Drug Administration (FDA) in the United States (Sec. 201 [f]) is "articles used for food or drink....", which does not help in defining the word food itself.

Table 18–1 APPROXIMATE SOURCES OF NUTRIENTS IN THE AVERAGE UNITED STATES DIET[a]

Food Groups	*Food Energy*	*Pro-tein*	*Fat*	*Car-bohy-drate*	*Cal-cium*	*Phos-phorus*	*Iron*	*Magne-sium*	*Vita-min A Value*	*Thia-min*	*Ribo-flavin*	*Nia-cin*	*Vita-min B-6*	*Vita-min B-12*	*Ascor-bic Acid*
	PERCENT OF TOTAL														
Meat (including pork fat cuts), poultry, and fish	21.0	42.9	36.1	.1	4.2	28.6	31.1	14.0	23.9	27.9	23.5	45.4	40.7	71.9	2.1
Eggs	1.8	4.9	2.7	.1	2.4	5.2	5.1	1.2	5.5	1.9	4.9	.1	2.1	8.2	0
Dairy products, excluding butter	9.9	20.2	11.2	5.7	71.6	32.6	2.4	19.8	12.2	7.2	36.3	1.2	10.7	18.4	3.2
Fats and oils, including butter	18.2	.1	43.0	[b]	.4	.2	0	.4	7.8	0	0	0	[b]	0	0
Citrus fruits	1.0	.6	.1	2.1	1.1	.9	.9	2.6	1.7	2.9	.6	.9	1.5	0	29.3
Other fruits	2.3	.7	.3	5.0	1.4	1.3	3.9	4.5	5.9	1.8	1.7	1.7	7.1	0	11.8
Potatoes and sweet potatoes	2.7	2.3	.1	5.1	1.0	3.6	4.4	7.1	5.0	4.5	1.4	5.9	9.5	0	13.5
Dark green and deep yellow vegetables	.2	.4	[b]	.4	1.5	.6	1.6	2.0	18.5	.7	1.0	.5	1.9	0	9.0
Other vegetables, including tomatoes	2.5	3.3	.4	4.7	5.2	5.1	9.9	10.7	16.7	6.2	4.7	5.7	10.7	0	27.8
Dry beans and peas, nuts, soya flour, and grits	3.0	5.5	3.7	2.1	3.1	6.4	6.8	12.3	[b]	5.0	1.9	6.8	5.0	0	[b]
Grain products	19.9	18.8	1.3	36.2	3.8	13.4	31.0	19.1	.4	41.7	23.3	28.4	10.6	1.6	0
Sugar and other sweeteners	17.0	[b]	0	38.1	3.3	.7	.6	.2	0	[b]	[b]	[b]	[b]	0	[b]
Miscellaneous[c]	.6	.3	1.0	.5	.8	1.5	2.1	6.4	2.2	.1	.6	3.3	.1	0	3.3

[a]From USDA Washington, D.C., U.S. Department of Agriculture, 1980. Percentages were derived from nutrient data that include quantities of iron, thiamin, and riboflavin added to flour and cereal products; quantities of vitamin A value added to margarine and milk of all types; and quantities of vitamin C added to fruit juices and drinks. These are based on food *available* before processing and cooking.

[b]Less than 0.05 percent.

[c]Including chocolate liquor equivalent of cocoa beans.

try and fish), fruit, grain products, and fats, oils, and sweeteners about in this decreasing order by weight (see Table 3 of Appendix).

In the United States the major sources of energy are meat, poultry, fish, grain products, fats and oils, and sugar and other sweeteners, as shown in detail in Table 18–1. The table also shows major sources of protein, fat, and many other nutrients.

In addition to common foods directly derived from plant and animal products that reach food markets, there are new, specific foods manufactured according to new technology by the competitive food industry in developed countries. From 6,000 to 10,000 different kinds of specific foods, mostly packaged, are on supermarket shelves from which the consumer may choose. Many of these were developed to fill a consumer need or demand. Thus, many new terms describing foods have been added to our vocabulary of older terms that go back for centuries. Examples of terms used to describe food are listed in Table 18–2. They stress the impor-

Table 18–2 THE COMPLEXITY OF HUMAN FOODS
(Examples of adjectives describing food, from the food and nutrition literature)[a]

← *Nutrition Related Adjectives* →			
	← *Food Science Related Adjectives* →		
Based on Nutritional Values of Foods[b]	Based on Food Sources and Composition	Based on Manufacturing Processes and Usage of Foods	
Basic	Animal	Baby	Infant
Empty-calorie	Carbohydrate	Bakery	Hospital
Fattening	Cereal	Canned	Institutional
Health	Dairy	Convenient	Kosher
High-energy	Dietetic	Cooked	Liquid
High-quality	Energy-rich	Dehydrated	Manufactured
High-value	Fatty	Dessert	Organic
Imitation	High-carbohydrate	Dried	Packaged
"Junk"	High-fat	Engineered	Prepared
Light	High-fiber	Enriched	Preserved
Low-energy	High-protein	Ethnic	Processed
Low-quality	Legume	Extruded	Puréed (or strained)
Low-value	Low-ash	Fabricated	Raw
Muscle-building	Low-fat	Fast	Reduced-calorie
Natural	Low-fiber	Fermented	Restaurant
Nourishing	Low-protein	Foreign	Snack
Nutrient-dense	Low-sodium	Formulated	Solid
Nutritious	Plant	Fortified	Standardized
Protective	Protein	Fresh	Stored
Real	Sea	Freeze-dried	Substitute
Snack	Soybean	Frozen	Textured
Supplementary	Starchy	Functional	Toxic
Traditional	Vegetable	Geriatric	Vegetarian
Wholesome	Wheat	Gourmet	Vended

[a]Not including descriptions of food based on socioeconomic, marketing and cultural usages (such as "cold," "hot," expensive, economical, low-cost, soul, spiritual, farm, etc.).

[b]The nutritional values may be presumed, or based on specific foods rather than on a whole meal or on a total day's intake of foods (which is a better way to judge the nutritive value of foods).

tance of the consumer's knowing about not only nutritional values but also processing technology, nonnutrient content, additives, safety, labeling, and marketing.

TECHNOLOGY OF PRESERVATION AND PROCESSING

Plant material is the source of most food, either directly or indirectly. Farmers and ranchers raise crops, breed fish and poultry, and herd cattle. This food ultimately leaves the farm in the form of plants, seeds, fruits, milk, eggs, or meat. The farmer's first concern is to produce, at a profit, the food that will be purchased in the marketplace by the consumer. Marketability, not nutrition, is the major determinant in the farmer's choice of foods to produce.

For most of the world's population, food must be either produced at home or purchased at a marketplace—or both. At its simplest, a market can be someone sitting by a roadside selling surplus food, that he or she has raised, to passing neighbors.

Food on an American table is a result of a very complex market system. It might include a melon grown in Texas, toast made from bread baked in a nearby city from wheat grown in Kansas, coffee from Latin America, and sugar from cane or beets grown in Louisiana, Hawaii, or California. Other foods might be potatoes from Idaho or Maine, beef from Colorado or Nebraska, poultry from Georgia, pork from Iowa, oranges from Florida, cheese from Wisconsin, or seafood from Alaska or Louisiana.

All this food reaches the consumer through a long chain of middlemen—food brokers, food processors, shippers, and truckers—until it appears in shops, supermarkets, restaurants, fast-food outlets, institutions, or homes, where it is consumed (see Fig. 18–1). The interaction of consumer and producer influences what the middleman offers for sale. In a free, market economy, consumers want products and producers seek profit; thus, whether a food appears in a market depends on what price the consumer is willing to pay and on what the middleman has to offer.

A producer will be discouraged from raising crops that cannot be readily sold or easily processed. In many agricultural communities, including those in the United States, it has often been more profitable to raise nonfood crops—such as tobacco, cotton, trees, and flowers.

Even foods that we buy in their "natural" state, such as eggs, fresh fruits, and vegetables, are usually routed through various middlemen. They undergo processing such as cleaning, sorting, and packaging. Inedible portions, such as husks and pods, are removed. Naturally occurring toxins are inactivated. Filth and impurities such as twigs, pebbles, and dirt are washed out.

Other processing operations are performed to preserve food products so that they can remain free of microbial spoilage, rancidity, flavor loss, destruction by enzymes present in the food, and other types of deterioration over the period of time necessary for transportation and storage. Such processing helps ensure economical, digestible, safe, and clean products that can be transported, stored, and made available to consumers throughout the year, even when the food is out of season. Without a food industry the American population, especially in large cities, could not provide food for itself. The food industry is an essential and acceptable part of American life.

The following sections outline the major types of basic food-processing procedures in use today before food is even packaged, stored, or brought to the marketplace. Some of these date back to ancient times (3,4).

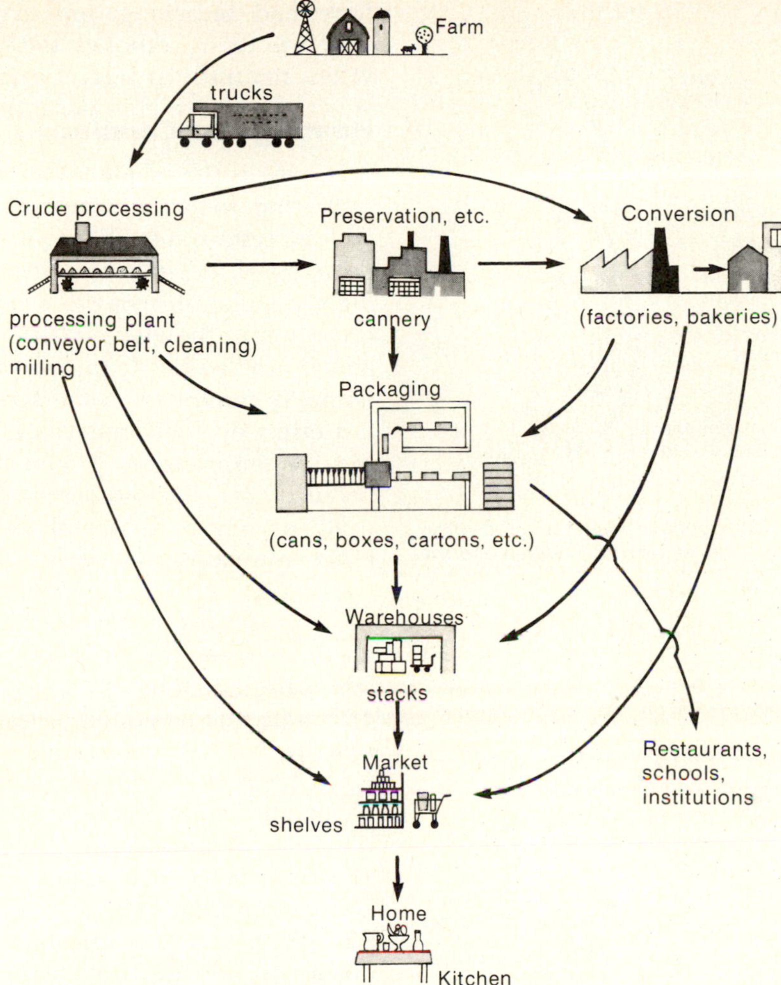

Figure 18–1 *Diagram of food channels from farm to consumer.*

Milling

Grains are milled to flour by removing the bran and germ of the kernel and crushing the endosperm (see Fig. 18–2). The products are separated by a series of sifters and rollers. The degree of milling will vary with the grade of flour desired. In the United States about 30 percent of the wheat kernel, mainly the bran and the germ, is removed to make common white flour. Thus, about 70 percent of the wheat is recovered as white flour—which is called in the trade an "extraction rate" of 70 percent. It has less nutritional value than whole-wheat flour (Table 18–3). White flour keeps better over long periods than does ground whole wheat, since most of the germ and bran is removed. Federal standards at present prevent an intermediate grade of flour of about 80 to 85 percent extraction rate. Such a flour would be nutritionally superior to the present white flour.

Most white flours in the United States

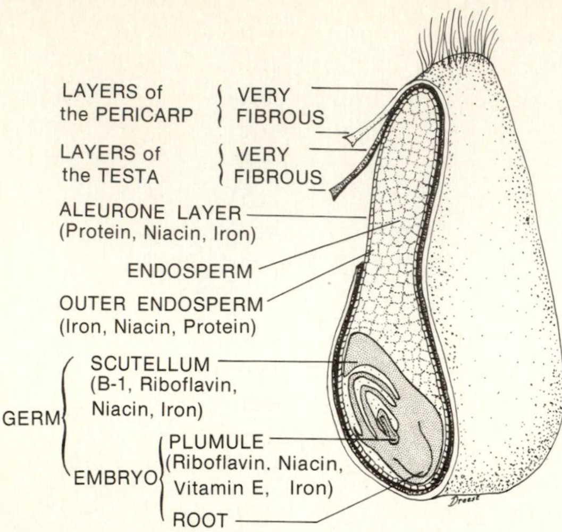

Figure 18–2 The distribution of nutrients in the wheat grain. (Courtesy of Sir J. Drummond, Dr. T. Moran, and *The Lancet.*)

Table 18–3 LOSSES OF NUTRIENTS IN THE REFINING OF WHEAT[a]

	Composition		
Nutrient	Wheat mg/kg	White Flour mg/kg	Loss in Refining %
Thiamin	3.5	0.8	77
Riboflavin	1.5	0.3	80
Niacin	50	9.5	81
Vitamin B-6	3.4	1.0	71
Pantothenic acid	10	5	50
Folacin	0.3	0.1	67
α-Tocopherol	16	2.2	86
Choline	1089	767	30
Manganese	46	6.5	86
Iron	43	10.5	76
Zinc	35	7.8	78
Calcium	450	180	60
Phosphorus	4330	1260	71
Magnesium	1830	280	85
Potassium	4540	1050	77

[a]Adapted from Schroeder, H. A.: Amer. J. Clin. Nutr., *24*:562, 1971 (before enrichment).

have had bleaching and maturing agents added to them, although the white color develops naturally to a great extent in storage.

Heating and Canning

Heating is the major traditional method of preparing foods for consumption at home and in restaurants. It requires a fireplace, oven, stove, or, in recent years, the increasingly popular microwave oven (5). Heating can result in the loss of nutrients such as the amino acid lysine. It can also reduce the vitamin B content of some foods, but it has less effect on food minerals (3). Some foods may be improved nutritionally by heating because heat destroys certain inhibitors naturally present in food, such as the trypsin inhibitors in various legumes.

Canning, a more sophisticated form of heating, is a major means of maintaining an adequate food supply throughout the year. The canning industry started in France in 1809 with the invention of the canning process by Nicolas Appert and began in the United States in 1819. It gained steadily in volume after the introduction of processing under steam pressure in sealed tins (cans) in 1874. Under steam pressure, processing is accomplished at higher temperatures and in a much shorter time and results in a better-quality product. The high temperature, along with the presence of acid in some foods, is important to inactivate microbes that may produce toxins in the sealed can. For many foods, including some that have been concentrated by removal of water, the sealed can offers a convenient way to transport and store food without refrigeration.

A recent variation on canning is the increasingly popular *retort pouch.* It is a sealed, laminated, plastic (sometimes aluminum foil) bag in a shape that allows food to be heated to 250°F (121°C) for shorter periods of time. Its use results in improved flavor, energy content, convenience, quality, and often, nutritional value (6). The pouches do not require refrigeration or freezing.

Another related preservation process is *aseptic canning,* in which food is canned under aseptic, or near sterile, conditions. In this way levels of harmful bacteria are kept as low as possible. This process requires much less heat than is otherwise necessary.

Pasteurization is another process employing heat. Milk, for example, is heated to a high temperature of 161°F (71.5°C) for fifteen seconds and immediately cooled. Insignificant amounts of nutrients are lost.

Considerable attention is being given in the United States and countries where refrigeration is not readily available to *sterilization* of milk for a few seconds at *ultrahigh temperatures* (UHT) from 205° to 307°F (96° to 153°C) (7). Aseptically packaged UHT milk will keep at room temperature for many months with very little loss in flavor, but it is more expensive than regular pasteurized milk.

Dehydration

Dehydration (reduction in water-activity by removal of some or all of the water) is a time-honored method of food preservation that goes back to the beginning of human society. It is still one of the best ways of preserving foods and reducing transportation costs (8).

Technological advances have made possible products of much-improved quality at lower cost. New methods include quick drying at low temperatures under vacuum or reduced pressure, with controlled temperature and fans for removal of the water vapor.

If the product is in liquid form, it may be blown in small droplets into a heated chamber, where it dries almost instantly to a fine powder, a process called *spray drying*. The resulting product has excellent keeping qualities and can later be "reconstituted" by the addition of water. This process has given us the very useful dried milk, which is the least expensive and most transportable form of milk solids. Other products made by spray drying are cream substitutes for use in coffee, citrus products, other fruit beverages, and instant coffee, all of which are ready for use merely by adding suitable amounts of water.

Partial dehydration, as in "intermediate-moisture foods" or in condensed or evaporated milks, has long been in use. Solid foods may be dehydrated by being cut in thin slices that are passed on a conveyor belt through an oven, or they may be finely mashed and placed on a perforated tray or mat. A current of heated air is blown up through the perforations. Such processes have been successfully used in drying fruits (for use in prepared cereals), and vegetables (for casserole dishes and soup mixes). Macaroni, spaghetti, and dried fruit, cheeses, eggs, and meat are other examples of commonly dried foods.

Dehydrated foods, precooked or raw, have been developed for activities that require lightweight foods (for example, for hiking or camping trips). These keep without refrigeration over long periods and can be reconstituted with the mere addition of hot or cold water. Such foods, specially packaged, are readily adapted for air drop in emergency situations or for space travel.

Cooling and Freezing

Since earliest times people in cold climates have cooled or frozen foods to preserve their quality and prevent spoilage by microorganisms. Today in those areas this principle, generally by some sort of mechanical refrigeration, is still the most common method of keeping food fresh.

Until well into the twentieth century people in rural areas kept perishable food in root cellars, or cold cellars, dug in the earth or near cold spring water. Houses in villages and cities had an "ice box," to which ice was delivered regularly. Some had cold pantries or used an outdoor shelf in winter. These methods are still used in areas in this country and around the world where mechanical refrigeration is not available. In commercial processing of poultry billions of pounds are still chilled rapidly by immersion in ice water, a cooling process more efficient than refrigeration.

In the early 1930s, especially in developed countries, mechanical home *refrigerators* became common. They are now considered a necessity wherever possible. Their temperatures of about 40°F (4°C), or below, are most effective in preserving food without freezing.

Frozen foods came into wide use in the 1940s when freezer compartments in refrigerators and separate freezers for quantity storage became available. Their propularity has gradually increased. Home freezers are kept at temperatures of −10°F (−23°C) up to 10°F (−12°C). Commercially, foods may be frozen at still lower temperatures for maximum effectiveness.

Meats, poultry, fish, fruits, and vegetables are the foods most commonly preserved by freezing. The variety and quality of frozen foods continue to improve, and one can purchase them in packages of different sizes to suit the customer's need. Also, complete frozen dinners and other meals are now widely available.

Because of their acceptable flavor and the saving of labor in preparation, frozen foods are strong competitors with fresh varieties. Frozen fruits and vegetables are especially valuable for variety in the diet during the seasons when fresh produce is scarce or high in price. Frozen fruits and vegetables must often be *blanched* first, by heating in water, in order to destroy enzymatic activity. Blanching usually results in some flavor and nutrient losses.

Most frozen foods must constantly be kept refrigerated in storage, in transport, and finally in the grocer's display counter, all of which adds to their cost. Those frozen foods that sell in very large volume are competitive in price with fresh products, or they may even be cheaper. For example, frozen, concentrated orange juice usually is cheaper than fresh orange juice. Other frozen foods that entail considerable labor in preparation and expense in packaging and refrigeration tend to be luxury items, which the consumer may buy, regardless of cost, in order to save time and labor in preparing meals.

Freeze-Drying

Foods may be frozen raw or precooked and may be partially dehydrated either before or after the freezing process. In the latter process, *freeze-drying,* raw food is quickly frozen, then passed into a special vacuum chamber, where the moisture is removed from the food by *sublimation*—that is, ice crystals go directly into the vapor state without passing through the liquid state. Freeze-dried foods have a spongy texture but retain their shape and flavor, require no refrigeration in storage, and can be reconstituted readily by being placed in warm water. The reconstituted product looks and tastes very much like its fresh counterpart. Many products, including instant coffee, onions, chives, and other vegetables, are freeze-dried.

Modified-Atmosphere Storage and Vacuum Packing

The freshness and nutritive value of foods are preserved longer during refrigeration when the atmosphere (air) is modified or removed entirely.

Commercially, fish, seafood, meat, and other fresh products may still be sold as "fresh" after a week if they have been transported and kept under refrigeration and in *modified-atmosphere storage.* When the conditions are still more rigidly controlled, they are in controlled-atmosphere storage. The atmosphere consists of high levels of carbon dioxide (CO_2) and/or nitrogen (N_2) along with some air or oxygen. Other mixtures of gases may be used depending on the product and length of storage. The method was developed for practical use in the 1930s but has gained considerable popularity recently (9).

Vacuum packing, in which all air is removed from a container, serves a similar purpose and is widely used today for a number of perishable food products. Plastic, airproof containers used for snacks and other cereal products are a modified version of vacuum packing.

Fermentation and Pickling

Although yeast and bacteria are generally considered to cause spoilage of foods, *fermentation* of food by desirable microorganisms is a common method of preserving and processing. In some instances it may even improve the nutritive value. Yogurt, most breads, cheese, buttermilk, olives, wine, beer, certain sausages, sauerkraut, fermented pickles, and tempeh (a soybean preparation) are examples of foods preserved or made with microorganisms. Lactic acid, acetic acid, and ethyl alcohol are the major products of fermentation that aid in the making of these foods.

In the past, cabbage, cucumbers, and other vegetables were often preserved by fermentation. Today they are often preserved by *pickling,* by being put directly into vinegar (mainly dilute acetic acid) and salt.

Food Additives: Salt, Sugar, Spices, and Smoke

Foods have been preserved by *salt* since earliest times. Salt effectively lowers the water-activity, thus preventing microbial spoilage. Vegetables, fish, and meats are still salted in many parts of the world. Salt is used in modern pickling procedures of cucumbers and olives. Salt is now less commonly used in processing foods in the United States because of the availability of refrigeration and the recent concern about excessive salt in foods. Sugar is used in much the same way as salt—to control microbial growth. Sugar preserves fruit and fruit flavors in jams, jellies, and candy and helps keep cookies, sweet rolls, and certain desserts "fresh" for extended periods. Spices also preserve food and enhance its flavor. Allowing foods to absorb wood smoke is another time-honored method of preservation still practiced today. Smoked ham, fish, and other sea foods are common examples of smoked foods.

Many other food additives are used today for a variety of reasons. They are discussed later in the chapter.

Radiation

Preservation of foods by *radiation* is being tested and used to some extent as a means of decreasing spoilage. Bombarding foods with electromagnetic waves that create ions appears to be most effective when the foods are dehydrated and/or vacuum packed. The most practical use of radiation processing today is administration of low dosages to destroy insects that infest cereals and to inhibit sprouting of onions and potatoes. These applications, though approved, are not used commercially in the United States at present and general approval of radiation processing with all foods has not been given. Legally, it is considered a "food additive" by the Food and Drug Administration (FDA) since it is still controversial (10).

Fabricated, Imitation, and Substitute Foods

The manufacture of fabricated, imitation, and substitute foods (also called engineered or manufactured foods) is another method of modern food processing. Unlike the previous methods, however, its purpose is not so much to preserve basic foods as it is to make available new types of food that will sell better, keep longer, have improved functional properties, or be more economical than the original product. Margarine, imitation fruit drinks, meat analogues, imitation dairy products (cheese, milk, and cream), and pancake syrups are examples. They represent an ever-increasing share of the food market (11). Manufacturers of such foods are not always concerned with better nutrition. Many fabricated foods are not nutritionally equivalent to the natural food they imitate. Some, however, have less fat or salt or higher levels of certain vitamins than the original product.

Some of these foods are manufactured from textured or extruded proteins (usually soybean proteins), which can be modified in many ways to imitate meat, dairy, egg, or other protein-rich foods. Various thickeners (gums or modified starches), colors, flavors, and other additives are often used to make the imitation resemble the original as closely as possible. In some instances such foods imitate no particular traditional food (cola drinks, calorie-free drinks, candies, and some desserts are examples) but are new kinds of foods.

In summary, preservation or processing by these methods or combinations of them, along with adequate packaging and storage procedures, allows for the transport of foods to areas where they are not produced or are in short supply. Although processing may decrease nutrient content, the loss may be made up, at least in part, by enriching the food and by more careful selection of other foods by the consumer. Also, it should be kept in mind that additional losses of vitamins and minerals can occur during final preparation of foods in the home or in food establishments just prior to eating.

NONNUTRIENTS AND TOXINS THAT OCCUR NATURALLY IN FOODS

As mentioned previously, in relation to the few essential nutrients in foods, thousands of chemicals that occur naturally in plants and animals have no known nutritional value to humans (4,12). The common potato, alone, has hundreds of such compounds. Many hundreds of these nonnutrients are known to be toxic when consumed in large amounts. Many have become useful drugs.

Nonnutrients encompass many categories of chemicals. Some may be antinutrients, such as avidin in raw egg whites (see Chap. 11) and thiaminases found in some raw fish, bracken fern, and blueberries. Some are plant pigments, such as chlorophyll. Some nonnutrients in food are *mycotoxins,* metabolites produced by fungi, including the toxins in poisonous mushrooms such as *Amanita phalloides,* the "death cup."

Nonnutrients in Common Foods

Many people think that if a substance is naturally present in a plant food it must be important to humans in some way. Some health-food stores encourage this mistaken belief by selling products rich in "bioflavonoids," chlorophyll, nucleic acids, para-aminobenzoic acid, inositol, and other nonnutrients present in natural foods.

Table 18–4 lists the major categories of the many nonnutrients in such foods as fruit, berries, onions, cheese, fermented foods, herbs, and spices. Some are formed in the processing of foods and so do not necessarily occur in the raw, fresh form. As far as is known, the compounds are nontoxic at the usual levels of foods eaten.

Inhibitors and Toxins in Foods

Many hundreds of compounds in foods are inhibitors, toxins, drugs, and, in some

Table 18–4 MAJOR CATEGORIES AND TYPES OF NONNUTRIENTS NATURALLY PRESENT IN COMMON FOODS, OR PRODUCED IN PROCESSING
(Not Considered Toxic at Usual Intake Levels in Mixed Diets)[a]

Categories and types of compounds (with some specific examples and with rough estimates of numbers of compounds)
I. NATURAL FOOD PIGMENTS (> 400)
Anthocyanins, betalaines and betacyanins, caramels, carotenoids, chlorophylls, terpenoids (gossypol), and tumeric pigments (curcumen).
II. NATURAL FOOD FLAVORS AND VOLATILE COMPOUNDS (>1500)
Aldehydes (propanol, hexanal, furfural), alcohols (methanol, ethanol, hexanol), cinnimates, esters (acetates, butanoates), ethylene, hydrocarbons (cymene, limonene), isothiocyanates, ketones (acetone), oxazoles, pyrazines, pyridines, pyrroles, sulfides, terpenes, and thiols.
III. NATURAL FLAVONOIDS AND OTHER PHENOLICS (> 1000)
Chalones, coumarins, flavones, flavonoids (rutin, hesperidin, quercetin), lignins, phenols (propyl-gallate, chlorogenic acid), quinones, serotonins, and tannins.
IV. NATURAL HORMONES, HORMONE-LIKE COMPOUNDS, AND STEROIDS (> 50)
Estrogens and estrogen-like substances, prostaglandins, steroidal alkaloids (solanine), and sterols and methyl steroids (cholesterol, sitosterol, and stigmasterol).
V. NATURAL NITROGEN CONTAINING COMPOUNDS (> 3000)
Alkaloids, amines (histamine, tyramine), benzo(a)pyrenes, carnitine, creatine and creatinine, cyanogenic-glycosides, enzymes and coenzymes, methyl-amines, nitrosamines, nucleosides and nucleotides, non-essential amino acids, nucleic acids (DNA, RNA), peptides, polyamines (cadaverine, putrescine, spermidine, spermine), pterins, purines (adenine, guanine, xanthine, caffeine, theobromine, uric acid), pyrimidines (uracil, orotic acid, thymine, cytosine), ammonia, indole, skatole, urea, and others.
VI. SPECIFIC NATURAL INHIBITORS AND TOXINS IN CERTAIN FOODS—NORMALLY PRESENT IN DIETS IN NON-TOXIC AMOUNTS (> 500)
See Table 18–5 and text (some are destroyed on cooking).
VII. OTHER CATEGORIES AND TYPES OF COMPOUNDS NATURALLY PRESENT IN FOODS (> 1000)
Coumarins, glucosinolates-goitergens, gums, heavy metals, maillard-reaction compounds, mutagens, organic acids (lactic, pyruvic, benzoic, oxalic), phytates, salicylates, saponins, non-nutrient sugar and sugar derivatives (glucuronic acid, raffinose, inositol, heptulose, stachyose), trace elements—non-essential, and waxes.
VIII. CONTAMINANTS (HUNDREDS ARE POSSIBLE AT NON-TOXIC LEVELS)[b]
Aflatoxins and other mycotoxins, agricultural chemicals (fertilizers, pesticides, and feed additives), industrial chemicals, migrants from processing agents and packaging materials, and nitrates and nitrites.

[a]Not an all-inclusive listing: We consume these hundreds of nonnutrients daily in less than 1 to 2 percent of our intake of foods. Roughly, over 90 percent or more of these types of compounds occur naturally in foods, up to 5 to 9 percent are released or formed during food processing, and less than 1 percent are contaminants. (Also see Table 18–5 for examples of food toxins, and Table 18–6 for food additives.)

No one has attempted to count all the different natural compounds in foods. There are thousands of different enzymes alone. Over 225 flavors have been found in potatoes, for example, over 70 compounds in cinnamon, over 220 volatile compounds in grapes and wine, over 180 in cooked chicken, with countless more in raw or cooked berries, vegetables, grains, fruit, milk, animal products, eggs, fish, spices and herbs and other common foods (most compounds are found in many different foods—there is much overlapping).

Also see supplementary readings and current issues of J. Food Sci., J. Agric. Food Chem., Food Chem., and the many other peer-reviewed food science journals from this and other countries. This is a constantly unfolding field.

[b]Often, non-toxic trace levels of contaminants can be found in foods by modern analytical techniques—levels considered insignificant. In rather rare situations, contamination of foods with high levels of toxins has occurred. Examples are mold growth in food storage facilities with moisture problems, in bakeries or processing plants with inadequate quality control procedures, or when animal foods have become contaminated with toxic substances passed on into meats, milk, or eggs.

instances, mutagens or even carcinogens. Some of these are natural compounds, and some are produced during normal processing procedures. The severity of their effect depends on the amount consumed (4,13,14,15,16). (See Fig. 18–3.)

Foods contain compounds that may inhibit enzymes, interfere with the central nervous system, give hallucinogenic effects, or promote goiter. Some have the capacity to increase blood pressure. *Safrole,* a natural component of sassafras, was used as a food additive to flavor root beer until it was reported to produce cancer in laboratory animals. *Glycyrrhizic acid,* a component of licorice, may cause electrolyte imbalance if ingested daily in large enough quantities.

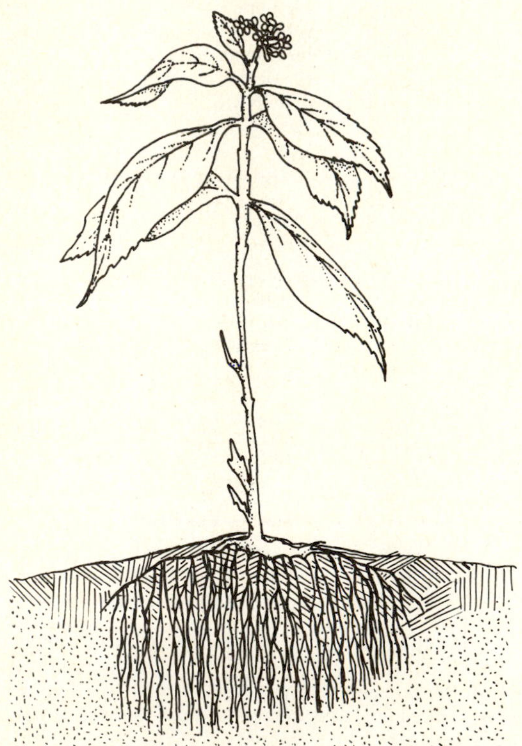

Figure 18–3 Some naturally occurring nonnutrients serve as therapeutic drugs. The root of the Rauwolfia plant is a source of reserpine, a tranquilizer. The root has been used in India for centuries to treat many diseases, including mental disorders.

Pressor amines, compounds found in fermented foods such as cheese, wine, and salami, when eaten with some prescribed tranquilizers may lead to an increase in blood pressure. (See Table 18–5.)

Thus, in some instances the consumption of certain naturally occurring nonnutrients may have adverse effects ranging from mild discomfort to serious consequences. In fact, many common natural components of food probably would never be allowed as food additives, since they would fail strict U.S. safety regulations. In addition, many naturally occurring substances, if allowed as food additives, would not be permitted in foods at the levels found naturally. The margin of safety for putting such substances into food is about 100 times less than the highest level that produced no adverse effects on subjects in animal studies. The margin of safety for many naturally occurring toxicants, however, is less than that permitted for food additives.[2] For example, the margin of safety for goitrogenic (goiter-promoting) substances is estimated as less than ten (17). It should also be noted that the margin of safety for some naturally occurring nutrients in our diet is much lower than 100. The margin of safety for sodium is estimated at less than 5; for iron, zinc, copper, and fluorine at 5 to 10; and for vitamins A and D at 25 to 40 or so for adults (17).

It is hypothesized that early humans discovered which foods were toxic by trial and error; thus foods associated with ill effects that occurred soon after ingestion were

[2]A lower margin of safety is not, in itself, necessarily hazardous but depends on the conditions of ingestion. This disparity between the levels of some naturally occurring substances and those of permitted food additives points up the strictness of regulations concerning food additives. As pointed out by P. B. Addis (Food Technol., *33* (Oct.):126, 1979), "The natural selection process has probably developed a tolerance toward naturally occurring toxicants which would not exist in the human population for food additives."

Table 18–5 EXAMPLES OF NATURALLY OCCURRING TOXINS, THEIR SOURCES AND TOXIC ACTIONS

Nonnutrient	*Food Source*	*Mode of Action*
Safrole	Sassafras, mace, nutmeg	Carcinogen
Myristicin	Nutmeg, dill, parsley	Hallucinogen
Methylmercury	Swordfish, tuna	Neurotoxin
Cyanogenic glycosides	Fruit seeds, cassava, legumes	Cyanide poisoning
Solanine	Potato shoots and skin	Acetylcholinesterase inhibitor
Aflatoxin	Mold-contaminated farm products	Carcinogen, liver toxin
Avidin	Raw egg whites	Biotin antagonist
Goitrogens	Brussels sprouts, broccoli, kale, soybeans	Promote goiter
Carototoxin	Carrots	Nerve poison
Benzo(a)pyrene	Smoked and charcoal-broiled meats	Carcinogen
Thiaminase	Bracken fern, raw clams and mussels, tea	Thiamin deficiency
Ergot alkaloids	*Claviceps purpurea*–infested grain	Gangrenous syndrome, CNS syndrome
Glycyrrhizic acid	Licorice plant	Hypertension
Genistein (estrogen)	Soybeans	Decreased weight and reproductive failure in rats
Amanitans	Amanita mushrooms	Liver and kidney damage
Tetrodotoxin	Liver and sex organs of puffer fish	Respiratory paralysis

avoided. This procedure exposed foods that produce short-term toxic effects but revealed very little about long-term effects of eating nonnutrients. Humans also discovered that some foods containing toxic substances could be prepared in ways that would detoxify or remove such substances. American Indians leached poisons out of acorns, and in Africa and South America people prepare *cassava,* a major food, by a water-soaking and fermentation process that releases *hydrogen cyanide* before the cassava is eaten. In addition, merely the usual heat used in cooking will inactivate many natural toxins, such as the *thiaminase* in fish; the *avidin* in egg; and the *enzyme inhibitors, hemagglutinins,* and *goitrogens* in legumes and other plants. Thus, staying clear of some foodstuffs and methods of food preparation has allowed humans to avoid the toxic effects of many natural nonnutrients.

In more recent times, new strains of plants have been developed so that the content of toxic substances is lessened. Thus, lima beans in the United States have a low content of hydrogen cyanide–releasing substances; and *gossypol,* a toxic substance present in cottonseed, has largely been eliminated from cottonseed oil. An example of plant breeding that led to a mixture of both desirable and undesirable qualities was the development of a potato that had excellent chipping and browning properties. Unfortunately, this newly developed strain also contained high levels of *solanine, an acetylcholinesterase inhibitor,* and could not be permitted on the market by federal regulations.

Hazards of Ingesting Naturally Occurring Food Toxins

All substances have an intrinsic toxicity; that is, if they are ingested at a certain level for a specified length of time, adverse effects will result. Even water is toxic if taken in excess quantities. However, humans can ingest small amounts of many substances of varying toxicity with no ill effects because of the remarkable detoxifying and defense mechanisms in the body. It is when the body's mechanisms become overwhelmed that we see most of the obvious toxic reactions. Therefore, the hazard of eating naturally occurring toxins is a relative phenomenon, depending on the context in which the food is eaten. Conditions of ingesting a food or naturally occurring toxin that might pose a hazard to the consumer (including amount, pattern, and interactions with other compounds in the diet) are more important to consider than the intrinsic toxicity of a compound.

On a worldwide basis, toxins in food that result from microorganisms and naturally occurring components of food have contributed the greatest number of food-related injuries to humans. Inadvertent or accidental contaminants of both natural and man-made toxins have contributed a lesser amount to food-related injuries, while food additives, agricultural chemicals, and chemicals produced in food during food processing reportedly have not led to adverse effects on human health when used according to good manufacturing and agricultural practices and when their intake is not grossly excessive (4,14,16,18).

Raw soybean meal, for example, is known to contain a pancreas-stimulating factor, a trypsin inhibitor, goitrogenic substances, saponins, estrogenic factors, hemagglutinins, and anticlotting factors. Upon heating, however, which is now common practice in making soybean foods, many of these potentially hazardous substances are inactivated.

It is a wonder how we can safely eat any foods, given the large number of naturally occurring toxins. Although many potentially harmful substances occur in our diet, usually no significant threat is posed. As previously mentioned, development of new strains of plants and improved methods of preparation of foods have helped to minimize the hazard. Additionally, proper storage of food reduces the hazard from microbial toxins, and the fact that many substances are present in such minute amounts, relative to their toxic level, insures safety. Notably, the interaction between substances in foods often reduces risk, or at least does not contribute to it. The toxicity of most chemicals is not additive, and interactions of some trace minerals are known to reduce the toxicity of other trace minerals. An example of the latter is the protective effect of zinc against cadmium toxicity. Also, the fact that food is transported throughout the world has helped to eliminate hazards deriving from local geochemical imbalances in the environment.

Circumstances occur, however, in which naturally occurring substances in the diet pose a threat. Certain foods usually avoided owing to their toxicity may accidentally or unavoidably be eaten, as has occurred in the misidentification of mushrooms and other plants. Also, foods generally avoided may be eaten in times of famine. *Lathyrism,* a neurological disorder involving weakness and paralysis of the lower limbs, has occurred periodically in parts of India and is associated with the consumption of a chickling vetch pea, *Lathyrus sativus,* during times of famine.

Ingestion of poisonous seafood and food

containing sufficient bacterial or fungal toxins will also lead to ill health, as will overconsumption of food that is not hazardous when eaten in "normal" quantities. Other conditions influencing the danger of ingesting certain foods include malnutrition, allergies, inborn errors of metabolism, and disease. Thus, some people may not be able to tolerate more than small amounts of lactose, and some may develop *hemolytic anemia* from the ingestion of cooked faba beans *(Vicia faba)* owing to a genetic predisposition.

A diverse and varied diet is the best way to eliminate any problems that arise from ingesting naturally occurring nonnutrients. This includes avoiding prolonged "fad" diets that involve an excess intake of any one food or an unbalanced food consumption.

Several examples of naturally occurring toxins are briefly discussed in the remainder of this section to illustrate their diverse nature and common occurrence in our food supply. Microbial infections and toxins are not discussed, although the greatest number of food-toxicity problems by far are due to bacterial infections of food (*Clostridium botulism, Clostridium perfringens, Staphylococcus aureus, Bacillus cereus, Escherichia coli* (a cause of many diarrheas), *Salmonella* organisms, *Shigella* organisms, and others). One should note, however, that bacteria are natural inhabitants of all external surfaces, including soil, air, water, plants, and even our skin, mouths, and gastrointestinal tracts. Thus, some bacteria, including some harmful ones, are usually present in all our foodstuffs. It is the amount and type of microbes that determine whether beneficial or ill effects result from their presence. The level of our resistance, including nutritional status, is also a factor.

Aflatoxins

One of the most potent liver carcinogens known in animals is *aflatoxin* B_1, one of a group of mycotoxins (fungal metabolites) collectively known as *aflatoxins. Aspergillus flavus,* a mold, contamination of foodstuffs including peanuts and maize appears to be the main source of aflatoxins. Wheat, rice, jowar, cottonseed, and grain sorghum also support the growth of *A. flavus,* as well as any food product in which the proper growing conditions prevail. Tropical areas with their high humidity and warm ambient temperatures favor the growth of *A. flavus.* There has been concern that unusual mold appearing on bread, cheese, jam, and other food products may signal danger of aflatoxin contamination; those who eat them should exercise caution (19).

Human susceptibility to carcinogenesis from aflatoxin consumption is still controversial. The removal of all aflatoxin-containing foods from the diet would greatly decrease the available food supply, resulting in malnutrition or starvation in some regions of the world. In the United States, corn, thought to be the greatest source of aflatoxin in the United States, and peanut products with more than 20 parts per billion (ppb) aflatoxins are illegal for interstate commerce. Fluid milk products with more than 0.5 ppb aflatoxin M_1 are not permitted by the FDA to be used in the manufacture of other dairy products. As yet, we do not know the hazard to humans, but the possibility exists that this unavoidable contaminant in the world food supply contributes to the occurrence of cancer.

Solanine

Solanine, a naturally occurring toxin and pesticide found in potatoes and tomato leaves, is an inhibitor of acetylcholinesterase, an enzyme needed for proper nerve transmission. In humans an oral dose of 2.8 milligrams (mg) per kilogram (kg) (about 200 mg total) has led to drowsiness and itchiness behind the neck. Greater consumption has resulted in vomiting and diarrhea. Lower levels appear to have no effect.

Potatoes are not allowed on the U.S. market if they contain an excess of 200 parts per million (ppm) of solanine. When bought fresh from the store, they usually contain less than 100 ppm of solanine. When potatoes are stored (even in dark places), their solanine content increases, being concentrated mainly in the shoots and to a lesser extent in the skin. About 4.5 pounds (2 kg) of whole potatoes with 100 ppm solanine, the highest levels found normally, would have to be eaten at one sitting to produce the initial effects (20).

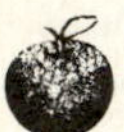

health considerations

Caffeine

The amount of caffeine in about two 5-ounce cups of coffee (about 200 mg) has a pharmacological effect. At this level it is known to stimulate the central nervous system, decrease fatigue, have a diuretic effect on the kidneys, increase heart rate, dilate blood vessels, and perhaps elevate levels of free fatty acids and glucose in the plasma. About 1 gram (gm) of caffeine will lead to insomnia, nervousness, and nausea. Larger amounts, taken at one time can, lead to convulsions and respiratory failure; a lethal dose is estimated at more than 10 gm (about 100 cups of coffee). Caffeine is found in coffee, tea, cocoa, cola, and many drugs.

Caffeine has been proposed as a weak *mutagen* and a *teratogen,* a cause of birth defects. This is an important consideration because caffeine crosses the placenta, and the blood concentration found in the fetus is the same as that in the mother. Also, caffeine can move freely into human ovaries and testes, so that it would have a chance to cause mutations at crucial sites if it were mutagenic.

Caffeine appears to be a weak mutagen in at least some nonmammalian systems; however, its significance to the human population is still unknown. Restrospective studies of women and their caffeine intake during pregnancy have shown no association between caffeine and birth defects. It has been suggested that humans may be protected from ill effects of caffeine because of their rapid metabolism of this chemical. There is no convincing evidence that the amount of caffeine in several cups of coffee a day is harmful to normal adults (including pregnant women) in any way.[3]

FOOD ADDITIVES

As the list of unfamiliar ingredients on a package grows longer so does the concern of the consumer. After all, how many people are able to recognize most chemical names and associate them with their function and safety? Chemical pollutants in our environment, industrial chemical accidents, and the emergence of newly recognized carcinogens, mutagens, and teratogens has sensitized the public to regard all "chemicals" as potentially hazardous. It should be recognized by most informed consumers that all foods are naturally made up of chemicals. Many persons remain perplexed, however, about which of the added and already present chemicals may contribute to adverse health.

The use of food additives has been traced to ancient times. The traditional use of salt, sugar, spices, and smoke in food preservation has already been noted. Ancient Egyptians used food coloring made from vegetables and insects; the Romans preserved fruit in honey and considered it a delicacy. Marco

[3]Good information about caffeine exists (21). Readers wishing more information about food toxins, food safety, nonnutrient compounds in food, and food additives should use the supplementary readings list in the Appendix and see current issues of food-science journals.

Polo and other European voyagers to the Orient sought food additives in the form of precious spices. Today food additives are routinely used, so that even a meal made from "scratch" in the home contains spices and herbs added to enhance color and flavor, and leavening to make bread rise (4, 14, 18, 22).

Nature of Additives

Many substances may be considered food additives, but for our purposes *food additives* will be defined as small amounts of substances intentionally added to a food for a specific effect or substances that become part of the food during processing or packaging. By this definition *direct additives* include substances used commonly at home, such as vanilla, salt, and garlic, as well as ingredients added during industrial processing, such as *propyl gallate* and *butylated hydroxylanisole* (BHA), which are used as antioxidants. Such a definition excludes, quite arbitrarily, added substances that provide a major caloric contribution to the food, such as sugar, corn syrup, unmodified starch, oils, and fats in the forms of shortening, butter, or margarine.

In addition to direct *additives,* which are intentionally added to foods for technical effects, there are *indirect additives,* which inadvertently become part of a food during handling. Examples of indirect additives are lubricants from processing machinery, plastics and BHA in packaging, and minerals from cooking vessels, Indirect additives such as these are present in such tiny amounts that they are generally negligible. In terms of this definition, it is estimated that there are about 2,000 to 2,600 direct additives and many thousands more of indrect additives in the United States alone.

Food additives may be pure or impure, products of nature or synthesized in factories. Spices are examples of impure, naturally occurring food additives. Calcium propionate (naturally found in Swiss cheese), sodium benzoate (a natural part of cranberry juice), and many vitamins are examples of pure chemicals that are added to foods but that occur naturally in them. Pure chemical substances synthesized but not found in nature include BHA and the coal tar dyes, such as FD&C Yellow No. 5.

Food additives were first legally defined in the United States in 1958. This official definition excludes pesticide residues and food colors, which are regulated by separate amendments, and substances that are generally recognized as safe (GRAS). A list of GRAS substances was first established in 1958 as a result of a major regulatory amendment, the 1958 Food Additives Amendment. This list represents substances that generally were in use prior to 1958 and whose safety was widely accepted by a surveyed sector of the scientific community. A few examples of the many food additives used in the United States are listed in Table 18–6 (4, 14, 18, 22). (Also see supplementary readings in Appendix.)

Purpose of Additives

There are technical, time-saving, and economic reasons—some essential, some not—for using food additives.

Technical reasons are that additives enable the manufacturer to achieve an aesthetically pleasing product with an increased shelf life and to supplement the nutritional value of the product. Food additives also allow the manufacturer to "improve" various food properties. Technical reasons for using food additives include the following:

1. Preservatives prevent spoilage and wastage of food by extending its keeping quality.
2. Aesthetic value is imparted to foods by the addition of colors, flavors, emulsifiers, stabilizers and thickeners, and acid-base adjusters. These add not only to eye appeal but also to the texture or "mouth feel." Aesthetic value is, perhaps, the most important function of food additives from the standpoint of the food industry since it has a large bearing on sales. For

Table 18–6 MAJOR CATEGORIES OF FOOD ADDITIVES, WITH EXAMPLES
(A listing of those added directly to one or more foods in the U.S.—examples of GRAS list substances also included.)[a]

Colors and Pigments

1. *Natural:* Annatto apo-8-carotenal, beet pigments, caramel, carotene, carrot oil, cochineal, grape skin extract, fruit juice, paprika, saffron, tomato paste, tumeric, and vegetable juice.
2. *Synthetic:* Citrus Red No. 2 (for orange skins only), orange B, certain FD & C colors (including Blue No. 1, Red No. 3 and 40, and Yellow No. 5).

Favors, Seasonings, and Flavor Enhancers

1. *Spices and Other Natural Sources of Flavors:* Allspice, almond, anise, balm, basil, bay leaf, caraway, cardamom, celery (salt and seed), chives, chili, chocolate, cinnamon, citrus oils, citron, cloves, cola, cumin, curry, dill, fennel, garlic, ginger, herbs (various ones), horseradish, lemon, licorice, lime, mace, mint, monosodium glutamate, mustard, nutmeg, onion, oregano, paprika, pepper, poppyseed, protein hydrolysates, rosemary, saffron, sage, salt, sesame seeds, smoked flavors, soy sauce, strawberry, terragon, thyme, vanilla, and wintergreen.
2. *Sweeteners* ("nonnutritive" and "nutritive")[b]: Aspartame, corn sweeteners (syrup, etc.), fructose, glucose (dextrose), polydextrose, saccharin (approval temporarily extended), sorbitol, sucrose ("sugar"), and xylitol.
3. *Synthetic Flavors (other than sweeteners—most also occur in nature):* Acetaldehyde, benzaldehyde, butyric acid, citric acid, citral, diacetyl, ethylacetate, isoamyl alcohol, lactic acid, limonene, malic acid, maltol, methyl butyrate, methyl disulfide, methyl propionate, and vanillin.

Leavening Agents (in dough and bread formation)

Monocalcium phosphate, sodium acid phosphate, sodium aluminum phosphate, and yeast (also see pH control).

Nutrients

Minerals and vitamins, etc. (see various nutrients in text and refs. 4, 14, 18, and 22).

pH Control—Acids, Alkaline Substances, and Buffers

Acetic acid, calcium carbonate, calcium oxide, citric acid, dicalcium phosphate, disodium phosphate, hydrochloric acid, phosphoric acid, sodium bicarbonate, sodium carbonate, sodium citrate, sulfuric acid, and tartaric acid.

Preservatives

1. *Acidity Control:* (see pH control above).
2. *Antimicrobial Agents:* Benzoic acid, calcium lactate, calcium propionate, citric acid, lactic acid, methyl paraben, nitrates, propionic acid, propylene glycol, sodium benzoate, sodium propionate, sorbic acid, sulfur dioxide, and wood smoke.
3. *Antioxidants:* Ascorbic acid, BHA (butylated hydroxyanisole), BHT (butylated hydroxytoluene), EDTA (a chelate), erythorbic acid, propyl gallate, and vitamin E (tocopherols).
4. *Other Preservatives:* Calcium ascorbate, calcium sorbate, carbon dioxide, gum guaiac, potassium bisulfite, sodium bisulfite, and sulfur dioxide.

Stabilizers, Emulsifiers, Thickeners, and Texture Enhancers

Agar-agar, alginates, carageenan, cholic acid, dextran, eggs, gelatin, gums (arabic, guar, locust bean, etc.), glycerides (di- and mono-), lecithin, median chain fats, modified starch, pectin, polysorbates, starch, and yeast.

Other Additives (miscellaneous)

1. *Anti-caking Agents (anti-stickiness):* Calcium silicate (and various other silicates), cornstarch, magnesium carbonate, mannitol, and silicon dioxide.
2. *Bleaching Agents:* Hydrogen perioxide, and potassium bromate.
3. *Humectants (to preserve moistness):* Glycerol, honey, and sorbitol.
4. *Pickling Agents:* Potassium nitrite and sodium nitrite.
5. Sequestants (to bind undesirable metal impurities): EDTA, citric acid, and phosphates (various ones).
6. *Others:* Effervescent agents (carbon dioxide), enzymes (lactase, papain), processing aids (calcium sulfate), surface acting agents, waxes and glazes, etc.

[a]Added during processing of foods (including packaged foods, snacks, candy, desserts, etc.) or in home preparation. Many additives have several overlapping functions. About 3000 to 4000 food additives are used in the United States, the largest category being about 1800 flavoring agents.

[b]A nonnutritive sweetener provides no calories or nutrients. An "artificial" sweetener, a term commonly used, is generally considered a synthetic one that does not exist in nature (though the distinction is hazy). One of these, cyclamate, is banned for use in the United States but approved for use in Canada as a nonnutritive sweetener.

this reason, more attention is often given to these aspects than to nutritional value.

3. Nutrients are added to food to improve or maintain preprocessing nutritional value. This important use of food additives has virtually eliminated the occurrence of such nutritional diseases as goiter as a result of soils poor in iodine, and pellagra, which was chiefly a result of niacin deficiency. Enrichment of foods with nutrients is discussed in a later section.
4. Maturing agents and agents that promote antifoaming, firming, hardening, drying, crisping, antisticking, anticaking, and whipping "improve" various characteristics of a food and enable the manufacturer to produce a uniform product. For example such food additives allow salt to pour freely and improve the baking characteristics of wheat flour.

A practical reason for buying foods with additives is convenience in food preparation. The lifestyle in more developed countries has changed rapidly during this century, and now many individuals prefer to spend less time preparing food and devote more time to other activities.

Economically speaking, food additives generally either help cut production costs for the manufacturer or aid in generating sales. For instance, preservatives make possible fewer deliveries to the store and less wastage. This saving to the manufacturer also often results in a lower product price to the consumer.

Amounts of Additives Consumed

Consumption of food additives is on the rise, accompanying the increased production of convenience foods, snack foods, and vitamin-supplemented foods. The amount of food additives consumed by the average American per year is an elusive figure because of lack of a uniform definition of additives and lack of accurate quantitative production and consumption data. An estimate was made by the President's Science Advisory Committee in 1973, based on the amount of food additives purchased by industry. On this basis, slightly more than 9 pounds of food additives were ingested per capita, excluding salt, dextrose, corn syrup, added fat, and sucrose. Of these 9 pounds, 7.5 to 8 are accounted for by thirty-two of the most commonly used chemicals, including flavoring agents such as mustard, pepper, and monosodium glutamate; gases for carbonating beverages; nutrient supplements such as calcium salts and sodium caseinate; and eighteen agents for leavening and the control of pH. The remaining 1.5 to 2 pounds is made up of all the rest of the hundreds of food additives.

Regulation of Additives

In the latter half of the nineteenth century, adulteration of food through the addition of harmful food additives in the United States was not uncommon. (See Fig. 18–4.) No federal laws governing food additives existed at that time. A sampling of candy in Boston in 1880 revealed 46 percent containing one or more toxic mineral pigments, chiefly lead chromate. Cheese was colored with red mercuric sulfide (HgS) and red lead (Pb_3O_4) compounds in some cases.

Adulteration was a deep concern of Harvey Wiley, a chemist for the U. S. Department of Agriculture (USDA) from 1883 to 1930, whose influence helped bring about the legislation of the Federal Pure Food and Drugs Act of 1906. This act prohibited the adulteration of foods. It was followed in 1938 by the U.S. Federal Food, Drug, and Cosmetic Act, which included further provisions against adulteration and also required the certification of coal tar dyes. Later, three amendments to this act shifted the burden of proof for safety of food additives, pesticide residues, and food colors to industry before their use could be approved. Thus, it was not until the U.S. 1958 Food Additives Amendment that a manufacturer had to

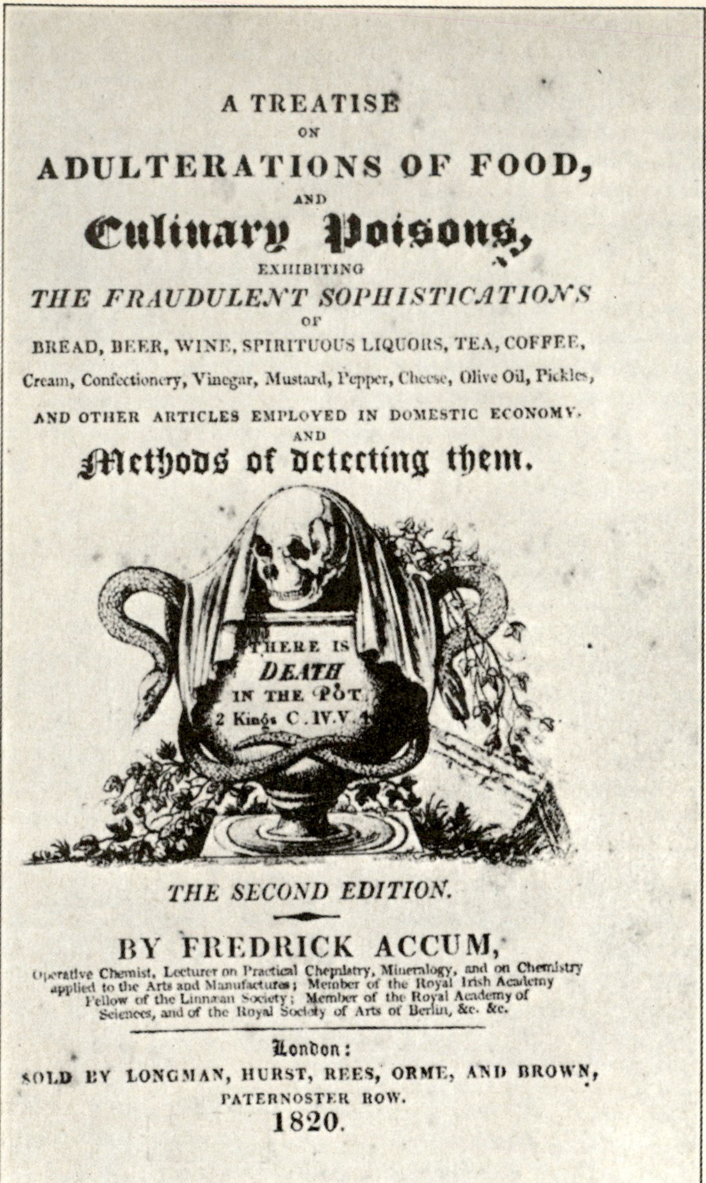

A TREATISE
ON
ADULTERATIONS OF FOOD,
AND
Culinary Poisons,
EXHIBITING
THE FRAUDULENT SOPHISTICATIONS
OF
BREAD, BEER, WINE, SPIRITUOUS LIQUORS, TEA, COFFEE,
Cream, Confectionery, Vinegar, Mustard, Pepper, Cheese, Olive Oil, Pickles,
AND OTHER ARTICLES EMPLOYED IN DOMESTIC ECONOMY.
AND
Methods of detecting them.

THE SECOND EDITION.

BY FREDRICK ACCUM,
Operative Chemist, Lecturer on Practical Chemistry, Mineralogy, and on Chemistry applied to the Arts and Manufactures; Member of the Royal Irish Academy Fellow of the Linnæan Society; Member of the Royal Academy of Sciences, and of the Royal Society of Arts of Berlin, &c. &c.

London:
SOLD BY LONGMAN, HURST, REES, ORME, AND BROWN,
PATERNOSTER ROW.
1820.

Figure 18–4 Prior to their regulation, food additives often constituted food adulteration. Fredrick Accum was a pioneer in exposing food adulteration in England. Authorship of this book led to the loss of his business and his friends. (From Chemistry, 46(5): 16, 1973.)

prove the safety of an additive to the FDA *before* its use in food, rather than the FDA proving that an additive was unsafe *after* it had already been added to foods.

The 1958 Food Additives Amendment also includes a provision known as the Delaney Clause. This clause states that "No additive shall be deemed to be safe if it is found to induce cancer when ingested by man or animals, or if it is found, after tests which are appropriate for the evaluation of the safety of food additives, to induce cancer in man or animals."

This clause has become controversial,

since some scientists think there is a "no risk" level of ingestion of carcinogens; hence, they think the clause interferes with the exercise of scientific judgment. Others are of the opinion that a low risk of cancer is outweighed by the benefits of some food additives. Still to be proven, however, is whether in fact carcinogenic substances have a no-effect ingestion level or merely present a lower risk when eaten in trace amounts. For this reason, other scientists prefer the clause as it is stated, based on the unknown rather than on our present knowledge, which is incomplete (23).

The regulation of additives and colors in food for interstate commerce in the United States falls under the jurisdiction of the Federal Drug Administration, while the regulation of pesticide residues, which remain on agricultural produce in interstate shipment, is controlled by the Environmental Protection Agency. International food standards, including those concerning food additives, are in part regulated by the Codex Alimentarius Commission, a joint Food and Agriculture Organization (FAO)/World Health Organization (WHO) commission. The commission was set up to protect the consumer against health risks and fraud and to facilitate international trade. More than ninety-nine countries have become members of the commission, and more than two-thirds of them are developing countries.

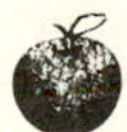

health considerations

The Safety of Additives

A chemical cannot be judged for safety on the basis of whether it is naturally occurring or artificially synthesized. There are many naturally occurring toxins and carcinogens, just as there are safe synthesized food additives. In addition, most consumers are not familiar with chemical names, so that reading a chemical name on the label does not tell them if it is natural or artificial, safe or toxic. Background information is needed for each substance before such judgments may be made.

In most developed countries, at least, food additives must now go through a rigorous testing procedure for safety before they will be approved. That was not true prior to 1958 in the United States and was not required for GRAS substances. Since 1958, methodology and testing procedures have continually improved; thus the government has imposed stricter regulations. Consequently, the number of new food additives (excluding flavors) approved by the FDA comes at a very slow rate. GRAS substances are under review at present (14,18,24).

Requirements for Safety Testing. Before being approved in the United States, a prospective additive must undergo safety testing, which generally follows certain accepted procedures of the National Research Council. Most often, the prospective additive goes through acute, subacute, and chronic (two-year) oral toxicity tests in at least two species of animals (usually rats and dogs), both male and female, to take into account interspecies and sex differences. Evaluations of possible reproductive, teratogenic, and mutagenic effects are made through multigeneration studies. Also, evaluations are made of possible subtle, long-term effects, including cancer, with lifetime studies. In some instances psychological or behavioral effects are evaluated. Investigations also determine the metabolic pathway of the additive and make sure that there is a practical method for determining the quantity of the additive in food (25).

Furthermore, an additive will not be approved by the FDA unless it has been shown to give the intended effect at the proposed level of use. Generally, as mentioned earlier, the amount approved for addition to foods includes a margin of safety of at least 100 times less than the highest level that caused no toxic effects in animal studies.

Problems in Evaluating Safety. There will always be problems involved with testing a compound for its safety. Direct extrapolation of data from animal experiments to humans is not possible, and investigators may not recognize subtle effects from feeding studies. Behavioral effects are particularly difficult to assess in animals. Interpretation of data is often not clear cut, and, owing to human error, experimental procedures may not always be optimal.

Industry has been known to influence the interpretation of some experiments, and the lobbying of industries and consumer groups may decide whether a substance is banned or not, even when scientific evidence is inconclusive for such a decision. Subjective evaluation plays a large part in such decision making, since inconclusive data and lack of scientific agreement often prevail.

It is important to weigh the biological risks against the benefits of each food additive and of the use of food additives in general. Weighing includes looking at how an additive may affect the total food, energy, and environmental system. For instance, if deleting a food additive results in abandonment of one processing method for a new method that increases the amount of carcinogenic air pollutants, is it more of a risk to eat the food additive or to breathe the pollutants? Ideally, it would be best to eliminate both sources, but we are not often given this choice.

A potential problem in the use of food additives may not be the safety of the additives themselves, but rather the nutritional safety of the fabricated foods that food additives make possible. These foods do not usually supply all of the vital known and unknown micronutrients and often contain high levels of sugar and fat. With the increasing consumption of fabricated foods, the possibility of diluted, imbalanced, and less nutritious diets may become a greater concern.

ENRICHMENT OF FOODS

Foods may be enriched to improve their nutritional value. *Restoration* is the addition to foods of nutrients lost in food processing, such as the vitamin C added to instant mashed potatoes. *Fortification* is the addition of nutrients to foods that may be replacing former common sources of certain nutrients (such as vitamin C in noncitrus fruit drinks), or the enhancement of the nutritional and economic value of a product (such as vitamins added to snack bars).

Enrichment is a legal term in the United States referring, for example, to the FDA program that requires thiamin, riboflavin, niacin, and iron to be added back to refined cereals (see Table 18–7). Fortification, enrichment, and restoration are terms often used interchangeably, as for example the first two are now legally indistinguishable in the United States (26). Meanings attached to them may vary, however, from country to country.

Foods may also be enriched for preservation rather than for improvement of nutrient composition. For example, ascorbic acid (as an antioxidant) can prolong the shelf life of products.

Technical Considerations

Once enrichment is deemed necessary, the first technical consideration is which foods should carry the nutrient in question. The choices are determined, in part, by who constitutes the target group. The eating habits of those in the group must be known, so that the food supplying the nutrient will be consumed in sufficient quantity to make a contribution to the diet.

A second technical consideration is the chemical form in which the nutrient is added. The nutrient should be in a utilizable form and should not change the appearance, flavor, odor, or keeping qualities of the food. For example, food technologists had to contend with the unfamiliar yellow color that

Table 18–7 COMPARISON OF THREE B VITAMINS AND IRON IN POUND LOAVES OF WHEAT BREAD[a]

Wheat Bread	*Thiamin mg*	*Riboflavin mg*	*Niacin mg*	*Iron mg*
Unenriched	0.40	0.36	5.6	3.2
Enriched[b]	1.8	1.1	15.0	8.0 to 12.5
Whole-wheat	1.17	0.56	12.9	10.4

[a]From U.S. Department of Agriculture: *Handbook 8,* according to 1980 standards (26).
[b]Enriched bread may also contain added calcium salts (including milk solids) in such quantity that each pound of the finished bread contains 600 mg of calcium (1320 mg/kg).

riboflavin imparted to rice. Adding the fat-soluble vitamins A and D to nonfat milk also posed a challenging technical problem. In order to keep bread volume high in protein-fortified loaves, dough conditioners and emulsifiers have been added along with the protein.

A third consideration is the manner in which food will be prepared. Coating rice with water-soluble vitamins, when the rice is cooked in water that is then discarded, does not increase the nutrient intake of the population. A more useful method of fortification of rice is the addition of a white, rice-shaped vitamin-mineral preparation in a ratio of 1 to 200 rice grains.

Nutrients found to be low in the diet of a population can be added to almost any product that is used widely. Staples such as wheat, rice, and maize have served as vehicles for niacin, riboflavin, thiamin, iron, calcium, and vitamin D. Vitamin D was first added to milk in the United States in 1929, and since 1924, salt has been fortified with iodine in the United States. Adding fluoride to water to bring it up to public health standards is another form of enrichment.

Enrichment of food with nutrients is an important source of these particular nutrients for the American public—at least for those who eat enriched products. Fig. 18–5 shows approximate percentages of these nutrients contributed to the total supply of nutrients. The cost of food-enrichment programs is very small. Enriching a whole loaf of bread, for example, costs only a fraction of a cent.

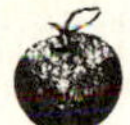

health considerations

Desirability of the New Enrichment Programs

Food enrichment is carried out as a public health measure. Sometimes a population or members of a subgroup are deficient in a nutrient. They may suffer gross deficiency symptoms (such as goiter in iodine deficiency) or exhibit biochemical signs of deficiency (such as low levels of iron in hemoglobin in iron deficiency). A change in a population's food habits may eliminate a source of vital nutrients. With food-enrichment programs, diets can be nutritionally improved without interfering with food habits. This is important, it can be argued, because people are generally averse to changing their habits. When habits do change, fortification may help keep the population's nutrient intake at an acceptable level. For example, with the increasing use of margarine in preference to butter in the United States, it became necessary to fortify margarine with vitamin A normally present in butter.

Persons responsible for the quality of our

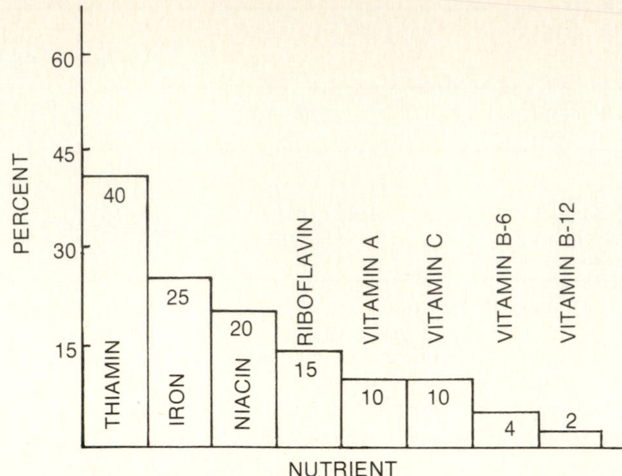

Figure 18–5 Approximation of food supply nutrients from enrichment or fortification supplementation. These are 1972 data but there is little reason to expect large changes since then.

food supply need to respect eating habits and preferences, be they culturally or individually determined. Food is viewed in many ways, only one of which is its role as a vehicle for nutrients. All of our nutrient requirements cannot be insured with any food-enrichment program unless the diet is properly chosen. Hence, it would seem that a more appropriate long-term goal is the provision of sound nutrition education so that populations will wisely change to more healthful eating habits.

When wholesome food adequate for a balanced diet is available, it may be difficult to see the reason for fortification. This is especially true when "unwholesome" vehicles such as sugar are chosen for fortification. Such vehicles as sugar, however, have served as expedient means in some countries of reducing some nutritional deficiencies such as that of vitamin A, but they should be viewed as only short-term stopgap measures.

Stopgap Measure? A potentially great problem with food-enrichment is the danger of its mushrooming from stopgap measure to the major means of coping with malnutrition. It could well stifle efforts of nations to implement long-range agricultural and nutritional improvement programs. There is the danger that an expedient fortification program will give a false sense of security when conducted at the expense of slower but more farsighted measures. Nutrients come from food, and it is impractical to provide them through fortification alone.

Aside from these advantages and disadvantages of enrichment, there are some practical problems with long-term fortification programs. As people's eating habits change, so do their nutrient intakes. Constantly adjusting enrichment levels to meet changing trends is cumbersome; not to do so, however, would defeat the public health objective of food enrichment. In the United States, bread enrichment standards were first established in 1943 to provide thiamin, riboflavin, niacin, and iron because the population was deficient in these nutrients. But with today's decreased bread consumption, the population is not receiving the amounts of these nutrients from bread, as planned. Also, additional nutrients have been shown to be low in American diets. Our needs change, but fortification levels often do not change as quickly, owing to a lag in legislation.

Fortifying at High Levels. The idea of fortifying a food to make it self-sufficient presents another problem. No food but human milk for the infant is the "perfect" food, and even that needs supplementation for infants after several months (see Chap. 23). Each food needs to be complemented by different types of foods to make an adequate diet. According to what we now know about nutrition, dependence on one so-called complete food, such as totally fortified breakfast cereal, would be unwise.

The addition of vitamins to foods with low nutritional value may cause the consumer to rationalize that it is legitimate to eat them in sizeable quantities, since they are obtaining some added nutrients by doing so. The high-caloric and less nutritive aspects of the food may offset this benefit, however, and may prevent the consumer from eating sources of other needed nutrients not included in the fortification. Another problem for the consumer is industry's manipulation of food fortification for economic benefit without true concern for the consumer's health. Advertisements and articles in food technology and food product journals speak of the benefits of "new markets" and increased sales of foods that result from food fortification. They usually say nothing about the increased cost for the consumer. In spite of these serious questions, the United States is approaching nearly unrestricted food-fortification programs.

FOOD LABELING

Food labeling, ideally, aids the consumer in making informed food purchases. Labels, to be read in the store or, less hurriedly, at home, are vehicles for both nutrition education and product information.

In the United States, food labels are required to list (1) the name of the product; (2) the name and place of business of the manufacturer, packer, or distributor; and (3) the net contents or net weight (Fig. 18–6).

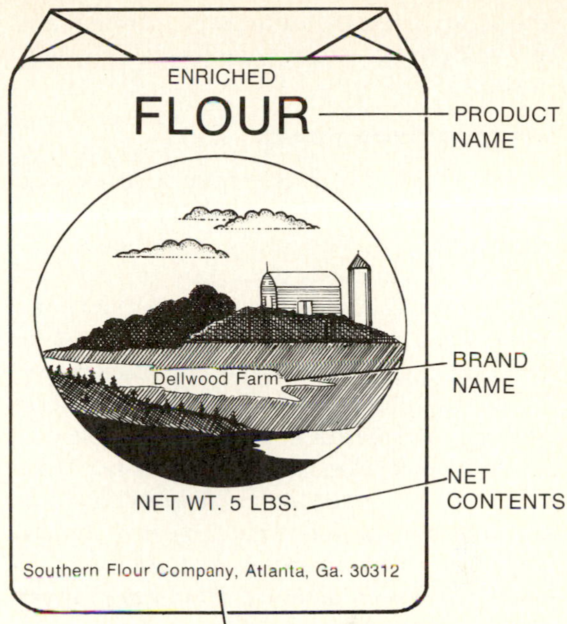

Figure 18–6 Food label with product name, net contents, and name and address of the manufacturer. Ingredients are not listed, since enriched flour is a standardized product. If a list of ingredients appears on the package, they are given in order of descending weight.

The net weight includes the liquid in which canned products are packed.

Most food labels in the United States also require a listing of the ingredients in order of descending weight. Fats or oils must be listed by their common or usual name (for example, coconut oil) rather than by a generalized name such as vegetable oil. At present, colors and flavors do not have to be listed by name but may simply be listed as "color" or "flavor," and the label must indicate if they are artificial. Federal law does not require the listing of coloring agents added to butter, cheese, and ice cream.

At the present time many changes in American food labeling rules are being made or are under debate. Many consumer groups want more nutrition information on food labels. Consumers, in general, want all labels to include a listing of all ingredients with their common name; the level, source, and kind of fat; the calories per serving; and the amount of sodium, cholesterol, and potassium (27).

Standardized Foods

More than 275 foods have a *standard of identity,* which is a standard "recipe" specifying limits of mandatory ingredients in a food. The standards also allow for optional ingredients. The mandatory ingredients of a food with a standard of identity need not be listed on the label; however, optional ingredients must be listed. All of the ingredients in some standardized foods have been designated as optional and, therefore, these particular foods require full ingredient labeling. Margarine, ice cream, peanut butter, jelly, soda water, macaroni and noodle products, and mayonnaise are examples of foods with standards of identity.

When the standards of identities were devised in the 1930s, it was still not uncommon to prepare such foods at home. Therefore, purchasers anticipated the presence of certain familiar ingredients in the purchased versions. The standards of identity insured that products would contain the expected ingredients in appropriate proportions. The FDA is considering requiring foods with standards of identity to list all ingredients, since consumers are now often out of touch with what goes into many of these products. Many manufacturers are doing this voluntarily with the encouragement of FDA.

USDA Grades

The USDA is responsible for the labeling and grading of most animal food products in the United States. Food labels of some 300 food products may bear a USDA grade (for example, USDA Grade A), which is voluntary but widely used, since the grade affects the price of these products. Products so graded include meats, eggs, and fresh, canned, and frozen fruits and vegetables. These grades are not based on the nutritional value of the food but primarily on appearance or texture, or both. The grade on milk and milk products is based on FDA recommended sanitation standards for the production and processing of these products.

Open Dating

Food labels may also include *open dating,* which indicates any one of the following: (1) the date when the product was packaged or processed, or the "pack date," such as appears on fresh meats in some markets; (2) the last day on which a retail store may offer a food for sale (which still allows for a reasonable time for product use before spoilage occurs), or the "pull date," which may appear on milk and refrigerated dough products; (3) the "use by" or "quality assurance date," after which the quality of a food has passed its peak but the product still may be used, which may appear on flour packages; or (4) the "expiration date," which denotes the last day a product should be used. This last is used, for example, on yeast and baby formula. Although these dates are potentially useful to the consumer, there is confusion about which meaning is to be attributed to a date on the product. No standardized format exists to indicate the meaning of the date or to specify the location of dates on the product.

Nutrition Labeling and the USRDAs

If a food is fortified with a nutrient or if a nutritional claim such as "low in cholesterol" is made for the food, then nutrition labeling is required; otherwise, nutrition labeling is voluntary. *Nutrition labeling* must include information specifying per serving size (Fig. 18–7): the amount of protein, carbohydrate, and fat in grams; the number of calories; and the percent of the *United States recommended daily allowances* (USRDA) fulfilled by seven vitamins and minerals. Information for twelve other vitamins and minerals and

CANNED FRUIT

NUTRITION INFORMATION

(PER SERVING)

SERVING SIZE = ½ CUP

SERVINGS PER CONTAINER = 4

CALORIES 120

PROTEIN .... 0 GRAM

CARBOHYDRATE ... 30 GRAMS

FAT .... 0 GRAM

PERCENTAGE OF U.S. RECOMMENDED DAILY ALLOWANCES (U.S. RDA)

VITAMIN C 2

THIAMINE 2

IRON 4

CONTAINS LESS THAN 2% OF U.S. RDA OF PROTEIN, VITAMIN A, RIBOFLAVIN, NIACIN, AND CALCIUM

Figure 18–7 A nutritional label panel containing the minimum information allowed.

for cholesterol, fatty acids, and sodium content is optional (4,27,28).

USRDAs are the Food and Drug Administration's simplified version of the recommended dietary allowances (RDAs) set by the Food and Nutrition Board in 1968, more than fifteen years ago.[4] The USRDAs (Table 18–8) usually represent the highest recommendation for a nutrient for nonpregnant and nonlactating females and males above four years of age. Therefore, the USRDAs actually may overestimate nutrient recommendations for some age and sex groups according to the Food and Nutrition Board RDAs, so that consumption of less than 100 percent of the USRDA does not necessarily result in a deficient diet. (This is also true for an individual eating less than 100 percent of the Food and Nutrition Board RDAs.)

The consumer needs to keep in mind that eating 100 percent of the USRDA for the seven listed vitamins and minerals does not insure an adequate diet, since these seven are just a few of the many nutrients essential to humans. In addition, the consumer should be conscious of the serving size for which the percent of USRDAs are listed. The serving size may be much smaller or larger than that which is normally eaten and therefore the consumer would be eating either less or more of the USRDA values listed on the label.

USRDAs should be used to compare one food with another for nutrient density (to relate the ratio of nutrients to calories or the ratio of nutrients to weight of the product), to learn which foods are good sources of the different nutrients, and as a guideline for eating a balanced diet—but not as the last word on an optimum diet plan (29).

Importance of Information on Labels

No one claims that present labeling regulations allow for as much product information as is desirable or that the format is without confusion. The FDA is at present considering changes in labeling with the hope that consumers will benefit from a more pertinent and informative format (27).

One consideration is the listing of food colors by individual names, since a small portion of the population may be allergic to specific food colorings. It has been claimed, for example, that 47,000 to 94,000 persons in the United States may be allergic to FD & C Yellow No. 5, or tartrazine (30). This estimate is based on the number of people who are allergic to aspirin, since these same people are often allergic to tartrazine. Many

[4]Because of legal restraints it is very difficult for the FDA to routinely update their "USRDAs." The 1968 RDAs were about 2 times as high then for vitamin E and for vitamin B-12. Otherwise there are no major differences.

Table 18–8 USRDAs*

	Used for Conventional Food or "Special Dietary Foods"	*Used for "Special Dietary Foods" Only*	
	Adults and Children 4 or More Years of Age	Infants and Children Under 4 Years of Age	Pregnant or Lactating Women
	*Nutrients That Must Be Declared on Label**		
Protein†	45 gm "high quality protein" 65 gm "proteins in general"		
Vitamin A	5000 IU	2500 IU	8000 IU
Vitamin C (ascorbic acid)	60 mg	40 mg	60 mg
Thiamin (vitamin B-1)	1.5 mg	0.7 mg	1.7 mg
Riboflavin (vitamin B-2)	1.7 mg	0.8 mg	2.0 mg
Niacin	20 mg	9 mg	20 mg
Calcium	1.0 gm	0.8 gm	1.3 gm
Iron	18 mg	10 mg	18 mg
	Nutrients That May Be Declared on Label		
Vitamin D	400 IU	400 IU	400 IU
Vitamin E	30 IU	10 IU	30 IU
Vitamin B-6	2.0 mg	0.7 mg	2.5 mg
Folic acid (folacin)	0.4 mg	0.2 mg	0.8 mg
Vitamin B-12	6 μg	3 μg	8 μg
Phosphorus	1.0 gm	0.8 μg	1.3 gm
Iodine	150 μg	70 μg	150 μg
Magnesium	400 mg	200 mg	450 mg
Zinc	15 mg	8 mg	15 mg
Copper	2 mg	1 mg	2 mg
Biotin	0.3 mg	0.15 mg	0.3 mg
Pantothenic acid	10 mg	5 mg	10 mg

*These figures are utilized for label information on any food that is enriched to provide more than 50 percent of the RDA of any given nutrient, plus any food that is said to be a special dietary food. If the dietary food is for young children or pregnant or lactating women, RDAs from the appropriate columns are used. (From the Food and Drug Administration, USDHEW.)

†"High quality protein" is defined as having a protein efficiency ratio (PER) equal to or greater than that of casein (a milk protein). "Proteins in general" are those with a PER less than that of casein. Proteins with a PER less than 20 percent that of casein are considered "not a significant source of protein" and may not be expressed on the label.

consumer groups would like to see the use of special symbols on labels that would indicate the presence of artificial colors or other food additives that may be of importance to consumers for other health reasons as well as allergies.

Nutrition labeling is being sought for nearly all the food on the market. Such labeling would greatly increase the amount of nutritional information available to the consumer, but it is not without its drawbacks. Nutrition labeling is especially difficult for fresh agricultural products, since the nutrient content varies with strain, weather, storage conditions, and a host of other circumstances.

In respect to nutrient content, nutrition labeling favors fabricated foods to which precise amounts of nutrients can be added. Also, in fabricated foods more of the specific nutrients identified on the label may be added to make the product appear, often unjustifiably, more nutritious than natural products. Furthermore, nutrition labeling may be more difficult for small companies that have no laboratories to analyze their products.

Nutritional-Quality Guidelines

The U.S. government is proposing voluntary nutritional-quality guidelines for certain classes of foods such as frozen dinners, breakfast cereals, and meat replacements. These guidelines would indicate appropriate levels and ranges of nutrients that should occur in these products. A guideline for frozen heat-and-serve dinners has already been established. A product that meets these guidelines may include on its label a statement that the contents abide by the U.S. government's stipulated nutritional guidelines for that class of food.

In the authors' opinion, guidelines should take into account trace elements and vitamins lost during processing, and fiber, as well as proportions and types of protein, fat, and carbohydrates. Guidelines not encompassing such a wide range of considerations may instill a false confidence in the consumer, who may feel that the statement of compliance with federal guidelines insures that the product is as healthful and nutritious as the original food.

FOOD BUYING

Consumers are concerned about higher food prices both at home and away from home. Such prices in the early 1980s averaged more than $1400 yearly per person in the United States. About 38 percent of the food dollar was spent on meals away from home in 1981, 12 percent higher than in 1960. This change has kindled renewed interest in the home preparation of food.

Food Costs

Our food supplies on the whole are less expensive today than they would be without present preservation methods. But in some instances, services built into a product add to the price the consumer pays. The advertising necessary to sell products and to make consumers aware of the availability of new products also adds to the price. The largest corporate food organizations spend about 5 percent of their income from sales on advertising (31,32).

For each dollar the consumer spends in the market for farm foods, the farmer receives about 30 cents. The farmer's share varies with the product.

Many marketing factors affect the cost of food. Foods that are scarce or out of season are often relatively higher priced. Those that are staples, have good storage life, and are in constant demand are cheaper. Choice cuts of meat are more costly because the amount of them is small in proportion to the whole carcass.

The cost of transporting the food to the consumer in good condition must be added to the total cost. Precooked and fancily packaged foods (especially in small portions) are usually more expensive. Advertised brands are no assurance of a higher quality than brands produced by smaller firms that do not advertise widely. Large chain stores often package and market their own "house brands" of staple foods, known as *generic foods,* at economical prices. Many stores offer special bargain days for certain foods they wish to "move" in quantity or for "loss leader" items, which can serve to draw people into the stores.

In spite of increased costs and rapidly growing inflation, the food budget of most American families is still only a relatively small part of their disposable income—about 17 percent for the average family. Low-income families spend up to about 40 percent for food and sometimes more.[5]

[5]These average figures exclude alcoholic beverages, which when included would add significantly to some food budgets. Also, the percentage of income spent on food varies widely according to area of the country, number in the family, and income level.

Consumer Demand

Items on the grocery shelf generally appear in response to *consumer demand.* But in modern marketing, this "demand" is often created. Usually a new product is devised, promoted through advertising campaigns, and then put to the test of *consumer acceptance.* For example, the change in preference from preparing cakes from basic ingredients at home to using mixes has come about primarily as a result of convenience coupled with advertising.

Consumers are constantly being urged to try new products. Those the consumer likes and continues to buy survive. The others join the several thousand new food products doomed to failure each year. It is the consumer's vote in the market place, influenced by advertising, that determines the long-term success of any food product or new convenience. That is why we need educated consumers to distinguish the nutritionally sound products from those with little or no nutritional value. The consumer should keep in mind that the major role of the food industry is not to make certain that the public is eating a nutritious diet. On the other hand, the industry is dedicated to making certain that abundant choices of tasty and nutritious foods are available in the market place (32).

Planning the Budget

The exact nature of the food budget depends on a number of factors. Among them are the following:

1. the number of members in the family and their food habits
2. where the family lives and how conveniently located the shopping areas are
3. the amount of food produced or preserved at home
4. special dietary needs, as in pregnancy and disease states
5. the availability of free or low-cost school foodservice programs
6. overall income and eligibility for food stamps or commodities

When a family budget is relatively liberal, certain foods of relatively high cost having nutritional value may be provided more easily. These foods include the so-called protective foods—milk, eggs, fruits, vegetables, and probably either more or higher-cost meats. The greater freedom of choice insures a better diet nutritionally only if wisely exercised, for the higher-cost foods are not necessarily those best for health. A so-called luxury consumption of foods rich in fat or salt, alcohol, and sweets does not insure health, and many cases of malnutrition still occur in families in which there is plenty of money for food. However, there is certainly less chance of malnutrition and its resultant ill health when the money spent for food is liberal than when it is scarce.

The size of a family is also a determinant of the food budget. A family of two adults usually has the most leeway on the amount to be spent for food, while the larger family, especially if there are several growing children, must spend not only a larger amount but also a greater proportion of its income for food. Young children and rapidly growing teenagers need a larger allowance of certain foods that are relatively more expensive (such as fresh whole milk, meat, and eggs for good quality protein; and fruits and vegetables for minerals and vitamins).

In certain sections of the country, such as the North Atlantic, Midwestern, and Pacific Coast states, the cost of living is higher than in other parts. City food costs vary more than in small towns, and when one lives on a farm and can produce part of the family food supply, the money spent for food is naturally less. If the food is produced locally and the homemaker has the time, equipment, and storage facilities, then home freezing, canning, drying, or other methods of preserving foods plentiful only in certain seasons may prove economical in the long run.

Efficient Buying

Efficient buying of food is one of the most satisfactory means of all to reduce food costs, because it involves no lessening in the variety, attractiveness, or nutritive value of the menu. By merely "stopping the leaks," enough saving may be effected to provide a better diet at less cost.

Considerable money savings can be effected by thrifty marketing. Some suggestions for efficient food buying practices are discussed in Table 18–9. In general, buying in larger quantities, watching for special bargains on certain foods, going to the market to select perishable foods that are of good quality, and selecting less expensive types or brands of food when these are suitable all result in lowering the food bill. One should plan to use some of the cheaper cuts of meat as often as feasible, for they may be just as nutritious as more expensive ones and are made very palatable if properly cooked. One should plan to use the organ meats, fish, legumes, or cheese in place of meat occasionally. Also, smaller amounts of meat may be "extended" by combining them with a starchy food, such as bread crumbs, noodles, or rice.

Table 18–10 gives suggestions of inexpensive food sources of various nutrients, helpful in connection with the information in Table 18–9.

Read package labels to know what you are paying for. Ingredients are listed in descending order of amount present. The consumer should look for the total contents in canned foods. Often a can with twice the quantity does not cost very much more than the smaller one. With fruits and vegetables, higher price is usually based on appearance and size rather than nutritional value. Those of lower size and price may well be suited for one's use, such as small, tart apples for applesauce.

Efficient Preparation with Minimal Loss of Nutrients

Proper preparation of foods can reduce costs and preserve nutritional value. Waste in the kitchen may occur in many ways. Some of the chief ones are (1) discarding portions of food that have nutritive value (vegetable trimmings, meat trimmings, cooking water, liquid from canned vegetables) and that are suitable for cooking; (2) burning foods or carelessly scraping them from cooking utensils in serving; (3) failing to utilize leftover foods properly; (4) wasting food at the table by taking individual portions that are too large or, rendering what is not eaten unfit to serve again; and (5) allowing food to spoil through improper care in storage.

Planning the menu ahead will help insure more efficient marketing. The buyer should keep in mind family food habits, preferences, and needs, and design meals that he or she knows will be enjoyed. The nutrients in food and the food in the market are of no value to anyone if the food is not eaten.

Some rules for minimizing the loss of nutrients in home storage and preparation are as follows:

1. Store perishables in a cool, dark place, preferably in the refrigerator. Buy no more than can be used.
2. Prepare perishables shortly before serving.
3. Save the water used in cooking vegetables, and use it for soup stock or in other foods.
4. Cook vegetables in a small amount of water, or steam them until just tender. To shorten cooking time, add the vegetables to boiling water.
5. Leave on skins of vegetables, if clean.

Nutrients must travel a long road before they reach the body. Food, which carries the nutrients, must be grown or raised on the farm, and then distributed, processed, and marketed through complex economic channels. It must then be bought at a store and prepared into appetizing meals. At every link of the chain, the nutrients in the food

Table 18–9 THE ECONOMY OF SUBSTITUTING CHEAPER FOODS IN THE SAME FOOD GROUP (or, how to save money in buying food)

Grain products—Even in this relatively inexpensive food group some foods are cheaper than others.
Corn and *rice* are usually cheaper than wheat.
The processed, fancy *ready-to-serve cereals* are relatively expensive.
Uncooked cereals bought in large quantity are usually cheaper than in small packages.
Oatmeal and *whole-wheat cereals* give especially good value because of their higher content of protein, minerals, and B complex vitamins.
Homemade *breadstuffs* are cheaper than some bakery products, and plain breads are cheaper than those with special flavor appeal. Crackers, sweet buns, cake, cookies, and doughnuts are relatively expensive.

Sweets—*Sugar* is one of the cheapest fuel foods but should not furnish more than about 10 percent of total calories.
Granulated white sugar is cheapest; *powdered* sugar, *loaf* sugar, *brown* sugar and *maple* sugar are considerably more expensive.
Molasses, corn syrup, and *cane* syrups are relatively inexpensive; blended syrups are of moderate cost; maple syrup and honey are expensive.
Jellies, jams, marmalades, and preserves are relatively expensive, but may be useful to make bread and other inexpensive starchy foods more acceptable. Homemade jams and jellies are least expensive.
Candy, except for simple hard candies, is an expensive form of sweets. All candies are high in calories.

Fats—*Meat fats, vegetable shortening* (from cottonseed, corn, or peanut oils), and *margarines* are relatively inexpensive; *butter* and *cream* are relatively expensive. *Olive oil* is an expensive fat.

Protein-rich foods—Cereal grains and legumes are the cheapest sources of protein, but should not be the only protein-bearing foods in the diet. Nuts are an excellent source, including peanuts and peanut butter. American (cheddar) cheese, milk (dried milk is one of the cheapest sources of complete protein), and *fresh* or *canned fish,* and poultry provide excellent quality protein at moderate cost. Eggs are a more economical protein source than most cuts of meat. Meats and shellfish are usually the most expensive of the protein-rich foods.

Flesh foods—Within this group cost levels differ greatly. Certain *fatty meats* may be relatively inexpensive, next come the *cheaper cuts* of red meats and the less expensive *fish,* next the more *tender cuts* of lean meats and cuts that may involve considerable waste, along with the more expensive forms of seafood such as shellfish. *Poultry* is usually moderately priced the year round. *Dried or canned fish* may offer good protein at low cost; canned *salmon* is valuable for vitamins A and D, and costs less than fresh salmon. *Frozen fish* are of excellent quality and have little waste.

Fruits—*Dried fruits* (raisins, dates, figs, apricots, prunes, peaches, and apples), an excellent source of minerals and some vitamins, were formerly inexpensive but have recently become high-cost. Any of them that are relatively inexpensive (e.g., prunes) should be used in the low-cost dietary. *Canned* or frozen *fruits* are usually less expensive than fresh, but they may not be when a fresh fruit is in season and plentiful. Of the *fresh fruits, apples, bananas* and *oranges* are apt to be the least expensive, though some of the others may be relatively cheap at the height of their season. The *citrus fruits* and *tomatoes* are especially valuable for their vitamin C content. Canned or frozen orange and grapefruit juices are usually the least expensive sources of vitamin C. Most expensive are the less common fruits and fresh fruits which are out of season.

Vegetables—*Potatoes* and the *root vegetables* are usually the least expensive.
Cabbage and some of the other *leafy vegetables* in their season are relatively inexpensive.
Leafy, green and *yellow vegetables* have the highest vitamin A value.
Dried legumes are relatively inexpensive. *Canned vegetables* are often moderately priced, and *canned tomatoes* are especially useful for adding flavor and vitamins to a low-cost diet.
Frozen vegetables (and fruits) afford variety in moderate-cost diets. They have the full nutritive value of fresh vegetables without having any of the waste.
Most *fresh vegetables* (especially the succulent ones) are at least fairly expensive, except at the height of their season.
The *less frequently used vegetables* and those that are out of season are generally the most expensive of all.

are subject to reduction. Careful processing, handling, and preparation of food, with an awareness of the instability and value of the nutrients within, can help insure that the money spent on food buys the nutrients necessary for a healthy life.

QUESTIONS

1. Choose five different kinds of food listed in Table 18–2 and give four examples of each. Give three adjectives to describe foods not in Table 18–2 and give two examples of each.

Table 18–10 INEXPENSIVE SOURCES OF VARIOUS NUTRIENTS

Nutrients	*Food Sources*
Energy	Fats, oils, flour, cereals, breads, potatoes, sugar, dried beans or peas, and peanut butter.
Protein	Dried beans or peas, peanut butter, whole-grain cereals or breads, milk (especially dried skim milk), cheaper cheeses, eggs, poultry, and less expensive meats and fish.
Calcium	Milk (especially dried skim milk), ice milk (dessert), cheese, dark green, leafy vegetables, whole-grain products, and legumes.
Iron	Dried beans or peas, liver, whole-grain or enriched breads or cereals, dark green, leafy vegetables, eggs, less expensive meats, potatoes and sweet potatoes, and prunes.
Vitamin A	Dark green and deep yellow vegetables, liver, fortified margarine, canned tomatoes, prunes, and less expensive cheeses.
Vitamin C	Canned or frozen citrus fruit juices, canned tomatoes, raw cabbage, some dark green, leafy vegetables, and potatoes.
Thiamin	Dried legumes, whole-grain or enriched bread and cereals, liver, inexpensive cuts of pork, and potatoes.
Riboflavin	Milk, ice milk (dessert), cheese, whole-grain or enriched breads, eggs, dried legumes, and dark green, leafy vegetables.
Niacin	Dried beans or peas, peanuts or peanut butter, whole-grain and enriched cereal products, meat, poultry, fish, and some dark green, leafy vegetables.

2. What motivated the development of so many new, processed foods since 1945? Name five methods of food preservation or processing that are now commonly used and two food products prepared by each type of processing. To what extent has the introduction of "convenience foods" changed our food habits and the consumption of different food groups? What are the advantages and disadvantages of extensive use of ready-to-serve and precooked foods?

3. List, and give the source, of five chemicals you eat regularly that are nonnutrients. Do you regularly eat any compounds known to be toxic? Explain.

4. Read the labels of various foods you have eaten in the past week and list five food additives present in them. What is the purpose of each additive? Discuss whether any of these have been useful in any way to you.

5. What is the difference between a GRAS substance and a regulated food additive (as legally defined in the United States)? Give examples of each.

6. List at least four considerations you would make before approving the fortification of a widely used candy with iron and folic acid. Which considerations are technical and which are nontechnical?

7. What arguments would you use to support the Delaney clause? To refute it?

8. What is the difference between the hazard and the toxicity of a compound? Under what conditions might the consumption of a naturally occurring toxin be hazardous? In general, does eating naturally occurring toxins in your diet pose a great threat? Explain.

9. Locate the following on a food label: (a) name and place of business of the manufacturer, packer, or distributor; (b) net contents or net weight; (c) list of ingredients; (d) nutritional infor-

mation (is this information required or voluntary for this label?); (e) open dating. What other information is given on the label?

10. List the differences between the USRDAs and the Food and Nutrition Board RDAs for your sex and age using the tables in the Appendix of this book.

11. Give examples of five foods you eat that are enriched. Estimate what percent of your total daily intake of these particular vitamins and minerals is supplied by these enriched foods.

12. Name four factors that influence the cost of foods. Name four factors, other than food prices, that affect the amount a family must spend to be adequately fed.

13. Give three principal ways to save money in the food budget. Which are especially useful for families of low income, moderate income, and high income? Why?

14. Calculate the grams of protein yielded by a dollar's worth each of legumes, milk, eggs, chicken, and whole-wheat bread using today's prices. How many calories would a dollar's worth of each of these foods provide?

References

1. Stefferud, A. (ed.): *Food, The Year Book of Agriculture.* Washington D.C., USDA, 1959 (see section by E. N. Todhunter, pp. 7–22, which outlines some of the problems in defining food in the early years).
2. Sims, J.: When is a food not a food? Nutr. Today, *13* (No. 3):11, 1978.
3. Lund, D. B.: Influence of processing on nutrients in food. J. Food Protect., *45*:367, 1982; Roberts, T.: Food preservation and nutrition. Nat. Food Rev. (USDA), *NFR–20* (Fall):2, 1982.
4. Ensminger, A. H., et al.: *Foods and Nutrition Encyclopedia.* Clovis, Calif., Pergus Press, 1983 (see sections on additives, bacteria in food, food composition, labeling, preservation of food, processed foods, and information about specific foods).
5. (On microwave cooking) Mai, J., et al.: J. Food Sci., *45*:1753, 1980 (effect on fatty acids); Klein, B. P., et al.: J. Food Sci., *46:*640, 1981 (effect on vitamins); Cross, G. A., and Fung, D. Y. C.: J. Environ. Health, *44:*188, 1982 (a review); Baldwin, R. E.: J. Food Protect., *46*:266, 1983 (a review).
6. Retort pouches. Consumer Rept., *46*:641, 1981; Rizvi, S. S. H., and Acton, J. C.: Nutrient enhancment of thermostabilized foods in retort pouches. Food Tech., *36* (April):105, 1982 (a review); Tuomy, J. M., and Young, R.: Retort-pouch packaging of muscle foods for the Armed Forces. Food Tech., *36* (Feb.):68, 1982; Potter, K. M., Tung, M. A., and Kitson, J. A.: Quality of processed peach slices stored in flexible pouches. Canad. Inst. Food Sci. Tech. J., *15*:96, 1982.
7. Arnold, S., and Roberts, T.: UHT milk: nutrition, safety, and convenience. Nat. Food Rev. (USDA), *NFR–18* (spring):2, 1982.
8. Chung, D. S., and Chang, D. I.: Principles of food dehydration. J. Food Protect., *45*:475, 1982; Cunningham, F. E.: Practical applications of food dehydration: a review. J. Food Protect., *45*:479, 1982; Maggard, P. D.: Practical approaches to home food dehydration. J. Food Protect., *45*:492, 1982.
9. Ogrydziak, D. M., and Brown, W. D.: Temperature effects in modified-atmosphere storage of seafoods. Food Tech., *36* (May):86, 1982; Finne, G.: Modified- and Controlled-Atmosphere storage of muscle foods. Food Tech., *36* (Feb.):128, 1982; Richter, E. R., and Banwart, G. J.; Evaluation of packaged fresh fish. J. Food Protect., *46*:245, 1983.
10. Niemand, J. G., et al.: Radurization of prime beef cuts. J. Food Protect., *44*:677, 1981; Thompson, R.: Purifying food via irradiation. FDA Consumer, *15*(Oct.):25, 1981; Maxcy, R. B.: Irradiation of food for public health protection. J. Food Protect., *45*:363, 1982; Giddings, G. G., and Welt, M. A.: Radiation preservation of foods. Cereal Foods World, *27*(Jan.):17, 1982; *Irradiated Foods.* Summit, N.J., American Council on Science and Health, Oct., 1982; Arnold, S. R.: Food irradiation hinges on approval, feasibility, and acceptance. Nat. Food Rev. (U.S.D.A.), NFR–20 (Fall):7, 1982; Elias, P.S., and Cohen, A.J. (eds.): *Recent Advances in Food Irradiation.* New York, Elsevier Biomedical Press, 1983.
11. Charalambous, G., and Inglett, G. (eds.): *Chemistry of Foods and Beverages: Recent Developments.* New York, Academic Press, 1982; Imitation and substitute dairy foods. Dairy Council Digest, *54* (No. 1):1, 1983; Kotula, K., and Briggs, G. M.: The nutritional aspects of imitation and substitute products. Nutrition News (National Dairy Council), Feb. 1983.
12. (On nonnutrients in food) Maga, J. A.: Pyrroles in food; Pyridines in food (reviews). J. Agric. Food Chem., *29*:691 and 895, 1981; Scheuer, P. J. (ed.): *Marine Natural Products.* Vol. 4. New York, Academic Press, 1981; Conn, E. E. (ed.): *Biochemistry of Plants.* Vol. 7. New York, Academic Press, 1981; Markakis, P. (ed.): *Anthocyanins as Food Colors.* New York, Academic Press, 1982; *List of Propietary Substances and Nonfood Compounds* (authorized for USDA inspection and grading programs). Washington D.C., USDA Misc. Pub. 1419, 1983. Also see current issues of J. Natural Products.
13. (On naturally occurring food toxins) Liener, I. E. (ed.): *Toxic Constituents of Plant Foodstuffs.* 2nd Ed. New York, Academic Press, 1980; Singleton, V. L.:

Naturally occurring food toxicants: phenolic substances of plant origin common in foods. Adv. Food Res., *27*:149, 1981; Elkowicz, K., and Sosulski, F. W.: Antinutritive factors in eleven legumes. J. Food Sci., *47*:1301, 1982; Hafez, Y. S., and Mohamed, A. I.: Presence of nonprotein trypsin inhibitor in soy and winged bean. J. Food Sci., *48*:75, 1983.

14. Roberts, H. R. (ed.): *Food Safety.* New York, John Wiley and Sons, 1981 (see Chapter 5—Food hazards of natural origin, by J. V. Rodricks and A. E. Pohland, p. 181).
15. (Other toxins in processed foods) Somogyi, J. C. (ed.): Foreign substances in foods. Bibl. Nutr. Diet., No. 29:1–148, 1980; Ayres, J. C., and Kirschman, J. C. (eds.): *Impact of Toxicology on Food Processing.* Westport, Conn., Avi Publishing Co., 1981; Gray, J. I., and Morton, I. D.: Some toxic compounds produced in food by cooking and processing. J. Human Nutr., *35*:5, 1981; Taylor, S. L. (Chairman): Interaction between nutrients and toxicants (a symposium, 5 papers). Food Tech., *36* (Oct.):89, 1982; Hathcock, J. N.: *Nutritional Toxicology.* Vol. 1. New York, Academic Press, 1982; Bjeldanes, L. F.: Hazards in the food supply: lead, aflatoxins, and mutagens produced by cooking. Nutr. Update (John Wiley and Sons, New York), *1*:105, 1983.
16. Goodhart, R. S., and Shils, M. E. (eds.): *Modern Nutrition in Health and Disease.* 6th Ed. Philadelphia, Penn., Lea and Febiger, 1980 (see Newberne, P. M.: Naturally occurring food-borne toxicants, p. 463).
17. Institute of Food Technologists' Expert Panel on Food Safety and Nutrition: J. Food Sci., *40*:215, 1975.
18. Gilchrist, A.: *Foodborne Disease and Food Safety.* Chicago, American Medical Association, 1981.
19. (On aflatoxin and other mycotoxins) Diener, U. L.: Aflatoxins. In Ayres and Kirschman: *Impact of Toxicology on Food Processing* (see ref. 15), p. 122; Wilson, B. J.: Mycotoxins in sweet potatoes. In Hathcock: *Nutritional Toxicology* (see ref. 15), p. 239 Bjeldanes, L. F.: Hazards in the food supply (see ref. 15); Labuza, T. P.: J. Food Protect., *46*:260, 1983 (on federal laws and regulations on mycotoxins—a review).
20. (On solanine) Jadhav, S. J., et al.: Naturally occurring toxic alkaloids in foods. CRC Crit. Rev. Toxicol., *9*:21, 1981.
21. (On caffeine and coffee) Relaxing over coffee. Food Chem. Toxicol., *20*:341, 1982; Linn, S., et al.: No association between coffee consumption and adverse outcomes of pregnancy. New Eng. J. Med., *306*:141, 1982 (also see p. 1548); Heany, R. P., and Recker, R. R.: Effects of nitrogen, phosphorus, and caffeine on calcium balance in women. J. Lab. Clin. Med., *99*:46, 1982; Morrison, A. S., et al.: Coffee drinking and cancer of the lower urinary tract. J. Nat. Cancer Inst., *68*:91, 1982; Dews, P. B.: Caffeine, Ann. Rev. Nutr. *2*:323, 1982; Nightingale, S. L., and Flamm, W. G.: Caffeine and health: current status. Nutr. Update (John Wiley and Co., New York), *1*:3, 1983; Expert Panel on Food Safety and Nutrition: Caffeine. Food Tech., *374*:87, 1983.
22. (On food additives, general) Oser, B. L.: Chemical additives in food. In Goodhart and Shils (eds): *Modern Nutrition in Health and Disease* (see ref. 16), p. 506; Fulton, K. R.: Surveys of industry on the use of food additives. Food Tech., *35* (Dec.):80, 1981; Freydberg, N., and Gortner, W. A.: The Food Additives Book. Box C-719, Brooklyn, N.Y., Consumers Reports Books, 1982.
23. Garfield, E.: Risk analysis. Parts 1 and 2, Current Contents, Aug. 23 and 30, p. 5, 1982.
24. Smith, M. V., and Rulis, A. M.: FDA's GRAS review and priority-based assessment of food additives. Food Tech., *35*(Dec.):71, 1981; Safety of 415 food ingredients assessed for the FDA. Public Health Rept., *96*:284, 1981; Yesterday's additives-generally safe. FDA Consumer, *15* (March):14, 1981.
25. Oser, B. L.: The rat as a model for human toxicological evaluation. J. Toxicol. Environ. Health, *8*:521, 1981; Bureau of Foods: Toxicological principles for the safety assessment of direct food additives and color additives used in food. U.S. Food and Drug Administration, 163 pages, 1982.
26. (On enrichment of foods) Hutt, P. B.: FDA food fortification policy. Cereal Foods World, *25*:396, 1980; Food and Drug Administration: Nutritional quality of foods: addition of nutrients. Federal Reg., *45* (Jan. 25):6314, 1980 (also see Code of Fed. Regulations, 101.9 and 104.20, 1981); Vetter, J. L. (ed).: *Adding Nutrients to Foods.* St. Paul, Minn., Amer. Assoc. Cereal Chemists, 1982; Amer. Med. Assoc.: The nutritive quality of processed foods: general policies for nutrient additions. Nutr. Rev., *40*:93, 1982; Ensminger, A. H., et al.: *Foods and Nutrition Encyclopedia* (see ref. 4), p. 667; Anon.: Enriched special formula bread-temporary permits granted. Food Chem. News, *25*(No. 21):55, 1983.
27. (On food labels) FDA, USDA, and FTC: Food labeling: tentative positions of agencies, Federal Reg., *44* (Dec. 21):75990, 1979; Heimbach, J. T., and Stokes, R. C.: Nutrition labeling and public health: survey of American Institute of Nutrition members, food industry, and consumers. Amer. J. Clin. Nutr., *36*:700, 1982. Also see J. Amer. Dietet. Assoc., *77*:70, 1980 (ADA position on FDA proposals); Food Tech., *35* (Feb.):61 and 65, 1981 (on frozen food labeling) and *35* (Feb.):89, 1981 (on open shelf-life dating of foods); FDA Consumer, *16* (July-Aug.):22, 1982 (on store-shelf labels); and Cereal Foods World, *27*(Feb.):55, 1982 (on net-weight labeling); Public Health Rept., 97:385, 1982 (new FDA proposals for sodium labeling); National Nutrition Consortium (Washington, D.C.): Nutr. Alert, *5*(No. 5):1, 1983 (statement on nutrition labeling); Reidy, K.: A new nutrient label? National Food Rev., USDA, NFR-22, p. 14, 1983.
28. (On the U.S. RDAs) Lecos, C.: RDAs: key to nutrition. FDA Consumer, *16* (Nov.):24, 1982.
29. Mohr, K. G., et al.: Aiding consumer nutrition decisions. Home Econ. Res. J., *8*:162, 1980.

30. HEW News, U.S. Dept. of Health, Education, and Welfare, Feb. 3, 1977.
31. Gallo, A. E., and Conner, J. M.: Advertising and American Food Consumption Patterns. Nat. Food Rev. (USDA), *NFR-19*(summer):2, 1982; Anon.: Beer advertising: Coming through for you. Consumer Rept., *48*:348, 1983.
32. Stillings, B. R.: The food industry's responsibilities in food and nutrition education. Food Tech., *34* (Dec.):64, 1980; Bender, A. E.: The appearance and the nutritional value of food products. J. Human Nutr., *35*:215, 1981; Moyes, P. V.: The response of the food industry to the nutrition information and education needs of consumers. J. Canad. Dietet. Assoc., *42*:24, 1981; Meister, K. A.: The food industry and nutrition. Amer. Council Sci. Health (newsletter), *2* (No. 3):4, 1981; Mogren, H. (Chairman): Nutrition and the food industry (a symposium with 8 articles). Nutr. Rev., *40* (Suppl., Jan.):5, 1982; Schwecke, W. M., Engstrom, A. M.: Corporate Nutrition policies—at General Mills, Inc., Cereal Foods World, *28*:145, 1983; Kohlhaas, H.:—at Kraft, Inc., *Ibid,* p. 146, 1983.

19 Food Beliefs and Eating Patterns

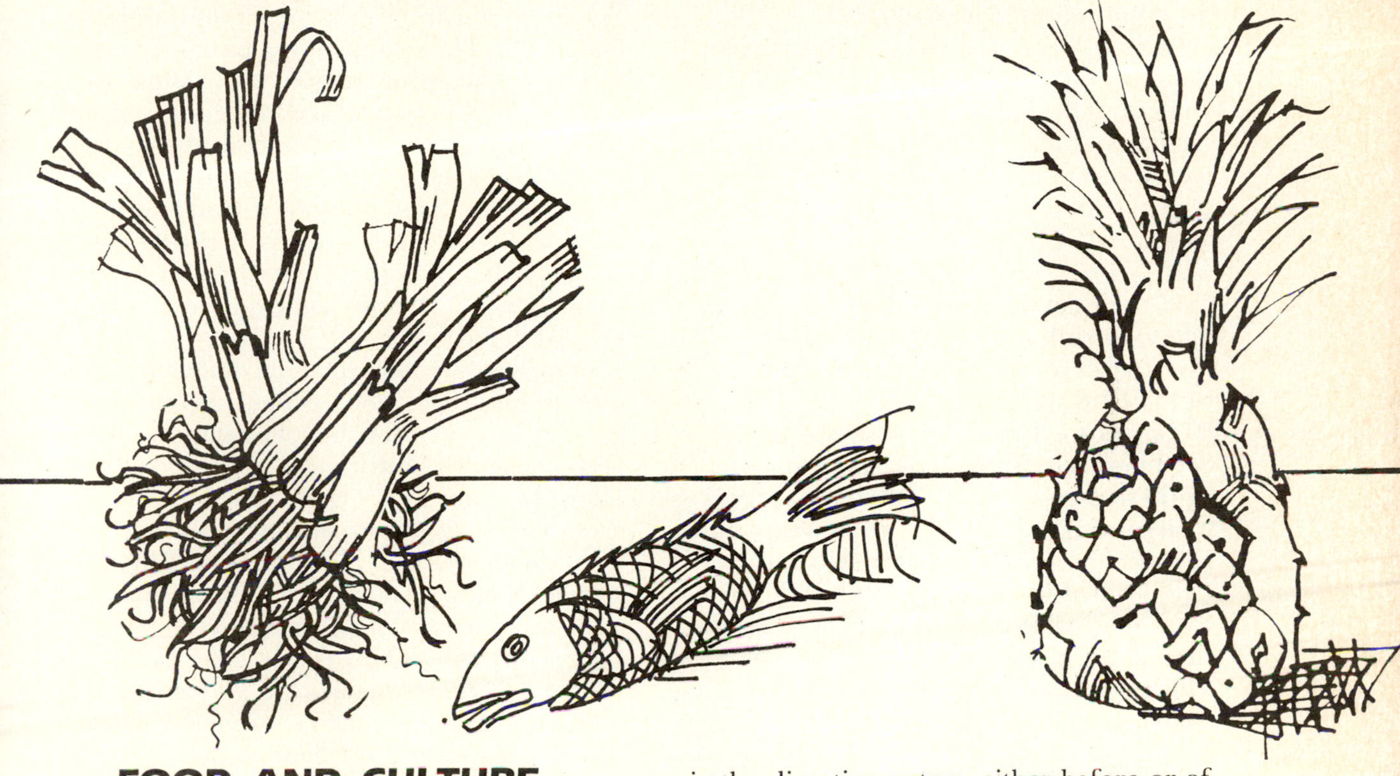

FOOD AND CULTURE

Food and eating are essential to existence. While human beings share this need with all living things, only humans—with their faculties of imagination and language—have endowed the act of eating with beliefs and rituals that they oblige themselves and others of their kind to observe. These beliefs seem to have come from an intuitive recognition that the food we put in our mouths literally becomes us, our blood, bones, and sinews. The hesitancy with which unfamiliar foods are sometimes greeted reflects this attitude, as do the beliefs of people such as rural Thais, for whom the staple rice becomes the body and its tissues. Conversely, the autonomic nervous systems can reinforce a hesitation at incorporating unknown substances into the body by causing physical rejection via the digestive system, either before or after the unwelcome new food is ingested.

If everyone everywhere ate the same foods there would be few problems for dietitians, physicians, and other nutrition educators who wish to redirect the food choices of patients for better health. However, the same foods are not all available everywhere, and those that may be are often prohibitively expensive in lands where they do not grow readily but must be transported over long distances. Thus both economic and ecologic factors, such as soil and climate, affect the kinds of foods available for eating in a given region.

Human factors also control what people eat. These are the ideas people have about the qualities of foods and what is edible. Not all these definitions regarding food are held by all people. They vary from one society to another, and may even differ for different types of individuals, such as old people or children, in the same population. These ideas or beliefs are usually determined by the culture in which people live.

Humans are relatively undifferentiated physiologically, compared with some other animals. They are physically capable of digesting and absorbing nutrients from a variety of potential edible items, as may be deduced from the wide range of viands consumed by people in different parts of the world. Few, however, eat every potential food their environment offers.[1] Instead they select, according to the "rules" of their culture, what to eat, when, where, how, and with whom. It has been said that the expedition trapped by snow at the Donner Pass need not have starved to death had they recognized insects and small rodents as food.

Culture is the sum of a given population's approach to life. It includes objects of material technology and spoken and written ideas, and directives for behavior in given situations. Individuals learn much of their culture early in life, so that it becomes an unconscious part of the self. The term "culture" is sometimes used interchangeably with "society." Culture can also be understood to be the customs of a given society of people, including their shared and often tacit assumptions as to how one is to respond to a given situation. The customs are purposive, that is, they help those who observe them live harmoniously with others who hold similar beliefs. Customs thus serve as checks and balances for the greater good of the greater number. Anthropologists—social scientists who study culture—see it as a functional whole of many parts in dynamic equilibrium, which may change from time to time as do biological organisms. Since a culture is made up of interrelated and interdependent parts, disruption of one part may affect other seemingly remote segments (1).

[1]One group that did was the Otomi Indians of the Mezquital Valley of Mexico, studied by a group of nutrition scientists from MIT(2).

The purpose of some customs may not readily be apparent to someone of a different culture. For example, in a particular culture, there may be reasons functional for that society why a child may not get as much of a nutritionally valuable food as growth would normally require: In many cultures people share food beyond kin and neighbors, a custom that spreads available nutrients widely if rather sparsely, and helps assure that the hunger of many will be allayed if not avoided.

In the past decade, research on behavioral aspects of food and eating has grown greatly. As a scientific discipline this area has been termed "nutritional anthropology." More than anthropology is involved, however: The fields of psychology, history, folklore, ethnobotany, archeology, and pharmacology also contribute to wider understanding of the meanings of food to humans and why as well as how they elect to eat (3).

Researchers on behavioral and sociocultural aspects of food and its utilization, when speaking or writing on these subjects, often use as illustrations examples from societies remote from technologically developed Western ones. Students of nutrition in North America may wonder why they should concern themselves with the food behaviors of such "exotic" cultures, as anthropologists term them. Most of us in Western lands no longer hunt and gather, or toil in a field for our food. It comes in neat, uniform packages, preweighed, premeasured, and often prepared for immediate consumption. The magicoreligious connotations food held for less sophisticated people seem no longer to apply to us, divorced as we are from obtaining it by efforts that would be aided or hindered by whims of nature, such as drought, flood, or pests.

Food still has meanings for eaters, however, which it is the purpose of this chapter to explore. We who live in technologically developed countries are less aware of these meanings than the so-called "primitive" peoples, partly because the reasons and beliefs have become somewhat muted and partly because our reasons and beliefs are part of our accepted, unquestioned culture. We are often unaware that our behavior—whether related to food or other things—has meanings rooted in the past.

Emotional and cultural values are still attached to foods by many populations that are more traditional in outlook, or by those considered to be in transition from traditional to modern ways. In recent years increasing numbers of immigrants from less technically modernized societies have been coming to our shores. These newcomers bring with them attitudes toward food and cooking practices that may cause difficulties for them if they cannot find foods they are accustomed to, or afford them if they can. These people's beliefs about inherent qualities of foods and their appropriateness in illness or indisposition may cause conflicts with their children's schoolteachers or with doctors or other health workers who do not understand the cultural bases for the beliefs.

For all people, the basic meanings of food are part of their culture and logical to them. Awareness of this fact should help persons from different cultures toward courteous consideration of each other's views.

Some of the widely held meanings attached to food are linked to powerful emotions, perhaps because of the intimacy of eating and its association with loving attention in earliest life. Such beliefs about food qualities may have nutritional consequences. In some areas of Latin America, milk and other protein-rich foods are thought to be too "strong" for infants and pregnant women, who are seen by their culture to be weak and susceptible. In some Latin and Asian countries such foods are forbidden to small children because they are believed to irritate prevalent intestinal parasites, thereby causing them to migrate to the eyes and cause blindness. The drying and clouding of the scleral coat of the eyeball in young children, due to insufficient intake of vitamin A-precursors, is blamed by Malays on the rising of these "eye worms" from the gut (4). Ironically, papaya, a fruit rich in carotene, is thought to be as potent a stimulant of the intestinal worms as meat or eggs, and so it, too, is forbidden to those who need it most.

Women in the reproducing years and young children are the objects of many taboos or prohibitions regarding food. Most often the foods are good animal-protein sources, which are also more scarce than staples and, therefore, more expensive. (Meat is also more costly to produce than vegetable crops, requiring longer periods to reach maturity and greater input in terms of animal feeding.) Thus meat is customarily reserved first for the able-bodied males, and has come to be a prized food in many cultures. Since the digestion of meat is slower than that of carbohydrate foods, meat "stays with you," allaying hunger pangs for longer periods.

Magic, meaning supernatural outcomes believed unsought by ordinary efforts, is often associated with food. Even today's individual is not immune to magical beliefs about meat, similar to those mentioned above. The belief that eating beef will build muscles or make better ball-players is an example of such magic. This idea may be traced to the nineteenth-century physiologist Liebig, who in the early days of nutritional science noted that muscle was high in protein, and thought eating animal muscle would contribute to human muscle enhancement. We know now this "targeting" does not occur. Eating meat won't make anyone fierce or aggressive, either.

Modern and traditional women alike have semimagical beliefs about foods that could harm or "mark" the fetus. While a non-

Western woman may be more concerned not to eat rabbit or hare for fear of causing harelip in her offspring, some Western women think that not eating foods "craved" during pregnancy can give the baby a birthmark resembling the object, for example, cherries, strawberries, or chocolate (5). Others, however, believe eating craved foods can cause such marks.

Both the ways in which food is perceived and used and the ways in which it is physically handled and processed may also be considered cultural manipulations. Some cultural manipulations of food are nutritionally beneficial. Since pre-Columbian times people in large parts of Latin America who subsist on maize have soaked the kernels in an alkali solution to soften them so they may be more easily ground into grain to make the basic flat bread, tortillas. Laboratory research showed that this practice releases the niacin in the corn that was chemically bound and otherwise unavailable to consumers. (See Chap. 10.) In most of the countries where maize is so treated, tortillas are eaten together with beans. These two items are considered the basis of a meal, forming what may be termed the "cuisine." They are perceived to "go together" and, in fact, the amino acids in the beans complement those in the maize. (See Chap. 4.) These two cultural practices have contributed to absence among maize-eating Latin Americans of the niacin-deficiency disease, pellagra, that was prevalent in cultures where corn was an introduced food.

Beliefs about Food Qualities and Their Effects

For some two thousand years the populations of China and India have believed that certain foods are "heating" or "cooling" to the body when eaten. These beliefs were systematized by the second-century A.D. Greek physician named Galen, who related them to certain bodily "humors" such as anger or phlegm, which were "hot" and "cold," respectively, or to disease states, also considered "hot" or "cold." Beliefs that certain foods, disease states, or careless behavior could cause harmful "airs" or "wind" to enter the body were a component of the system. Health was thought to result from proper balancing of "heating" and "cooling" foods or activities, and illness was treated with foods of properties opposite to those of the disease. These beliefs were carried first by Arab traders to Southeast Asia and Europe, and then brought to the New World, particularly Latin America. The Chinese beliefs in *yin* and *yang* are closely akin, as are the *doshas* (humors) of the people of India. These ideas were part of the scientific beliefs of Europeans until the rise of modern science about the seventeenth century, as an examination of some of Shakespeare's plays will show. Traces of these ideas remain in North America in what medical anthropologists call contemporary folk medicine (1). The stomach is seen as a kind of stove that recooks food, thus raising body temperature for an hour or more after eating. Some people in the United States still say "feed a cold, starve a fever" and "catch a cold."

Such descriptions of food qualities are only occasionally the same as the actual temperature of the food, although, depending on the culture, cooking may change the perceived quality of a raw food (6). (See Fig. 19–1.) Certain cultures would say that the food makes the eater feel "hot" or "cold." Not all foods, however, are held to be "hot" or "cold": A considerable number—generally the staple foods—are usually defined as "neutral."

Some traditional beliefs and folk practices may have bases in fact (see below, Modern Food Beliefs). Food pharmacology—the study of complex chemicals in foods and their physical effects on eaters—is a rather new field. (See Chap. 18.) As an example, potatoes contain two dozen identified non-

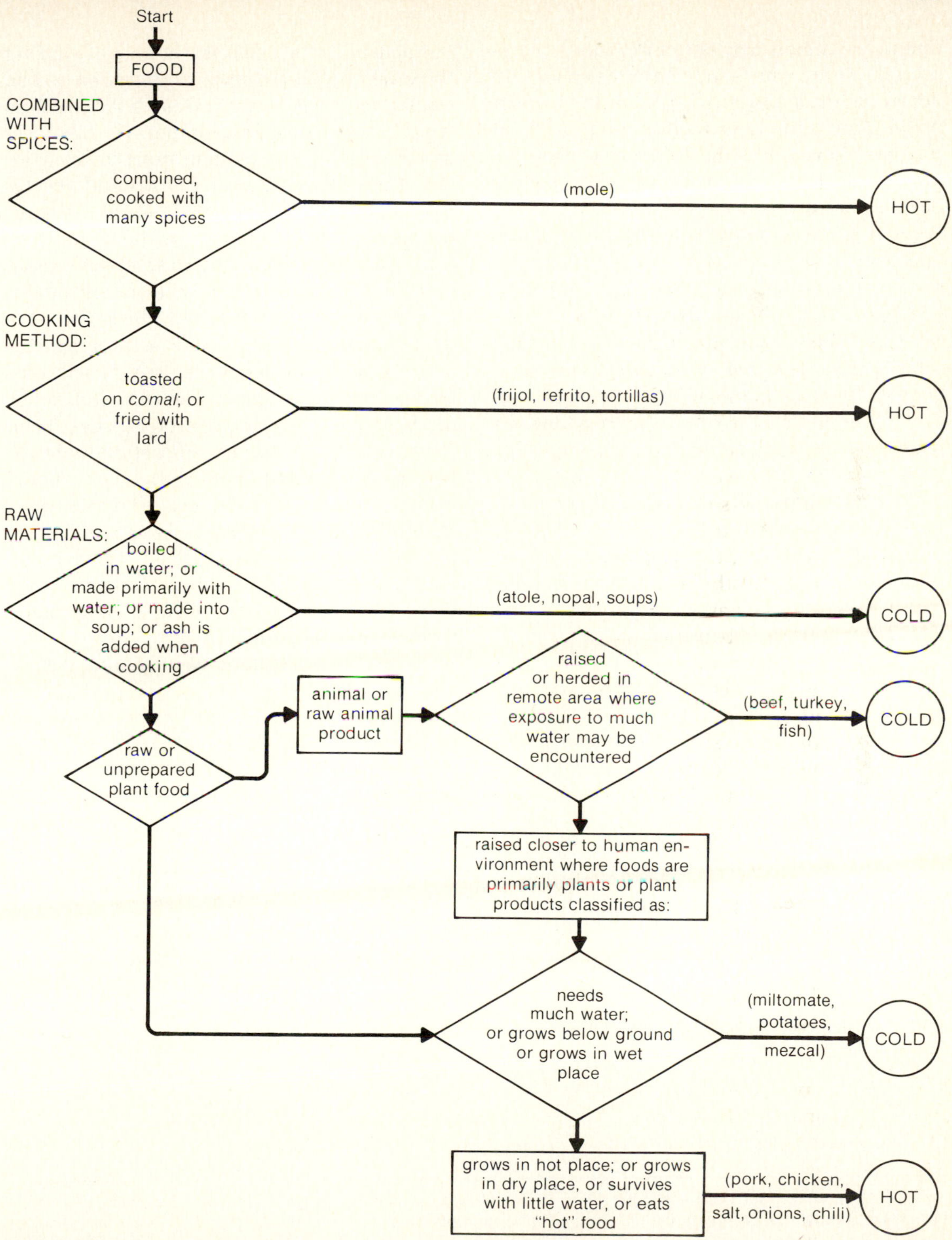

Figure 19–1 Cultural code of Spanish-Zapotec people for determining whether a given food is "hot" or "cold" (village Diaz Ordáz, Oaxaca, Mex.). (From Molony, C. H.: Ecol. Fd. Nutr., *4:* 67, 1975, with permission.)

nutritive chemicals and 200 more compounds as yet uncharacterized. Scientists do not know the physiologic roles in the human body of many compounds identified in plants, or even their function in the plants' life processes. However, anthropologists have pointed out that certain "hot" foods (animal protein sources) have satiety value, and that "cold" foods (fruits and vegetables for the most part) have a larger water content (7). It has also been postulated that compounds present in foods deemed "cold" may cause physiologic reactions that could have been defined as "cold" or "cooling" centuries ago (8). Legumes, for example, are known to produce "air" (flatulence) in the digestive system.

Whatever subsequent research determines on the question of foods as "hot" or "heating" and "cold" or "cooling," such beliefs are found among Puerto Ricans, Mexicans, Central Americans, Chinese, Vietnamese, Thais, and other minority groups in North America. The people most affected nutritionally by these beliefs are pregnant women, infants, and preschool children. Pregnancy is usually considered a "hot" state, so "hot" foods, such as eggs, may need to be avoided. (Eggs may also be considered to be dangerous abortifacients, that is, capable of causing the child to be aborted prematurely.) The woman who has just given birth is "cold," so "cold" foods must be avoided. As the foregoing suggests, the woman must in this condition abstain from eating fruits and vegetables until the time that her society decrees her period of lying-in or withdrawal from active participation in group activities is at an end. (See Table 19–1.) The duration of this confinement may vary, but thirty to forty days is common. The restrictions on vegetable foods may be harmful, particularly with frequent, recurring pregnancies. Deficiency of folacin, iron, and carotene has been found in Malay women undergoing these ritual dietary prohibitions (9). The Malay women, whose mothers and midwives prescribed what they should eat from beliefs handed down for generations, were afraid that "air" would enter their bodies if they flouted the taboos, thereby causing tissue damage and bleeding.

Some cultures extend postpartum dietary taboos for considerably longer periods: In South India, poor women eat only what is given them, because they are not considered to be expending energy (10). This society sees lactation as illness, and feeds the woman

Table 19–1 PERCENTAGE OF WOMEN IN CENTRAL MEXICO REPORTING THAT SPECIFIED FOODS WERE PERMITTED OR RESTRICTED POSTPARTUM OR DURING LACTATION (N = 125)

Permitted	*Percent*	*Restricted*	*Percent*
Soups (chicken broth, sopa aquada)	86	Avocado	54
Atoles (thick, maize-based drinks)	85	Fruits (all kinds)	50
Toasted tortilla	83	Pork	43
Boiled milk	56	Red beans	41
Chicken	50	Vegetables (all kinds)	15
Black bean broth	47	Red meat	12
Charcoal broiled cheese	45	Milk, cheese, eggs	17

From Sanjur, D.: Sociocultural approach to the study of infant feeding practices and weaning habits in a Mexican village. Doctoral dissertation, Cornell Univ., 1968, with permission.

sparingly. When her nursling is sick, she must also limit her diet.

Traditionally, the Chinese woman was somewhat better fed after giving birth than a South Indian woman. She is offered wine and a "chicken a day," along with ginger and other "hot" foods to cure the imbalance of yin ("hot") and yang ("cold") caused by pregnancy (11). This practice, called "doing the month," was to rid the body of dirty blood and assure future well-being. Chinese women, too, could eat no "cold" or raw foods for the thirty-day confinement period. Although adherence to these kinds of beliefs is less among ethnic groups after they leave their homeland, similar food and eating behaviors are still found among Mexican-Americans in the United States, Chinese in Canada, and Vietnamese in Australia.

Other reasons given by mothers for honoring these beliefs include one that "cold" or otherwise improper food choices for this period of life could cause a toxic factor to get into their milk and harm the newborn. In some cultures, for example Latin America and Ethiopia, new babies are thought to have "dirty" stomachs, and the *meconium* (the mucus in the baby's intestines at birth) is purged. Other beliefs about feeding babies affect their nutritional state chiefly when they are sick—in which case food may be withheld, herb teas being substituted—and when they are weaned from the breast. Many societies lack special foods for children, and introduce them gradually to adult foods. In the United States, meat was considered too "stimulatory" for children in the last century (12). The beliefs that meat and other protein foods would give children worms or cause inborn worms to rise, or are "too strong" for them, deprived them of needed protein. Eggs are sometimes forbidden to children because they are "hot," because they might make a person in an inappropriate age category fertile, or because they represent a source of supplemental cash income to the household. There is often little concept that pregnant women or growing children have special diet needs. In Latin America children are fed well when they are healthy, deprived of food when ill.

Modern Food Beliefs

Beliefs about qualities of foods that may be imparted to or otherwise affect the eater are not confined to people who live in or come from more traditional settings. Students of folklore find examples in rural areas such as Appalachia—sauerkraut made under the sign of Pisces will be slippery like a fish. Observers have said that in urban clinics "high blood" is believed by some to be caused by too much red meat or rich food. The belief that red beets or red wine are good for the blood are rather common examples of sympathetic magic wherein the colors of the food and blood indicate some imputed affinity. Certain foods or nutrients, bread, potatoes, and calories are considered "fattening" when taken in any amount. Some foods, such as fruits, are thought to cause "acid stomach," but the stomach can only function properly at an acidic pH. There is no known scientific reason for not eating fish and ice cream at the same meal, once feared to cause poisoning, and foods cooked in aluminum will not harm the consumer.

Some modern beliefs about properties of foods may be harmful. In the 1960s and 70s, as part of a general revolution in cultural attitudes, cults of vegetarianism and natural or organically grown foods came into being. Adherence to group precepts gave participants a sometimes spiritual sense of belonging to a community. The dietary code also sets them apart from nonpractitioners. (See Table 19–2.) Some of the dietary recommendations are probably beneficial: reduction of intake of expensive meat as well as of some highly processed foods. The dangerous

Table 19–2 FOOD FADDISTS AND THE SELF-NEEDS THEIR FEEDING PRACTICES SERVE

Type of Food Faddist	*Need Served by the Fad*
1. Miracle-seeker	Patterning need to establish stability regarding health, energy, etc. Accomplished by diets intended to forestall aging or restore organism to health. Ego defense need to reestablish positive self-concept and feeling of self-worth.
2. Antiestablishmentarian	Self-realization need to express self in a manner consistent with self-concept and value system.
3. Super health-seeker	Ego defense need to forestall aging process. Accomplished by diet intended to give super health. Self-realization need to present front of strength and health.
4. Distruster of medical profession	Ego defense need to establish control over own destiny and not be dependent on unknown others.
5. Fashion-follower	Ego defense and patterning need to establish an identity to gain approval and acceptance from others.
6. Authority-seeker	Self-realization need for recognition of self-competency, provided by apparent knowledge in area of food information.
7. Truth-seeker	Patterning need to process existing claims concerning nutrition.
8. One concerned about uncertainties of living	Patterning need for anchors and stability concerning the world.

From Beal, A.: Food faddism and organic and natural foods. Paper presented at NDC Food Writers Conf., Newport, R.I., 1972.

diets, however, are those in which all animal foods are abjured or in which the kinds of foods eaten are severely limited, as among fruitarians, or during frequent fasting. Observance of such zealous behavior, of course, limits amounts and kinds of needed nutrients consumed.

As the above discussion should suggest, the groups are not homogeneous, although health is the explanation usually given for the diet practices. The cult-believers' devotions range from macrobiotics, raw foods, and yoga to health foods and antislaughter motives. The adherents are alike in believing some particular benefit will come to them from following the diet. In this they are not much different from those who feel they must supplement their daily food intake with vitamin pills to "get enough." In Western countries those with actual needs for supplemental vitamins are the exception, a nonhealthy minority. Industry and advertising have taken advantage of this belief to urge purchase of pills and vitamin-enriched foods. All sorts of foods—some that could by no stretch of the imagination be produced naturally—and even cosmetics have acquired "natural" as part of their brand name, to entice more buyers.

There may be some truth in a number of beliefs held about foods. For centuries garlic has been thought to have almost magical properties to ward off colds and cure other ills. Recent research has indicated that it lowers blood levels of glucose and lipids in experimental animals due to the presence of some volatile oils that may be associated with characteristic odors (13). Onions possess the same properties and oils to a lesser degree. A researcher at the University of California, examining folk remedies for iron deficiency, has verified a belief that inserting a few iron nails into apples leads to a measurable amount of iron in the apple after one day. It is enough (15 mg) to meet current recommended intakes for children, for whom the treatment is intended (14). Research on fiber indicates that pectin, a constituent of apples, lowers blood cholesterol levels, suggesting that an apple a day really might help keep certain kinds of doctors away.

CULTURAL SIGNIFICANCE OF FOOD

What is food is a cultural definition. What is a meal is also culturally defined, as are the foods suitable for postpartum women and children discussed earlier. Foods may also be used culturally in nonfood ways, that is, the primary intent of the manipulation may not be to nourish but to say something, to make a point. One of these uses is symbolic. The Christian or Jewish sacraments, in which bread and wine are taken after being blessed, are examples. Food is offered to gods in many religions, from American Indian to Hindu Balinese. Fasting, either total or only from specific foods, is another example, done to symbolize an altered status or for religious or political reasons.

What foods a person is allowed to eat is another symbolic use of food. As suggested, diets prescribed for pregnant women, new mothers, and for their children usually differ from those for nonpregnant adults and older children. This is a way of setting people apart so others may see that they belong to a different category. A few societies also treat widows in this way. The transition to another recognized status is often accompanied by rituals, such as feasting or other ceremonies using foods. The food and the ceremony are the "markers" of the transition. (See Fig. 19–2.) Across cultures people so recognize the end of a woman's confinement, a child's naming, puberty or coming of age, marriage, and death. These people may then be gradually or abruptly incorporated into the eating ways of the rest of the group (15).

Another symbolic use of food is to define status. Just as pregnant women or babies are marked as being in altered states by being given different foods to eat, people use the foods consumed to show their relative status to their peers. This behavior refers both to public eating and to food purchasing. In either case they may select more expensive items to impress others. Eating of lower-status foods may take place behind closed doors.

We are all familiar with the prestige attached to scarce items that are therefore expensive, such as caviar, truffles, and berries grown out-of-season in hothouses. Such "exotic" foods may have lower status in locales where they are plentiful, however. Such was once the case with salmon in North America, or wild strawberries among European peasants. The status of fish is inferior to that of meat nearly everywhere, which accounts in part for its considerably lower consumption. Wild greens—often of better nutritional value than commercial substitutes—are considered the food of the poor. They may be relished for flavor, however, and do add variety to diets; examples are the purslane and lamb's quarters or pigweed (a pot herb of the Amaranth family, akin to a highly nutritious Andean plant, called *quinoa*). These foods are regular diet components for Mexicans and other people of Latin extraction. The low status of wild food plants has led to their being called "famine" or "emergency" foods, and probably reflects the fact that, being free for the picking, their cost and value are negligible.

Chicken dinner used to be a rather special meal in the United States, before the introduction of factory-like farms with their large, wire-bottomed enclosures. As availability increased, the price and prestige—and flavor—of these birds decreased. Perhaps the chicken served at banquets and tes-

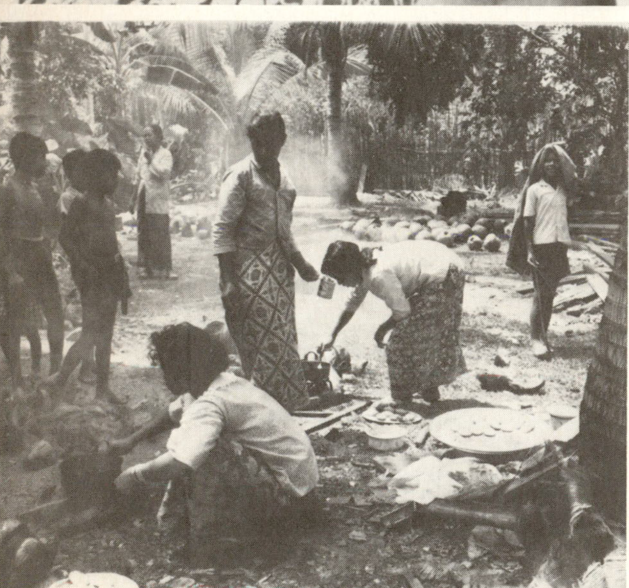

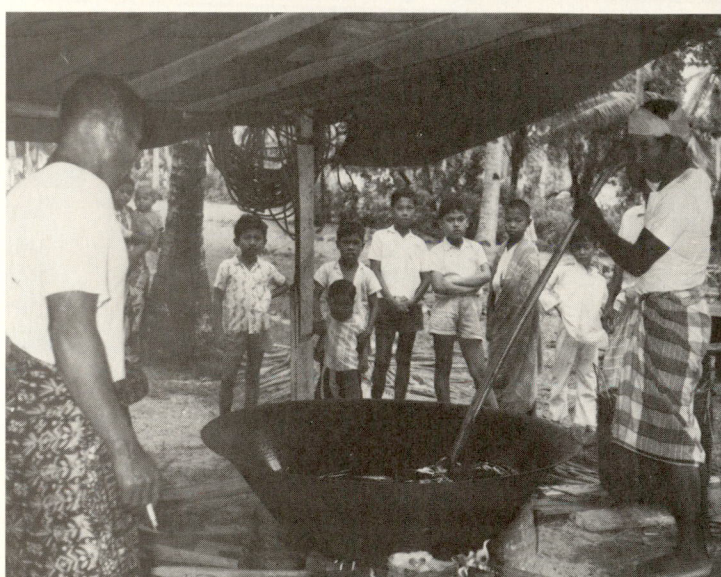

Figure 19–2 On feasting occasions, food preparation is part of the social event in which the whole family may participate. Top: Mexican family preparing for holiday visitors. Bottom: A Malay village prepares for a wedding feast. In this culture, only men cook the meat dishes. (Courtesy of C. S. Wilson, Univ. of California.)

timonial dinners is an echo of the earlier higher value once assigned it.

Nutritional problems related to status of foods are of greatest concern with respect to the refined foods of Western peoples—white flour, white sugar, sweetened condensed milk, and foods made from them such as white bread, cakes, cookies, pies, and soft drinks. People in developing countries see the inhabitants of the more industrialized countries as well-to-do, and seek to imitate their foods whenever possible, despite higher prices than those of indigenous, often more nutritionally worthy counterparts. The effect of these substitutions has been to increase alarmingly the rate of tooth decay and obesity in these lands. Foods that appear prestigious to traditional and emerging peoples are not limited to carbohydrate sources, however. Southeast Asians, for example, have access to a host of delicious, vitamins C- and A- and mineral-rich fruits, many of which the rest of the world can only sample upon visiting these regions, since most do not transport or grow readily elsewhere. In their local markets these indigenous products vie for the attention of high-status buyers with less nutritious but more expensive apples and pears imported from Australia and New Zealand.

Among Western people a food with lower-status connotations is the leftover, which causes problems for the thrifty homemaker. The problem, and the definition, appear to have come with the advent of year-round mechanical refrigeration. In the early part of this century refrigerators were iceboxes, stocked in summer with ice cut from ponds or lakes in winter and stored in straw in icehouses until needed in warm weather. In colder places winter refrigeration was merely storage in unheated pantries, cellars, or between the outside storm window and inner window. Leftovers are a more common occurrence in North America than in Europe, where refrigerators, when present, are small. This is related to the homemaker's tendency to buy fresh food daily, as do women in developing regions, where refrigerators are scarce and what is cooked for the midday meal also serves as the evening meal, thus conserving scarce fuel.

The term leftover has a somewhat derogatory association, implying that the food wasn't good enough to be finished at one sitting. Paradoxically, some foods considered gourmet items make imaginative use of leftovers: Cream soups, quiches, aspics, and souffles are examples.

Another kind of leftover is the food left on plates, as well as that thrown away by the cook. The term for these leftovers is waste, destined for the kitchen garbage disposal or the garbage can. In the non-Western world, edible and inedible waste (pits, bones, and peelings) is fed to chickens, pigs, or other domestic animals to be recycled for eventual human consumption as eggs or meat. Anthropologists at the University of Arizona have systematically studied food and related discards from urban households in several U.S. cities (16). The amount of uneaten food thrown away in one locale represented up to $100 per family per year.

Snacks are foods that people everywhere consider less important than meals. Their status may vary, but their emotional content is lower than that of any regular food eaten at a time defined as a "meal." Snacking is called between-meal eating by Westerners, whereas other populations may not consider a snack a food, but "something to keep the mouth busy." Snacking has contributed to the growth of fast-food outlets, and perhaps the reverse is also true. (See Fig. 19–3.) Certainly it has led to complaints on the part of parents and health educators about consumption of "junk" foods of little nutritional worth. However, analysis of between-meal foods of teenagers studied in the U.S. Ten-State Nutrition Survey revealed that these contributed substantial amounts of nutrients

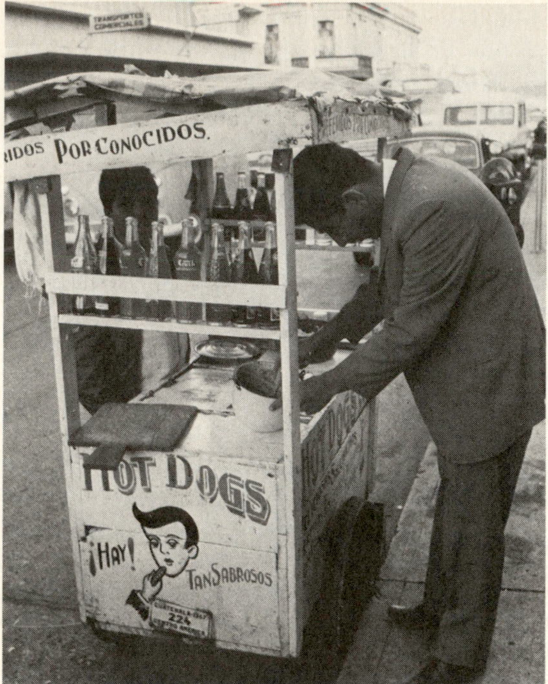

Figure 19–3 Quick snacks and between-meal foods form a significant part of the daily diet almost everywhere. Sanitation is not always what it might be. (Courtesy of WHO.)

to their daily diet. (See Chap. 20.) The nutritional quality of snack foods varies of course: In developing regions fruits are almost universally taken casually at nonmeal times, sometimes picked from the tree or bush in passing. Nuts are another nutritionally worthwhile snack, as well as various legume products of the Middle East and India, such as *hummus* (thick pea paste) and *poppadom* (legume chips).

EATING PATTERNS AND CHANGE

People's choices of things they believe are appropriate to eat and their consumption patterns have long been called "food habits." A better term might be "eating patterns," because "habits" suggests repetitive behavior of long standing. There are fashions in foods as there are in dress, and styles change over time due to political and other social causes as well as to economic and technological ones. This may be seen by examining menus in old cookbooks, or by noting references to meals and food use in literature. Some foods now frequently encountered in North America were earlier known only to world travelers and affluent households with paid cooks until modern manufacture and transportation introduced them or their replicas more widely. Vegetable souffles and croissants are relative newcomers but increasingly common in the average household. The current burgeoning interest in fine cooking may be an indication that the next popular food cult will be that of the creative gourmet.

Spontaneous food-habit changes happen all the time, although they most often involve one or a few foods. Contact between different cultures causes exchange, and European diets would be much less varied if North and South America had not been discovered: They would not have included the potato, maize, chocolate, cassava (tapioca), tomatoes, cashew nuts, or the later-introduced tea and coffee.

Food habits appear to evolve, usually slowly, unless some catastrophe causes abrupt change. Study of preferences for particular foods or flavors suggests that taste plays some part, but a taste for a particular flavor is often acquired—that is, if a culture introduces a strong, bitter, or hot substance at a young-enough age, the child will gradually turn from rejection to acceptance. Chili peppers, for example, have a burning quality to the mucous membrane that appears also to be addicting.

Culture teaches people to feel squeamish at the thought of eating certain protein sources, such as locusts, dogs, or horses. Beef, pork, or shellfish, while presented as legitimate foods to some, are categorized for others as items to avoid for religious or esthetic reasons.

Some changes in food and eating patterns may be brought about by introduced foods that have high-status appeal. This is the apparent reason for the popularity of refined carbohydrate foods and soft drinks nearly everywhere around the globe. Other disadvantageous change may occur in a cuisine, where items traditionally accompany each other in a meal and are often nutritionally complementary. Beans and tortillas, or bread and cheese for example, are pairs that may be disrupted due to disappearance or change in price of one of their components.

Food innovations may be resisted because their acceptance would be incompatible with the cultural framework: The required different fuel or cooking equipment may be hard to find. Such attempts at change are resisted because change itself is uncomfortable, requiring a consciously different mental attitude. The foods may not be given to the person for whom they were intended if the culture perceives them as inappropriate for the recipient. This happened following World War II, when dry milk was donated for malnourished children in the early days of nutrition interventions in developing countries.

Although there are disagreements about the influence of advertising in changing food choices, successful ways of gaining acceptance of new foods do exist. Since meals have varying emotional contents, foods to be introduced have a better chance of success if they are presented as components for meals about which people feel less strongly. This may explain the proliferation of snack foods and the changes in breakfast patterns that have taken place in Britain and North America in recent decades. Bland, neutral foods are more readily incorporated—even into meals with greater meaning for the eater—than those with strong flavors. This fact may account for the widespread acceptance of bread, which may be eaten along with the more traditional staple (such as tamales or rice) rather than replacing it. A new object or behavior has to be integrated into the existing system, so time is needed to allow for changed, accepting perceptions. A marketing message treating involvement of the actual consumer in the buying decision improves the chance that the new food will be accepted.

New foods may be accepted if they resemble some already-liked item in taste or texture. Foods already eaten by leaders or other prestigious persons, or foods with a money value, are more likely to be incorporated into diets. It also is likely that, once people have begun to change, it is futile to try to hold them to more traditional ways of eating. When attempts are made to change food habits, it should be remembered that what is really being changed is part of the culture. Both have a better chance of success when changes in the culture accompany changes in food practices so as to reinforce and encourage the latter.

Food habits learned very early in life in a pleasant home environment are the most resistant and difficult to change. The food habits of some people do change more readily, however, when they move to a different cultural setting. At present there are no formulas that would permit prediction about whether or not a particular habit or group of attitudes will respond to efforts to change them.

Finally, acceptance of a food does not imply merely trying and liking, as food manufacturers have learned. Instead it means that the food is incorporated into the diet thereafter, actively sought, becoming part of the menu, in accord with the cultural context into which the community has put it. Once fully accepted, the new food may later be displaced by another, for reasons some of which are suggested above.

Change agents also need to be alert to the possibility that an existing diet, although quite different from those to which the observer is accustomed, may still be fully satisfactory nutritionally.

QUESTIONS

1. From references in this book and other sources available to you, make a list of nutritionally valuable foods or combinations of foods that may be superior to snack foods or meals you are accustomed to. Would you eat them if they were available to you? Why or why not? Can you think of any food preparation practices or food combinations that we or our forebears have had that were nutrient-enhancing? (Example: Scottish households cooked porridge (oatmeal) slowly, overnight, on a low fire. The process reduced the amount of phytic acid that, if cooked for much shorter periods, normally complexes calcium in the milk taken with the porridge. Longer cooking, therefore, makes the milk calcium more biologically available to the consumer.)

2. Choose an ethnic group with which you are familiar. After determining, as best you can, whether their diet in normal amounts would meet their specific needs for a specific critical nutrient (e.g., protein, iron, or vitamin A), select a food to introduce that would enhance their nutrient intakes, and plan what methods you might use to ensure acceptability. Outline your proposed procedures, and speculate on the possible outcomes.

3. Make a list of as many beliefs and sayings regarding "hot" and "cold" qualities of foods, people, or other objects as you can find in current literature. You can also use the terms "humors," and "air" or "windy" or synonyms for them (i.e., "so-and-so is full of hot air"). Newspapers and magazines may be consulted. Investigate modern folk-medical lore by making a similar list of foods that are believed to affect health or disease states.

References

1. Foster, G. M., and Anderson, B. G.: *Medical Anthropology.* New York, John Wiley & Sons, 1978.
2. Anderson, R. K., et al.: A study of the nutritional status and food habits of Otomi Indians. Amer. J. Pub. Health, *36:*883, 1946.
3. Wilson, C. S.: Food—custom and nurture: an annotated bibliography on sociocultural and biocultural aspects of nutrition. J. Nutr. Ed., *11*(4) (Suppl. 1): October 1979.
4. McKay, D. A.: Food, illness, and folk medicine: Insights from Ulu Trengganu, West Malaysia. Ecol. Food Nutr., *1:*67, 1971.
5. Newman, F.: Folklore of pregnancy: Wives' tales in Contra Costa County, California. Western Folklore, *28:*112, 1969.
6. Ingham, J. M.: On Mexican folk medicine. Amer. Anthropol., *72:*76, 1970.
7. Ferro-Luzzi, G. E.: Temporary female food avoidances in Tamilnadu. Interpretations and parallels. East and West (New Series) *25*(3–4):471, 1975.
8. Wilson, C. S.: *Proposed: That "Hot" and "Cold" Food Beliefs Have Pharmacological Bases in Fact.* Cambridge, Cambridge Univ. Press, in press.
9. Wilson, C. S.: Food beliefs affect nutritional status of Malay fisherfolk. J. Nutr. Ed., *2:*96, 1971.
10. Katona-Apte, J.: The socio-cultural aspects of food avoidance in a low-income population in Tamilnad, South India. J. Trop. Pediatr. Environ. Child Health, *23:*83, 1977; Katona-Apte, J.: The relevance of nourishment to the reproductive cycle of the female in India. In Raphael, D. (ed): *Being Female: Reproduction, Power and Change.* The Hague, Mouton Pub., 1975, p. 43.
11. Pillsbury, B. L. K.: "Doing the month": Confinement and convalescence of Chinese women after childbirth. Soc. Sci. Med., *12:*11, 1978.
12. Jefferson, D. L.: Child feeding in the United States in the nineteenth century. J. Amer. Dietet. Assoc., *30:*335, 1954.
13. Chi, M. S., Koh, E. T., and Stewart, T. J.: Effects of garlic on lipid metabolism in rats fed cholesterol or lard. J. Nutr., *112:*241, 1982.
14. Rosanoff, A.: unpublished data, Univ. of California, Berkeley, 1982.
15. Sanjur, D., Cravioto, J., Rosales, L., and van Veen, A. G.: Infant feeding and weaning practices in a rural preindustrial setting. Acta Pediat. Scand., Supplement 200, 1970.
16. Rathje, W. L., and Harrison, G. G.: Monitoring trends in food utilization: application of an archeological method. Fed. Proc., *37:*49, 1978.

20 Applied Nutrition: Theory into Practice

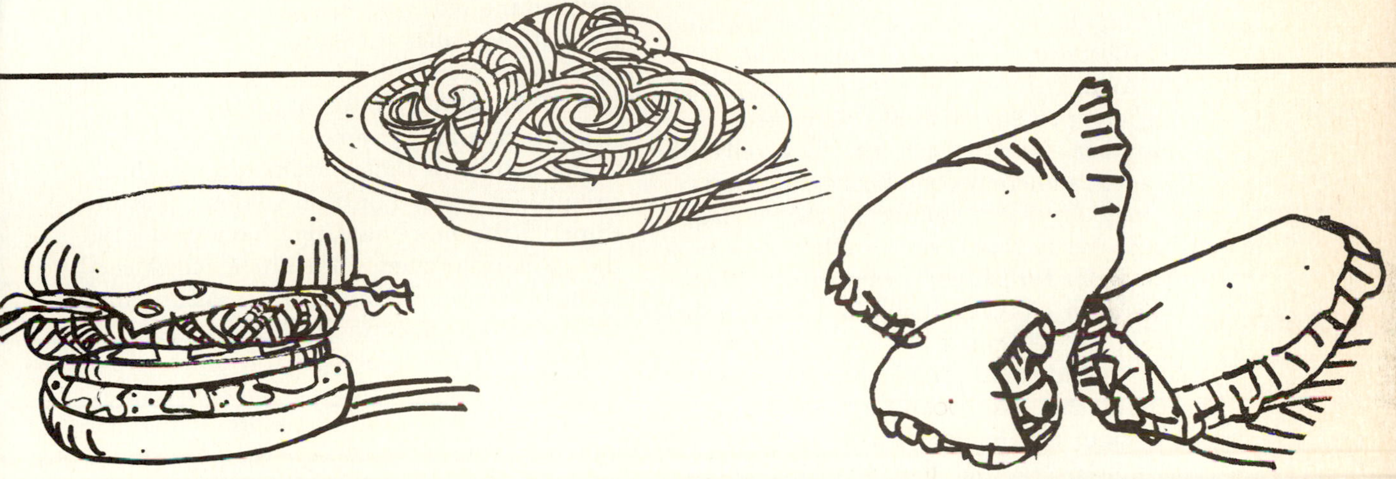

There is a rather broad range of intakes (depending on the nutrient in question) that can maintain a positive state of health with relatively little of the body's adaptive ability being brought into play. This may be illustrated as follows:

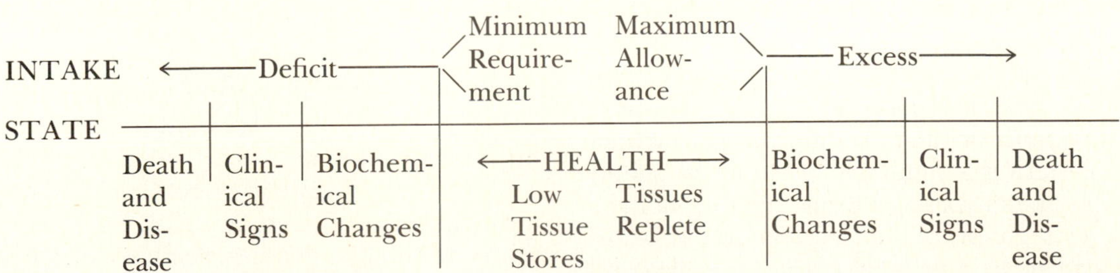

At the upper portion of the allowable range of intakes, all tissue reserves will be filled and daily output in the excreta will be high. If intake exceeds a certain upper limit, adaptive biochemical or physiological processes that can be detected by sophisticated laboratory techniques then develop; at the next stage of excess intake, there will be clinical signs and symptoms of the disordered state, and beyond that, manifest disease and death. The same sequence of events, beginning with depleted reserves, occurs with nutrient intakes at the lower end of the spectrum.

Taking iron as an example, inadequate intake leads first to lowered concentration of iron-transport substances in the blood, then to diminished hemoglobin, and finally to pallor, fatigue, decreased work capacity, and death because of lack of oxygen at the tissue level. With chronically excessive iron intake, transport protein becomes saturated, iron accumulates in the liver, the liver cells are damaged, sometimes the heart, and the person may die from failure of the damaged liver or heart. The range of safe intakes is much wider for some nutrients than for others because the body has more ways to dispose of excess and adapt to deficits, or because the nutrient does not participate in reactions that are as important to survival. Body state is affected by both present and past intakes, so that diagnosis of malnutrition is more difficult than a single example may indicate. What is important to know is that the body has some capacity to adapt to altered intakes, that there may be hidden evidence of malnourishment before it is clinically noticeable, and that not all body functions may be equally affected by a given degree of deficit or excess at a given time in the life history. Individuals in a borderline state—with adaptive mechanisms operating at near capacity and biochemically detectable but minimal changes in function—may be said to be *at risk* of malnutrition or to be in a subclinical state of malnutrition. The number of persons in this category is many times the number who show clinical signs. Whenever there is a significant number of people with unequivocal clinical malnutrition, a larger segment of the population can be assumed to be at risk. For these people a reduction of intake—or even continued low intake or increase in stress—may lead to open manifestation, or clinical signs, of malnutrition.

JUDGING NUTRITIONAL ADEQUACY

We usually detect malnutrition by certain outward signs that are the effects produced by that condition. It would seem to be an easy matter to tell whether or not a person is well nourished, and it is true that to the trained eye such differences in nutritional condition seem obvious and are quickly noted. However, there are all degrees of malnutrition and people are not apt to look at themselves or their own children with unprejudiced eyes. For this reason, a list of some of the more striking characteristics of the well-nourished individual, contrasted with those usually found in undernourished individuals, is given in Table 20–1.

There are physical signs of deficiency of protein, vitamins, and some minerals. An examiner will evaluate the quality of the skin and hair as well as observe the eyes for inflammation about the cornea that may be the result of riboflavin deficiency, and for Bitot's spots and evidence of difficulty in seeing in dim light, indicative of vitamin-A deficiency. The mucous membranes of the mouth and the tongue will be examined for signs that indicate a lack of niacin or riboflavin. Inquiries concerning appetite, and tests of nerve reflexes provide clues to deficiency of thiamin. The presence of an enlarged thyroid gland suggests iodine deficiency. Unsatisfactory bone development indicates lack of vitamin D or calcium, or both. Much can be learned from simple anthropometric measures such as height, weight, arm and head circumferences, and skinfold thickness (a measure of fatness).

The visible signs of severe or long-standing malnutrition, then, are easily noted, but more refined tests are needed to detect milder grades of malnutrition.[1] Examination

[1]Standard values used to determine nutritional state (i.e., below-normal levels of hemoglobin, etc.) will be found in the Appendix, Table 14.

Table 20–1 CHARACTERISTICS OF GOOD NUTRITION AND POOR NUTRITION*

Good Nutrition	*Poor Nutrition*
About average *height* for age	Body undersized or poorly developed
About ideal *weight* for height	Thin (more than 10 percent underweight) or fat and flabby (more than 20 percent overweight)
Good layer of *subcutaneous fat*	Subcutaneous fat lacking or in excess
Muscles well developed and firm	Muscles small; pot belly
Skin turgid and of healthy color	Skin pale, sallow, or rough (hyperkeratosis); edema; seborrhea; dermatitis
Gums firm and *mucous membranes* of mouth reddish pink	Mucous membranes pale; tongue abnormally red or smooth; lesions at corners of mouth; gums swollen or bleeding
Hair smooth and glossy	Hair rough and without luster; thin; easily plucked
Eyes clear, good night vision	Angular lesions of eyelids; reddened or thickened, opaque conjunctivae; night blindness
Legs straight	Bowed legs; knock-knees; beaded ribs
Appetite good	Appetite poor; diminished taste acuity
General health excellent	Susceptible to infections; lack of endurance and vigor
Good-natured and full of life	Irritable, overactive; or phlegmatic, listless, unable to concentrate

*A number of these signs are nonspecific; that is, they may relate to more than one nutrient and to other conditions of health besides nutritional state. Taken in conjunction with a good history, however, they provide a reasonable index of nutritional state.

of the blood cells and chemical analyses of the blood may be made to determine the presence of nutritional anemia or unacceptably low levels of certain vitamins and minerals. A so-called "loading" test may be performed in which a test dose of a vitamin is administered, after which its excretion in the urine is measured. Excretion of an abnormally small proportion of the given vitamin indicates that it has been taken up avidly by depleted blood and tissues, resulting from previous lack of that vitamin in the diet. The albumin content and ratios of amino acids in the plasma are commonly used indexes of protein nutrition. Other tests measure metabolic functions, enzyme activities, and the like.

Conditions of nutrition vary in different sections of a country and at different economic levels. The estimation of the amount of malnutrition that exists in a country depends on the standards set for good nutrition. If only those who are actually examined and found to be markedly underweight or those who show gross signs of poor physical condition are classified as malnourished, the number may be reassuringly small. At the other extreme, if everyone for whom chemical tests show that the body is not saturated with certain vitamins is classed as undernourished, a lot of apparently healthy people will be included and the numbers will be alarmingly large.

Estimates based on food availability and consumption at the national levels are of little value because the figures do not take into account uneven distribution of food among people, or even loss of nutrients that occur in the period between production and consumption. When surveys are made of foods consumed by individuals (dietary records), and the results are judged by comparison with the yardstick of recommended allowances for the U.S. National Research Council's Food and Nutrition Board, the conclusions still may be misleading, for reasons now to be discussed.

Assessment Based on Food Consumption Figures

Almost no one eats exactly the same amount and kind of food each day of the week and at all seasons of the year. A single 24-hour record of intake can be quite unrepresentative, but this is the only type of individual intake information deemed feasible to collect in population surveys. Two particularly troublesome deficiencies of such surveys have been identified, in addition to the question of the representativeness of the 24-hour intake. One is the reliability of the information: People may fail to remember or to report accurately; this is particularly true of adults who attempt to recall food intake of their children and of aged or distracted individuals. Generally, there is a tendency to underestimate food intake (Fig. 20–1). A second concern is with the validity of conventional population samples. This is an especially serious problem when conclusions are to be drawn about the relationship of nutrient intake to other conditions of life. In a Quebec study, for example, out of a sample of 340 households, 104 were absent, 59 refused to participate, and 177 completed the inquiry (1). However, 63 percent of those from the higher socioeconomic group participated and only 42 percent from the lowest group. The refusal rate of the low economic group was less than that of the more affluent group (14 percent vs. 24 percent), but a much larger number of the low economic group were absent from their homes (44 percent vs. 13 percent). There is no way to determine the extent of bias introduced in the results by low participation rates, but it is likely that the very households one is most concerned about are least well represented

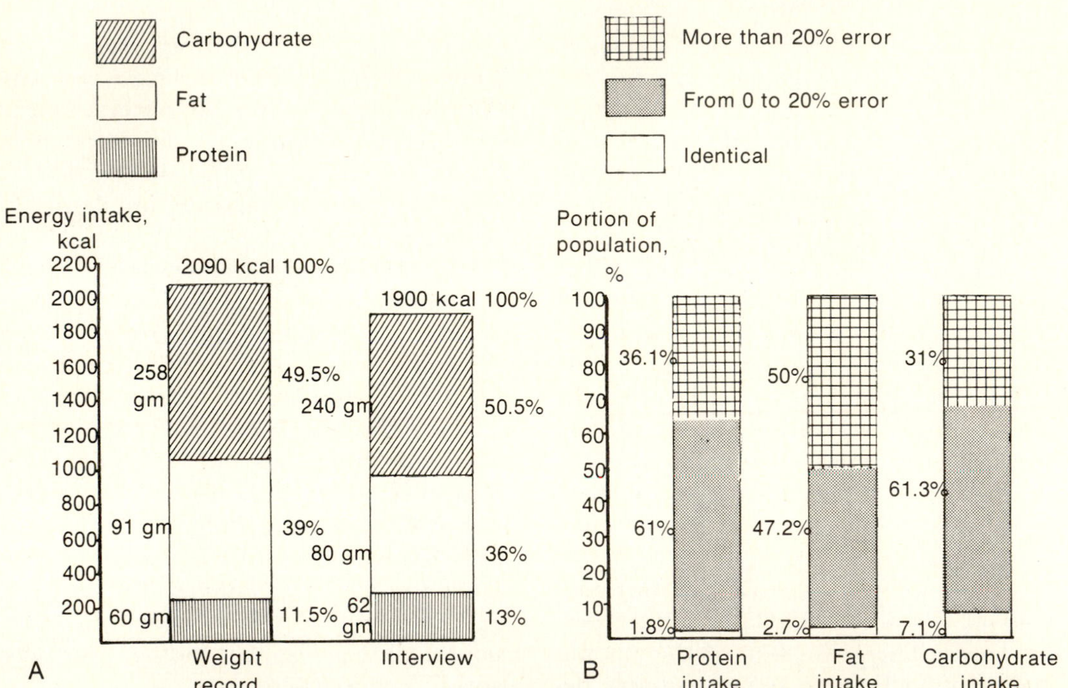

Figure 20–1 Comparison of data on a food intake obtained by weighing food and by recall interview. A, Mean values for energy, protein, fat, and carbohydrate intake. Note that weighed food intake was 10 percent higher than the interview findings. B, Correspondence of the two sets of data for individuals, showing that the estimated intake figure differed from the weighed intake by more than 20 percent in one-third (protein, carbohydrate) to one-half (fat) of the diets examined. (From Debry, G.: Validity of methods of dietary surveys. Ann. Nutr. Alim., *30:*115, 1976, with permission.)

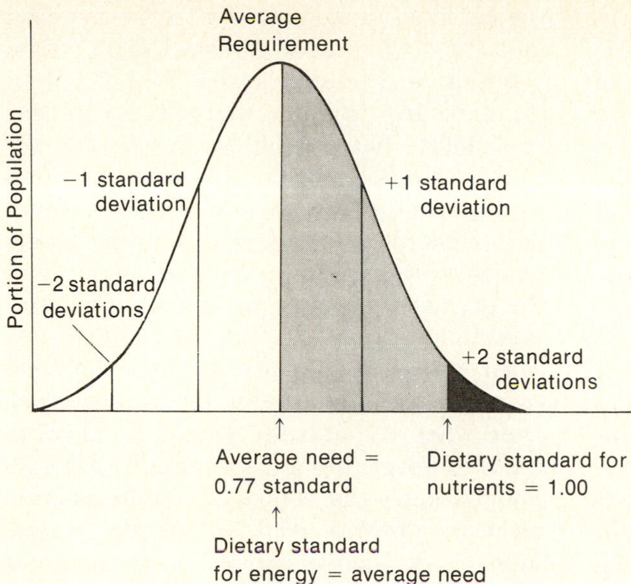

Figure 20–2 Dietary standards for protein, vitamins, and minerals are intended to cover the needs of almost all healthy people in a population; they are set at two standard deviations above the mean requirement where that is known. Thus, only 2 1/2 percent of a normally distributed population (the darker-colored area) will fail to meet their needs if their diets meet the standard. The standard deviation is about 0.15 of the mean requirement in the few instances where valid information exists. Thus the average need is about 77 percent of the standard, and the requirement of half the individuals will be met by intakes at this level. However, the standard for energy is set at the mean requirement, so the needs of half a population are not met (the lighter-colored area) by intakes that equal the standard.

in the sample. This problem is, of course, vexing no matter what method of nutritional assessment is used.

Nutritional status is governed by the quality of foods eaten over time, individual requirements, and environmental factors. However, 24-hour intake data for population groups are of value in that they do indicate the range of foods eaten and the overall quality of customary diets of that population.

Use of Recommended Allowances

Even when intake data are accurate and representative, there are problems in interpretation. Intake must be evaluated in relation to need.

Obviously, there are wide variations in energy requirements, according to sex, age, size, and especially the amount of physical activity. The protein requirement also varies with the amount of lean body tissue and the need to build new tissues. The recommended energy and protein allowances are given in terms of average or reference adults and are meant to be adapted to individual needs. Criteria for adjusting the mineral and vitamin allowances are not usually indicated, except for the obvious scaling of some of the vitamin B allowances for energy expenditure. However, we know there are differences between individuals in the efficiency with which they utilize these nutrients, so that some function well on smaller amounts while others require larger amounts to meet body needs.

The U.S. National Research Council's Recommended Dietary Allowance (RDA)(2) for all nutrients, except energy, is based on the average requirement plus two standard deviations (about 30 percent) above the mean requirement, if these figures are known.[2] (See Fig. 20–2.) The RDAs are placed at a high level with the idea that this covers the needs of even those with especially high requirements. For energy, the average figure is

[2]Average daily requirements of many nutrients have not been established. For these nutrients, RDAs are based on customary intakes of apparently healthy people, evaluated in light of requirements of other animals.

used as the RDA because both over- and under-consumption present problems, in contrast to the nutrients, modest excesses of which are harmless.

Allowances set for the United Kingdom are also intended to be "sufficient or more than sufficient for the nutritional needs of practically all healthy persons in a population" (3). Canadian standards are "considered adequate . . . to meet the physiological needs of practically all healthy persons . . . [and] exceed the minimum requirements of most individuals" (4).

Because we know that the majority of the population have their nutritional requirements met by lesser amounts than the U.S. RDAs, it is a mistake to assume that anyone whose intake falls below these levels is necessarily getting an inadequate diet. All that this comparison can indicate is the degree of risk of inadequacy at a given intake; the further below the RDA the intake falls, the greater becomes the chance that an individual's needs are not met. (See Fig. 20–3.) If the habitual intake is far below the standard (about 54 percent of standard for protein, vitamins, and minerals and 70 percent of standard for energy), there is a very low probability that the intake is adequate because only 2.5 percent of the population would have needs that low. When the number of people at any level of nutrient intake less than mean requirement is larger than the predicted number, then there is a corresponding risk that people are undernourished, *if* high intakes are consumed by high requirers and low intakes by low requirers. Even when the individual has free access to food, however, physiological mechanisms do not guarantee that intake, except for energy, meets or exceeds need. Hence, the magnitude of deficiency may actually be larger than the indicated statistical risk; it cannot be lower, if the estimate of needs is reliable and if requirement is normally distributed.

The body has some ability to adjust to somewhat lower levels of various nutrients. Adults have been maintained satisfactorily

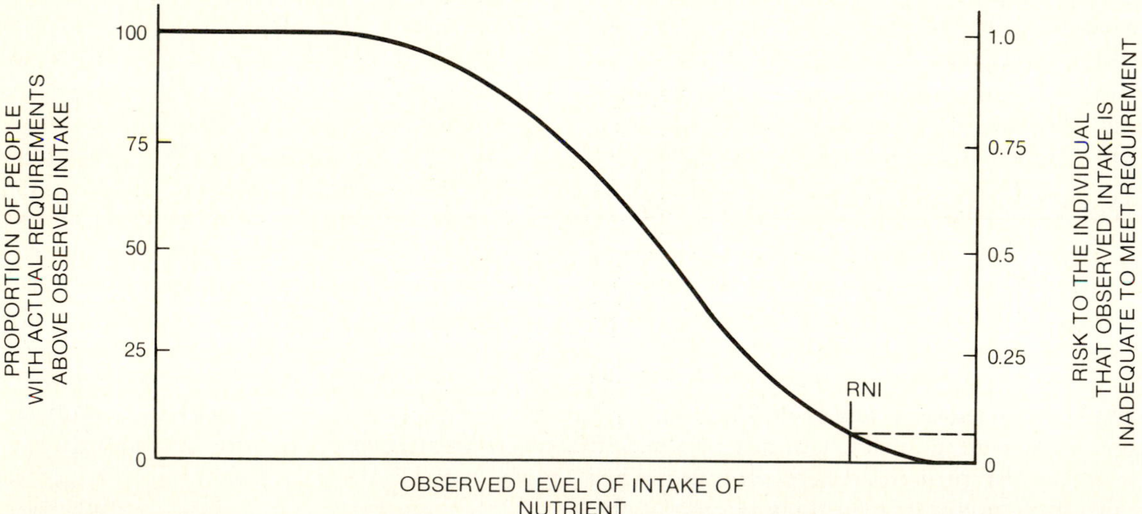

Figure 20–3 Probability approach to assessment of nutrient intake: inferred risk distribution curve describing probability of inadequacy associated with particular intakes of nutrients. For purposes of this illustration, the distribution of requirements is portrayed as gaussian. This is not always valid (e.g., the distribution of iron requirements in menstruating females is skewed). The distribution curves may vary for individual nutrients, but the conceptual approach continues to be applicable. The approach is not applicable to energy. From *Recommended Nutrient Intakes for Canadians* (1983) (4).

over long periods on as little as 40 to 50 gm of protein, 400 to 600 mg of calcium, and only a few milligrams of iron per day. For the world population as a whole, the World Health Organization (WHO) and the Food and Agricultural Organization (FAO) have established somewhat lower standards than the U.S. Food and Nutrition Board. For example, the international calcium allowance is 400 to 500 mg per day in contrast to the U.S. allowance of 800 mg. FAO/WHO standards, however, conform to the expectation of smaller body size and a limited degree of adaptation to habitually lower intakes.

Many nutritionists in this country believe that a substantial amount of protein, minerals, and vitamins over the minimum required levels will promote better health for all individuals of our varied population. However, this is by no means proved. Recommended allowances are revised as new information comes to light, and diets judged adequate or below standard on the basis of 1958 figures may be rated differently when measured against present allowances. (For instance, 12 mg of iron daily was recommended for adult women in 1958, 15 mg in 1963, and 19 mg in 1974.) A person whose diet meets the lower British standard for vitamin C might be judged poorly nourished if the U.S. Food and Nutrition Board allowances were used as the standard. Thus, final evaluation of the nutritional status of an *individual* must be determined by the condition of the person consuming the diet, not by comparison of calculated nutrient intake against standards intended for population groups and not necessarily applicable to an individual whose needs may vary from the norm.

Recommended allowances are intended to be a help in planning well-balanced diets for *groups of people*. They should not be regarded as a rigid standard that the diet must meet every single day. Slight shortages or surpluses cancel out from day to day. However, over a span of several days the diet should conform to accepted nutritional standards. The RDA should be met to prevent any continued shortage of protein, minerals, or vitamins. The energy intake must be adjusted to individual needs, for even a slight excess, if long continued, leads to overweight.

COMMON DIETARY DEFICIENCIES

Several surveys of the U.S. population (5–7) and the Canadian National Nutrition Survey (8) have evaluated nutrient intakes from food eaten in one 24-hour period as recalled by the respondents. These findings, as we have noted, may or may not be indicative of an individual's habitual intake. The USDA has also reported 24-hour intakes augmented by a two-day self-administered record (9).

In all surveys, a large number of substandard intakes was recorded, particularly among young women, pregnant women, the aged, ethnic minorities, and the poor. Only a very small proportion of populations examined had average energy intakes as high as American and Canadian standards. Even the three-day data from the USDA study indicate that only about one-fourth of the diets of individuals studied meet or exceed what is believed to be the *average* requirement for energy. This frequent finding of low energy-intake is particularly troubling in the further analysis of food-intake information. If the energy intakes are valid, many people are living on extremely low planes of intake. As the population generally tends to overweight more than underweight, intake must be reasonably adequate; people, therefore, must be far less active than is both assumed and physiologically desirable. If, on the other hand, intake has been underestimated, it is important to know if energy sources have been missed entirely (principally fats and

Table 20–2 MEAN 24-HOUR ENERGY INTAKES AND NUTRIENT INTAKE PER 1000 KCAL OF FOOD EATEN BY POOR PEOPLE AGED 60 YEARS AND OVER (U.S. TEN-STATE NUTRITION SURVEY) COMPARED WITH RECOMMENDED DIETARY ALLOWANCES(6)[a]

		Intake by Males				*Intake by Females*		
Nutrient	*NRC RDA*	White	Black	Spanish-American	*NRC RDA*	White	Black	Spanish-American
Energy, kcal/day	2400	1937	1508	1812	1800	1442	1174	1623
			per 1000 kcal				*per 1000 kcal*	
Protein, gm	23	40	43	43	26	40	41	42
Calcium, mg	333	449	358	255	444	433	416	361
Iron, mg	4	6	7	8	6	7	7	7
Vitamin A, IU	2083	2652	3334	1851	2222	2630	4997	2120
Vitamin C, mg	26	30	37	28	33	46	52	47

[a]Note that the *quality* (nutrients per 1000 kcal) of food selected generally met nutritional standards, except for calcium in diets of black men and Spanish-Americans of both sexes. If people had eaten *enough* of this same mixture of foods, nutrient intakes would have been satisfactory. Intakes of about three-fourths of the population were below the RDA for energy. Similar findings were recorded in the 1971–1972 HANES survey, and persons with incomes below the poverty level had lower energy intakes than did those living above poverty.

sugar added to foods), or if portion sizes have been underestimated. Should the problem be portion sizes, then the question of nutrient deficiency might be examined by looking at the nutrient density of diets; that is, the amounts of essential nutrients per 1000 kcal. (See Table 20–2.) If less visible energy sources, however, have not been recorded, then finding these and correcting the energy intakes would not affect estimates of essential nutrient intake to any great extent. Nutrients that commonly fail to be provided at RDA levels are: calcium, magnesium, and iron; thiamin, riboflavin, and vitamins B-6, B-12, A, and C. Remembering that the RDAs for nutrients are set well above average requirements, the amounts of these provided appear to come closer to meeting average needs than does the energy supplied. For example, three-day diets of the bottom 30 percent of energy consumers in the USDA study met 55 percent of the average requirement for energy (the RDA) and 57 percent of the RDA for calcium. Since the RDA for calcium is presumed to be about 130 percent of the average requirement for calcium, the diets met 74 percent of the average requirement (130 × .57) for calcium.

Two items have been omitted from the survey data cited, which bear importantly on these issues—alcoholic beverages and nonfood nutritional supplements. Consumption of alcohol in the United States is reported to be about 150 to 200 kcal per capita and would account for about half the difference between reported average adult intakes and the RDA. Alcohol consumption, however, could hardly contribute significantly to the deficits in the six-to-fourteen age groups. Information from small studies on use of such things as vitamin pills indicates that those people most likely to use supplements regularly are least likely to need them. Supplements tend to push intakes above 100 percent of the RDA, but probably do not affect the validity of findings at the lower end of the intake scale.

None of the surveys cited has examined dietary intakes of other trace elements, B-complex vitamins, or fat-soluble nutrients. Failure to include these nutrients is due to lack of adequate, reliable information on their presence in foods as consumed, and on the absence of reports of deficiency symptoms in human populations.

Based on the three-day data from the USDA, the nutrients of most concern are calcium, iron, magnesium, vitamin B-6, and, for some groups, vitamins A and C. A number of smaller surveys have identified zinc, folacin, and, possibly, copper as nutrients at risk of deficiency. Ratios of polyunsaturated to saturated fatty acids generally do not conform to prudent diet recommendations.

CHOOSING A BALANCED DIET

It is sometimes argued that dietetic advice is unnecessary, that left to our innate tendencies, we would select a nutritionally adequate diet. And it is true that animals in nature somehow must manage to select diets that are nutritionally adequate, or they could not live and reproduce. Adequacy could be coincidental with satisfaction of energy needs because, in nature, nutrients are not found singly. Food plants and animals are all mixtures of organic compounds and minerals, and animals come to occupy an ecological niche where the food available to them matches their needs for energy and nutrients. However, animals are, to some extent, able to choose the better of nutritional alternatives. For example, given a choice of mixed diets that are protein-free or that contain an adequate amount of protein, rats eat very little of the poorer one. Rats will also eat a reasonable balance of two diets that have widely different protein qualities, but they do not make very fine discriminations between proteins that are marginally different. When they are required to select among pure foodstuffs (pure protein, pure fat, and sugar), some animals are able to do so, but others within the same strain and age group are not.

Certain "specific hunger"—the situation in which an animal is deficient in one nutrient and seeks out that specific nutrient—is thought to be genetically determined. Animals can recognize a substance in which they are deficient and will go to it selectively, even if they have never before been deficient in that nutrient. Salt is thought to be in this class.

Other specific hungers are learned, as illustrated in Harris's classic experiments with rats deficient in B vitamins. The general pattern of experiments was to deprive rats of thiamin. The animals were then offered diets flavored with easily recognizable substances that were thought to mask the vitamin odor. The deficient rats reliably learned to select the diets containing the vitamin, but nondeficient rats showed no such preference among the diets. However, if animals made deficient were given a large number of diets (six to ten), only one of which contained the missing vitamin, they were unable to pick the correct one. The rats could be taught to choose the correct diet by giving them a training period when only that diet was given; later, when all the different diets were offered again, the rats would continue to choose the one they had learned contained the vitamin. If the vitamin was then removed from that diet and added to a diet with a different flavor, the rats continued to eat the previously learned, but now deficient, diet. They could be re-educated to accept the new flavor of diet by repeating the process of offering only one choice while they were in a deficient state. This indicates that the ingestion of the vitamin that had been lacking caused some reaction in the animal's body that provided a sufficient cue to establish learning of an associated flavor. Animals sense well-being, but there is nothing innate about vitamin recognition per se.

Perhaps nutritional food habits are formed by a comparable learning process. Animals that are deficient in one or more nutrients may try eating something in their environment, and if they feel better according to some internal cue, they learn that this is what animals should eat, and they develop a taste for it. That this mechanism is faulty is well known, because animals will eat things they like that are to their detriment. Animals will founder in a cornfield; birds will eat fermented fruit to the point of drunkenness, endangering their lives if predators are handy; and people seem to prefer sweet, rich foods over the simpler ones, in spite of internal cues that signal satiety and intellectual awareness of too much body fat. Animals, including humans, develop an aversion to foods that are associated with illness and thus learn to avoid toxins. Sensitivity to these is part of the process of gustation, but the aversion will develop in animals even if they are anesthetized at the time of ingestion, indicating that this regulatory process is quite different from usual associative learning. Many toxins have a bitter taste, which probably contributes to the low preference for bitter substances. Certainly, liking for such items as olives and quinine (tonic) water is a learned response.

One famous experiment is usually cited as proof that humans can choose their diet wisely. Davis allowed three newly weaned infants to choose their own diets from among thirty common, natural food materials (10). The choice was restricted to foods thought suitable for infants, and neither mixed dishes nor sweets were offered. Two of the infants were studied for six months and the other for a year. At first the babies tried anything in their mouths—inedible plates as well as edible foods—but they became selective and developed definite tastes. Their food preferences were erratic and unpredictable, and their diets were not balanced within a day. Sometimes the babies would indulge in binges, eating many oranges a day for several days and then none, for instance. Some of the babies' choices did suggest specific selection. They ate salt only rarely and obviously did not enjoy it, even crying when they took it, but they did go back for more. In retrospect, Davis regarded her experiment as flawed because she had limited the possible choices the babies might make to what her knowledge dictated they should have, and she thought the test might otherwise have failed. The infants did, however, balance a diet from among thirty options daily, and their health and growth were acceptable by 1928 standards, when the study was done.

The fact that nutritional deficiency states are seen is incontrovertible evidence that if we have an inherent regulator of intake, it is overridden by cultural and environmental factors. (See Chap. 19.)

The underlying causes of faulty nutrition have been stated to be *poverty, disease, advertising, peer-group pressures,* and *lack of home control.* Left to their own discretion, inadequately informed and motivated, children and adolescents often spend their lunch money on "soda pop," French-fried potatoes, and sweets—or spend it for other purposes entirely. These will be purchased in preference to a more adequate but less socially acceptable school or home-packed lunch. Disorganized households in which full meals are rarely prepared and in which the family does not eat together provide no protection against poor eating behavior outside the home and offer no guidance in food selection by parental example. In our affluent cultures, we often fail to notice that some people are poor. If one doesn't have the means to obtain enough food or the more expensive but essential foods such as milk and vegetables, it is impossible to prevent undernutrition.

Dietary Guides

It would be an almost impossible task to calculate and balance the diet with respect to forty or more nutrients every day (not to mention flavor, cost, and availability) without access to sophisticated computer programs. For this reason, one needs some general rule or set of rules that assure adequacy if followed in planning the diet.

The most commonly accepted food selection plan is one sponsored many years ago by the U.S. Department of Agriculture, and one that most children have been taught in elementary school—the "Basic Four Food Groups." This plan specifies the inclusion in the diet each day of foods from each of four groups—milk, meat, cereals, and vegetables and fruits—in a foundation diet. The basic diet is intended to provide practically the full allowances of all nutritive essentials except energy. The basic plan provides about 1200 kcal, to which more of the same foods or other foods are to be added to increase energy to the desired level. The number and size of servings from each of the groups included in the foundation diet are:

Milk Group: 3 servings per day for child, 4 for adolescent, and 2 for adult. Serving defined as 1 c milk, yogurt, or calcium equivalent (1½ oz cheddar cheese, 2 c cottage cheese, 1¾ c ice cream).

Meat Group: 2 servings per day, defined as 2 oz lean meat, fish, poultry, or protein equivalent (2 eggs, 2 oz cheese, 1 c cooked dry beans or peas, 4 Tbsp peanut butter, 2 oz nuts).

Vegetable and Fruit Group: 4 servings, including one rich in vitamin C and one rich in provitamin A. Servings are ½ c cooked or juice, or 1 c raw.

Cereal Group: 4 servings whole-grain or enriched products. Serving is 1 slice bread, 1 tortilla, 1 c ready-to-eat cereal, ½ c cooked cereal, rice, pasta, or grits.

This simple plan based on four food groups is by no means foolproof even for populations whose preferred style of eating fits the categories specified. It is quite easy to defeat the system by consistently making poorer choices within the group alternatives, by skimping on serving sizes, or by cooking or processing a food in such a way that its nutrient content is substantially lowered. This latter problem becomes increasingly important with the development of substitute foods that mimic but do not match the original.

Any simplified eating plan is based on the assumptions that (1) there are a *few key nutrients* that *must be monitored* out of the more than forty possible; and (2) the *nutrients not being monitored inevitably follow* in the variety of foods selected for the key or index nutrients. The Basic Four has oversimplified the indices. For example, legumes are accepted alternatives in the protein-index "Meat" Group of the Basic Four food plan. Almost the only thing all these foods have in common is protein of good quality. Meats contain vitamin B-12 and beans do not; most legumes are rich in folacin and most meats are only fair. Even the "meats" are not alike; marine fish provide iodine, but cattle and poultry flesh contribute very little of this nutrient. The consequences of these differences in composition depend upon all the other choices one makes. The absence of vitamin B-12 from the "Meat" Group alternative is irrelevant if the person selects the Milk Group as specified. The iodine in fish is of no importance to the inlander who uses iodized salt. On the other hand, a person who is allergic to milk or one who wishes to forego all animal food might carefully provide for his or her calcium needs elsewhere (remember that calcium is the key nutrient in the Milk Group), but conclude by having a diet deficient in vitamin B-12. Similarly, the person who has no marine food, whose native soil is low in iodine, and who does not use iodized or sea salt may develop a goiter.

Substitute foods are even more likely to defeat an index system. Vitamin C–fortified, orange-flavored sugar is a far cry from a fresh orange, in terms of both vitamin and, especially, mineral content. Again, the consequences of its use will vary. The impact will be minimal if the rest of the diet is of high quality; the juice substitute might be an improvement if it replaced a sugared drink without any vitamins at all or if the diet were lacking in vitamin C and nothing else. In a poor-quality diet, however, the substitution could be the final poor choice that changes a diet from marginal to deficient.

In time, food technologists will probably be able to develop substitute foods that more nearly match their natural counterparts, provided that nutritionists are well able to give advice about which nutrients to add and in what amounts. Unfortunately, knowledge is not this far advanced. Several of the B vitamins were scarcely recognized at the time the original legislation on enrichment of refined cereals was drafted, and they are not, to this date, restored in milled grains and their products. We are rapidly expanding our knowledge of trace minerals but have not yet proved the essentiality of some of them for man, and for only a few can we say how much is needed. As you have learned in earlier chapters, in some instances, the risk of too much of a nutrient is as great as the hazard of too little, and the balance between some of them is critical. Under these circumstances, food fabrication is difficult and carries a high nutritional risk.

We cannot plan for what we do not recognize or know to be essential. This has been a weakness in all food plans proposed thus far. The Basic Four made no certain provision for, among other nutrients, vitamin E, folacin, magnesium, or zinc—and with reason. When the plan was devised, there was no adequate information on the amount that should be included in the diet of all age groups, nor was there knowledge of the distribution of these nutrients in foods. The situation is not a great deal improved today in regard to two of those four nutrients, and we have even added new ones to the list.

Dietary Goals and Guidelines

In the decades since the Basic Four Food Groups Guide was developed, not only have nutrition knowledge, food supply, and intake patterns changed, but so have life-styles and health conditions. People are less active physically, and obesity is common; they die far more often from heart disease and cancer than from infectious diseases, the scourge of earlier generations. In 1976 and 1977 the U.S. Senate Select Committee on Nutrition and Human Needs considered the evidence linking health states and dietary intakes of the American public, and on the basis of this study and the testimony of experts, the Committee elaborated a set of "U.S. Dietary Goals." Although these goals did not provide a menu or food-selection guide, they suggest changes in eating habits intended to reduce the risk of the most common degenerative diseases.

Recommendations were patterned after those of the American Heart Association. The goals were to: avoid overweight; increase consumption of complex carbohydrates to 48 percent of energy; reduce intake of refined sugars to 10 percent of energy, fat to 30 percent, and saturated fat to 10 percent of energy; and reduce cholesterol to 300 mg and salt to 5 g per day. The issuance of these goals by a legislative body led to lively scientific debate. The Food and Nutrition Board discussed controversial points (principally cholesterol and saturated fats) and amplified others in a pamphlet entitled "Toward Healthful Diets." Finally a joint committee of the U.S. Departments of Agriculture and Health and Human Services issued a set of "Dietary Guidelines." The seven features emphasized are:

1. *Eat a variety of foods.* To assure an adequate diet, eat a variety of foods daily, including selections of fruits, vegetables, whole-grain and enriched breads, cereals and grain products, milk, cheese, yogurt, meats, poultry, fresh eggs, and legumes (dry peas and beans).
2. *Maintain ideal weight.* To lose weight, increase physical activity; eat less fat and fatty foods, sugar and sweets; and avoid too much alcohol.
3. *Avoid too much fat, saturated fat, and cholesterol.* Choose lean meat, fish, poultry, dry beans and peas as protein sources; moderate use of eggs and organ meats (liver, for example); limit intake of butter, cream, hydrogenated margarines, shortenings and coconut oil; trim excess fat from meat; and broil, bake, or boil rather than fry.
4. *Eat foods with adequate starch and fiber.* To eat more complex carbohydrates daily, substitute starches for fats and sugars; select foods that are good sources of fiber and starch, such as whole-grain breads and cereals, fruits and vegetables, beans, peas, and nuts.
5. *Avoid too much sugar.* Use less sugars of all kinds, including honey and syrups; eat less foods containing sugars, such as candy, soft drinks, ice cream, cakes, and cookies; select fresh fruits or fruits canned without sugar or in light syrup; and reduce amounts of sugar consumed between meals as snacks to aid in reducing dental caries.
6. *Avoid too much sodium.* Cook with only small amounts of added salt; learn to enjoy the unsalted flavors of foods; add little or no salt to food at the table; and limit intake of such salty foods as potato chips, pretzels, salted nuts, popcorn, cheese, pickled foods, cured meats, and condiments (for example, soy sauce, steak sauce, garlic salt).
7. *If you drink alcohol, do so in moderation.* Alcoholic beverages tend to be high in calories and low in nutrients. One or two drinks daily appear to cause no harm to adults. Pregnant women should avoid alcohol or at least limit intake to two ounces or less in a single day.

Unfortunately, there is little hope of the average consumer being able to follow these Guidelines unless he or she is exceptionally well informed as to food composition, and is able to store and accumulate the needed information from each meal and snack as the day wears on. For the Guidelines to be effective, they must be linked to a simple food guide.

A number of food group guides have been suggested that either add or refine groups, or recommend additional servings from some groups, or both. A radically different approach relates the amount of a given nutrient per 1000 kcal of a food to the RDA for that nutrient, per 1000 kcal (called the "Index of Nutritional Quality"). The revised guide presently in use was developed by the USDA to implement the Guidelines. It uses the same Basic Four Food Groups plus a Fifth Group consisting of fats, sweets, and alcohol. Philosophically, this represents no change at all from the original four-groups plan. (See Table 20–3.)

What the revised food groups guide attempts to do is combine scientific knowledge with Western cultural wisdom. Flawed though it is, there is not now an equally simple, equally workable alternative plan for Western food patterns. Our goal, then, will be to add to the scientific basis of the Four Food Groups, making finer discriminations among the group alternatives based on newer knowledge of nutrients and the foods in which they occur.

Selection of foods within groups to meet the needs for nutrients identified as being low in United States diets will be considered as will ways to modify the Basic Four Food Groups Plan to suit other preferred patterns of eating. The one rule to be emphasized is that *the family diet should include a wide variety of natural foods chosen from among a number of food classes.*

Foundation Diet from the Four Food Groups

Table 20–4 presents an evaluation of some of the nutrients provided by a conventional Basic Four foundation diet compared with

Table 20–3 REVISED BASIC FIVE FOOD GROUPS GUIDE[a]

Group	*Function*
Vegetable and Fruit 4 servings/day	Contributes vitamins A and C, potassium and fiber. Dark green and deep yellow vegetables are excellent sources of vitamin A. Most dark-green vegetables, if not overcooked, are also reliable sources of vitamin C. So are melons, berries, tomatoes, and citrus fruits (oranges, grapefruit, tangerines, lemons, and so forth). Dark-green vegetables in addition are valued for riboflavin, folacin, iron, magnesium, and vitamins E and K. Certain greens—collards, kale, mustard, turnip, and dandelion—provide calcium.
Bread and Cereal 4 servings/day	Whole-grain and enriched breads and cereals are important sources of thiamin, riboflavin, niacin, iron, and protein. Whole-grain products also contribute magnesium, folacin, vitamins B-6 and E, and fiber. Yeast used in making bread adds substantial amounts of several B vitamins, especially folacin and vitamin B-6. Lime used in making maize tortillas is a rich source of calcium. Baking powder and soda add sodium.
Milk and Cheese 2–4 servings/day	Milk and most milk products are calcium- and protein-rich foods. They contribute phosphorus, potassium, sodium, riboflavin, and vitamins A, B-6, and B-12, too. Some are fortified with vitamin D. Milk has more B vitamins per serving than cheese does, including folacin and riboflavin.
Meat, Poultry, Fish, Beans, and Nuts 2 servings/day	These foods are valued for protein, phosphorus, iron, zinc, copper, vitamin B-6, and other vitamins and minerals. It is a good idea to vary choices in this group. Fish, poultry, and meats are good sources of highly absorbable zinc. Liver and egg yolks are valuable sources of vitamin A. Fish fat is high in polyunsaturated fatty acids, and marine fish are rich in iodine. Beans, peas, and nuts are moderate sources of magnesium. All foods of animal origin contain vitamin B-12; foods of vegetable origin do not.
Fats, Sweets, and Alcohol in Moderation	Most foods in this group provide relatively low levels of vitamins, minerals and protein in relation to energy. Vegetable oils generally do supply essential fatty acids and vitamin E. Butter and fortified margarines contribute vitamin A. Other foods in this group are mayonnaise, salad dressing, sugar, honey, syrups, jelly, sugar-sweetened beverages, and other sweets; alcoholic drinks; and unenriched refined flour and meal and baking products.

[a]Serving sizes as defined on page 505. Adapted from *USDA Hassle-free Guide to a Better Diet,* Leaflet No. 567, 1980.

the total amounts specified as the recommended allowance. The nutrients tabulated are the well-studied ones, around which the Basic Four Food Groups plan was designed. The foundation diet is intended to be supplemented by other foods but does in itself provide almost enough of most of the listed nutrients to meet the recommended allowances, except for energy, iron for women, and thiamin for men. (Although 30 percent low for men in preformed niacin, it probably meets the need for this vitamin by synthesis from tryptophan in the protein.) The foundation diet furnishes only about 1200 kcal, so supplementary food is needed for energy: for the man a considerable amount, 1500 kcal, and for the woman perhaps 800 kcal. *The final quality of the diet will depend heavily on the food choices made to provide the extra energy.*

To understand this better, let us consider a typical North American menu that might be devised from the foods listed in the basic

Table 20–4 WELL-KNOWN NUTRIENTS IN A DIET PLANNED ACCORDING TO THE BASIC FOUR FOOD GROUPS[a]

Adult Plan	*Grams*	*Approximate Measure*	*Energy (kcal)*	*Protein (gm)*	*Calcium (mg)*	*Iron (mg)*	*Vitamin A (IU)*	*Thiamin (mg)*	*Riboflavin (mg)*	*Niacin (mg)*	*Vitamin C (mg)*
Milk Group, 2 servings											
Milk (3.3% fat)	488	2 glasses (1 pt)	300	16	580	0.2	610	0.18	0.80	0.4	4
Meat Group, 2 servings											
Meat, fish, or poultry[b]	100	1 av. serving, cooked, lean only	295	24	11	2.2	178	0.16	0.21	6.0	2
Egg	50	1 medium	80	6.1	28	1.0	260	0.04	0.14	<0.1	0
Vegetable and Fruit Group, 4 or more servings											
Vegetables:											
Deep green or yellow[c]	100	½ c cooked	29	2.0	5	1.1	3900	0.07	0.11	0.6	29
Potato	100	1 medium, baked	93	2.6	9	0.7	Trace	0.10	0.04	1.7	20
Other[d]	100	½ c cooked	42	2.1	22	0.8	220	0.07	0.06	0.7	13
Fruits:											
Citrus or tomato[e]	185	6 oz juice	55	1.1	20	0.7	519	0.09	0.04	0.7	50
Other[f]	100	1 avg. serving	75	0.7	13	0.7	550	0.04	0.05	0.5	11
Cereal Group, 4 or more servings											
Bread, white, enriched milk solids added	100	4 slices	267	8.3	126	2.8	Trace	0.47	0.31	3.8	Trace
Total nutrients in foundation diet			1236	63	814	10.2	6237	1.22	1.76	14.4	130
Recommended Allowances:										Niacin Equivalents[g] (mg)	
Man, 70 kg, moderately active, 23–50 yrs.			2700	56	800	10	5000	1.4	1.6	18	60
Woman, 55 kg, moderately active, 23–50 yrs.			2000	44	800	18	4000	1.0	1.2	13	60

[a]Solid boxes indicate that 25 percent or more of the daily need of that nutrient is expected to be derived from that food group; dashed boxes indicate an expectation of 10 to 25 percent of the nutrient from that group. Compositional data are all from USDA.

[b]Average of the ten 100-gm servings of lean, edible portion of meats, including beef, lamb, pork, poultry, and fish.

[c]Average of ten 100-gm servings, one each of asparagus, broccoli, Brussels sprouts, carrots, green snap beans, green lettuce and romaine, spinach, yellow (winter) squash, and sweet potato.

[d]Other vegetables: average of ten 100-gm servings of beets, cauliflower, celery, corn, green peas, lima beans, onions, summer squash, turnips, and zucchini.

[e]Daily average based on three servings of orange juice, two servings of grapefruit juice, three servings of tomato juice, and two servings of fresh raw tomatoes.

[f]Other fruits: daily average based on one average serving each of fresh apple, banana, peach, pear; one serving each of canned applesauce, apricots, peaches, and pineapple, plus one serving of dried or stewed prunes.

[g]Includes niacin as such and from tryptophan conversion.

plan. The menu given in Table 20–5 allows for a lunch carried from home and includes more servings from the Vegetable–Fruit Group than the plan demands. Listed in the table below this in the Supplement are foods typically added to the foundation diet. Except for larger servings of some of the basic foods, most of the usual supplements add little in the way of essential nutrients. It is small wonder, then, that iron deficiency is a common finding in women and girls, who are likely to forego the increased portions of ordinary foods to "save calories" for desserts and sweets. Men, with their higher energy requirements, are able to eat both larger servings and high-energy foods having little other nutritive value and so may be better nourished than women.

Even the man's nutritional status may be in jeopardy with this diet, however. Table 20–6 compares the content of lesser-studied nutrients in the typical menu plan with the allowances for them. With the exception of phosphorus, in which the diet is disproportionately high, this menu provides one-half to two-thirds, or less, of the recommended allowances. For some of the nutrients tabulated, especially folacin and zinc, the compositional data are not as reliable as one would like, but the discrepancies between content and recommended intake are so sizable that this does not negate the conclusions that must be drawn. Either the Basic Four diet is marginal to inadequate *as commonly followed,* or allowances are unrealistically high, or both.

If the extra foods listed in Table 20–5 were chosen mainly from the Fifth Food Group (e.g., 5 tsp sugar, 5 tsp butter, 1 Tbsp jam, 4 cookies, 20 potato chips, 12 oz cola, 2 glasses wine, 1 oz mints) they could provide about 125 gm refined sugar, and 45 gm fat. In the total diet 13 percent of energy would be derived from protein, 30 percent from fat, and 57 percent from carbohydrate, with 23 percent coming from refined sugar. Without knowing the composition of fat used in the processed foods, the amounts of

Table 20–5 TYPICAL NORTH AMERICAN MENU FOR THE FOOD GROUPS DIET IN TABLE 20–4

Breakfast	***Carried Lunch***	***Dinner***	***Snacks***
	Four Food Groups Foundation, 1200 kcal		
Small glass of orange juice Cornflakes with milk	Egg sandwich on white bread Raw tomato	Small chicken breast Baked potato Yellow summer squash Pickled green beans Hot bread or roll	Raw apple and cheese
	Supplement, 800–1500 kcal		
Coffee, tea, or hot chocolate Larger serving of juice Sugar for coffee, cereal Cream in lieu of milk Toast, butter, jam	Coffee or tea Butter or margarine and mayonnaise on sandwich Cookies Potato chips Soft drink Fruit	Larger serving of chicken Butter for potato, roll, and squash Sweet dessert Coffee or tea Alcoholic beverages Sugar and cream in coffee More rolls and butter	Coffee or tea Sugar and cream in coffee Soft drink or alcoholic beverages Candy Crackers

Table 20–6 LESSER-STUDIED NUTRIENTS[a] IN A DIET BASED ON THE MENU IN TABLE 20–5

Foods	*Grams*	*Phosphorus (mg)*	*Sodium (mg)*	*Potassium (mg)*	*Magnesium (mg)*	*Zinc (mg)*	*Vitamin E (mg TE)*	*Folacin (μg)*	*Vitamin B-6 (mg)*	*Vitamin B-12 (μg)*	*Pantothenic Acid (mg)*
Milk Group											
Milk	244	228	120	370	33	0.9	0.1	12	0.10	0.9	0.77
Cheddar cheese	28	145	176	28	8	0.9	0.1	5	0.02	0.2	0.12
Meat Group											
Chicken breast	100	228	74	256	29	1.0	0.4	4	0.60	0.3	0.96
Egg	50	90	69	65	6	0.7	0.2	24	0.06	0.7	0.86
Vegetable and Fruit Group											
Green beans	100	25	4	162	20	0.2	0.1	46	0.05	0	0.13
Summer squash	100	26	2	193	12	0.2	<0.1	2	0.06	0	0.11
Potato	100	32	6	355	13	0.3	<0.1	12	0.09	0	0.25
Tomato, raw	100	18	3	227	10	0.2	1.0	18	0.10	0	0.25
Orange juice, fresh	100	17	1	200	11	<0.1	<0.1	35	0.04	0	0.19
Apple, raw	100	17	0	115	5	<0.1	0.31	3	0.05	0	0.06
Cereal Group											
Bread, enriched, white	70	76	360[b]	78	15	0.4	0.1	24	0.02	trace[c]	0.30
Corn flakes	28	18	350[b]	26	3	0.1	0.1	2	0.02	0	0.02
TOTAL		857	1400[b]	2142	178	5	~3	148	1.2	2.1	3.78
Recommended Allowance											
Men		800	d	d	350	15	10	400	2.2	3	d
Women		800	d	d	300	15	8	400	2.0	3	d

[a]Compositional data for these nutrients (except for phosphorus and potassium) are not as reliable as one would wish and are tabulated only to indicate the order of magnitude of a nutrient. Methods are poor for the vitamins, and minerals vary by a factor of 10 to 100, depending on soil composition and processing contaminants. Entries are mainly from USDA Tables.

[b]Sodium added to these cereal products in manufacture. Other foods would have salt added in cooking. The expected daily total would be about 5 gm of sodium, with these additions and use of salted butter or margarine.

[c]Vitamin B-12 due to added milk in recipe.

[d]Recommended daily allowances of these have not been established. Potassium need is on the order of 2.5 gm a day, and a ratio of about 1:1 of sodium to potassium and of calcium to phosphorous is desirable.

saturated and polyunsaturated fatty acids cannot be calculated.

An Improved Menu

How might these defects be rectified? In part, the missing nutrients can be added by selecting different foods from within the categories and by taking larger servings of some of them. Others are best handled by adding more servings or different types of foods.

Had liver been chosen instead of chicken, the contribution of one serving from the Meat/Bean Group would have been: iron, 8.8 mg; zinc, 5.1 mg; vitamin A, 16,000 μg RE; thiamin, 0.26 mg; riboflavin 4.19 mg; niacin, 16.5 mg; vitamin C, 27 mg; vitamin E, 1.62 mg TE; free folacin, 82 μg; vitamin B-6, 0.8 mg; vitamin B-12, 80 μg; and pantothenic acid, 7.7 mg. (Amounts of the other nutrients tabulated would not differ appreciably, but there would be major added contributions of copper, molybdenum, manganese, and all other substances that are stored in the liver.) The *difference* in iron yields a 12 percent improvement in the *daily average intake* if the liver were eaten only once weekly. Vitamin A content would meet the full allowance for ten days. Liver would add a two-week supply of vitamin B-12 and a full two-day allotment of riboflavin. Half of a daily allowance of folacin, vitamin B-6, and vitamin C (ascorbic acid) would be provided. Its high content of ascorbic acid makes liver almost unique among animal foods. (Fish roe is also high in vitamin C, and breast milk, while not high in this nutrient, contains enough to meet all the needs of an infant.)

Not everyone will eat liver, liver sausage, or paté de foie gras, and a great improvement can be made in the diet from a few simple changes that are perhaps easier to practice on a day-to-day basis. (Considering the relative amounts of muscle and liver in a carcass, it is evident that the whole population could not have liver every week in any case.) Substitution of whole-grain cereals for refined milled ones—in our example, three slices of whole-wheat bread and a serving of oatmeal instead of enriched white bread and cornflakes—would increase the magnesium contribution from the Cereal Group sixfold, quadruple the amount of zinc and vitamin B-6, and double the folacin derived from this group. Vitamin E content is ten times higher in the whole grains. Note that potato is quite a good food and contributes nutrients that suggest it could well be classified with the Cereal Group with vitamin C as a bonus.

Another key change is to include larger and more frequent servings of dark-green, leafy vegetables. Products such as mustard and turnip greens, kale, dandelion greens, and collards all have about one-third more of all the essential nutrients than do the substitutes presently allowed (other green and yellow vegetables). A 100-gm serving of mustard or other greens meets almost the entire daily allowance of ascorbic acid and vitamin E. Addition of a generous serving of a raw leafy green, such as romaine, cos, or leaf lettuce, will go far toward guaranteeing the adequacy of folacin in the diet. These vegetables also contribute much calcium and magnesium. The 1982 U.S. NRC Diet, Nutrition and Cancer study stressed the importance of carotene and vitamin C, and suggested additional emphasis on vegetables of the cabbage family (cabbage, broccoli, kale, turnip greens, and so on). Fruits are generally more expensive than vegetables as a source of vitamins A and C, for which we rely on the Vegetable/Fruit Group, and many are lower in content of B vitamins. Note, however, that fresh or frozen orange juice contributes folacin, and so do bananas.

It is worth considering addition of a third serving of food from the Meat/Bean Group every day, and for this serving, choosing frequently fish (for iodine and other trace minerals) and dry beans or nuts (for more thiamin and folacin). This change would have the effect of increasing the spectrum of foods and thereby increasing the probability of including the nutrients we know very little about today. Fish (including shellfish), meats, and poultry, but not the alternative legumes or nuts, are the only recognized rich source of biologically available zinc habitually included in the diet of the United States resident. Fish, legumes, and nuts would also improve the ratio of saturated to polyunsaturated fatty acids in the diet.

In the United States the Milk Group contributes most of the calcium in the typical diet and makes good contributions of protein and B vitamins. Since calcium is the key nutrient in this group, cheese is an accepted substitute for milk. However, the bulk of the water-soluble nutrients present in milk are lost in the whey, so cheese compares unfavorably with milk with respect to all the B vitamins, magnesium, and potassium. Owing to the lactose present, some persons experience intestinal gas or softening of the stools when they drink milk. (See Chap. 2 and 5.) Cheese, which lacks the offending sugar, will be a good source of calcium for them. Lactose-intolerant persons may also be able to tolerate traditional yogurt or soured milk (see Chap. 5).

Other calcium sources do exist, of course. The dark leafy greens are one (excepting those that are high in oxalic acid, Chap. 15), and they provide as much riboflavin as does cheese. Fish bones eaten in sardines, smelt, salmon, or dried fishes are another. Another source commonly used in the Near and Middle East is whole sesame seed or sesame seed paste, the tahini of Egyptian cookery and a basic ingredient in the Oriental candy halvah. The plant sources of calcium are lacking in vitamin B-12, which will need to be added from other sources.

To raise the vitamin E content of the diet, it is necessary to turn to another food group, fats and oils. A few foods such as peanuts and soybeans are high in vitamin E, and oil expressed from these foods is a still more concentrated source of this fat-soluble vitamin. Peanuts contain about 7 mg of alphatocopherol per 100 gm of nuts or 14 mg per 100 gm of crude fat. Potato chips, because they are fried in vegetable oil, have about the same concentration of this vitamin as do peanuts. Salad oils and mayonnaise made from vegetable oil have 5 to 40 mg of vitamin E per 100 gm, depending on which oil is used. The amount taken with a salad, about one tablespoon (15 gm), would provide about 1 to 6 mg of vitamin E. Margarines have about 13 mg of vitamin E per 100 gm and butter only 1 mg. Vegetable oils (except coconut) and margarines and salad dressings made from them would augment the intake of polyunsaturated fatty acids. (See Chap. 3 for composition.)

Vitamin D is not found in popular North American foods in significant amounts, except for fatty marine fish (see Chap. 9). Vitamin D adequacy is assured by the use of fortified milk and exposure to sunlight. Iodine nutrition has been approached in the same way, by selection of salt fortified with iodine if marine foods are not eaten regularly. It is difficult today to give clear advice about this issue because more iodine is creeping into our food supply than was formerly the case. Much of the common, cheaper white bread is made by a continuous dough process that sometimes uses iodate as a dough conditioner; another potential source is iodine-containing antiseptics used to cleanse commercial food equipment and to treat dairy cattle. We know little about the trace minerals, and their concentrations in foods will surely depend on the soil conditions where the vegetables and fruits, cereals, and legumes are grown and on the processes through which the food has passed.

After the needs for essential fatty acids and vitamin E are met, which can be accomplished with one or two tablespoons of oil, there is no nutritional reason to add more energy in the form of fat. There is no nutritional basis for use of sugar and alcohol except as alternative energy sources. How much of fats, sugars, and alcohol the diet can tolerate depends on how well the other items are selected and prepared in the home and how much energy the individual needs. *A reasonable plan is to take at least the first 1600 kcal (6700 kJ) from wholesome basic foods* to provide a margin of safety for variation in food composition and preparatory losses.

Sweet desserts containing milk (puddings or ice cream) or milk and eggs (custard-filled pastries, cakes) or fruits and nuts (compote, fruit pastries) have some nutritional advantages over those that are mainly whipped cream or sugar. If sugar is added, brown sugar is a slightly better choice than white. Honey has only very small amounts of essential nutrients, and its physiological properties are not superior to those of other sugars. A diet that included not more than 1 Tbsp jam or 3 tsp sugar and one small serving of a dessert or sweet would meet the Dietary Guidelines.

If alcohol is used, beer is the best choice, because it contains appreciable amounts of B vitamins and minerals; wine is second choice. Distilled spirits are the poorest possible choice in terms of nutritive value.

Other Dietary Components

Some foods usually classed as nonnutritive substances are included in diets the world over. Tea is the favored beverage throughout the Orient and in the British Isles, while coffee and cocoa are more widely used in Europe and the Americas. These beverages do contain minerals because they are extracts of plant materials, but the steps through which they are processed leaves them without significant amounts of vitamins, except for some niacin in coffee (about 0.5 mg in a 6-oz cup). All three beverages add 10 to 20 mg of magnesium per cup of fluid and 45 to 65 mg of potassium. Tea makes a significant contribution of fluoride (0.3 to 0.5 mg per cup). By themselves they yield no energy, but each *level* teaspoon of sugar used with them adds 16 kcal (67 kJ) and each tablespoon of light cream about 32 kcal (134 kJ). Dry cream substitutes may contain some cream or only a substitute fat, usually coconut oil, which has a higher percentage of saturated fatty acids than does milk fat; the other usual ingredients are isolated milk protein (casein) or nonfat milk solids, corn syrup solids, and chemical additives. At equal "whiteness" in the beverage, cream substitutes may have negligibly lower energy yield than does light cream. Cocoa powder may be mixed with water or milk, and the total nutritional content of the beverage will vary accordingly. These contributions from beverages are not trivial in view of the large amount taken in the day. A not-uncommon intake of five servings of beverage would add about 100 mg of magnesium, a nutrient in which diets tend to be low, plus whatever minerals are present in the local water.

Coffee, tea, and cocoa all contain a related group of stimulants, the one highest in concentration in each being caffeine, theophylline, and theobromine, respectively. Caffeine is added to most cola-flavored beverages. Caffeine is the most active of the three compounds and when taken in excess may cause sleeplessness. It has also been reported to increase the levels of glucose and fatty acids in the blood, particularly of persons with diminished or diabeticlike tolerance for glucose. Caffeine is a weak diuretic (Chap. 13). Tea also contains tannins, which have astringent properties, and it has enough thiaminase (thiamin-splitting) activity to be of concern if the diet is marginal in this vitamin. All these beverages are taken without apparent untoward side-effects in most healthy people, but tea is usually much better tolerated than coffee when there are digestive upsets. Herbal teas have been less well studied, but several are known to contain pharmacologically active compounds; some caution regarding them is warranted, since there is not as yet even the test of long cultural use to help prove their safety.

Herbs, spices, and condiments are plant material and do contain nutrients; the significance of these depends on the amounts used. Chili peppers are high in vitamins C and A, and enough chili is used to make a real difference in Spanish-American and Oriental cookery. Kimchee, a Korean condiment, is also a rich source of vitamin C. Dried kelp and other seaweeds used in Asiatic cookery are high in calcium, magnesium, iodine, and other minerals found in sea water.

Other substances quite casually added in cookery or in preserving foods can make important differences in the diet: About half of the folacin in home-baked bread comes from yeast added for leavening, and the yeast and other bread ingredients add more B vitamins, an array of minerals, and some protein. Baking powders add substantial amounts of sodium (potassium tartrate type is an exception) and usually phosphate or sulfate and calcium, but no vitamins. All but about ½ gm of the sodium present in the diet is there because it has been added as salt or one of the other sodium-containing compounds used in preserving or cooking the food, such as sodium nitrite in corning beef, brine for pickles, salt in butter, monosodium glutamate (MSG), and soy sauce in cooking.

THE ROLE OF COOKING IN NUTRITION

Some foods can be eaten raw, but most require cooking to improve their digestibility and to insure food safety. Providing that sanitary methods of fertilization and watering are practiced (unprocessed fecal matter harbors bacteria, amebae, and other parasites), most vegetables and fruits can be eaten raw after thorough washing in clean water. Potatoes, cereals, and legumes all should be cooked in order to improve digestibility of the starch; the legumes should be cooked to destroy antidigestive and potentially toxic materials as well. Meats, fish, and poultry can be eaten raw but are better cooked if there is the least question of parasitic, bacterial, or viral infections. Fish, pork, and beef muscle may carry parasites that may be killed during prolonged storage at home freezer temperatures; but for absolute certainty of kill, the muscle should reach an internal temperature of 180° F (82.2° C). Mollusks pick up hepatitis virus from infected water, and poultry and eggs are subject to salmonella infection. Milk must be pasteurized for safety, and this has little effect on nutritive values.

If foods are to be cooked in water, loss of water-soluble nutrients will be lessened if the food is left in large pieces and cooked quickly in a small amount of water. However, traditional Chinese and Japanese cookery sets another excellent example, in which vegetables are stir-fried for a short period of time and all the juices are included in the final product. Another way of coping with the problem of loss of nutrients in cooking water, especially good for coarse vegetables that require a fairly long period of cooking, such as collards and other greens, is to use the cooking water as a soup or soup base. "Pot liquor" from greens is a standard item of diet in the rural southern part of the United States; and in northern Chinese cookery, small bits of food are cooked in broth at the table, and the cooking broth is eaten last, as a soup.

Dry heat is also detrimental to many vitamins, and there is some damage to protein if such treatment is excessive. Well-controlled roasting, broiling, and frying, according to the directions in any good cookery text, will cause only modest losses. Again, juices should be salvaged and used in soup and gravy stock, but unless energy needs are large, it is prudent to skim off and discard the rendered fat.

Some nutrients are susceptible to oxidation, but this is more a problem in commercial food processing than in home preparation. However, unsaturated fatty acids and vitamin E do deteriorate when oils are opened to the air and the products become rancid. Even in frozen storage, prepared foods lose much of their vitamin E content through oxidative changes that continue to occur at these low temperatures. Little vitamin E or unsaturated fatty acid is lost in deep-fat frying in fresh oil, but there is substantial loss of vitamin content on storage. When fats are heated to very high temperatures (250° C) or when oils are reused for long periods of time, damaged and potentially toxic products are formed. Thus both palatability and nutritional considerations dictate that only fresh fats be used in food preparation.

The only common home food preparation in the United States that involves fermentation with microorganisms is yeast leavening of doughs, to which we have referred earlier. Various bacterial and mold processes are employed quite commonly in Africa and Asia, such as manufacture of oggi from cassava, kefir and yogurt from milk, and tempeh from soybeans. Microorganisms are able to synthesize many nutrients required in the diet, but some have a definite requirement for vitamins that are essential to the human being. For this reason it is difficult to guess what the net effect of a fermentation process will be in terms of vitamin and amino acid content of the food. Generally, food processing organisms add more vitamins than they use up in their growth, and some bacteria and molds, but not yeast, even make the "animal" vitamin B-12.

Dill pickles are often cited as a good source of iron (about 1 mg per large pickle), which seems odd because cucumbers are not a good source of iron. The extra iron in pickles is present adventitiously, as a contaminant from processing in metal equipment that is no longer much used by commercial food processors. Pickles packed at home in earthenware crocks would not have much iron either.

Unintentionally, we used to add iron in the home by slowly cooking foods such as tomato sauce or greens in iron pots. Also, we made extensive use of foods packed in tinned containers that often took up tin and iron by corrosion of the can on long-term storage.[3] With the introduction of frozen and ready-to-eat foods, and aluminum, stainless steel, and special nonstick pots and pans, these beneficial additions of iron have been lost. Zinc is also taken up from galvanized containers,[3] and such contamination may account in part for the high concentration of zinc in maple syrup. The mineral content of household water depends not only on the composition of the main water supply, but also upon the kinds of pipes and softening systems through which it flows.

The food that finally reaches the table reflects a host of factors: soil, water, harvesting, processing, transportation, and storage, as well as personal selection and home preparation. No amount of care in the household can make up for damage that has occurred in other steps of the food distribution chain. These other factors are discussed in Chapter 18.

SPECIAL NUTRITIONAL CONSIDERATIONS

The Vegetarian Diet

A diet that avoids animal flesh but that does include milk and eggs poses no particular nutritional problems. One simply

[3]Zinc and tin are essential nutrients, but both are toxic at high levels. For this reason storage of acid products in open tinned or galvanized containers is very hazardous: Poisoning has occurred from party punches made ahead and stored in metal pails.

changes the source from which protein is derived by adding more cheese, eggs, milk, dry beans, peas, and nuts, plus the needed amounts of fruits and vegetables, cereals, oils, and other energy sources. Some caution will be required in selection of iron- and zinc-rich alternative foods, and generous intakes of these trace elements are required because they are not well absorbed from vegetable foods. (See Chap. 16.)

Nutritional planning, however, becomes virtually impossible if all animal products are eliminated from the diet, especially for people accustomed to Western styles of food preparation. Protein is not a problem, as there are many adequate combinations of legume, cereal, and vegetable proteins. Such a diet, however, lacks vitamin B-12 and has only a limited spectrum of calcium sources in addition to the problem areas mentioned above. Traditional cultures that have maintained themselves on strict vegetarian diets have done so by unintentionally finding a source of vitamin B-12, a universal requirement for life. Some possibilities for synthesis are found in microbial processes applied to foods and unintentional contamination with animal matter, such as insects or their eggs, or with soil microorganisms. There is perhaps some intestinal synthesis of this vitamin, but it is not certain enough to be relied upon, for ample evidence of vitamin B-12 deficiency has been found in strict vegetarians. Without generous use of oils, nuts, and fat-rich seeds, even energy intake may be a problem, particularly for children.

Vitamin Supplements

Vitamin pills will not be needed by people who regularly eat a good diet, except under very unusual conditions. People who have been well nourished in the past will have ample reserves of vitamins in the liver and other tissues that will carry them through the ordinary minor illnesses and occasional periods of dietary indiscretion. Supplements will be needed if intestinal absorption is impaired by disease and sometimes during and after prolonged illness.

If a daily supplement is to be taken, it should contain the same balance of water-soluble vitamins as one would wish to have in the regular diet; that is, *all* of the vitamin B complex and ascorbic acid in amounts suggested in the recommended daily allowances. Only for therapeutic purposes and under competent medical advice should a pharmaceutical vitamin preparation be taken that exceeds the recommended allowances.

The fat-soluble vitamins must be treated cautiously, for vitamins D and A are toxic at high dosages (Chap. 9). If the diet includes vitamin D–fortified milk, as it should, then no other supplement of this vitamin should be taken by normal persons. Quite commonly vitamins D and A are added to products such as ready-to-eat cereals, flavoring agents for milk, and "instant" meals, so there is some risk of increasing the intake unduly.

If a person suspects that his or her diet may not be adequate, the best procedure is to improve the diet, because if vitamins are low, chances are that minerals will be inadequate also. At the present stage of knowledge, we know of no sensible way to prepare an all-round mineral supplement. However, a modest, well-balanced vitamin supplement will do no harm unless the practice of taking it tempts one to ignore the necessity of choosing foods wisely.

Meal Spacing

The times at which meals are eaten and the intervals between them are usually determined by the convenience of the family and the accepted pattern of a culture. All patterns have existed, from a very large number of very small meals (a nibbling pattern) to a single large meal daily. The body's metabolic machinery adapts to any habitual pattern so that we are able to cope with a flood of nutrients at one time and maintain critical functions in the intervals, or vice versa. However, in both human studies and animal experiments, a pattern of frequent small meals leads to more satisfactory levels of blood lipids and deposition of more lean and less fat in the body than if one or two large meals are eaten daily.

Other investigations of the effect of omitting meals have centered on (1) the maintenance of blood-sugar level as a physiological parameter indicating homeostasis, or (2) the efficiency with which some mental or physical work is performed. In persons accustomed to eating three or more meals a day, blood sugar begins to fall about 2½ to 3 hours after breakfast, with the fall occurring somewhat later if protein-rich foods are included in the meal; blood sugar continues to fall unless a second meal is given about that time. Lessened efficiency coincided with the blood sugar changes in subjects who were not habituated to skipping meals and so were ill-adapted to this pattern of eating. In a University of California study that examined this issue, reaction time was measured in college students who habitually eat or skip breakfast. Breakfast-eaters performed less well when breakfast was omitted, but those who usually skipped breakfast performed equally well with or without breakfast.

An English study raises a question about the desirability of lunch, at least for people who do not take an afternoon siesta (11). Groups of twenty students either ate a "standard three-course meal" in the university cafeteria or had no lunch and walked for an hour. (Tea and coffee consumption was not controlled, and there was no lunch/exercise group.) The ability to discriminate between events (signal detection) was significantly impaired in the fed group and unaltered in the exercise group. The investigators interpret their data as indicating that "operational efficiency and safety may be at risk" after lunch. A physiological basis for postprandial drowsiness might exist if the lunch were relatively high in carbohydrate and led to an increased proportion of the amino acid tryptophan in the blood and serotonin production in the brain. (See Chap. 4 and 7.) Anecdotal evidence suggests, however, that many people become drowsy in the afternoon (when listening to lectures, reading texts, and so on) with or without lunch.

People do seem to prefer a nibbling pattern, at least early in life. Infants eat at 2- or 3-hour intervals for the first days or weeks of life and only gradually are accustomed to long periods of sleep between bouts of eating. Most people have two or three main meals a day interspersed with two to four small ones (morning and afternoon coffee or tea, snacks in the evening, an occasional piece of fruit or candy, and so on). Data from the 1977–1978 USDA Food Consumption Survey show that both men and women in the United States eat about 20 percent of their total daily energy intake at breakfast, 24 percent at lunch, 44 percent at dinner, and 12 percent between meals (12). The distribution varies a little among age groups: Preschoolers have the most even distribution among meals; adults have slightly smaller breakfasts and larger dinners; older adults are the lowest consumers of between-meal foods. (See Table 20–7.)

In the United States Ten-State Survey of low-income populations, the diet histories indicated that both black and white youths age twelve to sixteen consumed about 20 to 25 percent of their total daily energy intake as between-meal snacks and beverages; the value was 13 to 16 percent for Hispanic teenagers. Snacks eaten by upper- and middle-income children, however, provide about 8 to 23 percent of energy intake. (See Fig. 20–4.) During one week, on days when no snacks were eaten (18% of child-days), energy intake was 77 percent of the RDA; it was 90 percent of the RDA with one snack (35% of days), 103 percent with two snacks (37% of days), and 118 percent with three snacks (10% of days). Energy and nutrient intake from meals was only slightly more on

Table 20–7 PERCENTAGE OF DAILY ENERGY INTAKE BY AGE GROUPS, PROVIDED BY SPECIFIC WEEKDAY MEALS[a]

Age Group	*Breakfast*	*Lunch*	*Dinner*	*Other*
Preschoolers	26.5	23.3	34.9	15.0
School-age	23.0	27.2	28.2	11.6
Teenagers	20.1	23.9	42.2	13.8
Adults	17.3	24.0	46.6	12.0
Older adults	21.5	22.1	47.3	9.1

[a]From Kennedy, E. T., Harrell, M. W. and Frazao, B.: Distribution of nutrient intake across meals in the United States population. Ecol. Fd. Nutr., *11*:217, 1982.

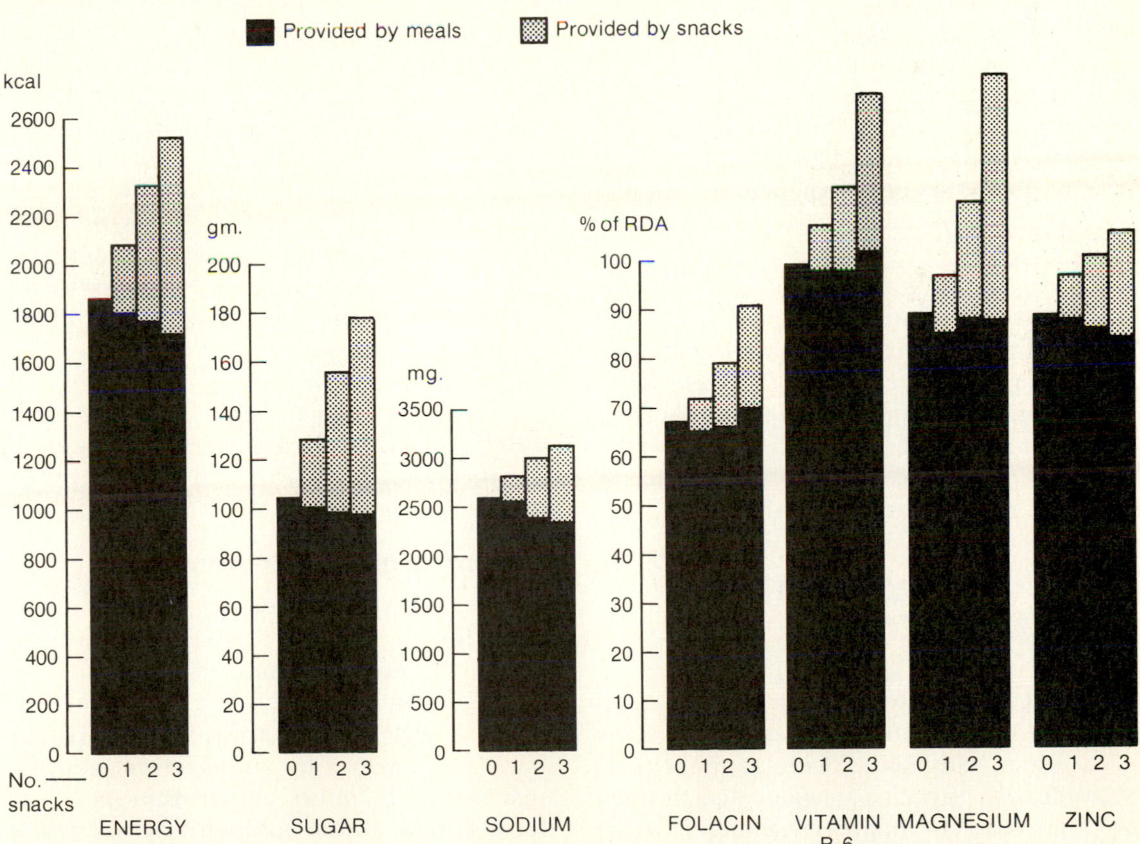

Figure 20–4 Contribution of meals and snacks to the nutritional intake of 657 middle- and upper-income children aged 5 to 12 years in the United States. At the three-snack-per-day frequency, snacks contributed an average of 81 gm sugar, 35 gm fat, and 645 mg sodium. (Data from Cala, R. F., Morgan K. J., and Zabick, M. E.: Home Econ. Res. J., *10*:150, 1981.)

days without snacks, indicating that snacks are simply added on to meals (also true of alcoholic beverages among adult social drinkers). Except for folacin and possibly magnesium and zinc, food at meals met nutrient allowances but snacks provided needed energy and significant amounts of some nutrients. The most commonly consumed snacks were beverages other than milk; fruits and vegetables; and milk and cookies.

A pattern of large, infrequent meals is customary in countries where food is in short supply and obesity is infrequent. In richer parts of the world, a larger number of small meals, five or six a day, seems to be preferred and physiologically desirable. However, nibbling is a good practice only if all the food forms part of a well-balanced diet. A midmorning, small meal of juice or milk is an asset, but one of a doughnut and black coffee is probably not. This pattern of food consumption can be adapted to a frequent meal schedule without sacrificing nutritional value.

Equally important is the need to arrange mealtimes, at whatever frequency, so that the family or living group eat together at least once and preferably twice a day. Disorganization in the household and lack of commensality contribute heavily toward development and practice of the poor food habits that lead to poor nutritional status.

NUTRITION OF THE ADOLESCENT

At about ten to twelve years of age, well-nourished girls enter the period of *pubescence,* which culminates with attainment of reproductive capacity at about age thirteen to fourteen. Comparable changes occur about two years later in boys. Both sexes experience a spurt in growth with the onset of puberty. Because the change occurs earlier in girls, they are taller and heavier than boys between the ages of ten and thirteen. Growth of boys then overtakes that of girls, and males are on the average taller and heavier than females during adolescence and adulthood. Growth continues, at a slower rate, however, during the period of *adolescence,* which is from ages thirteen to seventeen years in girls and fifteen to twenty-one years in boys. The onset of puberty is delayed about two years in underfed populations, but the pubescent growth spurt—a phenomenon peculiar to the human being—allows a final opportunity for catch-up body growth if enough food is available then.

Body composition also changes with puberty. During the pubescent growth spurt and adolescence, boys, under the influence of the anabolic male sex hormones, gain proportionately more lean tissue than fat, develop a heavier skeleton, and increase their pool of red blood cells. Mineralization of the skeleton is also completed at this time in girls, but the female sex hormones promote the deposition of proportionately more fat than lean tissue, and the red blood cell pool of females remains lower than that of males throughout adolescence and adulthood. For these reasons, boys need more energy and more of the body-building nutrients than girls do during pubescence and adolescence, but needs for both sexes are increased during this period.

Recommended Allowances

The U.S. recommended dietary allowances for boys and girls aged eleven to fourteen years are quite similar except for energy, for which the RDA is 2200 kcal (9.2 MJ) for girls and 2700 kcal (11.3 MJ) for boys. The reasons for this difference are (1) that the girls' pubescent growth spurt will have ended at the midpoint age (thirteen years), whereas the boys' growth spurt is just beginning; and (2) that after puberty many girls tend to reduce their customary levels of physical activity, while boys remain active. At ages fifteen to eighteen years, the disparity between usual activity patterns remains, and some boys are completing the accelerated growth phase. The RDA for energy at this age is 2100 kcal (8.8 MJ) for young women and 2800 kcal (11.8 MJ) for young men. Allowances for protein drop from 1 gm per kg body weight at ages eleven to fourteen to the mature allowance of 0.8 gm per kg at ages nineteen to twenty-two years. During the pubescent and adolescent periods, the RDAs for calcium and phosphorus are increased to 1200 mg per day, and 18 mg of iron per day is suggested for both sexes.

Canadian boys and girls engaged in their usual school activities are thought to require 2800 and 2200 kcal, respectively, between ages thirteen and fifteen years. Between sixteen and eighteen years of age, girls reach adult size and are thought to become less active, whereas boys continue to grow and engage in very active sports. The Canadian allowances for this age span are 3200 kcal for boys, which is 107 percent of the young (19–24 yr) adult men's value; and 2100 kcal for girls, which is the same as the young adult women's allowance. Protein, mineral, and vitamin intakes are adjusted upward for girls at the appropriate earlier age of ten years and lowered to mature values at age sixteen; for boys, the increase occurs at age thirteen and lasts until age nineteen.

Adolescence is a time of great physical, biological, and emotional adjustment. The teenager may exhibit immature judgment and uncertain behavior. The demand for independence may lead to abandonment of dietary practices taught in the family and to acceptance of fad diets and food patterns decreed by the peer group. School, work, and social activities take teenagers away from home a great deal, with the result that food habits, frequently not good before, become even poorer. Young people living continuously on diets providing suboptimal amounts of nutrients are in poor condition to withstand the stresses of their hectic life, let alone prepare their bodies for later productive career work and reproduction.

Dietary studies in the United States consistently show that intakes of calcium, magnesium, iron, vitamins A and B-6, and sometimes riboflavin and vitamin C, often fall far short of the recommended allowances for teenagers. Energy intakes of low-income, white girls and low-income, black boys and girls often were substandard, which coincides with findings of reduced growth in these groups. An Australian survey found that 16- to 19-year-old youths who were employed had poorer dietary intakes than those who remained in school, particularly the girls. The diets of only 3 percent of employed sixteen-year-old girls and 33 percent of the boys met Australian standards for all of eight nutrients tabulated. The Canadian National Nutrition Survey also found the diets of teenagers commonly to be substandard with respect to iron; calcium; vitamins A, D, and C; and riboflavin. The situation was worse for Eskimos and Indians than for the rest of the population, but some diets were at risk levels in all groups.

Usually, boys offer less problem than girls because their energy need is large so they can afford to eat more, and they are not so concerned about fatness. Girls of this age frequently have a capricious appetite, and if they develop an obsession about remaining slender, they rarely eat all the protective foods they need. The less food eaten, the more important it is to make all of it count. Fast-food establishments often become an important feature of the social scene, and a combination of limited spending money and teen subculture style may lead to selection of foods high in sugar and fat rather than of those with more needed protein, minerals, and vitamins. A soft drink and an order of "fries" or "chips" is relatively cheap and satisfying.

The family meal pattern is satisfactory for the teenager, with larger-size servings needed to provide additional calcium, iron, and energy. However, teenagers are often not at home for some of the family meals, which places on them the responsibility of knowing how to select nutritious foods.

Because snacks account for one fourth of the teenager's energy intake, these items should make a significant contribution of nutrients. If attractive, nutritious snacks are available at home, the teenager is able to choose food that contributes nutrients known to be at risk. Even when eating away from home, there are many nutritious snacks available. Snack foods that provide significant amounts of needed nutrients are: green vegetables and fruits (magnesium, folacin, vitamins A and C); nuts (magnesium, vitamin B-6); dry fruits, cereal and bran items; meat (iron); and cheese and milk (calcium).

Many young people are troubled by acne, a skin condition ascribed to effects of sex hormones on the sebaceous glands. There is no proven association of this disorder with nutritional deficiency or with specific foods, but physicians often recommend elimination of cola beverages and chocolate from the diet and reduction of fat intake. The net effect of such instruction, if followed, would be to reduce the amount of poor-quality foods and to increase the intake of other good foods to keep energy intake constant. Such an improved diet could benefit overall health, irrespective of its relevance to the skin disorder. Vitamin A has often been prescribed for skin conditions but has not been effective in treating common acne. Prolonged use of vitamin A at a prescribed dose of 16,000 μg RE per day for acne was the cause of clinically severe hypervitaminosis-A in a sixteen-year-old boy (13), so this nutritional therapy is not only ineffective but dangerous. There is also increasing prescription of zinc for skin disorders; the doses used generally are well above nutritional levels and should not be continued indefinitely.

Obesity is a common finding in teenagers: Most studies report a prevalence of the order of 15 percent of highschool students, as judged by body weight and anthropometric measurements. A key factor in juvenile obesity is inactivity, and the problem is better prevented or treated by increased energy expenditure than by food restriction at a stressful time of life. Participation in sports is recommended strongly for this reason and for establishing habits that promote life-long health.

NUTRITION OF THE OLDER ADULT

A marked change in life-style often occurs at about age sixty-five or with retirement from business. Changes in activity patterns are apt to be much more profound and abrupt for employed men than for women, who often continue with household tasks much as in earlier life. The bodily condition known as "old age" invariably develops sooner or later, but it is not simply the inevitable result of living a certain number of years. The rate of aging is affected by inheritance, nutrition, and other environmental factors. In animals, it is possible to show that aging may be postponed by the right dietary regimen. Some people are "older" in body at age fifty than others are at age seventy. Those who succeed in retaining their youthful vigor in the later years of life are usually not inactive people but, on the contrary, are those who are active mentally and physically.

Currently held concepts suggest that aging begins early in life and that procedures to alter the rate of decline need to begin equally early. However, most people are little concerned about aging until they themselves reach the middle years of life, when processes are well under way. Evidence from human populations is always epidemiological and retrospective because the life span of an investigator is no longer than the subject he needs to examine. Thus, animal systems provide our only model for research into methods to interrupt the processes of senile change. Current nutritional research focuses on two principal hypotheses. The first is that aging is due to oxidative changes that can be modified by increased dosages of vitamin E and other antioxidants. (There is no adequate proof for the antioxidant theory to date.) The second, more recognized theory is that delayed growth and maturation rate brought about by restriction of dietary energy early in life leads to a longer life span, or conversely, that overfeeding, with accelerated rates of growth and accumulation of adipose tissue, shortens it. Investigators have found that rats and mice receiving a lower energy intake in the early postweaning period lived longer than those that are liberally fed. However, there is no evidence that the same results would be true for humans, for in parts of the world where food intake and growth are low, average life span is shorter than in richer countries with more generous food supplies but also better public health practices. A diet that provides energy in *excess* of human needs, resulting in overweight, is definitely known to be associated with an increased incidence of heart and circulatory diseases, diabetes, and earlier mortality. (See Chap. 7.) When the overweight person reduces to normal or even slightly below normal weight, the risk of heart disease decreases. In many cases, adult diabetes may also be controlled simply by reducing body weight to normal, together with moderate restriction of dietary carbohydrate and judicious exercise.

A long-standing faulty diet may also be associated with *osteoporosis,* a disorder commonly seen in aged individuals in which there is thinning of the skeleton and lack of bone matrix. It occurs especially frequently in older women, and it may lead to spontaneous fracture of the spinal column and loss of height. The principal causes of osteoporosis are thought to be inactivity, lack of hormones, and decreased ability to absorb calcium from the intestine, coupled with chronic low intake of calcium and vitamin D.

In the later years of life, physical disabilities may lead to impaired nutrition. The loss of teeth frequently results in inability to masticate hard or coarse foods. Inadequately chewed foods may cause digestive discomfort, while the omission of all coarse foods from the diet may lead to a diet of poorer quality. Blood flow to the alimentary tract, secretion of digestive juices, particularly gastric acid, and intestinal absorption may be diminished. There are fewer active cells in the body, and various organs and tissues are either less active or less able to do extra work. Drugs taken for typical illnesses such as arthritis and hypertension may affect nutrient utilization or other requirements.

Nutritional needs of the older person differ from those of the younger adult, but not to the extent of a sparse and abstemious diet. The idea of such a diet for later life has gone out of style and for good reason. The same nutritive essentials (energy, protein, minerals, and vitamins) are required in adequate quantities to nourish the body throughout life, and too little of any of them does harm at any age.

The most significant change in the diets of aging persons is that less energy is needed. The energy requirement of older adults is materially reduced because (1) less energy is used in muscular activity; and (2) the basal metabolism is lowered.

Recommended Allowances

It is estimated that the basal metabolic rate between ages sixty and seventy is about 10 percent less than at age twenty-five. It is 20 percent less by age seventy to ninety, and about 25 percent less after age ninety. The resting metabolism of a man of average weight and in middle life requires about 1600 to 1700 kcal per day. Requirements of the same man at age sixty to seventy would be about 1440 to 1530 kcal, and at seventy to eighty years, 1280 to 1360 kcal. These differences in basal energy needs are due to a reduction in the amount of lean body mass, as the requirement *per unit of lean tissue* is nearly the same in young and old adults.

Few men in their seventies do enough muscular work to raise their total energy requirement to more than 2400 kcal a day. Small, aged women may have surprisingly low energy needs, but the average need between ages fifty and seventy is about 1800 kcal. It is thus apparent that the total amount of food—especially foods of high energy value—should be somewhat curtailed after age sixty years (slightly so even at forty to sixty), and considerably reduced after seventy. A Baltimore study of 252 men, age twenty to ninety-nine years and from upper-income groups, found that energy intake declined from about 2700 kcal for ages twenty to forty-four, to 2300 kcal for ages fifty-five to seventy-four, and 2100 kcal over age seventy-five. Body weight was 74 kg for ages twenty to thirty-four, 77 to 78 kg for ages thirty-five to seventy-four, and only 71 kg for men who lived beyond that age. If the weight factor is taken into account, the sharpest drop in energy intake occurred at about age sixty. Over the total age range, energy intake fell by 12.4 kcal per day per year, and the decrease in measured basal metabolism was 5.2 kcal per day per year. The difference (7.2 kcal) would be due to diminished activity. At all ages there is marked variation in energy need, and active older adults have much higher needs than the average. (See Fig. 20–5.)

Another variation in the needs of older adults compared with those of younger persons may be in protein requirement. Some studies have indicated that the requirement for total protein and for essential amino acids is higher in men over age fifty than in younger adult males, but in other studies no such age difference was apparent. In no case is there any suggestion of a decreased protein requirement with increasing age.

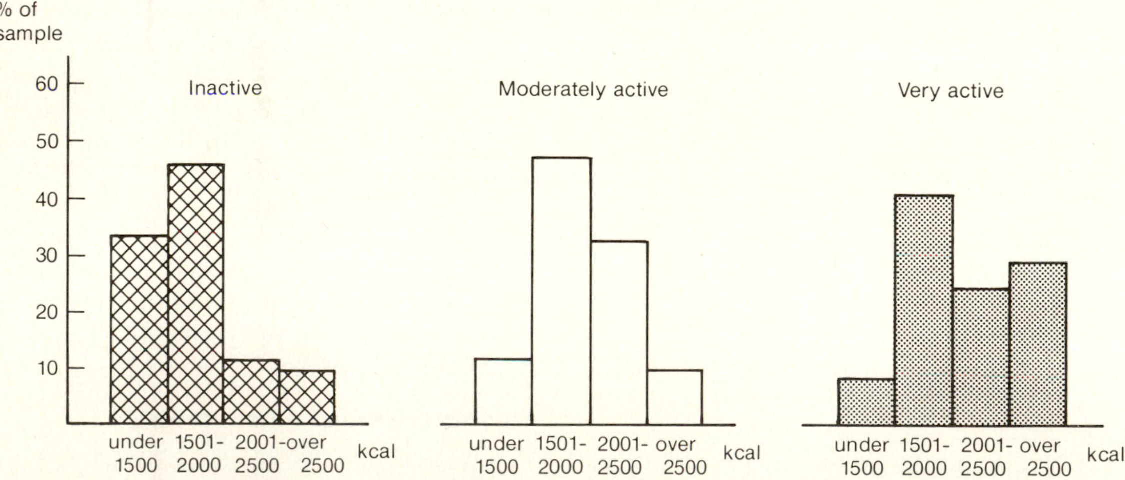

Figure 20–5 Distribution of mean daily energy intakes of 216 elderly French women, according to level of activity. (*Inactive* = light or little activity; *moderately active* = housework, shopping, daily walk; *very active* = moderate plus physical work, paid or unpaid.) Proportions of women in the three respective activity groupings were 30, 50, and 11 percent in the urban population and 25, 37, and 38 percent in the rural group. (From Debry, G., Bleyer, R., and Martin, J. M.: J. Human Nutr., *31*:195, 1977, with permission.)

Surveys of the diets of the elderly have indicated inadequate nutrient intakes. Studies in Britain, Australia, New Zealand, Canada, and the United States all concur in finding inadequate intakes of energy, protein, vitamins C and D, calcium, and iron. Although old people living alone are often in reduced financial circumstances, partially disabled, and without sufficient motivation to prepare foods for their solitary meals, residence in a care center does not guarantee an adequate intake of nutrients. (See Fig. 20–6.) A small group of women in an Australian hostel had unsatisfactory levels of vitamin C in the blood even though the diet was calculated to contain enough of this nutrient; analysis of the food as served showed that 99 percent of the vitamin C had been lost because of poor institutional food practices. Food transported to old people in their homes ("Meals

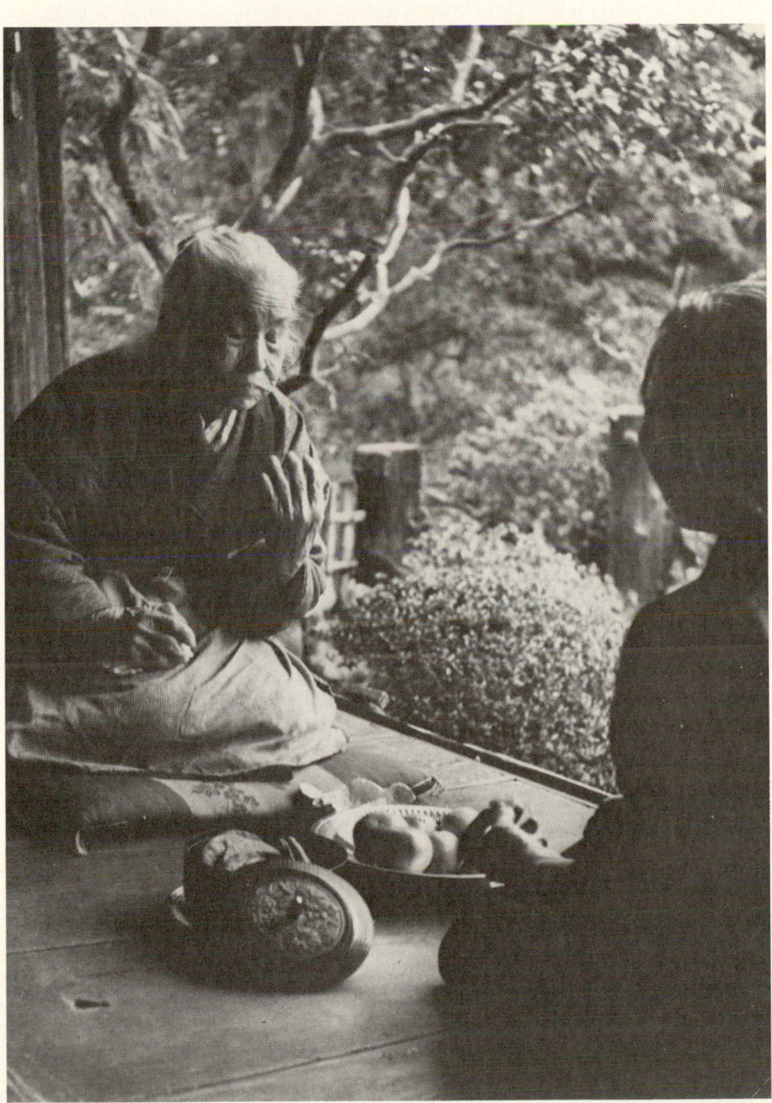

Figure 20–6 A grandmother enjoys a traditional meal with her daughter. The best possible protective environment, where an old person can live respected and loved by the family, is his or her own home. (Courtesy WHO/E. Schwab.)

on Wheels") is also prepared in quantity and held warm for some time in the trucks, leading to loss of vitamin C and other heat-sensitive vitamins, thiamin, and folacin. Unacceptable blood levels of thiamin and folacin have been found frequently in old people, in addition to ascorbic acid, as noted previously.

In planning diets for the aged person, all aspects of limited functional capability should be considered. Meals should be evenly spaced, with perhaps smaller amounts of food taken at more frequent intervals in view of diminished digestive and absorptive capacity. Adjustment of energy intake to achieve desirable body weight will relieve the strain imposed on the heart and on arthritic joints and an osteoporotic skeleton. The following physical conditions may impair the physical capability to ingest an adequate diet unless it is suitably prepared: (1) crippling joint disease; (2) muscular tremor; (3) poor vision; (4) missing teeth, badly fitting dentures; (5) reduced senses of smell and taste; (6) difficulties in swallowing.

Many workers in the field of geriatrics believe that lack of useful work or leisure activity and isolation from other people are the two most prominent factors that lead older people to take an inadequate amount of food. Other factors that have been found to influence food consumption of this group are: (1) social situation; (2) income; (3) cooking and refrigeration facilities; (4) food faddism; (5) long-standing erroneous concepts of good nutrition.

Planning a diet that is not too high in energy value, yet that at the same time furnishes plenty of high-quality protein, minerals, and vitamins may be difficult. The daily food intake should consist mainly of milk, meats, eggs, whole-grain bread or cereals, vegetables, and fruits, with restricted amounts of concentrated sweets and fats. Some raw fruits and vegetables should be included because of the question of nutrient loss in holding food for service. If the old person cannot chew these, fresh juices can be substituted. At this age in life, modest vitamin supplements may be advantageous. Because constipation is a common complaint, addition of prunes or bran to the diet may be recommended, but some caution is needed. Studies have shown that addition of 10 to 20 gm of unprocessed bran to the diet of old people significantly lowers levels of ionized calcium and iron in the blood, and these levels often are already abnormally low in the elderly. It would be safer to increase bran intake only to the extent of substituting whole-grain cereals and breads for refined products.

Foods included in the menu should be chosen from well-liked foods and presented in attractive, appetizing forms. Many old people have little to anticipate with pleasure in the day except their meals. They should not be deprived of this simple enjoyment by

Table 20–8 Caffeine Content of Beverages[a,b]

Item and serving	*mg caffeine per serving*
5-ounce cup	
Coffee, drip method	110–150
percolated	64–124
instant	40–108
decaffeinated	2–5
Tea, 1-minute brew	9–33
3-minute brew	20–46
instant	12–28
Cocoa, from mix	6
12-ounce container	
Tea, iced	22–36
Coca Cola, TAB	46
Shasta, all colas	44
Dr. Pepper, regular or diet	40
Pepsi, diet or light, RC cola	36

[a]Data abstracted from "Caffeine", a Scientific Status Summary by the Institute of Food Technologists, April, 1983.

[b]Milk chocolate candy contains 6 mg caffeine/oz and baking chocolate, 35 mg.

arbitrary insistence on fixed rules of food selection.

A word may be in order concerning the place of mild stimulants such as tea and coffee or the moderate use of alcoholic beverages. Most elderly persons experience comfort and cheer from hot drinks, and hot coffee or tea slightly stimulates the motility of the digestive tract. Their stimulating effect may be welcome to those whose bodily processes are slow. They also help to keep up fluid intake. Except in certain abnormal conditions, there is no reason to forbid their use. Much the same may be said of alcoholic beverages. Alcohol dilates the capillary blood vessels and thus may improve circulation temporarily. The abuse of alcoholic beverages by some persons should not rule out their proper use by others.

QUESTIONS

1. Plan a day's menu using Table 2, Nutritive Value of Foods, in the Appendix and, as far as possible, foods that you commonly use. Estimate how much of each essential nutrient is furnished by the foods in your menus. Compare the total with the recommended daily allowance of needs for a person of your sex, body weight, and degree of physical activity. What changes would be needed to adapt this diet for a boy of sixteen? A woman of seventy?

2. Consult Table 20–4, which gives the nutritive evaluation of the foundation diet. Determine for each of the individual nutrients listed what proportion of the total values for nutrients in the basal diet comes from certain classes of foods. What are the strengths and weaknesses of the Basic Four Food Group's pattern of menu planning? How may adequacy of lesser-studied vitamins and minerals be assured?

3. Outline briefly the types of dietary pattern characteristic of the following countries: Italy, Mexico, China, and Japan. In each case, what nutrients might be provided in insufficient amounts and what foods are in use or could be used to supply those nutrients?

4. If the diet does not furnish the full amount of the allowance recommended by the U.S. Food and Nutrition Board (the RDA), does it necessarily indicate that a person will suffer a deficiency of the nutritive essential that is provided in lower-than-recommended quantity? Explain your answer.

5. What is meant by specific hunger? Is specific hunger genetic or learned? Do human beings have the ability to select an adequate diet? Justify your answer.

6. At what age does the pubertal growth spurt occur in boys and girls? How do nutrient requirements of adolescents differ from those of adults? What features of teenagers' life-style and food habits affect quality of their intake?

7. According to the U.S. Food and Nutrition Board, how much should the total energy intake of a sixty-year-old man be reduced below that recommended for him at age thirty? Are protein needs of older people also reduced? What is the evidence? What factors in the social environment of elderly people tend to prevent the consumption of a balanced diet even if finances are adequate?

References

1. Beaudry-Darisme, M., et al.: J. Canad. Dietet. Assoc., *35*:274, 1974.
2. Food and Nutrition Board: *Recommended Dietary Allowances,* 9th Ed. Washington, D.C., National Research Council, National Academy of Sciences, 1980.
3. *Recommended Intakes of Nutrients for the United Kingdom.* Rept. on Public Health and Medical Subjects, No. 120, London, 1969.
4. Committee for the Revision of the Dietary Standards for Canada, Bureau of Nutritional Sciences, Food Directorate: *Recommended Nutrient Intakes for Canadians.* Ottawa, Dept. of Natl. Health and Welfare, 1983.
5. U.S. Dept. of Agriculture: *Food and Nutrient Intakes of Individuals in One Day in the United States. Spring 1977.* USDA Consumer Nutrition Center, Hyattsville, Maryland, Prelim. Rept. No. 2, 1980.
6. U.S. Dept. of Health, Education, and Welfare: *Ten-State Nutrition Survey, 1968–1970.* Vol. V, Dietary.

Dept. of Health, Education, and Welfare Pub. No. (HSM) 72–8133, 1972.

7. U.S. Dept. of Health, Education, and Welfare: *Preliminary Findings of the First Health and Nutrition Examination Survey, United States, 1971–1972; Dietary Intake and Biochemical Findings.* Dept. of Health, Education, and Welfare Pub. No. (HRH) 74–1219–1, 1974.
8. Sabry, Z. I.: *Nutrition Canada: National Survey.* Information Canada, Cat. No. H58–36, 1973.
9. Pao, E. M., and Mickle, S. J.: Problem nutrients in the United States. Food Techn., *35*:58, 1981.
10. Davis, C. M.: Self-selection of diet by newly weaned infants. Amer. J. Dis. Child. *36*:651, 1928.
11. Craig, A., Baer, K., and Diekmann, A.: The effects of lunch on sensory-perceptual functioning in man. Internat. Arch. Occup. Environ. Health, *49*:105, 1981.
12. Kennedy, E. T., Harrell, M. W., and Frazao, B.: Distribution of nutrient intake across meals in the United States population. Ecol. Food Nutr., *11*:217, 1982.
13. Farris, W. A., and Erdman, J. W., Jr.: Protracted hypervitaminosis following long-term, low level intake. J. Amer. Med. Assoc., *247*:1317, 1982.

21 Nutrition, Sports, and Physical Activity

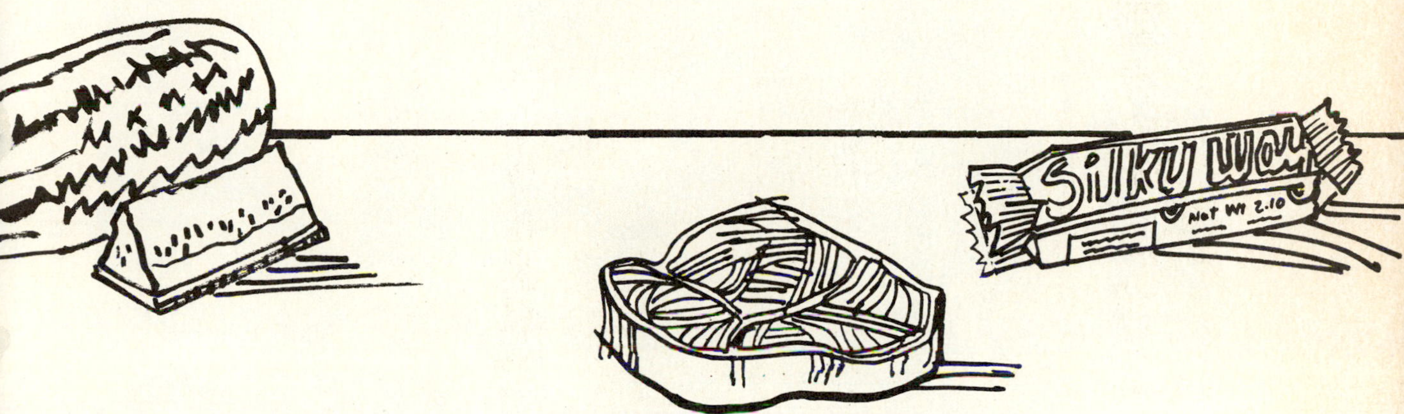

Sound nutrition and a sensible program of physical activity are two of the chief requirements for health. (See Fig. 21–1.) Most people are aware of the need for a good diet, whether or not they have one, but fewer people seem to realize how important exercise is to their general well-being. Exercise is a dominant variable in energy balance (total energy expenditure). Energy intake is not adequately regulated to prevent obesity unless enough physical work is done (Chap. 7).

Even a modest but diligently followed program of training has been shown to alter the body composition of sedentary middle-aged men. In one study the men were required to walk only forty minutes at a speed of 4 to 5 miles per hour four times a week, and yet their weight and body fat were somewhat reduced and their cardiovascular fitness was significantly improved. Measurements of old men showed that among those in the eighth decade of life the ones who were most active had the highest amount of lean body tissue and their muscle strength was equal to that of inactive men who were ten years younger. Physical activity (defined as any amount of habitual running) was also shown to be equivalent to a difference of ten years of age as regards parameters of physical fitness in middle-aged men. Fitness is also related in a desirable way to a number of factors associated with risk of heart disease including decreases in total blood cholesterol and shifts in the form in which the cholesterol is carried. (See Chap. 3.) In addition, inclusion of physical activity as a part of a weight-control program may lead to a greater proportion of the total weight loss being fat than when exercise is not included. Inactivity is associated with loss of bone substance (osteoporosis),

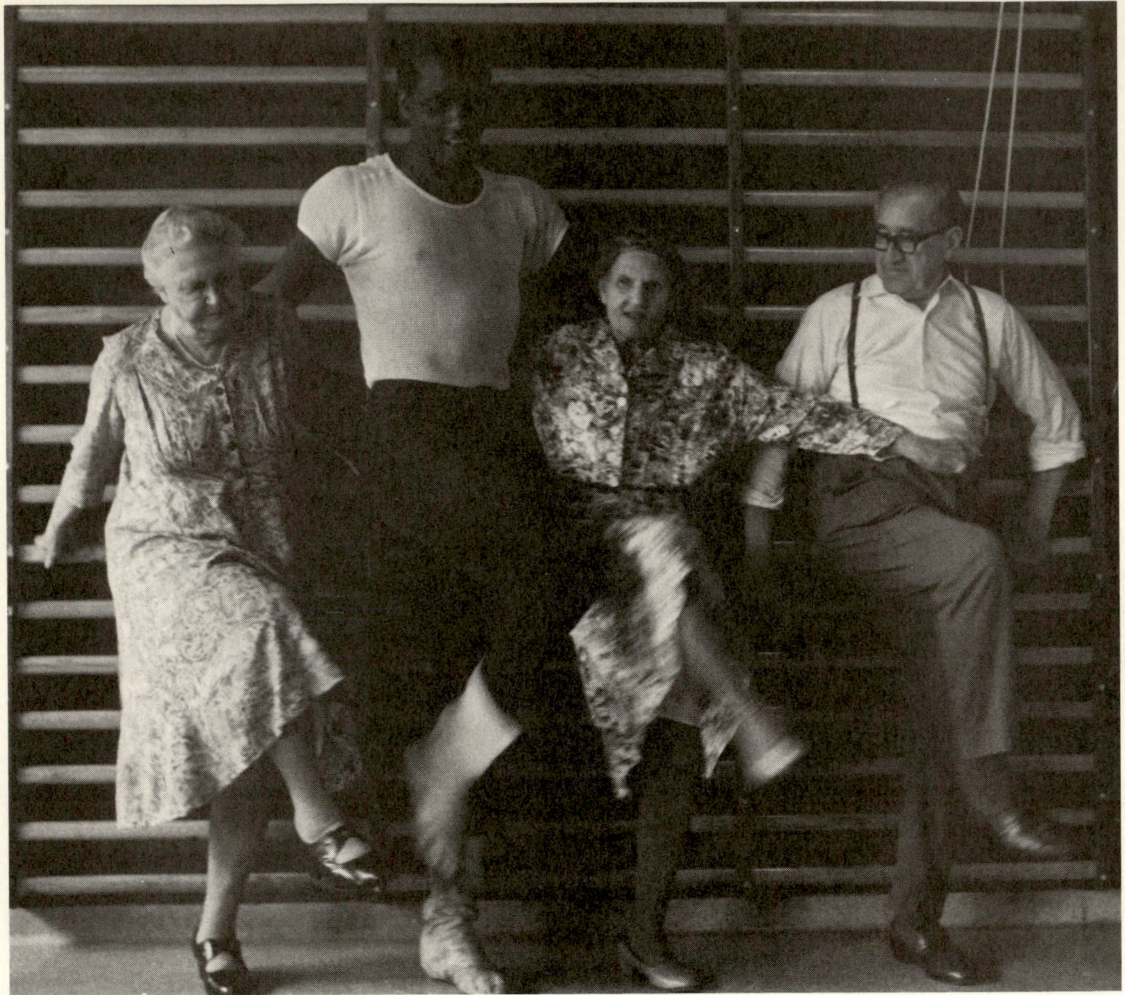

Figure 21–1 Exercise that is fun is good for everyone. Participants in these jazz-ballet classes, age 80 and over, said they "felt as if they were in their twenties again." (Photo courtesy of WHO/E. Mandelmann.)

and the epidemiology of hip fracture suggests that hard physical work throughout life protects against it.

It has been suggested that lack of physical activity and sports in childhood leads to underdeveloped abdominal muscles and weak connective tissue sheaths that then contribute to chronic low back pain in women after pregnancy. Women often restrict physical activity owing to the old-fashioned notion that menses are made difficult by vigorous movement. In most women, fitness is slightly reduced two to six days before the onset of menstruation, yet women athletes perform superbly throughout the menstrual cycle.

Psychologists also point out beneficial effects of physical activity. Exercise is said to be an outlet for unconsumed, accumulated energy and so reduces "free floating tension" and channels aggression outward. Fretfulness, restlessness, and insomnia are outcomes ascribed to failure to relieve tension by physical activity.

Neither adults nor teenagers are very active in typical Western cultures. Although teenagers in the United States were found to spend a bit more time in moderate and strenuous activity than adults of the same sex, girls spent 95 percent of their time either asleep or in activities classed as very light (2.5 kcal per minute or less) or light (2.5 to 4.9 kcal per minute); boys spent over 90 percent of their time in light activities. Urban Australian youth spent 78 to 80 percent of their time lying or sitting, 14 to 20 percent in very light activity, and only 1.5 to 4.4 percent in any activity that involved greater energy expenditure than walking.

WORK CAPACITY AND METABOLISM

The ability to perform work is dependent on energy-yielding processes in muscle cells. To work, muscle cells must have oxygen, which comes from the lungs via the blood and is taken up by the muscle cell. The ability to work can be limited by failure of any one of these processes: inadequate lung capacity, inadequate capability of the heart to pump blood, inadequate oxygen-carrying power of the blood, or failure of the peripheral circulation to supply enough blood to the working muscle. In some disease conditions or in very heavy smokers, lung power may be limiting, but generally, it is cardiovascular factors that limit work. During exercise blood is diverted from the organs to the maximum extent feasible to supply the working muscles and the heart. As illustrated in Figure 21–2, the combined effect of diversion of blood circulation and increased heart pumping action augments the blood supply to the muscles by thirtyfold. Anemia is one condition in which oxygen transport is limited. Low blood hemoglobin levels in anemic patients and the sharp drop in hemoglobin occasioned by blood donation in healthy women reduce blood buffering power and capacity to transport oxygen and have a detrimental effect on work performance. In sedentary but normal persons, limitation is usually due to poor cardiovascular fitness, and the heart then has to work very hard to pump blood at levels of work that are well tolerated by persons who are more fit.

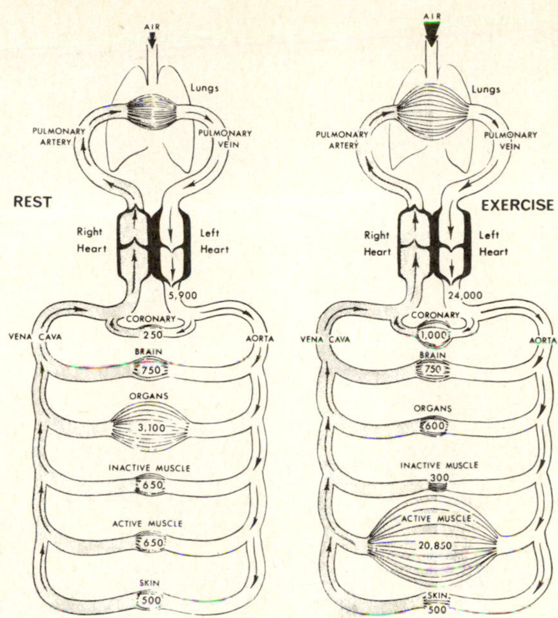

Figure 21–2 Schematic representation of the blood circulation of a sedentary man during standing rest and during exercise at the maximal oxygen uptake. Organs include kidneys, liver, gastrointestinal tract, and others. Blood flow is given in milliliters per minute. (From Mitchell, J. H. and Blomqvist, G., *New England J. Med. 284:*1018, 1971, with permission.)

Since work requires energy expenditure involving oxygen, higher work levels are always associated with higher tissue uptake of oxygen and more oxygen removal in respiration. *Maximal oxygen uptake* is the greatest amount of oxygen a person can take in during exercise and so reflects the ability to transport oxygen to the tissues (Fig. 21–3). Thus, maximal oxygen uptake is one index of fitness. For average, middle-aged men the maximal oxygen uptake is 35 to 40 ml per kg of body weight per minute, or about 2.5 liters of oxygen per minute. In well-trained young athletes, maximal oxygen uptake is about 70 ml per kg per minute.

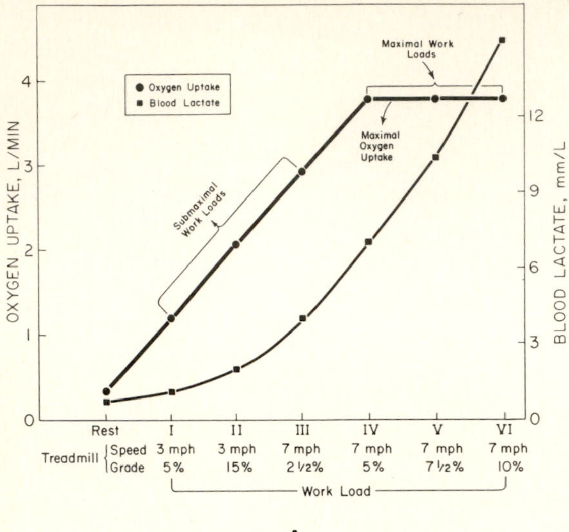

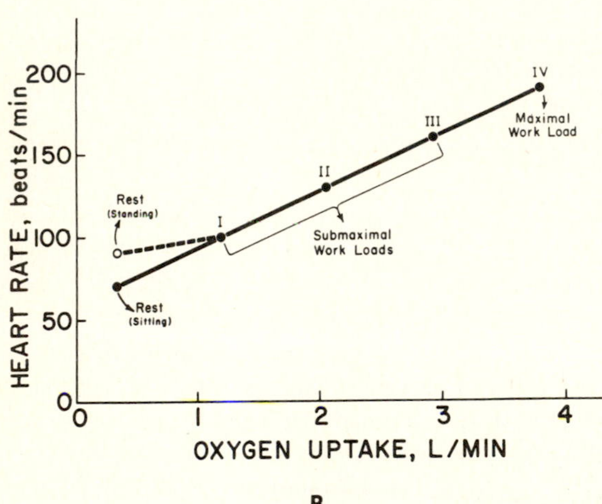

Figure 21–3 *A,* Maximal oxygen uptake determined by means of a motor-driven treadmill. The man does increasingly harder work until the capacity to take in oxygen reaches its limit. After this point, lactic acid rises because there is not enough oxygen to metabolize glycogen completely. *B,* With progressively increasing exercise loads there is a linear relation between heart-rate and oxygen uptake. (From Mitchell, J. H. and Blomqvist, G. *New England J. Med. 284:* 1018, 1971, with permission.)

When people work at very high rates, oxygen supplied to the tissues is not sufficient to oxidize muscle glycogen completely, and an intermediate compound, lactic acid (see glycolysis, Chap. 6) is produced. Some of this lactate is metabolized during exercise, but some accumulates. Expending energy at such an intensity is referred to as *anaerobic work.* After such work is completed, the person continues to breathe heavily and maintains an oxygen consumption greater than that at rest until the body's metabolic processes return to the pre-exercise level. This oxygen is used not only to metabolize the accumulated lactate to CO_2, amino acids, and glycogen, but also to help re-establish intracellular equilibrium and proper body temperature. The total amount of oxygen consumed in recovering from an anaerobic work situation may amount to as much as 2 to 5 liters.

Work at lower intensity that is performed without building up lactic acid in the tissues is called *aerobic work.* For most healthy people, the limit of aerobic work capacity approximates the energy expenditure of a brisk walk and corresponds to use of just over 1 liter of oxygen or 5 kcal per minute. This is about four to five times the resting metabolic rate (Chap. 6). Work at or below the aerobic capacity is called *steady state work* because it can be continued steadily for long periods without fatigue.

How long a person can work at a time without a break obviously varies according to the work rate. This is an important consideration in industry, where rest periods must be established, and in endurance sports events, where the work must be paced. If the work task is at or below the aerobic capacity, rest periods are not needed. Durnin and Passmore suggest that rest periods can be calculated simply according to multiples of the aerobic capacity (1). If the work task requires 7.5 kcal per minute and the aerobic capacity is 5 kcal, then thirty minutes of rest will be needed for every hour worked; if the task is one requiring 10 kcal per minute, then the rest periods will have to be the same length as the work periods. For maximum work output it is best to work and rest for short periods—ten minutes of work and five

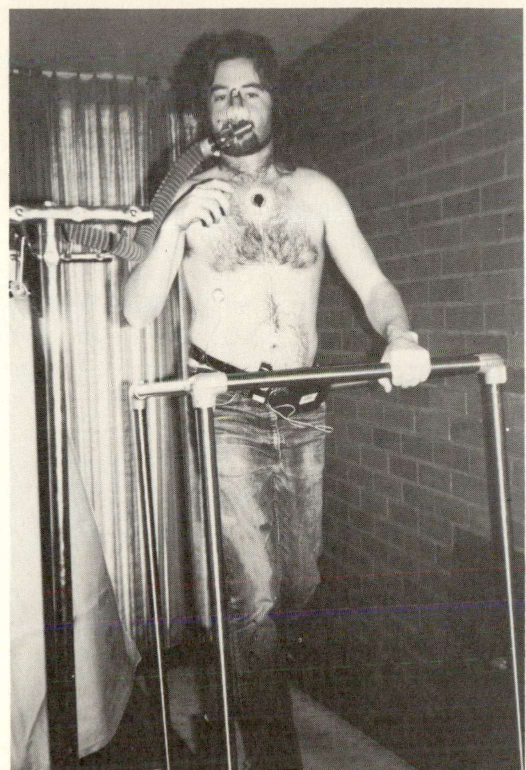

Figure 21–4 Stimultaneous measurement of heart-rate and oxygen uptake of a subject walking on a motor-driven treadmill. There is a linear relationship between these two parameters and, therefore, between heart-rate and energy cost of work at heart-rates above 90 beats per minute; at lower heart-rates and energy expenditures (sedentary or very light work), the slope is minimal and the error term is large. (Courtesy of D. Armstrong, University of California, Berkeley.)

minutes of rest in climbing a hill, for instance. Otherwise, the work pace must be slowed so that expenditure rate does not exceed the aerobic capacity of the workers. The value of 5 kcal per minute suggests a maximum work output of 2400 kcal per eight-hour work-shift and coincides well with actual observations of sustained hard industrial work, such as coal mining and nonmechanized agriculture. The trained athlete is capable of sustained work at about ten times his resting rate, but he does become fatigued and does accumulate lactate during this load of work.

In a study of the energy needs of college football players, food eaten at the training table and between meal snacks amounted to 5600 kcal per day during playing season, and the men were not gaining weight. They averaged 80 kg (small, perhaps, but it was the Harvard team), which would indicate an expected energy requirement of the order of 3200 kcal per day if the men had pursued a usual collegiate pattern of moderate activity rather than sports. The difference between ordinary needs and those of the team, 2400 kcal, should be ascribable in some way to football practice and competition. This activity occupied only two hours a day, indicating an energy expenditure rate of 1200 kcal per hour, nearly twenty times the basal metabolic rate, which is above a level that is usually sustainable for an extended period. The extra energy need of the team probably reflects in part a continued high rate of metabolism after the exercise was concluded.

Benedict's classic research on energy metabolism in the early 1900s included an observation that metabolism during sleep was 25 percent higher when very severe work had been performed one hour earlier than when the sleep followed a day of rest; sleeping metabolic rate was still 10 to 15 percent higher as long as seven hours after severe work. This continued effect of exercise on resting metabolism serves as a reminder that calculations of total energy need based on activity categories are only rough approximations. The only satisfactory basis for judging energy need is by maintenance of ideal body weight, because physical work affects the body in ways that have not yet been adequately explained.

Fuel for Muscular Work and Performance Capacity

The source of energy for muscular work is ATP generated from the common metabolic pathways (Chap. 6) or, in short term, from creatine phosphate stored in the muscle. Creatine is a nitrogen-containing compound synthesized in the body from amino acids. It combines with phosphate from ATP in a high-energy linkage, forming creatine phosphate and ADP. When ATP is needed for the initial stages of muscular work, the reverse reaction of creatine phosphate with ADP yields ATP for muscle contraction, and creatine. The latter is again regenerated to creatine phosphate when ATP is abundant.

Theoretically, the nature of the substance undergoing metabolism can be determined by measuring the amount of oxygen used and the amount of carbon dioxide formed during metabolism. (See Chap. 6.) An RQ of 1 indicates the burning of pure glucose; an RQ of 0.7 suggests the metabolizing of pure fat. However, when measuring RQ in an exercising individual, interpretation of the values obtained is complicated because the CO_2 in the exhaled air is a sum of that produced by cellular metabolism and nonmetabolic CO_2. This latter CO_2 is pushed out of the blood at the lungs as a consequence of hyperventilation and of changes in the buffering capacity of the blood caused by the buildup of lactate. Thus, under such circumstances, the ratio of CO_2 exhaled to O_2 consumed is referred to as the *respiratory exchange ratio,* or R, rather than the metabolic measure RQ. During high-intensity exercise, R may exceed 1.0 and is not useful in establishing the fuels being burned. The energy equivalent of oxygen in such circumstances is assumed to be that associated with burning a "usual" mixture of fuels, or 4.8 kcal per liter.

Formerly carbohydrate was thought to be the only energy source for physical work, but present information indicates that carbohydrate plays a dominant role only in heavy exercise when oxygen supply to the muscle becomes limiting. During steady state work, fat provides about half of the energy; with prolonged work (four hours or more), fatty acid metabolism may reach 60 to 70 percent of the total. The fat utilized comes from lipid pools in the muscle tissue and fatty acids mobilized from adipose tissue and transported to the working muscle by the blood. In the past, protein was not considered a significant fuel source for muscular activity. Recent evidence, however, suggests that, at rest, amino acids may supply as much as 14 percent of the total energy expended in an untrained person, and 10 to 12 percent in an individual adapted to strenuous exercise. The proportion of the total energy expended that is supplied from amino acids during physical activity is considerably less (3 to 5 percent). This energy contribution from protein seems to arise from the metabolism of specific amino acids.

At rest, the output of the amino acids alanine and glutamine exceeds the input to muscle, and as glucose utilization increases during exercise, there is a parallel rise in muscle alanine output (derived from pyruvate; see Chap. 6). The source of the amino groups used in this synthesis is primarily the branched-chain amino acids (leucine, isoleucine, valine), and their carbon skeletons may contribute importantly to the ATP supply for exercise. The alanine formed is carried to the liver, where it is used for synthesis of glucose (with amino groups disposed of via urea formation and transamination reactions) to help maintain blood sugar during prolonged exercise and to replenish liver glycogen after exercise. The contribution of such amino acid metabolism to the overall body need for protein has not as yet been established. Individuals exercising daily while consuming as little as 40 gm of protein, a value well below the RDA for protein, have been found to be able to maintain nitrogen balance, provided the energy needs for the added exercise are met by nonprotein foods.

To determine if the metabolic mixture utilized during work does affect work performance, two types of studies have been made. In one, persons were fed a normal diet or one very high in either of the work-energy sources (fat or carbohydrate) for some period of time to foster preferential use of that source during work. Other studies emphasized the composition of meals taken just prior to an event. Carbohydrate has more oxygen in its composition than does fat, and about 10 percent less oxygen is needed per unit of energy when carbohydrate is metabolized, so theoretically preferential utilization of carbohydrate should be beneficial when oxygen limits work.

Diets containing little or no carbohydrate have adverse effects on performance in every study. One experiment compared a diet containing less than 5 percent with one supplying over 90 percent of energy as carbohydrate. Capacity for hard physical work was reduced by one half with the high-fat diet and increased by one fourth with the high-carbohydrate regimen, as compared with performance during normal diet periods. Other studies confirm these findings and indicate that one factor involved is the amount of glycogen present in the muscle. Swedish investigators measured performance capacity (work to exhaustion in a standard bicycle test) and obtained samples of muscle by needle biopsy from a group of men fed three diets. Time to exhaustion was 114 minutes for those with a normal diet, 57 minutes when the diet was made up exclusively of high-protein and high-fat foods, and 167 minutes when the diet was high in carbohydrate. After the normal mixed diet, glycogen content was found to be 1.75 gm per 100 gm wet muscle before exercise; after 3 days of carbohydrate-free diet it was 0.63 gm, and after the same period of high-carbohydrate feeding, 3.51 gm.

When men fed a normal mixed diet worked at a rate of about 75 percent of their maximum oxygen uptake, glycogen content of muscle was almost completely depleted in 90 minutes, but blood sugar was satisfactorily maintained. Past this point, evidence indicates that blood sugar falls and constitutes a final limit to performance. (See Fig. 21–5.) Administration of glucose at the point of exhaustion allows work to proceed for an additional period of time.

Diets based on the principle of improving the fuel for muscular work have been developed and enthusiastically adopted in Europe in the past. It is difficult to say if this has a significant effect on the outcome of athletic competition, because there are uncontrollable differences in skills and training between

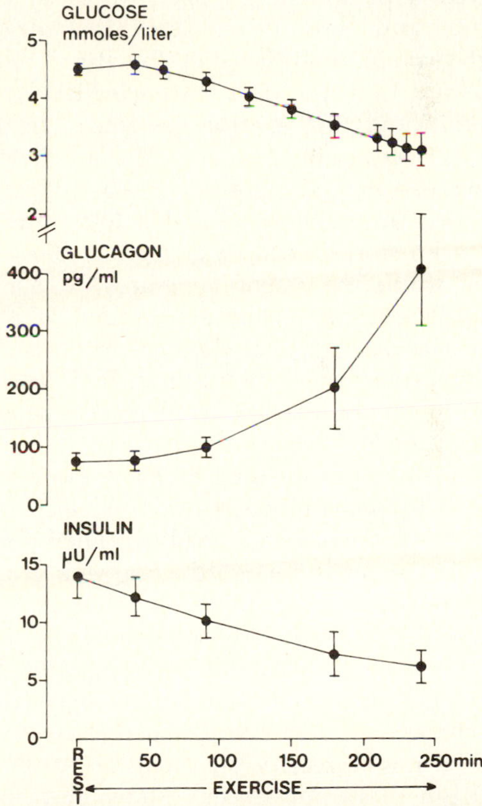

Figure 21–5 Exercise induces a fall in plasma insulin and a rise in plasma glucagon; levels of other hormones that favor maintenance of blood glucose (pituitary growth hormone, epinephrine, norepinephrine, cortisol) also are elevated. In spite of these hormonal responses, in prolonged heavy exercise, hepatic gluconeogenesis and glycolysis fail to keep pace with the accelerated utilization of glucose, and the blood glucose level falls. (From Felig, P. and Wahren, J. *New England J. Med. 293:*1078, 1975, with permission.)

competitors and in environmental factors between events. Also, strength of belief in the efficacy of a treatment may be sufficient to make the treatment effective, a point that is difficult to rule out even in laboratory studies involving subjective acknowledgment of "fatigue." However, this treatment does have a sound basis in theory and a reasonable body of experimental evidence in support of it.

The preparation recommended by Åstrand for competition in endurance events exceeding 30 to 60 minutes' duration involved depletion of glycogen stores by exercise and use of a low-carbohydrate, high-protein, high-fat diet for three days, followed by three days during which large quantities of carbohydrate are added to the diet (2). Åstrand's tests show that muscle glycogen can exceed 4 gm per 100 gm of muscle with this regimen and that total muscle glycogen stores could be as high as 700 gm. This would represent a reserve of about 2800 kcal if completely metabolized or half that if lactic acid were the end-product due to anaerobic work metabolism. This is approximately double the usual reserve capacity in trained athletes.

Some notes of warning have been sounded by physicians concerned over possible side-effects of carbohydrate loading. They point out that water is deposited along with glycogen, which may cause the muscles to feel heavy and stiff. In addition, the high fat–high protein period is often accompanied by irritability and other signs of hypoglycemia or changes in acid-base balance (this effect can be minimized by the inclusion of 80 to 100 gm of carbohydrate). The high-carbohydrate period is associated with transient diarrhea in some individuals, leaving them dehydrated and lacking in appropriate levels of electrolytes at the start of a competitive event. Others suggest that the inclusion of an exhaustive depletion activity may not be appropriate just before competition, leading perhaps to injury or early "peaking" (3).

In an older marathon runner, chest pain and changes in the electrocardiogram occurred when carbohydrate loading was used; although there is no proof that the diet was the specific causative agent, it was speculated that accumulation of cardiac glycogen might have been a factor (4). Those who wish to try this method for improving performance would be well advised to do so under supervision and before a competition, so that they and their advisers can determine what the probable effects will be.

A modified version of this dietary regimen is now recommended for those individuals who exercise strenuously on a regular basis. Costill finds that glycogen stores can be elevated 2.5 times above those found in nonexercising muscle, an elevation more than adequate to cover the increased needs of most endurance activities, simply by eating a diet high in complex carbohydrate (70% of calories) for the three days before an event. He also finds that such a diet is best to replenish the glycogen stores used in daily exercise bouts (see Fig. 21–6) (3). Even this regimen, however, does not totally replete those stores in one day, and a rest day now and then is necessary for total repletion of the anaerobic fuel supply. Such an "off" day thus becomes an important part of a regular training schedule.

Nutritional Deficiency and Performance

Among factors known to be detrimental to performance, two are outstanding: *dehydration* and *food deprivation.* Evidence on these points comes from careful laboratory studies and abundant field experience. Of the two, dehydration is the more immediate and serious risk. Normally, voluntary drinking is stimulated when the body water content drops by 1 percent, but during exercise voluntary intake is inhibited and water balance may not be attained until hours or days after a severe bout of work with high rates of water loss as sweat.

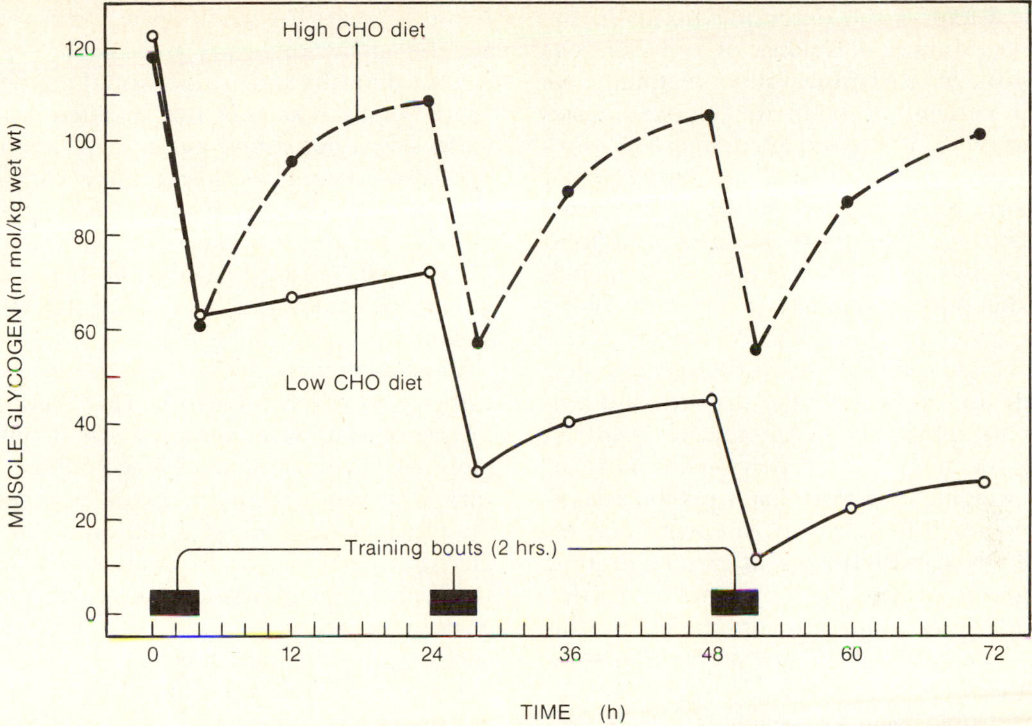

Figure 21–6 *Muscle glycogen content during three successive days of heavy training with diets containing 40 percent carbohydrate (low CHO) and 70 percent carbohydrate (high CHO). (From Costill, D. L., and Miller, J. M.: Intl. J. Sports Med., 1:2, 1980, with permission.)*

In fact, individuals exercising daily may only replace about 50 percent of their water losses when allowed to drink at will. Conscious attention to increasing water intake above appetite is required to insure adequate hydration over the long run. In a comfortable environment water loss due to sweating during moderate exercise will be about 1 liter per hour; at higher work output or in the heat, loss may be two to four times that rate (Chap. 13). Physical performance begins to deteriorate when the water deficit exceeds 3 percent of body weight.

In spite of this evidence, extremely ill-advised practices are used to meet weight ranges in competitive sports such as wrestling—practices that include withholding water, wearing rubberized apparel, and inducing vomiting. The American College of Sports Medicine (ACSM) lists the following as some of the possible consequences associated with acute food and fluid restriction: (1) reduction in muscle strength; (2) decreased work performance; (3) decreased blood volume; (4) decreased output of the heart; (5) impaired ability to regulate body temperature; (6) decreased kidney function; and (7) increased losses of electrolytes from the body. The ACSM further states that "Since it is possible for these changes to impede normal growth and development there is little physiological or medical justification for the use of the weight reduction methods currently followed by many wrestlers."

There is, therefore, a serious question as to how much weight (other than water) an athlete can safely lose without impairing his performance. Any amount of *excess* fat can be trimmed off to advantage, and reducing weight to the desirable level for height and age is a logical and defensible point. In the famous Minnesota studies of conscientious objectors on a semistarvation regimen, loss of 25 percent of body weight over a six-month period resulted in diminished work performance, endurance, and strength of the large muscles. Later studies in the same laboratory tested more severely restricted diets of 580 and 1010 kcal per day. The 580-kcal diet was inadequate to maintain blood sugar levels for work and can be dismissed from further consideration. With the higher energy intake, loss of hand strength and lowering of maximal oxygen uptake occurred when the men lost 10 percent or more of body weight. Low work loads can be accomplished for a few days in an emergency, especially if at least 100 gm of carbohydrate, a few grams of salt (such as bouillon cubes), and adequate water are consumed, but this is not compatible with top performance capability.

A sensible plan of weight control, suggested by the AMA Committee on Medical Aspects of Sports, is to undertake "an intensive conditioning program related to the demands of [the sport] for at least four weeks, preferably six, without emphasis on [body] weight. . . . At the end of this period and without altering the daily training routine, [record] weight in a pre-breakfast, post-micturition state. Consider this weight the minimal effective weight for competition as well as certification purposes." A program of this kind that includes sound nutrition education is ideal and is especially important for young people who participate in more than one sport according to the season and for which weight advantages differ, such as football and wrestling. Alternating attempts to gain and lose weight cannot help but be detrimental. Weight can be reduced to a very small extent—at most 200 to 300 gm—by changing to a low-residue diet for 72 hours before an event so that the large bowel is more nearly empty. This means substituting refined cereals for whole grains and reducing the intake of beans and coarse vegetables. Ordinarily, such a diet would not be advised, but a few days of this regimen will not harm a well-nourished person. At this time, it is also reasonable to eliminate from the diet foods that are *highly* salted (chips, ham, pickles) to prevent excess water retention (Chap. 10). However, normal salt intake should be maintained to allow for sweat losses.

Vitamin deficiencies of all kinds are damaging to work performance. How long performance can be maintained when one or more vitamins are omitted from the diet will vary with the amount of tissue reserves of the nutrient the individual has and the role that the specific nutrient plays in work metabolism. On the basis of their participation in the metabolic pathways, lack of the B vitamins would be expected to have the most immediate effects, and this is borne out by investigations of the subject. Lack of thiamin is evident in a few days or weeks, and the symptoms of deficiency appear earlier in men fed a deficient diet who are actively working than in those who are sedentary. This early damage to performance is probably true of most of the B complex vitamins, while effects of lack of vitamin A do not appear for months in previously well-nourished subjects.

Deficiencies of minerals other than sodium and iron have not been well studied, but because of their important role in neuromuscular transmission and as enzyme cofactors, detrimental effects would certainly be expected. The skeleton provides an essential reserve of calcium, which is withdrawn to maintain blood levels of ionized calcium; the liver holds some stores of the trace minerals, but these are variable according to the quality of the usual diet. When effects of mineral deficiencies other than the electrolytes are examined, one would expect them to appear only after periods of weeks or months, or when there are abnormal losses due to diarrhea or vomiting.

As indicated earlier in this chapter, lack of adequate iron stores as manifested in anemia is a condition associated with diminished oxygen transport and decreased work performance. Anemia has also been associated with increased heart-rate, elevated blood lactate, and decreased work time in response to a specific exercise task. Recovery from anemia seems to correct these parameters. The widespread need for iron in energy release in muscle (as an oxygen-transfer molecule, myoglobin, and as a part of the energy-capturing machinery, the cytochromes) suggests the possibility of nonhematological effects of iron deficiency on performance as well. Davies has shown that length of performance is affected most by reduced energy-releasing capacity of muscle, and maximal oxygen uptake is most affected by oxygen-carrying capacity of the blood (5).

Total deprivation of protein with adequate energy intake for two weeks has not been shown to alter performance of fixed work tasks in a laboratory nor to reduce muscular strength. The men do complain of feeling less "fit" subjectively, and the blood volume is reduced somewhat, which would be disadvantageous in high-performance work situations and competitive sports. However, lower levels of protein intake, 50 to 60 gm a day, which are much below intakes of athletes and men engaged in hard physical labor, have not been shown to affect adversely the performance of persons who are *already trained.*

RECOMMENDATIONS

Diets During Physical Training

Nutrition is an important feature of any training program. Education of coaches and athletes is needed in regard to both nutritional needs and the role of different foods in the diet. A study of Australian Olympic athletes showed great variability in their diets and in their nutrition knowledge. Intakes of some nutrients were much higher than required, particularly protein, calcium, and vitamin C, and although these are usually harmless, the diets would not be economical. Some diets were below recommended levels of thiamin if the large energy need of the athletes is taken into account. Records in the competition showed that those whose thiamin intake was adequate placed better, some winning medals, in comparison with the ones whose diets were suboptimal in thiamin content. American athletes generally express a concerned awareness, and many resort to excessive and unnecessary supplementation of the diet with vitamins, minerals, and protein powders.

It has been a common belief that athletes have an increased need for protein, especially during training. Muscle tissue must be built, and there is an increase in plasma proteins and in iron-containing muscle and blood proteins. In fact, during the initiation of strenuous physical work, there may be a transient (12 to 14 days) period of negative nitrogen balance. This period of negativity has been shown in studies in which the exercising individuals consumed 1 gm of protein per kilogram of body weight. The magnitude of that negativity was diminished, however, by increasing the protein intake to 2 gm per kilogram of body weight (6). Other investigators, however, have shown that on protein intakes as low as 0.57 gm per kilogram of body weight this transient period can be weathered without significant loss of muscle tissue, provided energy intake is adequate to cover the increased activity (7). The efficiency with which protein is converted to muscle tissue is greater at the lower intakes, and that efficiency falls off rapidly above 2 gm of protein per kilogram of body weight—the approximate amount of protein many inactive people in North America consume daily. Thus, protein intakes above this amount are really not necessary for athletes, and in fact they may do perfectly well on much lower intakes.

The higher energy needs of physical activity must be met, but there is often some loss of body weight and a shift in body composition toward more lean and less fat. This is seen in both military recruits and athletes in training. On the other hand, body weight is apt to increase in persons who are below average weight at the time training begins. Along with increased energy requirements there are increased needs for the B vitamins. (See Chap. 8.)

The diet must be adequate in all essential nutrients, but there is no evidence that supernormal intakes of nutrients (except as cited previously) will do anything to improve work capacity. There have been hopeful claims for exotic foods such as royal jelly or bee pollen; mysterious benefits have been ascribed to wheat-germ oil, "octacosanol" (a long-chain alcohol present in wheat-germ oil) and lecithin; and a number of "ergogenic" substances have been tested with a view toward expanding the creatine phosphate pool (glycine, gelatin—which is one-fourth glycine—and creatine per se). Salts of the nonessential amino acid, aspartic acid, have also been suggested as improving neuromuscular excitability. None of these has proved to be of benefit in carefully controlled studies. A good diet—one based on meat, milk, fish, poultry and eggs, whole-grain cereals, legumes and nuts, leafy, green vegetables, and other vegetables and fruits—will meet all the nutritional requirements of athletes and persons engaged in hard physical labor. Vitamin pills and special supplements are not needed and should not be relied upon because they may lull the individual into thinking that all nutritional needs have been met when in reality protein and minerals or some as-yet-unidentified essential factor may still be lacking.

Eating Just Before and During Work

Industrial experience indicates that frequent feeding is beneficial to work output, which may be due either to meal spacing or to the physical and psychological benefit of rest periods. In any case, more frequent intake of smaller amounts of food may be desirable. (See Chap. 20.) In someone used to taking breakfast, omission does lead to poorer work performance, and blood sugar falls to undesirably low levels with continued deprivation of food.

Eating before athletic competitions has been a subject of lively controversy. Small, balanced meals of 500 to 800 kcal taken three to four hours before the event have not been shown to have any adverse effect on a variety of athletic performances conducted in a test situation. The tension and stress of game competition may be another matter, and the experience of seasoned coaches and athletes is a good practical guide. There is general agreement that high-protein meals are undesirable before competition. The usual recommendation is to eat a light, balanced meal high in complex carbohydrate, which seems to be a sensible approach.

The American Alliance for Health, Physical Education, and Recreation offers the following suggestions for a meal to be eaten 3 to 4 hours before competition (8): 1 serving of roasted or broiled meat or poultry; 1 serving of mashed potatoes or a baked potato or ½ cup of macaroni, rice, or similar; 1 serving of vegetables; 1 cup of skim milk; 1 teaspoon of fat spread; 2 teaspoons of jelly or other sweets; 1 serving of fruit or juice; 1 serving of sugar cookies or plain cake. Take 1 or 2 cups of extra beverages and salt the food well.

This group also suggests that a commercial or home-prepared formula may be substituted for a normal meal and is preferred by some athletes. However, these formulas are usually based on milk plus added milk solids, and so are high in lactose content, which is a sugar not well tolerated by many Oriental and African populations and some others. (See Chap. 2 and 5.)

Note again that it is recommended that precompetition meals or formulas be eaten three to four hours in advance. Eating, especially foods high in carbohydrate within 1.5 to two hours of an event should be discouraged; such ingestion of carbohydrates elevates blood glucose, which then calls forth insulin from the pancreas. The surge of insulin promotes the storage of the various body fuels, resulting in lowering blood glucose and inhibition of fat or glycogen breakdown in the tissues. The result of such a practice may be low blood sugar at the beginning of an event (see Fig. 21–7) with more rapid depletion of muscle glycogen and more rapid fatigue (3). Whereas the more rapid utilization of muscle glycogen is of greatest concern to endurance athletes, the low blood sugar at the initiation of an event may leave any athlete feeling a little "sluggish" and less apt to put out a maximal effort.

Coffee and tea are best omitted due to their stimulating effect on the sympathetic nervous system. The use of caffeine to promote the release of free fatty acids from adipose tissue, first proposed by Costill (9), has little effect in short- or medium-duration events. In long-term events, this practice provides a fuel source alternative to muscle glycogen, thus maintaining that store, but the ethical considerations involved in use of such central nervous system stimulants must be noted. Alcohol is quite deleterious to coordination and judgment.

During competition that involves much sweating, it is essential that water losses be replaced as the activity continues. Sweat is less concentrated in minerals than is plasma, and the fluid used to replace it should be also (Chap. 13). In short-term sports, salt is not a problem, and the fluid given could be

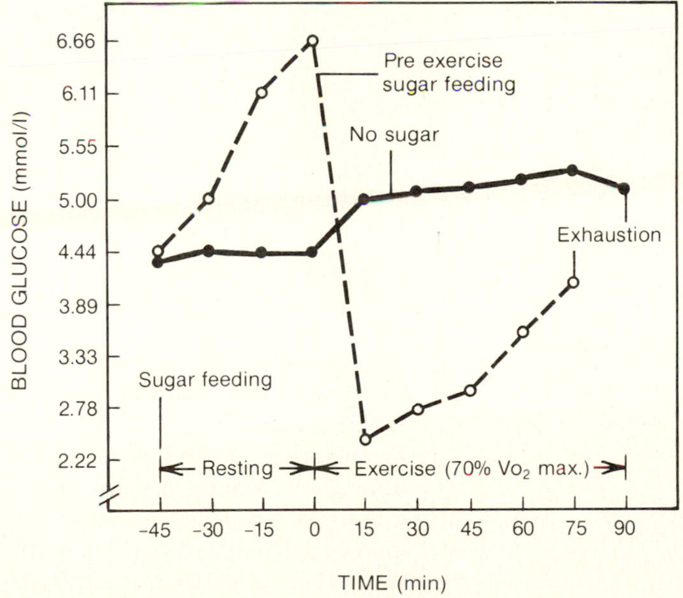

Figure 21–7 Effects of pre-exercise CHO feedings on blood glucose and on work time to exhaustion. (*From* Costill, D. L., and Miller, J. M.: Intl. J. Sports Med. 1:2, 1980, with permission.)

water or sweetened lemonade. However, for continued high work output or in severe heat, salt will be needed. Since salt absorption is improved if glucose is present for absorption at the same time, workers and athletes in endurance events should take some carbohydrate as well as salt and water. For this purpose the ACSM recommends a solution that contains small amounts of sugar (less than 2.5%) and electrolytes (about 0.2% salt). They further recommend that the athlete consume this fluid frequently throughout an athletic event, beginning with 400 to 500 ml (about one pint) just before the event (10). The ingestion of 150 ml (a little more than one-half cup) of a cool fluid of the composition mentioned above every ten to fifteen minutes throughout an event has been found to maintain blood volume in an exercising individual. (See Fig. 21–8.) Workers and climbers may prefer a snack of dried fruits and salted crackers or chips with water or an accustomed beverage. The important consideration is continued replacement of water and salt, not the form in which these are given.

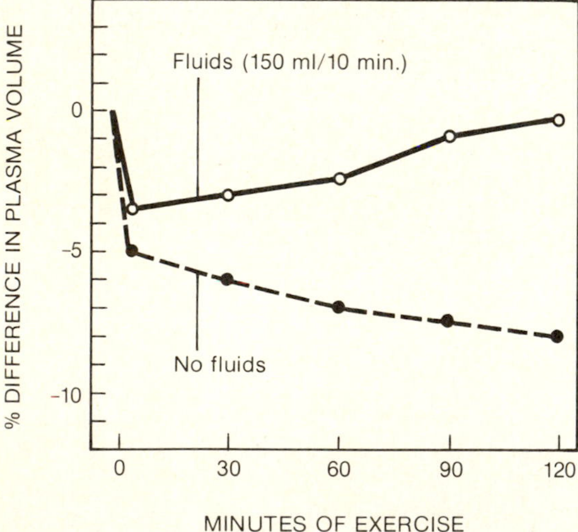

Figure 21–8 Changes in plasma volume during two hours of cycling in the heat (38° C, 35% R.H.) with and without fluid intake. (From Costill, D. L., and Miller, J. M.: Intl. J. Sports Med., *1*:2, 1980, with permission.)

Special Considerations for the Physically Active Woman

More and more girls are participating in strenuous physical activities in high school, and many women continue to swim, run, play tennis, and participate on athletic teams in their adult years. The recent surge in the study of the female athlete has illuminated some elements of particular concern to these women.

The most noteworthy and well-documented concern is the delay by one to three years of first menstruation (menarche) in some young female runners, swimmers, and ballet dancers, and the development of irregular periods or cessation of menstrual periods (secondary amenorrhea) in women who increase their physical activity beyond some ill-defined critical point (11). The physiological basis for this delayed menarche and secondary amenorrhea is not known. One theory states that a relationship exists between the lean/fat ratio of these women and their menstrual patterns: Women who exercise strenuously generally do have a lower body fat and greater muscle mass than sedentary women of the same age. Since fat tissue is known to be one site of conversion of circulating steroid precursors to the female hormones (estrogens), some think that those women who have low body fat do not produce appropriate levels of hormones to promote and maintain normal menstrual function. Others feel this is a simplistic answer, and that the many hormonal changes that accompany strenuous physical activity must contribute to the condition. The long-term effects of this menstrual dysfunction are not as yet determined, but among them is loss of bone mineral with increased tendency to fracture. Women who have been amenorrheic are reported to develop normal periods upon cessation or diminution of their exercise, even before there is significant weight gained.

In light of the possibility that it is her lean/fat ratio that predisposes the female athlete to amenorrhea, it is interesting to note that the energy intake of young women runners reportedly is not greater than that of less active women of the same age. Only in a group of women who ran more than thirty to forty miles per week was energy intake increased significantly above that of controls (2300 kcal per day vs. 1900 kcal), and even then the difference reported did not seem commensurate with the activity performed (12).

Iron is a nutrient considered to be at risk for the general population of women in the United States. Present reports on iron status in young women are complicated by differences in intensity of activity performed and blood parameters measured, by lack of information on dietary or supplementation practices of participants, and lack of control groups. One study of the 1968 Olympic athletes found 5 percent of the women to be anemic as assessed by hemoglobin levels and 20 percent to be iron deficient as defined by transferrin saturation (13). Serum ferritin levels, the most sensitive measure of iron status, have been measured in women runners (14). No significant difference was found between mean values in women who ran more than thirty miles per week and those who ran less, and the percentage of individuals with low iron stores was no different than in a population of controls. Thus, iron status in these women did not seem to be adversely affected by their activity.

A growing controversy for active women is the continuation of exercise and sports during pregnancy. Many physicians recommend against it, yet there is little actual information, pro or con, in the literature. The last months of pregnancy place a great burden on the woman's circulation. When the mother does physical work, her muscles compete with the placenta for blood, and if her heart is small or untrained, it may not adequately cope with this dual burden. In fact, women with small hearts are at increased risk for premature delivery (15). However, women who have participated in an active exercise program before pregnancy do not show during pregnancy the increased cost of controlled exercise (riding a stationary bicycle) as women do who have not exercised before pregnancy (16). Also, the increase in fetal heart-rate found to accompany maternal physical activity is less pronounced in the previously trained women. A study of Hungarian athletes suggests that the complications of pregnancy and delivery may be lower in athletes than in the general population (17).

Women who are in good physical health and who have exercised regularly prior to pregnancy can probably continue moderate activity, with adequate prenatal supervision. On the other hand, women who have complicating conditions, such as diabetes or hypertension, or who smoke or have been inactive before pregnancy, should not undertake a strenuous activity program during pregnancy (18). In all circumstances the pregnant woman must increase her energy intake to cover not only the needs of the growing fetus (see Chap. 22) but also the increased needs of her activity, given the extra weight being moved.

QUESTIONS

1. *What are the advantages of exercise? How does exercise affect body weight? Food intake? Fitness? Weight loss?*

2. *What factors affect work capacity? What is meant by maximal oxygen uptake? Distinguish between aerobic and anaerobic work. How should work and rest cycles be spaced?*

3. How much additional energy intake will be required by an athlete? A worker in heavy industry? (Consult the tables in Chap. 6.) Do all sports have high energy demands? Make a list of high- and low-energy cost recreations. How much of your time is spent in activities requiring more energy than in walking?

4. What is the fuel for muscular work? How is this determined? How much glycogen is present in muscle and what affects this amount? Of what importance is muscle glycogen? Liver glycogen?

5. What effect does nutritional deficiency have on work performance? On fitness and training? Why does dehydration have serious effects on performance? How is dehydration prevented?

6. Make up a menu for a meal to be eaten three to four hours before a sports event. Devise a liquid formula from inexpensive ingredients that would provide about the same nutrients.

References

1. Durnin, J. V. G. A., and Passmore, R.: *Energy, Work and Leisure.* London, Heinemann Educational Books, Ltd., 1967.
2. Åstrand, P. O.: Diet and athletic performance. Fed. Proc., *26:*1772, 1967, and Nutr. Today, *3(2):*9, 1968.
3. Costill, D. L., and Miller, J. M.: Nutrition for endurance sport: carbohydrate and fluid balance. Internat. J. Sports Med., *1*:2, 1980.
4. Nelson, R. A., and Gastineau, C. F.: Nutrition for athletes. In Craig, T. T. (ed.): *The Medical Aspects of Sports: 15.* Chicago, American Medical Association, 1974; Mirkin, G.: J. Amer. Med. Assoc., *223*:1511, 1973.
5. Davies, K. J. A., et al.: Bioenergetics in iron deficiency and repletion. Amer. J. Physiol., 1981.
6. Gontzea, I., Sutzescu, R., and Dumitrache, S.: The influence of adaptation to physical effort on nitrogen balance in man. Nutr. Rept. Internat., *11*:231, 1975.
7. Butterfield, G. and Calloway, D. H.: Protein utilization in men under two conditions of energy balance and work. Fed. Proc. *36*: 1166, 1977.
8. American Alliance for Health, Physical Education, and Recreation: *Nutrition for Athletes: A Handbook for Coaches.* Washington, D.C., 1971.
9. Costill, D. L., Dalsky, G. P., and Fink, W. J.: Effects of caffeine ingestion on metabolism and exercise performance. Med. Sci. Sports, *10*:155, 1978.
10. Amer. College Sports Med.: Position statement on prevention of heat injuries during distance running. Med. Sci. Sports, 7:vii, 1975.
11. Rebar, R. W., and Cumming, D. C.: Reproductive function in women athletes. J. Amer. Med. Assoc., *246*:1590, 1981.
12. Nerad, J.: Nutritional and biochemical differences between physically active and inactive women. MS Thesis, Univ. Calif., Berkeley, 1980.
13. DeWijn, T. F., deJongste, J. C., et al.: Hemoglobin, packed cell volume, serum iron and iron binding capacity of selected athletes. J. Sports Med., *11*:42, 1971.
14. Hamilton, S.: Evaluation of iron stores in physically active women. MS Thesis, Univ. Calif., Berkeley, 1982.
15. Karvonen, M. J.: Women and men at work. World Health, Jan., 1971, p. 3.
16. Edwards, M. T., et al.: Accelerated respiratory response to moderate exercise in late pregnancy. Respir. Physiol., in press.
17. Pomerance, J. J., Buck, L., and Lynch, V. A.: Maternal exercise as a screening test for uteroplacental insufficiency. Obst. Gyn., *44*:383, 1974; Bullard, J. A.: Exercise and pregnancy. Canad. Family Physician, *27*:977, 1981.
18. Metcalf, J., McNulty, T. H., and Neland, K.: Cardiovascular physiology. Clin. Obst. Gyn., *24*:693, 1981.

22 Nutrition, Pregnancy, and Lactation

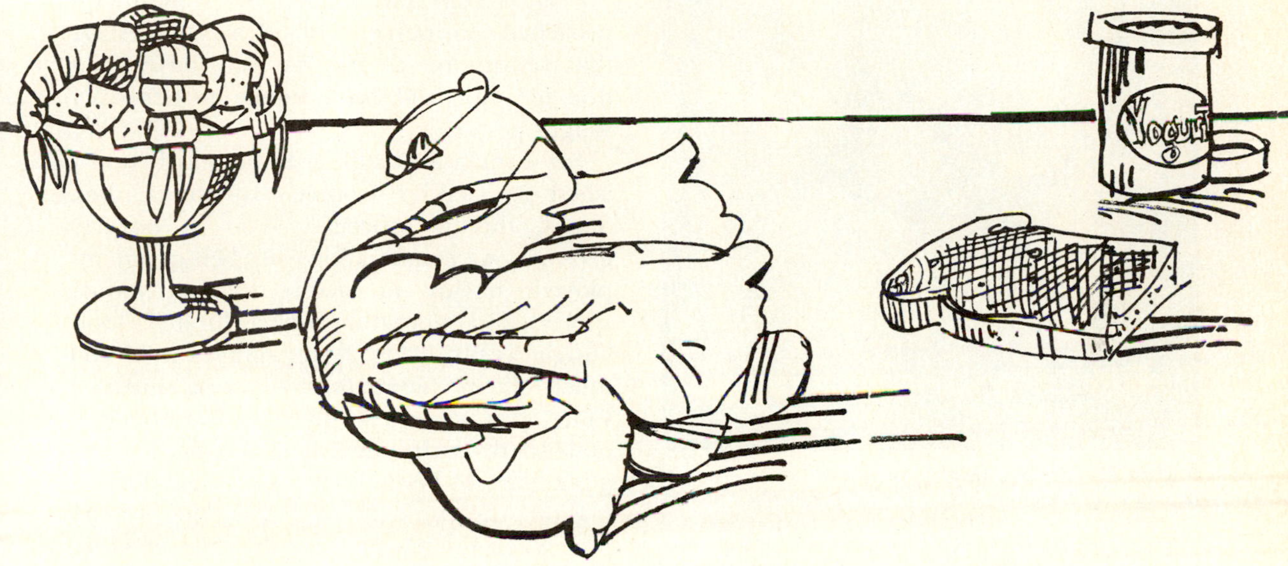

MATERNAL NUTRITION

Diet is especially important for pregnant and nursing mothers because the woman is nourishing the child through her own body, in the uterus before birth or through the milk she secretes. The nutrients needed by the child must be furnished in the mother's food—they may be drawn to some extent from her own tissues, but with the result that the mother will be depleted and the infant not adequately nourished. Pregnancy in teenage girls presents a situation of particular stress, because the needs of the developing infant are superimposed on the mother's own needs for adequate growth and development. Maternal and infant complications occur about twice as frequently among early teenage mothers as among mature women. Pregnancy hazards are also greater in American nonwhite populations than in white, and in women from lower socioeconomic groups.

A young woman who has good food habits and is well nourished when she becomes pregnant has little cause for concern. (See Fig. 22-1.) She will need to alter her diet only by increasing intake of some of the foods she is already accustomed to eating. Unfortunately, too many young women have not formed good food habits and thus enter pregnancy in a poorly nourished condition. A borderline deficiency may become apparent at this time. If previous intake of iron or folacin has been low, anemia may develop during pregnancy because of the extra demands of the fetus. In goitrous regions, latent iodine deficiency is likely to be manifested by enlargement of the thyroid gland during pregnancy.

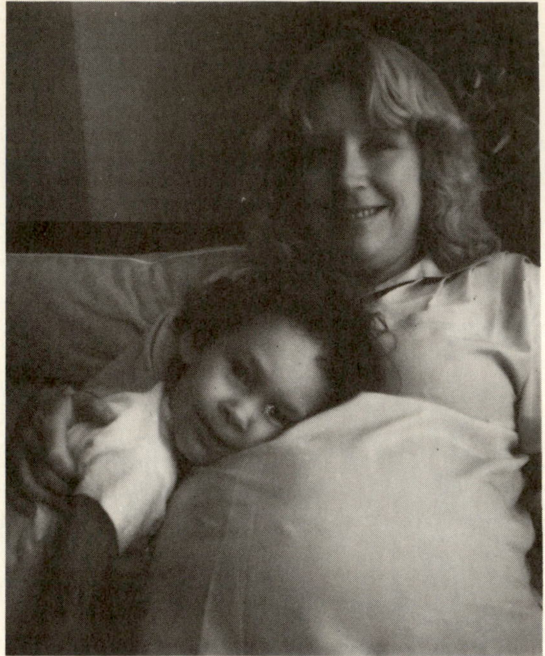

Figure 22–1 For a healthy, well-nourished woman, repeated pregnancies impose no special physiological hazard, but repeated cycles of pregnancy and lactation in the face of chronic food deprivation deplete the maternal body, contributing to early menopause and premature aging. (Photo courtesy of D. H. Calloway, II, Woodland Hills, CA)

Nutritional Status of Women of Child-Bearing Age

In the United States, the prevalence of adolescent females (ages 11 to 16 years) whose nutrient intakes are below standard increases with age, and those in the lowest socioeconomic group tend to have lower nutrient intakes than others. Being fat or being anxious about keeping slim leads to chronic self-imposed dieting that may further lower body stores of essential nutrients. Menstrual irregularity and amenorrhea occur commonly in women whose body fat content is severely reduced by chronic dieting or, as discussed in Chapter 21, by very high levels of physical activity such as marathon running. In some, this leads to reproductive failure. A recent study of women who kept their body weights well below ideal weight (91 ± 1%) by self-imposed food restriction, found that 73 percent of those who had been infertile conceived without treatment when they followed a dietary regimen designed to increase their weight to normal (1). Conception occurred when average weight gain was only 3.7 kg (8.2 lb) and when body weights approached 95 percent of ideal, suggesting that restoration of fertility may have been due to improved food intake rather than weight per se.

Fat women are as likely to be poorly nourished as slender women. In the United States, this is especially true in poverty groups. A combination of being unemployed, having no access to recreational sports, and operating on a limited food budget easily leads to consumption of too much cheap, filling food of poor nutritive value. Just when a woman needs to be well nourished, at the time of conception, she is quite likely to be in a poor or marginal state.

From the moment of fertilization to the time when the placenta is fully developed, at about eight weeks, the embryo receives its nutrition mainly from nutrients present in the uterine tissues and secretions. Thus, the prior nutritional status of the mother, as reflected in these tissues, is especially important during this early period, when most of the organs are being formed in the fetus.

After menarche, monthly blood loss increases the need for iron. Iron lost in menstrual flow averages 15 to 30 mg, or 0.5 to 1.0 mg per day over the monthly cycle. Because only 10 to 20 percent of dietary iron is absorbed, iron intake should be increased by 5 to 10 mg per day after menarche, yet older girls and women usually take less iron in the diet than do boys and men. Folacin status is also unsatisfactory in many women, including those who are affluent. This important B vitamin is low in many diets and is commonly omitted from vitamin pills, so the frequency of folacin deficiency is perhaps not surprising. Diets of people living in poverty and those of people eating little or no animal foods are also low or deficient in vitamin B-12. Thus, anemia and undesirably low iron stores are common in women on a worldwide basis (Fig. 22–2). The situation becomes worse during pregnancy when the maternal blood volume must expand and the placenta must be supplied to support the fetus.

In all age and economic groups, dietary histories indicate unsatisfactory intakes of calcium, iron, and vitamin A, and often of B vitamins, vitamin C, and iodine. It is likely that intake of the lesser-known nutrients such as zinc and copper is also low, but this point has not been well studied. Previous use of oral contraceptive pills may have increased the need for vitamin B-6 and, in some cases, folacin; or the presence of an intrauterine contraceptive device may have led to large monthly losses of blood. Normal or increased needs coupled with poor diets lead inevitably to an undesirable state of nutrition.

Effect of Malnutrition on the Outcome of Pregnancy

In poor human populations, mixed deficiencies are common because what people generally lack is food rather than a single nutrient. Birth rates are high in poorer, less-developed countries, where food intakes are chronically low, so it is apparent that the prevalent undernutrition is not so severe as to impair fertility. However, surveys of poor women in India show that 28 to 32 percent

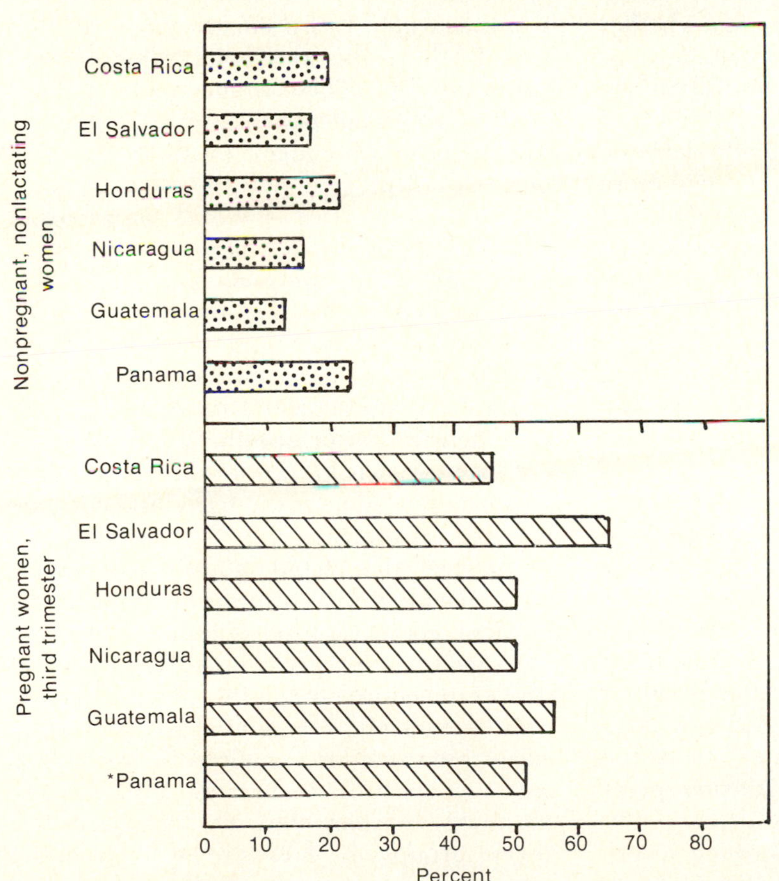

Figure 22–2 Percent of pregnant women with deficient transferrin saturation (15 percent), in Central America and Panama (1965–1966). Transferrin is a protein that transports iron. (From Arroyave, G.: Nutrition in pregnancy. Archivos Latinamer. Nutr. *26*:129, 1976.)

of pregnancies end in spontaneous abortion or stillbirth (2). An undernourished mother, however, may still be able to produce a healthy child, though there is evidence that a larger percentage of babies in poor condition are born to groups of mothers in poor nutritional condition (3).

Illustrative evidence that the nutritional condition of the mother during pregnancy frequently influences not only her own health but also the well-being of her child comes from investigations in Canada (4) and the United States (5) during the 40s. In each case, pregnant women from low-income groups were studied during the later months of pregnancy, and for some time after birth of the children. At the Boston Lying-In Hospital, 216 women attending the prenatal clinic were classified according to whether their diets were considered good, fair, or poor. No attempt was made to influence the diet, and records were kept of condition of mother and baby at and after delivery. Mothers in the poorest diet group had more complications and difficult types of delivery; moreover, all the stillborn babies and all but one of those who were premature or died soon after birth were born to mothers in this group. Conversely, a higher proportion of babies whose condition was rated at birth as superior or good was born to mothers who had had good or excellent diets during pregnancy.

In the Toronto studies (4), the women in one group, whose diets were poor, received supplementary food. Another group were given neither food nor instruction and served as controls. Those who received supplementary food had better health, both before and after delivery, fewer complications at delivery, and fewer miscarriages, stillbirths, or premature deliveries, than the mothers who ate poor diets during pregnancy.

Studies made in Europe following severe food restriction during World War II documented various reproductive difficulties—premature births, stillborn infants, infants below normal weight, and high neonatal death rate. In the Netherlands, food available to pregnant women provided on the average 1925 kcal and 61 gm of protein in 1944; by the spring of 1945, these allowances had fallen to 800 kcal and 35 gm of protein. About 50 percent of women became infertile, and there is an indication that the women who became pregnant were the better nourished. Birth weights of infants were decreased, but rose after relief feeding. The situation was much worse during the siege of Leningrad, where the principal food available was rye bread of very poor quality. The total daily allowance for a working man was 300 to 350 gm of bread. At the height of the seige, the stillbirth rate rose to 56 percent, and the incidence of prematurity was 40 percent. Birth weights were low and infant mortality was high. These women were stressed in many ways, but poor nutrition is thought to have been a dominant factor in the poor outcomes of pregnancy.

Ample supportive evidence is available from animal studies in which poor diets were consumed during pregnancy (3). Not only do restricted laboratory and farm animals bear undersized young, but under severe conditions there is permanent stunting of growth and poor mental development. Severe deficiencies of specific nutrients have also been shown in animal studies to cause sterility, resorption of the fetus, and congenital malformations.

On the other hand, some investigators have failed to find a relationship between the nutrient content of self-selected diets and the quality of pregnancy (6–10). In some studies the entire population appears to have been reasonably well-nourished, so differences due to minor variations in diet would not have been expected. In others, confounding variables were not the same between groups of pregnant women being compared.

Investigators have turned to supplementation trials to determine if dietary improvement does affect the outcome of pregnancy. Again, results are mixed (6, 11). One major difficulty with these studies is that the supplement does not always raise intake sufficiently, either because the extra food is shared with others, only part of the supplement is consumed, or the supplement displaces other food from the diet. In general, benefit has been seen where the initial food intake was very low or the women were noticeably undernourished.

In the United States, a Special Supplemental Feeding Program for Women, Infants and Children (WIC), introduced in 1972, offers a monthly food supplement to low-income pregnant, breastfeeding, and postpartum women, infants, and preschool children who meet certain medical and nutritional criteria. In addition to a monthly food package (through delivery of the actual foods or in the form of vouchers for the purchase of specified foods), participants receive nutrition and diet counseling. WIC foods include milk, eggs, cheese, iron-fortified cereals, and vitamin C–rich juices. Evaluation of the program found that, initially, the average birth weight was lower and the infant mortality rate was higher than is usual in well-nourished populations. WIC participants showed increased weight gain during pregnancy, and heavier infant birth weights (12).

In animal studies, protein appears to be particularly important for reproduction. Human experience is more difficult to evaluate because when protein intake is low, the diet is also low in energy and usually lacking in other nutrients, notably B vitamins, iron, and zinc. In the United States, Dieckman (13) showed that there was an increased incidence of abortion when mothers were on a low-protein intake and, on the positive side, that the number of infants born in excellent condition increased steadily as the protein intake of the mothers was on a progressively higher level. Burke and her associates also found a positive relationship between maternal protein intake (up to 90 gm per day) and infant weight, length, and physical well-being.

A note of caution was recently sounded by Rush and associates who found a slightly poorer pregnancy outcome (a small excess of premature deaths and neonatal deaths) in a large group of women in Harlem, New York, who were offered a high-protein supplement (40 gm protein, 470 kcal, vitamins, and minerals lacking zinc) than in the group given a supplement low in protein (6 gm protein, 322 kcal, vitamins, and minerals). Several hundred infants born in this study were later examined at one year of age (6). There were no significant differences in height and weight between maternal supplement groups. The psychological performance of the high-protein group was significantly better than that of infants born to women given the low-protein supplement during pregnancy. This finding coincides with data from supplementation trials in Guatemala that show beneficial effects of maternal protein supplementation on intellectual performance of children (15).

While it is true that pregnancy outcome is often satisfactory in spite of seemingly limited food intake, and that hormonal changes due to pregnancy do lead to more efficient utilization of nutrients, the weight of evidence indicates that superior performance is associated with generous intake of a well-balanced diet during pregnancy.

PREGNANCY

How the Child Is Nourished

There is no direct connection, either nervous or circulatory, between the mother and the fetus, but interchange between the blood streams of mother and child takes place through the placenta. This is a vascular organ on the inner surface of the uterus, in which the blood from the mother and the fetus are brought closely together so that interchange of constituents from one to the other is possible. Thus, the fetal blood takes up nutrients processed in the placenta from the mother's blood, and carries them to the fetus (through the umbilical cord), where they are built into the more complex substances forming the organs, muscles, and other tissues of the child.

Stages of Pregnancy

During the first trimester of pregnancy, the daily need of materials for the growth of the fetus is so small as to be practically negligible. (The fetus gains hardly more than 1 gm of weight per day.) Maternal tissues are growing during this time. The uterus and breasts enlarge, the placenta and amniotic fluid are formed, and the maternal blood volume expands (Fig. 22–3). This is the period during which many women experience nausea or digestive disturbances. Nausea in early pregnancy is due usually to adjustments in establishing relationships between the fetus and the mother, not primarily due to misfunctioning of the digestive tract itself, and it should soon disappear. Food may be better tolerated in smaller meals at shorter intervals. Eating a few salted crackers before rising may help and certainly will do no harm. If vomiting is severe and prolonged, medical attention is advisable. In spite of optimistic claims, there is no clear evidence that administration of vitamins alleviates the nausea of early pregnancy in the well-nourished patient. In fact, some vitamin-mineral supplements are not well tolerated, and *if prescribed,* these should be taken with, or immediately after, meals.

During the second trimester, the mother stores a substantial amount of fat, which protects the fetus against possible maternal food deprivation and constitutes a physiological reserve energy supply for lactation later. By the sixth month the fetus is gaining about 10 gm daily, but about half the total weight increase of the fetus during gestation occurs in the last two months. (See Table 22-1.) Therefore, during the final months of pregnancy it is especially important that the diet be unusually rich in all the nutritive factors needed for the growing child. The extra energy needs should be met in the form of foods that also provide high-quality proteins, minerals, and vitamins.

The National Research Council recommends increased allowances for almost all the essential nutrients during pregnancy. These recommended allowances, as well as those of the Canadian Department of National Health and Welfare, are found in Table 22–2. The extra energy allowance suggested by the NRC is not large (300 kcal or 1.26 MJ per day). The energy value of new tissue formed in pregnancy is about 50,000 kcal, of which a substantial portion is maternal fat. The basal metabolic rate is increased, owing to the energy requirement of fetal and supporting tissues and the added burden on the maternal heart and lungs (Table 22–3). The total energy cost of a pregnancy is about 80,000 kcal of metabolizable energy, or 285 kcal per day for the 280 days of gestation. The United States standards allow for this full amount. Previously, the NRC RDA was set lower on the basis of the observation that women in the later months of pregnancy are often not very active physically. However, the RDA for nonpregnant women assumes that there is only light activity, and it is now recognized that pregnant women cannot be appreciably less active in ordinary households. If the woman is active, and she should be to maintain fitness, her needs will be great because of the higher energy cost of moving a heavier, awkward body mass.

Many women continue working and exercising much as before pregnancy until near term, and their needs consequently will be large. The additional energy allowance should be adjusted to the needs of the individual, so that the energy costs of building

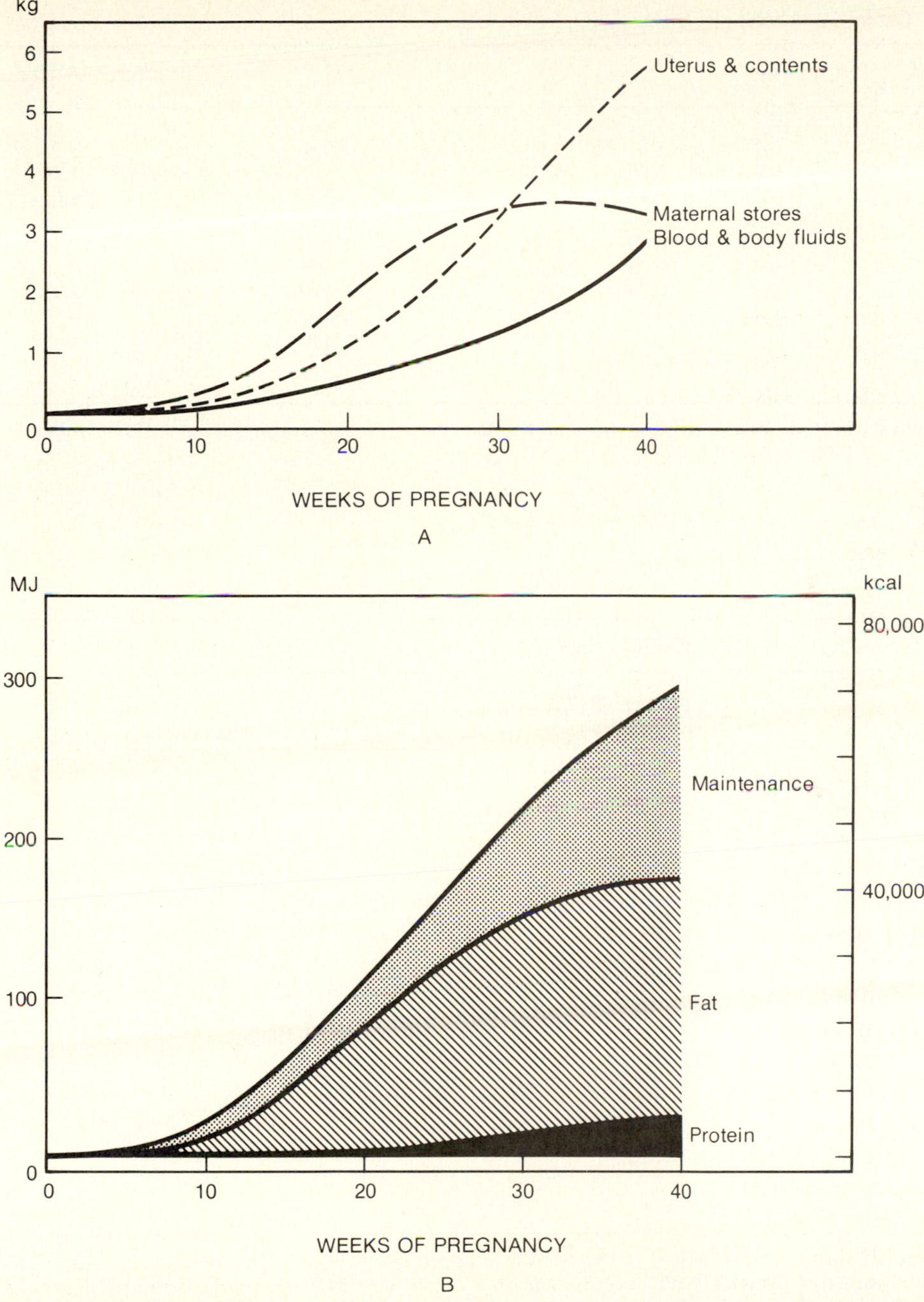

Figure 22–3 The components of weight gain during pregnancy (*A*, above) and its energy cost (*B*, below). In the first ten weeks, little weight is gained; during the next 20 weeks, maternal stores increase at a faster rate than the fetus; fetal growth is dominant in the last ten weeks. Energy cost of pregnancy is due to growth of fetus, maternal tissues, including fat, and to increased basal metabolism and other maintenance costs. (From Hytten, F. E., in *Maternal Nutrition during Preganancy and Lactation*, Hans Huber, 1980, with permission.)

Table 22–1 NITROGEN AND MINERAL CONTENT OF THE HUMAN FETUS[a]

Fetal age (weeks)	*12*	*16*	*20*	*24*	*28*	*32*	*36*	*40*
Weight (kg)	*0.02*	*0.1*	*0.3*	*0.75*	*1.35*	*2.0*	*2.7*	*3.4*
Total N (g)	0.18	1.0	3.6	10.4	19.6	30.2	44.3	64.3
Na (g)	0.06	0.26	0.75	1.63	2.74	3.85	4.89	5.56
K (g)	0.03	0.16	0.48	1.22	2.22	3.29	4.65	6.14
Cl (g)	0.06	0.29	0.84	1.92	3.00	4.32	5.14	5.85
Ca (g)	0.03	0.36	1.38	4.44	8.86	13.7	20.1	28.1
Mg (g)	0.002	0.02	0.05	0.13	0.26	0.41	0.58	0.76
P (g)	0.03	0.25	0.90	2.59	5.34	8.46	12.5	16.4
Fe (mg)	—	5.0	17.4	45.9	91.2	141	208	278
Cu (mg)	—	—	1.05	2.74	5.21	8.08	11.0	14.0
Zn (mg)	—	—	5.4	13.3	23.5	33.8	44.0	52.6

[a]Adapted from Widdowson, E. F., in *Maternal Nutrition during Pregnancy and Lactation,* Hans Huber, 1980.

Table 22–2 RECOMMENDED DIETARY ALLOWANCES FOR PREGNANCY AND LACTATION[a]

	United States		*Canada*	
Nutrient	Pregnancy	Lactation	Pregnancy	Lactation
Energy, kcal	300	500	300	450
Protein, g	30	20	25	20
Calcium, mg	400	400	500	500
Phosphorus, mg	400	400	500	500
Magnesium, mg	150	150	25	80
Iodine, μg	25	50	25	50
Iron, mg	*b*	*b*	6	0
Zinc, mg	5	10	8	6
Vitamin A, μg RE	200	400	100	400
Thiamin, mg	0.4	0.5	0.12	0.18
Riboflavin, mg	0.3	0.5	0.15	0.22
Niacin, mg equiv.	2	5	2	3
Folacin, mg	0.4	0.1	0.3	0.12
Vitamin B-6, mg	0.6	0.5	0.4	0.3
Vitamin B-12, μg	1	1	1	0.5
Vitamin C, mg	20	40	20	30
Vitamin D, μg	5	5	2.5	2.5
Vitamin E, mg TE	2	3	2	3

[a]Amounts of nutrient to be added to the allowance appropriate to the maternal age, as recommended by the U. S. National Research Council, 1980, and the Canadian Department of National Health and Welfare, 1983.

[b]The NRC states that the increased iron requirement during pregnancy cannot be met by the iron content of habitual American diets nor by the existing stores of many women. They recommend that supplemental iron be taken, 30–60 mg per day, during pregnancy and for 2–3 months after delivery. This recommendation lacks strong experimental support and a more modest supplement of 15 mg seems adequate, if any is needed. This, of course, depends on the quality of the habitual diet.

Table 22–3 ENERGY COST OF VARIOUS ACTIVITIES DURING PREGNANCY AND POSTPARTUM*

Activity	*Energy Cost*†			
	20–28 Weeks	29–36 Weeks	37–40 Weeks	Post-partum
Mature women:		←*calories/kg/min*→		
basal metabolic rate	15	15	15	12
quiet sitting	17	17	17	15
quiet standing	19	19	19	18
work involving upper torso	–	–	28	–
walking, 3.0 mph, 0° grade	64	67	62	61
bicycling, 300 kpm.	61	62	62	61
personal care, eating, child care, child feeding	26	26	26	26
typing and office work	29	29	29	26
driving car	32	32	32	29
housecleaning	46	46	46	46
gardening	64	64	–	–
shopping	–	–	–	62
swimming	–	91	–	–
			Last Trimester	***Postpartum***
Teen-agers:				
basal metabolic rate			16	16
knitting			20	20
combing hair			24	22
cooking			28	26
dishwashing			28	23
sweeping			44	43
climbing stairs			44	60
making beds			48	47
walking stairs with load			73	85

*From Blackburn, M. W., and Calloway, D. H.: J. Amer. Dietet. Assoc., *69*:29, 1976.

†Note that the values are given in small calories. To convert to kcal, divide by 1000. For example, the basal rate of a reference woman who weighs 70 kg (58 kg nonpregnant + 12 kg gain) at 37 to 40 weeks is (15 × 60 × 24) (70) ÷ 1000, or 1512 kcal/day.

new tissues, of higher metabolic rate and of physical workload are met. In a University of California study, while mature women were found to require 2300 kcal per day in mid-pregnancy, they required about 2500 to 2600 kcal per day in the last ten weeks (16). Women in active occupations or with young children in the household have higher needs than the minimum 36 kcal per kg recommended by the NRC. Pregnancies involving twins also impose much greater demands. It is more important that the woman gain weight at an appropriate rate than that she have any particular energy intake.

A normal and desirable weight gain during the forty weeks of pregnancy is 24 to 28 pounds (12.5 kg) (see Fig. 22–4). Maternal complications are more frequently associated with marked over- or underweight at the time of conception and with wide deviation from normal rate of weight gain during pregnancy. Some studies have suggested an

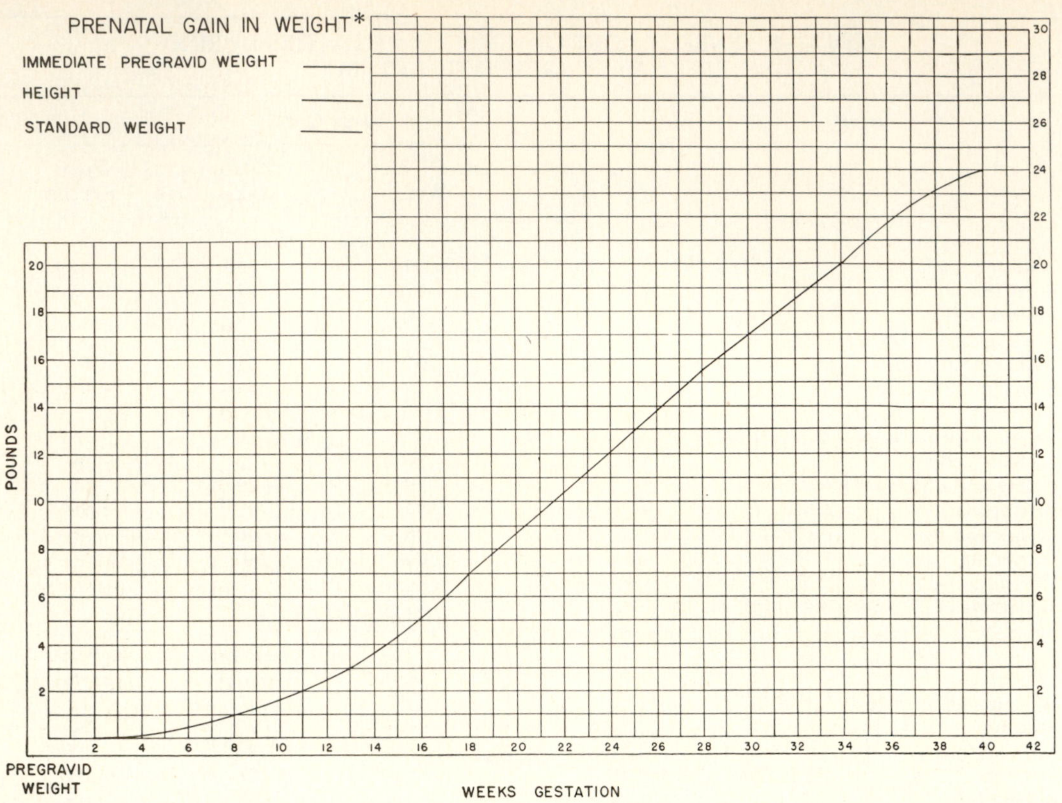

Figure 22–4 *Desirable prenatal gain in weight. Women who are underweight may need to gain more than average and overweight women slightly less. (Reprinted with permission from Lull, C., and Kimbrough, R.: Clinical Obstetrics. Philadelphia, J. B. Lippincott Company, 1953.)*

increased incidence of toxemia[1] in obese pregnant women, but others have not. Large early weight gain has also been regarded as a bad omen of maternal complications. This fear has led to excessive concern with weight gain, especially in the obese woman. With family planning, the obese woman can lose weight prior to pregnancy, but while she is pregnant she should not attempt to correct the preexisting condition. If there is a tendency to excessive weight gain, it is far wiser to increase physical activity than to restrict food intake.

Many slender women will need to gain more than the average 25 pounds. A study of 10,000 births showed that higher maternal weight gain was related to higher birth weight, a lower incidence of prematurity, and better growth and performance during the infant's first year of life (17). The key consideration is that healthy tissue be formed at a smooth progressive rate, irrespective of the total gain, and that the mother's health remain good. Some suggest that the weight gain may be spaced at about 4, 10, and 10 pounds in each of three trimes-

[1]Toxemia usually refers to a condition of blood poisoning that results from growth of microorganisms in the tissues or blood or from the absorption of noxious materials from food and water, or both. Toxemia of pregnancy differs and is a disorder of unidentified cause that is characterized by high blood pressure, protein in the urine, edema, headache, visual disturbances, and, in severe cases, convulsions and death.

ters, but healthy women vary widely in this regard. Women carrying twins will gain about twice as much as those with single babies.

Diet During Pregnancy

The nutritive needs during pregnancy are best met by a simple, wholesome diet, the basis of which is cheese, milk, eggs, meat, legumes, nuts, whole grains, vegetables, especially the dark green, leafy ones, and fruits. If the diet consumed before pregnancy was adequate, only simple modification is required to meet all additional nutrient allowances. Addition of two glasses of milk or cheese equivalent, one egg or larger amounts of fish, poultry, or legumes and one serving of dark green leafy vegetables, with frequent substitution of fruit for rich dessert and organ meats for other meat, fish, or poultry, is sufficient. In general, the more fruits and vegetables eaten the better, because these foods help to ensure the surplus of vitamins and minerals that is so very advantageous, without appreciably increasing energy intake.

The nutritional recommendations for pregnancy that are most difficult to meet are those for iron, zinc, folacin, and calcium. A diet that meets the allowances for these four nutrients *from food sources* will provide much more protein than the specified RDA and will meet other requirements, as well. The daily diet during pregnancy should be built around the following foods, in regard to types and amounts of foods daily:

Milk: 1 quart of whole or skimmed milk or yogurt.

Milk powder or canned milk may be substituted either as beverage or in cooking; 1½ oz (45 gm) of cheddar cheese may be substituted for one glass of milk. Alternative sources of calcium are discussed in Chapter 20.

Meat: Eight oz (250 mg) cooked weight of meat, fish, or poultry. Weekly use of liver is desirable. Eggs, cheese, dry legumes (beans, peas, lentils), and nuts may be substituted with cautions as noted in Chapter 20.

Vegetables and Fruits: Four large servings.

At least one serving should be a dark green, leafy vegetable. One serving should be a vegetable or fruit high in vitamin C content, such as green or red peppers, a citrus variety of fruit (orange, lemon, lime, grapefruit), papaya, melon, cabbage, or tomato.

Breads and Cereals: Four slices of whole-grain bread.

Cereal, ½ to ⅔ cooked, may be substituted for one slice of bread. Potatoes and whole-grain or enriched rice, corn meal, macaroni, spaghetti, barley, or wheat (bulgur) may also be used. Ready-to-eat cereal should be made from whole grain or have added bran or germ. Additional servings from this food group should be taken as required to meet energy needs.

Fat: 2 Tbsp of soft margarine or vegetable oil. If whole milk or milk products are used, 1 Tbsp of vegetable oil may be sufficient, depending on proportion of poly-unsaturated fatty acid in the fats selected.

Vitamin D: 10 μg from fortified milk or dietary supplement.

Fluid whole milk, canned evaporated milk, and some dry and skimmed milks are fortified with vitamin D at the level of 10 μg (400 IU) per quart. Some milk powder is not fortified, nor are cheese and ice cream. Package labels specify the addition of vitamin D.

Iodine: Iodized salt should be used in cooking and at the table. The normal intake of salt should be maintained throughout pregnancy.

It is difficult to assure adequate intakes of calcium and iron if a strict vegetarian ("vegan") diet is followed during pregnancy, and there is the further complication of the relatively poor absorption of iron, zinc, and possibly other trace elements from plant sources. Such diets are lacking in vitamin B-12, and supplementation is *mandatory* to prevent damage to the central nervous system of the infant. A more liberal vegetarian diet that includes milk and eggs and perhaps fish can meet the RDA if good selections are made from the food groups listed.

The woman should supplement the foods listed above to furnish energy sufficient for her individual needs and desired weight gain. The energy needs vary with weight and especially with degree of activity, so the energy allowance should be estimated individually, then increased in the second trimester of pregnancy by about 300 kcal. A moderately active 55 kg woman who needs 2000 kcal normally should have 2300 kcal or more in the latter part of pregnancy. But an active woman whose ordinary daily energy need is about 2400 kcal requires at least 2700 kcal in late pregnancy. Also, a woman who begins pregnancy in an undernourished condition may need a more liberal energy allowance in order to gain some weight. Teenagers must add the pregnancy allowance to the higher energy values recommended for nonpregnant girls of the same level of maturity.

A woman who is overweight when she becomes pregnant will need to keep her physical activity level high, or increase it, in order not to add to her obesity. The diet should not be too restrictive, that is, not below 36 kcal per kg of ideal pregnant body weight. Foods containing large amounts of sugar and fats should be the ones eliminated, rather than the more nutritious foods; skim milk, for example, may be substituted for whole milk. However, fat intake cannot be greatly reduced because of the need to have about 8 to 10 gm of essential fatty acid in the diet (about 3 to 4% of energy).

Enough energy must be supplied so that there will be no need to burn protein merely as fuel. Obviously, all the essential amino acids are required for fetal growth, so it is advisable that about half the protein in the diet should be from foods of high-quality (milk, meats, eggs, beans, nuts).

Extra calcium for the mother during pregnancy (and lactation) goes far toward insuring teeth of good quality and well-calcified bones in the child. The teeth of the child are formed and in large part calcified during the latter half of fetal life and the first few months after birth. About 28 gm of calcium is present in the body of a full-term infant, which means that the mother must supply an average of 100 mg of *absorbed* calcium daily. If the diet is adequate, calcium is also stored in the maternal skeleton during pregnancy, another physiological adaptation to the needs of lactation.

If the mother's diet is rich in iron and copper during pregnancy, the child will be born with a liver well stored with these trace elements, often a reserve sufficient to last through the months when it will be fed chiefly milk—a food low in iron and copper content. The newborn infant body has about 0.2 to 0.3 gm of iron and another 0.5 gm is present in the placenta and extramaternal tissues. The average woman has about 0.3 gm of storage iron, and another 150 mg will be spared because she is not menstruating. This is only about half the amount needed even if maternal stores were to be totally depleted. Unless the diet is rich in iron, the baby will be born without a good iron reserve, and the woman will become anemic. In accordance with our present state of knowledge, routine supplementation of the diet with salts of trace elements other than iron is not recommended. We know that the *balance* of trace elements is important, not just the amount of each one, and information regarding many of the micronutrients is quite incomplete. The safest course is to eat well. However, supplementary iron is often prescribed at dosage levels (30 to 60 mg/day) well above probable requirement. The Canadian recommendation is to add 6 mg per day. It seems that a supplement of 15 mg per day should be ample. A folacin supplement may also be needed; 0.3 to 0.4 mg will meet the additional allowance for pregnancy.

Women are sometimes advised to restrict their salt intake when their weight gain is judged excessive and they are accumulating tissue fluid. Some gain in blood volume and in other extracellular fluid, however, is perfectly normal under the hormonal influences of pregnancy. Salt is a dietary essential, and neither maternal nor fetal tissues can be maintained satisfactorily without it (18, 19). The association of sodium, edema, and hypertension (Chap. 14) led to the practice of salt restriction as a medical measure in threatened toxemia, but a careful study of over 2000 women showed that there were fewer complications in the group instructed to take more salt than in the one told to restrict it (19).

If digestion is upset or if there is difficulty in taking enough food, the regular meals may be reduced in size and extra nourishment taken between meals in the form of easily tolerated foods, such as milk, eggnog, cheese, crackers, fruit, or fruit juice. Meals may easily be made to fit into the family schedule, if foods for the family are wisely chosen—that is, planned to be of high nutritive value and cooked simply.

The extra allowances of all the essential nutrients recommended for pregnancy are a protection for both mother and child. They provide an abundance of building materials for growth and development of the infant without any need to deplete the stores of these substances in the mother's body; and in the baby they help to build reserves of such nutrients as can be stored before birth.

Pregnancy is also a time to avoid nonnutritious substances in foods and to restrict the use of tobacco and drugs, including caffeine and alcohol. A characteristic pattern of malformation (small head size, subnormal mentality, facial abnormalities, growth deficiency) has been reported with increasing frequency in babies born to women who drink heavily (20). Smoking is associated with low birth weights. The question of caffeine and coffee is still under investigation, but it is better to restrict intake until safety is proved.

LACTATION

During lactation, there is increased need for energy, protein, minerals, and vitamins: (1) to cover the amounts secreted in the milk; (2) to cover the cost of secreting the milk; and (3) to protect the mother's body (Table 22–2). Energy requirement varies with the amount of milk produced, and intake must be regulated to the individual woman. A woman who is meeting all the needs of a 5-kg infant (11 pounds) must secrete about 850 ml of milk, providing about 600 kcal daily. Human milk is produced with about 80 percent efficiency, so the requirement for lactation is about 750 kcal per day. If the woman has gained properly during pregnancy, about one-third of the extra need can be met from body fat reserves over a 100-day period of lactation. Thus, the RDA is an extra 500 kcal. If the period of lactation extends beyond 4 months, as it should ideally, then energy intake should be increased to the full amount required.

These recommendations accord with the experience of lactating women. A study compared Scottish women who were breastfeeding their infants with those who gave bottle feedings, in terms of energy intake, physical activity level, and loss of body fat (21). Energy intakes of the two groups were 2716 and 2125 kcal, respectively; both were losing weight and the lactating women negligibly more. Energy available for milk formation was 618 kcal per day, and the calculated energy content of milk was 597 kcal. Body weights of lactating and nonlactating women have been found to be the same eight to twelve weeks postpartum (16,22), but reported energy intakes of the lactating women were higher by 600 to 900 kcal per day. Thus, an adequate fat reserve is a real benefit during the first few weeks postpartum when a mother is physically active and short on sleep, a period when her food intake does not keep up with her needs. Body weight will be normalized without need for special effort at slimming, and the woman who carries through the whole of the reproductive cycle should not become fatter with each pregnancy. There is evidence that lactation performance can be maintained in spite of what appear to be inadequate intakes of energy (23) sufficient to support low-normal infant weights. However, the diet always should be of good quality to prevent depletion of the maternal lean tissues and to guarantee adequate content of vitamins and trace minerals in the milk.

Human milk contains about 12 gm of protein per liter. In arriving at the recommended allowance of an additional 20 gm of protein per day during lactation, the National Research Council has assumed that the dietary protein is of lower quality than milk protein so that conversion is not 100 percent efficient; and that milk production may exceed 1 liter per day. Successful lactation is achieved on lower protein intakes, but there is no clear evidence that this is not detrimental to the mother. The essential amino acids incorporated in milk proteins must be furnished, so it is advisable to obtain the extra protein allowance from high-quality sources. The lipid composition of breast milk is affected by diet, and the milk will be richer in essential fatty acids if the maternal diet contains a liberal amount of polyunsaturated fats.

Because milk is so high in calcium and phosphorus content, its secretion makes great demands for these mineral elements. Nursing mothers are often found to be in negative calcium and phosphorus balance. This causes a drain on the mother's body, but it does not affect milk secretion. If a mother increases her own milk intake by the amount she is providing to her child (an additional 1 pint to 1 quart daily), she will meet the high calcium needs, as well as the need for some other nutrients. Extra vitamin D (5 μg) is also needed to insure good utilization of calcium and phosphorus.

The vitamin content of human milk, especially the water-soluble vitamins, is largely dependent on the vitamin intake of the mother. Lactation, like pregnancy, is a period when borderline nutritional status may develop into frank deficiency. Allowances recommended for vitamins are about 50 percent more than those for nonpregnant women. Relatively little iron is secreted in milk (0.5 to 1.0 mg per day), and lactating women usually do not menstruate, so there is no added allowance for iron in lactation.

Diet for Nursing Mothers

Recommendations for the diet in the nursing period are almost identical with those given for pregnancy, except that the need for almost all nutritive essentials is greater during lactation, especially as the infant grows and takes larger quantities of milk. The *quality* of the diet required remains essentially the same—a diet containing liberal amounts of milk, eggs, fruits, and vegetables to furnish the extra protein, mineral salts, and vitamins needed.

Milk is the best food for protecting against any drain on calcium and phosphorus reserves to supply these elements in her milk. At least 1 quart of milk should be taken daily, or its equivalent in cheese or yogurt. If a woman cannot or will not use dairy products, then alternative calcium sources must be included. It is a good thing to take supplementary nourishment just before nursing the baby in the middle of the morning and afternoon, and at bedtime. It is essential to have a plentiful intake of *fluids* (about 3 l from all sources) to provide the water in the milk secreted, in addition to that needed by the mother. Fruit and vegetable juices are useful to give added fluids, as well as vitamins and minerals.

Many constitutents other than nutrients are passed into milk. Excessive use of alcohol and artificially sweetened products is to be avoided during nursing periods for this reason. Drugs, including those sold without prescription, such as aspirin, laxatives, and sedatives, pass into the milk and should be taken only on the advice of a physician. Oral contraceptive agents affect lactation adversely, but injected preparations have been used with no detected detriment (24).

Breastfeeding Technique

During the latter weeks of pregnancy, the mother should use extra care in cleansing the nipples, preferably without soap, and massage them as needed to assure protractility. Following delivery, the infant should be offered breastfeeding as early and at as frequent intervals as possible, using both breasts. It is important that the infant receive the first flow (*colostrum*), as it contains many of the immune substances. The infant should not be given supplementary feedings because they decrease the appetite and vigor of sucking. If there is difficulty in the beginning, boiled water should be given from a spoon.

Milk is secreted continuously but it does not flow easily. When the baby suckles, sensory impulses are transmitted to the hypothalamus, causing secretion of the hormone *oxytocin,* which causes cells in the breast to contract and "let down" the milk. Psychogenic factors can inhibit oxytocin secretion and consequently interfere with nursing.

Advantages of Breastfeeding

Breastfeeding is an emotionally satisfying experience, important to the bonding of mother and baby. Child abuse is relatively rare among women who have nursed their infants. Physiologically, breastfeeding leads to more rapid readjustment of the uterus after delivery and acts for some weeks or months as a natural contraceptive.

In addition to the warmth, closeness, and emotional satisfaction of breastfeeding for

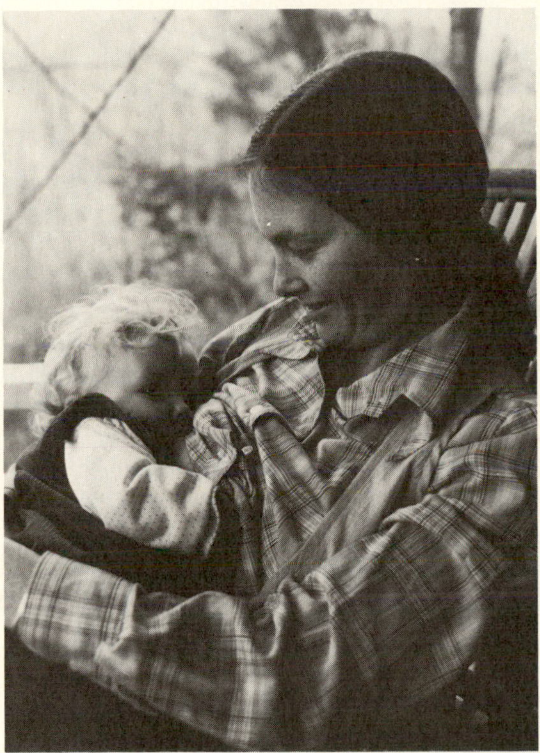

Figure 22–5 Until about the 1920s, almost all infants were breastfed. Advancing technology and increased employment of women were accompanied by a decline in breastfeeding in the United States, and women received little social or medical support for nursing their babies. Attitudes are now changing and increasing numbers of women, especially those in upper income and educated groups, recognize the advantages of breastfeeding and are doing so for at least some weeks. Assistance and advice are available from the LaLeche League in most cities, as well as from experienced grandmothers.

both mother and child, human milk for human infants is clearly superior to other kinds of milk (see Chap. 23). Most mothers can nurse their babies adequately, and the advantages certainly warrant serious effort to do so, at least for the first three to six months of the child's life.

To insure good milk flow, dietary practices should be sound throughout pregnancy, as well as after the birth of the child. Successful nursing is promoted when the mother is relaxed, has an adequate and satisfying diet, and enjoys exercise, rest, sunshine, fresh air, and the happy company of her infant. Breastfeeding is most often a very happy and rewarding experience for both mother and child.

QUESTIONS

1. Discuss the special problems and energy needs of the different periods of pregnancy. Do the needs for protein, mineral elements, and vitamins differ in early and late pregnancy and, if so, how?

2. By what selection of food groups could the higher energy need of the later months of pregnancy be satisfied and at the same time a diet rich in good quality protein, mineral elements, and vitamins be provided? What food groups should be prominent in the diet during pregnancy?

3. How much weight should be gained in a pregnancy involving a single child? With twins? What tissues are formed in pregnancy? Is a reserve of body fat advantageous or disadvantageous? Why?

4. Compare the allowances for each of the nutritive factors in pregnancy with those for a woman who is nursing a baby (see Table 22–2). In what respects do the requirements in lactation differ from those in pregnancy, and why? Why are more energy, protein, and calcium, needed than are passed on to the baby in the mother's milk? What factors in the diet, if taken in plentiful amounts, favor milk secretion? What environmental factors tend to suppress milk secretion?

5. Plan a day's meals for a woman in the last 2 months of pregnancy. Calculate the energy and protein in this diet, and compare with the allowances given in Table 22–2 to see if the diet is adequate in these respects. Can you make any suggestions regarding how it might be altered to provide more liberal intake of mineral elements and vitamins? Does the woman need some vitamin D supplement, and why?

6. Plan a day's diet for a nursing mother, and calculate the amount of calcium and vitamin A supplied to see if they are adequate. For meeting the calcium allowance, why are cacium pills not an adequate dietary supplement to use in place of milk? If the diet needs to be improved in these respects, what changes would you suggest?

References

1. Bates, G. W., Bates, S. R., and Whitworth, N. S.: Reproductive failure in women who practice weight control. Fertility and Sterility, *37*:373, 1982.
2. Rao, 1972, cited by Raman, L.: Nutrition supplement studies in India. p. 158 in ref. 11 below.
3. Committee on Maternal Nutrition, Food and Nutrition Board: *Maternal Nutrition and the Course of Pregnancy.* Washington, D.C., NAS/NRC, 1970.
4. Ebbs, J. H., Tisdall, F. F., and Scott, W. A.: The influence of prenatal diet on the mother and child. J. Nutr., *22*:515, 1941.
5. Burke, B. S., Beal, V. A., Kirkwood, S. B., and Stuart, H. C.: The influence of nutrition during pregnancy upon the condition of the infant at birth. J. Nutr., *25*:569, 1943.
6. Metcoff, J., Klein, E. R., and Nichols, B. L. (eds.): Maternal nutritional status and fetal outcome. Amer. J. Clin. Nutr., *34*:653, 1981.
7. Thomson, A. M.: Diet in pregnancy. III. Diet in Relation to course and outcome of pregnancy. Brit. J. Nutr., *13*:509, 1959.
8. McGanity, W. J., et al.: The Vanderbilt cooperative study of maternal and infant nutrition. VI. Relationship of obstetric performance to nutrition. Amer. J. Obst. Gyn., *67*:501, 1954.
9. Bagchi, K., and Bose, A. K.: Effect of low nutrient intake during pregnancy on obstetrical performance and offspring. Amer. J. Clin. Nutr., *11*:586, 1962.
10. Campbell, D. M., Campbell-Brown, B. M., Jandial, L., and MacGillivray, I.: Maternal energy intake in

pregnancy and its relation to maternal fetal factors. Proc. Nutr. Soc., *41*:30A, 1982.

11. Lechtig, A. (ed.): Effects of maternal nutrition on infant health. Archivos Latinamer. Nutr., *29* (suppl. 1):155, 1979.
12. Edozian, J. C., Switzer, B. R., and Bryan, R. B.: Medical evaluation of the special supplemental food program for women, infants and children. Amer. J. Clin. Nutr., *32*:677, 1979.
13. Dieckman, W. J., et al.: Observation on protein intake and the health of mother and baby. I. Clinical and laboratory findings. II. Food intake. J. Amer. Dietet. Assoc., *27*:1046, 1951.
14. Rush, D., Stein, Z., and Susser, M.: *Diet in Pregnancy. A Randomized Controlled Trial of Nutritional Supplements.* Natl. Foundation Original Articles Series. Vol. 16, No. 3. New York, Alan R. Liss Co., 1979.
15. Balderston, J. B., Wilson, A. B., Freire, M. E., and Simonen, M. S.: *Malnourished Children of the Rural Poor.* Boston, Auburn House Publ. Co., 1981.
16. Blackburn, M. W., and Calloway, D. H.: Energy expenditure and consumption of mature, pregnant, and lactating women. J. Amer. Dietet. Assoc., *69*:29, 1976.
17. Singer, J. E., Westphal, M., and Niswander, K.: Relationship of weight gain during pregnancy to birth weight and infant growth and development in the first year of life. Obst. Gyn., *31*:417, 1968.
18. Palomaki, J. F., and Lindheimer, M. D.: Sodium depletion simulating deterioration in a toxemic pregnancy. New Eng. J. Med., *282*:88, 1970.
19. Robinson, M.: Salt in pregnancy. Lancet, *1*:178, 1958.
20. Hanson, J. W., Jones, K. L., and Smith, W. D.: Fetal alcohol syndrome: experience with 41 patients. J. Amer. Med. Assoc., *235*:1458, 1976.
21. Thomson, A. M., Hytten, F. E., and Billewicz, W. Z.: The energy cost of human lactation. Brit. J. Nutr., *24*:565, 1970.
22. Naismith, D J., and Ritchie, C. D.: The effect of breast-feeding and artificial feeding on body weights, skinfold measurements and food intakes of forty-two primiparous women. Proc. Nutr. Soc., *34*:116A, 1975.
23. Gopalan, C., and Belavady, B.: Nutrition and lactation. Fed. Proc., *20*:177, 1961.

23 Nutrition in Infancy and Childhood

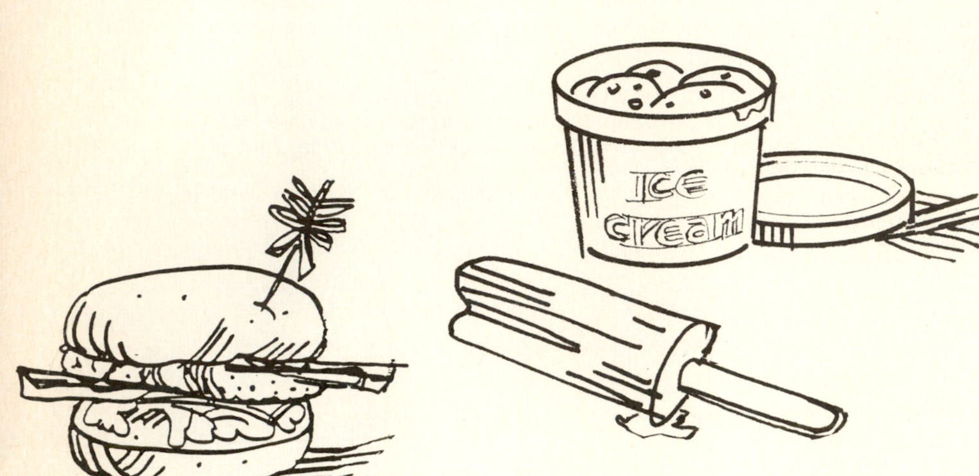

It is essential that infants and children receive a good diet to insure that they grow and develop normally. All body tissues as they form, including the cells of the brain, must receive minimal levels of each nutrient so that each child's full physical and intellectual potential may be reached. This need begins at the moment of conception, continues throughout pregnancy (see Chap. 22), and is no less important after the baby is born.

This chapter will center on the nutritional needs of children from infancy through the early school years. Knowledge of the "basics" of childhood nutrition allows parents to make informed choices regarding healthy diets for children. In addition, those concerned with day-to-day care of children inside or outside the home (teachers, nurses, daycare staff, etc.) need to be competent in the area of proper nutrition for the young growing child (see Fig. 23–1).

FEEDING OF THE INFANT AND CHILD: GENERAL CONSIDERATIONS

Growth

The normal infant's rate of growth in the first year is truly remarkable (see Fig. 23–2). The birth weight is doubled by age four to six months and tripled by the age of one year. If the rate of weight gain of the first six months (doubling every six months) were to continue, the child would weigh about 7000 pounds, or 3.5 tons, by his or her fifth

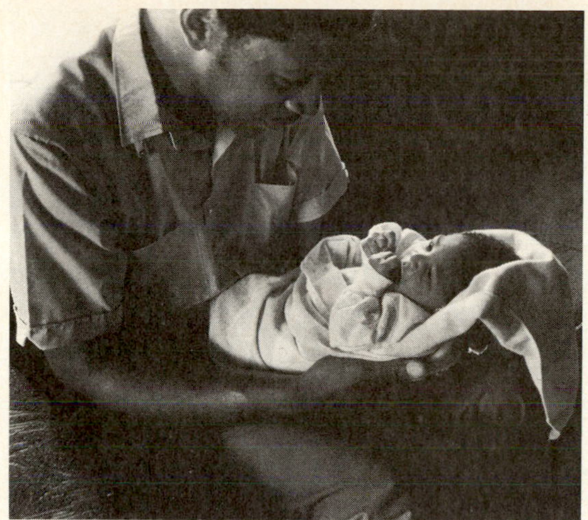

Figure 23–1 Good nutrition along with loving nurture from parents will help this baby grow and develop to full potential. (From Livingston, S. K.: J. Nutr. Ed., *3*:18, 1971. Courtesy of the National Dairy Council.)

birthday! Instead, of course, the average weight by age five is a more reasonable 40 to 42 lb (18-19 kg), and, with a relatively steady growth in the early school years, reaches approximately 70 lb (32 kg) by age ten.

The average birth weight in the United States is 3.4 kg (7½ lb). Ninety-five percent of full-term newborns weigh between 2.5 kg (5½ lb) and 4.6 kg (10 lb). The average length is about 50 cm (20 in), and head circumference averages about 35 cm (14 in).

Babies commonly lose 5 or 6 percent of their body weight in the first 24 to 48 hours due to water loss. Full-term babies can be expected to regain their birth weight by about ten days.

Most physicians schedule the first check-up visit by about two weeks of age; this is an important opportunity to evaluate the infant's weight gain. (See Table 23–1 for average weight gains during the first year of life.) Growth records of the infant and child are important indicators of nutritional adequacy and general health. Growth patterns of individual children can be recorded on growth charts. See Fig. 23–3 for nationally used growth charts of children of the United States (1). Such charts are based on growth records of large samples of normal children. Similar charts show head circumference for age, and weight for length, which are generally used in conjunction with the charts shown in Figure 23–3.

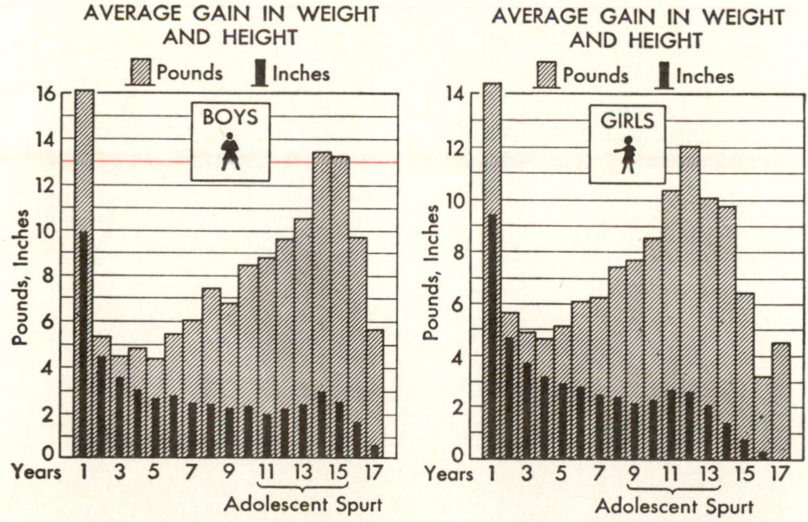

Figure 23–2 Growth increment graphs for boys and girls. (Courtesy of the Metropolitan Life Insurance Co.)

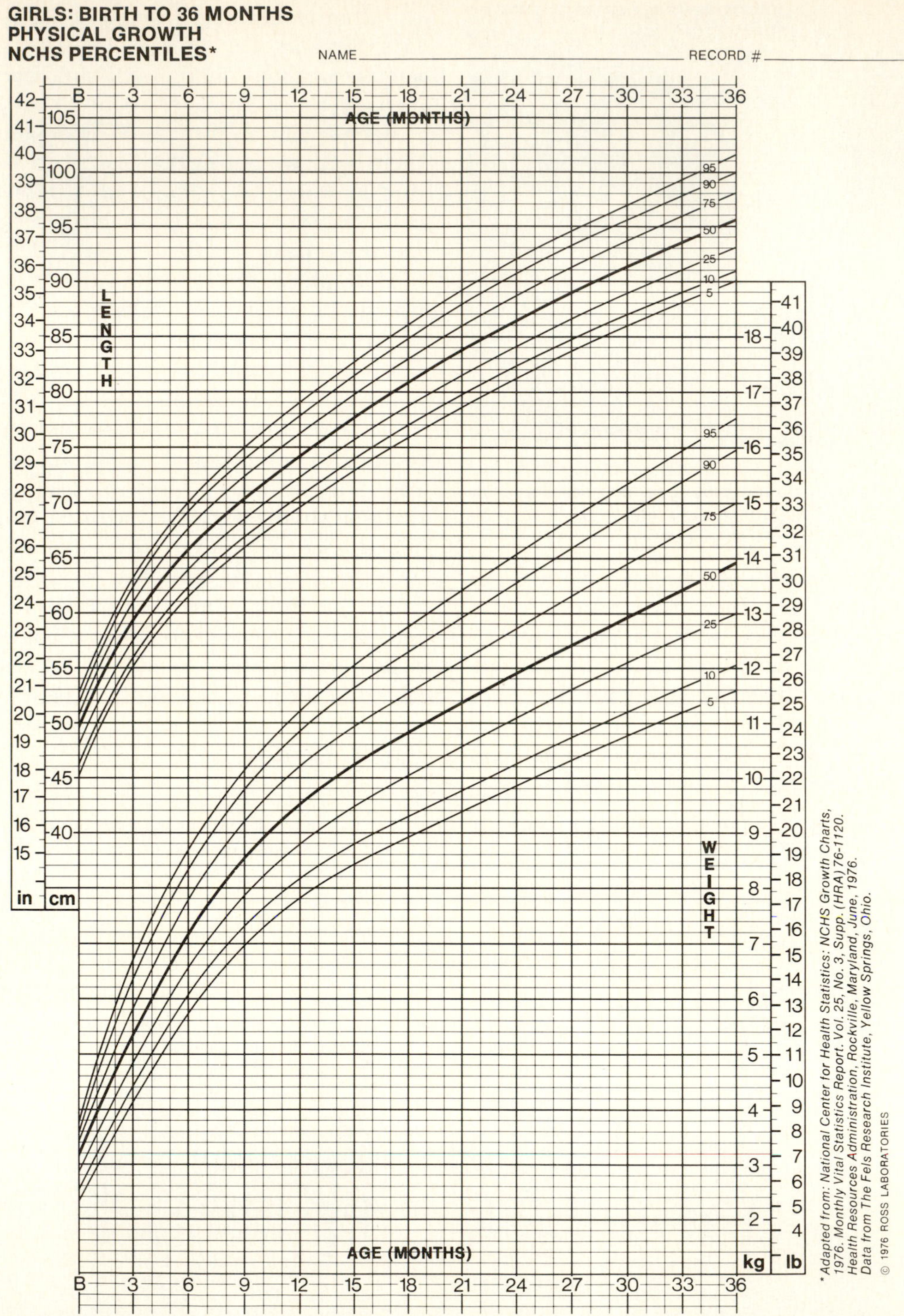

Figure 23–3 National Center for Health Statistics: NCHS Growth Charts, 1976 (1). The 50 percentile line is the average weight or length for children at any given age. A weight plotted on the 75 percentile line, for example, means that 74 percent of normal children are *below* that weight. The 5th and 95th percentiles represent unusual although not necessarily abnormal weights and lengths. There are similar charts showing head circumference for age, and weight for length, which are generally used in conjunction with the charts pictured. (From the U.S. Dept. of Health and Human Services.)

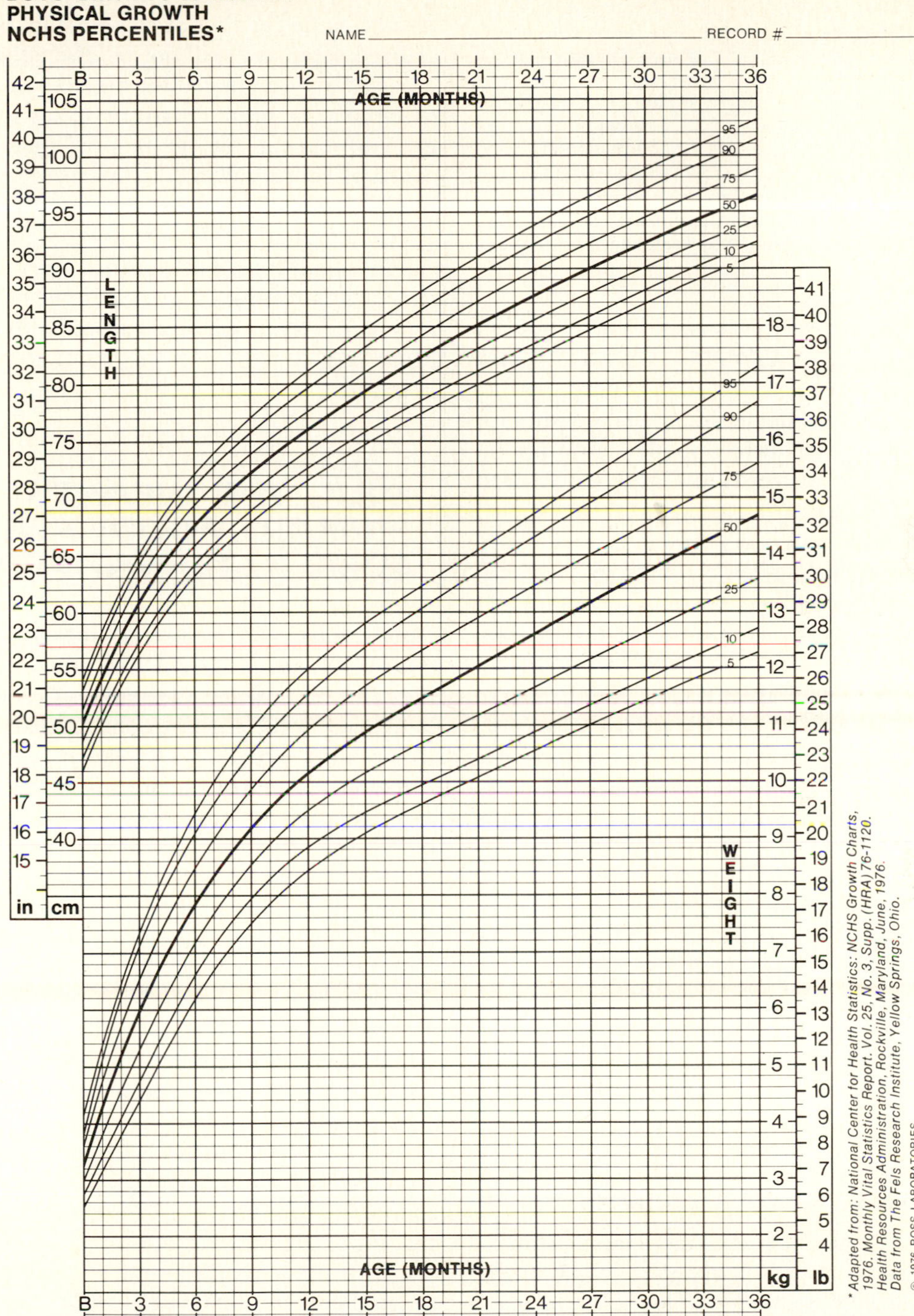
BOYS: BIRTH TO 36 MONTHS
PHYSICAL GROWTH
NCHS PERCENTILES*
NAME
RECORD #
AGE (MONTHS)
B 3 6 9 12 15 18 21 24 27 30 33 36
LENGTH
WEIGHT
95 90 75 50 25 10 5
in
cm
kg
lb
* Adapted from: National Center for Health Statistics: NCHS Growth Charts, 1976. Monthly Vital Statistics Report. Vol. 25, No. 3, Supp. (HRA) 76-1120. Health Resources Administration, Rockville, Maryland, June, 1976. Data from The Fels Research Institute, Yellow Springs, Ohio.
© 1976 ROSS LABORATORIES

Table 23–1 GROWTH DURING INFANCY

Age	*Weight Gain per Week*
Birth–3 mo	200 gm (6–7 oz)
4–6 mo	140 gm (5 oz)
7–9 mo	85 gm (3 oz)
10–12 mo	70 gm (2½ oz)

Weight gain during the first year. Note the normal decrease in the rate of weight gain by the end of the first year.

A child's growth generally follows one of the percentile curves on the chart, and if this pattern changes it is a sign that there may be a nutritional problem. Metabolic conditions and diseases that affect intake, absorption, or utilization of nutrients also can affect growth patterns.

Undernutrition is a major reason for impaired physical growth, and growth increases are seen when nutrition is improved. Perhaps the best example is the increase in height by nearly 6 to 7 cm (3 in) noted in Japanese children after World War II, when their heights were compared with pre-war Japanese average heights. This growth increase is attributed to an improvement in nutritional intake (2). There is also a phenomenon of "catch-up growth" seen in certain individual children who have been malnourished and then are rehabilitated (3). The growth rates of these children increase when nutrition is improved.

In addition to energy needs for growth, the child has continual basal metabolic needs as well as energy needs of physical activity (see Chap. 6). The satisfaction of these needs is critical to the child's present and future health, growth, and development.

The Low-Birthweight Infant

About 7 percent of American newborns weigh less than 2500 gm (5½ lb) at birth. These babies are termed "low birthweight" infants and are at higher risk for health problems. They are, therefore, generally given special medical and nutritional attention (4). The feeding of these babies is a specialized topic and will not be discussed here.

Low-birthweight babies may be small due to either (1) prematurity or (2) inadequate growth during the gestational period because of maternal malnutrition or placental insufficiency. Babies in this second category, born at term yet underweight, are called "small for dates" infants; the effects of the early stunting of growth tend to persist into later years when these individuals are often found to have a shorter than average height (5).

MILK, THE INFANT'S PRIMARY FOOD, AND SOME ALTERNATIVES

Breast milk and prepared infant formula both fulfill an important function by providing the complete spectrum of nutrients known to be required by the human infant. Breast milk alone offers a second important function, that of protecting the infant against certain infections. The multiple health benefits of breast milk have been more completely described and understood within the past several years, and during this time there has also been a resurgence of interest in breastfeeding as the preferred method of infant feeding (see Fig. 23–4). In 1971 in the United States, only 20 percent of all infants leaving hospital nurseries were breastfed, whereas a recent survey showed that over half, or 55 percent of all infants, are now started on the breast (6). For those who use substitute milk preparations, commercially prepared formulas have been more popular than evaporated milk formulas since the early 1960s.

Of the formulas marketed in the United States at the present time, ready-to-feed prepackaged formulas constitute about 40 per-

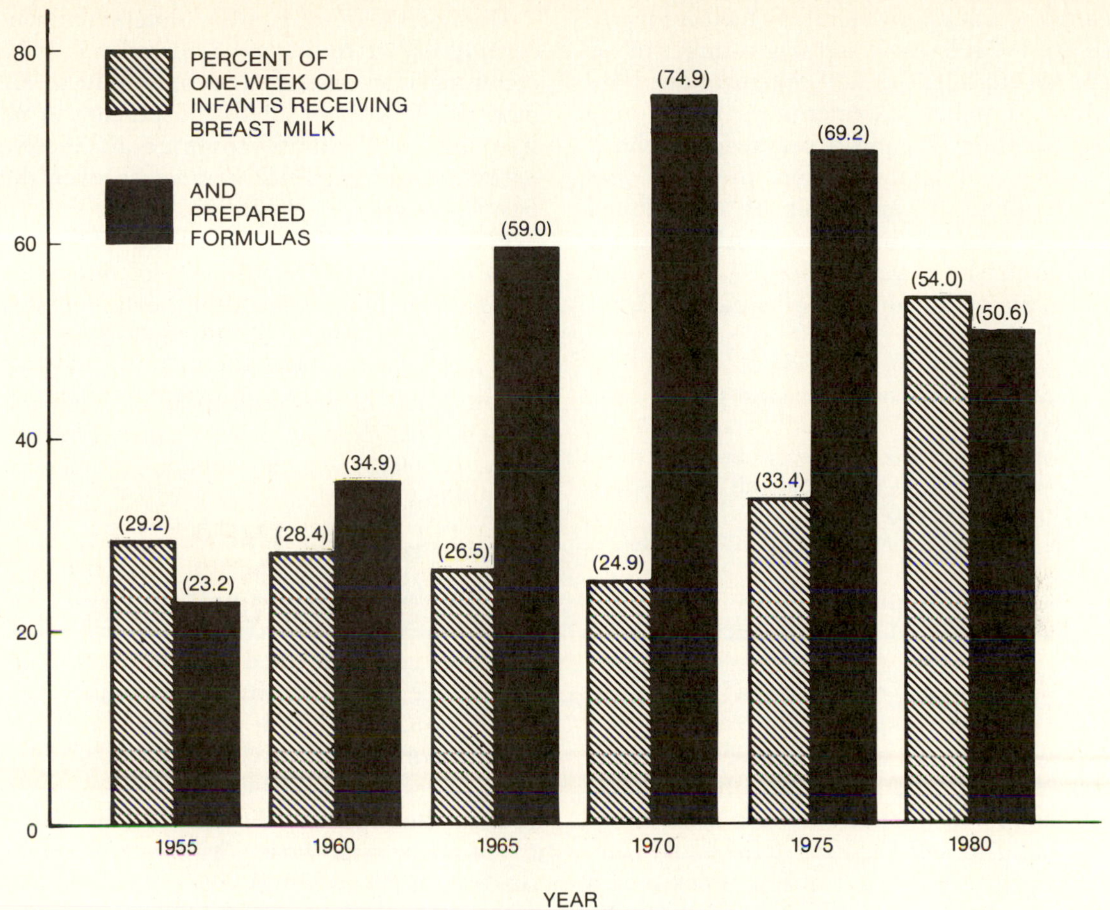

Figure 23–4 Changes in the use of breast milk and prepared formulas for feeding of one-week-old infants. (Figures may add up to over 100 percent since some infants receive both.) The use of evaporated milk is not included in the graph; it has declined in usage as an infant formula from 46 percent in 1955 to 0.2 percent in 1980. The use of whole cow's milk at this age was 4 percent in 1955 and its use is justifiably rare in 1980, at 0.1 percent; it is not a recommended food for infants. Interest in breastfeeding reached a low point in about 1970 and has been renewed since, with the use of prepared formulas showing a resultant decline since then (6).

cent; concentrated liquids over 50 percent; and powdered forms less than 10 percent.

Breast milk has always been the most readily available and natural food for infants. Historically, artificial feeding of infants (that is, with animal milk or concocted formula rather than with breast milk) had very poor results. It has been estimated that artificially fed babies in the period of the Industrial Revolution, before any of the important bacteriological studies of Pasteur and Koch, had a mortality rate at least three times as high as breastfed babies. Even today, in the less developed regions of the world, an increase in the practice of bottle feeding can result in an increased infant sickness and death rate.

Benefits of Human Milk

There is a wealth of scientific evidence to indicate that breastfeeding is the best way to feed the infant during the first year of life. Human milk is the reference standard against which all other infant feeding methods are judged. An increasing number of official health agencies and organizations have published policy statements recommending breastfeeding (7), and a pediatrician who is a recognized authority on nutrition has stated, "The dietary goals of the United States might well include breastfeeding for all infants who can nurse" (8).

The major advantages of breast milk for the infant are:

1. Its nutrient composition is ideal for the term newborn.
2. Protective, anti-infective factors are present.
3. The absorption of trace minerals such as iron and zinc is enhanced.
4. The biologic value of breast milk protein is high.
5. There is a lower risk of allergies.
6. There is enhanced mother–infant bonding.

Babies fed breast milk have a lower incidence of gastrointestinal infections, and probably fewer, or at least less severe, respiratory infections as well. They are less likely to develop constipation, and are more likely to be able to self-regulate their intake successfully (9). There are many reports of a decreased tendency toward allergic problems for babies who are breastfed, although this is probably not a permanent protection. The trace minerals iron and zinc are absorbed especially well from breast milk. Recently, a growth-promoting factor has been identified in human milk which is not present in prepared formulas (10). In addition to all the physical benefits, many mothers feel that breastfeeding helps to promote an exceptionally close and harmonious relationship with the child.

Some concern has arisen about possible environmental pollutants in breast milk. Experts at this time agree that the benefits of breastfeeding outweigh possible hazards of contaminants in almost all cases (11).

Most of the recent policy statements concerning breastfeeding recommend that it be continued for at least the first four to six months. At present, about 25 percent of all six-month-old infants continue to receive breast milk, a significant increase over the past few years.

Breastfeeding is an acquired skill; for some infants and mothers it comes easily and for others it takes a little work. To assist new mothers who wish to breastfeed, the La Leche League International is an organization of mothers willing to help. Their address is 9616 Minneapolis Avenue, Franklin Park, IL 60131; their telephone number is (312) 455-7730.

Infant Formulas

A sensible alternative to breastfeeding exists, if necessary, in the form of commercially available iron-fortified infant formulas (see Table 23–2). (Evaporated milk is still an option for infant feeding, with the addition of sugar and vitamins, but is rarely used.) Cow's milk is the basis for most formulas, although soy protein isolate is also a common milk base. There are special soy-free and cow's milk–free formulas prescribed mainly for allergy-prone infants who are not breastfed.

Cow's milk is modified for infant formulas in the following ways:

1. It is diluted, since the salt and protein content of whole cow's milk is too high for the young infant.
2. More carbohydrate (lactose) is added since the dilution has now decreased the calories per volume.
3. Unsaturated vegetable fats are substituted for saturated fats so that fat absorption by the infant's digestive system will be improved.
4. The milk is heat processed, which tends to decrease the incidence of allergic reactions and increase the absorption of cow's milk protein.
5. Essential vitamins and minerals are added.

Table 23–2 NUTRIENTS IN HUMAN MILK, COW'S MILK, AND FORMULAS*

			Examples of:		
	Mature Human Milk	*Cow's Milk, Fresh, Whole*	Modified Infant Formula, Based on Cow's Milk	Soy-Based Formula	Hydrolyzed Protein Formula
Calories/100 ml	75	66	67	67	67
Linoleic acid as percent of fatty acids	10.6	2.1	a	a	a
Gm/100 ml of:					
Protein	1.1	3.3	1.6	2.0	2.2
Carbohydrate	6.8–7.2	4.8	7.2	6.8	8.5
Fat	4.5	3.7	3.6	3.6	2.6
Water	87	87	87	87	87
Calcium: phosphorus ratio (mg/liter)	340:140	1170:920	550:440	800:630	1000:700
Vitamins/liter					
A, IU[b]	1898	1025–1690	2500	2100	1500
C, mg	43	11	55	50	50
D, IU	22	14–33[c]	400	400	400
Thiamin, mg	0.16	0.44	0.65	0.5	0.46
Riboflavin, mg	0.36	1.75	1.0	1	1.8
B-6, mg	0.1	0.64	0.4	0.4	0.5
B-12, μg	0.3	4	1.5	2	4.5
Pantothenic acid, mg	1.8	3.4	3	2.5	3.2
Niacin, mg	1.5	0.94	7	7	4
Folacin, μg	52	55	100	100	50
K, μg	15	60	35	90	18
E, mg/IU	1.8 mg	0.4 mg	17 IU	9 IU	10 IU
Iron, mg/l	0.5	0.5	1.4 (with iron — 8–12 mg)	8–12	12

*Adapted from: Fomon (12), manufacturers' data, and Vaughan, V. C., McKay, R. J., and Behrman, R. E.: *Nelson: Textbook of Pediatrics.* Philadelphia: W. B. Saunders, 1979. (Also see Feeley, R. M., et al., Amer. J. Clin. Nutr., *37*:443, 1983 for copper, iron, and zinc content of human milk at early stages of lactation, and see Lönnerdal, B., et al., Amer. J. Dis. Child., *137*:433, 1983 for iron, zinc, copper, and manganese content of 94 infant formulas.)

[a]Present, but amount not available.

[b]For conversion to retinol equivalent, see Chap. 9.

[c]400 IU when fortified. To convert IU of vitamin D to μg divide by 40.

Milk Intake

The total volume of milk required varies from infant to infant, with an average intake of about 3 oz per pound (or 175 to 200 ml per kg) of body weight in the first weeks of life, reduced to 1½ or 2 oz per pound in the later months of infancy. (A premature baby may need up to 4 to 5 oz per pound.) Milk intake will vary with such factors as individual appetite, growth rate, body size, and the amount of solids and of other liquids taken. Most infants over a few weeks of age will consume a total of about one quart, or about one liter, of milk in 24 hours, with a standard deviation of intake of approximately 25 percent.

The average quantity per feeding ranges from 60 to 90 ml (2–3 oz) until the second week; 150 to 180 ml (5–6 oz) at 2 to 3 months; to 210 to 240 ml (7–8 oz) at 5 to 12 months.

Milk intake is not easy to measure in a breastfed baby, but it is useful to know that most infants take 80 percent of the milk in the first four minutes on each breast. Usually, nutritive suckling is complete within a 15-minute total feeding time, with each breast generally given at each feeding.

The frequency of breast or bottle feedings begins at about seven to ten times per 24 hours, and gradually decreases to five to six times at two months, by which time many infants will be content to sleep throughout the night. Then feedings average about every four hours during the day. There is no virtue in fixing rigid feeding times, as most infants will develop their own fairly regular schedules according to individual needs.

Water Needs

After the newborn period, the growing child requires over 100 ml per kg of water each day (see Table 23–3). The majority of this water will come from milk, but after solids are started less milk may be given. The first signs that an infant is taking in less water than needed are decreased urinary output and constipation. Dehydration results if there is severe water deprivation or excess loss of unreplaced water. Such difficulties are usually prevented if the infant is allowed self-regulated "demand" feedings. To be certain, it makes sense to offer extra water occasionally, especially when the child is ill or in hot temperatures. The healthy, older child will generally be able to independently increase water or juice intake when thirsty.

Table 23–3 AVERAGE WATER REQUIREMENT OF HEALTHY CHILDREN*

Age	Average Body Wt in kg	Total Water in 24 hrs	Water per kg Body Wt in 24 hrs
		ml	ml
3 days	3.0	250–300	80–100
10 days	3.2	400–500	125–150
3 months	5.4	750–850	140–160
6 months	7.3	950–1100	130–155
9 months	8.6	1100–1250	125–145
1 year	9.5	1150–1300	120–135
2 years	11.8	1350–1500	115–125
4 years	16.2	1600–1800	100–110
6 years	20.0	1800–2000	90–100
10 years	28.7	2000–2500	70– 85

*Adapted from: Vaughan, V. C., McKay R. J., and Behrman, R. E.: *Nelson: Textbook of Pediatrics.* Philadelphia: W. B. Saunders, 1979.

INTRODUCTION OF SOLID FOODS

When the infant reaches five or six months of age, nutritional needs increase to a point at which they are not entirely met by milk alone. The process of adding foods other than milk to the infant's diet and acquainting the infant with a spoon and a cup is called "weaning," or the "transitional period." The weaning transition best occurs gradually, often over a period of months. Neither breast nor bottle feedings should be discontinued suddenly.

Foods other than milk for infants have been termed supplemental foods, "beikost" (12), and "transitional foods." Medical and nutritional authorities recommend that the introduction of foods to supplement milk is best begun at around four to six months of age (12), depending on the infant and its needs (see Fig. 23–6). Earlier feedings are not necessary nutritionally for most healthy infants. In addition, an effective swallowing mechanism is not developed until between the ages of 2½ and 3½ months (13).

General guidelines for the introduction of solids include (14):

1. Start with small serving sizes of 1 to 2 teaspoonfuls, increasing gradually according to the infant's appetite.
2. Introduce single-ingredient foods one at a time and continue for about a week before introducing another food.
3. There are no hard and fast rules as to the order in which foods are introduced. It is common practice to introduce rice cereal first, then fruits, then vegetables, and finally meat. If solids are started at about six months, meats can be started as one of the first foods.
4. Introduce juices (apple, orange, etc.) one at a time also, preferably from a cup.
5. For the older infant, establish a diet plan for balance and diversity, including the milk group, the meat group, the bread/cereal group, and the fruit/vegetable group.
6. Provide solid food of a texture compatible with the infant's ability to chew and swallow. Start with semiliquid and purèed, and progress to foods of a larger particle size when teeth are present.
7. Avoid developing the infant's taste for excessive salt or sugar.
8. When the infant starts chewing, it is ready to try mashed foods from the family table.
9. Unmodified foods directly from the table should not be given until about a year.
10. In the second year of life, a child no longer needs a special infant diet and should be ready to begin sharing the family meals that are reasonably modified.

Most infants will give clues when they are full, and parents soon learn to recognize these. Signs of satiety include clamping the mouth shut and turning the head away. By responding to these signals, overfeeding can be avoided.

A blender is a useful and practical addition to a household with a growing infant. Most fresh vegetables and fruits, as well as meats or beans, may be ground or blended to the consistency enjoyed by the infant. This method assures a greater variety of foods earlier in the child's life as well as enabling the family to know exactly what the infant is receiving. Improved labeling of commercial infant foods also allows more complete knowledge of ingredients. Most infant foods are now being prepared without added sugar or salt.

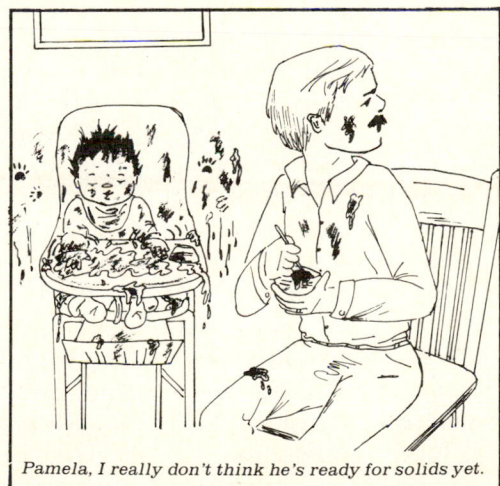

Pamela, I really don't think he's ready for solids yet.

Figure 23–5 Authorities in infant feeding agree there is no need to start solid foods for the healthy growing infant until around the middle of the first year. (Courtesy La Leche League.)

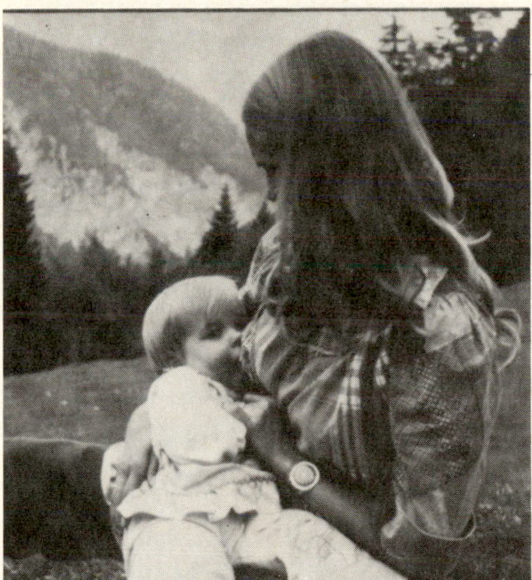

Figure 23–6 In addition to the nutritional and immunological advantages of breastfeeding, it is also no doubt the most convenient infant feeding method. This mother does not have to carry bottles and worry about their possible bacterial contamination while she is traveling with her baby. (Courtesy La Leche League.)

Table 23–4 CALORIC DISTRIBUTION IN VARIOUS TYPES OF MILK*

Type of Milk	*Percent of Total Calories*		
	PROTEIN	FAT	CARBOHYDRATE
Human milk	6–7	56	38
Commercial formulas (standard)	9–13	47–48	40–43
Cow's milk			
Whole milk	22	48	30
Low-fat (2%)	28	31	41
Skim	40	3	57

*The difference in the proportion of protein content found in human milk (and in formulas manufactured to simulate human milk) and that found in cow's milk is clearly seen here. The level found in human milk and in formulas is considered to be the safest level for the young infant.

Composition of Typical Infant Diets

Studies on the diets of infants in the United States show that by four months, about 20 to 30 percent of calories come from foods other than milk or formula, and by twelve months, 60 to 70 percent of the total caloric intake is from foods other than milk (12).

The typical selection of strained foods fed to infants contains approximately 80 percent of calories from carbohydrates. They are generally low in fat content, and the amount of protein is usually low unless meat is present. Water makes up from 70 to 90 percent of the composition of most varieties of prepared strained and junior foods.

It can be seen that early feeding of solids adds mainly water and carbohydrates to the infant's diet. This helps to explain why it is recommended that solids be delayed until after early infancy when breast milk or a prepared infant formula best meets the baby's needs.

The distribution of calories in milk is shown in Table 23–4. From this table, it is clear how markedly different cow's milk, and skimmed milk in particular, are from human milk and commercial formulas. In fact, the feeding of skim milk to infants results in diets that are calorically inadequate for growth and are undesirably low in fat and undesirably high in protein. It is also deficient in iron, ascorbic acid, and essential fatty acids, and it has no role in the diet of a normal, healthy infant.

Feeding the Older Infant and Toddler

At around eight months the infant may begin to use a cup rather than, or in addition to, the bottle or breast. By this time he or she should be taking, in addition to milk, a varied diet including cereal, cooked and mashed vegetables, egg yolk, puréed meats, fruit juices, and fruit. The child of this age will usually enjoy chewing on bread and toast products. More solid, chewy foods direct from the table should not be introduced until after twelve months of age, as there is a danger of choking.[1]

During the second year of life, the child should complete the transition to the cup and to table foods. He or she should be drinking three cups of milk a day and eating a balanced diet with products from all four

[1]Snack foods such as nuts, raw carrots, and small hard candies should never be fed to toddlers; food inhaled into the trachea and lung can have serious consequences.

food groups. The mother will often complain about her child's "loss of appetite" during this year; but when the normal decline in the child's rate of growth after the first twelve months is understood, it will be clear that the decreased appetite has a physiological basis. In fact, this has been termed the *physiologic anorexia* (loss of appetite) of the one-year-old, and mothers should be reassured that this is normal. The toddler should continue to be offered a balanced diet suitable for his or her age, with an emphasis on easily self-fed foods ("finger foods"), because this is a time at which the child is developing a sense of independence. Some examples of protein-rich "finger foods" are peanut butter on crackers, toddler meat-sticks, cheese squares, and hard-boiled eggs. These may be offered as midmorning or mid-afternoon snacks or as part of a meal.

The toddler will usually acquire the skill of self-feeding by age eighteen months to two years. The younger one-year-old will still need to be fed some foods, but will wish to participate in the process by using the spoon. This is an important developmental stage and should be encouraged; often two spoons, one for each participant in the meal, are very helpful.

By age two, most children can manage a normal adult diet.

Feeding the Preschool Child

A common complaint about preschool children is that they won't eat vegetables (see Table 23-5). In this case, one can attempt to encourage the use of a variety of vegetables—such as cherry tomatoes, carrots, zucchini, and green beans—that can be easily picked up by the child. (See Fig. 23–7.)

Familiarity with food helps to increase its acceptance. Even if once refused, a new food should be reoffered at a later time. Considerations of food attractiveness and periods of enjoyment and comfort related to eating times are also important.

Table 23–5 CONCERNS OF MOTHERS REGARDING EATING BEHAVIOR OF PRESCHOOL CHILDREN*

	Age Group	
Concerns	1–2 YR (% OF 497 SUBJECTS)	2–3 YR (% OF 551 SUBJECTS)
1. Chooses limited variety	35.9	40.3
2. Dawdles with food	30.0	36.8
3. Eats too little fruits and vegetables	22.6	27.2
4. Eats too many sweets	6.2	26.3
5. Eats too little meat	26.4	22.3
6. Eats too little food	14.3	21.6
7. Drinks too little milk	13.7	20.1
8. Drinks too much milk	11.9	10.0
9. Eats too much food	4.4	2.7

*Adapted from: Eppright, E. S., et al.: Eating behavior of preschool children. J. Nutr. Ed., *1(#1)*:16, 1969.

Quantities eaten by preschoolers will seem small. A useful rule of thumb regarding minimal serving sizes for preschoolers is "one tablespoonful for each year of age" of each separate food served. Preferred foods often include those at room temperature and foods served separately rather than mixed or creamed. Finger foods continue to be popular.

Three further guidelines which apply to preschoolers, as well as to older children, are: (1) concentrated sweets such as cake, cookies, pie, and candy should be fed only rarely, if at all, since they are high in calories and low in needed nutrients; (2) nutritious snacks are important in this age group since it is easier for children to adapt to smaller amounts of food five or so times a day than to a strict regimen of three large meals; and (3) milk continues to be the usual and primary source of calories, protein, fat, and calcium as well as other nutrients, so continued use of three cups of milk a day is strongly recommended.

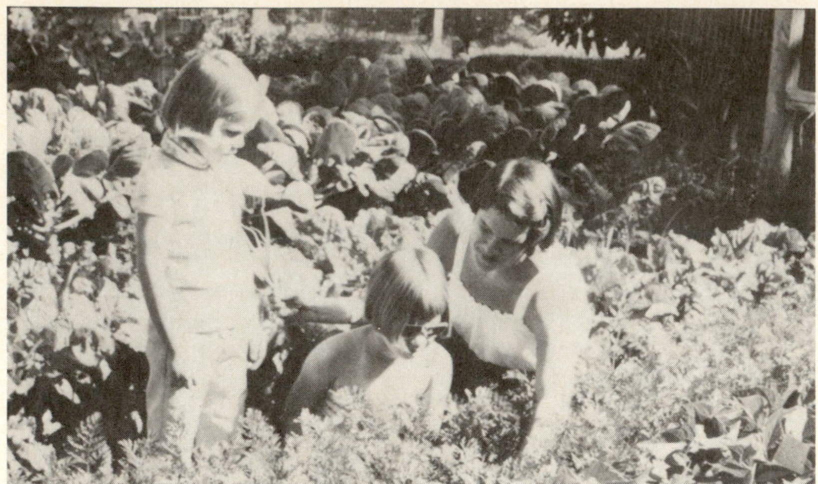

Figure 23–7 Preschool and school-age children are often eager to help out in growing and preparing foods. Participation in food growing and preparation should be encouraged, as this very often increases interest at mealtimes. (Photo reproduced with permission of La Leche League International.)

In the preschool years the child continues to strive to assert his new feelings of individuality and independence. Consistency, some adaptability to whims, and creativity on the part of the parents should continue to insure that the child receives the nutritional intake required for his activity and growth needs. For recommended servings and their nutrient values and for menu suggestions, see Tables 23–7 and 23–8.

NUTRITION OF THE SCHOOL-AGE CHILD

The healthy, active school-age child generally has fewer feeding problems than the toddler or preschooler. The child going to school needs a nutritious breakfast to start the day, a complete lunch that satisfies approximately one-third of the daily nutritional requirements and a satisfying third meal at the end of the day. Snacks are also a way of life with schoolchildren, and are popular for their energy needs. Midmorning and midafternoon nutritious snacks are appropriate. Attractively presented food and an enjoyable eating environment are just as important for school-age children as for preschool children. The normal, healthy child will naturally increase his or her intake if good nutrition habits are encouraged.

The elementary school child's growth rate is slower than the rate during infancy or adolescence. Meeting nutrient needs continues to be critical to the development of the child during this time, with peak nutritional requirements coinciding with maximum growth. The average increment in weight per year is steady until nine or ten years of age, averaging about 2.5 kg (5.5 lb) a year. Then the weight increment curve shows a slow, steady increase which represents the beginning of the adolescent growth spurt.

NUTRITIONAL REQUIREMENTS OF, AND RECOMMENDATIONS FOR, INFANTS AND CHILDREN

Needs for most types of nutrients for infants and children are proportionately (per unit of size) higher than the needs of an adult. For example, human infants need more calories per unit of body weight than at any other time of life, with the newborn requiring

Table 23–6 RECOMMENDED DAILY DIETARY ALLOWANCES FOR INFANTS AND CHILDREN FOR VITAMINS AND MINERALS, 1980

Nutrient	*Age 0–6 mos.*	*Age 7–12 mos.*	*Age 1–3 yrs.*	*Age 4–6 yrs.*	*Age 7–10 yrs.*
VITAMINS					
Vitamin A (μg RE)[a]	420	400	400	500	700
Vitamin D (μg)[b]	10	10	10	10	10
Vitamin E (mg of αTE)[c]	3	4	5	6	7
Vitamin C (mg)	35	35	45	45	45
Thiamin (mg)	0.3	0.5	0.7	0.9	1.2
Riboflavin (mg)	0.4	0.6	0.8	1.0	1.4
Niacin (mg NE)[d]	6	8	9	11	16
Vitamin B-6 (mg)	0.3	0.6	0.9	1.3	1.6
Folacin (μg)	30	45	100	200	300
Vitamin B-12 (μg)	0.5[e]	1.5	2.0	2.5	3.0
MINERALS					
Calcium (mg)	360	540	800	800	800
Phosphorus (mg)	240	360	800	800	800
Magnesium (mg)	50	70	150	200	250
Iron (mg)	10	15	15	10	10
Zinc (mg)	3	5	10	10	10
Iodine (μg)	40	50	70	90	120

[a]Retinol equivalents: 1 retinol equivalent = 1 μg retinol or 6 μg β carotene. See Chap. 9 for calculation of vitamin A activity of diets as retinol equivalents.

[b]As cholecalciferol: 10 μg cholecalciferol = 400 IU of vitamin D.

[c]α-tocopherol equivalents: 1 mg *d*-α tocopherol = 1 αTE. See Chap. 9 for calculation of vitamin E activity of the diet as α-tocopherol equivalents.

[d]1 NE (niacin equivalent) is equal to 1 mg of niacin or 60 mg of dietary tryptophan (or any combination thereof).

[e]The recommended dietary allowance for vitamin B-12 in infants is based on average concentration of the vitamin in human milk. The allowances after weaning are based on energy intake (as recommended by the American Academy of Pediatrics) and consideration of other factors, such as intestinal absorption.

about 100 to 120 kcal per kg (2.2 lb) of body weight compared to the average young adult's need for 35 to 40 kcal per kg. This also applies to the need for water, protein, vitamins, and minerals.

The Recommended Dietary Allowances (RDAs) for infants are derived from estimated intakes of breastfed babies, with an additional safety factor added for infants fed on cow's milk formulas. See Table 23–6 for 1980 RDAs for infants and children.

Protein

Protein allowances of the infant are in the range of 2 to 4 gm per kg of body weight per day. Breast milk provides approximately 2 gm of protein per kg of the child's weight per day, and countless infants have thrived on this level of protein intake for the first 5 to 6 months of life. Most commercial formulas have followed the general composition of breast milk, but with a slightly higher protein content (see Table 23–2). Protein allowances as recommended for infants and children are: 23 gm for ages one to three; 30 gm for ages four to six; and 34 gm for ages seven to ten. Infants' protein recommendations are set by body weight: 2.2 gm per kg from birth to six months and 2 gm per kg for seven to twelve months. See Appendix for values for older children and adults.

Carbohydrates

Carbohydrates make an essential contribution to meeting energy requirements of

Table 23–7 RECOMMENDED FOOD INTAKE FOR GOOD NUTRITION ACCORDING TO FOOD GROUPS AND THE AVERAGE SIZE OF SERVINGS AT DIFFERENT AGE LEVELS*

Food Group	*Servings per Day*	*Average Size of Servings*			
		1 YR	2–3 YR	4–5 YR	6–9 YR
Milk and cheese 1.5 oz cheese = 1 c milk) (c = 1 cup – 8 oz or 240 gm)	4	½ c	½–¾ c	¾ c	¾–1 c
Meat group (protein foods)	3 or more				
Egg		1	1	1	1
Lean meat, fish, poultry (liver once a week)		2 tbsp	2 tbsp	4 tbsp	2–3 oz (4–6 tbsp)
Peanut butter			1 tbsp	2 tbsp	2–3 tbsp
Fruits and vegetables	At least 4, including:				
Vitamin C source (citrus fruits, berries, tomato, cabbage, cantalope)	1 or more (twice as much tomato as citrus)	⅓ c citrus	½ c	½ c	1 medium orange
Vitamin A source (green† or yellow fruits and vegetables)	1 or more	2 tbsp	3 tbsp	4 tbsp (¼ c)	¼ c
Other vegetables (potato and legumes, etc.) or	2	2 tbsp	3 tbsp	4 tbsp (¼ c)	⅓ c
Other fruits (apple, banana, etc.)		¼ c	⅓ c	½ c	1 medium
Cereals (whole-grain or enriched)	At least 4				
Bread		½ slice	1 slice	1½ slices	1– slices
Ready-to-eat cereals		½ oz	¾ oz	1 oz	1 oz
Cooked cereals (including macaroni, spaghetti, rice, etc.)		¼ c	⅓ c	½ c	½ c
Fats and carbohydrates	To meet caloric needs				
Butter, margarine, mayonnaise, oils: 1 tbsp = 100 calories (kcal)		1 tbsp	1 tbsp	1 tbsp	2 tbsp
Desserts and sweets: 100-calorie portions as follows: ⅓ c pudding or ice cream 2–3 cookies, 1 oz cake, 1½ oz pie, 2 tbsp jelly, jam, honey, sugar		1 portion	1½ portions	1½ portions	3 portions

*Adapted from Vaughan, V. C., III, and McKay, R. J.: *Nelson Textbook of Pediatrics.* 11th Ed. Philadelphia, W. B. Saunders Co., 1979, p. 187.

†Green, leafy vegetables should be eaten every day because of their folic acid content. See text.

infants and children (see Table 23–7). If insufficient carbohydrate is ingested to meet daily energy needs, the body must break down a certain portion of dietary and body protein to meet these needs.

In the newborn, the most usual carbohydrates ingested are lactose (from milk), glucose, and sucrose. Nearly all infants can digest and absorb these sugars adequately. However, if they are given in high concentrations, diarrhea is likely to occur.

Fats

Fats contribute about half the energy requirement of the infant who is fed on milk alone. Infant formulas should provide at least 15 percent of the total calories as fat in order to meet the energy needs.

The essential fatty acid, linoleic acid, is important in promoting optimal health in infants. Without it, poor growth and a severe skin rash will result (15). Rich sources of linoleic acid are corn oil, cottonseed oil, soybean oil, and whole-grain cereals. The minimal recommended level of linoleic acid is from 1 to 3 percent of the total amount of calories. Human milk contains 6 to 9 percent of calories as linoleic acid. Skim milk contains only traces of this important fatty acid, and this is one of the reasons it should not be used as an infant food. (Also see Chap. 3.)

Distribution of Calories in the Diet

The distribution of calories in the infant's and child's diet does not differ markedly from that recommended for the adult. Protein should provide at least 7 percent of calories, or growth needs will not be met. A general guideline would be that 7 to 15 percent of total calories come from protein, 35 to 55 percent from fat, and the remainder (about 30 to 60 percent) from carbohydrate (12).

Vitamins

Growing, active children have a special need, relatively higher than adults, for a complete supply of the known vitamins. Some details about the more important ones are given here. (See Table 23–6 for complete vitamin requirements according to age; also see individual chapters on each vitamin.)

Vitamin D. The recommended level of 10 μg (400 IU) per day is intended to prevent rachitic symptoms (rickets) in all babies, small or of normal size. This is also the level recommended for growing children and adults. Sunlight (certain ultraviolet wavelengths) is an alternative way to meet the need for vitamin D, through conversion of 7-dehydrocholesterol in the skin to vitamin D_3 (cholecalciferol).[2] An infant wearing a normal amount of clothing would probably receive an antirachitic dose of sunlight in approximately a 30-to-60 minute exposure each day, or less if more skin were exposed.

Vitamin D is not present in significant quantities in human or unenriched cow's milk. Breastfed infants should receive supplemental vitamin D unless safe exposure to sunlight is assured *every* day as just described. There have been recent cases of rickets reported in the United States that resulted from inadequate vitamin D intake (16). Vitamin D is now a routine supplement in all commercial infant formulas, including evaporated milk. It is not, however, found in all brands of nonfat dry milk.

Vitamin A and D Toxicity. The adverse effects of excess quantities of vitamins A and D cannot be overemphasized. An infant who repeatedly receives more than 45 to 75 μg (1800 to 3000 IU) of vitamin D per day is in danger of toxicity, which may lead to hypercalcemia and other complications. Thus, the RDA of 10 μg (400 IU) of vitamin D should not be consistently or significantly exceeded. This is sometimes a difficult task, because of the multiplicity of vitamin D–fortified foods. Vitamin A may be toxic if an infant is given dosages of 465 μg (18,500 IU) per day for one to three months (17).

Vitamin C. The recommended daily allowance of vitamin C, 35 mg, is found in 850 ml of breast milk of well-nourished mothers. Most infant formulas are fortified with vitamin C. Pediatricians will sometimes recommend that the infant avoid citrus fruits and juices up to the age of a year or so in order to prevent the development of possible allergic reactions to these foods. In these cases,

[2]Reasonable caution should be exercised in exposing small infants to sunlight in order to prevent sunburn.

supplemental vitamin C should be given in the form of vitamin drops if the infant is taken off prepared formulas or breast milk and started on regular milk.

Vitamin B-Complex. All the B vitamins are usually present in milk formulas or breast milk in sufficient amounts to meet the recommended daily allowances for infants and toddlers who are on a normal milk intake. However, a woman who is vitamin B-12 deficient may not form milk with a sufficient vitamin B-12 supply for the baby, and the deficiency may also be passed on to the infant (18). In general, however, B vitamin deficiency states in infants and small children are rare in the United States.

Folacin. Folacin is essentially absent in goat's milk, which is occasionally used as the primary milk for an allergy-prone infant or child (although commercially prepared, fortified, nonallergenic formulas are replacing it in most cases). Thus any infant on goat's milk as a primary food should receive folacin supplementation at the recommended level of 30 to 45 μg per day (depending on the age) to prevent the deficiency state characterized by megaloblastic anemia. Also, it has been shown that commercially prepared baby foods contain significantly lower amounts of this vitamin than do fresh foods.

Minerals

The infant's diet should include all the minerals essential for normal metabolism and growth. Most of the minerals needed by the infant occur in generous amounts in human milk, cow's milk–based formulas, and many other foods common in the infant's diet. (Only a few minerals are highlighted here. For a review of each mineral and its specific role, see Chap. 15 to 17; for 1980 RDAs, see Table 23–6. For "safe and adequate" intakes of other minerals see inside back cover.)

Calcium and Phosphorus. Calcium is extremely important in the growth and development of bones and teeth in children. During increased periods of growth, such as in infancy, the calcium absorption rate is higher than when the growth rate slows. Vitamin D is necessary for this absorption. The advisable intake for calcium is set at twice the calculated requirement of a breastfed baby, because calcium absorption may be different in infants given nourishment other than human milk, and the phosphate allowance is approximately the same.

A child who is not receiving the required intake of calcium and phosphorus, both of which are found primarily in milk and milk products, will still continue to grow, but the mineralization of bones and teeth will not be optimal.

Sodium. Healthy infants can tolerate a reasonable range of sodium intakes without serious consequences. Sodium intake is relatively low in human milk, prepared formula, and infant foods. Intake climbs when table foods and cow's milk are consumed. Authorities feel that no special efforts are presently warranted to further decrease infants' salt intakes, other than watching that table foods for the infant and the family do not contain unnecessarily high or added salt content (19).

Iron. The importance of this mineral in the diet of infants and children has long been recognized. Recently, definite recommendations have been made to insure that youngsters will be protected from the anemia that results from lack of iron in the diet.

The anemia of iron deficiency, if present, usually begins to appear at age six to twelve months. Up to six months of age, the full-term infant's iron stores, which were deposited in fetal life, are generally adequate for the production of hemoglobin. After that age, body stores must be resupplied by the diet to insure proper blood formation. The highest incidence of iron-deficiency anemia in children is in those under thirty-six months of age, and those most often affected are children of low-income families.

The usual hemoglobin level at birth is high, at 16 to 18 gm per 100 ml of blood, and falls normally to a level of 10 to 11 gm when the child is three to four months of age. The level of hemoglobin should be maintained thereafter at 11 gm or higher.

The use of iron-fortified infant formulas has been shown to decrease significantly the incidence of iron-deficiency anemia in later infancy. Milk formulas fortified with iron cost little or no more than nonfortified formulas.

The daily requirement for iron in infancy, according to Fomon, is at least 6 mg a day beginning at birth, or 8 mg a day if supplements are begun at three months of age (12). This requirement can best be met in the formula-fed infant by (1) an iron-supplemented formula or (2) iron drops. Iron-fortified infant cereal is useful in later months. Another method of calculating iron recommendations is by body weight, and these recommendations are 1 mg per kg per day for term infants and 2 mg per kg per day for low birth-weight infants.

The relatively small amount of iron in breast milk is very efficiently absorbed by the infant (20). Fresh cow's milk can cause microscopic blood loss in the infant's gastrointestinal system (21), which then adds to the problem of deficient iron stores in the young child. This is one of the many reasons why the use of fresh cow's milk in the young infant's diet is not recommended.

Strained, prepared infant foods have generally not provided generous amounts of iron for infants' diets. Most prepared infants' dinners, for example, contain less than 1 mg of iron per 100 gm of food.

Fluorine. This element is particularly important in early infancy and childhood because of its role in the prevention of dental caries (see Chap. 17 and Chap. 24).

If there is fluoridation of the water supply at approximately 1 part per million, the baby whose powdered formula is made with that water will receive the recommended fluoride intake per day, and the infant receiving equal parts water and formula will also receive the recommended fluorine. However; if the infant is on "ready-to-serve" formula or is breastfed,[3] he or she may not take in sufficient quantities of water to provide the necessary fluoride, and thus may need a supplemental dosage. (Supplemental fluoride preparations are available only on prescription.) Baby foods, which usually are composed of 70 to 80 percent water, may have varying quantities of fluoride.

Zinc. In some areas of the United States, serum levels of zinc have been found to be low in certain recent studies of otherwise normal children, particularly preschoolers (22). Zinc levels appear to be lower in children from low-income groups than in those from middle-income groups. The effects of zinc deficiency are discussed in more detail in Chapter 17 and include growth retardation and loss of appetite.

Measures to prevent zinc deficiency, which include breastfeeding and an adequate intake of animal protein, are wise in infancy and early childhood. Such measures are also likely to be beneficial in respect to other trace elements, knowledge of which is more limited at this time.

Selenium. Selenium concentrations in infants fed breast milk appear to be higher

[3]Breast milk contains less than 0.03 ppm of fluoride, regardless of the mother's fluoride intake. Cow's milk contains slightly more, but still not nearly enough to meet the infant's requirement.

than infants on formulas. The exact role this element may play in infant health and growth is not yet determined (see also Chap. 17). It has been recently reported that malnourished infants treated with selenium may show improvements in weight gain and anemia (23). Such improvements could result if they were actaully selenium deficient—this is an active area of research.

Table 23–8 gives some practical menu suggestions for providing nutritional requirements of young children.

Fortification

The essential vitamins and minerals have been incorporated into processed formulas with the aim of providing a complete food for infants. Specific nutrients deemed

Table 23–8 PRACTICAL MENU SUGGESTIONS FOR CHILDREN AT VARIOUS AGES

1–2 yr	*3–6 yr*	*7–12 yr*
Breakfast	*Breakfast*	*Breakfast*
Orange juice Oatmeal with milk Whole wheat toast Milk to drink	Orange juice Cereal with milk Whole-wheat toast Milk to drink	Banana Omelette – plain Toast Milk to drink
Midmorning	*Midmorning*	*Midmorning*
Juice	Raisins	Apple
Lunch	*Lunch*	*Lunch*
Egg, soft poached Peas Zwieback or toast Milk to drink Rice pudding	Egg salad sandwich with lettuce Milk to drink Oatmeal cookies (1–2) Custard pudding	Vegetable soup with rice Peanut butter and jelly sandwich Milk Fresh peaches
Midafternoon	*Midafternoon*	*Midafternoon*
Milk Crackers with soft cheese spread	Juice Apple and cheese wedges	1–2 molasses cookies Fruit juice or milk
Dinner	*Dinner*	*Dinner*
Fish sticks Spinach or carrots Rice Bread and butter Applesauce Milk	Hamburger with tomato and lettuce, buttered bun Squash Carrots and celery Milk Stewed prunes	Spaghetti with meat sauce Carrots and peas Shredded cabbage salad Milk Orange wedges

A meal plan for a child for a day should be based on a knowledge of the "Basic 4" (Chapter 20). For example: *Breakfast:* milk group, 1; fruit-vegetable group, 1; bread-cereal group, 2. *Lunch:* meat-protein group, 1; bread-cereal group, 1; milk group, 1; vegetable-fruit group, 1. *Dinner:* meat-protein group, 1; milk group, 1; vegetable-fruit group, 2; bread-cereal group, 1. Additional servings may easily be added as midmorning or midafternoon snacks.

likely to be lacking from the diet of older infants and children are also used to fortify certain common food products for these ages, such as the addition of iron in infant cereals.

Supplementation

The normal breastfed infant of the well-nourished mother has not been shown conclusively to need any specific vitamin or mineral supplement, presuming adequate exposure to ultraviolet light, one dose of vitamin K at birth, and fluoridated water. Similarly, there is no evidence that supplementation is necessary for the full-term infant fed prepared formula and for the properly nourished normal child (24). These statements may not apply to infants and children at special nutritional risk due to life-style, economic disadvantage, or illness. With this in mind, vitamin and mineral supplements might be recommended in the following cases (24):

1. For children from economically disadvantaged families, since surveys done in the United States showed some deficiencies in children living in these conditions.
2. For children and adolescents with anorexia, with poor or changeable appetities, or poor eating habits, and those on weight-reduction diets.
3. For pregnant teenagers.
4. For children and adolescents on vegetarian diets without adequate dairy products.
5. For conditions of ill health and disease.

The supplements indicated in these situations are commercially available multivitamin, multimineral preparations and are meant to be given only in the doses recommended on the label. For any questions, a physician should be consulted. See text for discussion of specific vitamin/mineral needs in infancy.

Some authorities are in favor of providing vitamin D as a routine supplement during the first six months of life, and iron is often recommended from six to twelve months either as a supplement or in infant formula. Fluoride is usually recommended when there is no intake of fluoridated water; see Chapter 24 for current fluoride recommendations.

NUTRITIONAL STATUS

Several surveys of the health of infants and children in the United States reveal the following (25–27):

1. The overall nutritional status of infants and young children was reasonably good.
2. Nutritional status correlated directly with economic status.
3. Iron deficiency was the major nutrient deficiency disorder.
4. Six to 8 percent of children ages two to four years were classified as obese.
5. Vitamin A levels were low in 30 to 50 percent of Spanish-American children and in 10 percent of black children, compared with 2 percent of white children.
6. Ascorbic acid intakes were low in 10 to 15 percent of children.
7. Calcium intakes were low in 10 to 30 percent of children.

SPECIAL CONCERNS IN INFANT AND CHILDHOOD FEEDING

Several topics of special concern in infant and childhood feeding are given in these sections.

Food and Milk Allergies

Allergies caused by foods are not as common as inhalant (pollen, etc.) allergies; however, they do occur more frequently in infants and young children than in adults. The infant has a greater tendency to absorb unaltered protein in the gastrointestinal tract and thus to have a greater potential for setting up antigen–antibody reactions, which constitute the allergic response.

Foods that may act as allergens include chocolate and cola (kola nut), cow's milk, corn, eggs, peanuts, citrus fruits, tomatoes, wheat and other small grains, nuts, seafood, and in rare cases certain food colors such as amaranth (red) and tartrazine (yellow).

It is frequently recommended that infants with a family history of allergy avoid, at least in the first few months, foods that may frequently cause allergies at early ages, including cow's milk in some cases.

There are two types of allergic reactions to foods. One is immediate, with the rapid occurrence of symptoms, and may be seen after the ingestion of fish, other seafood, eggs, or nuts. The other, a more common type, is a delayed response that may occur hours or days after the allergenic food (commonly wheat, milk, corn, oranges, or chocolate) is eaten. Examples of possible allergic responses are listed in Table 23–9.

A child who is suspected of having a food allergy should be on a trial period of elimination of the food for about three weeks to see if symptoms will clear. Then a "challenge" (reintroduction) of the suspected food may be made, on the advice of the physician, to see if symptoms recur. In this way, the diagnosis of food allergy can be made. Treatment consists of avoidance of the identified food or foods. A child with a known food allergy will require special menu planning to allow for a balanced, palatable, and enjoyable diet.

Milk Allergy. This has also been termed *milk sensitivity* or *milk intolerance.* Milk intolerance is a term best reserved for the rare condition resulting from a congenital deficiency of *lactase,* the enzyme that digests the milk sugar lactose. It is not based on an antigen–antibody reaction and thus is not a true allergy. Cow's milk is probably the most common food allergen in the United States. Estimates of the incidence of cow's milk allergy in the population range from 0.3 to 3 percent. It tends to run in families, and an infant who has an allergy to milk may also be allergic to other common food allergens such as citrus fruits or egg whites.

Cow's milk allergy in susceptible children may be manifested by frequent loose stools, stomach aches, respiratory symptoms, or allergic skin reactions. Other signs may include asthma, headache, tension, fatigue, and possibly hyperactivity. More serious problems, such as shock (cardiovascular collapse), rarely occur. The symptoms may occur as early as two to four weeks of age, or later during the preschool years. Symptoms will begin in a susceptible, breastfed

Table 23–9 ADVERSE REACTIONS ATTRIBUTED TO FOOD ALLERGY*

Systemic: Shock, malaise, fever, failure to grow
Gastrointestinal: Stomatitis, colic, abdominal pain, flatulence, diarrhea, malabsorption, colitis
Central nervous system: Headache, irratability, hyperactivity, tension and fatigue
Muscular: Leg pains
Respiratory: Hay fever, asthma
Skin: Hives, eczema, other skin rashes
Ear: Serous otitis media

*Adapted from Vaughan, V. C., III, and McKay, R. J.: *Nelson Textbook of Pediatrics.* 10th Ed. Philadelphia, W. B. Saunders Co., 1975, p. 519.

child soon after the first cow's milk feedings are given.

It may sometimes be necessary to eliminate cow's milk and milk products from the diet. Excellent cow's milk substitutes that provide essentially all nutrients normally found in milk are available.[4] It has been shown that the growth of infants given these milk substitutes is no different from the growth of infants given breast milk. However, the older child may refuse the milk substitutes, and in these cases care must be taken that a proper diet including a source of calcium is given.

Cow's milk that has been heat-treated, or substitution of milk of another species (e.g., goat's milk) is occasionally helpful in decreasing allergic symptoms for some individuals.

Vegetarian Diets for Children

Can a child be fed successfully on a vegetarian diet? The answer is a qualified yes. It is true that a diet excluding meat protein will allow for adequate growth and development of a child, *provided* it is based on sound nutritional knowledge. There are different types of vegetarian diets, ranging from *lacto-ovo-vegetarian,* which includes dairy products and eggs, to *vegan,* or strictly vegetarian. The lacto-ovo-vegetarian diet is acceptable for children *if* the following criteria are met:

1. The protein sources are complemented (that is, come from correct combinations of legumes, grains, and vegetables) in order to supply the essential amino acids, all of which are not found in any *one* vegetarian food.
2. There is an adequate supply of folacin and zinc (sometimes low in these diets).
3. A form of iodized salt is used.
4. The diet does in fact include allowances of milk, cheese, and eggs. These foods are important because they would be the sole source of vitamin B-12 in this meatless diet, and they also help supply important amino acids, minerals such as calcium and iron, and other vitamins such as vitamin A.

[4]Examples include formulas based on hydrolyzed casein; strained, homogenized lamb product; and soybean (a food that may itself cause allergic responses).

Vegetarian diets other than this carefully selected lacto-ovo-vegetarian type would not be advised for children. To try to raise infants and children without some form of milk or its complete equivalent, such as soy milk substitute, is very difficult and nutritionally unwise. (Also see Chap. 11 and 20.)

Overnutrition in Infancy and Childhood

Obesity, in children as well as in adults, is very hard to resolve successfully. Prevention is far easier than cure, and is dependent upon early detection of children who are exhibiting an excess rate of weight gain, as well as early identification of factors in the infant or child or in his or her environment that may predispose to obesity.

Overweight in children can result from increased lean body mass, adipose tissue, or both. Skinfold measurements are an important adjunct to the classic measurements of weight and height, since they may help to differentiate children who are overweight owing to increased muscle mass from those in the early stages of obesity who need preventive interventions.

Factors that may predict later obesity include the following:

1. Family history of obesity
2. Weight at age four to seven
3. Weight during infancy
4. Birth weight (and weight/height ratio)

Family history of obesity is at present the best predictor of later obesity in an infant or child. It has been shown that with one obese parent, there is a 40 percent chance that the child will be overweight, and with two obese parents, the risk increases to the range of 70 to 80 percent (28). Similar risks have also been demonstrated in children who have been adopted by obese parents (29). Thus, the definite increased incidence of obesity in children with obese parents may be a combination of a genetic disturbance and the family's eating habits.

The importance of the early weight history of a child has been the subject of conflicting reports and opinions. Conclusions of different studies include the following (30–32):

1. The predictive value of obesity in infancy ranges from 10 to 40 percent in different studies.
2. A British report states that infants who gained weight rapidly in infancy attained a greater height and weight at the age of six years.
3. In one study, nearly all children overweight by age four were also heavy at age seven.
4. For those children overweight later in childhood, 80 percent will remain overweight later in life.

Thus, it appears that not all overweight babies are marked for a later bout with obesity, but the risk is somewhat greater than for infants of average weight. Childhood obesity has a more definite correlation with adult obesity than does infant obesity. It also appears that the earlier the onset of obesity the greater the number of adipose (fatty) cells; yet correlation of number of fat cells with later obesity is uncertain.

The relationship of energy expenditure to overweight is also relevant: obese infants and children are often less active than their slimmer companions. Lack of activity with resultant low calorie expenditure may cause obesity in some children whose intakes of food are not particularly high. There is no doubt that a vigorous activity program has an important part in the prevention, as well as the treatment, of obesity.

What are some practical recommendations for weight control in overweight children? First, it should be realized that weight *loss* is not a goal for children; rather, the goal is a weight that is kept relatively constant while linear growth continues normally. Total calories should not drop below 1200 to 1400 a day, or growth requirements may be compromised.

A balanced, varied diet should be maintained. Family meals may have to be altered to include fewer foods with excess calories, such as fried foods, gravy, fatty meats, and rich desserts. Sugary snacks between meals should be eliminated, with more nutritious snacks substituted. Parents should learn to recognize the child's cues for satiation and not feed them beyond that point.

The use of food for nonnutritive reasons should be explored with parents, and decreased if possible. Nonnutritive uses of food (rewards for desired behavior, comforting of a frustrated child, etc.) teach children to rely on food to compensate for emotional and social difficulties. This pattern may continue throughout life if begun early in childhood.

The problem of overweight is much better prevented early, and suggestions for prevention are summarized in Table 23–10. (Also see Chap. 7 and supplementary readings.)

TABLE 23–10 SUGGESTED MEASURES FOR THE PREVENTION OF OVERWEIGHT PROBLEMS IN CHILDREN

1. Breast-feed if possible, and introduce other foods at 4 to 6 months of age.
2. Recognize when the infant or child is satisfied with a meal (the feeding) and STOP there.
3. Try not to use food as a reward, or its withholding as a punishment.
4. Encourage an energetic program of physical activity for all children.
5. Children with overweight parents should have special attention given to the development of good eating and exercise habits, since they are at much higher risk for becoming overweight.

Hyperlipidemia

Certain inborn diseases that involve high cholesterol and lipid levels in the blood (*hyperlipidemia*) are associated with an early onset of atherosclerosis. This condition of the blood vessels in turn greatly increases the risk of coronary heart disease.

It is not practical at the present time to test all children for hyperlipidemia, since this condition affects only a very small proportion of the population. Physicians are generally using this testing procedure for "high risk" children; that is, those with (1) diabetes, (2) obesity, or (3) a family history of close relatives with early heart disease before age 50 (33).

Dental Caries Prevention

Dental disease is probably the most prevalent disorder found in routine health exams of children in the United States today. See Chapter 24 for a complete discussion of nutritional preventive measures, which include, briefly, (1) decreasing the amount of sugary foods eaten by children, especially sticky, sugary foods eaten between meals and (2) insuring a proper intake of fluorine.

INFANT AND CHILD MALNUTRITION

Severely malnourished infants and children are rarely seen in the United States. However, an occasional report of an infant with *marasmus* or *kwashiorkor* (see Chap. 4) does appear, sometimes linked to familial–social problems or to a lack of information on nutrition or food products. Examples of the latter include overdilution of formulas and inappropriate decrease in protein intake (34, 35).

Many countries around the world, often those with very low per capita incomes and high population growth rates, have problems of infant and child nutrition not touched upon here (see Fig. 23–8). The infant and childhood mortality rates in these countries are generally high—for the most part as a result of the combined effects of malnutrition, infection (see Fig. 23–9), poor economic conditions, and lack of accurate information about nutrition and health.

Most critical to the development of symptoms of malnutrition in most areas is currently an overall insufficiency of calories (36). (See also Chap. 25.) Thus an increasing prevalence of marasmus compared with kwashiorkor has been noted worldwide. Significant protein-energy malnutrition results from maldistribution of food within a family as well as from overall food shortages.

Some specific examples of problems that contribute to childhood malnutrition are:

1. Sudden weaning from the breast of a toddler at the arrival of a new baby demanding all the mother's breast milk. This toddler is then deprived of this already minimal supply of the only high nutrient food, with other portions of the typical weaning diet consisting of foods high in mainly carbohydrate content. This train of events is particularly common in the causation of kwashiorkor.
2. Lack of sufficient supplemental foods for the breastfed baby after about six months of age.
3. Traditional customs, such as those demanding that the few high nutrient foods available go first (and often, only) to the adult males of the tribe and family. In some areas, cultural food taboos effectively deny certain protein-rich foods, such as eggs, to pregnant women and young children.

The increasing practice of bottle feeding, considered to be the "modern method" in some underdeveloped areas, is also a subject of serious concern. The advantages of breastfeeding in these areas are very high, because (1) there are inherent advantages to human milk, (2) the facilities for safe, sterile preparation and storage of bottle formulas are limited, and (3) the milk substitutes are

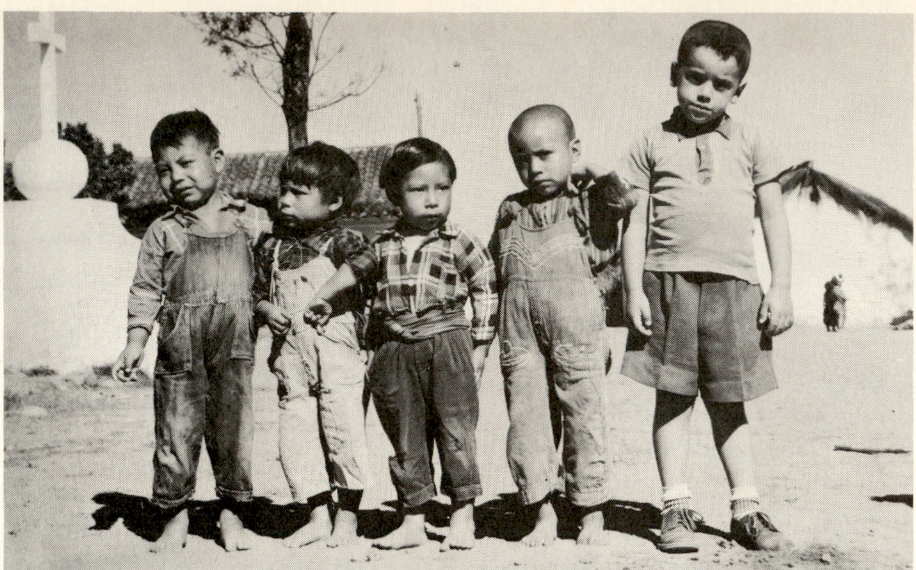

Figure 23–8 Marked difference in growth and general nutritive condition of Guatemalan boys age four to five, contrasting village children reared on the native diet (corn and beans as chief food staples) with a boy of the same age-group from a professional's family, in which the diet was superior. The latter boy (at right) is of normal height and weight for this age group; the others show stunted growth and other evidence of poor nutrition. Supplementing the poor diets to meet nutritive needs results in better growth and condition, but tissue damage caused by early deprivation may persist into later life. (Courtesy of Dr. Miguel A. Guzman, Institute of Nutrition for Central America and Panama.)

subject to overdilution with water due to misinformation or poverty, with consequent loss of nutritive value. In one location, rice water was given because it resembled the European pictures of bottled formulas. Halting the decline in breastfeeding in developing countries is a current objective of international health organizations. Statistics have shown that when breastfeeding is low in these countries, infant death rates are high.

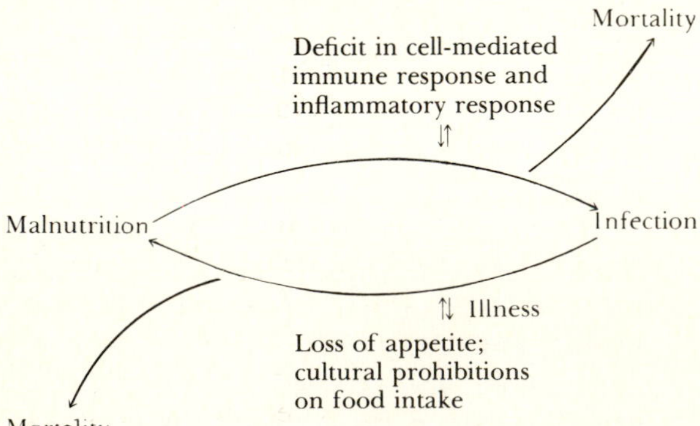

Figure 23–9 The "vicious cycle" of malnutrition and infection, which leads to high mortality in infants and preschool children in developing countries.

The importance of breastfeeding as viewed by the international community was evident in 1981 at the World Health Assembly (37). At this meeting the assembly endorsed an international code of marketing of breast milk substitutes directed at the infant formula industry. The code was designed to carefully regulate marketing practices that promote commercial formulas to new mothers.

PROGRAMS FOR IMPROVING CHILDHOOD NUTRITION IN THE UNITED STATES

WIC Program

The objective of the WIC Program[6] is to insure optimal nutrition for pregnant women and for children up to age five who otherwise might not be able to meet their nutritional requirements. Vouchers are given, and the parent can buy milk, eggs, cheese, cereals, and other nutritious food products for themselves and their children.

Evaluations of this program have demonstrated nutritional and health benefits to participating women and children.

School Food Programs

An understanding of child nutrition programs is important to parents and teachers who influence the child's eating habits. The food that students get in the cafeteria can reflect the nutrition training they get in the classroom along with the guidance they receive at home.

Planning the school lunch menu is a challenge for the nutritionist, who must take into consideration government specifications, cost limitations, physical set-up of the school kitchen, cultural, religious, and racial background of the children, inclusion of a wide variety of foods, and, most important, acceptance of the meal by the children.

The National School Lunch Act was passed in 1946 "to safeguard the health and well-being of the nation's children and to encourage the domestic consumption of nutritious agricultural commodities and other food, by assisting the states through grants-in-aid and other means, in providing an adequate supply of foods and other facilities for the establishment, maintenance, operation, and expansion of nonprofit school lunch programs."

The current National School Lunch Program is based on the original act, and a number of amendments have been added to the original legislation. For example, in 1970, an amendment stipulated that every needy American schoolchild should be given a free or reduced-price meal. Also, in 1973, the School Breakfast Program became available to all schools wishing to apply.

The school-lunch meal requirements are designed to provide a simple and easy-to-follow framework for planning nutritious and well-balanced lunches. The lunch pattern is flexible so that it may provide children with a wide variety of foods and allow consideration of their regional, cultural, ethnic, and special dietary needs and food practices in menu planning. The National School Lunch Program regulations specify that a school lunch must contain a specified quantity of each of four food components (see Fig. 23–10 for specific quantities by age/grade group).

The nutritional goal for school lunches is to provide approximately one-third of the Recommended Dietary Allowances. It is not expected that each lunch each day will provide one-third of the RDA for all nutrients, but that, when averaged over a

[6]Women, Infants, and Children (WIC), a supplemental feeding program, began in 1972. It is administered by the USDA on the Federal level and by health departments on the state and local levels.

period of time—in which a wide variety of foods are served—the goal will be met.

Menu planners are advised to include the following in each day's menu: (1) a vitamin A vegetable or fruit at least twice a week; (2) a vitamin C vegetable or fruit at least 2 or 3 times a week; and (3) several foods for iron each day.

To help reduce the amount of food wasted in school lunches, an "offer versus serve" provision has been mandated for high schools (see Fig. 23–10). This allows students to choose less than all of the food items within the lunch pattern. The program guidelines include that the school cannot mandate that any specific food item be required, although five items are offered and the acceptance of all five is encouraged. Meat alternates include cheese; eggs; cooked, dry beans or peas; and peanut butter. Bread alternates include rice, macaroni, and noodles. Because of the success of this provision in high schools, it can now be used as an option in junior and/or middle schools.

National School Lunch Program regulations *require* school food authorities to promote activities to involve students and parents in the school lunch program. Such activities may include menu planning, enhancement of the eating environment, program promotion, and related student community support activities. The establishment of parent and student school food-service committees to assist in menu planning and other activities may greatly improve the overall acceptability of school lunches.

Nutrition Education of Children

The preschool and elementary grades are an important time to emphasize nutrition education in the classroom. The school meal can ideally be used as a "learning laboratory" for classroom instruction. An imaginative approach, with field trips, cooking activities, games, use of audiovisual materials, and the involvement of children in evaluating and planning their own eating habits can promote an effective nutrition education program.

The subject can be reinforced throughout the school year by integrating nutrition education with other subject areas. For example, in a social studies unit, different cultural

Components:	Preschool		Grades K-3	Grades 4-12$_1$	Grades 7-12
	ages 1-2 (Group I)	ages 3-4 (Group II)	ages 5-8 (Group III)	age 9 & over (Group IV)	age 12 & over (Group V)
MEAT OR MEAT ALTERNATE	1 oz.	1½ oz.	1½ oz.	2 oz.	3 oz.
	1 oz.	1½ oz.	1½ oz.	2 oz.	3 oz.
	½	¾	¾	1	1½
	¼ cup	⅜ cup	⅜ cup	½ cup	¾ cup
	2 Tbsp	3 Tbsp	3 Tbsp	4 Tbsp	6 Tbsp
VEGETABLE AND/OR FRUIT	½ cup	½ cup	½ cup	¾ cup	¾ cup
BREAD OR BREAD ALTERNATE	5 per week	8 per week	8 per week	8 per week	10 per week
MILK	¾ cup (6 fl oz)	¾ cup (6 fl oz)	½ pint (8 fl oz)	½ pint (8 fl oz)	½ pint (8 fl oz)

Figure 23–10 School lunch patterns for various age groups. Group V (Grades 7–12) are recommended quantities, the other groups (Preschool through Grades 4–12) are minimum quantities. Students age 12 and over may request smaller portions of Group V offerings, but not smaller than those specified in Group IV. The portions for the vegetable/fruit group represent two or more servings of vegetable or fruit or both. Bread alternates include rice, macaroni, and noodles.

food habits can be explored. Also, names of different varieties of foods may be introduced in spelling or mathematics lessons.

CONCLUSION

There is a developing consensus that nutrition is a major component of national and international efforts to promote health and prevent disease (38). It is an especially important factor in pregnancy, infancy, and childhood—the periods of rapid growth and development of the human organism.

Study and research continue on many questions involving issues of infant and childhood nutrition. Above all, however, there is a real need for *application* of nutritional knowledge already gathered to help insure optimal health and development for all the world's infants and children—from children in your own neighborhood to those in the farthest lands.

QUESTIONS

1. By what age will the newborn infant normally double its birth weight? Triple it?
2. List three advantages of breast milk as an infant food.
3. A neighbor asks you if you think his five-month-old baby should be put on skim milk since she is getting chubby. Your response?
4. What is your view of supplemental vitamins for infants fed breast milk or infant formula? Defend your point of view.
5. By what age should the infant be on a diet that includes a variety of foods in addition to milk?
6. Name three foods that might be suspected if a nine-month-old infant begins to develop signs of allergy.
7. What would you advise a vegetarian mother who asks you about the adequacy of the vegan diet that she feeds her two-year-old?
8. Prepare a day's sample menu (including snacks) for a day-care center for three- to five-year-olds, open from 7 A.M. to 6 P.M.
9. What would you say is the major nutritional problem of children in the United States today? In the developing countries? Discuss your choices.
10. Recall a typical high-school lunch from your own experience. Does it meet the school lunch recommendations as described in this chapter?

References

1. National Center for Health Statistics: NCHS Growth Charts, 1976. Monthly Vital Statistics Report, Vol. 25, No. 3, Supp. (HRA) 76–1120.
2. Mitchell, H. S.: Nutrition in relation to stature. J. Amer. Dietet. Assoc., *40*:521, 1962.
3. Prader, A., Tanner, J. M., and Von Harnack, G. A.: Catch-up growth following illness or starvation. J. Pediatr., *62*:646, 1963.
4. Committee on Nutrition, American Academy of Pediatrics: Nutritional needs of low birth-weight infants. Pediatr., *60*:519, 1977.
5. Postnatal growth of small-for-dates babies. Nutr. Rev., *31*:51, 1973.
6. Martinez, G. A., Dodd, D. A., and Samartgedes, J. J.: Milk feeding patterns in the United States during the first twelve months of life. Pediatrics, *68*:863, 1981; also see Ekwo, E. E., et al.: Factors influencing initiation of breast-feeding. Amer J. Dis. Children, *137*:375, 1983; Anon.: The dynamics of breast-feeding. WHO Chronicle, *37*(No. 1):6, 1983.
7. Food and Nutrition Board, National Research Council: *Nutrition Services in Perinatal Care.* National Academy Press, Washington D.C., 1981; Resolution of the 27th World Health Assembly (1974); Canadian Pediatric Society, Nutrition Committee: Infant feeding. J. Canad. Dietet. Assoc., *41*:46, 1981; Committee on Nutrition, American Academy of Pediatrics: Commentary on breast-feeding and infant formulas. Pediatrics, *57*:278, 1976.
8. Barness, L.: Formula manufacture and infant feeding (editorial). J. Amer. Med. Assoc., *243*:1075, 1980.
9. Ounsted, M., and Sleigh, G.: The infant's self-regulation of food intake and weight gain. Lancet, *1*:1393, 1975.
10. Carpenter, G.: Epidermal Growth Factor as a major growth-promoting agent in human milk. Science, *210*:198, 1980.
11. Rogan, W. J., Bagniewska, A., and Damstra, T.: Pollutants in breast milk. N. Eng. J. Med., *302*:1450, 1980.

12. Fomon, S.J.: *Infant Nutrition.* 2nd Ed. Philadelphia, W. B. Saunders Co., 1974.
13. Bordeaux, D., et al.: Infant nutrition. J. Fam. Prac., *14*:145, 1982.
14. American Academy of Pediatrics: *Pediatric Nutrition Handbook.* Evanston, Ill., American Academy of Pediatrics, 1979; Underwood, B. A., and Hofvander, Y.: Appropriate timing for complementary feeding of the breast-fed infant—a review. Acta Paediatr. Scand., Supplement 294 (179 refs.), 1982.
15. Hansen, A. E., et al.: Influence of diet on blood serum lipids in pregnant women and newborn infants. Amer. J. Clin. Nutr., *15*:11, 1964.
16. O'Connor, P.: Vitamin D deficiency rickets in two breast fed infants who were not receiving vitamin D supplementation. Clin. Pediatr., *16*:361, 1977.; Tsang, R. C.: The quandary of vitamin D in the newborn infant. Lancet, *I*:1370, 1983.
17. Mahoney, C. P., et al.: Chronic vitamin A intoxication in an infant fed chicken liver. Pediatrics, *65*:893, 1980.
18. Johnson, P. R., and Roloff, J. S.: Vitamin B-12 deficiency in an infant strictly breast-fed by a mother with latent pernicious anemia. J. Pediatr., *100*:917, 1982.
19. Report of Committee on Nutrition, American Academy of Pediatrics: Sodium intake of infants in the United States. Pediatrics, *68*:444, 1981.
20. Owen, G. et al.: Iron nutriture of infants exclusively breastfed in the first five months. J. Pediatr., *99*:237, 1981.
21. Woodruff, C. W., Wright, S. W., and Wright, R. P.: The role of fresh cow's milk in iron deficiency. Amer. J. Dis. Child., *124*:26, 1972.
22. Hambidge, K. M., Walravens, P. A., Brown, R. M., et al.: Zinc nutrition of preschool children in the Denver Head Start Program. Amer. J. Clin. Nutr., *29*:734, 1976.
23. Smith, A. M., Picciano, M. F., and Milner, J. A.: Selenium intakes and status of human milk and formula fed infants. Amer. J. Clin. Nutr., *35*:521, 1982.
24. Committee on Nutrition, American Academy of Pediatrics: Vitamin and mineral supplement needs in normal children in the United States. Pediatrics *66*:1015, 1980.
25. Dept. of Health, Education, and Welfare: *Ten-State Nutrition Survey 1968–1970.* Dept. of Health, Education, and Welfare Pub. No. (HSM) 72–1219, 1972.
26. Dept. of Health, Education, and Welfare: *Preliminary Findings of the First Health and Nutrition Examination Survey, U.S. 1971–1972.* Dept. of Health, Education, and Welfare Pub. No. (HRA) 74–1219–1, 1975.
27. Owen, G., and Lippman, G.: Nutritional status, U.S.A. Pediatr. Clin. North Amer., *24*:214, 1977.
28. Bruch, H.: *Eating Disorders.* New York, Basic Books, Inc., 1973, p. 26.
29. Weil, W. B., Jr.: Current controversies in childhood obesity. J. Pediatr., *91*:175, 1977.
30. Charney, E., Goodman, H. C., McBride, M., Lyon, B., and Pratt, R.: Childhood antecedents of adult obesity. Do chubby infants become obese adults? N. Eng. J. Med., *295*:6, 1976.
31. Pipes, P.: *Nutrition in Infancy and Childhood.* St. Louis, C. V. Mosby, 1977, Chapter 9.
32. Dine, M. S., et al.: Where do the heaviest children come from? A prospective study of white children from birth to 5 years. Pediatrics, *63*:1, 1979.
33. Heldenberg, D., et al.: Lipoprotein measurements—a necessity for precise assessment of risk in children from high-risk families. Arch. Dis. Child., *54*:695, 1979.
34. Chase, H. P., et al.: Kwashiorkor in the United States. Pediatrics, *66*:972, 1980.
35. Sinatra, F. R., and Merritt, R. J.: Iatrogenic kwashiorkor in infants. Amer. J. Dis. Children, *135*:21, 1981.
36. McLaren, D. S., and Burman, D.: *Textbook of Pediatric Nutrition.* New York. Churchill Livingstone, 1976, Chapter 6.
37. WHO Chronicle, *35*:112, 1981; Amer. J. Dis. Children, *135*:889, 1981.
38. Public Health Service, U. S. Department of Health and Human Services: *Better Health for Our Children: A National Strategy.* DHHS (PHS) Publication No. 79–55071, 1979, Chapter 4. Beaton, G. H., and Ghassemi, H.: Supplementary feeding programs for young children in developing countries. Amer. J. Clin. Nutr., *35* (Supplement, April): 864, 1982.

24 Dental Health, Nutrition, and Diet

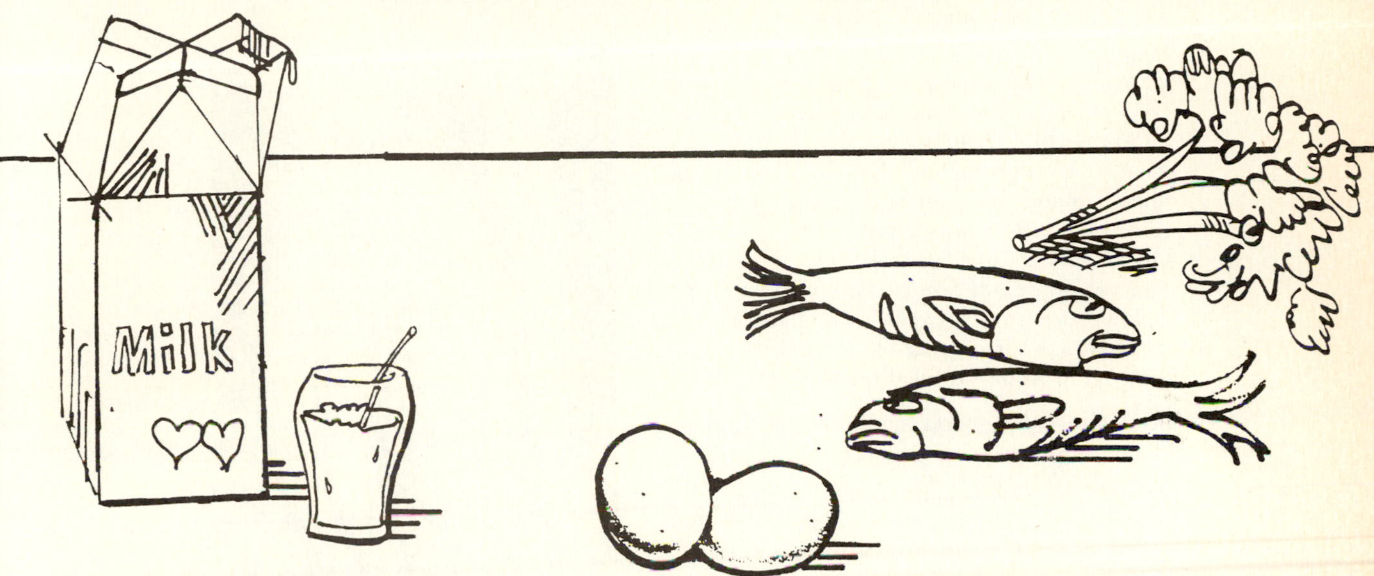

Dental disease is one of the most widespread and costly diseases in this country. For example, 90 percent of all American children already have dental decay by age four. The total cost of repairing the effects of tooth decay for this nation is at least $6 billion a year (1).

Understanding of the complex causes of the two most important types of dental disease, *dental decay* and *periodontal (gum) disease,* has increased greatly in the past few decades. Awareness of these causes is an important step toward obtaining all the personal benefits of healthy teeth and gums.

There are important interrelationships between oral health and nutrition. First, good nutrition is important for developing and maintaining healthy, sound teeth and gum structures. In turn, healthy dental structures are needed so that an adequate diet may be eaten (see Fig. 24–1).

What exactly is dental disease? Why are "permanent" teeth lost? How can tooth loss and cavities be prevented, and how does diet play a role? In order to answer these questions, this chapter reviews the current concepts regarding the causes of dental decay and periodontal disease, with special emphasis on the role of dietary factors.

The extent of some of the problems associated with dental decay and periodontal disease—and their secondary result, loss of nat-

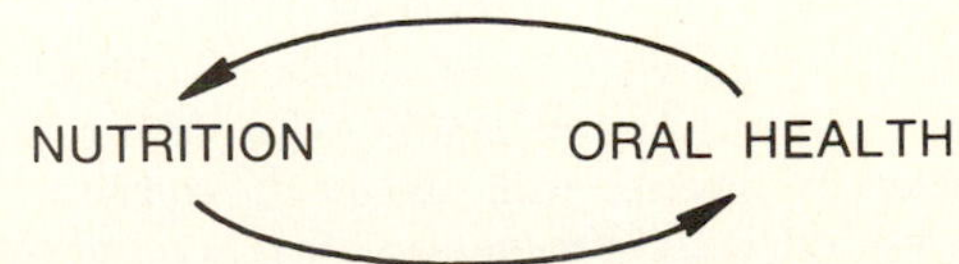

Figure 24–1 Good nutrition is necessary for oral health, and oral health is necessary for good nutrition.

ural teeth—is demonstrated by the following figures obtained from various sources in the last decade.

1. Over 20 million people—10 percent of the U. S. population—have lost all their teeth.
2. Over 95 percent of people in the United States have decayed teeth by the time they are adults.
3. People with low family income and minimal education tend to lose teeth earlier and more frequently than people with higher earnings and levels of education.
4. Nearly 40 percent of the children in the United States age four to seventeen have not visited a dentist within a year.
5. One-third of the entire U.S. population receives no dental care except, possibly, emergency procedures for relief from pain.
6. The average fifteen-year-old in the U.S. has 10 decayed, missing, or filled teeth.

Thus there has been a pattern of neglect, including nutritional neglect, surrounding oral health, leading to painful teeth and unhealthy gums. In turn, tooth-loss has resulted in the need for artificial replacements of teeth.

One hopeful note: Recent health surveys have recorded declines in caries (tooth decay) incidence in both children and adults in the last ten to twenty years, ranging from a "slight" decline in adults to a 32 percent decrease in children age five to seventeen (2).

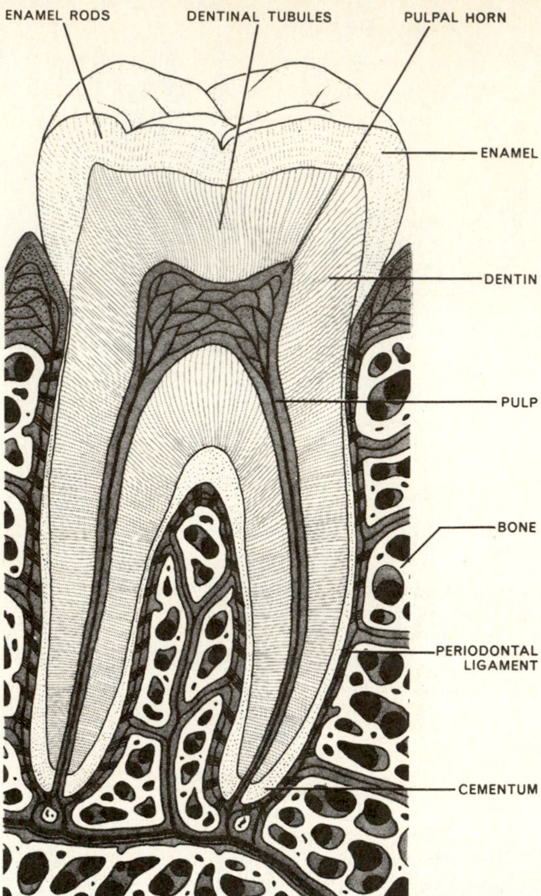

Figure 24–2 The anatomy of the tooth and surrounding structures. (From Morrey, L. W., and Nelson, R. J.: *Dental Science Handbook.* Washington, D.C., Superintendent of Documents, 1970. Copyright by the American Dental Association. Reprinted by permission.)

NUTRITION AND DEVELOPMENT OF THE TOOTH

The basic structure of the tooth and adjacent gum area is shown in Figure 24–2. The tooth is composed of four separate tissues:

Enamel, the outer layer, is the most durable of all body tissues. It is primarily (95 percent) inorganic in nature, with its major constituents being calcium, phosphorus, magnesium, and carbonate. It can function as a semipermeable membrane.

Dentin, the major part or core of the hard portion of the tooth, is 80 percent inorganic, composed mainly of calcium and phosphorus. It extends almost the entire length of the tooth, and is covered by enamel on the crown and by cementum on the roots. Unlike enamel, it is a very sensitive portion of the tooth.

Cementum is also a calcified tissue that is presumed to be similar in composition to bone and dentin. It acts as a surface for the attachment of the fibers (periodontal ligaments) that hold the tooth to the surrounding tissues.

Pulp, the soft part in the tooth's center, is a vital tissue containing nerves, lymph, blood vessels, and fibrous tissue. It extends for about four-fifths of the length of the tooth, with communication to the general nutritional and nervous systems through the root.

In addition, the *periodontal tissues* make up the gums and the tissues that hold the teeth in place; they contain much connective tissue. If the *deciduous* or *"baby" teeth* (the teeth that are lost before the permanent teeth erupt) are lost too early through neglect or any other reason, the spacing of the *permanent teeth* may be affected, and there may be irregularities in their proper positioning. Also, the deciduous teeth, like the permanent teeth, are important for eating normally, for a healthy appearance, and for proper speech development.

Nutrition plays an important part in future tooth development even prior to birth. The genetic make-up of the individual provides the pattern for the tooth and other oral development, but unless the environment supplies adequate nutrients, the genetic potential is not realized. Thus the pregnant mother must receive generous supplies of calcium, protein, iron, and vitamins, especially A, C, and D (see other sections on these subjects). Examples of how specific nutrients are related to tooth development are the following:

1. Vitamin D aids in absorption and utilization of calcium, promoting the deposition of both calcium and phosphorus in teeth. Excessive vitamin D in pregnant animals leads to badly shaped jaws in the offspring, with resultant *malocclusion,* or faulty bite.
2. Vitamins C and A affect the functional activities of the formative cells. Vitamin C is important for calcification of dentin, and vitamin A is necessary for optimal calcification and development of enamel.
3. In animal studies, specific nutritional deficiencies, or vitamin excesses in some cases, cause defective development of oral structures—for example, cleft palate is seen in offspring when maternal diets are deficient in vitamin E, vitamin A, a number of the B vitamins, and many minerals.
4. Low protein in the diet of pregnant rats has been shown to be associated with reduction in the size of molars, delay in the eruption of certain teeth, and increased susceptibility to carious lesions (3).

Thus in experimental animals, there are demonstrated relationships between nutritional factors and microscopic structure, chemical composition, tooth shape and size, eruption time, and susceptibility to caries, as well as to jaw malformations.

Although specific oral and dental malformations resulting from specific nutritional deficiencies have not been experimentally demonstrated in humans, optimal development of the teeth is undoubtedly related to the intake of a balanced and adequate diet. The important role of the nutrient fluoride in tooth development was discussed in Chapter 17, and will also be treated later in this chapter. There is some evidence that strontium and other trace elements may have some relationship to tooth development and in dental resistance to caries as well (4).

DENTAL CARIES AND NUTRITION

The two major causes of dental ill health and subsequent tooth loss are dental *caries,*[1] or "cavities" as they are generally known, and *periodontal disease,* which refers to disease of the gums and jaw structures that hold the teeth. The first stage of periodontal disease is *gingivitis,* or gum inflammation. A severe form of gum disease, involving the bone under the gums, is known as *periodontitis.*

Tooth-loss prior to age 35 years is primarily a result of dental caries (see Fig. 24–3). Dental caries does not have a single cause; it

[1]The word "caries" is derived from the Greek word for "rottenness."

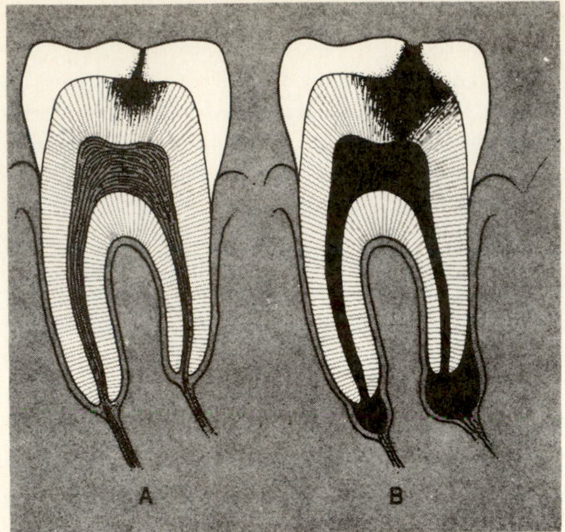

Figure 24–3 The progress of decay: A, the bacteria have penetrated the enamel and attacked the softer dentin. B, the bacteria have penetrated the dentin and killed the pulp, and infection has spread to the root. At this point the tooth may have to be removed. (From Morrey, L. W., and Nelson, R. J.: *Dental Science Handbook.* Washington, D.C., Superintendent of Documents, 1970. Copyright by the American Dental Association. Reprinted by permission.)

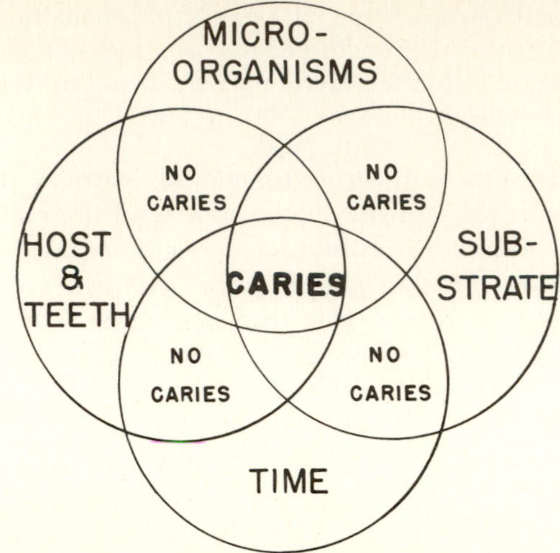

Figure 24–4 The four circles represent the factors involved in the formation of dental caries. All four factors must be acting together (where circles overlap) for caries to occur. (From Newbrun, E.: *Etiology of Dental Caries.* San Francisco, University of California, 1971.)

is a complex disease involving four major factors: (1) characteristics of the host where the teeth are present; (2) actions of specific *bacteria* in the mouth; (3) the presence of certain substrates (the material, such as sugar, acted upon by the bacteria) in the diet that are needed for the bacterial action; and (4) the passage of *time* necessary for the development of caries (see Fig. 24–4).

The carious lesion is initiated when enamel is decalcified by acids that are produced by bacteria present in dental plaque and progresses to cavitation when the dentin is invaded and destroyed by bacteria.

Dental caries has been termed one of the oldest diseases of man. Wall painting depicting dental problems of the Cro-Magnon race—22,000 years ago—have been found. Early theories on the cause of dental decay ranged from invasion by worms to "gangrene" beginning in the inside of the tooth to an imbalance of the four bodily "humours."

In 1600 an English writer noted a relationship between carbohydrate intake and poor teeth, with the following observation: "'Overuse" of most confections and sugar plummes . . . rotteth the teeth and maketh them look black" (5). In the early nineteenth century, a chemical theory on the origin of dental caries was postulated. It related carious teeth to "a chemical agent" (acid) produced when food "putrefied" on tooth enamel. Then in the mid-nineteenth century, with the advent of the microscope, bacteria were seen on teeth, and the groundwork was laid for understanding the actual cause of dental caries. It was Miller in 1890 who first demonstrated that the acid-producing action of salivary bacteria on ingested carbohydrates caused decalcification of enamel. An early study that provided proof of the effect of diet on this process was reported in 1938 and showed a significant difference in the number of dental caries between two groups of children—one group that had a balanced diet with no between-meal sweets and no caries; and a second group eating a poor diet, with small quantities of vegetables, fruits, and vitamin D and large amounts of sweets daily, that had an extremely high incidence of caries (6). This study is one of the many that have documented the role of dietary factors—such as type of food, clearance rate of food, frequency of eating, and "detergent" effects of foods—in the causation or prevention of caries.

Effect of Physical Properties of Foods

Physical properties of foods, such as adhesiveness, solubility, and viscosity, may modify the caries-producing potential of foods. Foods that are highly adherent to tooth surfaces and that are slowly soluble contribute to an increase in caries-promoting action (7). Thus, liquid foods tend to cause fewer caries than sticky or retentive foods.

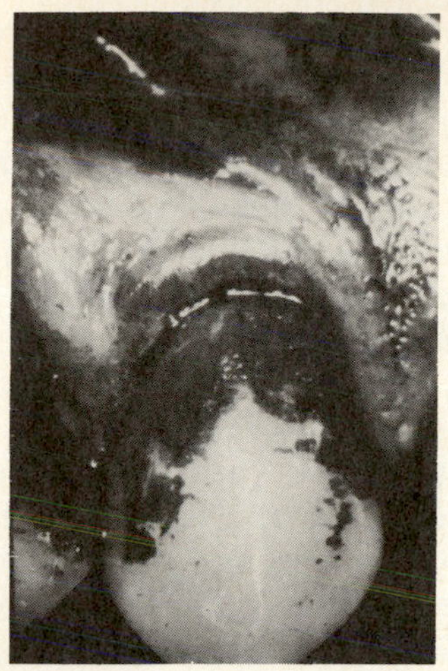

Figure 24–5 Microbial dental plaque (dark area on tooth) stained by a disclosing solution. Dental brushing and flossing is the best method for the removal of plaque. A diet limited in frequency of sucrose intake is important in the prevention of plaque formation. Bacterial plaque is the cause of most common forms of periodontal disease, as well as being involved in the development of caries. (From Moss, S. (Ed.): *Preventive Dentistry,* 1972. Courtesy of Medcom, Inc.)

Effect of Food on the Microbiology of the Oral Cavity

Plaque is an important factor in dental caries. It is a sticky, nearly colorless layer of gelatinous material that accumulates on a tooth surface, to which it develops a tenacious attachment (Fig. 24–5). It is composed primarily of microcolonies of bacteria and their by-products (see Fig. 24–6). The plaque is colonized by several types of bacteria, both *cariogenic* (those that cause caries and that live mainly on sucrose and other carbohydrates) and *noncariogenic.* The most important cariogenic bacteria are streptococcal types. These bacteria ferment dietary carbohydrates to form *organic acids,* which, at susceptible sites, initiate the carious lesion by demineralizing the enamel surface.

Caries do not develop in germ-free animals reared in the complete absence of bacteria. This is perhaps the most striking evidence that has linked the bacteria in plaque to dental caries. Even when germ-free animals are fed high-carbohydrate, special cariogenic diets, they do not develop caries unless cariogenic bacteria are established in their mouths. Antibiotics, when fed to animals, are effective in reducing the incidence and severity of caries. Children receiving ongoing antibiotic therapy effective against streptococcal bacteria (for example, in certain heart conditions) are known to have

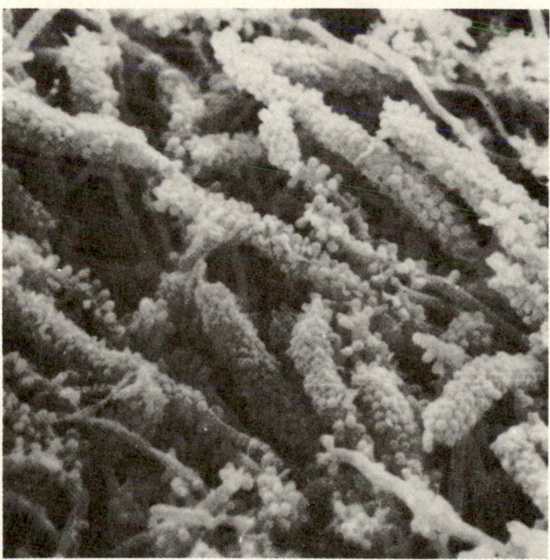

Figure 24–6 Dental plaque, shown here in a scanning electron micrograph, is composed of countless bacteria. (From Jones, S. J. Dent. Abstr., *17:* 8, 1972.)

fewer caries in their teeth than children not receiving such antibiotics (8).

Further evidence to implicate the role of bacteria in caries formation is that specific bacteria have been isolated and cultivated from carious lesions. By inoculating them in germ-free animals, caries have developed. *Streptococcus mutans* appears to be a primary culprit in caries formation (8). The organism can begin its role in the mouth as early as infancy, when the bacteria may be passed from parent to infant. It also has the ability to convert sucrose into extracellular polymers called *glucans*. These polymers then form a sticky, insoluble substance that causes plaque to adhere to the teeth and appears to serve as a barrier to buffer systems in the saliva that might otherwise neutralize the acids formed by the bacteria in the plaque. Production of these extracellular carbohydrate materials has been shown to be directly correlated with the ability of bacteria to produce caries.

Thus dental caries are basically a local disease of the teeth subject to the influence of those dietary components that provide the caries-causing bacteria with their necessary growth material, including a dietary source of essential amino acids, vitamins, and minerals in addition to carbohydrate. Caries are indeed a type of bacterial infection, and a vaccine against this type of dental disease may eventually be an effective preventive measure.

Role of Sucrose and Other Carbohydrates in Dental Caries

Plaque and its bacteria alone do not cause caries; a diet conducive to caries is also necessary. Sugar ingestion has now been clearly implicated as the major dietary factor contributing to dental caries.

The association of food and caries has been known for centuries, ever since it was observed that caries occur almost exclusively on tooth surfaces where self-cleansing mechanisms are least effective. Food is a necessary factor in allowing the cariogenic plaque bacteria to actually begin causing caries. Dietary carbohydrates, and sucrose in particular, are of primary importance in the processes of bacterial colonization of the tooth surface and production and support of dental decay.

With the aid of carbohydrates to ferment, the plaque bacteria will produce an acid medium with a pH of about 4.5 to 5.5 (quite acid), by the formation mainly of lactic acid. The drop in plaque pH may remain for up to two hours after sucrose ingestion. An example of the pH change observed in plaque after the ingestion of various foods is seen in Figure 24–7.

The important role of sucrose and, to a lesser extent, other fermentable carbohydrates in the etiology of dental decay has been demonstrated by epidemiological and chem-

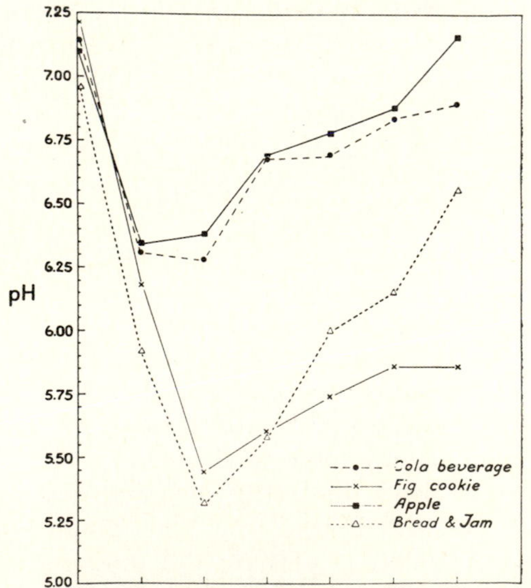

Figure 24–7 Some examples of the changes in plaque pH following eating of different foods. (From Ludwig, T.G., and Bibby, B.G. J. Dent. Res., *36*:56, 1957.)

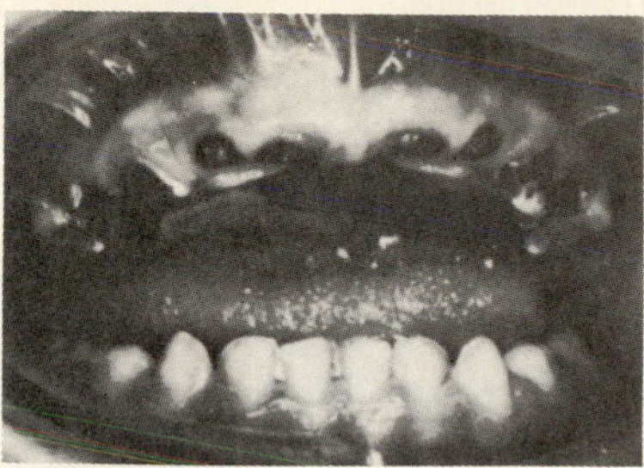

Figure 24–8 Teeth of a 2½-year-old child who frequently received apple juice in a baby bottle. Note the nearly complete destruction of upper teeth by caries. (Lower teeth are thought to have been protected because of the position of the tongue and lower lip during sucking.) (From Kaplan, H., and Rabbach, V. P. Apple juice and dental caries, Bambino. Children's Hospital Medical Center, Oakland, CA, Winter 1971.)

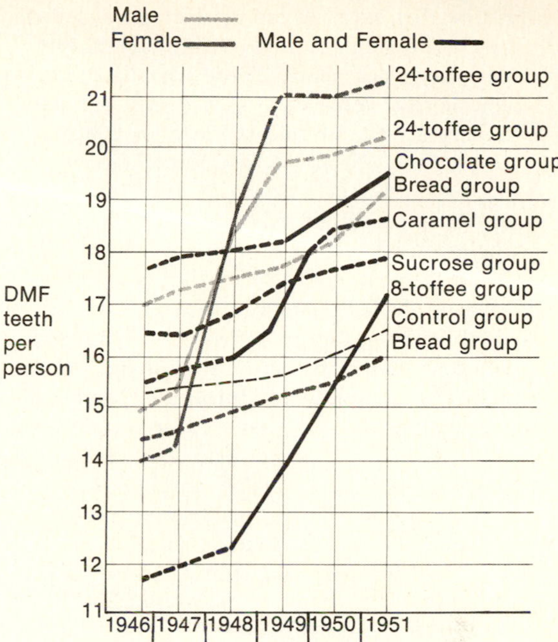

Figure 24–9 Graph of the Vipeholm study, showing the relationship of time of sugar consumption and of type of sugar-containing item to dental caries incidence over a period of 5 years: Key: -------- sugar consumed only at meals; ——— sugar consumed both at meals and between meals; DMF = decayed, missing, or filled. This study was important in demonstrating that increased frequency of consumption of sugar-containing items that are retained on tooth surfaces is a cause of caries. (From Sweeney, E. A. (Ed.): *The Food That Stays: An Update on Nutrition, Diet, Sugar and Caries,* 1977. Courtesy of Medcom, Inc.)

ical studies as well as by controlled studies on animals and humans. For example:

1. During World War II, sugar consumption in Europe was severely restricted, and caries dropped significantly two years thereafter. When the sugar intake increased again, caries recurred at previous levels.
2. Rampant caries (especially in the upper front teeth, a rare location) have been observed with frequency in children who fall asleep sucking a bottle of fruit juice or milk with sugar. This condition is known as the *nursing bottle caries syndrome*, and is one of the most crippling dental problems in young children (see Fig. 24–8).
3. A Scandinavian study (the Vipeholm study) is a classic that examined the cariogenicity of various diets in humans (9). For example, subjects who ate sticky toffee several times a day had twelve times as much caries development as control subjects who did not have this frequent exposure to sugar (see Fig. 24–9).
4. People with a genetic defect known as hereditary fructose intolerance tend to avoid all foods containing sucrose and fructose because eating such foods produces unpleasant symptoms (nausea, vomiting, etc.). Their dental health is excellent, and their teeth often show total absence of dental caries.[2]
5. In one small, South Atlantic island, dental decay was virtually nonexistent before the advent of Westernized foods and sweets. Twenty years later, after the inhabitants began consuming an average of 0.5 kg of sugar a week, one-half of permanent molars were carious in those 20 years old and under.
6. England has had a documented increase in sugar consumption of from 20 to 110 pounds per person over the last 100 years, and there has been a nearly parallel rise in caries prevalence.
7. Widely different cavity counts were found in eight countries, while sugar consumption followed the same pattern (with highest caries incidence and sugar intake found in the United States and Central and South America) (10).
8. An important Finnish study demonstrated that subjects ingesting an average level of sucrose

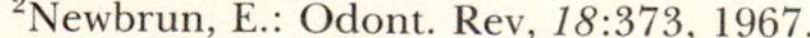

[2]Newbrun, E.: Odont. Rev, *18*:373, 1967.

in the diet experienced an average of 7.2 decayed, missing, or filled (DMF) teeth over a period of two years. Those who had sucrose completely replaced by fructose or xylitol experienced a 3.8 and 0.0 level of DMF teeth respectively. Xylitol is not fermented by oral bacteria, and the absence of caries on the sucrose-free, xylitol-replacement diet documents the essential role of fermentable carbohydrate in caries production (11).

9. Maltose, lactose, fructose, and glucose can be used by the plaque bacteria for synthesizing cell-wall, capsular, and intracellular polysaccharides, as well as for forming organic acids; but, unlike sucrose, they cannot be utilized in the creation of *extra*cellular polysaccharides. These other fermentable carbohydrates are not blameless in caries production. When they are available in the diet it may take only very low levels of sucrose to stimulate rapid decay.

Starches probably cannot diffuse into plaque, as sucrose so easily does, because of the relatively large size of the molecules. Starches may, however, be metabolized by certain (nonstreptococcal) oral bacteria to polysaccharides, which then may become part of the plaque matrix, undergo breakdown by caries-causing bacteria, and thus institute the decay process. See Figure 24–10 for a diagrammatic summary of the metabolism of ingested carbohydrates.

It is clear that the relationship of the consumption of sugar to the prevalence of caries is very strong. Areas of continued study concern the relationship of total sugar consumption, the frequency, and the form of sugar consumption to caries (12).

Cariogenic Potential

A food's potential to induce caries formation is called its *cariogenic potential,* or *cariogenicity.* Unfortunately, it is not a simple matter of using the amount of fermentable carbohydrates in a food to predict its precise cariogenic potential. If a sugary food is rapidly cleared from the mouth, or if it has other components that buffer the acid produced, its cariogenicity will be reduced.

There is much current interest in a "scoring system" for identifying relative cariogenic potentials, a system that would be useful to guide consumers in food selection (13). Present techniques used to set up cariogenic scores include pH measurements after a food is introduced into the mouth, and *in vitro* tests.

Until such time as a measure of exact cariogenic potential may become available, there is such strong evidence that the proportion of sucrose in a food is a major cariogenic determinant that the percentage of

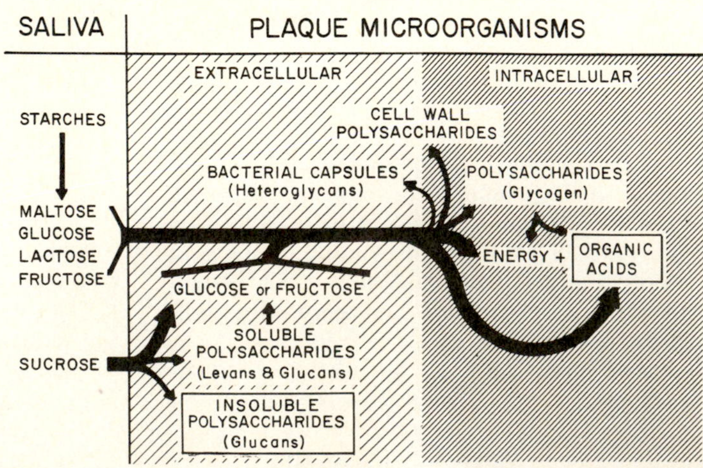

Figure 24–10 Metabolic fate of ingested carbohydrates in plaque showing both extracellular and intracellular end-products. Heavy arrows represent major pathways; end-products that are particularly harmful to the teeth are shown in the boxes. (From Newbrun, E.: *Etiology of Dental Caries.* San Francisco, University of California, 1971.)

sucrose alone can be used to approximate a food's potential cariogenicity (14). (See next section, however.)

Role of the Time Factor and the Frequency of Eating

A small area of decalcified enamel, just barely detectable, will generally progress to clinical caries in one or two years. If, however, careful preventive measures are immediately undertaken (dietary and oral hygiene measures), the development of the caries may be halted, although the eroded spot can never revert to normal.

The age of the tooth plays a part in caries susceptibility. A tooth is most likely to develop caries two to four years after eruption, when enamel is in the final stages of maturation. When complete enamel maturation has been attained (after two to four years) the tooth is more resistant to caries formation. This helps to explain why young children and teenagers (with fairly new deciduous and permanent teeth, respectively) have higher caries rates than individuals of other age groups.

In addition, timing of sugar exposure is related to caries development in that the more often sweets are in contact with the teeth, the longer the exposure to acid decalcification and the higher the caries incidence will be (see Fig. 24–11).

This overriding importance of the frequency of exposure to sweets was first documented by the Vipeholm study (9). Those who ate sweets between meals had more caries than those who ate sweets only at mealtimes, regardless of the total amount of sugar intake per day.

Thus, "snacking" on sugary foods plays a definite role in caries causation (15). The more frequently sugar is eaten between meals, the greater is the increase in caries. In addition, the longer the sugar substance stays in contact with the teeth, the greater the cariogenicity. Sticky candy such as taffy and regular chewing gum are examples of prime offenders.

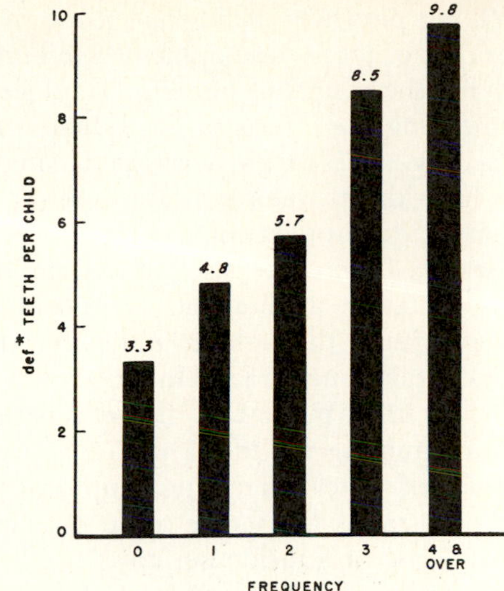

Figure 24–11 The effect of between-meal eating on caries activity in children. This shows that the more snacks children eat, the higher is the incidence of decay. (From Weiss, R. L., and Trithart, A. H.: Amer. J. Public Health, *50*:1097, 1960.)

If sucrose and sticky snacks cannot be avoided in the diet, they should be removed from the teeth as quickly as possible by proper oral hygiene measures, that is, by brushing and flossing.

Role of Fluoride

Fluoride is at present the only dietary trace element of proven effectiveness in producing decay-resistant teeth in humans. The beneficial effects of fluoride on teeth have been known for over 70 years, and there have been over 10,000 articles on fluoride and dental health printed in the world's scientific journals. At present, *fluoridated water* programs reach about 110 million people in the United States.

The incidence of dental caries in both the deciduous and the permanent teeth is reduced about 60 percent in children who drink water containing about 1 part per million (1 mg per liter) of fluorine throughout the period of tooth development. See Figure 24-12 for the results of one important study documenting the effects of fluoridation in a community. The caries decrease is smaller when fluoridated water consumption (or dietary fluoride supplementation) is started at a later age. There are also indications that caries inhibition attributable to fluoridated water continues throughout adult life. Most foods contain only trace amounts of fluorides, with the average U.S. diet, exclusive of water, containing 0.2 to 0.5 mg of fluoride. Inclusion of water containing 1 ppm of fluoride thus raises the intake to an estimated 1.5 to 2.0 mg of fluoride per day.

The safety of fluoridation has been well documented by the World Health Organization. Mild, harmless mottling of teeth may occur when water containing as little as 2 ppm or more of fluoride is ingested, but only at the ages from one to six. (See also Chap. 17.) Fluoride is cleared very rapidly by the kidneys; thus, small amounts do not accumulate in the body in sufficient quantities to produce any health hazard.

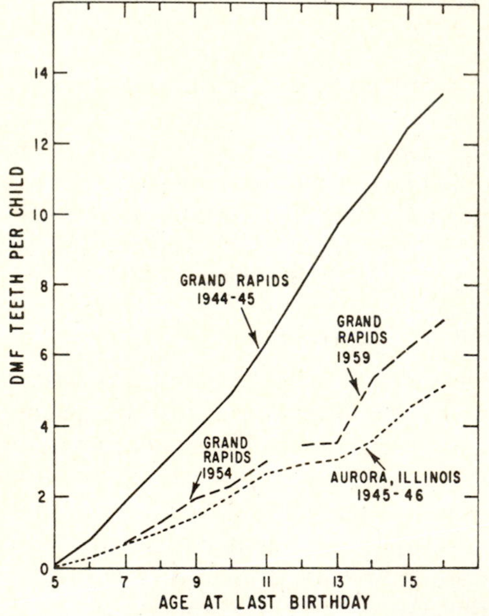

Figure 24–12 This diagram shows the beneficial results of a 15-year period of fluoridation in Grand Rapids, Michigan. It presents the dental caries experience in terms of decayed, missing, and filled teeth (DMF) per child for Grand Rapids, both before and 15 years after fluoridation, and includes caries data from Aurora, Illinois, a community with natural water fluoridation, for comparison. (From Arnold, F. A., Jr., et al.: J. Amer. Dent. Assoc., *65*:780, 1962.)

One mode of action of fluoride in preventing dental caries is related to its accumulation in enamel. It renders the structure of the enamel of the tooth more stable, less soluble to acid, and thus more resistant to demineralization and caries. In order to protect the deciduous teeth, fluoride should be ingested during the first year of life.

Fluoride appears also to directly inhibit the cariogenic effects of bacteria in dental plaque. In addition, frequent applications of fluoride have been shown to increase remineralization of precarious tooth lesions, thus preventing full-scale caries development (16–18).

With newer knowledge of fluoride's actions, it is clear that this mineral is beneficial not only to children and youth, but also to adults. Root surface caries, more prevalent in adults, have been reported to be 50 percent less frequent in a fluoridated than in a nonfluoridated community (19).

The use of fluorine tablets does not appear to be quite as effective as fluoridation of water, perhaps primarily because this method relies on daily cooperation of parent and child. In one study, only 50 percent of families continued giving the pills for the recommended number of years, and this is probably a generous estimate. Fluoride tablets are more costly than community water fluoridation, which costs only 5 to 15 cents per person per year.

The use of fluorides applied topically to the teeth is possible in a practical way by using fluoride-containing toothpastes and mouth rinses. Their use results in a significant preventive value, giving about 20 to 50 percent reduction in incidence of new carious surfaces.

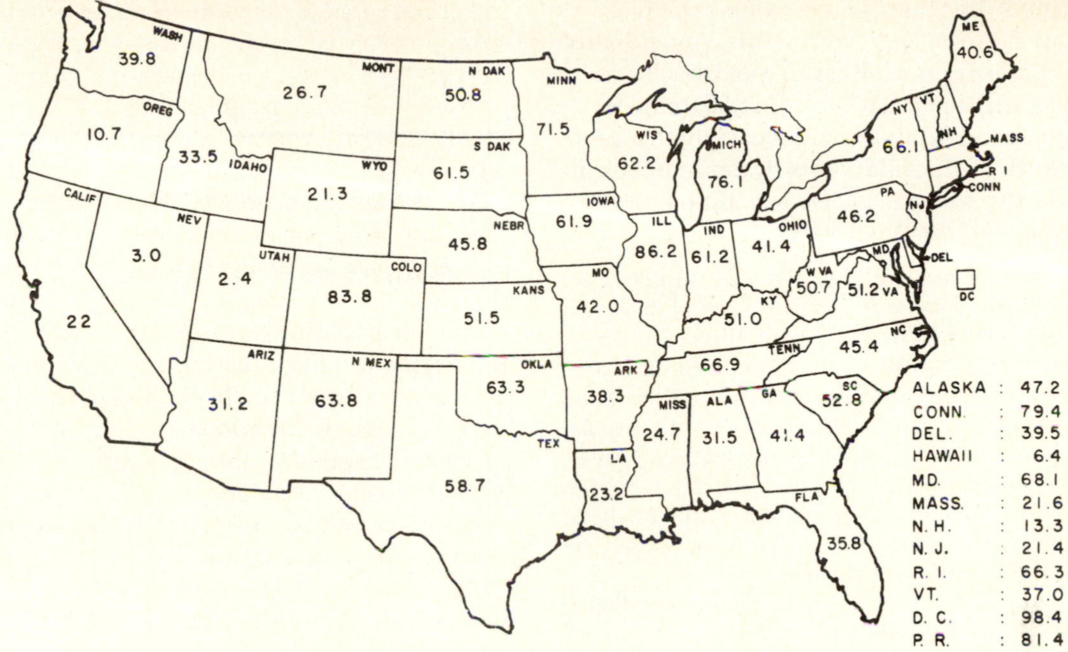

Figure 24–13 Percent of state populations using fluoridated water, 1975, as determined by a fluoridation census conducted by the Center for Disease Control. How does your state stand on fluoridation? (From Morbidity and Mortality Weekly Report, *26(27)*:1, 1977.)

The different uses of fluoride give additive benefits for dental caries prevention; for example, a child receiving fluoridated water supplies will also receive added protection from using fluoridated rinses in school as well as fluoridated toothpaste (20). Self-applied fluorides such as fluoride mouthrinse will probably have more and more use over the next decade (21).

Studies have shown that there are definite reductions in family dental bills after institution of water fluoridation programs at the levels recommended by the United States Public Health Service. For example, the cost of initial dental care for a typical child dropped from 32 dollars to 14 dollars after fluoridation was established in one community. The Head Start Program has found that it must pay from three to ten times as much for dental services for an enrolled child from a nonfluoridated area as it does for such services for a child from a community with fluoridation. It has been estimated that fluoridated water would mean a savings of $7 million a year in dental bills for the one-half million children in just one city in the eastern United States (22).

With so much evidence regarding the usefulness, safety, and economy of fluoridation, and its unanimous recommendation by scientific bodies,[3] to what extent is it used in the United States? Unfortunately, not anywhere near 100 percent. The utilization rate in the different states in 1975 is shown in Figure 24–13; the total number of persons

[3]The United States Public Health Service was the first to endorse fluoridation in 1945. Since then it has been endorsed by the American Dental Association, the American Medical Association, the World Health Organization, the American Public Health Association, the American Institute of Nutrition, and the Food and Nutrition Board, among others.

reached by fluoridated water supplies is about 50 to 60 percent of the United States population. Of cities with populations over 100,000, 70 percent have fluoridation.

Further considerations regarding the practicalities of fluoridation of water supplies include the following (also see supplementary readings in the Appendix):

1. Recommendations for fluoride supplements depend on fluoride concentration in the water supply as well as the age of the child. These recommendations are summarized in Table 24–1. For infants who are exclusively breastfed and do not receive fluoridated water, supplementation with fluoride is advised, since breast milk contains very little fluoride (23).
2. In hot climates, where there is a high intake of water, fluoridation concentration should be less than in colder climates.
3. The cost per year of community water fluoridation is approximately 20 cents (U.S.) per person.
4. At least eight states have passed legislation to require fluoridation in all community water supplies. Countries in addition to the United States that have fluoridation in a good number of communities are Australia, Brazil, Canada, Chile, Czechoslovakia, Ireland, the Netherlands, New Zealand, and the U.S.S.R. The further use of added fluoride for drinking water will probably be rapidly increasing throughout the world.

Table 24–1 THE FLUORIDE SUPPLEMENTATION SCHEDULE (MG/DAY) OF THE AMERICAN ACADEMY OF PEDIATRICS, CORRESPONDING ALSO TO THAT OF THE AMERICAN DENTAL ASSOCIATION (23)[a]

	Concentration of Fluoride in Drinking Water ppm		
Age	<0.3	0.3–0.7	>0.7
		mg per day	
2 wk–2 yrs	0.25	0	0
2–3 yrs	0.50	0.25	0
3–16 yrs	1.00	0.50	0

[a]2.2 mg sodium fluoride contains 1 mg fluoride.

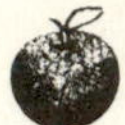

health considerations

The Politics of Fluoridation

The legal validity of fluoridation has been thoroughly tested in the United States in the last decades and has been invariably confirmed. Even so, opponents call it a "compulsory medication," and attempt to raise fears regarding its safety.

One issue sometimes raised is the relation between fluoridation and cancer; the few studies that reported relationships between fluoridated water and cancer in animals have not stood up under scientific scrutiny, and this claim has been refuted (24, 25). Similarly, claims linking fluoridation to birth defects, toxicity, and damage to internal organs or bone development have also been proven false.

It has been recently pointed out that new strategies for education on this issue must be developed, for out of nineteen referenda on water fluoridation in local communities in 1980, only two passed. Public health and dental experts feel that the public health importance of fluoride is so great that profluoridation groups must use political strategies to match their opponents, in addition to the traditional educational approach (26).

Role of Other Nutritional Factors

Other nutrients, such as molybdenum, vanadium, and vitamin B-6 have been reported to help protect against caries development in the experimental animal. A variety of studies suggest but do not conclusively prove that there are relationships between caries prevalence and a wide variety of trace elements other than fluorine in either humans or experimental animals. The mechanisms for the role of these minerals may have to do with increasing the resistance of enamel or with changing the properties of saliva or plaque.

In animals, phosphate supplementation of food helps to decrease caries susceptibility by lowering the solubility rate of enamel, but this has not been proven in humans. There is no evidence for any direct role of calcium in decreasing caries after the tooth is formed.

Highly acid foods, such as undiluted lemon juice or soft drinks with a high phosphoric acid content, are known to be able to dissolve or etch tooth enamel after long-term contact periods. The usual infrequent short-term exposure, along with the buffering effect of saliva, probably results in little or no damage, however.

PERIODONTAL DISEASE AND NUTRITION

Periodontal disease[4] (disease of the gums and other tissues surrounding the teeth), like caries, is an ancient malady and one still prevalent throughout the world. Tooth loss after the age of 35 years in this country is usually due to the effects of periodontal disease, because it results in the loss of healthy supporting tissues for viable teeth. Periodontal disease and its effects thus worsen with increasing age, but the potential for advanced disease may start early.

What are the factors that cause poor periodontal health? Local factors in the mouth, such as the state of oral cleanliness and hygiene, and the effect of foods that either encourage or discourage bacterial growth at gingival (gum) margins are all-important. Rates of periodontal disease incidence are highest in populations with the poorest states of oral hygiene.

There have been no consistent correlations between specific nutrient intake and periodontal disease. Vitamins A and E have shown some positive correlations, but firm evidence is lacking. Certain acute periodontal problems—for example, scurvy with its bleeding gums and diseased gums often found in niacin deficiency—do stem from a lack of nutrients in the diet, but these are not examples of classic periodontal disease.

Experimental studies have shown that protein starvation and magnesium deficiency may adversely affect the periodontium. An advanced stage of bone and periodontal destruction has been seen with protein deficiency. In addition to contributing to tissue growth and resistance, proteins are also important in the function of the endocrine system, whose hormones play a role in proper maintenance of periodontal tissue. Experimental magnesium lack in animals can cause imperfect development of the alveolar bone, widening of the periodontal membrane, gingival enlargement, and loosening of the teeth. In humans, iron deficiency has been shown to be related to unhealthy gingival tissues.

Bacterial masses in plaque are key culprits in periodontal disease. The bacterial accumulations on the tooth surfaces closest to the gingival margins are implicated in this case. In addition, the subsequent accumulation of calculus (a mixture of minerals) occurs on the teeth and under loosened gingival margins. These factors lead to *gingivitis,* the inflammation and infection of the periodontal tissues. This gingivitis, if untreated, is followed by loosening and destruction of the periodontal fibers or ligaments (see Fig. 24–2).

This last stage of periodontal disease is

[4]From the two Greek words peri and odont, meaning "around tooth."

gradual resorption of the alveolar bone that supports the tooth, with consequent tooth loosening and, finally, tooth loss. It is easy to see the detrimental effect that advanced disease will have on the diet. An affected individual will choose foods that are easy to chew but which, unfortunately, are often soft carbohydrates.

Good nutrition, then, is important in the prevention of gingival and periodontal disease because it helps to maintain optimally healthy tissues that are resistant to disease.

Dietary control of sugars and sticky snacks is particularly important because of the key role of bacterial plaque in the process of gingival inflammation as well as caries formation (Review Fig. 24–10.)

PREVENTION OF DENTAL DISEASE

Prevention must be the key to the problem of dental disease (see Fig. 24–14). The four most important factors in prevention are *plaque control, good nutrition, fluoridation,* and *nutrition education.*

Preventive oral hygiene measures are important in removing plaque and local irritants, and include proper tooth brushing

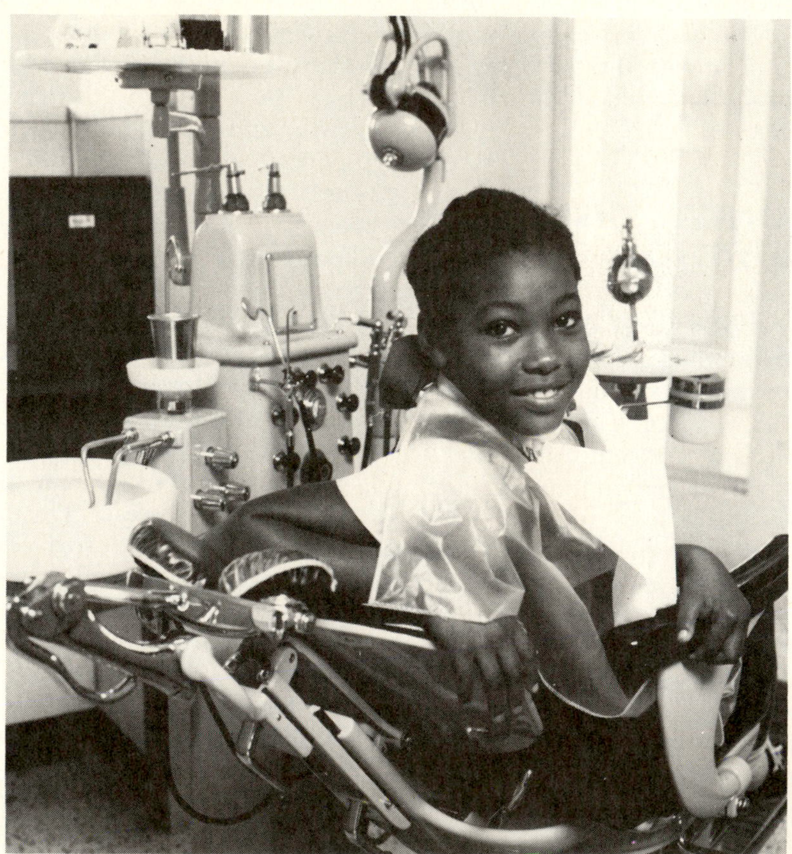

Figure 24–14 Foundations for good oral health are established in childhood. Preventive measures are most effective when instituted early, and these include good eating habits, as well as regular dental care for healthy smiles. (From World Health, Dec. 1973. Courtesy of WHO/P. Almasy.)

and use of dental floss. If plaque is thus broken up at least every 24 hours, the activity of the plaque bacteria will be stopped before the underlying enamel begins to decalcify. Tooth brushing is particularly important prior to sleep, for in sleep salivary production decreases, thus reducing the natural salivary buffers that help to partially counteract the effects of the acid-producing bacteria.

Preventive dietary measures include the following:

1. Avoid foods with the highest caries potentials (Table 24–2).
2. Use cheese, nuts, and raw vegetables and fruits instead of candy and cookies for snacks.
3. Avoid sticky and hard candy, sugared chewing gum, and frequent soft drinks.
4. Consume carbohydrates mainly at meals.

Table 24–2 "CARIES-POTENTIALITY" OF REPRESENTATIVE FOODS[a]

Food	*Total Sugar Content (Percent)*	*"Caries Potentiality"*
Caramel	64.0	27
Honey + bread + butter	19.0	24
Honey	72.8	18
Sweet cookies (biscuits)	9.0	18
Marmalade	65.3	10
Marmalade + bread + butter	16.3	9
Ice cream	2.4	9
Potatoes (boiled)	0.8	7
Potatoes (fried)	3.9	7
White bread + butter	1.5	7
Coarse rye bread + butter	2.3	7
Milk	3.8	6
Apple	7.5	5
Orange	6.5	3
Lemonade	9.3	2
Carrot (boiled)	2.4	1

[a]Adapted from Dunning, J. M.: *Principles of Dental Public Health.* Cambridge, Mass., Harvard University Press, 1970. Calculated from sugar concentrations in saliva and how long they remained high after eating each specific food. In general, those with the lowest scores should be used instead of those with highest scores if optimal dental health is desired.

5. Use a diet that provides good general nutrition, especially in children, for optimal developmental protection of the teeth.
6. Insure for all an adequate intake of fluoride in either water or supplement form.

Dental disease has been shown to be caused by factors that are accessible, controllable, and correctable. Improvement of individual dental health is within the reach of everyone, with the aid of the dentist. The amount of decay and gingival disease found is really an index of inadequate application of preventive procedures.

QUESTIONS

1. Name the parts of the tooth. What are some nutrients found in the tooth structures?

2. Describe how carbohydrates in the diet play a role in the formation of plaque. Why are the bacteria in plaque an important factor in causing dental caries?

3. Describe the "nursing bottle caries" syndrome and explain how it occurs.

4. Which foods are associated with a high incidence of dental caries?

5. Plan a lunch that may be carried from home, that provides approximately one-third of the daily nutrient needs of an 8-year-old child, and that will not foster dental caries.

6. How does fluoride aid in prevention of caries? How may fluoride be administered? Which method do you think is most practical? What is the fluoride level of the water in your community?

References

1. Sanders, H. J.: Tooth decay. Chem. Eng. News, *58*:30, 1980.
2. National Institute of Dental Research: *The Prevalence of Dental Caries in United States Children 1979–1980.* National Caries Program, Bethesda Maryland, 1982.
3. Menaker, L., and Navia, J. M.: Effect of undernu-

trition during the perinatal period on caries development in the rat. J. Dent. Res., *52*:680, 1973.
4. Strontium, other trace elements and dental caries Nutr. Rev., *36*:334, 1978; Curzon, M. E. J.: Combined effect of trace elements and fluoride on caries: changes over ten years in northwest Ohio (U.S.A.) J. Dental Res., *62*:96, 1983.
5. Hardwick, J. L.: Brit. Dent. J., *108*:9, 1960.
6. Read, T., and Knowles, E.: Brit. Dent. J., *64*:185, 1938.
7. Caldwell, R. C.: J. Dent. Res., *49*:1293, 1970.
8. Hamada, S., and Slade, H.: Biology, immunology, and cariogenicity of *Streptococcus mutans*. Microbiol. Rev., *44*:331, 1980.
9. Gustafsson, B. E., Quensel, C., Lanke, L., et al.: Acta Odont. Scand., *11*:232, 1954.
10. Dunning, J. M.: Principles of Dental Public Health. Cambridge, Mass., Harvard University Press, 1970.
11. Scheinin, A., and Makinen, K. K.: Turku Sugar Studies I-XXX. Acta Odont. Scand., *33*:1, 1975; also see papers on xylitol, sorbitol, and other sugar substitutes in Caries Res., *17*:335, 340, 365, and 369, 1983.
12. Sreebny, L. M.: The sugar-caries axis. Intern. Dent. J., *32*:1, 1982; Sreebny, L. M.: Sugar and human dental caries, World Rev. Nutr. Dietet., *40*:19, 1982; Scheiham, A.: Sugars and dental decay. Lancet, *I*:873, 1983.
13. Cooperative program on foods, nutrition and dental health. J. Amer. Dent. Assoc., *97*:239, 1978.
14. Caan, B.: Dietary recommendations for the maintenance of dental health. Med. Clin. No. Amer., *63*:1087, 1979; Newbrun, E.: Sugar and dental caries, Clin. Prev. Dent., *4*(no. 3):11, 1982.
15. Bibby, B. G.: J. Amer. Dental Assoc., *90*:121, 1975.
16. Kleinberg, I.: Prevention and dental caries. J. Prev. Dent., *5*:9, 1978.
17. Shern, R. J., Driscoll, W. S., and Korts, D. C.: Enamel biopsy results of children receiving fluoride tablets. J. Amer. Dent. Assoc., *95*:310, 1977.
18. Thylstrup, A., et al.: Enamel changes and dental caries in 7-year-old children given fluoride tablets shortly after birth. Caries Res., *13*:265, 1979.
19. Schrotenboer, G. H. Fluoride benefits—after 36 years. J. Amer. Dent. Assoc., *102*:473, 1981.
20. Horowitz, H. S.: Combinations of caries-preventive agents and procedures. J. Dent. Res., *59*:2183, 1980; Wei, S. H., and Kanellis, M. J.: Fluoride retention after sodium fluoride mouthrinsing by preschool children. J. Amer. Dental Assoc., *106*:626, 1983
21. Heifetz, S. B., Self-applied fluorides for use at home. Clin. Prev. Dent., *4*:6, 1982.
22. Walsh, D. C.: N. Eng. J. Med., *296*:1118, 1977.
23. Committee on Nutrition, American Academy of Pediatrics: Fluoride supplementation: revised dosage schedule. Pediatrics, *63*:150, 1979.
24. Erickson, J. D.: Mortality in selected cities with fluoridated and non-fluoridated water supplies. New Eng. J. Med., *298*:1112, 1978.
25. Rogot, E., et al.: Trends in urban mortality in relation to fluoridation status. Amer. J. Epidem., *107*:104, 1978.
26. Isman, R.: Fluoridation: strategies for success. Amer. J. Pub. Health, *71*:717, 1981; *Fluoridation.* Summit, N.J., American Council on Science and Health, 1983.

Dental Journals for Additional Reading[5]

Other reliable references to current dental health research and its application are most likely to be found in recent issues of such journals as:

Advances in Caries Research
American Journal of Orthodontics
Archives of Oral Biology
British Dental Journal
Caries Research
Community Dentistry and Oral Epidemiology
Dental Abstracts
Dental Clinics of North America
Fluoride
International Dental Journal
Journal of the American Dental Association
Journal Canadian Dental Association
Journal of Dental Research
Journal of Periodontology
Journal of Periodontal Research
Journal of Public Health Dentistry
Scandinavian Journal of Dental Research

[5]The American Dental Association, 211 E. Chicago Ave., Chicago, Ill. 60611, is a good source of additional applied information.

25 Malnutrition: A Global Perspective

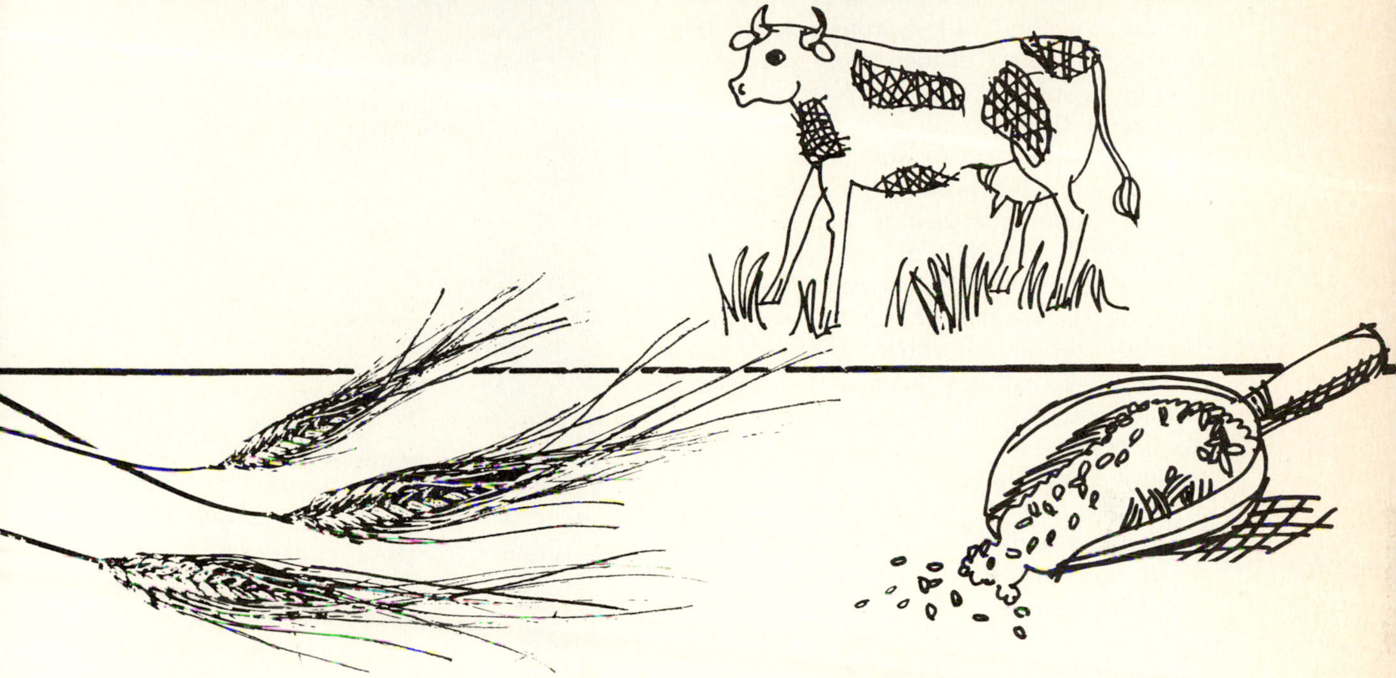

Two types of malnutrition can be found in all countries: the malnutrition of poverty and that of affluence—a convenient classification that calls attention to the characteristic extreme syndromes. At one extreme are the poor, often living in abject misery, for whom undernutrition is only one aspect of general deprivation. At the other extreme are the affluent, whose easy access to food and comfortable lifestyle lead to overnutrition and the diseases associated with it. While both types of malnutrition are found throughout the world, their prevalence and severity differ markedly from country to country. Furthermore, undernutrition is also to be found among people who are in a position to be adequately nourished, and overnutrition occurs among those who are less than truly affluent. Usually, however, discussion of world malnutrition focuses on the two extreme conditions that are readily recognizable and with which we have become familiar through television and other news media. Yet between the extremes of undernutrition and overnutrition, there is a continuum of deficiency, adequacy, and excess. Wherever malnutrition is manifest, there is usually a larger number of people whose intake is borderline and who are at risk of overt malnutrition if their life situation deteriorates at all.

WHO ARE THE MALNOURISHED?

Vulnerability to manifest malnutrition is conditioned by various characteristics of a person's situation. For example, all over the vast savannah areas of Africa, where the staple foods are cereals and legumes, the lives of millions of people are conditioned to the rhythm of the rains, the harvest, and the preharvest "hungry months," when grain is scarce and when they must look to the perenially available but low-protein cassava for their major source of food (see Fig. 25–1).

Some people are exposed to seasonal fluctuation in the amount and sources of nutrients available and to work stress and disease. Others are exposed to, or are at risk of, natural disaster, or their socioeconomic status makes them subject to loss of income and vulnerable because of poverty. Thus, for these reasons we may be able to identify sections of a population who in various ways are in danger of manifest malnutrition. Among them some will be undernourished to a lesser degree that will produce no clinical symptoms but that still may affect their reproductive and child-rearing capacity, their resistance to or recovery from disease, their activity and work output, and their attitudes and behavior.

Policies to reduce malnutrition must clearly aim at reducing the numbers who are at risk as well as treating those who are manifestly malnourished. Unless the at-risk population is reduced, malnutrition will continue to be manifest. Moreover, the consequences of less than severe malnutrition will have a continuing effect on those societies whose demography, disease patterns, work productivity, and social behavior are thus affected (see Fig. 25–2). There are clearly limits to the effectiveness of attempts to tackle specific aspects of this situation singly. Poverty and accompanying malnutrition have effects that can be inferred, but the evidence of causal relationships is diffuse, and the social effects of malnutrition have as yet hardly been researched (1).

There are problems in the assessment of nutrition status of populations. Some of the methods that might be used to evaluate the status of individuals—their tissue stores and

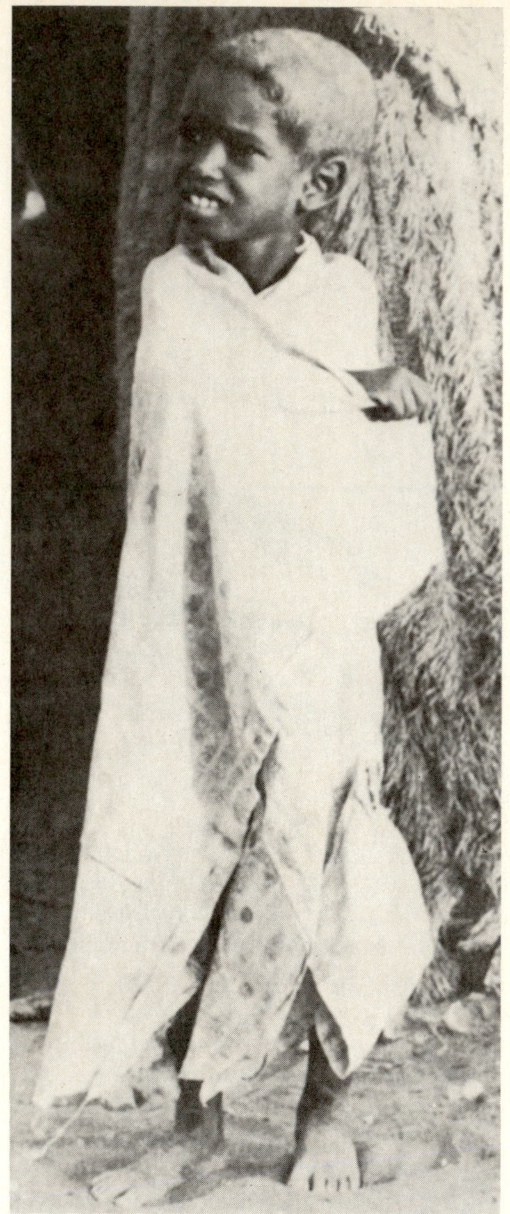

Figure 25–1 In the language of the Iteso people of Eastern Uganda, each month of the year is given a descriptive name. The preharvest month of May, when the granaries are empty, is called "the month when the children wait for food." It is in these hungry months, when the millet crop is growing, that many children, weakened by malnutrition, die of illnesses that well-nourished children would easily survive. (Courtesy of UNICEF/T. S. Satyan.)

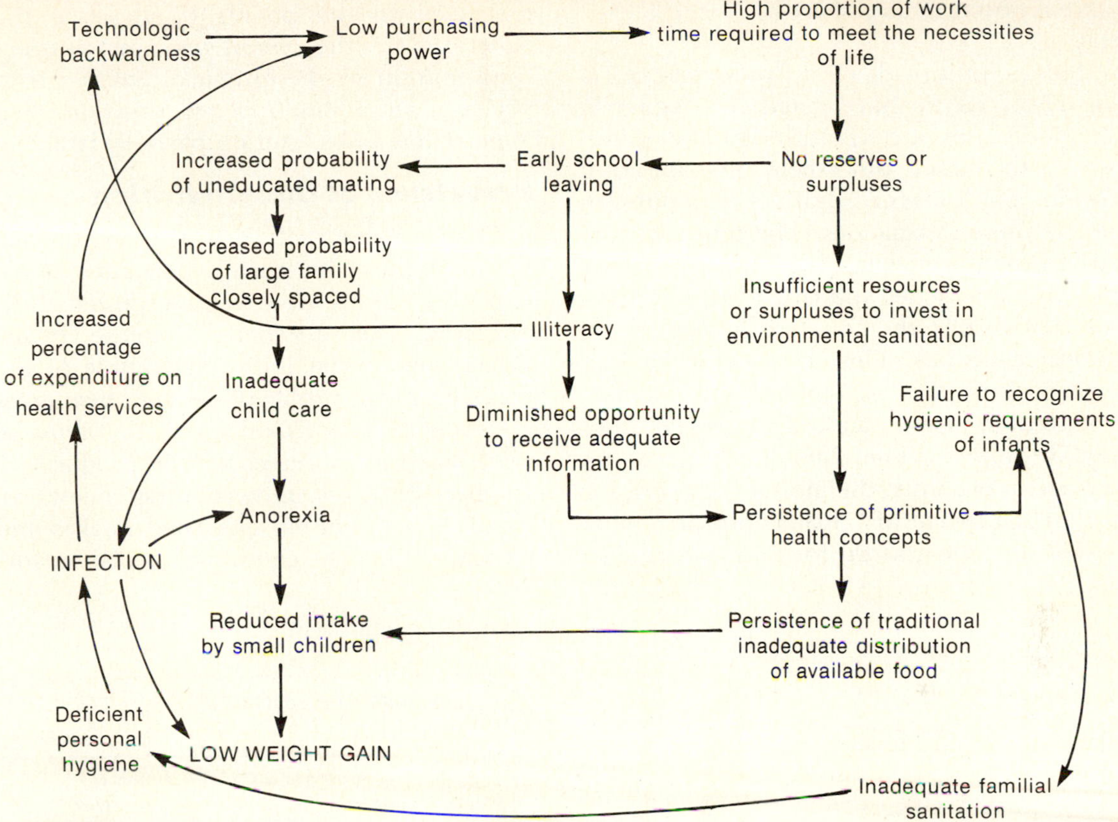

Figure 25–2 This flow chart brings out the interdependence of health, nutrition, and socioeconomic status and the mutually reinforcing and cumulative effects of the contribution of each element to sustaining the poverty condition. What this diagram does not illustrate is the impact of individual and family poverty, and its characteristic malnutrition, on the community as a whole—the overall impact on demography, disease, work productivity, social activity, attitudes, and social cohesion. (Redrawn from Cravioto, J., and DeLicardie, E. R. Malnutrition in early childhood, Food Nutr. No. 4, 1976.)

biochemical indicators especially—are expensive and impractical for application to large populations. Assessment of individual and household food intakes is also expensive.

Attempts are often made to assess the prevalence of malnutrition in a country by comparing national food consumption data with estimated per capita needs. Neither of the statistics being compared is fully accurate. For example, consumption statistics may be faulty owing to erroneous data on farm food yields, diversion of food to alcohol production, and so on; per capita needs may include wrong assumptions about physical activity and sizes and ages of the population—even the census figures may be in error. But even if the information were accurate, aggregative data could not provide an accurate diagnosis of malnutrition. These statistics can only indicate whether or not the food consumed would have been sufficient if it had been equitably distributed according to need—an assumption we know to be invalid. Even in affluent societies, foods such as steak and strawberries are not evenly divided among the people, and in the poor countries, the poorest segment does not receive a proportionate share of even the basic staples.

This point is made clear by the data in Table 25–1. As we have noted in Chapter 7, some diseases are characteristically associated with obesity and others with undernutrition. The causes of death in a population reflect these associations. The mortality rate from heart disease and hypertension is high in affluent societies and that from infectious diseases is low; the converse is true of the poorer countries. This contrasting situation is seen also within a country due to unequal distribution of food and of health and other welfare services. The Union of South Africa is such an example: the mortality pattern for whites is like that of Canada and the United States, and the pattern for nonwhites is like that seen in the poorer countries of the Americas. Yet the overall per capita nutrient consumption of the Union of South Africa places it in a much better situation than Mexico and Cuba, and on par with Israel.

Prevalence of Undernutrition

The limitations of such aggregative data for estimating the magnitude of the nutrition problem are now well recognized. Nevertheless, two questions continue to be posed. First, what is the magnitude of the undernutrition problem? Second, how great is the deficiency of food supply that must be made good by increases in food production? In attempting to answer these questions, comparisons between estimated intakes and estimated needs continue to be made,

Table 25–1 MORTALITY PATTERNS AND NATIONAL FOOD CONSUMPTION STATISTICS FOR REPRESENTATIVE COUNTRIES[a]

		Canada	*United States*	*Mexico*	*Guatemala*	*Union of South Africa*		
Food energy available, kcal/cap/day	1957–59	3040	3120	2410	2175	2620		
	1969–71	3307	3462	2701	2049	2767		
	1978–80	3358	3652	2803	2064	2827		
Causes of death: rate per 100,000 population						Asian	Colored	White
Diarrheal dis., enteritis	1966[b]	3.6	3.9	92.2	242.8	61.8	341.6	11.4
	1978[c]	0.9	0.9	86.2	209.4	279.5[d]		6.8
Measles	1966	0.2	0.1	18.2	105.8	9.8	21.1	1.1
	1978	0	0	9.9	70.0	25.2		0.4
Tuberculosis respiratory	1966	3.0	3.6	19.4	25.7	15.3	75.2	5.2
	1978	0.6	1.0	11.8	11.5	45.6		2.6
Heart disease, ischaemic	1966	240.8	320.0	18.8	15.2	78.1	67.6	205.5
	1978	215.6	294.3	20.4	9.6	87.8		205.3
Mortality: 1978 rate per 100,000 live births								
Maternal		6.4	9.6	108.2	83.9	90.1	150.4	14.5
Infant <1 year		11.9	13.8	52.0	76.9	35.6	122.1	20.9

[a]Data from FAO Production Yearbook and UN Demographic Yearbook.
[b]1966 statistics except Union of South Africa, 1964.
[c]1978 statistics for Canada and US, 1977 for Guatemala, 1976 for Mexico, and 1971 for Union of South Africa, as in 1980 Yearbook.
[d]Union of South Africa no longer lists causes of death separately for Asian and colored population.

Table 25–2 NUMBER OF PEOPLE CONSUMING INSUFFICIENT ENERGY, AND ENERGY DEFICITS IN DEVELOPING COUNTRIES, BY REGIONS, 1965*

Region	*Population with Daily Energy Deficits*				*Total Daily Energy Deficit (Thousand Millions) kcal*
	More Than 250 kcal		*Fewer Than 250 kcal*		
	Millions of People	Average Deficit	Millions of People	Average Deficit	
Low estimate:					
Latin America	55	450	58	131	32
Asia	563	364	173	116	225
Middle East	75	407	16	94	32
Africa	151	380	39	72	61
Total	844		286		350
High estimate:					
Latin America	87	783	26	211	74
Asia	563	503	0	0	283
Middle East	48	906	25	60	45
Africa	151	570	0	0	86
Total	849		51		488

*Adapted from Reutlinger, S., and Selowsky, M.: *Malnutrition and Poverty: Magnitude and Policy Options.* World Bank Occasional Papers, No. 23. Baltimore, Johns Hopkins University Press, 1976.

though on a more disaggregated basis. Thus, in a World Bank study (2), Reutlinger and Selowsky attempt to calculate the number of people with different levels of energy deficiency by using estimates of the relationship between income and energy consumption and estimates of numbers at different income levels in various countries. Such disaggregation leads to considerable upward revision of previous estimates of the numbers of undernourished based on more aggregative procedures. The estimates quoted here (Table 25–2, Fig. 25–3) have been challenged,[1] and there is as yet no general agreement about an appropriate definition of nutritional adequacy. Nevertheless, whatever criteria or calculation procedures are used, estimates of the numbers of undernourished in the world are measured in hundreds of millions. Moreover, while the methods used in attempting to predict the number of people who will be malnourished in future years are also crude and questionable, the general expectation is that the numbers, of moderately malnourished at least, will grow.[2]

Food Supply

While the magnitude of the numbers of malnourished poses problems in definition as well as in estimation, it may be necessary to reformulate the question, "How great is the deficiency of food supply that must be made good by an increase in food production?" (See Fig. 25–4.) In posing the question in this way, one makes the assumption that if the energy value of food supply were in-

[1]See the reviews by Sukhatme (3) and Payne (4) of Reutlinger and Selowsky. Sukhatme attempts to establish a new criterion of "inadequacy" with regard to energy intake. Using this criterion he reduces the estimate for the number of malnourished in one country for which the calculations are presented (Brazil) by half. It should be noted that the FAO (5), using different reasoning, produced an estimate of 460 million malnourished in the world in 1970—a figure more in line with Sukhatme's than with Reutlinger and Selowsky's.

[2]The FAO estimates that there will be 600 to 800 million malnourished in 1985, which corresponds to their estimate of 460 million in 1970 (5).

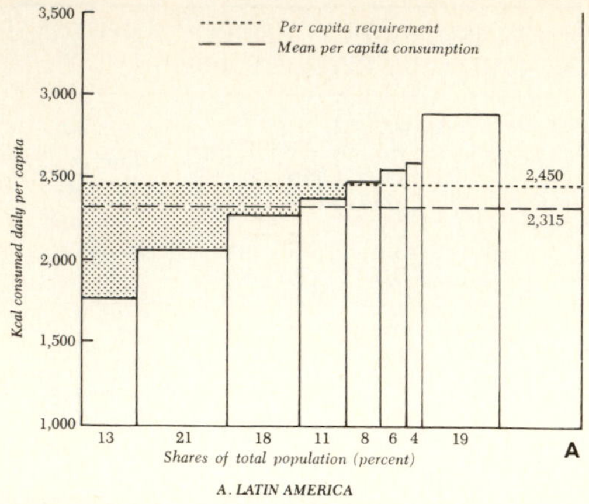

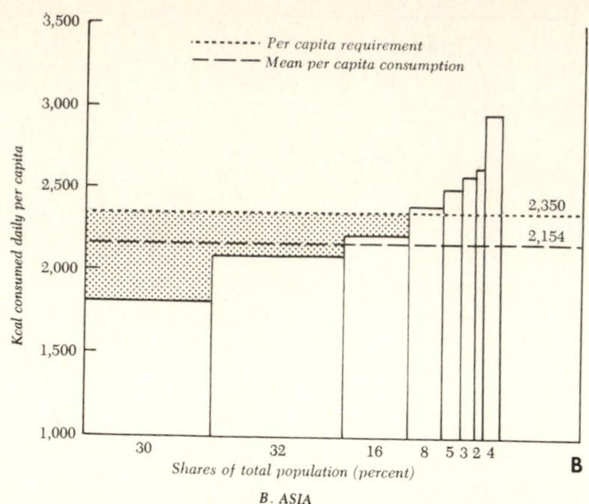

Figure 25–3 Income distribution and calorie consumption, Third World regions, 1965. The relationship between mean per capita consumption and per capita requirement gives only a rough indication of the extent of malnutrition. A, energy consumption by income groups, Latin America (low estimate); B, energy consumption by income groups, Asia (low estimate) (2).

creased by at least the sum of individual deficits, then these individual deficits would be corrected. But this is not necessarily so. Increasing food supply may not, in itself, reduce malnutrition.

Changing food supply implies changes also in the amounts of labor, fertilizer, and other inputs used in food production, which mean changes in people's incomes (farmers, farm laborers, and employees in fertilizer factories, marketing firms, etc.). This in turn produces changes in the demand for food, in food prices, and in people's consumption. If the increase in food supply is achieved without an accompanying rise in the employment rate, or perhaps even achieved by mechanization or technologies that displace people from employment, then increases in food supply may be associated with little or no reduction in the numbers of malnourished. Food prices may fall, and this will ease the position of those whose cash incomes are sustained. But a fall in food prices will adversely affect others: Farmers who normally sell some small percentage of their crop to meet cash needs will be worse off and may have to sell more food and keep less for themselves; farm laborers who find that there is less work being offered by small farmers may be quite badly affected (see Fig. 25–5). The most critical factor, therefore, is whether the purchasing power of the poorly nourished is increased.

While we need to increase food supplies, we need most critically to raise the incomes of the very poor. For this reason, the world food problems cannot be solved simply by increasing the food production of the rich nations. (Or by North Americans eating less meat!) Increasing the production of rich or even modestly comfortable farmers in poor countries may also not help much to reduce malnutrition if the increase in production does not create extra incomes for those who are extremely poor. Thus, there may be *no* increase in food supply that alone will eliminate malnutrition. A plan to eradicate malnutrition, however, will include an increased food supply, one that will be available for people to buy when they have enough income to meet their needs.

When people have more than enough to meet their needs, they will spend more on food than is necessary (6). People with higher incomes buy more expensive foods, including especially animal products whose pro-

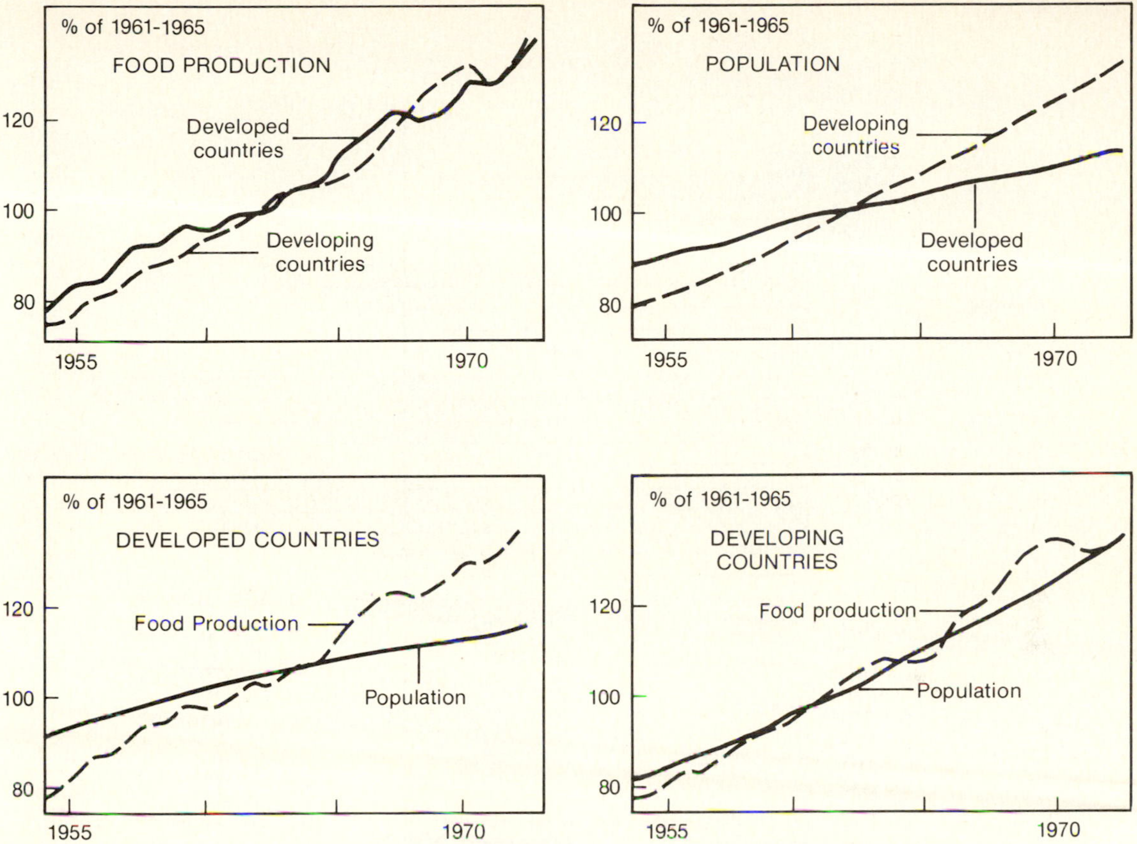

Figure 25–4 Peoples of the developed and developing countries have not fared equally from the roughly equal growth in food production. In the developed countries, production has increased much faster than population, boosting production per capita. In the developing countries, population gains have absorbed nearly all of the production increase; production per capita has improved only slightly. (From U. S. Department of Agriculture. Data exclude communist Asia.)

duction has often required considerable amounts of grain. Therefore, as incomes rise, the direct and indirect consumption of food also rises. In addition, as demand for foods increases as a result of rising incomes, so prices increase unless supplies keep pace.

In rich countries, governments are often more concerned about the prospect of falling food prices. Measures have been taken to discourage increases in U.S. food grain production, and many major food-producing countries adopt such measures. The fear is that without them prices would be depressed. In the world as a whole we can expect shortages in some places and at some times, and there is even a risk of recurrence of the temporary global shortfall in supply that occurred in 1972–1974; but *the problem of malnutrition is not a problem of the world's inability to produce food.* Even those poor countries where malnutrition is rife mostly have productive potential in excess of their present realized output. But measures to increase output must be related to those designed to raise the economic status of the malnourished. If they are not, there is likely to be only limited success in relieving malnutrition because, unless production is exported, there will be no market to absorb and sustain the increase in production.

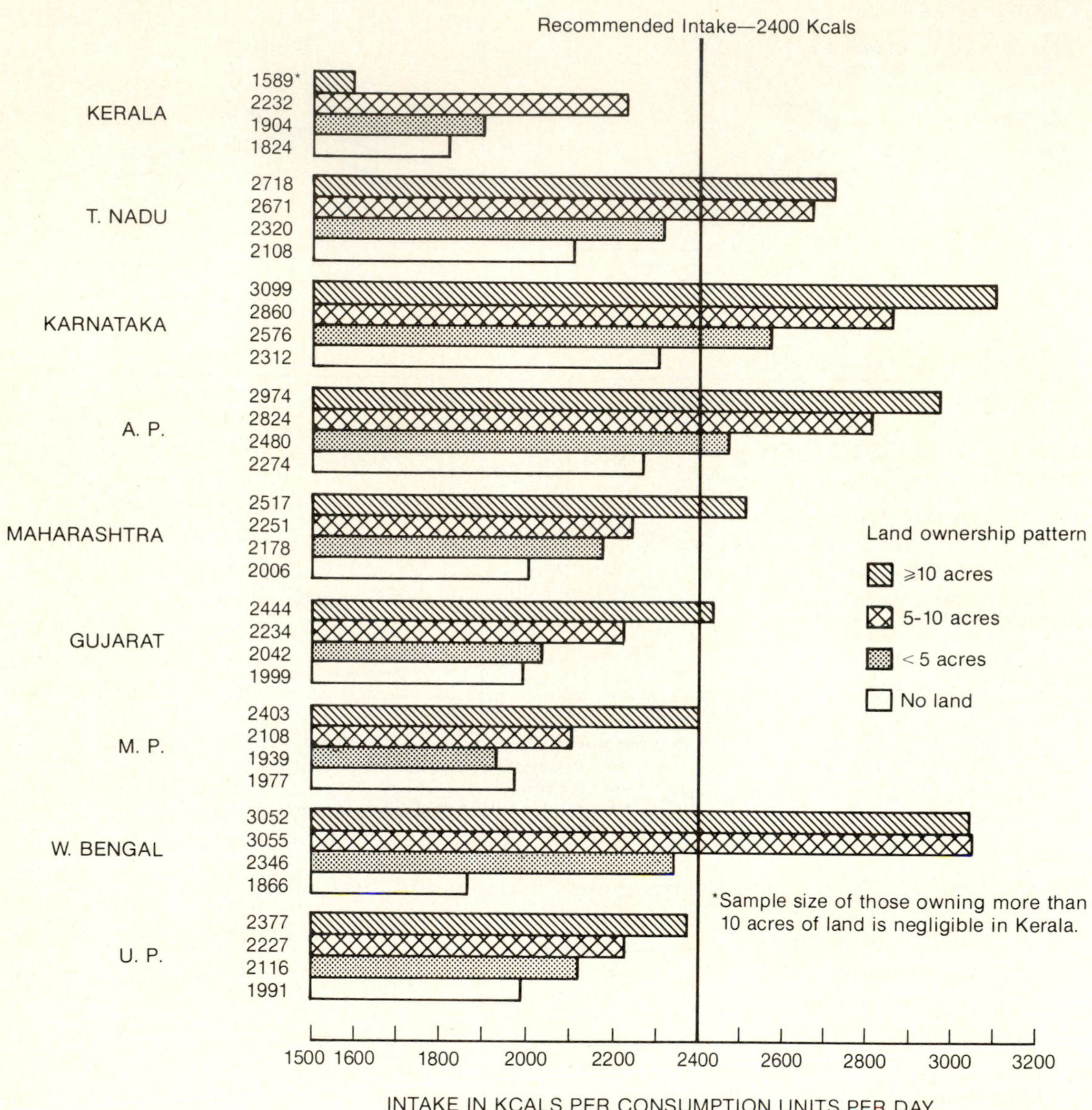

Figure 25–5 Energy intake according to land ownership in India. Regions differ in productivity, resources, and income, but in each case landless laborers and small landholders have the poorest food intakes. (From National Institute of Nutrition, Hyderabad–500 007, India.)

POLICIES AND PROGRAMS FOR REDUCING MALNUTRITION

Policies and programs for reducing malnutrition must address themselves to: (1) the correction of manifest malnutrition; (2) the prevention or amelioration of crises of famine and hunger, which produce episodes of malnutrition; (3) the improvement of the conditions of those who are at risk, in order to reduce their numbers; and (4) the reversal or attenuation of the social and economic trends that are creating at-risk groups.

Obesity is the present focus of concern with regard to the malnutrition of affluence, because the disorders associated with it diminish the enjoyment of life, shorten the life span, and impose heavy medical costs on the individuals affected and on the society (see Chap. 7). The basic condition of overeating in relation to need must be remedied. This is clearly a matter of bringing individual energy intake and expenditure into balance. Such a measure requires individuals to change their life-styles. The scope of present programs is limited to efforts to encourage and support individuals in achieving the necessary changes. If it were governmental policy to prevent obesity, then other programs might be devised. Greater emphasis might be placed on encouraging active participant sports and recreations in the school system and in the communities, in lieu of major investment in spectator sports arenas and diversions involving little or no activity. Measures designed to decrease use of personal vehicles might encourage walking. As far as intake is concerned, use of high-energy foods might be reduced by a number of coordinated actions involving taxation, advertising regulation, shelf placement in stores, and improved health education.

The correction of malnutrition which stems from inadequate intakes is a very different matter. While it is true that some individuals and families have more success in securing adequate diets than others in similar situations, there are often severe limits to what people can do to help themselves. Nevertheless, the first question to be asked in seeking to develop programs to improve nutrition is, "What can be done by the people themselves to improve their nutrition status?" The answers are likely to vary considerably, depending upon the situation being examined. For example, improvement in infant feeding may require different measures in different situations. While there are common classes of problems (e.g., overdilution of weaning foods), the specific measures designed to meet them will vary and will need to take account of such factors as available foods, mothers' preoccupations, conditions in which food is prepared, possibilities of regular visits to clinics, and so on.

Community health services have, potentially, a major role to play in preventing manifest malnutrition (see Fig. 25–6). As well as treating the most common ailments, they might do much by providing prenatal, perinatal, and infant care; this would include vitamin, mineral, and food supplements, especially during pregnancy; regular weighing and measuring of infants and advice to mothers; and immunization against common childhood diseases, whooping cough and measles especially. When accompanied by measures to improve sanitation and drinking water supplies, the net impact of these health services on morbidity and mortality—especially infant mortality—can be considerable. And the cost can be small. At the same time, it may not be easy to insure that the poorest people, those most susceptible to malnutrition, will be served. A general problem of applied nutrition programs is that it is much easier to reach people who have some resources (for example, access to transportation) than it is to get the program ben-

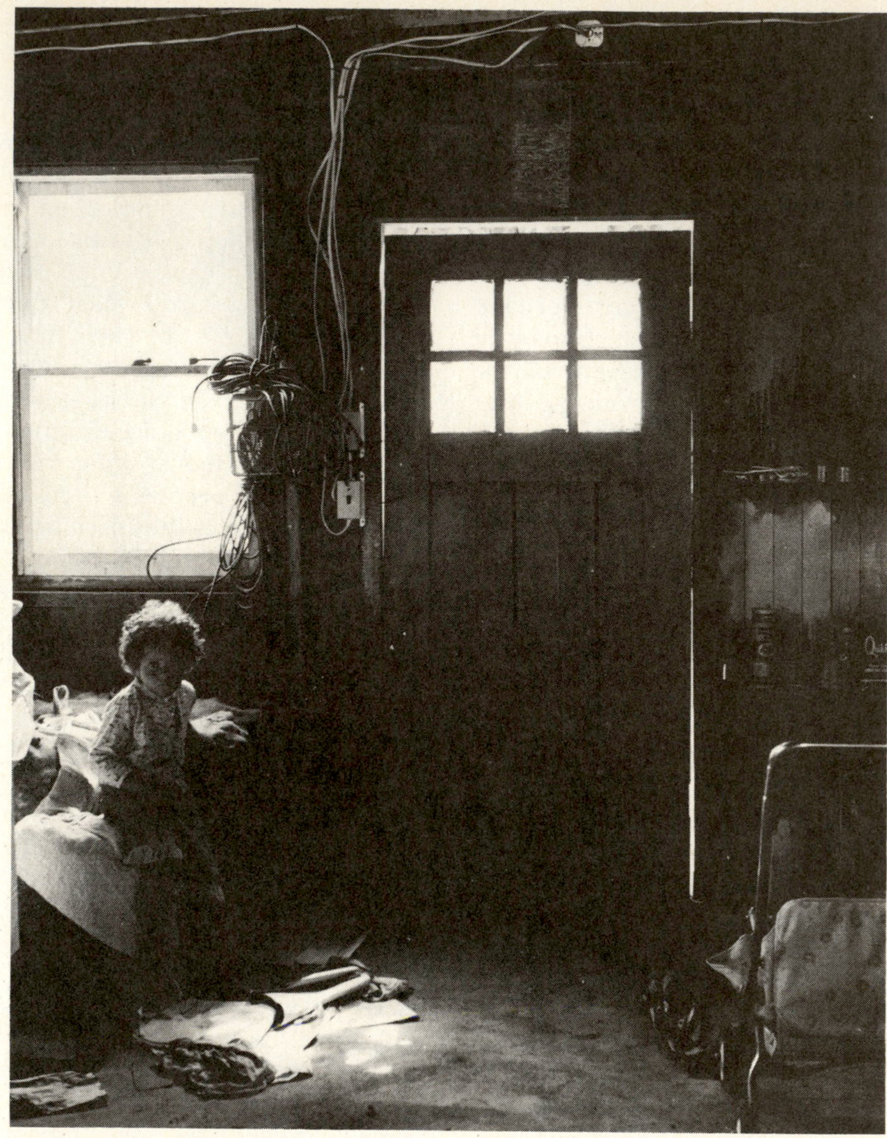

Figure 25–6 Migrant farm worker's housing, Tulare County, California, 1969. The WHO has observed that "Disease and sociopsychological problems are to a great extent determined by the immediate environment of the family—its home. A clean and functional house, not necessarily expensive but adapted to the environment and favoring a healthy way of life for its inhabitants, is an important factor in the prevention of many of the diseases and other problems now afflicting large population groups in rural areas, and even more so in city slums." (Courtesy of Donald Heiny, San Francisco, and University of California, Berkeley.)

efits to the poorest, especially those in remote rural areas.

For many households the key question will be how to manage resources in order to secure an adequate food supply through the year or how best to utilize and allocate an inadequate food supply over time and among household members. In some cases, understanding of nutritional requirements is poor and nutrition education is needed.

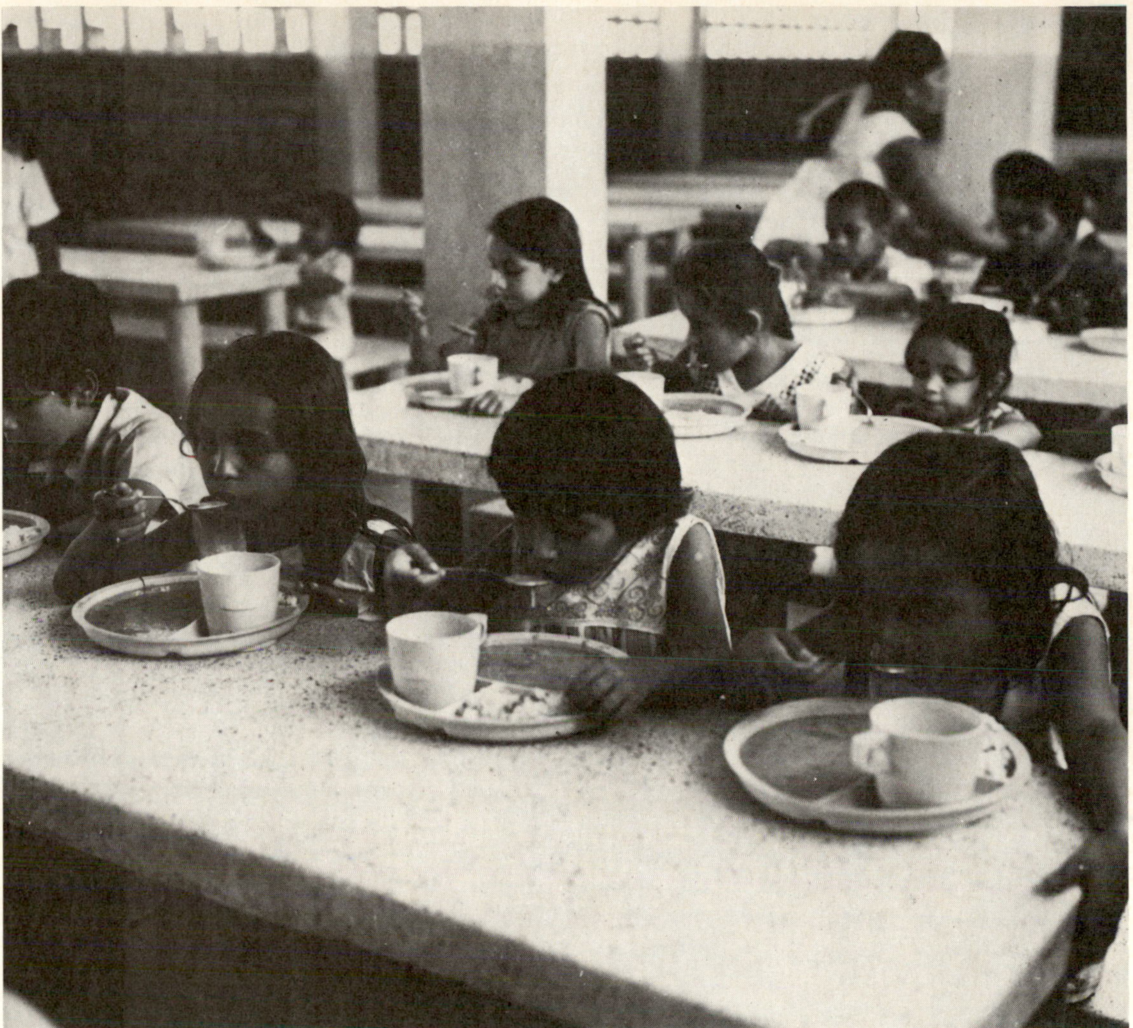

Figure 25–7 Colombian children eating a school meal supplemented by food from the World Food Programme. The supplementary food also serves as an object lesson in nutrition. (Photo WHO/P. Almasy.)

Usually this will be best related to other programs, for example, community health programs, school and literacy programs, and farmer education. (See Fig. 25–7.)

Not all households, with the resources and the employment opportunities open to them, will be able to provide for themselves adequately and continuously. Thus, the next step concerns the possibilities of social action to provide households with a basis for self-reliance. Clearly, the sorts of actions that might be considered again will vary. Households that have some land may be aided in ways different from those that are landless. But for the most part, the problem is one of how to help people so that they are capable of producing their own means of subsistence—that is, how to direct to them the resources and employment opportunities that will enable them to feed themselves.

Preventive Measures

It is necessary to examine the specific situations in which malnutrition becomes manifest in order to see what can be done. But there are, nevertheless, measures that can be applied not to specific groups of people but to whole communities or to large sections of the population. Where people eat purchased, centrally processed foods—flour, sugar, salt, tea—it is possible to fortify these with vitamins and minerals if there is a demonstrated need to do so (for example, in areas where specific deficiency diseases such as anemia, rickets, goiter, and so on are prevalent). The cost of adding iodine to salt, for example, is very low. Such programs can be very effective. A comprehensive world review of endemic goiter in 1960 produced an estimate of 200 million people suffering from this disease and although some progress has since been made, it remains a serious problem in central Africa, the Middle East, Southeast Asia and seventeen of the twenty-six countries of Latin America (7).

Protein–energy deficiencies are not readily tackled by such means, however. Generally, the diets that people traditionally eat, in the quantities usually eaten, provide enough of both protein and energy. When protein–energy malnutrition (PEM) is a problem among people eating traditional diets, it is usually because people are not eating enough to meet their energy requirement. They may not, therefore, be eating enough to meet their protein needs either.

When energy intakes are too low, there is usually little value in fortifying to increase protein intake. But there have been such fortification schemes, many of which have been based on the fortification of cereal grains with lysine. Such schemes have not been generally successful as measures to reduce PEM, however: In some cases the malnourished were precisely those who did not purchase flour; or, if the malnourished were energy-deficient, the improvement in protein quality did not significantly affect their status, or, in many cases, overall diets were found to be neither protein-deficient nor, specifically, lysine-deficient. A review by Gershoff of experience with cereal grain enrichment programs claims that they have disappointed expectations and concludes "that we lack considerable fundamental information concerning the etiology of malnutrition in developing countries and that this deficiency will have to be corrected before effective public health nutrition programs which will meet their needs can be developed" (8).

The shortcomings of lysine fortification programs apply in part also to attempts to improve the protein quality of food grains through breeding new high-protein or high-lysine varieties. Problems associated with the utilization of these varieties include the maintenance of recessive genetic traits in field crops, and increased vulnerability to disease during growth or to pests in storage. Costs may include reduced yield and the increased requirements of fertilizer. There is seldom reason for believing that there is any great value to strengthening cereal protein quality in this way. Generally, the protein levels of cereal staples are adequate for adults and even for school children. For very young children, the characteristics that often determine whether or not cereal gruels are nutritionally satisfactory are the stickiness and texture of the cereals and therefore the degree of dilution found necessary for feeding, and the bulkiness of a diet based largely on cereals. Thus, from the point of view of child feeding, these characteristics should receive the attention of plant breeders. But there may be better ways of approaching this problem than through plant breeding. What can and should be done will need to be determined for each situation.

In the past there have been many feeding programs designed to improve the protein intake of the malnourished. Often these have been based on the use of protein-rich foodstuffs provided as supplements—dried skim milk and soy protein especially have been the basis of cookies and biscuits for distribution to children of preschool and school age, or of weaning foods. Concern for the protein content of these foods may have been exaggerated, and such programs have been criticized for being too expensive for poor country governments to sustain independently, and for inducing new habits that are too expensive for poor people to be encouraged to follow. Above all, they have been said to be unnecessary, since, it is claimed, local, traditional diets offer the cheapest and most acceptable sources and are adequate in protein if sufficient food is eaten to meet energy requirements. Such arguments need to be reviewed in relation to specific situations, but there are undoubtedly cases in which the criticisms cited have been valid.

Strategies

Applied nutrition programs of various kinds[3] will be necessary in the attempt to cure manifest malnutrition, but malnutrition will continue to be manifest unless the at-risk population can be reduced. Reducing this group will call for measures to: (1) improve overall nutrition status of those who are marginal; (2) increase the resources of those who have insufficient means to meet the stresses to which they are exposed; and (3) eliminate or alleviate these stresses. Following the World Food Conference in November 1974,[4] several countries have instituted nutrition surveillance measures, one of the purposes of which is to give early warning of impending crises and the emergence of malnutrition. Such measures are clearly required if floods, droughts, and other natural and social disasters are to be forestalled and their consequences attenuated. Many countries have longstanding regular procedures to this end,[5] and the attempt to develop these and to provide international support for countries facing such crises is clearly desirable.

Helping people in emergencies is only one of many things that need to be done, however, for malnutrition is not associated simply with famines and disasters. Somehow the poor and the vulnerable must be made less poor and more self-reliant. To see this as primarily a matter of raising incomes, however, is to oversimplify and to miss the point of what has to be accomplished. If we attempt to forecast future trends in malnutrition, the most significant feature affecting these trends is likely to be the growth in the number of households with insufficient land from which to feed themselves and without employment and earnings adequate to support their families. In part, this is a consequence of growing populations, but the process of economic development itself tends to displace people from land, and, in many countries, the rate of growth of jobs is much less than the rate of growth of the labor force.[6] There is nothing new in this. What is new, however, is that whereas in the past the process promoted massive international migrations, such migrations can no longer occur.

[3]We have in mind here such programs as mother-child care schemes, school feeding programs, fortification programs, and nutrition education programs.

[4]See Resolution V of the United Nations World Food Conference, Rome, 1974 (Table 25–3).

[5]India, for example, has a Famine Code dating from the eighteenth century, which defines administrative duties and procedures for forewarning of disaster and for appropriate response.

[6]According to Lester Brown, if the 1982 rate of world economic growth (2 percent, which was less than half the 1968 rate) continues, nearly half the world people will have lower incomes and standards of living will fall. The majority of those most seriously affected live in third world countries where populations are expanding at 3 percent or more per year, far outstripping economic growth (9).

Table 25–3 RECOMMENDATIONS CONTAINED IN RESOLUTION V OF THE UNITED NATIONS WORLD FOOD CONFERENCE (ROME 1974)

The World Food Conference,

—*recognizing* that malnutrition is closely linked to widespread poverty and inadequate social and institutional structures, and that its effects are aggravated by infectious diseases and the lack of environmental sanitation; and that increased agricultural production and increased incomes may not by themselves lead to improved nutrition; and that to this end a more just and equitable distribution of food and incomes is essential, among nations as well as within countries among their various social categories, . . .

Recommends

1. That all governments and the international community as a whole, in pursuance of their determination to eliminate within a decade hunger and malnutrition, formulate and integrate concerted food and nutritional plans and policies aiming at the improvement of consumption patterns in their socioeconomic and and agricultural planning, and for that purpose assess the character, extent and degree of malnutrition in all socioeconomic groups as well as the preconditions for improving their nutritional status. . . .

3. That governments, . . . in close cooperation with agricultural production programmes, initiate new or strengthen existing food and nutrition intervention programmes, on a scale large enough to cover on a continuing basis a substantial part of the vulnerable groups;

4. That governments include nutrition education in the curricula for educational programmes at all levels . . .

5. That governments strengthen basic health, family well-being and planning services and improve environmental conditions, including rural water supplies and the elimination of water-borne diseases; and provide treatment and rehabilitation of those suffering from protein-energy malnutrition;

6. That governments consider the key role of women and take steps to improve their nutrition, their educational levels and their working conditions; and to encourage them and enable them to breast-feed their children;

7. That governments review special feeding programmes . . . to determine the desirability and feasibility of undertaking such new programmes, or improving existing ones, particularly among the vulnerable groups (children, pregnant and nursing mothers), but also for schoolchildren, workers and others; such programmes should promote increased local food production and processing thereby stimulating local initiative and employment and should also include an element of nutrition education . . .

9. That governments should explore the desirability and feasibility of meeting nutrient deficiencies, through fortification of staples or other widely consumed foods, . . . should establish a worldwide control programme aimed at substantially reducing deficiencies of Vitamin A, iodine, iron, folate, Vitamin D, riboflavine, and thiamine as quickly as possible; . . .

11. That governments take action to strengthen and modernize consumer education services, food legislation and food control programmes and the relevant aspects of marketing practices, aiming at the protection of the consumer (avoiding false and misleading information from mass media and commercial fraud), and that they increase their support of the Codex Alimentarius Commission . . .

13. That a global nutrition surveillance system be established by FAO, WHO and UNICEF to monitor the food nutrition conditions of the disadvantaged groups of the population at risk, . . .

14. That governments consider establishing facilities and funds for applied nutrition research related to economic, cultural, social and medical aspects of production, processing, preservation, storage, distribution and utilization of food. . . .

Thus, in the long run, the solution of the problem of malnutrition is to be found not in development itself but in the choice of development strategies that aim, as a prime objective, to absorb people productively on the land or in other employment—especially those who would otherwise be very poor. Unless we succeed in this, the numbers at risk will grow and so also will the prevalence of manifest malnutrition. If we succeed in reducing malnutrition in a way that contributes to improved life expectancy, then we may also make a significant contribution to creating the conditions in which birth rates might be reduced and populations brought into equilibrium.

As we have noted, the ideas just presented differ significantly from the current conventional opinions about the solution to the world's malnutrition problem. Conventionally, the problem continues to be viewed as a failure of food production to keep pace with the growth of population. In the last twenty years food supplies have grown faster than population. The increase in malnutrition during this same period is ascribable to the increase in the number of people neither contributing to nor having a fair share of this supply. Conventional solutions to the problem, as it is usually perceived, involve a massive transfer of technology from rich to poor countries in order to increase food production in the poor countries. To this end attempts are made to mobilize political support for rich countries to give, and poor countries to receive, technical assistance and material aid. While such assistance may help to reduce malnutrition, it is of utmost importance that the measures promoted should succeed in absorbing productively those people who cannot now produce, or afford to buy for themselves, the food that they need. If we do not succeed in this, extra food supplies will have little impact on reducing malnutrition. Indeed, if this is not done, the depression in food prices that would result from substantial increases in supply is likely to cause economic depression and the aggravation of malnutrition in many rural areas.

Recognition of these arguments could lead to the identification of new strategies for rural development and for increasing food supplies (10). Such strategies, when supplemented with community health programs, could have a major effect on reducing malnutrition. Malnutrition is not inevitable. There are enough food and resources to eliminate it now. When this is fully comprehended, when the full consequences of poor nutrition are recognized, and when it is more widely understood what needs to be done in order for people to be adequately fed, we can hope that governments, international agencies, and people will insist upon taking the action necessary to eliminate malnutrition.

In opening the Second World Food Congress (The Hague, 1970), A. H. Boerma, (11) then Director-General of the Food and Agriculture Organization, reminded the delegates of the continued existence of two contrasting worlds:

> There is a world of luxury foods, and another where food is the only luxury known.
>
> There is a world of well-appointed homes, and another where people sleep in rat-infested huts or sprawled in their thousands on city streets.
>
> There are those who are free to speculate—and lose—vast fortunes and those who are enslaved to the moneylender for pitifully small sums.
>
> There are those who live for the end of the working week and those who live in hopes of one beginning.

This theme was carried through the World Food Conference convened in Rome in 1974, from which emerged a series of resolutions calling for specific actions to eliminate hunger and malnutrition within a decade (Table 25–3). Little progress has been made in reaching the objective, and the time is nearly gone. The Food and Agriculture Organization's Boerma urged:

> As a first step, every effort must be made, every device must be used, to make as many people as possible—both the privileged majorities in the richer countries and the privileged minorities in the poorer ones—realize that development is something which is not just morally desirable but in their own best interests—and, even more, in the interests of their children and their children's children. For what future is there for a world of which by far the larger part is in misery and revolt? How can even the privileged enclaves live at ease surrounded by the constant threat—and the enactment—of violence? Where will the richer countries find the new markets they are now starting to scurry for if the others are too poor to buy from them?
>
> What is required is that people everywhere should see the value, not only to others but also to themselves, of thinking in wider terms

than those of their own immediate interests. Although for the majority this would amount to nothing less than an internal political revolution within their own minds, recent history has shown that it can be done and that it can produce successful results. Some of the richer countries of the world have now evolved into welfare states, with elaborate systems of social services. And this was as much the result of common sense as of compassion. What is now needed—only more urgently—is that the same kind of thinking that has prevailed in these societies should be applied to produce similar results in what is now a single world society.

In speaking of the changes that are needed in human attitudes toward development, I have so far been talking about individuals. But that is only part of the story. Equally essential are the changes needed in the attitudes of governments. For the structure of world society and the problems confronting it mean that, except for a handful of multinational corporations, it is only governments that are large enough to bring into play sufficient resources sufficiently fast to make a real impact.

Not only have these changes not been made, but we appear to be *losing* ground: The deteriorating economies and political forces of the United States and Mexico seem, at the time this is being written, to be worsening the lot of vast numbers of under- and unemployed people. In other places, such as Somalia, and Cambodia, natural and man-made disasters seem to be causes of the desperate circumstances many face. Aid from the richer to the poorer countries is less generous and perhaps more politically focused than it was ten or fifteen years ago. There is less support given to the international agencies for their important work. (See Table 25-4.)

Table 25–4 UNITED NATIONS FOOD AND NUTRITION PROGRAMS

United Nations Childrens Fund (UNICEF)

UNICEF is the largest agency in the world devoted exclusively to the welfare of children. Its purpose is to provide assistance in developing programs of long-range benefit to children, primarily in economically underdeveloped areas. Aid is supplied in the form of basic medical equipment for health centers and schools, vaccines and antibiotics to control disease, insecticides, clothing, multivitamins and powdered milk to combat malnutrition, and equipment for local dairy and food-processing industries. UNICEF's budget is based on a two-year allotment. Seventy-five percent (75%) of the funds come from contributions by the governments of 132 countries, with the remainder coming from the general public through donations and sale of Christmas cards and other items.

Food and Agricultural Organization (FAO)

The FAO endeavors to raise world food and nutrition standards through research, technical assistance, and the reallocation of surpluses. Work and funding are on a cooperative basis with the 136 member nations. Local governments share in the cost of the projects and provide facilities for the work. FAO pays salaries and travel expenses.

World Food Program

The World Food Program, a joint undertaking of the United Nations and the FAO, is an experimental program established as the food aid agency of the UN system. The program's assistance is provided exclusively on a project basis. Food aid has been used primarily to support developing countries in their efforts to implement economic and social development projects. Voluntary contributions to the regular resources of the program are required to make up a budget that exceeds $1 billion. Despite the steady growth of the World Food Program, requests for food aid in developing countries have only been partially met.

World Health Organization (WHO)

WHO serves as a research organization and as an information center on world medical developments. WHO assistance includes the strengthening of national health services, the training of health workers; disease control; maternal and child health; the improvement of sanitation and water supplies; and the organization of mental health services. WHO is financed primarily from annual contributions made by member governments on the basis of the ability to pay. The United States provides approximately ⅓ of the budget. Grants for special purposes have been made on occasion by private foundations and individual governments.

From Environmental Nutrition Newsletter.

In his 1980 Farewell Presidential Address to the Board of Governors of the World Bank, Robert McNamara (12) reminded them that:

> What these countless millions of the poor need and want is what each of us needs and wants: the well-being of those they love; a better future for their children; an end to injustice; and a beginning of hope.

He concluded with a quote from George Bernard Shaw:

> You see things, and say why? But I dream things that never were, and I say why not?

References

1. Calloway, D. H.: Functional consequences of malnutrition. Rev. Infect. Dis., *4*:763, 1982.
2. Reutlinger, S., and Selowsky, M.: *Malnutrition and Poverty: Magnitude and Policy Options.* World Bank Occasional Papers, No. 23. Baltimore, Johns Hopkins University Press, 1976.
3. Sukhatme, P. V.: *Measurement of Poverty Based on Nutritional Needs.* Proceedings, Indian Agricultural Economics Association Conference, 1977.
4. Payne, P. R.: Review of Reutlinger and Selowsky's article. Food Policy, *2*:164, 1977.
5. U.N. World Food Conference, 1974: Extracts of papers. Reprinted in Food and Nutrition, Vol. *1,* No. *1,* 1975. Rome, FAO.
6. Périssé, J., and Kamoun, A.: The price of satiety. A study of household consumption and budgets in Tunisia. Food Nutr., 7(2): 3, 1981.
7. Stanbury, J. B., et al.: Endemic goitre and cretenism: public health significance and prevention. WHO Chronicle, *28*:220, 1974.
8. Gershoff, S. N.: *Evaluation of Cereal Grain Enrichment Programs.* Paper, Western Hemisphere Nutrition Congress, Quebec, Canada, August 15, 1977.
9. Brown, L. R.: *Population Policies for a New Economic Era.* Worldwatch Institute, 1983.
10. Johnston, B. F., and Clark, W. C.: *Redesigning Rural Development. A Strategic Perspective.* Baltimore, Johns Hopkins University Press, 1982.
11. Boerma, A. H.: Keynote Address, Second World Food Congress, The Hague, June, 1970. In *FAO Studies in Food and Population.* FAO Economic and Social Development Ser., No. 1, p. 129. Rome, 1976.
12. McNamara, R. S.: Address to Board of Governors. World Bank, Washington, D.C., September 30, 1980.

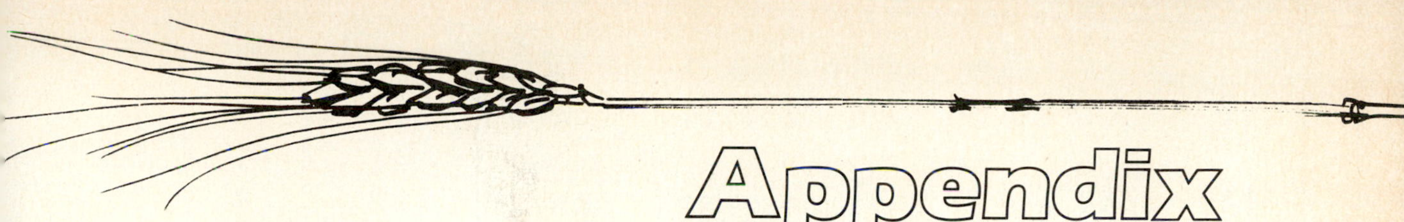

Appendix

CONTENTS

Table

Table 1A SUMMARY EXAMPLES OF RECOMMENDED NUTRIENT INTAKES FOR CANADIANS*[a][b]

				Fat-Soluble Vitamins			Water-Soluble Vitamins			Minerals				
Age	Sex	Weight (kg)	Protein (g/day)	Vitamin A (RE/day)[d]	Vitamin D (μg/day)[e]	Vitamin E (mg/day)[f]	Vitamin C (mg/day)	Folacin (μg/day)[g]	Vitamin B_{12} (μg/day)	Calcium (mg/day)	Magnesium (mg/day)	Iron (mg/day)	Iodine (μg/day)	Zinc (mg/day)
Months														
0–2	Both	4.5	11[h]	400	10	3	20	50	0.3	350	30	0.4[i]	25	2[j]
3–5	Both	7.0	14[h]	400	10	3	20	50	0.3	350	40	5	35	3
6–8	Both	8.5	16[h]	400	10	3	20	50	0.3	400	45	7	40	3
9–11	Both	9.5	18	400	10	3	20	50	0.3	400	50	7	45	3
Years														
1	Both	11	18	400	10	3	20	65	0.3	500	55	6	55	4
2–3	Both	14	20	400	5	4	20	80	0.4	500	65	6	65	4
4–6	Both	18	25	500	5	5	25	90	0.5	600	90	6	85	5
7–9	M	25	31	700	2.5	7	35	125	0.8	700	110	7	110	6
	F	25	29	700	2.5	6	30	125	0.8	700	110	7	95	6
10–12	M	34	38	800	2.5	8	40	170	1.0	900	150	10	125	7
	F	36	39	800	2.5	7	40	170	1.0	1000	160	10	110	7
13–15	M	50	49	900	2.5	9	50	160	1.5	1100	220	12	160	9
	F	48	43	800	2.5	7	45	160	1.5	800	190	13	160	8
16–18	M	62	54	1000	2.5	10	55	190	1.9	900	240	10	160	9
	F	53	47	800	2.5	7	45	160	1.9	700	220	14	160	8
19–24	M	71	57	1000	2.5	10	60	210	2.0	800	240	8	160	9
	F	58	41	800	2.5	7	45	165	2.0	700	190	14	160	8
25–49	M	74	57	1000	2.5	9	60	210	2.0	800	240	8	160	9
	F	59	41	800	2.5	6	45	165	2.0	700	190	14[k]	160	8
50–74	M	73	57	1000	2.5	7	60	210	2.0	800	240	8	160	9
	F	63	41	800	2.5	6	45	165	2.0	800	190	7	160	8
75+	M	69	57	1000	2.5	6	60	210	2.0	800	240	8	160	9
	F	64	41	800	2.5	5	45	165	2.0	800	190	7	160	8
Pregnancy (additional)														
1st Trimester			15	100	2.5	2	0	305	1.0	500	15	6	25	0
2nd Trimester			20	100	2.5	2	20	305	1.0	500	20	6	25	1
3rd Trimester			25	100	2.5	2	20	305	1.0	500	25	6	25	2
Lactation (additional)			20	400	2.5	3	30	120	0.5	500	80	0	50	6

*From *Recommended Nutrient Intakes for Canadians, 1983*.

[a]Recommended intakes of energy and of certain nutrients are not listed in this table because of the nature of the variables upon which they are based. The figures for energy are estimates of average requirements for expected patterns of activity. For nutrients not shown, the following amounts are recommended: thiamin, 0.4 mg/1000 kcal (0.48 mg/5000 kJ); riboflavin, 0.5 mg/1000 kcal (0.6 mg/5000 kJ); niacin, 7.2 NE/1000 kcal (8.6 NE/5000 kJ); vitamin B_6, 15 μg, as pyridoxine, per gram of protein; phosphorus, same as calcium.

[b]Recommended intakes during periods of growth are taken as appropriate for individuals representative of the mid-point in each age group. All recommended intakes are designed to cover individual variations in essentially all of a healthy population subsisting upon a variety of common foods available in Canada.

[c]The primary units are grams per kilogram of body weight. The figures shown here are only examples.

[d]One retinol equivalent (RE) corresponds to the biological activity of 1 μg of retinol, 6 μg of β-carotene or 12 μg of other carotenes.

[e]Expressed as cholecalciferol or ergocalciferol.

[f]Expressed as *d*-α-tocopherol equivalents, relative to which β- and γ-tocopherol and α-tocotrienol have activities of 0.5, 0.1 and 0.3 respectively.

[g]Expressed as total folate.

[h]Assumption that the protein is from breast milk or is of the same biological value as that of breast milk and that between 3 and 9 months adjustment for the quality of the protein is made.

[i]It is assumed that breast milk is the source of iron up to 2 months of age.

[j]Based on the assumption that breast milk is the source of zinc for the first 2 months.

[k]After the menopause the recommended intake is 7 mg/day.

TABLE 1B. Summary of Recommended Dietary Intakes for Young Men and Pregnant and Lactating Women*
(demonstration of diversity of RDAs of 41 countries)

Nutrient	Number of countries	RDI								
		For men, 26–29 years			Addition for women, 23–30 years, during pregnancy			Addition for women, 23–30 years, during lactation		
		Lowest	Highest	Mean	Lowest	Highest	Mean	Lowest	Highest	Mean
Energy (kcal x 10)	41	Japan (250)	Argentina, FRG, Poland, Portugal (320)	284.0	Hungary (+0)	USSR (+0–70)	+29.7	W. Pacific (+20)	USSR (+90–110) Poland (+110)	+63.0
Protein (g)	41	FAO/WHO (37)	Czechoslovakia (105)	66.1	Hungary (–5)	USSR (+23–56)	+13.5	FRG (+0/kg) Hungary (+5)	USSR (+36–43)	+23.5
Vitamin A (μg R.Eq. x 10)	41	Japan, Korea (60)	Poland, Portgual, USSR, W. Pacific (150)	91.0	14 countries (+0)	Bulgaria (+100)	+15.6	China (+20)	India (+192)	+51.6
Vitamin D (μg)	31	Australia, India, Korea, Poland, UK (0)	China, France, Hungary, NZ, Thailand (10.0)	4.40	Australia, China, Hungary, India, NZ, Thailand, W. Pacific (+0)	Korea, Poland, UK, USSR (+10.0)	+5.71	Australia, China, Hungary, India, NZ, Thailand, W. Pacific (+0)	Korea, Poland, UK, USSR (+10.0)	+5.71
Vitamin E (mg)	12	Canada (9)	Poland, USSR (20)	12.0	France, FRG, NZ (+0) USSR (+0–5)	USSR (+0–5)	+1.9	France, NZ (+0)	Czechoslovakia, FRG (+8)	+3.0
Thiamin (mg)	41	Bolivia, Colombia, Indonesia, Japan, Malaysia, Singapore, Thailand (1.0)	USSR (1.7–1.8)	1.26	Hungary, NZ (+0)	USSR (+0.6–1.5)	+0.21	Hungary, NZ, W. Pacific (+0.1)	USSR (+0.6–1.5)	+0.33
Riboflavin (mg)	41	Philippines (1.3)	USSR (2.2–2.4)	1.65	Hungary (+0)	USSR (+1.1–1.5)	+0.29	W. Pacific (+0.1)	USSR (+1.1–1.5)	+0.48
Niacin (mg)	40	FRG (9–15)	Mexico (24)	18.3	Hungary, NZ (+0)	China, Poland (+6)	+2.2	W. Pacific (+1)	Bulgaria (+10)	+4.6
Vitamin B6 (mg)	14	FRG (1.8)	France, Scandinavia, USA (2.2)	2.03	9 countries (+0.5)	USSR (+2.2–2.3)	+0.76	FRG (+0.4)	USSR (+2.2–2.3)	+0.65
Folate** (μg x 10)	27	India (10)	All others except UK (20)	19.4	Canada (+5)	NZ (+30)	+18.8	Poland (+0)	FRG (+30)	+9.4
Vitamin B12 (μg)	25	India (1.0)	FRG, Poland (5.0)	2.52	India (+0.5)	USSR (+8.0–13.0)	+1.58	16 countries (+0.5)	FRG (+2.5)	+0.81
Vitamin C (mg)	41	16 countries (30)	Bulgaria (95)	47.4	FAO/WHO, NZ, W. Pacific (+0)	USSR (+85–90)	+21.4	FAO/WHO, NZ, W. Pacific (+0)	Bulgaria (+100)	+27.4
Calcium (g)	41	W. Pacific (0.4)	Bulgaria (1.1)	0.61	Indonesia (+0.1)	Argentina (+1.4)	+0.55	Indonesia (+0.1)	China (+1.4)	+0.61
Phosphorus (g)	10	Taiwan (0.6)	USSR (1.6)	0.96	GDR (+0.2)	USSR (+0.4–1.4)	+0.48	Uruguay, USA (+0.4)	USSR (+2.2)	+0.68
Magnesium (mg x 10)	13	GDR (25)	USSR (50)	34.5	Canada (+3)	USSR (+43)	+12.2	France (+5)	USSR (+73)	+15.8
Iron (mg)	42	Finland, W. Pacific (5)	India (24)	10.0	9 countries (+0)	Chile (+18)	+3.7	Turkey (–3)	Hungary, Thailand, Uruguay (+10)	+3.1
Iodine (μg)	14	France (120)	USSR (100–200) NZ (200)	145.4	NZ (+0)	FRG (+50)	+23.8	NZ (+0)	Bolivia, Colombia, FRG, Poland, Uruguay, USA (+50)	+38.1
Zinc (mg)	9	Czechoslovakia (8)	USSR (10–15) Italy, NZ, Spain, Uruguay, USA (15)	13.1	GDR (+1–3)	Czechoslovakia (+8)	+4.8	Canada (+7)	GDR (+13)	+10.0

* From Truswell, A.S., et al.: Food and Nutrition Bull. (U.N.), *4*(4): 34, 1982. This reference lists the sources of RDA tables for 41 countries.

**Either the figure taken as free folate or 50 per cent of the figure given for total folate is used.

Table 1C FAO/WHO RECOMMENDED INTAKES OF SELECTED NUTRIENTS*

RECOMMENDED DAILY INTAKES OF VITAMIN C, VITAMIN D, VITAMIN B-12, AND FOLACIN

		Vitamin C (mg)	*Vitamin D[2] (μg)[3]*	*Vitamin B-12 (μg)*	*Folacin (μg)*
Infants	0– 6 months[1]	20	10	0.3	40
	7–12 months	20	10	0.3	60
Children,	1– 3 years	20	10	0.9	100
	4– 6 years	20	10	1.5	
	7– 9 years	20	2.5	1.5	
	10–12 years	20	2.5	2.0	
Boys, Girls	13–19 years	30	2.5	2.0	200
Adults,	men, women	30	2.5	2.0	200
	pregnancy	50[4]	10[4]	3.0	400
	lactation	50	10	2.5	300

[1]It is accepted that for infants aged 0–6 months breast-feeding by a well-nourished mother is the best way to satisfy the requirements of vitamin C, vitamin B-12 and folacin, but not of vitamin D.

[2]Adequate exposure to sunlight may partially or totally replace dietary vitamin D.

[3]2.5 μg of cholecalciferol are equivalent to 100 IU of vitamin D.

[4]For 2nd and 3rd trimesters.

*From FAO/WHO: *Requirements of Ascorbic Acid, Vitamin D, Vitamin B_{12}, Folate, and Iron.* WHO Technical Report Series No. 452. Geneva, WHO, 1970. Also see *Handbook of Human Nutritional Requirements,* Geneva, WHO, 1974 for a discussion of those values.

Table 1C—(*Continued*) RECOMMENDED DAILY INTAKES OF IRON

		Amount of Iron Actually Absorbed (mg)	*Recommended Intake According to Type of Diet*		
			Less Than 10% of Calories from Animal Foods (mg)	10–25% of Calories from Animal Foods (mg)	More Than 25% of Calories from Animal Foods (mg)
Infants,	0– 4 months	0.5	[1]	[1]	[1]
	5–12 months	1.0	10	7	5
Children,	1–12 years	1.0	10	7	5
Boys,	13–16 years	1.8	18	12	9
Girls,	13–16 years	2.4	24	18	12
Adults,	men, nonmenstruating women	0.9	9	6	5
	menstruating women, pregnancy, lactation	2.8	28	19	14
Assumed upper level of absorption by normal individuals			10%	15%	20%

[1]Breast-feeding is assumed to be adequate.

Table 1C—*(Continued)* FAO/WHO RECOMMENDED INTAKES OF SELECTED NUTRIENTS*

RECOMMENDED DAILY INTAKES OF THIAMIN, RIBOFLAVIN, AND NIACIN*

Age	*Thiamin (mg)*	*Riboflavin (mg)*	*Niacin[1] Equivalents (mg)*
0–6 months[2]	–	–	–
7–12 months	0.4	0.6	6.6
1 year	0.5	0.6	7.6
2 years	0.5	0.7	8.6
3 years	0.6	0.8	9.6
4–6 years	0.7	0.9	11.2
7–9 years	0.8	1.2	13.9
10–12 years	1.0	1.4	16.5
13–15 (boys)	1.2	1.7	20.4
(girls)	1.0	1.4	17.2
16–19 (boys)	1.4	2.0	23.8
(girls)	1.0	1.3	15.8
Adults (man)	1.3	1.8	21.1
(woman)	0.9	1.3	15.2

*From FAO/WHO: *Requirements of Vitamin A, Thiamine, Riboflavin, and Niacin.* Geneva, World Health Organization Tech. Rep. Series No. 362, 1967. Recommendations are based on the following intakes per 1000 kcal: thiamin 0.4 mg; riboflavin: 0.55 mg; niacin equivalents: 6.6.

[1]A niacin equivalent is 1 mg niacin or 60 mg L-tryptophan.

[2]For children 0 to 6 months it is accepted that breast-feeding by a well-nourished mother is the best way to satisfy the nutritional requirements for thiamin, riboflavin, and niacin.

Introductory Notes for Table 2: Nutritive Value of Foods in Average Servings or Common Measures

Values for foods and nutrients are taken mainly from revised volumes of U.S.D.A. Agriculture Handbook No. 8 (Vols. 1–9, 1976–1982) and from preliminary data made available through the courtesy of Dr. F. Hepburn and the staff of the U.S.D.A. Human Nutrition Information Service. Additional values are from Adams, C. F.: *Nutritive Value of American Foods in Common Units.* U.S.D.A. Agriculture Handbook No. 456, 1975. The following are primary sources used for values not included in those handbooks:

Polyunsaturated fatty acids: Paul, A. A. and Southgate, D. A. T.: *McCance and Widdowson's The Composition of Foods.* 4th rev. ed., London, HMSO, 1978.

Magnesium: Watt, B. K., and Merrill, A. L.: *Composition of Foods–Raw, Processed, Prepared.* U.S.D.A. Agriculture Handbook No. 8, 1963.

Zinc: Murphy, E. W., Willis, B. W., and Watt, B. K.: Provisional tables on the zinc content of foods. J. Amer. Dietet. Assoc., 66:345, 1975; Freeland, J. H., and Cousins, R. J.: Zinc content of selected foods. J. Amer. Dietet. Assoc., 68:526, 1976.

Copper: Pennington, J. T., and Calloway, D. H.: Copper content of foods. J. Amer. Dietet. Assoc., 63:143, 1973.

Vitamin B-6, pantothenic acid, and vitamin B-12: Orr, M. L.: *Pantothenic Acid, Vitamin B-6 and Vitamin B-12 in Foods.* U.S.D.A. Home Econ. Res. Rpt. No. 36, 1969.

Folacin: Perloff, B. P., and Butrum, R. R.: Folacin in selected foods. J. Amer. Dietet. Assoc., 70:161, 1977; Hoppner, K., Lampi, B., and Perrin, D. E.: The free and total folate activity in foods available in the Canadian market. Can. Instit. Food Sci. Tech. J., 5:60, 1972; Hurdle, A. D. F., Barton, D., and Searles, I. H.: A method for measuring folate in foods and its application to a hospital diet. Am. J. Clin. Nutr., 21:1202, 1968; Toepfer, E. W., Zook, E. G., Orr, M. L., and Richardson, L. R.: *Folic Acid Content of Foods.* U.S.D.A. Agriculture Handbook No. 29, 1951.

A few values were abstracted from Pennington, J. A.: *Dietary Nutrient Guide.* Westport, Conn., Avi Publishing Co., 1976, from Church, C. F., and Church, H. N.: *Bowes and Church's Food Values of Portions Commonly Used.* 12th Ed., Philadelphia, J. B. Lippincott Co., 1975, and from Chinese Academy of Sciences: Table of Food Composition. Peking, 1962.

Values for some commercial foods were taken from information published by manufacturers for professional use. This information did not generally include data on the lesser studied nutrients, and in many cases we have assigned values to these from counterpart items.

We have provided information on some food combinations that are widely used (sandwiches, salads). Data represent our summation of ingredients or values given by fast-food purveyors.

Most values have been rounded because these figures are, at best, merely representative of foods typically consumed. The exact nutrient yield is affected by serving size, variety and breed, animal diets and plant fertilizers, environmental factors, and conditions of processing, storage, and the like. The data provided here should be used with this in mind.

Explanatory Notes, Table 2

[a]Symbols used are: tr = trace; u = unknown but thought to be present; 0 = absent or below detection limit.

[b]In bleached asparagus, vitamin A activity is 8 RE.

[c]All canned foods listed, except fruits, have salt added according to commercial practice, unless otherwise noted.

[d]Made with yellow maize-corn meal.

[e]Based on green variety.

[f]If added, approximately 375 RE vitamin A and approximately 15 mg vitamin C per 1 oz portion.

[g]Yellow variety; white products have essentially no vitamin A activity.

[h]No salt added.

[i]Vitamin A-fortified fluid milk has 140 RE per cup.

[j]Buttermilk has 320 mg sodium per cup.

[k]Zinc content of oysters may vary from 6 to 100 mg/100 gm, probably as a result of environmental conditions. Ascorbic acid content also is variable, from traces to 30 mg/100 gm.

Table 2 NUTRITIVE VALUE OF FOODS IN AVERAGE SERVINGS OR COMMON MEASURES

Food	Weight gm	Approximate Measure	Energy Kcal	Protein gm	Fat gm	Total Carbohydrate gm	Calcium mg	Phosphorus mg	Magnesium mg	Sodium mg	Potassium mg	Zinc mg	Copper mg	Iron mg	Total Vitamin A Activity RE	Thiamin mg	Riboflavin mg	Niacin mg	Vitamin B-6 mg	Pantothenic Acid mg	Folacin Total μg	Vitamin B-12 μg	Vitamin C mg	Polyunsaturated Fatty Acids gm
Almonds, chopped	15	12–15 nuts, 2 tbsp	90	3.0	8.0	3	35	75	40	1	115	0.2	0.1	0.7	0[a]	0.04	0.1	0.5	0.02	0.07	15	0	tr[a]	1.6
Apples, raw with skin	140	1 medium 3/lb	80	0.3	0.5	20	10	10	6	1	159	0.05	0.01	0.3	7	0.02	0.02	0.1	0.07	0.1	75	0	8	0.1
Apple juice, canned, no sugar added	125	½ c	60	0.1	tr	15	10	10	4	4	150	0.04	0.03	0.5	0	0.03	0.02	0.1	0.04	0.07	tr	0	1	0.03
Applesauce, sweetened	125	½ c	100	0.2	0.2	25	5	10	4	4	80	0.05	0.06	0.5	1	0.02	0.04	0.2	0.03	0.07	1	0	2	0.07
Apricots																								
Fresh	100	2–3 medium	50	1.4	0.4	11	15	20	8	1	300	0.3	0.09	0.5	270	0.03	0.04	0.6	0.05	0.2	9	0	10	0.08
Canned, with skin heavy syrup	85	3 halves, 1¾ tbsp juice	70	0.4	0.1	18	5	10	6	3	120	0.09	0.07	0.3	110	0.02	0.02	0.3	0.05	0.08	1	0	3	0.02
water pack	85	3 halves, 1¾ tbsp juice	20	0.6	0.1	5	10	10	6	2	160	0.09	0.07	0.3	110	0.02	0.02	0.3	0.05	0.08	2	0	3	0.03
Dried, sulfured, raw	30	6–8 medium halves	75	1.2	0.2	20	15	40	15	3	480	0.3	0.15	1.5	250	tr	0.05	1.0	0.06	0.3	3	0	3	0.03
Apricot nectar, canned	125	½ c	70	0.4	0.1	18	10	10	7	4	140	0.1	0.09	0.5	165	0.01	0.02	0.3	0.05	0.08	2	0	1	tr
Artichokes, French, boiled	120	1 large (300 gm as purchased)	30	3.0	0.2	12	60	85	u[a]	35	360	0.4	0.4	1.3	20	0.08	0.05	0.8	0.30	0.60	150	0	10	tr
Asparagus,[b]																								
Fresh, green, cooked	100	½ c cut, 6–7 spears	25	3.0	0.2	4	20	65	15	7	270	0.6	0.1	0.7	85	0.1	0.1	1.3	0.13	0.2	190	0	30	tr
Canned, salt[c] added	100	½ c cut, 6–7 spears	15	2.0	0.2	3	20	45	9	373	195	0.5	0.1	0.6	65	0.06	0.1	0.7	0.06	0.2	85	0	18	tr
Avocados	100	½ fruit 4 in long	160	2.0	15	7	10	40	40	10	600	0.4	0.2	1.0	60	0.1	0.1	1.9	0.3	1.0	60	0	8	2.0
Baby foods																								
Dinners	130	Contents 4½ oz jar																						
beef-noodle			70	3.0	2.0	9	12	35	9	35	60	0.5	0.04	0.5	140	0.05	0.05	0.9	0.06	0.3	65	0.1	2.0	u
beef-vegetable			100	7.0	5.5	5	15	62	10	45	180	1.7	0.1	0.9	140	0.04	0.08	2.0	0.10	0.3	7	0.6	2.0	u
vegetable-beef-cereal			60	2.5	1.0	10	20	50	8	60	100	0.5	0.04	0.5	50	0.06	0.05	1.0	0.07	0.3	2	0.3	1	u
Fruits and desserts	130	Contents 4¾ oz jar																						
applesauce-pineapple			50	0.1	0.1	13	5	8	4	3	100	0.02	0.04	0.3	3	0.03	0.03	0.1	0.05	u	2.5	0	36	0
custard pudding			110	2.0	2.5	20	70	60	70	80	60	0.4	0.06	0.3	8	0.02	0.1	0.1	0.03	0.3	7.5	u	1	u
fruit pudding			105	1.5	0.4	25	40	40	11	25	100	0.2	0.04	0.2	5	0.05	0.06	0.1	0.05	u	u	0.08	35	u
Bacon, broiled, drained	25	2 strips, thick	140	6.5	12.5	1	3	55	5	245	60	1.2	0.1	0.8	0	0.1	0.08	1.0	0.03	0.08	0.5	0.2	0	1.0
Bagels	60	4 in diameter	175	6.5	1.5	34	25	40	12	215	45	0.3	0.05	1.6	0	0.2	0.2	2.1	0.03	0.2	14	0	0	u
Bamboo shoots	100	¾ c	25	2.5	0.3	5	13	60	45	25	530	u	u	0.5	2	0.15	0.07	0.6	u	u	u	0	4	u
Bananas	115	1 medium	105	1.2	0.6	27	10	20	35	1	450	0.2	0.12	0.4	9	0.05	0.1	0.6	0.7	0.3	22	0	10	0.09
Beans																								
Canned, with pork and tomato sauce	130	½ c	160	8.0	3.5	25	70	115	35	590	270	1.0	0.2	2.3	15	0.10	0.04	0.8	0.4	0.1	30	0	3	u
Canned, with pork and sweet sauce	130	½ c	190	8.0	6.0	25	80	145	35	485	u	1.0	0.3	3.0	u	0.08	0.05	0.7	0.1	0.1	10	0	3	u
Green, snap, fresh or frozen,	65	½ c	15	1.0	0.1	3	28	15	13	3	105	0.1	0.03	0.6	30	0.04	0.05	0.2	0.03	0.1	30	0	6	tr
canned	65	½ c	15	0.9	0.1	3	20	15	8	260	80	0.1	0.06	0.4	30	0.01	0.03	0.2	0.03	0.1	12	0	2	tr
Lima, fresh or frozen, boiled	85	½ c	90	5.5	0.3	17	20	60	32	64	405	0.4	0.5	1.2	20	0.07	0.06	1.0	0.1	0.2	75	0	17	tr
Red, canned	125	½ c	120	7.0	0.5	20	35	140	35	4	335	1.0	0.2	2.3	tr	0.06	0.05	0.8	0.4	0.1	35	0	0	tr
Refried	120	½ c	230	8.5	12.5	25	50	165	35	340	360	1.0	0.2	2.3	tr	0.30	0.07	0.8	0.2	0.2	20	0	0	u
Soybeans, mature, dry, cooked	90	½ c (1 oz, dry wt.)	120	10.0	5.0	10	65	160	80	2	490	0.6	0.3	2.5	2	0.20	0.08	0.6	u	u	70	0	0	3.0

Food	Weight gm	Approximate Measure	Energy Kcal	Protein gm	Fat gm	Total Carbohydrate gm	Calcium mg	Phosphorus mg	Magnesium mg	Sodium mg	Potassium mg	Zinc mg	Copper mg	Iron mg	Total Vitamin A Activity RE	Thiamin mg	Riboflavin mg	Niacin mg	Vitamin B-6 mg	Pantothenic Acid mg	Folacin Total µg	Vitamin B-12 µg	Vitamin C mg	Polyunsaturated Fatty Acids gm
Bean sprouts, See *Sprouts*.																								
Beef																								
Corned, canned	80	2 slices each, 3 in × 2 × ¼ in	170	20.0	9.5	0	15	85	20	u	u	2.5	u	3.4	tr	0.02	0.20	3.0	0.08	0.5	2	1.5	0	0.4
hash, with potatoes	110	½ c	200	10.0	12.5	12	15	75	20	595	220	1.4	u	2.2	tr	0.01	0.10	2.5	0.08	0.6	u	0.8	0	u
Dried, creamed	120	½ c	190	10.0	12.5	9	130	170	40	880	190	1.8	u	1.0	130	0.08	0.20	0.8	0.6	0.7	u	u	1	u
Hamburger, broiled, lean, 21% fat	85	4/lb, raw wt.	240	20.0	16.5	0	10	160	20	50	220	3.7	0.07	2.6	10	0.07	0.20	4.5	0.4	0.3	3	1.5	0	0.7
very lean, 10% fat	85	4/lb, raw wt.	190	23.0	9.5	0	10	195	20	60	260	4.9	0.09	3.0	7	0.08	0.20	5.0	0.4	0.3	3	1.5	0	0.4
Roast, chuck, braised	85	3 oz	240	23.0	16.5	0	10	115	20	40	185	3.7	0.07	2.9	10	0.04	0.20	3.5	0.4	0.3	3	1.5	0	0.7
rib, U.S. choice	85	3 oz	380	17.0	33.5	0	10	160	20	40	190	3.1	0.07	2.2	20	0.05	0.10	3.0	0.3	0.3	3	1.5	0	1.4
Steak, broiled																								
round with fat	85	3 oz	220	24.5	13.0	0	10	215	25	60	270	5.0	0.09	3.0	7	0.07	0.20	5.0	0.3	0.4	3	2.2	0	0.6
sirloin with fat	85	3 oz	330	20.0	27.0	0	10	160	20	50	220	3.7	0.07	2.5	15	0.05	0.20	4.0	0.3	0.4	3	1.5	0	1.2
Beef stew, with vegetables	245	1 c	220	15.5	10.5	15	30	185	50	90	615	2.4	0.05	2.9	250	0.15	0.15	4.7	0.3	0.2	7	1.6	15	u
Beer	360	12 oz container	150	0.9	0	13	15	50	35	18	115	0.2	0.3	0.1	0	0	tr	1.8	0.2	0.2	20	0	0	0
Beet greens, boiled	75	½ c	15	1.0	0.2	2	70	20	80	55	240	0.5	0.1	1.4	370	0.05	0.10	0.2	0.08	0.2	20	0	10	tr
Beets, sliced, canned	85	½ c	30	0.8	0.1	7	1	10	10	240	145	0.2	0.1	0.5	tr	0.01	0.03	0.4	0.04	0.1	25	0	2	tr
Beverages. See *Carbonated beverages*, individual entries, and Table 3–6.																								
Biscuits, from mix, enriched	30	1 of 2 in diameter	100	2.0	3.6	15	5	120	4	375	30	0.1	0.02	0.6	0	0.1	0.1	1.0	0.01	0.1	2	0	0	u
Blackberries, boysenberries, etc., raw	70	½ c	35	0.5	0.3	9	25	15	14	0	140	0.2	0.1	0.4	12	0.02	0.03	0.3	0.04	0.2	4	0	15	tr
Blueberries, raw	70	½ c	40	0.5	0.3	10	5	10	4	5	65	0.1	0.04	0.1	7	0.03	0.03	0.3	0.03	0.1	5	0	9	tr
Bokchoy. See *Pakchoy*.																								
Brazil nuts, raw	30	6 large nuts	180	4.0	19.0	3	55	195	65	tr	205	1.4	0.4	1.0	tr	0.30	0.03	0.5	0.05	0.1	tr	0	0	7.4
Bread																								
Boston brown, canned	45	1 slice, ½ in thick	95	2.5	0.6	20	40	70	u	115	130	u	u	0.9	3	0.05	0.03	0.5	u	u	u	0	0	u
Corn, from mix	55	2-½ in square	180	4.0	6.0	30	135	210	10	265	60	0.2	0.02	0.8	15[d]	0.10	0.10	0.8	0.03	0.2	5	0.1	0	u
Cracked wheat	25	1 slice	65	2.3	0.9	12	15	30	9	110	35	0.4	0.08	0.7	tr	0.09	0.09	0.9	0.02	0.1	u	0	tr	u
French, Vienna Italian, enriched	25	1 slice	70	2.4	0.9	13	25	20	5	140	20	0.2	0.04	0.8	tr	0.12	0.09	1.0	0.01	0.9	9	0	tr	u
Fry bread,																								
Indian enriched	60	1 piece, medium	200	4.0	7.5	28	80	80	u	305	35	u	u	1.0	0	0.10	0.09	1.3	0.02	0.2	10	0	0	u
Raisin, enriched	25	1 slice	70	2.0	1.0	13	25	20	6	95	60	0.2	0.03	0.8	tr	0.08	0.15	1.0	0.01	0.1	9	0	tr	u
Rye, American	25	1 slice	65	2.1	0.9	12	20	40	6	175	50	0.3	0.03	0.7	0	0.1	0.08	0.8	0.02	0.1	10	0	0	u
White, not enriched	25	1 slice	65	2.1	1.0	12	30	25	5	125	30	0.2	0.03	0.1	tr	0.03	0.02	0.03	0.01	0.1	9	0	tr	u
enriched	25	1 slice	65	2.1	1.0	12	30	25	5	125	30	0.2	0.03	0.7	tr	0.1	0.08	0.9	0.01	0.1	9	0	tr	u
Whole wheat	25	1 slice	60	2.4	1.1	11	20	65	25	160	45	0.4	0.09	0.9	tr	0.09	0.05	1.0	0.05	0.2	14	0	tr	u
Broccoli, fresh or frozen, boiled	85	½ c	25	2.4	0.2	4	45	45	14	2	190	0.2	0.03	0.7	170	0.04	0.09	0.4	0.11	0.2	50	0	50	tr
Brussels sprouts, fresh or frozen, boiled	85	4 large sprouts	30	3.1	0.2	6	25	50	17	12	290	0.3	0.03	0.6	60	0.1	0.1	0.5	0.16	0.3	130	0	60	tr
Burrito, beef, Taco Bell	184	one	465	30.0	21.0	37	85	290	u	325	320	u	u	4.6	335	0.3	0.4	7.0	u	u	u	u	15	u
Butter, salted	5	1 tsp or pat (90/lb)	35	tr	4.0	tr	1	1	tr	40	1	tr	0	tr	40	tr	tr	tr	0	0	0	tr	0	0.1
	15	1 tbsp	100	0.1	11.5	0.1	3	3	tr	120	3	tr	0	tr	115	tr	tr	tr	0	0	0	tr	0	0.3
Cabbage, green, headed																								
Raw, shredded	70	1 c	17	0.9	0.1	4	35	20	10	15	165	0.3	0.08	0.3	10	0.04	0.04	0.2	0.1	0.1	20	0	35	tr
Cooked, chopped	70	½ c	15	0.8	0.2	3	30	15	10	10	120	0.3	0.02	0.2	10	0.03	0.03	0.2	0.09	0.1	2	0	25	tr

Cakes																								
Angel food	40	2 in sector of 10 in cake	105	3.1	0.1	24	5	10	5	110	40	0.1	0.02	0.3	0	tr	0.1	0.4	tr	0.1	4	tr	tr	0
Cheese cake, frozen	85	1⁄10 of cake	255	4.6	16.0	24	50	75	8	190	85	0.4	0.05	0.4	65	0.03	0.1	0.4	0.05	0.5	15	0.4	4	u
Chocolate with chocolate icing	90	2 in sector of 8 in cake	350	3.9	16.0	51	75	95	30	160	130	0.6	0.2	1.3	15	0.08	0.1	0.8	0.03	0.3	6	0.1	tr	u
Gingerbread	65	2¾ in square	250	2.8	12.0	32	45	35	14	90	220	0.3	0.1	2.0	7	0.12	0.1	1.0	0.05	0.3	5	0.1	tr	u
Cupcake, iced	50	1 medium	190	2.0	6.0	30	60	95	10	160	55	0.2	0.06	0.4	25	0.02	0.05	0.1	0.01	0.1	4	0.1	0	u
Pound cake	30	3½ in × 3 in × ½ in	140	1.5	9.0	14	6	25	5	35	20	0.2	0.02	0.2	25	0.01	0.03	0.1	0.01	0.09	2	u	0	u
Yellow with chocolate icing	70	2 in sector of 8 in cake	270	2.9	12.0	41	60	60	13	195	75	0.3	0.08	0.3	15	0.08	0.1	0.7	0.02	0.2	6	0.1	tr	u
Candy																								
Caramels	30	1 oz	120	1.0	3.0	20	40	35	u	65	55	u	0.01	0.4	tr	0.01	0.05	0.1	tr	0	u	u	0	u
Chocolate bar																								
plain milk chocolate	30	1 oz	150	2.2	9.0	16	65	65	20	25	110	0.1	0.3	0.3	20	0.02	0.10	0.1	tr	0.03	2	u	0	u
with almonds	30	1 oz	150	2.5	10.0	14	65	75	u	25	125	0.1	u	0.5	20	0.02	0.10	0.2	tr	u	1	u	0	u
Fudge with nuts	30	1 oz	120	1.0	5.0	20	20	30	u	50	50	0.1	u	0.3	tr	0.01	0.03	0.1	u	u	u	tr	0	u
Hard	30	1 oz	110	0	0.3	30	6	2	0	10	1	0	0.03	0.5	0	0	0	0	0	0	0	0	0	0
Marshmallow	30	1 oz, 4 large	90	0.6	tr	25	5	2	u	10	2	0.01	0.06	0.5	0	0	tr	tr	u	u	0	0	0	0
Peanut brittle	30	1 oz	120	1.5	3.0	25	10	25	u	10	45	u	u	0.7	0	0.05	0.01	1.0	u	u	u	0	0	u
Cantaloupe. See *Melons*.																								
Carbonated beverages sweet, cola type	170	6 oz	70	0	0	19	5	30	2	5	3	0.01	0.1	0.1	0	0	0	0	0	0	0	0	0	0
Carrots																								
Raw	80	1 carrot 7½ in × 1⅛ in	35	0.9	0.1	7	25	25	10	35	155	0.3	0.05	0.6	880	0.03	0.04	0.6	0.04	0.2	24	0	4	0
Boiled	70	½ c diced	20	0.5	0.1	4	20	15	8	25	155	0.2	0.05	0.3	800	0.01	0.02	0.4	0.02	0.1	16	0	3	0
Cashews, roasted	30	1 oz	160	5.0	13.0	8	10	105	80	60	130	1.3	0.2	1.1	3	0.1	0.07	0.5	0.1	0.4	20	0	0	u
Cauliflower																								
Raw	50	½ c whole flower buds	10	2.0	0.1	2	10	20	6	10	100	0.1	0.01	0.3	1	0.02	0.04	0.2	0.06	0.1	30	0	25	0
Boiled	60	½ c	15	2.0	0.1	3	15	20	7	12	120	0.1	0.01	0.3	1	0.03	0.04	0.2	0.07	0.1	25	0	30	0
Celery																								
Raw	80	2 large stalks	15	0.8	0.1	3	30	20	17	100	270	u	0.09	0.2	20[e]	0.02	0.02	0.2	0.05	0.3	10	0	8	tr
Boiled	75	½ c diced	10	0.6	0.1	2	25	15	u	65	180	u	0.08	0.2	20[e]	0.02	0.02	0.2	0.05	0.3	u	0	4	tr
Cereals, breakfast																								
Ready-to-eat																								
bran flakes, 40% enriched	30	1 oz	90	3.5	0.5	22	15	140	50	260	180	3.7	0.2	8.1	375	0.4	0.4	5.0	0.5	u	14	1.5	0[f]	tr
corn flakes, enriched	30	1 oz	110	2.0	0.1	24	1	20	3	350	25	0.08	0.02	1.8	0[f]	0.3	0.4	3.0	0.02	0.05	3	0	0[f]	tr
granola	30	1 oz	150	3.5	7.7	16	20	115	35	3	140	1.0	0.2	1.1	1	0.17	0.07	0.5	0.10	0.2	14	0	0	u
rice, puffed, enriched	15	½ oz	60	0.9	0.1	13	1	15	3	0	15	0.2	0.03	0.2	0[f]	0.02	0.01	0.4	0.01	0.04	3	0	0[f]	tr
wheat flakes, enriched	30	1 oz	100	3.0	0.5	23	45	100	30	350	105	0.7	0.1	4.5	375[f]	0.4	0.4	5.0	0.05	0.2	9	1.5	15[f]	0.24
wheat, shredded	30	1 oz	100	3.0	0.6	23	10	100	40	3	100	0.9	0.2	1.2	0	0.07	0.08	1.5	0.07	0.2	12	0	0	tr
Cooked (1.3 oz dry wt., salt added)																								
cornmeal and grits, degermed																								
unenriched	240	1 c	145	3.5	0.5	31	1	30	10	520	55	0.2	0.03	0.2	14[g]	0.04	0.02	0.5	0.06	u	1	0	0	tr
enriched	240	1 c	145	3.5	0.5	31	1	30	10	520	55	0.2	0.03	1.5	14[g]	0.24	0.15	2.0	0.06	u	1	0	0	tr
cornmeal, bolted, whole	240	1 c	145	3.5	1.6	29	8	100	u	u	110	0.7	u	0.9	20[g]	0.15	0.04	0.8	u	u	9	0	0	0.8
oatmeal	240	1 c	145	6.0	2.4	25	20	180	55	380	130	1.2	0.13	1.6	4	0.26	0.05	0.3	0.05	0.5	7	0	0	1.0
wheat, farina light, enriched (e.g., Cream of Wheat)	250	1 c	135	4.0	0.5	28	50	40	10	330	45	0.3	0.08	10.3	0	0.2	0.1	1.5	u	0.2	9	0	0	tr
whole-meal (e.g., Ralston)	250	1 c	135	5.5	0.8	28	15	150	60	470	150	1.4	0.2	1.6	0	0.20	0.18	2.0	0.1	0.3	18	0.1	0	tr

Food	Weight gm	Approximate Measure	Energy Kcal	Protein gm	Fat gm	Total Carbohydrate gm	Calcium mg	Phosphorus mg	Magnesium mg	Sodium mg	Potassium mg	Zinc mg	Copper mg	Iron mg	Total Vitamin A Activity RE	Thiamin mg	Riboflavin mg	Niacin mg	Vitamin B-6 mg	Pantothenic Acid mg	Folacin Total µg	Vitamin B-12 µg	Vitamin C mg	Polyunsaturated Fatty Acids gm
Chard, Swiss, boiled	70	½ c	15	1.5	0.2	2	55	20	45	60	230	u	u	1.3	390	0.03	0.08	0.3	u	0.1	u	0	0	tr
Cheese																								
Natural																								
blue or Roquefort	30	1 oz	105	6.0	8.5	0.6	170	110	8	515	25	0.6	0.04	0.2	65	0.01	0.2	0.2	0.04	0.5	14	0.2	0	1.1
cheddar	30	1 oz	115	7.0	9.5	0.4	205	145	8	175	30	0.9	0.04	0.2	85	0.01	0.1	tr	0.02	0.1	5	0.2	0	0.27
cottage, creamed	110	½ c	120	14.0	5.0	3.0	70	150	6	455	95	0.4	0.02	0.2	50	0.02	0.2	0.1	0.1	0.25	15	0.7	0	0.12
cream	30	2 tbsp	100	2.0	10.0	0.8	25	30	2	85	35	0.2	0.01	0.3	120	tr	0.06	tr	0.01	0.1	4.0	0.1	0	0.36
Parmesan	30	1 oz	130	12.0	8.5	1.0	390	230	15	530	30	0.9	0.1	0.3	60	0.01	0.1	0.1	0.03	0.1	2.0	u	0	0.19
Swiss	30	1 oz	110	8.0	8.0	1.0	270	170	10	75	30	1.1	0.04	0.1	70	tr	0.1	tr	0.02	0.1	2.0	0.5	0	0.28
Pasteurized, processed																								
American	30	1 oz	110	6.0	9.0	0.5	175	210	6	405	45	0.8	0.05	0.1	80	0.01	0.1	tr	0.02	0.1	2.0	0.2	0	0.28
cheese spread	30	1 oz	80	4.5	6.0	2	160	200	8	380	70	0.7	u	0.1	60	0.01	0.1	tr	0.03	0.2	2.0	0.1	0	0.18
Cheese fondue	100	⅔ c	260	15.0	18.5	10	320	295	u	540	165	u	0.04	1.2	300	0.06	0.3	0.2	u	u	u	u	0	u
Cherries																								
Raw, sweet	75	10 cherries	50	0.8	0.6	11	10	15	8	0	150	tr	0.06	0.3	14	0.03	0.04	0.3	0.02	0.1	6	0	5	0.2
Red, canned heavy syrup	130	½ c with syrup	110	0.8	0.2	27	10	25	10	3	190	0.1	0.2	0.5	20	0.02	0.05	0.5	0.04	0.1	10	0	5	0.1
water pack	125	½ c with juice	55	1.0	0.2	15	15	20	10	2	160	0.1	0.1	0.5	20	0.03	0.05	0.5	0.04	0.1	10	0	3	0.1
Chestnuts, water	100		75	1.1	tr	19	4	35	16	95	380	u	u	2.1	0	0.05	0.04	0.9	u	u	u	u	6	u
Chicken																								
Canned, boned with broth	150	½ c	165	22.5	8.0	0	14	255	12	500	140	2	0.2	1.6	75	0.02	0.1	6.3	0.4	0.8	u	0.3	2	1.8
Creamed	120	½ c	210	17.5	12.0	7	85	140	u	u	u	u	u	1.1	100	0.04	0.2	4.0	u	u	u	u	tr	u
Fried																								
Breast, meat and skin, flour-coated	100	½ breast	220	31.0	5.0	2	16	230	29	75	255	1.1	0.1	1.2	15	0.08	0.1	13.5	0.6	1.0	4	0.3	0	1.9
Drumstick, meat and skin, flour-coated	50	1 medium	120	13.0	7.0	1	6	85	11	45	110	1.4	0.1	0.7	3	0.04	0.1	3.0	0.2	0.6	4	0.2	0	1.6
Thigh, meat and skin, flour-coated	60	1 medium	160	16.5	9.0	2	8	115	5	55	150	1.5	0.1	0.9	18	0.06	0.2	4.5	0.2	0.7	5	0.2	0	2.1
Kentucky-fried, Col. Sanders																								
Drumstick	54	one	135	14.0	8.0	2	20	u	u	u	u	u	u	0.9	10	0.04	0.1	2.7	u	u	u	u	0	u
Thigh	97	one	275	20.0	19.0	12	40	u	u	u	u	u	u	1.4	20	0.08	0.2	4.9	u	u	u	u	0	u
Roasted, light meat without skin	140	5 oz	240	43.5	6.0	0	21	300	40	110	345	1.7	0.1	1.5	12	0.09	0.2	17.4	0.8	1.4	5	0.5	0	1.4
Chicken curry	100		160	9.6	10.0	10	22	85	25	670	430	1.7	0.2	1.2	tr	0.02	0.09	0.9	0.1	0.3	5	1.0	5	u
Chick peas or *garbanzos*, cooked without salt	125	½ c (30 gm dry wt.)	110	6.0	1.0	18	45	106	u	10	240	2.7	u	2.1	2	0.1	0.03	0.6	0.2	0.4	125	0	0	u
Chili con carne, with beans, canned	255	1 c	340	19.0	15.5	30	80	320	65	1355	595	4.2	0.8	4.3	30	0.08	0.20	3.3	0.3	0.4	40	u	tr	u
Chili powder, chilis. See *Peppers*.																								
Chili relleno (stuffed pepper)	110	1 pepper	190	10.5	14.0	6	225	195	u	465	270	u	u	1.3	300	0.08	0.2	0.8	0.1	0.7	15	1.0	55	u
Chocolate, bitter or baking	30	1 oz	140	3.0	15.0	8	20	110	35	1	235	0.7	0.8	1.9	2	0.01	0.07	0.4	0.01	0.06	3	0	0	0.5
Sweet, milk. See *Candy*.																								
Chow mein, canned, chicken without noodles	250	1 c	95	6.5	0.3	18	45	85	45	725	420	1.2	0.3	1.3	30	0.05	0.10	1.0	0.4	1.2	10	1.6	15	tr
Clams, canned, with liquid	100	3½ oz, ½ c	50	8.0	0.7	3	55	135	115	u	140	1.2	0	4.0	u	0.01	0.1	1.0	0.08	0.3	3	20	0	tr
Cocoa, dry	5	1 tbsp	20	0.6	0.1	4	15	20	4	30	45	0.1	0.02	0.1	tr	0.01	0.03	tr	0.07	0.6	1	0.1	0	u
beverage w/milk	250	1 c	220	9.0	9.0	26	300	270	55	125	480	1.2	0.01	0.8	85	0.10	0.43	0.4	0.11	0.8	12	0.9	2	0.3
Coconut, dry, unsweetened	30	1 oz	180	2.0	17.5	6	5	50	u	u	160	u	0.2	0.9	0	0.02	0.01	0.2	0.01	0.06	8	0	0	tr

Coffee, instant, regular dry powder	2.5	1–2 tsp	4	tr	tr	1	4	10	10	1	90	0.03	0.01	0.1	0	0	tr	0.6	tr	tr	u	0	0	0
Collards, boiled	70	½ c	20	2.0	0.3	3	140	20	20	35	175	0.2	0.04	0.7	410	0.04	0.1	0.4	0.08	0.1	35	0	30	tr
Cookies																								
Commercial	35	4 cookies	170	1.5	7.0	25	10	55	5	125	25	0.2	0.05	0.2	10	0.01	0.02	0.1	0.02	0.1	1	0	0	u
Fig bar	55	4 cookies	200	2.0	3.0	40	45	40	30	175	160	0.4	0.2	1.3	15	0.08	0.07	0.7	0.05	0.2	3	0	tr	u
Oatmeal	50	4 cookies	235	3.0	10	35	45	70	20	170	120	0.5	0.06	1.5	7	0.10	0.07	0.6	0.02	0.3	7	0.05	0	u
Corn, sweet, yellow																								
Fresh or frozen, boiled	80	½ c	70	2.5	0.6	17	4	55	15	3	160	0.3	0.03	0.4	20	0.06	0.05	1.3	0.13	0.2	40	0	4	tr
Canned, whole kernel	80	½ c	50	1.4	0.3	12	2	45	15	200	135	0.4	0.06	0.3	10	0.03	0.05	0.6	u	u	30	0	5	tr
Cream style	130	½ c	95	2.5	0.5	24	3	80	30	355	235	0.8	0.10	0.6	20	0.04	0.08	1.2	u	u	30	0	8	tr
Corn fritter	35	1 fritter	130	2.5	8.0	14	20	55	u	165	45	u	u	0.6	15	0.06	0.07	0.6	u	u	u	tr	u	u
Corn syrup	20	1 tbsp	60	0	0	15	10	3	u	15	1	u	0.07	u	0	0	0	0	0	0	0	0	0	0
Cowpeas or *blackeye peas*																								
Immature	80	½ c	90	7.0	0.6	15	20	120	15	1	310	0.6	0.2	1.7	30	0.2	0.09	1.0	0.04	0.2	80	0	15	tr
Mature, dry, cooked	125	½ c (1 oz dry wt.)	95	6.5	0.4	17	20	120	u	10	285	2.0	0.2	1.6	1	0.2	0.05	0.5	0.07	0.3	100	0	0	tr
Crabmeat	100	½ c, packed	100	18.0	2.0	0.6	45	185	30	550	90	4.5	1.0	0.8	tr	0.2	0.08	3.0	0.3	0.6	2	10	2	0.9
Crackers																								
Butter (e.g., Ritz)	15	5 round	75	1.1	3.0	11	25	40	u	180	20	u	0.03	0.1	5	tr	tr	0.1	u	u	u	0	0	u
Graham	15	1 cracker 5 in × 2½ in	55	1.1	1.6	12	5	20	5	70	25	0.1	0.02	0.4	tr	0.05	0.04	0.5	0.01	0.1	2	0	0	u
Rye wafer (e.g., Rykrisp)	15	2 wafers	40	1.5	0.2	10	5	50	u	110	u	u	0.04	0.5	0	0.04	0.03	0.2	u	u	u	0	0	u
Saltines	10	4 each, 2 in square	45	0.9	1.0	7	5	10	3	135	15	0.1	0.02	0.3	0	tr	tr	0.6	tr	tr	2	0	0	u
Cranberry jelly, or *sauce*, canned	35	⅛ c	50	tr	tr	13	1	2	1	10	9	tr	tr	tr	1	tr	tr	tr	tr	u	u	0	tr	0
Cream																								
Half-and-half	60	¼ c or 4 tbsp	80	2.0	7.0	3	65	55	8	25	80	0.3	0.07	tr	60	0.02	0.08	0.02	0.02	0.2	1.5	0.2	tr	0.2
Heavy, whipping	60	¼ c; ½ c whipped volume	210	1.0	22.0	2	45	35	4	20	45	0.1	0.06	tr	250	0.01	0.08	0.02	0.01	0.2	0.4	0.1	tr	0.8
Light, for coffee	60	¼ c, 4 tbsp	120	1.6	11.6	2	60	50	5	25	75	0.2	0.06	tr	110	0.02	0.08	tr	0.02	0.2	1.5	0.1	tr	0.4
Sour	60	¼ c, 4 tbsp	130	1.9	12.6	2	60	50	5	25	80	0.2	0.06	tr	110	0.02	0.09	0.05	0.01	0.2	5	0.1	tr	0.5
Cream substitutes																								
Coffee whitener	3	1 tsp or packet	15	0.1	0.8	2	1	12	tr	5	20	0.02	u	tr	tr	0	0	0	0	0	0	0	0	tr
Whipped topping, frozen	10	2 tbsp	30	0.1	2.5	2	1	1	tr	2	2	tr	u	tr	6	0	0	0	0	0	0	0	0	tr
Cucumber, raw, peeled	80	½ small	10	0.4	0.1	2	15	15	5	4	125	0.08	0.04	0.2	tr	0.02	0.03	0.2	0.03	0.2	10	0	8	tr
Custard, baked	130	½ c	150	7.0	7.5	15	150	155	u	105	195	u	0.1	0.6	135	0.06	0.2	0.2	u	u	4	u	0	u
Dandelion greens, boiled	50	½ c	20	1.0	0.3	3	75	20	20	25	120	u	u	1.0	610	0.07	0.08	u	u	u	u	0	10	tr
Dasheen (Japanese taro), raw	100	1⅓ corms	100	2.0	0.2	25	30	60	u	5	515	u	u	1.0	2	0.1	0.04	1.1	u	u	u	0	4	tr
Dates, dried	80	10, pitted	230	1.6	0.4	61	25	35	30	2	540	0.2	0.2	1.0	4	0.07	0.08	1.8	0.16	0.6	10	0	0	tr
Doughnuts																								
Cake type	40	1 average	170	2.0	9.0	20	15	90	10	225	40	0.2	0.05	0.6	7	0.1	0.08	0.7	0.01	0.2	3	0	tr	u
Yeast, raised	40	1 average	180	2.5	11.0	16	15	30	5	100	35	0.3	0.04	0.6	8	0.07	0.07	0.6	0.02	0.2	4	0	0	u
Duck, pressed, salted	100		450	9.7	45.0	2	65	150	u	u	u	u	u	2.7	u	u	u	u	u	u	u	u	u	u
Eggnog	250	1 c	340	9.5	19.0	34	330	275	45	140	420	1.1	u	0.5	200	0.08	0.5	0.3	0.1	1.1	2	1.1	3	0.9
Eggs, chicken																								
Whole, raw or hard cooked	50	1 large	80	6.0	5.5	0.6	30	90	6	70	65	0.7	0.05	1.0	80	0.04	0.15	tr	0.06	0.9	25	0.6	0	0.7
white	33	1 white	15	3.5	tr	0.4	4	4	3	50	45	tr	0.01	tr	0	tr	0.09	tr	tr	0.07	5	0.02	0	0
yolk	17	1 yolk	65	3.0	5.0	tr	25	85	3	10	15	0.6	0.05	0.9	80	0.04	0.07	tr	0.05	0.8	25	0.6	0	0.7
Scrambled	140	2 eggs	190	12.0	14.0	3.0	95	195	15	310	170	1.4	0.07	1.9	160	0.07	0.30	0.1	0.1	1.8	50	1.3	tr	1.4
Eggplant, boiled	100	½ c diced	20	1.0	0.2	4	10	20	15	1	150	u	0.1	0.6	1	0.05	0.04	0.5	0.08	0.2	2	0	3	tr
Enchiladas, beef																								
Frozen, Campbell's	200	7 oz portion	240	15.0	8.5	25	20	190	u	725	155	u	u	2.5	120	0.1	0.2	3.0	u	u	u	u	u	u
Home recipe	190	2 enchiladas	365	32.0	16.7	22	450	480	u	510	585	u	u	5	1200	0.1	0.4	6.0	0.8	0.7	10	2	10	u

Food	Weight gm	Approximate Measure	Energy Kcal	Protein gm	Fat gm	Total Carbohydrate gm	Calcium mg	Phosphorus mg	Magnesium mg	Sodium mg	Potassium mg	Zinc mg	Copper mg	Iron mg	Total Vitamin A Activity RE	Thiamin mg	Riboflavin mg	Niacin mg	Vitamin B-6 mg	Pantothenic Acid mg	Folacin Total µg	Vitamin B-12 µg	Vitamin C mg	Polyunsaturated Fatty Acids gm
Fats, shortening, solid or oil	100	½ c	880	0	100.0	0	0	0	0	0	0	0	0	0	0	0	0	0	0	0	0	0	0	14.8
	12	1 tbsp	110	0	12.0	0	0	0	0	0	0	0	0	0	0	0	0	0	0	0	0	0	0	1.8
Figs, fresh	100	2 medium	75	0.8	0.3	20	35	15	15	1	230	0.1	0.07	0.4	14	0.06	0.05	0.4	0.11	0.3	u	0	2	0.14
Dried	30	2 small	75	1.0	0.3	20	40	20	20	3	225	0.2	0.1	0.7	4	0.02	0.03	0.2	0.07	0.1	2	0	tr	0.56
Fish																								
Cod, steak, sauteed	110	4 oz	180	30.0	6.0	0	30	285	30	115[h]	420	0.9	0.2	1.0	60	0.08	0.1	3.0	0.3	0.3	10	0.9	0	3.4
Fish sticks, breaded	110	4 sticks	200	19.0	10.0	7	10	190	20	u	u	0.3	0.2	0.4	0	0.04	0.08	2.0	0.06	0.3	10	1.1	0	u
Haddock, fried	110	4 oz	180	22.0	7.0	6	45	270	30	195[h]	385	1.1	0.2	1.3	tr	0.04	0.08	3.5	0.2	0.1	10	1.4	2	3.2
Mackerel, sauteed	105	3 average	250	23.0	17.0	0	5	295	30	u	u	1.0	0.2	1.3	165	0.2	0.3	8.0	0.7	0.9	10	9.4	0	4.6
Salmon, steak, broiled	145	1 average 6 in × 2 in	230	35.0	9.0	0	u	530	60	150[h]	565	2.4	1.2	1.5	60	0.2	0.08	12.5	1.0	1.9	30	5.8	0	2.4
canned, pink	110	½ c	160	23.0	6.0	0	215	315	30	425	395	1.0	0.3	0.9	25	0.04	0.2	9.0	0.3	0.6	20	7.6	0	1.6
red	110	½ c	190	22.0	10.0	0	285	380	30	575	380	1.0	0.3	1.3	75	0.04	0.2	8.0	0.3	0.6	20	7.6	0	2.6
Sardines canned in oil	85	3 oz drained	170	20.5	9.0	0	370	425	35	700	500	2.4	0.03	2.4	60	0.03	0.2	4.5	0.2	0.7	15	8.5	0	1.8
Sole or flounder, fillet, baked	100	3 oz	200	30.0	8.0	0	25	345	30	235[h]	585	1.0	0.07	1.4	u	0.07	0.08	2.5	0.2	0.8	15	1.2	2	3.8
Swordfish, broiled	100	3 oz	170	26.5	6.0	0	25	260	u	u	u	u	u	1.3	600	0.04	0.05	10.5	u	0.2	u	1.0	0	u
Tuna, raw	100	½ c	135	27.5	3.0	0	5	175	30	35[h]	180	0.5	0.5	1.3	15	0.02	0.05	6.6	0.9	0.5	u	3.0	7	1.1
canned in oil	100	½ c	200	28.0	8.0	0	10	230	25	u	u	1.0	0.1	1.9	25	0.05	0.1	12.0	0.4	0.3	15	2.2	0	3.0
in water	100	½ c	130	28.0	0.8	0	15	190	25	865	275	u	u	1.6	25	0.05	0.1	13.0	0.4	0.3	15	2.2	0	0.3
Flour, wheat																								
White, all purpose																								
unenriched	115	1 c	420	12.0	1.0	90	20	100	30	2	110	0.8	0.2	0.9	0	0.07	0.06	1.0	0.07	0.5	20	0	0	0.6
enriched	115	1 c	420	12.0	1.0	90	20	100	30	2	110	0.8	0.2	3.3	0	0.5	0.3	4.0	0.07	0.5	20	0	0	0.6
Whole-grain	120	1 c	400	16.0	2.5	85	50	445	135	4	445	2.9	0.6	4.0	0	0.7	0.1	5.0	0.4	1.3	35	0	0	1.6
French toast, frozen, Campbell's	65	1 slice	130	5.0	4.3	18	50	85	u	305	80	u	u	1.3	75	0.1	0.1	0.7	u	u	u	u	0	u
Frozen dinners																								
Chicken, fried with potatoes, mixed vegetables	310	11 oz dinner	570	28.0	29.0	48	70	350	60	1075	350	3.0	0.4	3.2	360	0.2	0.6	16.0	0.9	1.6	20	0.7	10	u
Meat loaf with tomato sauce, potatoes, peas	310	11 oz dinner	410	25.0	21.0	30	60	365	60	1225	360	3.5	0.5	4.0	260	0.3	0.4	5.5	0.7	0.9	20	1.1	10	u
Turkey with gravy, potatoes, peas	310	11 oz dinner	340	25.0	9.0	40	80	260	65	1200	530	3.0	0.4	3.3	80	0.2	0.3	7.0	0.8	1.8	30	0.6	10	u
Fruit cocktail, heavy syrup	130	½ c	95	0.5	tr	24	10	15	7	7	110	0.1	0.09	0.4	25	0.02	0.02	0.5	0.06	0.1	u	0	2	0.04
Gelatin, dry	8	1 tbsp or packet	30	7.0	0	0	u	u	2	1	u	u	0.1	u	0	0	0	0	0	0	0	0	0	0
Gelatin dessert, plain	120	½ c	71	2.0	0	17	u	u	2	u	u	0.02	0.03	u	0	0	0	0	0	0	0	0	0	0
Grapefruit, raw	100	½ medium	30	0.6	0.1	8	10	10	8	0	140	0.1	0.05	0.1	10	0.04	0.02	0.3	0.04	0.3	10	0	35	0.02
Grapefruit juice, canned																								
Unsweetened	250	1 c	95	1.2	0.2	22	20	25	25	3	380	0.2	0.09	0.5	2	0.1	0.05	0.6	0.05	0.3	25	0	70	0.06
Sweetened	250	1 c	115	1.4	0.2	28	20	25	25	4	405	0.1	0.12	0.9	0	0.1	0.06	0.8	0.05	0.3	25	0	65	tr
Grapes, raw																								
Slip-skin	100	20 grapes	65	0.6	0.3	17	15	10	5	2	190	tr	0.04	0.3	10	0.09	0.06	0.3	0.11	tr	4	0	4	0.10
Adherent skin	100	20 grapes	70	0.7	0.6	18	10	15	6	2	185	tr	0.09	0.3	8	0.09	0.06	0.3	0.11	tr	4	0	10	0.17
Grape juice	250	1 c	155	1.4	0.2	38	20	25	25	7	335	0.1	0.07	0.6	2	0.07	0.09	0.7	0.16	0.1	6	0	tr	0.06
Gravy, canned																								
Beef	15	1 tbsp	8	0.5	0.3	0.7	1	5	0	10	12	0.15	0.01	0.1	0	tr	tr	0.1	tr	u	u	tr	0	0.01
Chicken	15	1 tbsp	10	0.3	0.9	0.8	3	4	0	85	16	0.12	0.01	0.1	2	tr	tr	0.1	tr	u	u	u	0	0.2
Guacamole	120	½ c	140	2.1	12.8	7	15	40	u	165	565	u	0.3	0.7	55	0.10	0.2	1.6	0.4	0.9	30	0	35	2
Ham, baked	85	3 oz	250	18.0	19.0	0	10	145	15	635	200	3.4	0.3	2.2	0	0.4	0.2	3.0	0.3	0.3	1	0.4	0	2

Hominy grits. See *Cereal,* cooked.																								
Honey, strained	20	1 tbsp	65	0.1	0	17	1	1	1	1	10	0.02	0.03	0.1	0	tr	0.01	0.1	tr	0.04	0	0	tr	0
Ice cream, vanilla																								
Plain, 10% fat	65	½ c	135	2.5	7.0	15	90	70	10	60	130	0.7	0.02	0.05	65	0.02	0.2	0.05	0.03	0.3	1	0.3	0	0.3
Rich, 16% fat	75	½ c	175	2.0	12.0	16	75	60	8	50	110	0.6	0.02	0.05	105	0.02	0.15	0.05	0.03	0.3	1	0.3	0	0.4
Ice cream cone, Dairy Queen	142	1 dip, reg.	230	6.0	7.0	35	200	150	u	u	u	u	u	u	70	0.09	0.26	u	u	u	u	0.6	u	u
Ice milk, vanilla	65	½ c	90	2.5	3.0	15	90	65	10	50	130	0.3	u	0.09	25	0.04	0.2	0.05	0.04	0.3	1	0.4	0	0.1
Ices, water, lime	95	½ c	120	0.4	tr	30	tr	tr	u	tr	3	u	u	tr	0	tr	tr	tr	0	0	0	0	0	0
Jams and *Jellies*	20	1 tbsp	55	0.1	tr	14	4	2	1	2	20	0.1	0.02	0.2	tr	tr	0.01	tr	0.01	0.02	1	0	tr	0
Kale, boiled without stems	55	½ c, diced	15	1.4	0.2	3	75	15	10	8	185	0.1	0.03	0.5	375	0.03	0.6	0.3	0.05	tr	25	0	20	tr
Kidney, braised	100	3½ oz	250	33.0	12.0	0.8	20	240	20	250	320	2.4	0.1	13.0	330	0.5	4.8	10.5	0.4	3.8	60	30	u	u
Kohlrabi, boiled	80	½ c, diced	20	1.5	0.1	4	25	35	30	5	215	u	u	0.2	1	0.05	0.02	0.2	0.1	0.5	u	0	35	tr
Kumquat, raw	20	1 medium	10	0.2	tr	3	10	5	2	5	35	tr	0.02	0.1	6	0.01	0.02	u	u	u	u	0	7	0
Lamb, choice grade																								
Chop, loin, broiled lean and fat	95	1 average	340	21.0	28.0	0	10	165	15	50	235	u	0.1	1.2	tr	0.1	0.2	5.0	0.3	0.5	1	2.0	0	1.4
lean only	65	1 average	120	18.0	5.0	0	10	140	15	45	205	3.0	0.1	1.3	tr	0.1	0.2	4.0	0.2	0.4	1	1.4	0	0.25
Leg, roasted lean only	85	3 oz	160	24.0	6.0	0	10	200	15	60	275	3.6	0.05	1.9	tr	0.1	0.3	5.5	0.2	0.5	1	1.8	0	0.3
Shoulder, roasted lean and fat	85	3 oz	280	18.5	23.0	0	10	145	15	45	205	u	0.1	1.0	tr	0.1	0.2	4.0	0.2	0.5	1	1.8	0	1.1
Lard	12	1 tbsp	110	0	12.0	0	0	0	0	0	0	0	0	0	0	0	0	0	0	0	0	0	0	1.1
Lasagna, frozen, Sara Lee	225	8 oz serving	380	27.0	12.4	43	310	470	55	1100	740	1.4	u	5.6	185	0.4	0.4	4.5	u	u	50	u	15	u
Lemon juice, fresh	15	1 tsp	5	0.1	tr	1	1	1	1	0	15	tr	tr	tr	tr	tr	tr	tr	tr	tr	1.5	0	5	tr
Lemonade, from frozen concentrate	250	1 c	110	0.1	tr	30	2	3	2	1	40	0.02	0.02	0.1	1	0.01	0.02	0.2	0.01	0.03	5	0	15	0
Lentils, dried, cooked	100	½ c	110	8.0	tr	19	25	120	20	u	250	1.0	0.3	2.1	2	0.07	0.06	0.6	u	u	36	0	0	0
Lettuce, raw																								
Head, solid (iceberg type)	90	⅙ head	10	0.8	0.1	3	20	20	10	10	160	0.4	0.08	0.5	30	0.05	0.05	0.3	0.05	0.2	30	0	5	tr
Loose leaf, romaine, cos	55	1 c chopped	10	0.7	0.2	2	35	15	10	5	145	0.2	0.05	0.8	100	0.03	0.04	0.2	0.03	0.1	30	0	10	tr
Liver																								
Beef, fried	85	3 oz	200	22.5	9.0	4	10	405	15	155	325	4.3	2.5	7.5	9000	0.2	3.6	14.0	0.7	6.5	70	68.0	25	2.4
Calf, fried	85	3 oz	220	25.0	11.2	3	10	455	20	100	385	5.2	6.5	12.1	7000	0.2	3.5	14.0	0.6	6.5	70	51.0	30	3.5
Chicken, simmered	70	½ c, chopped	110	18.0	3.5	1	10	110	15	40	105	3.0	0.2	6.0	3500	0.1	1.9	8.0	0.5	4.2	160	17.5	10	0.67
Lobster, northern, cooked	95	⅔ c meat	90	18.0	1.5	0.3	65	185	20	205	175	2.1	1.6	0.8	tr	0.1	0.07	u	u	1.4	15	0.5	0	u
Lychee nuts, raw	150	10 nuts	60	0.8	0.3	15	5	40	u	3	155	u	u	0.4	0	u	0.05	u	u	u	u	0	40	tr
Macaroni and other pastas, cooked																								
Unenriched	130	1 c	190	6.5	0.7	40	15	85	25	1[i]	105	0.6	0.03	0.7	0	0.03	0.03	0.5	0.03	0.2	5	0	0	tr
Enriched	130	1 c	190	6.5	0.7	40	15	85	25	1[i]	105	0.6	0.03	1.4	0	0.2	0.1	2.0	0.03	0.2	5	0	0	tr
Macaroni with cheese, casserole, baked	200	1 c	430	17.0	22.0	40	360	320	50	1085	240	1.3	0.08	1.8	200	0.2	0.4	2.0	0.09	0.4	10	0.8	0	u
Mangos, raw	165	1 c, diced	110	1.0	0.5	28	20	20	15	3	255	0.1	0.18	0.2	640	0.1	0.1	1.0	0.22	0.3	u	0	45	0.11
Margarine	5	1 tsp, 1 pat (90/lb)	35	tr	4	tr	1	1	tr	50	1	0.01	tr	0	5	0	0	0	0	0	0	0	0	1.2
Melons																								
Cantaloupe	160	½ small melon or 1 c, cubed	60	1.4	0.4	13	20	25	15	15	495	0.2	0.07	0.3	510	0.06	0.03	0.9	0.18	0.2	27	0	65	tr
Honeydew	170	⅛ melon or 1 c, cubed	60	0.8	0.2	16	10	15	10	15	460	u	0.07	0.1	7	0.13	0.03	1.0	0.1	0.4	u	0	40	tr
Watermelon	480	1/16 melon (2 lb with rind)	150	3.0	2.0	35	40	40	50	10	560	0.3	0.15	0.8	175	0.4	0.1	1.0	0.7	1.0	10	0	45	tr

Food	Weight gm	Approximate Measure	Energy Kcal	Protein gm	Fat gm	Total Carbohydrate gm	Calcium mg	Phosphorus mg	Magnesium mg	Sodium mg	Potassium mg	Zinc mg	Copper mg	Iron mg	Total Vitamin A Activity RE	Thiamin mg	Riboflavin mg	Niacin mg	Vitamin B-6 mg	Pantothenic Acid mg	Folacin Total μg	Vitamin B-12 μg	Vitamin C mg	Polyunsaturated Fatty Acids gm
Milk, cow																								
Whole, fluid, 3.3% fat	245	1 c	150	8.0	8.2	11	290	225	30	120	370	1.0	0.08	0.1	75	0.09	0.4	0.2	0.1	0.8	10	0.9	2	0.3
2%, low-fat	245	1 c	140	10.0	5.0	14	350	275	40	145	450	1.1	0.08	0.1	140[i]	0.1	0.5	0.2	0.1	0.9	15	1.0	2	0.2
Skim, nonfat, or buttermilk	245	1 c	90	8.5	0.4	12	300	245	30	125[j]	400	1.0	0.08	0.1	140[i]	0.09	0.4	0.2	0.1	0.8	15	1.0	2	tr
Chocolate, low-fat	250	1 c	180	8.0	5.0	26	285	255	30	150	420	1.0	u	0.6	140[i]	0.1	0.4	0.3	0.1	0.7	10	0.8	2	0.2
Dried, instant whole	30	¼ c	160	8.5	8.5	12	290	250	25	120	425	1.0	0.06	0.1	90	0.09	0.4	0.2	0.09	0.7	10	1.0	2	0.2
nonfat	35	½ c	125	12.0	0.2	18	420	345	40	190	600	1.5	0.1	0.1	2	0.1	0.5	0.3	0.1	1.1	15	1.4	2	tr
Evaporated	250	1 c	340	17.5	20.0	25	660	510	60	265	765	1.9	0.2	0.4	140	0.1	0.8	0.5	0.1	1.6	20	0.4	3	0.6
Condensed, sweetened	40	1 fl oz	120	3.0	3.5	20	105	95	10	50	140	0.4	0.08	0.1	30	0.03	0.2	0.1	0.02	0.3	4	0.2	tr	0.1
Milk, human, U.S.	30	1 fl oz	21	0.3	1.3	2.1	10	4	1	5	16	0.05	0.01	0.01	20	0.004	0.01	0.1	0.003	0.07	2	0.02	2	0.2
Milkshakes, commercial	290	10 fl oz	320	10.0	8.0	52	345	265	35	250	500	1.0	0.06	0.2	100	0.12	0.66	0.6	0.12	u	u	0.9	tr	u
Molasses																								
Light	20	1 tbsp	50	0	0	13	35	10	9	3	185	u	u	0.9	0	0.01	0.01	u	u	u	u	0	0	0
Medium	20	1 tbsp	50	0	0	12	60	15	16	5	215	0.9	0.3	1.2	0	0.01	0.02	0.2	0.04	0.07	2	0	0	0
Blackstrap	20	1 tbsp	45	tr	0	11	135	15	52	20	585	u	u	3.2	0	0.02	0.04	0.4	u	u	u	0	0	0
Muffins																								
Bran	40	1 muffin	110	3.0	5.0	17	55	110	30	170	90	0.9	0.08	1.1	40	0.1	0.1	1.1	0.11	0.2	16	0.1	2	u
Cornmeal	40	1 muffin	130	3.0	4.0	19	40	70	20	190	55	u	u	0.7	20[d]	0.08	0.09	0.6	u	u	u	u	0	u
English	55	1 muffin	130	4.0	1.0	18	90	60	10	350	310	0.4	0.17	1.6	0	0.25	0.18	2.0	0.02	0.3	18	0	0	u
Plain or blueberry	40	1 muffin	125	2.5	4.0	20	15	80	5	200	50	0.2	0.03	0.5	8	0.1	0.1	1.0	u	u	u	u	tr	u
Mushrooms, raw	35	½ c, sliced	10	1.0	0.1	2	2	40	5	5	145	0.1	0.04	0.3	tr	0.04	0.2	1.5	0.04	0.8	7	0	1	tr
Mustard greens, boiled	70	½ c	15	2.0	0.2	2	80	20	10	20	120	0.2	0.05	0.9	360	0.03	0.04	0.2	0.11	tr	u	0	20	tr
Mustard, prepared, yellow	5	1 tsp	4	0.2	0.2	0.3	4	4	2	65	5	0.03	0.02	0.1	0	u	u	u	u	u	u	0	0	0
Noodles, egg, cooked																								
Unenriched	105	⅔ c	130	4.5	1.5	25	10	65	25	2	45	0.6	0.02	0.6	20	0.03	0.02	0.4	0.02	0.2	2	tr	0	u
Enriched	105	⅔ c	130	4.5	1.5	25	10	65	25	2	45	0.6	0.02	0.9	20	0.10	0.09	1.3	0.02	0.2	2	tr	0	u
Oils. See *Fats.*																								
Okra, boiled	105	10 pods	30	2.0	0.3	6	100	45	40	2	185	u	0.1	0.5	50	0.1	0.2	1.0	0.08	0.2	10	0	20	tr
Olives																								
Green	25	5 large	20	0.2	2.5	0.2	10	4	5	465	10	0.02	0.09	0.3	6	tr	tr	tr	0.01	0	3	0	0	0.3
Ripe	25	5 large	35	0.2	4.0	0.6	20	4	u	150	5	0.07	0.09	0.4	2	tr	tr	tr	tr	tr	3	0	0	0.5
Onions																								
Green, raw, bulb and top	25	¼ c, chopped or 3 onions	10	0.4	tr	2	15	10	3	1	60	0.07	0.01	0.3	50	0.01	0.01	0.1	u	0.4	10	0	8	0
Mature, dry	85	½ c, chopped	30	1.5	0.1	7	25	30	10	10	135	0.3	0.1	0.4	4[g]	0.02	0.04	0.2	0.1	0.1	8	0	8	tr
raw	10	1 tbsp, ⅛ onion	4	0.2	tr	0.9	3	4	1	1	15	0.03	0.01	0.1	tr	tr	tr	tr	0.01	0.01	1	0	1	0
boiled	105	½ c, sliced	30	1.0	0.1	7	25	30	10	10	115	0.6	0.08	0.4	4[g]	0.03	0.03	0.2	0.1	0.1	10	0	8	tr
Oranges, raw	130	1 medium	60	1.2	0.2	15	50	20	15	0	235	0.1	0.06	0.1	25	0.11	0.05	0.4	0.08	0.3	40	0	70	0.03
Orange juice, fresh or frozen	250	1 c	110	1.7	0.5	26	25	40	25	2	495	0.1	0.11	0.5	50	0.22	0.07	1.0	0.10	0.5	110	0	125	tr
Oysters, raw	120	6 oysters	60	13.0	1.0	tr	220	320	50	610	310	25[k]	9.0	7.2	75	0.1	0.2	1.6	0.04	0.6	12	17	10[k]	1.0
Pakchoy, raw	100	⅔ c	15	1.0	0.1	3	165	45	u	25	305	u	u	0.8	300	0.05	0.1	0.8	u	u	u	0	25	tr
Pancakes, plain	110	4, ea 4 in diameter	240	7.5	9.0	32	145	290	20	650	175	0.8	0.07	1.1	30	0.15	0.24	1.0	0.23	0.4	12	1.3	tr	u
Papaya, raw	140	½ fruit or 1 c, cubed	55	1.0	0.2	14	35	5	15	4	360	0.1	0.02	0.1	280	0.04	0.04	0.5	0.03	0.3	u	0	85	0.04
Parsley, raw	5	1 tbsp, chopped	2	0.1	tr	0.3	5	2	2	2	25	tr	0.02	0.2	30	tr	0.01	tr	0.01	0.02	2	0	6	tr
Peaches, without skin																								
Raw, yellow	115	1 medium	45	0.6	0.1	10	5	10	6	0	170	0.1	0.06	0.1	45	0.01	0.04	0.9	0.02	0.1	3	0	6	0.04
Canned, heavy syrup	160	2 halves, 3 tbsp syrup	120	0.7	0.2	32	5	20	8	10	150	0.1	0.08	0.4	55	0.02	0.04	1.0	0.03	0.1	5	0	4	0.04
water pack	155	2 halves and 3 tbsp juice	35	0.7	0.1	9	5	15	8	6	150	0.1	0.08	0.5	80	0.01	0.03	0.8	0.03	0.1	5	0	4	0.04
Dried, sulfured, uncooked	60	½ c (5 halves)	190	3	0.6	48	20	95	35	6	785	0.4	0.29	3.2	80	0.02	0.06	2.8	0.09	0.3	4	0	6	0.29

Peanuts, roasted, salted	30	1 oz, 30 nuts	165	7.5	14.0	5	20	115	50	120	190	0.9	0.1	0.6	0	0.09	0.04	4.9	0.1	0.6	8	0	0	4.1
Peanut butter	15	1 tbsp	95	4.0	8.0	3	10	60	25	95	100	0.4	0.09	0.3	0	0.02	0.02	2.4	0.05	0.3	3	0	0	2.1
Pears																								
Raw, with skin	165	1 3½ in × 2½ in	100	1.0	0.7	25	20	20	10	1	210	0.2	0.19	0.4	3	0.03	0.07	0.2	0.03	0.1	12	0	7	0.16
Canned, syrup	160	2 halves and 3 tbsp juice	115	0.3	0.2	30	10	10	6	8	100	0.1	0.08	0.3	0	0.02	0.03	0.4	0.02	tr	2	0	2	0.05
water pack	155	2 halves and 3 tbsp juice	45	0.3	tr	12	5	10	6	4	80	0.1	0.08	0.3	0	0.01	0.02	0.1	0.02	tr	2	0	2	0.01
Peas																								
Green, frozen, boiled	80	½ c	65	4.0	0.4	11	20	70	20	80	120	0.6	0.09	1.2	55	0.2	0.1	1.6	0.1	u	70	0	8	0.06
Canned, drained	85	½ c	75	4.0	0.4	14	20	65	10	200	80	0.7	0.1	1.6	50	0.08	0.05	0.7	0.04	0.1	20	0	7	0.06
Split, dry, cooked	100	½ c (1 oz, dry wt.)	115	8.0	0.3	20	10	90	8	15	295	1.1	0.07	1.7	4	0.2	0.09	0.9	0.04	0.6	5	0	0	0.05
Peas and carrots, frozen, boiled	80	½ c	50	2.5	0.3	9	20	50	15	65	155	0.4	0.07	0.8	80	0.13	0.1	1.1	0.09	0.2	10	0	10	tr
Pecans	30	1 oz, 20 halves	200	2.5	20.0	4	20	80	40	tr	170	u	0.3	0.7	4	0.2	0.04	0.3	0.05	0.5	4	0	1	u
Peppers, hot (chili)																								
Green, canned sauce	15	1 tbsp	3	0.1	tr	1	1	2	u	u	u	u	u	0.1	10	tr	tr	0.1	u	u	u	0	10	0
Red, dry, chili powder	3	1 tsp	10	0.3	0.4	1	5	10	4	25	50	0.1	u	0.4	90	tr	tr	0.2	u	u	u	0	2	tr
Peppers, sweet																								
Green, raw	75	½ c, chopped	15	0.9	0.1	4	5	15	15	10	155	0.2	0.07	0.5	30	0.06	0.06	0.4	0.2	0.2	15	0	95	tr
Red, raw	90	1 medium	25	1.0	0.2	5	10	20	u	u	u	u	u	0.4	330	0.06	0.06	0.4	u	0.2	20	0	150	tr
Pickles, cucumber																								
Dill	135	1 large	15	0.9	0.3	3	35	30	1	1930	270	0.4	0.03	1.4	15	tr	0.03	tr	0.01	0.3	4	0	8	tr
Sweet	35	1 medium	50	0.2	0.1	13	4	5	tr	u	u	0.05	0.07	0.4	3	tr	0.01	tr	tr	0.07	1	0	2	0
Relish, sweet	15	1 tbsp	20	0.1	0.1	5	3	2	u	105	u	0.01	0.05	0.1	u	0	0	0	u	u	0	0	tr	0
Pies																								
Apple, berry, rhubarb	160	⅙ of 9 in pie	400	3.5	17.5	60	15	35	5	475	125	0.1	0.1	0.5	5	0.03	0.03	0.6	0.06	0.2	8	0	2	u
Cherry, peach	160	⅙ of 9 in pie	410	4.0	18.0	60	20	40	u	480	165	0.06	0.1	0.5	70	0.03	0.03	0.8	u	u	u	0	tr	u
Cream, pudding type with meringue	150	⅙ of 9 in pie	380	7.5	18.0	50	105	150	u	390	210	u	u	1.1	75	0.05	0.2	0.3	u	1.4	14	u	tr	u
Custard	150	⅙ of 9 in pie	330	9.5	17.0	35	145	170	u	u	u	u	u	0.9	85	0.08	0.3	0.5	u	u	u	tr	0	u
Lemon meringue	140	⅙ of 9 in pie	360	5.0	14.5	55	20	70	u	395	70	u	u	0.7	60	0.04	0.1	0.3	u	u	14	u	4	u
Mince	160	⅙ of 9 in pie	430	4.0	18.0	65	45	60	u	710	280	u	0.1	1.6	tr	0.10	0.06	0.6	u	u	u	u	2	u
Pecan	140	⅙ of 9 in pie	580	7.0	31.5	70	65	140	u	305	170	u	u	3.9	20	0.20	0.1	0.4	u	u	u	0	tr	u
Pumpkin	150	⅙ of 9 in pie	320	6.0	17.0	35	80	105	10	325	245	0.6	0.08	0.8	380	0.05	0.2	0.8	0.06	0.8	5	u	tr	u
Sweet potato	150	⅙ of 9 in pie	325	7.0	17.0	36	105	130	u	330	250	u	u	0.8	360	0.08	0.2	0.5	u	u	u	u	6	u
Pineapple, diced or crushed																								
Raw	155	1 c	75	0.6	0.7	19	10	10	20	1	175	0.1	0.17	0.6	3	0.1	0.1	0.7	0.13	0.2	16	0	24	0.23
Canned, in heavy syrup	130	½ c solids and liquids	100	0.5	0.1	26	20	10	20	1	130	0.1	0.13	0.5	2	0.1	0.03	0.4	0.10	0.1	6	0	9	0.05
in juice	125	½ c solids and liquid	75	0.5	0.1	20	20	10	20	2	150	0.1	0.12	0.4	4	0.1	0.02	0.4	u	u	u	0	12	0.04
water pack	125	½ c solids and liquid	40	0.5	0.1	10	29	5	20	2	155	0.1	0.13	0.5	2	0.1	0.03	0.4	0.09	0.1	6	0	9	0.04
Pineapple juice	250	1 c	140	0.8	0.2	34	40	20	35	2	335	0.3	0.22	0.6	6	0.1	0.05	0.6	0.24	0.2	58	0	27	0.07
Pinenuts, pinon	30	1 oz, 4 tbsp	180	3.5	17.0	6	3	170	u	u	u	u	u	1.5	1	0.4	0.07	1.3	u	u	u	u	u	u
Pizza, cheese	65	⅛ of 14 in pizza	150	8.0	5.5	18	145	125	20	455	85	0.8	0.2	0.7	100	0.04	0.1	0.7	u	u	24	u	5	u
Sausage	65	⅛ of 14 in pizza	160	5.0	6.0	20	10	60	u	490	115	0.8	u	0.8	100	0.06	0.08	1.0	u	u	23	u	6	u
Plantain	275	1 banana 11 in × 2 in	220	2	0.7	57	5	60	65	7	895	0.2	0.14	1.1	200	0.1	0.1	1.2	0.53	0.5	39	0	33	tr
Plums, raw	70	1 medium	35	0.5	0.4	9	2	5	4	0	115	0.1	0.03	0.1	20	0.03	0.06	0.3	0.05	0.1	1	0	6	0.09
Canned, purple in heavy syrup	140	3 and 3 tbsp syrup	120	0.5	0.1	31	10	15	7	25	120	0.1	0.05	1.1	35	0.02	0.05	0.4	0.04	0.1	3	0	1	0.03
Popcorn with oil and salt	10	1 c	40	0.9	2.0	5	1	20	10	175	u	0.2	0.03	0.2	u	u	0.01	0.2	0.02	0.04	0	0	0	u

Food	Weight gm	Approximate Measure	Energy Kcal	Protein gm	Fat gm	Total Carbohydrate gm	Calcium mg	Phosphorus mg	Magnesium mg	Sodium mg	Potassium mg	Zinc mg	Copper mg	Iron mg	Total Vitamin A Activity RE	Thiamin mg	Riboflavin mg	Niacin mg	Vitamin B-6 mg	Pantothenic Acid mg	Folacin Total µg	Vitamin B-12 µg	Vitamin C mg	Polyunsaturated Fatty Acids gm
Pork																								
Chop, broiled lean and fat	80	1 medium	300	19.5	24.5	0	10	210	15	45	215	2.3	0.13	2.7	0	0.8	0.2	4.5	0.3	0.5	3	0.4	0	2.0
lean only	50	1 medium	110	13.0	6.5	0	5	135	10	30	145	1.5	0.04	1.6	0	0.5	0.1	2.9	0.1	0.2	2	0.2	0	0.5
Loin, roasted lean and fat	85	2½ in × 2¼ in × ½ in	310	21.0	24.0	0	10	220	20	50	235	2.2	0.05	2.7	0	0.8	0.2	4.8	0.3	0.5	4	0.5	0	2.0
Spareribs, braised	90	yield from 6½ oz as purchased	400	18.5	35.0	0	15	220	u	65	300	u	u	4.7	0	0.8	0.4	6.1	u	u	u	0.6	0	2.2
Potatoes																								
Baked	200	1 large	140	4.0	0.2	35	15	100	45	5[i]	780	0.4	0.3	1.1	tr	0.2	0.07	2.7	0.3	0.4	20	0	30	tr
Boiled, pared	135	1 medium	90	2.5	0.1	20	10	55	30	3[i]	385	0.4	0.1	0.7	tr	0.1	0.05	1.6	0.2	0.3	15	0	20	tr
French-fried, McDonald's	70	1 "order"	220	3.0	10.2	28	9	70	20	120	250	0.2	0.1	0.4	tr	0.1	0.04	2.4	0.2	0.1	15	0	9	u
frozen, reheated	100	20 strips	140	2.0	5.0	23	5	65	15	30[i]	365	0.3	0.11	0.6	0	0.07	0.02	1.1	u	u	15	0	11	u
Mashed with milk	100	½ c	100	2.0	4.5	13	25	50	15	350	260	0.1	0.1	0.4	45	0.08	0.05	1.0	0.2	0.2	10	0	10	u
Potato chips	20	10 chips, 2 in diameter each	115	1.0	8.0	10	10	30	10	200	225	0.2	0.04	0.4	tr	0.04	0.01	1.0	0.04	0.1	2	0	3	u
Potato salad. See *Salads.*																								
Pretzels	30	10, 3-ring pretzels	120	3.0	1.0	24	10	25	7	480	30	0.3	0.05	0.6	u	0.1	0.1	1.2	0.01	0.1	5	0	0	tr
Prunes, dried, raw	50	5–6	120	1.3	0.2	30	25	35	20	2	370	0.2	0.20	1.2	100	0.04	0.07	0.8	0.13	0.2	2	0	2	0.05
Cooked without sugar	110	½ c	115	1.2	0.2	30	25	40	20	2	355	0.2	0.20	1.2	30	0.01	0.11	0.8	0.23	0.1	tr	0	3	0.05
Prune juice, canned	255	1 c	180	1.5	0.1	45	30	65	35	10	705	0.5	0.17	3.0	1	0.04	0.18	2.0	u	u	1	0	10	0.02
Puddings																								
Almendrado	65	⅓ c and 2 tbsp sauce	100	2.7	4.3	14	35	50	u	35	50	u	u	0.3	60	0.02	0.08	0.03	0.02	0.3	8	0.4	tr	u
Apple Brown Betty	110	½ c	160	1.5	4.0	30	20	25	5	165	110	u	u	0.6	20	0.06	0.04	0.4	u	u	u	u	1	u
Capirotada	155	½ c	385	10.8	14.0	58	230	200	u	335	355	u	u	2.5	50	0.1	0.20	3.0	0.1	0.4	6	0.3	0	u
Chocolate, instant, packaged	130	½ c	160	5.0	3.0	30	185	120	u	160	170	u	u	0.4	40	0.04	0.20	0.2	u	u	u	u	0	u
Custard	130	½ c	150	7.0	7.5	15	150	155	u	105	195	u	0.1	0.6	135	0.06	0.2	0.2	u	u	4	u	tr	u
Rice with raisins	130	½ c	200	5.0	4.0	35	130	125	u	95	235	0.4	0.04	0.6	30	0.04	0.2	0.2	u	u	5	u	tr	u
Tapioca	80	½ c	110	4.0	4.0	14	85	90	u	130	110	u	0.04	0.4	60	0.04	0.2	0.1	u	u	2	u	0	u
Vanilla, home recipe	130	½ c	140	4.5	5.0	20	150	115	u	85	175	u	0.05	tr	45	0.04	0.2	0.2	u	u	u	u	0	u
Pumpkin, canned	245	1 c	80	2.0	0.7	19	45	90	60	10	535	0.4	0.26	1.8	8300	0.05	0.15	1.0	0.13	1.0	35	0	11	tr
Radishes, raw	45	5 large	7	0.4	tr	1	10	10	7	10	130	0.1	0.04	0.4	tr	0.01	0.01	0.1	0.03	0.08	10	0	10	0
Raisins	35	¼ c	105	1.0	0.2	28	15	35	10	4	265	0.1	0.10	0.7	tr	tr	tr	0.3	0.08	tr	1	0	1	0
Rhubarb, cooked with sugar	120	½ c	140	0.5	0.1	37	175	10	15	2	115	0.1	0.03	0.2	15	0.02	0.03	u	0.02	0.1	6	0	4	0
Rice cooked, salt added																								
Brown	130	⅔ c	160	3.5	0.8	35	15	95	40	370	90	0.8	0.1	0.7	0	0.1	0.03	1.8	0.2	0.5	20	0	0	0.3
White, enriched	135	⅔ c	150	3.0	0.1	35	15	85	10	515	40	0.5	0.07	1.2	0	0.2	0.01	1.4	0.05	0.3	12	0	0	tr
Precooked, instant	110	⅔ c	120	2.5	tr	25	3	20	u	300	u	0.2	u	0.9	0	0.1	u	1.1	u	u	3	0	0	0
Rolls and buns																								
Danish pastry	65	1, of 4 in diameter	250	4.0	14.0	29	70	65	10	250	60	0.6	u	1.2	15	0.16	0.16	1.5	u	u	u	u	tr	u
Hamburger or frankfurter bun, enriched	40	1 average	115	3.4	2.0	20	55	30	10	240	35	0.2	0.07	1.2	tr	0.20	0.13	1.6	0.01	0.2	15	0	tr	u
Hard rolls, enriched	50	1 large	135	4.3	1	28	10	40	12	285	50	0.3	0.05	0.6	tr	0.05	0.06	0.6	0.03	0.2	30	0	0	u
Plain pan rolls, white, enriched	30	1 small	85	2.5	1.5	15	20	25	10	140	25	0.4	u	0.5	tr	0.08	0.05	0.6	0.01	0.1	15	0	0	u
Rutabagas, boiled	85	½ c, cubed	30	0.8	0.1	7	50	25	12	4	140	u	u	0.2	50	0.05	0.05	0.7	0.08	0.1	15	0	20	0
Salads																								
Chef's (lettuce w/ham, cheese, dressing, Red Barn)		1 serving	285	13.0	24.0	3	150	185	u	u	u	u	u	2.2	125	0.2	0.2	1.2	u	u	u	u	13	u
Potato, home recipe	125	½ c	120	3.5	3.5	20	40	80	u	650	400	0.3	u	0.8	20	0.1	0.09	1.4	u	u	u	u	14	u
Tuna fish	100	½ c	170	15.0	10.0	4	20	145	u	u	u	u	u	1.3	50	0.04	0.1	5.1	u	u	u	u	1	u

Salad dressings																								
Blue cheese	15	1 tbsp	75	0.7	8.0	1.0	10	10	u	165	5	0.04	u	tr	6	tr	0.02	tr	u	u	u	tr	tr	4.3
French, regular	15	1 tbsp	65	0.1	6.0	3.0	2	2	2	220	15	0.01	u	0.1	u	u	u	u	u	u	u	0	u	3.4
low-calorie	15	1 tbsp	20	0	0.9	3.0	2	2	u	125	15	u	u	0.1	u	u	u	u	u	u	u	0	u	0.5
Italian, regular	15	1 tbsp	70	tr	7.0	1.0	1	1	2	115	2	0.02	0.1	tr	tr	tr	tr	tr	0	0	0	0	0	4.1
low-calorie	15	1 tbsp	15	tr	1.5	0.7	tr	1	u	120	2	u	u	tr	tr	tr	tr	tr	0	0	0	0	0	0.9
Mayonnaise	15	1 tbsp	100	0.2	11.0	0.3	3	4	tr	80	5	0.02	0.04	0.1	10	tr	0.01	tr	u	0.02	0	0	0	5.7
Salad dressing	15	1 tbsp	65	0.2	6.5	2.0	2	4	tr	90	1	0.08	u	tr	6	tr	tr	tr	0	0.02	0	0	0	3.1
Thousand Island	15	1 tbsp	60	0.1	6.0	2.5	2	3	u	110	20	0.02	u	0.1	10	tr	tr	tr	u	u	u	u	tr	u
Salmon. See *Fish.*																								
Sandwiches																								
Bacon, lettuce, tomato on white bread	150	1 average	280	7.0	15.5	30	55	90	u	u	u	u	u	1.5	85	0.2	0.1	1.5	u	u	u	u	15	u
Egg salad on white bread	140	1 average	280	10.5	12.5	30	70	155	u	u	u	u	u	2.4	100	0.2	0.02	1.0	u	u	u	u	2	u
Fish fillet, fried on bun, McDonald's	135	1 average	410	15.0	21.5	37	95	235	20	760	u	u	u	1.6	20	0.2	0.4	2.9	0.1	u	20	0.8	2	u
Ham and cheese on white bread, Red Barn		1 average	350	20.0	19.0	30	215	240	u	u	u	u	u	3.1	60	0.4	0.3	2.5	u	u	u	u	0	u
Hamburger on bun,	95	1 regular	250	13.0	9.6	28	50	120	15	540	u	u	u	2.6	30	0.2	0.4	3.7	0.1	u	20	0.8	4	u
"Big Mac," McDonald's	185	1 large	560	26.0	32.0	40	160	290	30	1060	u	u	u	3.8	40	0.8	0.6	6.5	0.2	u	30	1.5	5	u
Roast beef, Arby's	141	1 regular	350	22.0	15.0	32	200	u	u	1220	u	u	u	4.5	u	0.3	0.3	5.0	u	u	u	u	u	u
Tuna salad on white bread	105	1 average	280	11.0	14.0	25	50	135	u	u	u	u	u	1.2	50	0.1	0.1	4.0	u	u	u	u	1	u
Sashimi. See *Fish*, tuna, raw.																								
Sardines. See *Fish.*																								
Sauces																								
Butterscotch	45	2 tbsp	200	0.5	7.0	35	40	25	u	u	u	u	u	1.4	60	tr	tr	tr	u	u	u	0	0	u
Cheese	40	2 tbsp	65	3.0	5.0	2	90	65	u	u	u	u	u	0.1	45	0.01	0.08	0.1	u	u	u	u	tr	u
Chocolate																								
thin syrup	40	2 tbsp	100	0.9	0.8	25	7	35	u	u	u	u	0.2	0.6	tr	0.01	0.03	0.2	u	u	u	0	0	u
fudge type	40	2 tbsp	125	2.0	5.0	20	50	60	u	35	105	u	u	0.5	6	0.02	0.08	0.2	u	u	u	tr	0	u
Custard	70	¼ c	85	3.5	4.0	10	80	80	u	u	u	u	u	0.4	60	0.04	0.2	0.1	u	u	u	u	tr	u
Hard sauce	20	2 tbsp	95	0.1	5.5	12	2	1	u	u	u	u	u	tr	60	tr	tr	tr	0	0	0	0	0	u
Hollandaise	50	¼ c scant	180	2.0	18.5	0.4	25	80	u	u	u	u	u	0.9	300	0.03	0.04	tr	u	u	u	u	tr	u
Soy	35	2 tbsp	25	2.0	0.5	4	30	40	u	2665	135	u	u	1.7	0	0.01	0.09	0.1	u	u	u	0	0	0
Tartar	15	1 tbsp	75	0.2	8.0	0.6	3	4	u	100	10	u	u	0.1	3	tr	tr	tr	u	u	u	u	tr	u
Tomato catsup	15	1 tbsp	15	0.3	0.1	4	3	10	3	155	55	0.04	0.09	0.1	20	0.01	0.01	0.2	0.02	u	tr	0	2	u
White, medium	125	½ c	200	5.0	15.5	11	145	115	20	475	175	0.5	0.05	0.2	140	0.05	0.2	0.2	0.06	0.8	1	0.2	1	u
Sauerkraut, canned	120	½ c	25	1	0.3	6	40	25	20	800	235	0.2	0.12	1.9	3	0.02	0.02	0.3	0.16	0.1	u	0	18	0
Sausages																								
Bologna	30	1 slice 4¼ in × ⅛ in	90	3	8	0.5	3	25	5	285	45	0.6	0.01	0.4	0	0.02	0.04	0.7	0.05	0.1	1	0.4	5	0.3
Frankfurter (all meat)	45	1 average	145	5	13	1.0	5	40	5	505	75	0.8	0.04	0.5	0	0.09	0.05	1.2	0.06	0.2	2	0.6	12	1.2
Liverwurst	30	1 oz	95	4	8	0.6	5	65	u	u	u	u	u	1.8	1200	0.08	0.29	u	u	0.8	8	24.3	0	0.7
Luncheon meat, pork, cured	30	1 oz	100	3.5	9	0.7	5	25	5	370	60	0.5	0.01	0.2	0	0.09	0.04	0.8	0.06	0.2	2	0.4	4	1.1
Pork sausage links	50	3 links	185	11	15	1.0	15	80	10	720	160	1.4	0.03	0.6	0	0.3	0.1	2.2	0.2	0.4	7	0.7	tr	0.6
Salami, dry	30	3 small slices	125	7	10	0.8	5	40	6	560	115	1.0	0.03	0.4	0	0.2	0.09	1.5	0.2	0.3	u	0.6	tr	1.0
Vienna, canned	50	3 sausages	135	5	12	1.0	5	25	5	450	50	0.8	0	0.4	0	0.04	0.05	0.8	0.06	u	u	0.5	0	0.8
Scallops																								
Breaded, fried	95	3½ oz	180	17.0	8.0	10	u	u	u	u	u	u	0.1	u	0	u	u	u	u	0.1	15	u	0	u
Steamed	95	3½ oz	105	22.0	1.5	3	110	320	u	250	455	u	0.1	2.8	0	u	0.06	1.3	u	u	18	1.1	u	0.4
Sesame seeds, hulled	40	¼ c	220	7.0	20.0	7	40	220	7	u	u	u	0.6	0.9	0	0.07	0.05	2.0	u	u	25	0	0	u
Sherbet, orange	95	½ c	135	1.0	2.0	29	50	35	7	45	100	0.7	u	0.2	20	0.02	0.04	0.1	0.01	0.03	7	0.08	2	0.07
Shrimp, canned	85	3 oz	100	20.5	0.9	0.6	100	225	45	835	105	1.8	0.1	2.7	tr	0.01	0.03	1.5	0.05	0.2	10	u	0	0.4
French-fried	85	3 oz	190	17.5	9.5	8	60	160	40	160	195	0.8	0.3	1.8	u	0.03	0.06	2.5	0.05	0.3	5	0.6	0	u

Food	Weight gm	Approximate Measure	Energy Kcal	Pro-tein gm	Fat gm	Total Carbo-hy-drate gm	Cal-cium mg	Phos-pho-rus mg	Mag-ne-sium mg	So-dium mg	Po-tas-sium mg	Zinc mg	Cop-per mg	Iron mg	Total Vitamin A Activity RE	Thia-min mg	Ribo-flavin mg	Nia-cin mg	Vita-min B-6 mg	Panto-thenic Acid mg	Fola-cin Total µg	Vita-min B-12 µg	Vita-min C mg	Polyun-saturated Fatty Acids gm
Soups																								
Albondiga (meatballs in tomato broth)	240	1 c with 4 meatballs	340	18.5	21.4	17	25	175	u	180	460	u	u	3.6	50	0.2	0.2	5.0	0.6	0.7	10	1.2	8	u
Bean with bacon	250	1 c	170	8.0	6.0	22	80	130	45	950	400	1.0	0.4	2.0	90	0.1	0.03	0.6	tr	u	32	u	2	1.8
Bouillon, broth, consomme	240	1 c	15	3.0	0.5	0.1	15	30	u	780	130	u	u	0.4	u	tr	0.05	1.8	u	u	u	u	0	tr
Cream soups, canned																								
Chicken diluted with water	245	1 c	115	3.5	7.5	9	35	40	5	990	90	0.6	0.1	0.6	55	0.03	0.06	0.8	tr	u	2	u	0.2	1.5
Chicken diluted with milk	250	1 c	190	7.5	11.5	15	180	150	20	1050	275	0.7	0.1	0.7	95	0.07	0.26	0.9	0.06	u	8	u	1	1.6
Mushroom diluted with water	245	1 c	130	2.5	9.0	9	45	50	5	1030	100	0.6	0.1	0.5	0	0.05	0.09	0.7	0.01	0.3	7	0.1	1	4.2
Mushroom diluted with milk	250	1 c	200	6.0	13.5	15	180	160	20	1075	270	0.6	0.1	0.6	40	0.08	0.28	0.9	0.06	u	u	u	2	4.6
Chicken noodle, from dry mix	250	1 c	55	3.0	1.0	7	30	30	5	1285	30	0.2	0.03	0.5	6	0.07	0.06	0.9	tr	u	1	u	0.3	0.3
Clam chowder, Manhattan	245	1 c	80	4.0	2.5	12	35	60	10	1810	260	0.9	0.15	1.9	90	0.06	0.05	1.3	0.08	0.1	10	2.1	3.0	1.3
Onion	240	1 c	55	4.0	1.5	8	25	10	2	1050	70	0.6	0.12	0.7	0	0.03	0.02	0.06	0.05	u	15	0	1.0	0.6
Split pea with ham	250	1 c	190	10.0	4.5	28	20	210	48	1010	400	1.3	0.37	2.3	45	0.15	0.08	1.5	0.07	u	2	u	1.0	0.6
Tomato	265	1 c	100	2.5	2.5	19	50	65	15	945	295	0.2	0.09	0.4	80	0.06	0.05	0.8	0.1	u	7	u	5.0	0.2
Vegetable beef	245	1 c	80	5.5	2.0	10	15	40	6	955	175	1.5	0.18	1.1	190	0.04	0.05	1.0	0.07	u	10	0.3	2.0	0.1
Soybeans, mature, dry, cooked	90	½ c (1 oz dry wt.)	120	10.0	5.0	10	65	160	80	2	490	0.6	0.3	2.5	2	0.20	0.08	0.6	u	u	70	0	0	3.0
Spaghetti																								
Canned, with tomato sauce and meatballs, Franco American	210	1 can, 7½ oz	250	10.4	12.8	23	20	120	u	1035	375	u	0.3	2.2	100	0.15	0.2	3.4	u	u	u	u	u	u
Home recipe, with tomato sauce																								
with cheese	250	1 c	260	9.0	9.0	35	80	135	30	955	410	0.2	0.3	2.3	250	0.2	0.2	2.5	0.1	0.8	2	0.6	15	u
with meatballs	250	1 c	330	18.5	11.5	40	125	235	40	1010	665	3.5	0.4	3.7	300	0.2	0.3	4.0	0.4	0.5	15	0.6	20	u
Spinach, fresh or frozen, boiled	90	½ c	20	2.5	0.2	3	90	40	60	50	300	0.5	0.1	2.0	730	0.06	0.1	0.4	0.2	0.2	60	0	20	tr
Sprouts, raw																								
Alfalfa	100	1 c, packed	40	5.0	0.6	5	30	u	u	u	u	1.0	u	1.4	u	0.1	0.2	1.5	u	u	u	0	15	tr
Mung bean	100	1 c	35	4.0	0.2	7	20	65	u	5	235	0.9	u	1.4	2	0.1	0.1	0.8	u	u	u	0	20	tr
Soybean	100	1 c	50	6.5	1.5	6	50	70	u	u	u	1.6	u	1.1	8	0.2	0.2	0.8	u	u	u	0	15	tr
Squash																								
Summer, boiled	90	½ c	10	0.8	0.1	3	20	20	15	1	125	0.2	0.07	0.4	35	0.04	0.07	0.7	0.2	0.1	10	0	9	tr
Winter																								
baked	100	½ c	65	2.0	0.4	15	30	50	17	1	470	u	u	0.8	350	0.05	0.1	0.7	0.09	0.3	u	0	15	tr
boiled	120	½ c	45	1.5	0.4	10	25	40	17	1	315	u	u	0.6	350	0.05	0.1	0.5	0.1	0.3	u	0	10	tr
Strawberries																								
Fresh	150	1 c, whole	45	1.0	0.5	10	20	30	15	2	245	0.2	0.07	0.6	25	0.03	0.1	0.3	0.09	0.5	26	0	85	0.28
Frozen, sweetened	255	1 c	245	1.4	0.3	66	30	30	20	8	250	0.1	0.05	1.5	6	0.04	0.1	1.0	0.08	0.3	38	0	105	0.16
Sugar																								
Brown	220	1 c, packed	820	0	0	210	185	40	u	65	755	u	0.7	7.5	0	0.02	0.07	0.4	u	u	u	0	0	0
White																								
granulated	200	1 c	770	0	0	200	0	0	0	2	5	0.1	0.04	0.2	0	0	0	0	0	0	0	0	0	0
	4	1 tsp	15	0	0	4	0	0	0	tr	tr	tr	tr	tr	0	0	0	0	0	0	0	0	0	0
powdered	8	1 tbsp	30	0	0	8	0	0	0	tr	tr	tr	tr	tr	0	0	0	0	0	0	0	0	0	0
Sundaes, ice cream w/topping																								
Hot fudge, McDonald's	164	1 regular	310	7.0	11.0	46	215	236	35	175	410	1.0	0.13	0.6	50	0.07	0.3	1.1	0.1	u	u	0.7	2	u
Banana split, Dairy Queen	383	1 regular	540	10.0	15.0	91	350	250	u	u	u	u	u	1.8	150	0.6	0.6	0.8	u	u	u	0.9	18	u

Sunflower seed, raw	35	¼ c	200	8.5	17.0	7	45	305	13	10	335	u	0.6	2.6	2	0.7	0.08	2.0	0.4	0.5	80	0	0	8.9
Sweet potatoes																								
Baked in skin	145	1 potato, 5 in × 2 in	160	2.5	0.6	35	45	65	45	15	340	1.0	0.2	1.0	920	0.1	0.08	0.8	0.05	1.0	10	0	25	tr
Boiled in skin	130	½ c mashed	150	2.0	0.5	35	40	60	u	15	620	u	0.2	0.9	900	0.1	0.08	0.8	0.3	1.0	9	0	20	tr
Candied	105	½ medium	180	1.5	3.5	35	40	45	u	45	200	u	0.06	0.9	660	0.06	0.04	0.4	u	u	7	0	10	u
Syrup, maple-flavored, artificial	20	1 tbsp	50	0	0	13	20	2	u	2	35	tr	0.08	0.2	0	0	0	0	0	0	0	0	0	0
Tacos, beef	80	1 taco	160	11.0	8.5	9	135	160	u	200	210	u	u	2.0	60	0.07	0.1	2.3	0.3	0.3	25	0.7	3	u
Tamales, canned	100	3½ oz	140	4.5	7.0	14	20	40	10	665	u	0.9	0.05	1.2	u	u	u	u	u	u	u	u	u	u
Home recipe, chicken	130	2 tamales	275	8.3	23.7	8	100	60	u	60	90	u	u	0.9	300	0.05	0.1	2.7	0.2	0.3	1	0.1	7	u
Tea, instant	1	½ tsp	0	0	tr	tr	0	5	3	1	50	tr	0.01	tr	0	0	0.02	0.1	u	u	u	0	0	0
Tofu, soybean curd	120	1 piece, 2½ × 2¾ × 1 in	85	9.5	5.0	3	155	150	130	10	50	u	u	2.3	0	0.07	0.04	0.1	u	u	u	0	0	3.0
Tomatoes, raw	135	1 medium	25	1.5	0.2	6	15	35	20	4	300	0.3	0.10	0.6	110	0.07	0.05	0.9	0.1	0.4	25	0	30	tr
Canned	120	½ c	25	1.0	0.2	5	30	25	15	190	350	0.2	0.12	0.6	70	0.06	0.04	0.8	0.1	0.3	25	0	22	tr
Tomato juice, canned	180	¾ c	30	1.4	0.2	7	15	35	20	500	445	0.3	0.27	1.2	70	0.07	0.05	1.3	0.35	0.5	u	0	75	0
Tomato paste	130	½ c	110	4.4	0.5	26	45	115	75	40	1340	1.0	0.77	3.2	215	0.3	0.2	4.0	0.49	0.6	u	0	70	0
Tongue, beef, braised	100	3½ oz	250	21.5	17.0	0.4	5	120	16	60	165	u	0.07	2.2	0	0.05	0.3	3.5	0.1	2.0	u	u	0	u
Tortillas																								
Corn, lime-treated	30	1, of 6 in diameter	65	1.5	0.6	14	60	40	30	u	u	0.03	0.06	0.9	tr	0.04	0.02	0.3	0.02	0.03	tr	0	0	0.3
White flour	30	1, of 6 in diameter	110	3.0	1.0	20	4	50	15	250	30	u	u	1.0	0	0.08	0.04	0.5	0.02	0.03	5	0	0	0.6
Tostada with beans and small portion of cheese	210	1 tostada	335	11.6	17.6	35	195	245	u	350	425	u	u	3.2	170	0.3	0.2	1.3	0.2	0.4	10	0.2	10	u
Tuna. See *Fish.*																								
Turkey, roasted																								
Light meat	85	2 slices, each 4 in × 2 in × ¼ in	170	25	7	0	20	175	20	55	240	1.7	0.04	1.2	0	0.05	0.1	5.3	0.4	0.5	5	0.3	0	1.7
Dark meat	85	4 slices, each 2½ × 1½ × ¼ in	185	25	10	0	30	165	20	65	235	3.5	0.1	1.9	0	0.05	0.2	3.0	0.3	1.0	8	0.3	0	2.6
Turnips, boiled	80	½ c, cubed	20	0.6	0.2	4	25	20	10	25	145	0.07	0.03	0.3	tr	0.03	0.04	0.2	0.06	0.08	13	0	15	tr
Turnip greens, boiled	70	½ c	15	1.5	0.2	3	135	25	20	10	125	0.1	0.04	0.8	460	0.1	0.2	0.4	0.1	0.1	40	0	50	tr
Veal cutlet, broiled	85	3 oz	180	23.0	9.5	0	10	195	20	55	260	4.1	0.04	2.7	0	0.06	0.2	4.5	0.3	0.8	15	1.6	0	tr
Vinegar, cider	15	1 tbsp	2	tr	0	1	1	1	u	tr	15	0.02	0.01	0.1	0	0	0	0	0	0	0	0	0	0
Waffles																								
Made from mix	75	1, of 7 in diameter	210	6.5	8.0	25	180	260	20	515	145	u	u	1.0	60	0.1	0.2	u	u	0.5	u	u	0	u
Frozen, Aunt Jemina	45	2 sections	125	2.6	4.0	19	35	170	10	310	95	0.4	0.03	2.2	120	0.2	0.2	2.3	0.12	0.2	2	tr	tr	u
Walnuts, English	100	1 c halves	650	15.0	64.0	16	100	380	135	2	450	2.8	0.9	3.1	3	0.3	0.1	0.9	0.7	0.9	45	0	2	45.0
	15	2 tbsp, chopped	100	2.5	10.0	3	15	60	20	tr	70	0.4	0.1	0.4	1	0.06	0.02	0.2	0.1	0.1	5	0	tr	7.0
Watercress, raw	35	10 sprigs	5	0.8	0.1	1	55	20	5	20	100	u	0.03	0.6	170	0.03	0.06	0.3	0.04	0.1	70	0	30	tr
Wheat bran, crude	30	1 oz	60	4.5	1.0	17	35	355	135	3	315	2.7	0.4	4.2	0	0.2	0.1	6.0	0.2	0.1	80	0	0	0.6
Wheat germ, raw	30	1 oz	100	7.5	3.0	13	20	315	90	tr	230	4.7	0.7	2.6	u	0.6	0.2	1.0	0.3	0.9	80	0	0	1.5
Toasted	30	1 oz	110	8	3.0	14	15	325	90	1	270	4.7	0.18	2.6	0	0.5	0.2	1.6	0.28	0.4	100	0	2	1.84
Wine, dessert (18.8%)	105	3½ fl. oz	140	0.1	0	8	10	u	4	7	100	0.1	0.06	1.6	0	0.02	0.02	0.2	0.05	0.02	2	0	0	0
Table (12.2%)	100	3½ fl. oz	90	0.2	0	4	10	15	10	10	115	0.1	0.03	1.0	0	0.01	0.03	0.1	0.04	0.04	1	0	0	0
Yeast																								
Dry, active	5	1 tbsp	20	2.5	0.1	3	3	90	3	4	140	u	0.2	1.1	tr	0.2	0.4	2.5	0.1	0.6	7	0	0	0
Brewer's, debittered	5	1 tbsp	25	3.0	0.1	3	15	140	10	10	150	u	u	1.4	tr	1.2	0.3	3.0	0.1	0.6	9	0	0	0
Yogurt																								
Low-fat, plain	230	8 fl oz carton	145	12.0	3.5	16	415	325	40	160	530	2.0	u	0.2	35	0.1	0.5	0.3	0.1	1.3	25	1.3	2	0.1
fruit, sweetened	230	8 fl oz carton	225	9.0	2.6	42	315	245	30	120	400	1.5	u	0.1	25	0.08	0.4	0.2	0.1	1.0	20	1.0	1	0.1
Regular plain	230	8 fl oz carton	140	8.0	7.5	11	275	215	25	105	350	1.3	u	0.1	70	0.07	0.3	0.2	0.1	0.9	20	0.8	2	0.14

Table 3 PER CAPITA FOOD CONSUMPTION, SELECTED ITEMS,[1] SELECTED YEARS, 1960–81*

Food item	*1960*	*1970*	*1979*	*1980*	*1981*[2]
			Pounds		
All items	1400.1	1397.0	1415.1	1406.9	1399.8
Animal products	614.2	614.2	589.9	587.4	582.2
Crop products	785.9	782.8	825.2	819.5	817.6
Total red meat (excluding game and offal)	134.0	151.6	144.9	147.7	145.2
Beef	64.2	84.0	78.0	76.5	77.2
Pork	60.3	62.3	63.8	68.3	65.0
Lamb and mutton	4.3	2.9	1.3	1.4	1.4
Veal	5.2	2.4	1.7	1.5	1.6
Fishery products	10.3	11.8	13.0	12.8	13.0
Chicken	27.8	40.4	50.6	50.1	51.7
Turkey	6.2	8.0	9.9	10.5	10.7
Eggs	42.6	39.1	35.2	34.6	33.6
All dairy products	653.4	560.7	547.7	544.3	541.5
Fluid whole milk	263.9	213.3	150.1	143.5	137.9
Total cheese	8.3	11.5	17.2	17.6	18.2
Butter	7.5	5.3	4.5	4.5	4.3
Ice cream	18.3	17.6	17.1	17.3	17.2
Fats and oils—total fat food content (including butter)	45.1	52.6	55.8	55.8	56.9
Animal fats	18.1	14.1	11.0	11.0	10.8
Vegetable oils	27.0	38.5	44.8	44.8	46.1
Total fruit	139.4	134.5	136.2	141.2	142.3
Processed	50.3	55.6	55.5	55.4	55.0
Fresh	89.1	78.9	80.8	85.7	87.3
Total vegetables	146.6	152.1	160.8	159.2	154.3
Fresh (commercial)	96.2	91.4	96.4	99.0	97.1
Processed	50.4	60.9	64.4	60.2	57.2
Wheat flour	118.2	110.8	117.2	116.9	116.6
Rice	6.1	6.7	9.4	9.4	11.0
Sugar	97.6	101.7	89.3	83.7	79.4
Corn sweeteners	10.2	18.4	43.3	48.9	55.0
Coffee	11.6	10.4	8.5	7.8	7.7
Soft drinks (gallons)	13.6	23.7	36.8	37.8	38.0
Sprits	1.9	2.5	2.6	2.5	2.5
Beer	22.0	25.2	30.5	30.9	31.1
Wine	1.3	1.7	2.5	2.8	2.7

*From Nat. Food Review (USDA), 1983 (Feb). p. 11.
[1]Alcoholic beverages are in gallons of beverage volume for the drinking age population.
[2]Preliminary.

Table 4 PERCENTILES* FOR HEIGHT AND WEIGHT FOR BOYS 0–18 YEARS†

Age	Body Weight, kg			Height, cm		
	3*	50*	97*	3*	50*	97*
0–3 months	3.72	4.56	6.01	51.55	55.50	59.15
3–6 months	5.58	6.65	8.44	59.90	63.40	67.05
6–9 months	6.94	8.32	10.25	65.35	68.80	73.15
9–12 months	7.96	9.57	11.72	69.50	73.20	78.10
1–2 years	9.57	11.43	14.29	77.50	81.80	88.20
2–3 years	11.43	13.61	16.78	86.90	92.10	99.50
3–4 years	12.93	15.56	18.82	94.30	99.80	106.50
4–5 years	14.33	17.42	21.50	100.60	106.70	114.30
5–6 years	16.56	20.68	25.92	105.30	114.40	122.85
6–7 years	18.48	23.22	29.71	111.25	120.80	129.80
7–8 years	20.64	25.90	33.86	116.80	127.10	136.80
8–9 years	22.79	28.62	38.38	121.90	132.80	142.75
9–10 years	24.78	31.30	43.04	126.45	137.90	147.80
10–11 years	26.90	33.93	48.02	131.05	142.30	152.35
11–12 years	29.26	36.74	53.50	135.75	146.90	158.15
12–13 years	31.57	40.23	59.47	140.15	152.30	165.70
13–14 years	34.43	45.50	65.46	144.30	158.90	173.30
14–15 years	38.80	51.66	70.80	149.05	165.30	180.95
15–16 years	44.16	56.65	75.32	154.10	169.70	183.70
16–17 years	48.51	60.33	78.50	157.75	172.70	186.10
17–18 years	50.69	62.41	80.42	159.30	174.10	187.10

*The percentile refers to the percent of subjects below the given weight or height.
†From Nelson, W. E., et al. (eds.): *Textbook of Pediatrics.* 9th Ed. Philadelphia, W. B. Saunders Co., 1969.

Table 5 PERCENTILES* FOR HEIGHT AND WEIGHT FOR GIRLS 0–18 YEARS†

Age	Body Weight, kg			Height, cm		
	3*	50*	97*	3*	50*	97*
0–3 months	3.54	4.49	5.51	51.45	54.85	58.35
3–6 months	5.10	6.44	7.92	58.45	62.35	65.95
6–9 months	6.30	7.98	10.02	63.25	67.65	71.45
9–12 months	7.24	9.23	11.64	67.15	72.15	76.45
1–2 years	8.80	11.11	14.02	74.90	80.90	86.70
2–3 years	10.70	13.43	17.33	84.50	91.40	98.70
3–4 years	12.47	15.38	20.55	92.00	99.50	108.00
4–5 years	13.98	17.46	23.09	98.10	106.80	116.20
5–6 years	16.08	19.96	25.06	105.30	112.80	121.70
6–7 years	17.30	22.41	28.58	111.00	119.10	128.55
7–8 years	19.64	25.04	33.16	116.55	125.20	134.55
8–9 years	21.41	27.67	38.28	121.35	130.50	140.40
9–10 years	23.20	30.44	43.50	125.65	135.80	146.35
10–11 years	25.20	33.79	48.72	130.00	141.70	153.35
11–12 years	27.56	37.74	54.56	135.05	148.10	161.00
12–13 years	30.80	42.37	61.24	140.75	154.30	166.50
13–14 years	35.22	47.04	66.48	145.95	158.40	169.55
14–15 years	39.03	50.35	69.40	149.20	160.40	171.15
15–16 years	41.00	52.30	70.96	150.50	161.70	171.80
16–17 years	42.12	53.57	71.94	150.90	162.40	172.10
17–18 years	42.73	54.20	72.62	151.00	162.50	172.00

*The percentile refers to the percent of subjects below the given weight or height.
†From Nelson, W. E., et al. (eds.): *Textbook of Pediatrics.* 9th Ed. Philadelphia, W. B. Saunders Co., 1969.

Note: See Table 7-1, p. 160 for "Guidelines for Body Weight" for desirable weights of men and women. Also see following tables.

Table 6 1983 Metropolitan Height and Weight Tables: Men*

Height		Frame†		
Feet	**Inches**	**Small**	**Medium**	**Large**
5	2	128-134	131-141	138-150
5	3	130-136	133-143	140-153
5	4	132-138	135-145	142-156
5	5	134-140	137-148	144-160
5	6	136-142	139-151	146-164
5	7	138-145	142-154	149-168
5	8	140-148	145-157	152-172
5	9	142-151	148-160	155-176
5	10	144-154	151-163	158-180
5	11	146-157	154-166	161-184
6	0	149-160	157-170	164-188
6	1	152-164	160-174	168-192
6	2	155-168	164-178	172-197
6	3	158-172	167-182	176-202
6	4	162-176	171-187	181-207

*Source: Metropolitan Life Insurance Company

†Weights at ages 25-59 based on lowest mortality. Weight in pounds according to frame (in indoor clothing weighing 5 lb, shoes with 1″ heels).

Table 7 1983 Metropolitan Height and Weight Tables: Women*

Height		Frame†		
Feet	**Inches**	**Small**	**Medium**	**Large**
4	10	102-111	109-121	118-131
4	11	103-113	111-123	120-134
5	0	104-115	113-126	122-137
5	1	106-118	115-129	125-140
5	2	108-121	118-132	128-143
5	3	111-124	121-135	131-147
5	4	114-127	124-138	134-151
5	5	117-130	127-141	137-155
5	6	120-133	130-144	140-159
5	7	123-136	133-147	143-163
5	8	126-139	136-150	146-167
5	9	129-142	139-153	149-170
5	10	132-145	142-156	152-173
5	11	135-148	145-159	155-176
6	0	138-151	148-162	158-179

*Source: Metropolitan Life Insurance Company

†Weights at ages 25-59 based on lowest mortality. Weight in pounds according to frame (in indoor clothing weighing 3 lb, shoes with 1″ heels).

Note: See Knapp, T.R.: A methodological critique of the 'ideal weight' concept. J. Amer. Med. Assoc. *250*:506, 1983 (a discussion of these and other height weight tables). Also see RDA table inside front cover and the RDA booklet).

Table 8 INTRODUCTION TO SOME BASIC ORGANIC GROUPS AND COMPOUNDS

Classification and Distinguishing Chemical Group	***Examples***
Hydrocarbon Composed of only hydrogen (H) and carbon (C)	Methane; Ethane; Methyl group
Alcohol Oxygen = O (−OH) = alcohol group or hydroxyl group.	Methanol; Ethanol (in alcoholic beverages)
Organic acid (−COOH) = acid or carboxyl group.	Formic acid; Acetic acid; Propionic acid

```
    H            H  H            H
    |            |  |            |
 H—C—H       H—C—C—H         —C—H
    |            |  |            |
    H            H  H            H
 Methane       Ethane        Methyl group

    H             H  H
    |             |  |
 H—C—OH       H—C—C—OH
    |             |  |
    H             H  H
 Methanol     Ethanol (in alcoholic beverages)

       O          H    O          H  H    O
      //          |   //          |  |   //
 H—C          H—C—C          H—C—C—C
      \           |   \           |  |   \
       OH         H    OH         H  H    OH
 Formic acid   Acetic acid     Propionic acid
```

Table 8 *(Continued)* INTRODUCTION TO SOME BASIC ORGANIC GROUPS AND COMPOUNDS

Classification and Distinguishing Chemical Group	*Examples*
Ketone Carbonyl group = (–C=O) R, R, C=O *R = Remainder of the compound.*	H H H—C—C—C—H H O H Acetone
Aldehyde Carbonyl group with hydrogen attached, R, H, C=O (–CHO) = aldhyde group.	H—C(=O)—H Formaldehyde H—C(H)(H)—C(=O)—H Acetaldehyde
Examples of other common biological compounds containing more than one of the above groups:	
H O O H—C—C—C H H OH Lactic acid	H—C(H)—C(=O)OH HO—C—C(=O)OH H—C(H)—C(=O)OH Citric acid HO—C(=O)—C(=O)—OH Oxalic acid
Compounds with Nitrogen (N) $(-NH_2)$ = amino group (NH_3) = ammonia (a gas) $(-NH_4)$ = ammonium ion	NH_2, NH_2, C = O Urea (1st organic compound made) NH_2 R—C—COOH H an alpha amino acid
Purines and pyrimidines	N=C—NH_2 HC C—NH CH N—C—N Adenine (a purine) N=C—NH_2 O=C CH HN—CH Cytosine (a pyrimidine)

Table 9 STRUCTURAL FORMULAS OF THE MOST COMMON AMINO ACIDS*

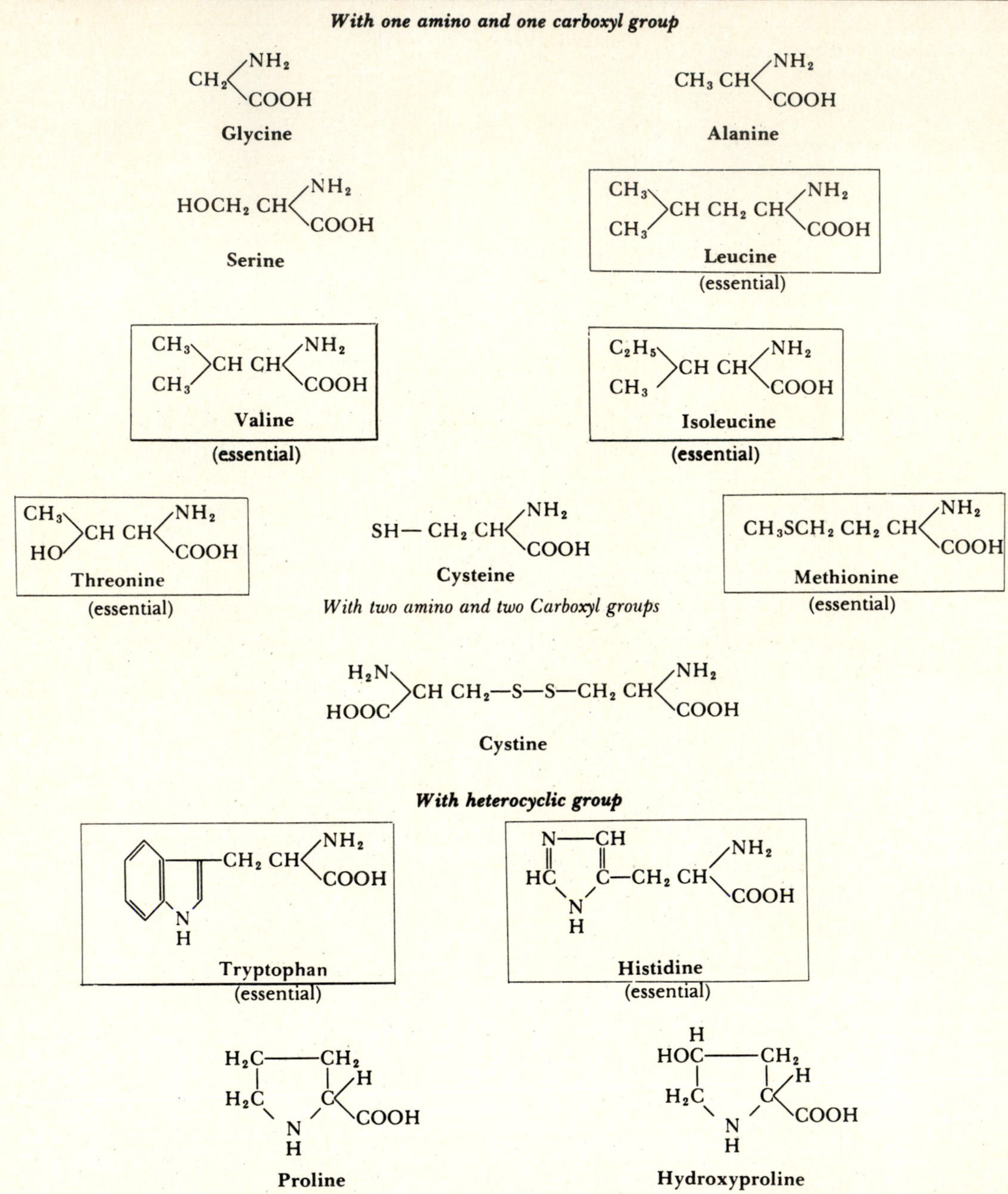

*Each of the essential amino acids is marked. Histidine and perhaps arginine are needed only by growing children, not by adults (see Chapter 4).

Table 9 STRUCTURAL FORMULAS OF THE MOST COMMON AMINO ACIDS (*Continued*)

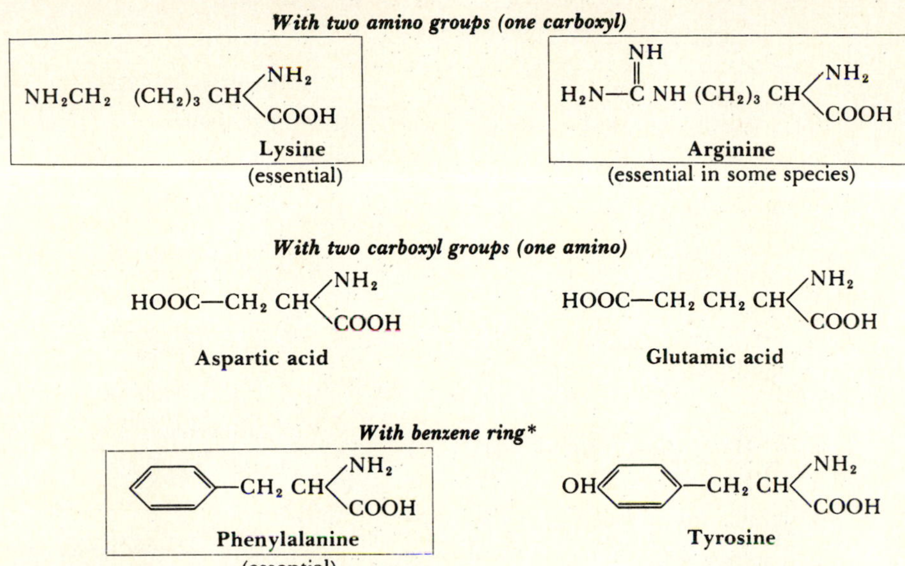

*For simplification, the benzene ring is often represented by a hexagon. It should be understood that there is a carbon atom (C) at each of the six points of the hexagon with hydrogen atoms attached, except where the valence bond is attached to the remainder of the molecule. The benzyl radical may also be represented as:

C_6H_5— or HC(CH=CH)(CH=CH)C— *or* ⬡—

In the heterocyclic groups, simplified representations of which are used in formulas on the following page, there are also carbon atoms at each point unless otherwise indicated (e.g., N), with hydrogen atoms attached as needed to satisfy valences.

Table 10 STRUCTURES OF WATER-SOLUBLE VITAMINS

Vitamin C: Ascorbic Acid

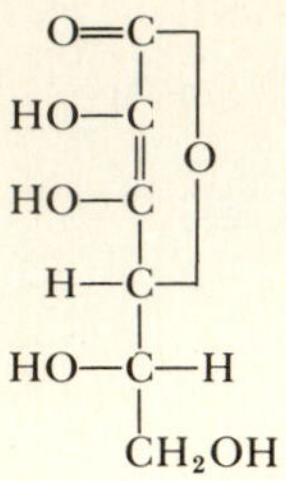

```
   O=C──┐
     |  |
 HO─C   |
    ||  O
 HO─C   |
     |  |
   H─C──┘
     |
 HO─C─H
     |
    CH2OH
```

Riboflavin

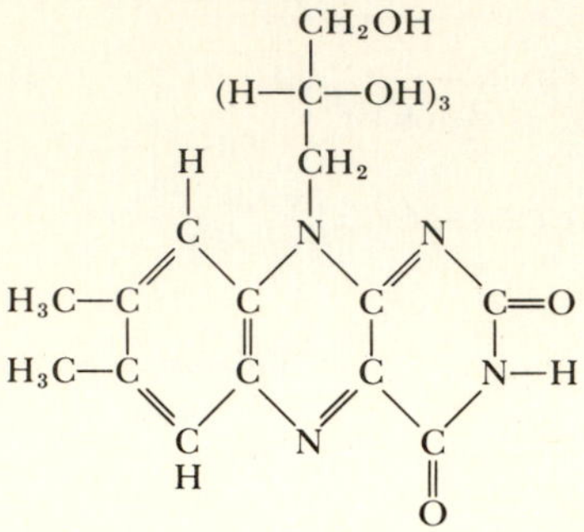

```
                 CH2OH
                  |
               (H─C─OH)3
                  |
          H      CH2
          |       |
          C       N       N
        //  \   /   \   // \
  H3C─C      C         C     C=O
       |     ||        |     |
  H3C─C      C         C     N─H
        \\  /   \   //  \   /
          C       N       C
          H               ||
                          O
```

Thiamin

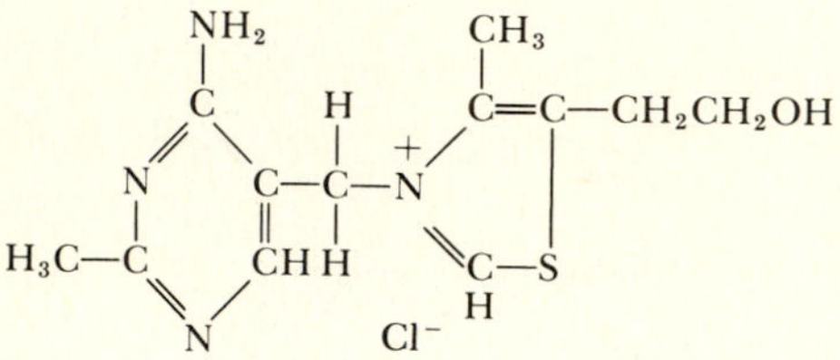

```
        NH2           CH3
         |             |
         C      H      C=C─CH2CH2OH
       //  \    |   + /   |
      N     C───C───N     |
      |     ||  |    \\   |
 H3C─C      CH  H     C──S
      \\   /          H
        N         Cl⁻
```

Niacin

Nicotinic Acid

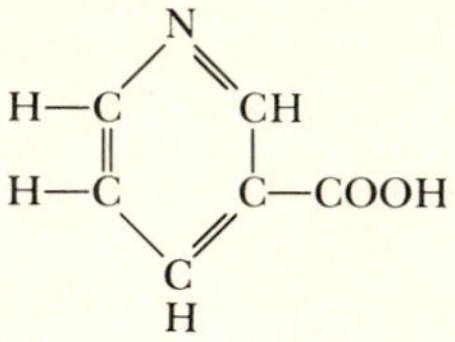

```
        N
      /  \\
  H─C      CH
    ||     |
  H─C      C─COOH
      \  //
        C
        H
```

Nicotinamide

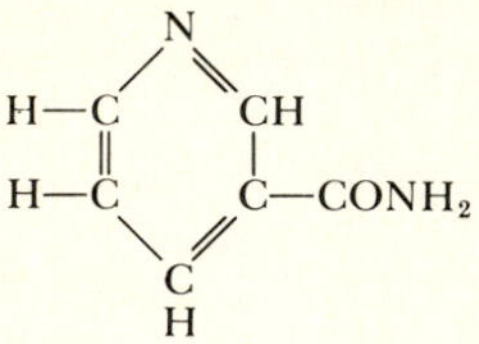

```
        N
      /  \\
  H─C      CH
    ||     |
  H─C      C─CONH2
      \  //
        C
        H
```

Vitamin B-6 Group

Pyridoxine

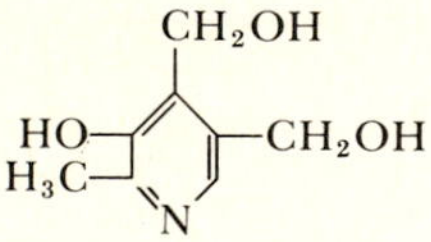

```
        CH2OH
         |
   HO─┐//  \┌─CH2OH
  H3C─┘\\  /
          N
```

Pyridoxal

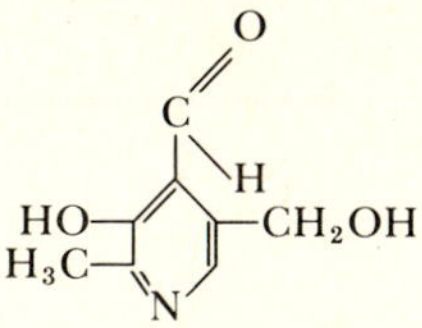

```
           O
          //
         C
         | \
         |  H
   HO─┐//  \┌─CH2OH
  H3C─┘\\  /
          N
```

Pyridoxamine

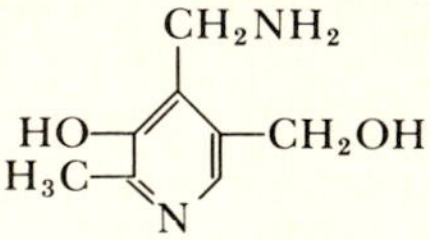

```
        CH2NH2
         |
   HO─┐//  \┌─CH2OH
  H3C─┘\\  /
          N
```

Pantothenic Acid

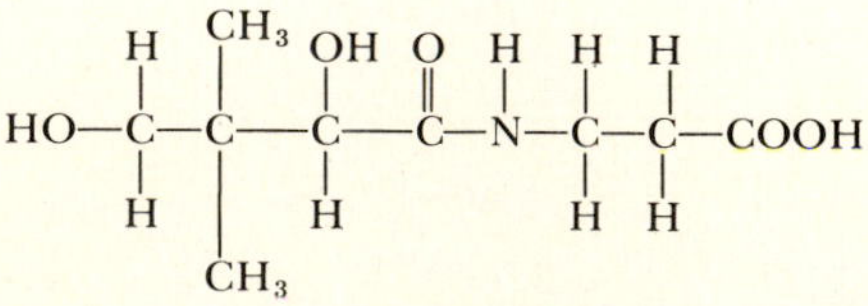

```
      H  CH3  OH  O   H  H  H
      |   |   |   ||  |  |  |
  HO─C───C───C───C───N─C──C─COOH
      |   |   |         |  |
      H   |   H         H  H
         CH3
```

Table continued on following page.

Folacin

(represented by monopteroylglutamic acid)

H H H N N

H H O C=C H H C C C—NH_2

HOOC—C—N—C—C C—N—C—C C N

H—C—H C—C H N C

HOOC—CH_2 H H OH

Biotin

O

C

HN NH

H—C——C—H

CH_2—CH_2—CH_2CH_2COOH

H_2—C C

S H

Vitamin B-12

(represented by cyanocobalamin)

CH_2CONH_2

CH_2 H CH_3 CH_3

—CH_2CONH_2

NH_2COCH_2 A B —$CH_2CH_2CONH_2$

CH_3 N CN N

CH_3 Co^+

N N CH_3

NH_2COCH_2— D C CH_3

$COCH_2CH_2$ CH_3 CH_3 $CH_2CH_2CONH_2$

NH

CH_2

$CHCH_3$

O O^-

P N CH_3

O O OH N CH_3

H C—C

C H H C

$HOCH_2$ H

O

Choline

CH_3 CH_2CH_2OH

CH_3—N

CH_3 OH

Table 11 STRUCTURES OF FAT-SOLUBLE VITAMINS

Vitamin A
(represented by retinol)

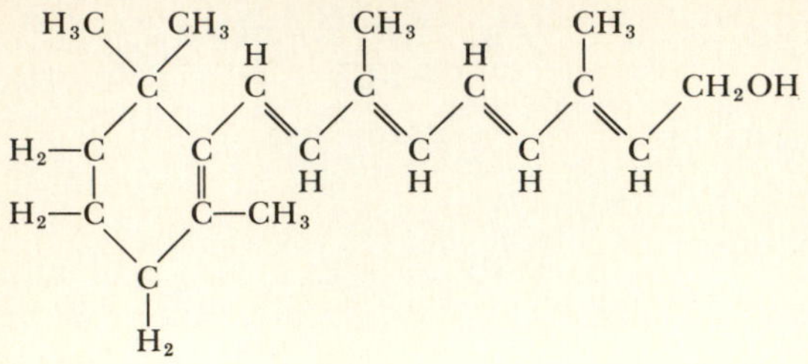

Beta-carotene
(provitamin A)

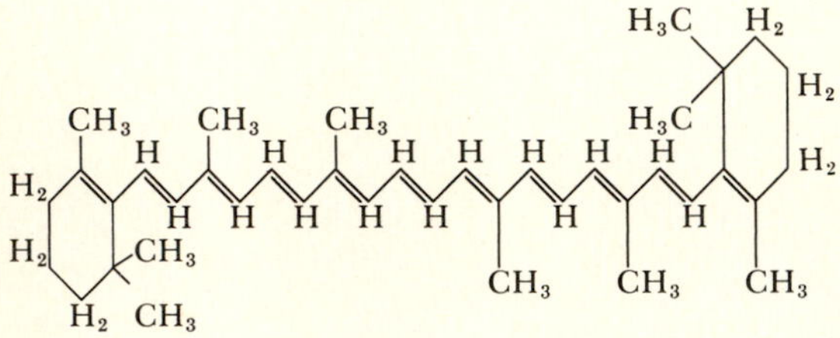

Vitamin D
(represented by cholecalciferol, vitamin D_3)*

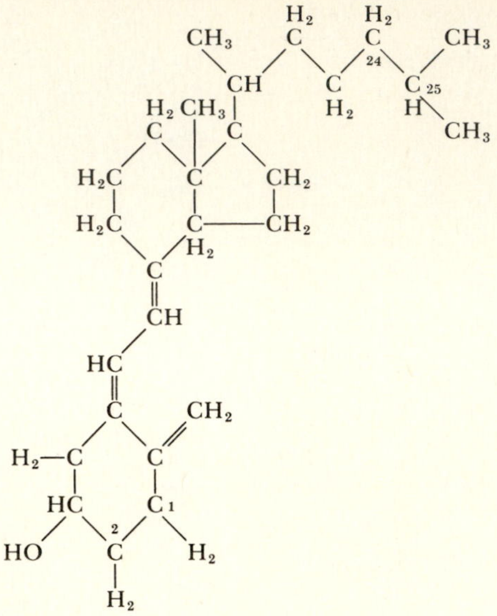

*The numbers of the carbon atoms involved in the biosynthesis of vitamin D hormone are shown.

Vitamin E
(represented by alpha-tocopherol)

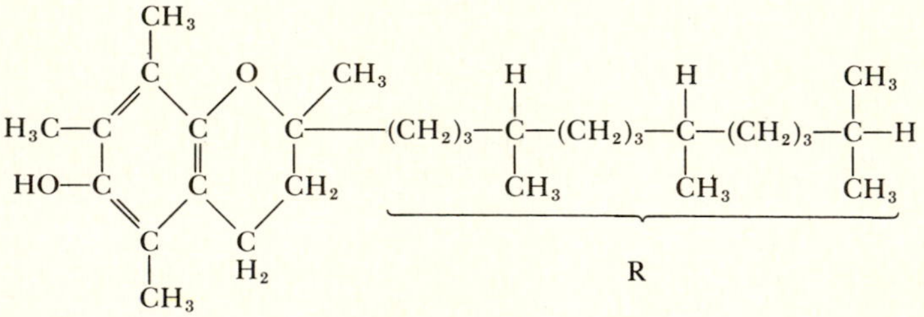

R

Vitamin K
(represented by phytylmenaquinone, vitamin K_1)

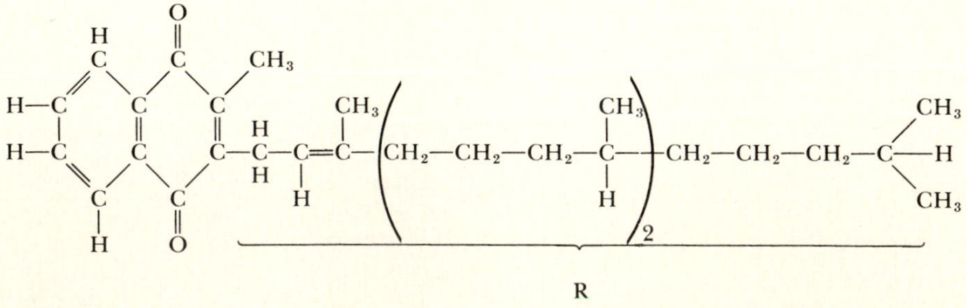

R

Table 12 TABLE OF CURRENT GUIDELINES FOR CRITERIA OF NUTRITIONAL STATUS FOR LABORATORY EVALUATION

Nutrient and Units	*Age of Subject (years)*	*Criteria of Status*		
		DEFICIENT	MARGINAL	ACCEPTABLE
*Hemoglobin (gm/100 ml)	6–23 mos.	Up to 9.0	9.0– 9.9	10.0+
	2–5	Up to 10.0	10.0–10.9	11.0+
	6–12	Up to 10.0	10.0–11.4	11.5+
	13–16M	Up to 12.0	12.0–12.9	13.0+
	13–16F	Up to 10.0	10.0–11.4	11.5+
	16+M	Up to 12.0	12.0–13.9	14.0+
	16+F	Up to 10.0	10.0–11.9	12.0+
	Pregnant (after 6+ mos.)	Up to 9.5	9.5–10.9	11.0+
*Hematocrit (Packed cell volume in percent)	Up to 2	Up to 28	28–30	31+
	2–5	Up to 30	30–33	34+
	6–12	Up to 30	30–35	36+
	13–16M	Up to 37	37–39	40+
	13–16F	Up to 31	31–35	36+
	16+M	Up to 37	37–43	44+
	16+F	Up to 31	31–37	37+
	Pregnant	Up to 30	30–32	33+
*Serum Albumin (gm/100 ml)	Up to 1	–	Up to 2.5	2.5+
	1–5	–	Up to 3.0	3.0+
	6–16	–	Up to 3.5	3.5+
	16+	Up to 2.8	2.8–3.4	3.5+
	Pregnant	Up to 3.0	3.0–3.4	3.5+
*Serum Protein (gm/100 ml)	Up to 1	–	Up to 5.0	5.0+
	1–5	–	Up to 5.5	5.5+
	6–16	–	Up to 6.0	6.0+
	16+	Up to 6.0	6.0–6.4	6.5+
	Pregnant	Up to 5.5	5.5–5.9	6.0+
*Serum Ascorbic Acid (mg/100 ml)	All ages	Up to 0.1	0.1–0.19	0.2+
*Plasma Vitamin A (μg/100 ml)	All ages	Up to 10	10–19	20+
*Plasma Carotene (μg/100 ml)	All ages	Up to 20	20–39	40+
	Pregnant	–	40–79	80+
*Serum Iron (μg/100 ml)	Up to 2	Up to 30	–	30+
	2–5	Up to 40	–	40+
	6–12	Up to 50	–	50+
	12+M	Up to 60	–	60+
	12+F	Up to 40	–	40+
*Transferrin Saturation (percent)	Up to 2	Up to 15.0	–	15.0+
	2–12	Up to 20.0	–	20.0+
	12+M	Up to 20.0	–	20.0+
	12+F	Up to 15.0	–	15.0+
**Serum Folacin (ng/ml)	All ages	Up to 2.0	2.1–5.9	6.0+
**Serum Vitamin B_{12} (pg/ml)	All ages	Up to 100	–	100+

Table continued on following page.

Table 12 TABLE OF CURRENT GUIDELINES FOR CRITERIA OF NUTRITIONAL STATUS FOR LABORATORY EVALUATION – (*Continued*)

Nutrient and Units	*Age of Subject (years)*	*Criteria of Status*		
		DEFICIENT	MARGINAL	ACCEPTABLE
*Thiamine in Urine (μg/g creatinine)	1–3	Up to 120	120–175	175+
	4–5	Up to 85	85–120	120+
	6–9	Up to 70	70–180	180+
	10–15	Up to 55	55–150	150+
	16+	Up to 27	27–65	65+
	Pregnant	Up to 21	21–49	50+
*Riboflavin in Urine (μg/g creatinine)	1–3	Up to 150	150–499	500+
	4–5	Up to 100	100–299	300+
	6–9	Up to 85	85–269	270+
	10–16	Up to 70	70–199	200+
	16+	Up to 27	27–79	80+
	Pregnant	Up to 30	30–89	90+
**RBC Transketolase-TPP-effect (ratio)	All ages	25+	15–25	Up to 15
**RBC Glutathione Reductase-FAD-effect (ratio)	All ages	1.2+	–	Up to 1.2
**Tryptophan Load (mg Xanthurenic acid excreted)	Adults (Dose: 100 mg/kg body weight)	25 + (6 hrs.) 75 + (24 hrs.)	– –	Up to 25 Up to 75
**Urinary Pyridoxine (μg/g creatinine)	1–3	Up to 90	–	90+
	4–6	Up to 80	–	80+
	7–9	Up to 60	–	60+
	10–12	Up to 40	–	40+
	13–15	Up to 30	–	30+
	16+	Up to 20	–	20+
*Urinary N'methyl nicotinamide (mg/g creatinine)	All ages	Up to 0.2	0.2–5.59	0.6+
	Pregnant	Up to 0.8	0.8–2.49	2.5+
**Urinary Pantothenic Acid (μg)	All ages	Up to 200	–	200+
**Plasma vitamin E (mg/100 ml)	All ages	Up to 0.2	0.2–0.6	0.6+
**Transaminase Index (ratio)				
†EGOT	Adult	2.0+	–	Up to 2.0
‡EGPT	Adult	1.25+	–	Up to 1.25

From Christakis, G. (ed.): Nutritional assessment in health programs. Amer. J. Pub. Health, 63 (Suppl.): 34–35, 1973.

*Adapted from the Ten State Nutrition Survey.
**Criteria may vary with different methodology.
†Erythrocyte Glutamic Oxalacetic Transaminase.
‡Erythrocyte Glutamic Pyruvic Transaminase.

Table 13 STANDARDS FOR DIETARY INTAKE* AND BLOOD† DATA

Age, sex, and physiological state		*Calories (per kg)*	*Protein (gm per kg)*	*Calcium (mg)*	*Iron (mg)*	*Vitamin A‡ (IU)*	*Vitamin C (mg)*	*B Vitamins (All Ages)*	*Acceptable Hemoglobin (gm/100 ml)†*	*Acceptable Hematocrit (%)†*
AGE AND SEX										
1–5 years:										
12–23 months,								Thiamin,		
male and female		90	1.9	450	15	2000	40	0.4 mg	≥10.0	≥31
24–47 months,								per 1000		
male and female		86	1.7	450	15	2000	40	calories	≥11.0	≥34
48–71 months,										
male and female		82	1.5	450	10	2000	40		≥11.0	≥34
6–7 years, male and female		82	1.3	450	10	2500	40		≥11.5	≥36
8–9 years, male and female		82	1.3	450	10	2500	40	Riboflavin,	≥11.5	≥36
10–12 years	Male	68	1.2	650	10	2500	40	0.55 mg	≥11.5	≥36
	Female	64	1.2	650	18	2500	40	per 1000	≥11.5	≥36
13–16 years	Male	60	1.2	650	18	3500	50	calories	≥13.0	≥40
	Female	48	1.2	650	18	3500	50		≥11.5	≥36
17–19 years	Male	44	1.1	550	18	3500	55	Niacin,	≥14.0	≥44
	Female	35	1.1	550	18	3500	50	6.6 mg	≥12.0	≥38
20–29 years	Male	40	1.0	400	10	3500	60	per 1000	14.0	≥44
	Female	35	1.0	600	18	3500	55	calories	≥12.0	≥38
30–39 years	Male	38	1.0	400	10	3500	60		≥14.0	≥44
	Female	33	1.0	600	18	3500	55		≥12.0	≥38
40–49 years	Male	37	1.0	400	10	3500	60		≥14.0	≥44
	Female	31	1.0	600	18	3500	55		≥12.0	≥38
50–54 years	Male	36	1.0	400	10	3500	60		≥14.0	≥44
	Female	30	1.0	600	18	3500	55		≥12.0	≥38
55–59 years	Male	36	1.0	400	10	3500	60		≥14.0	≥44
	Female	30	1.0	600	10	3500	55		≥12.0	≥38
60–69 years	Male	34	1.0	400	10	3500	60		≥14.0	≥44
	Female	29	1.0	600	10	3500	55		≥12.0	≥38
70 years and over	Male	34	1.0	400	10	3500	60		≥14.0	≥44
	Female	29	1.0	600	10	3500	55		≥12.0	≥38
PHYSIOLOGICAL STATE										
Pregnancy (5th month and beyond), add to basic standard		200	20	200		1000	5§			
Lactating, add to basic standard		1000	25	500		1000	5			

*Standards for evaluation of dietary intake used in the Health and Nutrition Examination.
Survey, by age, sex, and physiological state: United States, 1971–1974. DHEW. Pub. No. (HRA) 77-1647, July, 1977, p. 74.

†Guidelines for classification and interpretation of group blood data collected as part of the Ten State Nutrition Survey: 1968–1970.

‡Assumed 70 percent carotene, 30 percent retinol.

§For all pregnancies.

Table 14 PERIODIC CHART OF THE ELEMENTS

From Masterson, W. L., E. J. Slowinski, and C. L. Stanitski: *Chemical Principles*, 5th ed. Philadelphia, Saunders College Publishing, 1981.

PERIODIC CHART OF THE ELEMENTS

TRANSITION METALS (groups 21–30 columns below)

1	2											3	4	5	6	7	8
1 H 1.0079																1 H 1.0079	2 He 4.00260
3 Li 6.941	4 Be 9.01218											5 B 10.81	6 C 12.011	7 N 14.0067	8 O 15.9994	9 F 18.998403	10 Ne 20.179
11 Na 22.98977	12 Mg 24.305											13 Al 26.98154	14 Si 28.0855	15 P 30.97376	16 S 32.06	17 Cl 35.453	18 Ar 39.948
19 K 39.0983	20 Ca 40.08	21 Sc 44.9559	22 Ti 47.90	23 V 50.9415	24 Cr 51.996	25 Mn 54.9380	26 Fe 55.847	27 Co 58.9332	28 Ni 58.70	29 Cu 63.546	30 Zn 65.38	31 Ga 69.72	32 Ge 72.59	33 As 74.9216	34 Se 78.96	35 Br 79.904	36 Kr 83.80
37 Rb 85.4678	38 Sr 87.62	39 Y 88.9059	40 Zr 91.22	41 Nb 92.9064	42 Mo 95.94	43 Tc (98)	44 Ru 101.07	45 Rh 102.9055	46 Pd 106.4	47 Ag 107.868	48 Cd 112.41	49 In 114.82	50 Sn 118.69	51 Sb 121.75	52 Te 127.60	53 I 126.9045	54 Xe 131.30
55 Cs 132.9054	56 Ba 137.33	57 ★La 138.9055	72 Hf 178.49	73 Ta 180.9479	74 W 183.85	75 Re 186.207	76 Os 190.2	77 Ir 192.22	78 Pt 195.09	79 Au 196.9665	80 Hg 200.59	81 Tl 204.37	82 Pb 207.2	83 Bi 208.9804	84 Po (209)	85 At (210)	86 Rn (222)
87 Fr (223)	88 Ra 226.0254	89 ʼAc 227.0278	104 § (261)	105 § (262)	106 § (263)												

★ Lathanoid Series

58 Ce 140.12	59 Pr 140.9077	60 Nd 144.24	61 Pm (145)	62 Sm 150.4	63 Eu 151.96	64 Gd 157.25	65 Tb 158.9254	66 Dy 162.50	67 Ho 164.9304	68 Er 167.26	69 Tm 168.9342	70 Yb 173.04	71 Lu 174.967

ʼ Actinoid Series

90 Th 232.0381	91 Pa 231.0359	92 U 238.029	93 Np 237.0482	94 Pu (244)	95 Am (243)	96 Cm (247)	97 Bk (247)	98 Cf (251)	99 Es (252)	100 Fm (257)	101 Md (258)	102 No (259)	103 Lr (260)

§ The International Union for Pure and Applied Chemistry has not adopted official names or symbols for these elements.

Note: Atomic masses shown here are 1977 IUPAC values.

Table 15

From Masterson, W. L., E. J. Slowinski, and C. L. Stanitski: *Chemical Principles*, 5th ed. Philadelphia, Saunders College Publishing, 1981.

TABLE OF ATOMIC MASSES* (Based on Carbon-12)

The following values apply to elements as they exist in materials of terrestrial origin and to certain artificial elements. When used with the due regard to footnotes, they are reliable to ±1 in the last digit, or ±3 when followed by an asterisk (*). Value in parentheses is the mass number of the isotope of longest half-life.

	Symbol	*Atomic No.*	*Atomic Mass*
Actinium	Ac	89	227.0278
Aluminum	Al	13	26.98154
Americium	Am	95	[243]†
Antimony	Sb	51	121.75
Argon	Ar	18	39.948
Arsenic	As	33	74.9216
Astatine	At	85	[210]
Barium	Ba	56	137.33
Berkelium	Bk	97	[247]
Beryllium	Be	4	9.01218
Bismuth	Bi	83	208.9804
Boron	B	5	10.81
Bromine	Br	35	79.904
Cadmium	Cd	48	112.41
Calcium	Ca	20	40.08
Californium	Cf	98	[251]
Carbon	C	6	12.011
Cerium	Ce	58	140.12
Cesium	Cs	55	132.9054
Chlorine	Cl	17	35.453
Chromium	Cr	24	51.996
Cobalt	Co	27	58.9332
Copper	Cu	29	63.546
Curium	Cm	96	[247]
Dysprosium	Dy	66	162.50
Einsteinium	Es	99	[252]
Erbium	Er	68	167.26
Europium	Eu	63	151.96
Fermium	Fm	100	[257]
Fluorine	F	9	18.998403
Francium	Fr	87	[223]
Gadolinium	Gd	64	157.25
Gallium	Ga	31	69.72
Germanium	Ge	32	72.59
Gold	Au	79	196.9665
Hafnium	Hf	72	178.49
Helium	He	2	4.00260
Holmium	Ho	67	164.9304
Hydrogen	H	1	1.0079
Indium	In	49	114.82
Iodine	I	53	126.9045
Iridium	Ir	77	192.22
Iron	Fe	26	55.847
Krypton	Kr	36	83.80
Lanthanum	La	57	138.9055
Lawrencium	Lr	103	[260]
Lead	Pb	82	207.2
Lithium	Li	3	6.941
Lutetium	Lu	71	174.967
Magnesium	Mg	12	24.305
Manganese	Mn	25	54.9380
Mendelevium	Md	101	[258]
Mercury	Hg	80	200.59
Molybdenum	Mo	42	95.94
Neodymium	Nd	60	144.24
Neon	Ne	10	20.179
Neptunium	Np	93	237.0482
Nickel	Ni	28	58.70
Niobium	Nb	41	92.9064
Nitrogen	N	7	14.0067
Nobelium	No	102	[259]
Osmium	Os	76	190.2
Oxygen	O	8	15.9994
Palladium	Pd	46	106.4
Phosphorus	P	15	30.97376
Platinum	Pt	78	195.09
Plutonium	Pu	94	[244]
Polonium	Po	84	[209]
Potassium	K	19	39.0983
Praseodymium	Pr	59	140.9077
Promethium	Pm	61	[145]
Protactinium	Pa	91	231.0359
Radium	Ra	88	226.0254
Radon	Rn	86	[222]
Rhenium	Re	75	186.207
Rhodium	Rh	45	102.9055
Rubidium	Rb	37	85.4678
Ruthenium	Ru	44	101.07
Samarium	Sm	62	150.4
Scandium	Sc	21	44.9559
Selenium	Se	34	78.96
Silicon	Si	14	28.0855
Silver	Ag	47	107.868
Sodium	Na	11	22.98977
Strontium	Sr	38	87.62
Sulfur	S	16	32.06
Tantalum	Ta	73	180.9479
Technetium	Tc	43	[98]
Tellurium	Te	52	127.60
Terbium	Tb	65	158.9254
Thallium	Tl	81	204.37
Thorium	Th	90	232.0381
Thulium	Tm	69	168.9342
Tin	Sn	50	118.69
Titanium	Ti	22	47.90
Tungsten	W	74	183.85
Uranium	U	92	238.029
Vanadium	V	23	50.9415
Xenon	Xe	54	131.30
Ytterbium	Yb	70	173.04
Yttrium	Y	39	88.9059
Zinc	Zn	30	65.38
Zirconium	Zr	40	91.22

*Atomic masses given here are 1977 IUPAC values.

†A value given in brackets denotes the mass number of the longest-lived or best-known isotope.

SUPPLEMENTARY READINGS

Chapter 1 Food and Its Relation to Physical Fitness

Books and Reviews (General)

(Also see ref. 5 to 9, this chapter.)

Adams, C. F.: *Nutritive Value of American Foods in Common Units.* USDA, Agriculture Handbook No. 456, 1975 (also see Handbook 8, revised, issued in looseleaf sections, No. 1–9, 1976 to 1983).

Alfin-Slater, R. B., and Kritchevsky, D.: *Human Nutrition: A Comprehensive Treatise.* Vols 1, 2, 3A, 3B, 4. New York, Plenum Press, 1979 and 1980.

Beal, V. A.: *Nutrition in the Lifespan.* New York, John Wiley & Sons, Inc., 1980.

Committee on Diet, Nutrition, and Cancer, National Research Council: *Diet, Nutrition, and Cancer.* Washington, D.C., National Academy Press, 1982, 350 pp.

Committee for the Revision of the Dietary Standard for Canada: *Recommended Nutrient Intakes for Canadians.* Ottawa, Canadian Govt. Pub. Center, 1983.

Ellenbogen, L. (ed.): *Controversies in Nutrition.* Vol. 2: *Contemporary Issues in Clinical Nutrition.* New York, Churchill Livingston, Inc., 1981

Fieldhouse, P., and Lennon, D.: *Social Nutrition.* London, Forbes Publications Ltd., 1982.

Harper, A. E., and Davis, G. K. (eds.): *Nutrition in Health and Disease and International Development* (Symposia from the XII International Congress of Nutrition, San Diego, California). 95 articles. New York, Alan R. Liss, Inc, 1981.

Herbert, V.: *Nutrition Cultism—Facts and Fictions.* Philadelphia, Penn., George F. Stickley Co., 1980.

Herbert, V., and Barrett, S.: *Vitamins and "Health Foods": The Great American Hustle.* Philadelphia, Penn., George F. Stickley Co., 1981.

Hui Y. H.: *United States Food Laws, Regulations, and Standards.* New York, John Wiley and Co., 1979.

Marshall, C. W.: *Help or Harm? Vitamins and Minerals.* Philadelphia, Penn., George F. Stickley Co., 1983.

McLaren, D. S.: *Color Atlas of Nutritional Disorders.* Chicago, Ill., Year Book Medical Publishers, Inc., 1981.

Pennington, J. A. T., and Church, H. N.: *Bowes and Church's Food Values of Portions Commonly Used.* 13th Ed. Philadelphia, Penn., J. B. Lippincott Co., 1980.

Section on Clinical Nutrition: Symposium on Assessing Therapeutic Dietary Claims. Bull. N.Y. Acad. Med. *58*:219 (10 articles), 1982.

Wurtman, J. J., and Wurtman, R. J.: *Nutrition and the Brain* (in 4 volumes). New York, Raven Press, 1979.

Zeman, F. J.: *Clinical Nutrition and Dietetics.* Lexington, Massachusetts, Collamore Press, D. C. Heath and Company, 1983.

(Note: There are now well over 100 reliable professional and popular books on nutrition published annually in North America, so the above listing represents only a selected few. See the book review sections of the Journal of Nutrition Education, the Journal of the American Dietetic Association, the Journal of the Canadian Dietetic Association, and Food Technology, among others, for coverage and evaluation of the most important current books in nutrition, foods, and in the nutritional aspects of physical fitness. Also see the list of recommended books by the Chicago Nutrition Association.

For books published in Canada see "Nutrition books—made in Canada," J. Canad. Dietet. Assoc., *42*:30, 1981, and current issues.

Nutrition Education and Training

Aronson, V.: You can't tell a nutritionist by the diploma. FDA Consumer, 17(6):28, 1983.

Dwyer, J. (ed.): National Conference on Nutrition Education—directions for the 1980s. J. Nutr. Educ. *12* (Supplement): 79–137, 1980.

Federally supported human nutrition research, training, and education: update for the 1980s. Nutr. Rev., *41*:22, 1983.

Fieldhouse, P.: Nutrition and education of the schoolchild. World Rev. Nutr. Dietet., *40*:83, 1982.

Frank, R. C.: Information resources for food and human nutrition. J. Amer. Dietet. Assoc., *80*:344, 1982.

Long, J. M.: Opening the closet door: the key is education. J. Parenter. Ent. Nutr., *6*:280, 1981 (on the nutrition training of physicians).

Nutrition For Everybody: An Annotated List of Resources. Oakland, Calif., Society for Nutrition Education, 1981.

Oace, S. M. (ed.): Perspectives on nutrition education instrumentation. J. Nutr. Educ., *13*:83–114 (10 articles), 1981.

Olson, C. M., and Gillespie, A. H.: Proceedings of the workshop on nutrition education research. J. Nutr. Educ., *13* (Supplement No. 1): S1–S119 (20 articles), 1981.

Sims, L. S., and Light, L. (eds.): *Directions for Nutrition Education Research—the Penn State Conferences, a Proceedings.* The Pennsylvania State University, 1981.

St. Pierre, R. G., and Rezmovic, V.: An overview of the National Nutrition Education and Training Program evaluation. J. Nutr. Educ., *14*:61, 1982.

Food Consumption Surveys and Nutrition Status

(Also see refs. 9, 12–14, this chapter.)

Crocetti, A. J., and Guthrie, H. A.: Food consumption patterns and nutritional quality of the U.S. Diets, a preliminary report. Food Tech., *35* (Sept.):40, 1981 (part of a symposium—also see pp. 50, 58, 70, and 110).

Hoover, L. W.: Computerized nutrient data bases I and II. J. Amer. Dietet. Assoc., *82*:501 and 506, 1983.

Kennedy, E. T., Harrell, M. W., and Frazo, B.: Distribution of nutrient intake across meals in the United States population. Ecol. Food Nutr., *11*:217, 1982.

Kerr, G. R., et al.: Relationships between dietary and biochemical measures of nutritional status in Hanes I data. Amer. J. Clin. Nutr., *35*:294, 1982.

Krantzler, N. J., et al.: Methods of food intake assessment—an annotated bibliography. J. Nutr. Educ., *14*:108, 1982.

Mitchell, M. E., et al.: *Nutritional Status and Food Acceptance of Women in the Western Region.* Bulletin 0891, Washington State Univ., Pullman, 1981.

Rewko, S. L., et al.: A comparison of two methods of evaluating food intakes. J. Canad. Dietet. Assoc., *41*:137, 1980.

Rizek, R. L., and Jackson, R. M.: *Current Food Consumption Practices and Nutrient Sources in the American Diet.* USDA Consumer Nutrition Center, Hyattsville, Maryland, June 1980.

Swan, P. B.: Food consumption by individuals in the United States: two major surveys. Ann. Rev. Nutr., *3*:413, 1983.

Windham, C. T., et al.: Alcohol consumption and nutrient density of diets in the nationwide food consumption survey, J. Amer. Dietet. Assoc., *82*:364, 1983.

Windham, C. T., et al.: Consistency of nutrient consumption patterns in the United States. J. Amer. Dietet. Assoc., *78*:587, 1981.

National Nutrition Policies and Guidelines

(Also see ref. 10, this chapter and Chapters 20 and 25.)

Cleveland, L. E., et al.: Recommended dietary allowances as standards for family food plans. J. Nutr. Educ., *15*:8, 1983.

Dwyer, J.: Dietary recommendations and policy implications: the U.S. experience. Nutr. Update, *1*:315, 1983.

Food and Nutrition Board: *Toward Healthful Diets.* National Academy of Sciences, Washington D.C., 1980.

Hansen, R. G., Wyse, B., and Windham, C.: Balancing nutrition intake with calories. Cereal Foods World, *26*:674, 1981.

Harper, A. E.: Dietary guidelines for Americans. Amer. J. Clin. Nutr., *34*:121, 1981.

McNutt, K.: Dietary advice to the public. Nutr. Rev., *38*:353, 1980 (also see National Nutrition Consortium statement on a national policy, Nutr. Rev., *38*:96, 1980; and comments from Stare, F. J.: Nutr. Rev., *39*:192, 1981).

Nestle, M., Lee, P. R., and Baron, R. B.: Nutrition policy update. Nutr. Update, *1*:285, 1983.

Oace, S. M. (ed.): Perspectives on food guidance. J. Nutr. Educ., *13*:46–66 (7 papers), 1981.

Peterkin, B. B., et al.: Changes in dietary patterns: one approach to meeting standards. J. Amer. Dietet, Assoc., *78*:453, 1981.

Schwerin, H. S., et al.: Food, eating habits, and health: a further examination of the relationship between food eating patterns and nutritional health. Amer. J. Clin. Nutr., *35*:1319, 1982 (also see p. 1479 for a critique).

Swenerton, H., and Dunkley, W. L.: Recent activities of public agencies to assure healthful diets for Americans. J. Dairy Sci., *65*:484, 1982.

USDA and USDHEW: *Nutrition and Your Health, Dietary Guidelines for Americans.* Home and Garden Bulletin No. 232, 1980.

Wretlind, A.: Standards for nutritional adequacy of the diet: European and WHO/FAO viewpoints. Amer. J. Clin. Nutr., *36*:366, 1982.

Nutrition History

(Also see readings in previous editions)

Benham, H.: *Man's Struggle for Food.* Washington D.C., University Press of America, 1981.

Cosman, M. P.: A feast for Aesculapius: historical diets for asthma and sexual pleasure. Ann. Rev. Nutr., *3*:010, 1983.

Day, H. G., and Prebluda, H. J.: E. V. McCollum: "lamplighter" in public and professional understanding of nutrition. Agric. History, *54*:149, 1980.

Guggenheim, K. Y.: *Nutrition and Nutritional Diseases: The Evolution of Concepts.* Lexington, Mass., The Callamore Press, D. C. Heath and Co., 1981.

Hill, F. W., Williams, H. H., and Morgan, A. F. (eds.): The American Institute of Nutrition: a history of the first 50 years, 1928–1978. J. Nutr., *109* (Supplement, Dec.):1, 1979.

Hoch, S. L.: Serf diet in nineteenth-century Russia. Agric. History, *56*:391, 1982.

Todhunter, E. N.: Some aspects of the history of dietetics. World Rev. Nutr. Dietet., *18*:1, 1973.
Todhunter, E. N. (ed.): Special topics in the history of nutrition. Fed. Proc., *37*:2504 (4 papers), 1977.
Whorton, J.: Sex, diet, and debility in Jacksonian America: Graham Sylvester and health reform. J. Hist. Med. Allied Sci., *36*:358, 1981.

Other General Readings, Chapter 1

Akin, J., et al.: Who benefits from school feeding? An analysis of participation in the National School Lunch Program. Food Tech., *35* (Sept.):70, 1981.
Cala, R. R., Morgan, K. J., and Zabik, M. E.: The contribution of children's snacks to total dietary intakes. Home Econ. Res. J., *10*:150, 1981.
Dubick, M. A., and Rucker, R. B.: Dietary supplements and health aids—a critical evaluation. J. Nutr. Educ., *15*:47, 1983.
Foss, S. B., and Keith, R. E.: Food habits and dietary adequacy of single professional women. Nutr. Rept. Internat., *26*:613, 1982.
Frank, R. C.: Information resources for food and human nutrition. J. Amer. Dietet. Assoc., *80*:344, 1982.
Glantz, S. A.: Biostatistics: how to detect, correct and prevent errors in the medical literature. Circulation, *61*:1, 1980.
Granzin, K. L., and Bahn, K. D.: Personal values as an explanation of food usage habits. Home Econ. Res. J., *10*:401, 1982.
Hepburn, F. N.: The USDA National Nutrient Data Bank. Amer. J. Clin. Nutr., *35*:1297, 1982.
Hou, H. C.: Concerning the study of nutrition in China. Proc. Soc. Exp. Biol. Med., *171*:1, 1982.
Johnson, S. R., Burt, J. A., and Morgan, K. J.: The food stamp program: participation, food cost, and diet quality for low-income households. Food Tech., *35* (Oct.):58, 1981.
Lowenthal, J. P. (ed.): Workshop conference on nutrition in cancer. Cancer Res., *43* (No. 5) (Supplement):2389s–2515s, 1983.
O'Hanlon, P., et al.: Socioeconomic factors and dietary intakes of elderly Missourians. J. Amer. Dietet. Assoc., *82*:646, 1983 (inadequacies of energy, calcium, iron, thiamin, and riboflavin).
Read, M. S.: Malnutrition and behavior, Occasional Paper series, Inst. Nutr., Univ. N. Carolina, *2*(No. 9):1, 1982.
Revlin, R. S., and Young, E. A., (eds): Symposium on evidence relating selected vitamins and minerals to health and disease in the elderly population in the United States. Amer. J. Clin. Nutr., *36* (Supplement, Nov.): 977–1086 (8 papers), 1982.
Vermersch, J. (ed): Nutrition services in state and local public health agencies. Public Health Reports, *98* (1): 7, 1983.
Watt, B. K.: Tables of food composition: uses and limitations. Contemp. Nutr. (General Mills), *5* (Feb.):1, 1980.
White, P. L., and Selvey, N.: Nutrition and the new health awareness. J. Amer. Med. Assoc., *247*:2914, 1982.
Wise, A.: Nutrient interrelationships (134 references). Nutr. Abstr. Rev. (Series A), *50*:319–332, 1980.

Additional Scientific Journals with Many Important Nutrition Articles

These are generally peer reviewed and/or generally reliable, but less readily available in college libraries in North America than those listed at end of Chapter 1.*

Acta Nutrimenta Sinica (China)
Annals of Nutrition and Metabolism (Switzerland) (new title in 1981)
Appetite (U.K.) (new in 1980)
Archivos Latinoamericanos de Nutrición (Guatemala)
Arteriosclerosis (U.S.) (new in 1981)
Atherosclerosis (Ireland)
Baroda Journal of Nutrition (India)
Biological Trace Element Research (U.S.)
Canadian Institute of Food Science and Technology Journal
Cereal Chemistry (U.S.)
Food and Chemical Toxicology (U.K.)
Food and Nutrition (F.A.O.—United Nations)
Food and Nutrition Bulletin (United Nations University)
Food Policy (U.S.)
International Journal for Vitamin and Nutrition Research (Switzerland)
International Journal of Eating Disorders (U.S.) (new in 1981)
International Journal of Obesity (U.K.)
Journal of Agricultural and Food Chemistry (U.S.)
Journal of Chronic Diseases (U.K.)
Journal of Dairy Science (U.S.)
Journal of Food and Nutrition (Australia) (new title in 1981)
Journal of Food Protection (U.S.)
Journal of Lipid Research (U.S.)
Journal of Nutrition for the Elderly (U.S.) (new in 1980)
Journal of Nutritional Science and Vitaminology (Japan)
Journal of Plant Foods (U.K.) (new title in 1982).
Journal of Studies on Alcohol (U.S.)
Journal of The American College of Nutrition (U.S.) (new in 1982)
Korean Journal of Nutrition
Lipids (U.S.)
Medicine and Science in Sports and Exercise (U.S.)
Metabolism (U.S.)
Nutrition and Health (U.K.) (new in 1982)
Nutriton and Metabolism (Switzerland)

*Because of space limitations a number of reliable non-English-language and foreign publications, food journals, and clinically oriented journals with nutrition coverage had to be omitted from this list.

Nutrition Planning (U.S.)
Philippine Journal of Nutrition

Scientific Societies with Nutrition Concerns

The most reliable journals with nutrition-related papers generally are those sponsored by leading scientific organizations, which in North America are:

American Association for the Advancement of Science
American Association of Cereal Chemists
American Chemical Society
American Dietetic Association
American Institute of Nutrition
American Physiological Society
American Society of Animal Science
American Society of Biological Chemists
American Society of Clinical Nutrition
American Society for Parenteral and Enteral Nutrition
Canadian Dietetic Association
Canadian Institute of Food Science and Technology
Home Economics Association
Institute of Food Technologists
Society for Nutrition Education

Additional Sources of Nutrition Information

These are generally reliable but not necessarily peer reviewed. Also see list at end of Chapter 1.

ACSH News and Views (bimonthly). American Council of Science and Health, 1995 Broadway, New York, N.Y. 10023.

American Diabetic Association, 600 Fifth Ave., New York, N.Y. 10020.

American School Food Service Association, 4104 E. Iliff Ave., Denver, Colorado 80222 (publishes *School Food Service Journal* and *School Food Service Research Journal*).

Campbell Soup Company, 375 Memorial Ave., Camden, New Jersey 08101.

CAST Reports. Council for Agricultural Science and Technology, 250 Memorial Union, Ames, Iowa 50011.

Chicago Nutrition Association, 8158 Kedzie Ave., Chicago, Illinois 60652 (source of a list of reliable nutrition books).

Consumer Reports (monthly). P.O. Box 1949, Marion, Ohio 43305.

Cooperative Extension Service, USDA, Washington D.C. 20250. (Offices in every land grant university and in most every county of the country. A good source of reliable information about food and nutrition.)

Environmental Nutrition (10 issues/yr.). 52 Riverside Drive, 15–A, New York, N.Y. 10024.

H J. Heinz, Consumer Relations, P.O. Box 57, Pittsburgh, Pennsylvania 15230.

Health (formerly *Family Health*) (monthly). Portland Place, Boulder, Colorado 80302 (also publishes *Health's Nutrition News,* [weekly] starting in 1983).

Institute of Nutrition, University of North Carolina, Chapel Hill, North Carolina 27514 (publishes *Occasional Paper Series*).

La Leche League International, Inc., 9616 Minneapolis Ave., Franklin Park, Illinois 60131.

National Foundation/March of Dimes, Box 2000, White Plains, N.Y. 10605.

Nutrition and Food Science (bimonthly). Forbes Publications Ltd., 120 Bayswater Road, London W2 3JH.

Nutrition and the M.D. (monthly). Box 2160, Van Nuys, California 91404-9983.

Nutrition Quarterly. Nutrition Division, Dairy Bureau of Canada, 20 Holly St., Toronto, Ontario, Canada M4S 2E6.

Obesity and Bariatric Medicine (quarterly). 5200 S. Quebec, St., Englewood, Colorado 80111.

Professional Nutritionist (quarterly). Foremost-McKesson, Inc., One Post St., Suite 3275, San Francisco, California 94104.

Ross Laboratories, 625 Cleveland Ave., Columbus, Ohio 43216 (publishes *Dietetics Currents* and provides other information).

United Fresh Fruit and Vegetable Association, North Washington St., Alexandria, Virginia 22314.

(Note: most large food processing companies supply consumer information about their products on request. Addresses are generally available on package labels.)

Popular Magazines with Nutrition Information

(generally reliable)*

50 Plus
Good Housekeeping
Newsweek
Parents
Readers Digest
Redbook
Time
U.S. News and World Report

Chapter 2 Carbohydrates

Carbohydrate

Akrabawi, S. S., Saegert, M. M., and Salji, J. P.: Studies on the growth and changes in metabolism of rats fed carbohydrate-deficient, fatty-acid based diets supplemented with graded levels of maize stach. Brit. J. Nutr., *32*:209, 1974.

*Adapted from Hudnall, M.: ACSH News and Views *3* (Jan.1:1, 1982 (except the weekly news magazines, which were not rated). The magazines *Mademoiselle, Essence, Cosmopolitan, Harper's Bazaar, Organic Gardening,* and *Prevention* were rated as "unreliable" in terms of nutrition coverage in this survey. Other popular magazines such as *Woman's Day, Family Circle* and *McCalls* were rated as "inconsistent."

Anderson, J. W., Herman, R. H., and Zakim, D.: Effect of glucose and high sucrose diets on glucose tolerance of normal men. Amer. J. Clin. Nutr., *26*:600, 1973.

Anderson, T. A.: Recent trends in carbohydrate consumption. Ann. Rev. Nutr., *2*:113, 1982.

Bierman, E. L., and Nelson, R.: Carbohydrates, diabetes and blood lipids. World Rev. Nutr. Dietet., *22*:280, 1975.

Birch, G. G., and Green, L. F. (eds.): *Molecular Structure and Function of Food Carbohydrate.* New York, Halsted Press, Div. of John Wiley & Sons, Inc., 1973.

Danowski, T. S., Nolan, S., and Stephen, T.: Hypoglycemia. World Rev. Nutr. Dietet., *22*:288, 1975.

Demigne, C., and Remesy, C.: Influence of unrefined potato starch on cecal fermentation and volatile fatty acid absorption in rats. J. Nutr., *112*:2227, 1982.

Garn, S. M., Solomon, M. A., and Cole, P. E.: Sugar food-intake and the obese. Ecol. Food Nutr., *12:* 1982.

Grande, F.: Sugar and cardiovascular disease. World Rev. Nutr. Dietet., *22*:248, 1975.

Gray, G. M.: Carbohydrate digestion and absorption. Gastroenterology, *58*:96, 1970.

Hyams, J. S.: Sorbitol intolerance: an unappreciated cause of functional gastrointestinal complaints. Gastroenterology, *84*:30, 1983.

Holloway, W. D., Tasman-Jones, C., and Lee, S. P.: Digestion of certain fractions of dietary fiber in humans. Amer. J. Clin. Nutr., *31*:927, 1978.

Jenkins, D. J. A., Taylor, R. H., and Wolever, T. M. S.: The diabetic diet, dietary carbohydrate and differences in digestibility. Diabetologia, *23*:477, 1982.

Kanarek, R. B., and Orthen-Gambill, N.: Differential effects of sucrose, fructose and glucose on carbohydrate-induced obesity in rats. J. Nutr. *112*: 1546, 1982.

Kelsay, J. L., et al.: Effect of fiber from fruits and vegetables on metabolic responses of human subjects: fiber intakes, fecal excretions, and apparent digestibilities. Amer. J. Clin. Nutr., *34*:1849, 1981.

Kritchevsky, D.: Dietary fiber and disease. Bull. N.Y. Acad. Sci., *58*:230, 1982.

Marlett, J. A., and Bokram, R. L.: Relationship between calculated dietary and crude fiber intakes of 200 college students. Amer. J. Clin. Nutr., *34*:335, 1981.

Morgan, K. J., and Zabik, M. E.: Amount and food sources of total sugar intake by children ages 5 to 12 years. Amer. J. Clin. Nutr., *34*:404, 1981.

Passmore, R., and Swindells, Y. E.: Observations on the respiratory quotient and weight gain of man after eating large quantities of carbohydrates. Brit. Med. J., *17*:331, 1963.

Reiser, S., et al: Serum insulin and glucose in hyperinsulinemic subjects fed three different levels of sucrose. Amer. J. Clin. Nutr., *34*:2348, 1981.

Richardson, J. F.: The sugar intake of businessmen and its inverse relationship with relative weight. Brit. J. Nutr., *27*:449, 1972.

Ritzel, G., and Brubaker, G. (eds): *Monosaccharides and Polyalcohols in Nutrition, Therapy and Dietetics.* Berne, Hans Huber, 1976.

Sipple, H. L., and McNutt, K. W. (eds.): *Sugars in Nutrition.* New York, Academic Press, 1974.

Southgate, D. A. T.: Fibre and the other unavailable carbohydrates and their effects on the energy value of the diet. Proc. Nutr. Soc., *32*:131, 1973.

Spiller, G. A., and Kay R. M. (eds): *Medical Aspects of Dietary Fiber.* New York, Plenum Press, 1980.

Stephen, A. M.: Should we eat more fibre? J. Human Nutr., *35*:403, 1981.

Story, J. A.: Dietary carbohydrate and atherosclerosis. Fed. Proc., *41*:2797, 1982.

Trowell, H. C.: *Dietary Fibre in Human Nutrition: A Bibliography.* London, Libbey Publ., 1979.

Vahouny, G. V.: Dietary fiber, lipid metabolism, and atherosclerosis. Fed. Proc., *41*:2801, 1982.

Wright, E., and Hughes, R. E.: Dietary critic acid. Nutrition (Lond.), *29*:367, 1975.

Chapter 3 Fats, Other Lipids, and Alcohol

Lipids

Akesson, B., et al.: Content of trans-octadecenoic acid in vegetarian and normal diets in Sweden. Amer. J. Clin. Nutr., *34*:2517, 1981.

Burr, M. L., et al.: Plasma cholesterol and blood pressure in vegetarians. J. Human Nutr., *35*:437, 1981.

Buzzard, I. M., et al.: Effect of dietary eggs and ascorbic acid on plasma lipid and lipoprotein cholesterol levels in young men. Amer. J. Clin. Nutr., *36*:94, 1982.

Chemoweth, W., et al.: Influence of dietary cholesterol and fat on serum lipids in men. J. Nutr., *111*:2080, 1981.

Eastwood, M. A., et al.: A study of diet, serum lipids, and fecal constituents in spouses. Amer. J. Clin. Nutr., *36*:290, 1982.

Glueck, C. J., et al.: Sucrose polyester and covert caloric dilution. Amer. J. Clin. Nutr., *35*:1352, 1982.

Gordon, E. T., et al.: Lipoproteins, cardiovascular disease and death: The Framingham Study. Arch. Inter. Med., *141*:1128, 1981.

Holman, R. T., et al.: Essential fatty acid deficiency in malnourished children. Amer. J. Clin. Nutr., *34*:1534, 1981.

Kritchevsky, D.: Trans fatty acid effects in experimental atherosclerosis. Fed. Proc., *41*:2813, 1982.

Liu, K., et al.: Dietary lipids, sugar, fiber, and mortality from coronary heart disease. Bivariate analysis of international data. Arteriosclerosis, *2*:221, 1982.

Masson, L.: Relative nutritional value of various fats and oils. J. Amer. Oil Chem. Soc., *58*:249. 1981.

O'Dea, K., and Sinclair, A. J.: Increased proportion of arachidonic acid in plasma lipids after 2 weeks on a diet of tropical seafood. Amer. Clin. Nutr., *36*:868, 1982.

Symposium: Lecithin. J. Amer. Oil Chem. Soc., *58*:885, 1981.

Thomas, L. H., et al.: Hydrogenated oils and fats: the presence of chemically modified fatty acids in human adipose tissue. Amer. J. Clin. Nutr., *34*:877, 1981.

Vahouny, G. V., et al.: Comparative lymphatic absorption of sitosterol, stigmasterol, and fucosterol and differential inhibition of cholesterol absorption, Amer. J. Clin. Nutr., *37*:805, 1983.

Vessby, B., Lithell, H., and Boberg, J.: Reduction of low density and high density lipoprotein cholesterol by fat-modified diets. A survey of recent findings. Human Nutr.: Clin. Nutr., *36C*:203, 1982.

Wiggins, R. C.: Myelin development and nutritional insufficiency. Brain Res. Rev., *4*:151, 1982.

Wood, J. L., and Allison, R. G.: Effects of consumption of choline and lecithin on neurological and cardiovascular systems. Fed. Proc., *41:*3015, 1982.

Alcohol

Australian Med. Assoc.: Statement on alcohol consumption and abuse. J. Food Nutr., *38*:75, 1981.

Baker, H., et al.: Inability of chronic alcoholics with liver disease to use food as a source of folates, thiamin and vitamin B-6. Amer. J. Clin. Nutr., *28*:1377, 1975.

Barboriak, J. J., Anderson, A. J., and Hoffman, R. G.: Smoking, alcohol and coronary artery occlusion. Atherosclerosis, *43*:277, 1982.

Barboriak, P. N., et al.: Blood pressure and alcohol intake in heart patients. Alcoholism: Clin. Exp. Res., *6*:234, 1982.

Bebb, H. T., et al.: Calorie and nutrient contribution of alcoholic beverages to the usual diets of 155 adults. Amer. J. Clin. Nutr., *24*:1042, 1971.

Bennion, L. J., and Li, T. K.: Alcohol metabolism in American Indians and whites. New Eng. J. Med., *294*:9, 1976.

Edwards, G.: Alcohol and advice to the pregnant woman. Brit. Med. J., *286:* 247, 1983.

Glueck, C. J., et al.: Effects of alcohol ingestion on lipids and lipoproteins in normal men: isocaloric metabolic studies. Amer. J. Clin. Nutr., *33*:2287, 1980.

Hanson, J. W., Jones, K. L., and Smith, D. W.: Fetal alcohol syndrome. J. Amer. Med. Assoc. *235*:1458, 1976.

Hartung, G. H. et al.: Effect of alcohol intake on high-density lipoprotein cholesterol levels in runners and inactive men. J. Amer. Med. Assoc., 249:747, 1983.

Majchrowicz, E., and Noble, E. P. (eds.: *Biochemistry and Pharmacology of Ethanol.* New York, Plenum, 1979.

McDonald, J., and Margen, S.: Wine vs. ethanol in human nutrition. I. Nitrogen and calorie balance. Amer. J. Clin. Nutr., *29*:1093, 1976.

Smith, R.: The politics of alcohol. Brit. Med. J., *284*:1392, 1982.

Topping, D. L., et al.: Adaptive effects of dietary ethanol in the pig: changes in plasma high-density lipoproteins and fecal steroid excretion and mutagenicity. Amer. J. Clin. Nutr., *36*:245, 1982.

Windham, C. T., Wyse, B. W., and Hansen, R. G.: Alcohol consumption and nutrient density of diets in the Nationwide Food Consumption Survey. J. Amer. Dietet. Assoc., *82*:364, 1983.

Chapter 4 Protein and Amino Acids

Proteins

Anderson, G. H.: Control of protein and energy intake: role of plasma amino acids and brain neurotransmitters. Canad. Physiol. J. Pharm., *57*:1043, 1979.

Arroyave, G.: Comparative sensitivity of specific amino acid ratios versus "essential to nonessential" amino acid ratio. Amer. Clin. Nutr., *23*:703, 1970.

Ballard, F. J., and Gunn, J. M.: Nutritional and hormonal effects on intracellular protein catabolism. Nutr. Rev., *40:*33, 1982.

Beaton, G. H., and Swiss, L. D.: Evaluation of the nutritional quality of food supplies: prediction of "desirable" and "safe" protein:calorie ratios. Amer. J. Clin. Nutr., *27*:485, 1974.

Bodwell, C. E., and Marable, N. L.: Effectiveness of methods for evaluating the nutritional quality of soybeans. J. Amer. Oil Chem. Soc., *58*:475, 1981.

Bounos, G., and Kongshavn, P. A. L.: Influence of dietary proteins on the immune system of mice. J. Nutr., *112*:1747, 1982.

Calloway, D. H.: Nitrogen balance of men with marginal intakes of protein and energy. J. Nutr., *105*:914, 1975.

Calloway, D. H., and Kurzer, M. S.: Menstrual cycle and protein requirements of women. J. Nutr., *112*:356, 1982.

Carroll, K. K.: Hypercholesterolemia and atherosclerosis: effects of dietary protein. Fed. Proc., *41*:2792, 1982.

DeAngelis, R. C., Elias, L. G., and Bressani, R.: Mixtures of rice and beans (55:45 and 77:23). I. Nutritional value of the mixed proteins. Archivos Latinoamer. Nutr., *32:*47, 1982.

Fernstrom, J. D., and Wurtman, R. J.: Effect of chronic corn consumption on serotonin content of rat brain. Nature (New Biol.), *234*:62, 1971.

Fiorotto, M., and Coward, W. A.: Pathogenesis of oedema in protein-energy malnutrition: the significance of plasma colloid osmotic pressure. Brit. J. Nutr., *42:*21,1979.

Gibney, M. J.: Hypocholesterolaemic effect of soya-bean proteins. Proc. Nutr. Soc., *41*:19, 1982.

Hegsted, D. M.: Balance studies. J. Nutr., *106*:307, 1976.

Hill, C. H.: Interaction of detary amino acids with the immune response. Fed. Proc., *41*:2818, 1982.

Inoue, G., Fujita, Y., and Niiyama, Y.: Studies on protein requirements of young men fed egg protein and rice protein with excess and maintenance energy intakes. J. Nutr., *103*:1673, 1973.

Irwin, M. J., and Hegsted, D. M.: A conspectus of research on protein requirements of man. J. Nutr., *101*:385, 1971.

Irwin, M. I., and Hegsted, D. M.: A conspectus of research on amino acid requirements of man. J. Nutr., *101*:539, 1971.

Johnson, A. A., Latham, M. C., and Roe, D. A.: An evaluation of the use of hair root morphology in the assessment of protein-calorie malnutrition. Amer. J. Clin. Nutr., *29*:502, 1976.

Johnson, D. J., and Anderson, G. H.: Prediction of plasma amino acid concentration from diet amino acid content. Amer. J. Physiol., *243*:R99, 1982.

Leverton, R. M., Schlaphoff, D., and Huffstetter, M.: Blood regeneration in women donors: II. Effect of protein, vitamin and mineral supplements. J. Amer. Dietet. Assoc., *24*:480, 1948.

MacLean, W. C., and Graham, G. G.: Growth and nitrogen retention of children consuming all of the day's protein intake in one meal. Amer. J. Clin. Nutr., *29*:78, 1976.

Nicol, B. M., and Phillips, P. G.: The utilization of protein and amino acids in diets based on cassava *(Manihot utilissima),* rice or sorghum *(Sorghum sativa)* by young Nigerian men of low income. Brit. J. Nutr., *39:*271, 1978.

Olson, R. E. (ed.): *Protein-Calorie Malnutrition.* New York, Academic Press, 1975.

Pant, K. C., Rogers, Q. R., and Harper, A. E.: Food selection studies of rats fed tryptophan-imbalanced diets with or without niacin. J. Nutr., *102*:131, 1972.

Porter, J. W. G., and Rolls, B. A.: *Proteins in Human Nutrition.* New York, Academic Press, 1973.

Prothro, J., et al.: Utilization of nitrogen, energy, and sulfur by adolescent boys fed three levels of protein. J. Nutr., *103*:786, 1973.

Shaw, S. N., et al.: Effects of increasing nitrogen intake on nitrogen balance and energy expenditure in nutritionally depleted adult patients receiving parenteral nutrition. Amer. J. Clin. Nutr. *37:*930, 1983.

Simmons, W. K.: Urinary urea nitrogen:creatinine ratio as indicator of recent protein intake in field studies. Amer. J. Clin. Nutr., *25*:539, 1972.

Torun, B., Cabrera-Santiago, M. I., and Viteri, F. E.: Protein requirements of preschool children: obligatory nitrogen losses and nitrogen balance measurements using cow's milk. Archivos Latinoamer. Nutr., *31*:571, 1981.

Uauy, R., et al.: The changing pattern of whole body protein metabolism in aging humans. J. Gerontology, *33*:663, 1978.

Waslien, C. I.: Unusual sources of proteins for man. Crit. Rev. Food Sci. Nutr., p. 77, June, 1975.

Waterlow, J. C., and Stephen, J. M. L.: *Nitrogen Metabolism in Man.* Essex, England, Applied Sci. Publ., 1982.

Yanez, E., et al.: Capacity of the Chilean mixed diet to meet the protein and energy requirements of young adult males. Brit. J. Nutr., *47*:1, 1982.

Chapter 5 Digestion and Absorption

Digestion and Absorption

Adibi, S. A.: Intestinal phase of protein assimilation in men. J. Amer. Clin. Nutr., *29*:205, 1976.

Brown, K. H., Khatum, M., and Ahmed, M. G.: Relationship of the xylose absorption status of children in Bangladesh to their absorption of macronutrients from local diets. Amer. J. Clin. Natr. *34*:1540, 1981.

Bueno, L., and Ferre, J. P.: Central regulation of intestinal motility by somatostatin and cholecystokinin octapeptide. Science, *216*:1427, 1982.

Calloway, D. H., and Chenoweth, W. L.: Utilization of nutrients in milk- and wheat-based diets by men with adequate and reduced abilities to absorb lactose. 1. Energy and nitrogen. Amer. J. Clin. Nutr., *26*:939, 1973.

Carey, M. C., Small, D. M., and Bliss, C. M.: Lipid digestion and absorption. Ann. Rev. Physiol. *45,* 1983.

Carlson, G. L., et al.: A bean α-amylase inhibitor formulation (starch blocker) is ineffective in man. Science, *219:*393, 1983.

Chernow, B., and Castell, D. O.: Diet and heartburn. J. Amer. Med. Assoc., *241*:2307, 1979.

Cornu, A., and Delpeuch, F.: Effect of fiber in sorghum on nitrogen digestibility. Amer. J. Clin. Nutr., *34*:2454, 1981.

Davenport, H. W.: *A Digest of Digestion.* 2nd Ed. Chicago, Year Book Med. Publ., Inc., 1978.

Floch, M. H. (ed): Symposium: Diet, bacteria and the colon. Amer. J. Clin. Nutr., *29*:1409, 1976.

Grieg, P. D., et al.: Metabolic effects of total parenteral nutrition. Ann. Rev. Nutr., *2*:179, 1982.

Gupta, M. C., Basu, A. K., and Tandon, B. N.: Gastrointestinal protein loss in mild hookworm and roundworm infections. Amer. J. Clin. Nutr., *27*:1386, 1974.

Gustafsson, B.: The physiological importance of the colonic microflora. Scand. J. Gastroenterol., *17*:117, 1982.

Holdstock, D. J., et al.: Propulsion (mass movements) in the human colon and its relationship to meals and somatic activity. Gut, *11*:91, 1970.

Jenkins, D. J. A., et al.: Combined use of guar and acarbose in reduction of postprandial glycaemia. Lancet, *2*:924, 1979.

Kien, C. L., et al: Fecal characteristics in healthy young adults consuming defined liquid diets or a free-choice diet. Amer. J. Clin. Nutr., *34*:357, 1981.

Lebenthal, E., Antonowicz, I, and Schwachman, H.: Correlation of lactase activity, lactose tolerance, and milk consumption in different age groups. Amer. J. Clin. Nutr., *28*:595, 1975.

McArthur, K., Hogan, D., and Isenberg, J. I.: Relative stimulatory effects of commonly ingested beverages on gastric acid secretion in humans. Gastroenterology, *83*:199, 1982.

Morley, J. E.: Food peptides. A new class of hormones? J. Amer. Med. Assoc., *247*:2379, 1982.

Munro, H. N. (Chairman): *Symposium:* Iron absorption and nutrition. Fed. Proc., *36*:2016, 1977.

Paul, D., and Hoskins, L. C.: Effect of oral lactobacillus feedings on fecal lactobacillus counts. Amer. J. Clin. Nutr., *25*:763, 1972.

Ravich, W. J., Bayless, T. M., and Thomas, M.: Fructose:incomplete intestinal absorption in humans. Gastroenterology, *84*:26, 1983.

Rosenberg, I. H., and Scrimshaw, N. S. (eds.): Symposium: Workshop on malabsorption and nutrition. Amer. J. Clin. Nutr., *25*:1045, 1972.

Taylor, I. L., et al.: Effect of individual L-amino acids on gastric secretion and serum gastrin and pancreatic polypeptide release in humans. Gastroenterology, *83*:273, 1982.

Walcher, D. N., and Kretchmer, N. (eds.): *Food, Nutrition and Evolution.* Chap. 14–18. New York, Massn Publ. USA, Inc., 1981.

Young, E. A., et al.: Gastrointestinal response to nutrient variation of defined formula diets. J. Parenter. Ent. Nutr., *5*:478, 1981.

Chapter 6 Energy I

Energy, Part 1: Basics

Bouchard, C., et al.: A method to assess energy expenditure in children and adults. Amer. J. Clin. Natr. *37*:461, 1983.

Bradfield, R. B. (ed.): Symposium: Assessment of typical daily energy expenditure. Amer. J. Clin. Nutr., *24*:1111 and 1405, 1971.

Brooke, O. G., and Ashworth, A.: The influence of malnutrition on the postprandial metabolic rate and respiratory quotient. Brit. J. Nutr., *27*:407, 1972.

Buskirk, E. R., Thomson, R. H., and Whedon, G. D.: Metabolic response to cold air in men and women in relation to total body fat content. J. Appl. Physiol., *18*:603, 1963.

Consolazio, C. F., et al.: Energy requirements in extreme heat. J. Nutr., *73*:126, 1961.

Fulton, D. E.: Basal metabolic rate of women. J. Amer. Dietet. Assoc., *61*:516, 1972.

Galton, D. J., and Wallis, S.: The regulation of adipose cell metabolism. Proc. Nutr. Soc., *41*:167, 1982.

Garrow, J. S., and Hawes, S. F.: The role of amino acid oxidation in causing "specific dynamic action" in man. Brit. J. Nutr., *27*:211, 1972.

Hurni, M., et al.: Metabolic effects of a mixed and a high-carbohydrate low-fat diet in man, measured over 24 h in a respiration chamber. Brit. J. Nutr., *47*:33, 1982.

Krebs, H. A.: The history of the tricarboxylic acid cycle. Perspect. Biol. Med., *14*:154, 1970.

McGandy, R. B., Barrows, C. H., et al.: Nutrient intakes and energy expenditure in men of different ages. J. Gerontology, *21*:581, 1966.

NAS/NRC: Biological Energy Interrelationships and Glossary of Energy Terms. Pub. 1411, 1966.

Pike, R. L., and Brown, M. L.: *Nutrition: An Integrated Approach.* 2nd Ed. New York, John Wiley & Sons, Inc., 1975.

Pirola, R. C., and Lieber, C. S.: Hypothesis: energy wastage in alcoholism and drug abuse: possible role of hepatic microsomal enzymes. Amer. J. Clin. Nutr., *29*:90, 1976.

Reeds, P. J., Wahle, K. W. J., and Haggarty, P.: Energy costs of protein and fatty acid synthesis. Proc. Nutr. Soc., *41*:155, 1982.

Richardson, M., and McCracken, E. C.: Energy expenditures of women performing selected activities. U.S. Department of Agriculture Home Econ. Res. Rept. No. 11. Washington, D.C., Government Printing Office, 1960.

Schuster, J. A., and Levitsky, D. A.: Insensible weight loss as an indicator of metabolic rate. Physiol. Behavior, *28*:381, 1982.

Shambaugh, G. E.: Urea biosynthesis. IV. Normal and abnormal regulation. Amer. J. Clin. Nutr., *31*:126, 1978.

Skubic, V., and Kodgkins, J.: Energy expenditure of women participants in selected individual sports. J. Appl. Physiol., *21*:133, 1966.

Solomon, S. J., Kurzer, M. S. and Calloway, D. H.: Menstrual cycle and basal metabolic rate in women. Amer. J. Clin. Nutr., *36*:611, 1982.

Southgate, D. A. T.: Assessing the energy value of the human diet. Nutr. Rev., *29*:131, 1971.

Southgate, D. A. T., and Durnin, J. V. G. A.: Calorie conversion factors. An experimental reassessment of the factors used in the calculation of the energy value of human diets. Brit. J. Nutr., *24*:517, 1970.

Swindells, Y. E.: The influence of activity and size of meals on caloric response in women. Brit. J. Nutr., *27*:65, 1972.

Symposium: The application of human and animal calorimetry. Proc. Nutr. Soc., *37*:1, 1978.

Thompson, A. M., and Billewicz, W. Z.: Height, weight and food intake in man. Brit. J. Nutr., *15*:241, 1961.

Torun, B., McGuire, J., and Mendoza, R. D.: Energy cost of activities and tasks of women from rural region of Guatemala. Nutr. Res., *2*:127, 1982.

Wallace, R. K., and Benson, H.: The physiology of meditation. Sci. Amer., *226*:84, 1972.

Webb, P.: Energy expenditure and fat-free mass in men and women. Amer. J. Clin. Nutr., *34*:1816, 1981.

Chapter 7 Energy II

Energy, Part 2

Arteaga, P., DosSantos, J. E., and Dutra de Oliveira, J. E.: Obesity among schoolchildren of different socioeconomic levels in a developing country. Internat. J. Obesity, *6*:291, 1982.

Borkan, G. A., et al.: Assessment of abdominal fat content by computed tomography. Amer. J. Clin. Nutr., *36*:172, 1982.

Bray, G. A.: Effect of caloric restriction on energy expenditure in obese patients. Lancet, *2*:397, 1969.

Bullen, B. A., Reed, R. B., and Mayer, J.: Physical activity of obese and nonobese adolescent girls appraised by motion picture sampling. Amer. J. Clin. Nutr., *14*:211, 1964.

Cronk, C. E., and Roche, A. F.: Race- and sex-specific reference data for triceps and subscapular skinfolds and weight/stature. Amer. J. Clin. Nutr., *35*:347, 1982.

Crisp, A. H., et al.: Reproductive hormone profiles in male anorexia nervosa before, during and after restoration of body weight to normal. Internat. J. Eating Disorders, *1*(3):3, 1982.

Dalrit, S. P.: The effect of the menstrual cycle on patterns of food intake. Amer. J. Clin. Nutr. *34*:1811, 1981.

DeWaard, F., Poortman, J., and Collette, B. J. A.: Relationship of weight to the promotion of breast cancer after menopause. Nutr. Cancer, *2*:273, 1981.

Duncan, K. H., Bacon, J. A., and Weinsier, R. L.: The effects of high and low energy density diets on satiety, energy intake, and eating time of obese and nonobese subjects, Amer. J. Clin. Nutr., *37*:763, 1983.

Garn, S. M., Bailey, S. M., and Higgins, I. T. T.: Fatness similarities in adopted pairs. Amer. J. Clin. Nutr., *29*:1067, 1976.

Garrow, J. S.: Energy stores in man, their composition and measurement. Proc. Nutr. Soc., *41*:175, 1982.

Hirsch, J., Knittle, J. L., and Salans, L. B.: Cell lipid content and cell number in obese and nonobese human adipose tissue. J. Clin. Invest., *45*:1023, 1966.

Houpt, K. A.: Gastrointestinal factors in hunger and satiety. Neurosci. Biobehav. Rev., *6*:145, 1982.

Huse, D. M., et al.: The challenge of obesity in childhood. Parts I and II. Mayo Clinic Proc., *57*:279 and 285, 1982.

Kahle, E. B., et al.: Moderate diet control in children: the effects on metabolic indicators that predict obesity-related degenerative diseases. Amer. J. Clin. Nutr., *35*:950, 1982.

Lewis, S., et al.: Effects of physical activity on weight reduction in obese middle-aged women. Amer. J. Clin. Nutr., *29*:151, 1976.

Lincoln, J. E.: Weight gain after cessation of smoking. J. Amer. Med. Assoc., *210*:1765, 1969.

Mallick, M. J.: Health hazards of obesity and weight control in children: a review of the literature. Amer. J. Pub. Health, *73*:78, 1983

Metzner, H. L., et al.: The relationship between frequency of eating and adiposity in adult men and women in the Tecumseh Community Health Study. Amer. J. Clin. Nutr., *30*:712, 1977.

Miller, D. S., and Mumford, P.: Gluttony. 1. An experimental study of overeating low- or high-protein diets. Amer. J. Clin. Nutr., *20*:1212, 1967.

Miller, D. S., Mumford, P., and Stock, M. J.: Gluttony. 2. Thermogenesis in overeating man. Amer. J. Clin. Nutr., *20*:1233, 1967.

Mirkin, G. B., and Shore, R. N.: The Beverly Hills diet. Dangers of the newest weight loss fad. J. Amer. Med. Assoc., *246*:2235, 1981.

Naismith, D. J., et al.: Carbohydrate conservation in the obese: a theory to explain the ease of weight gain. Ann. Nutr. Metab., *26*:18, 1982.

Newsholme, E. A.: The interrelationship between metabolic regulation, weight control and obesity. Proc. Nutr. Soc., *41*:183, 1982.

O'Sullivan, J. B.: Body weight and subsequent diabetes mellitus. J. Amer. Med. Assoc., *248*:949, 1982.

Payne, P. R., and Dugdale, A. E.: Mechanisms for the control of body weight. Lancet, *1*:583, 1977.

Pradelier, A., et al.: Relationship between pain and obesity: an electrophysiological study. Physiol. Behavior, *27*:961, 1981.

Pugliese, M. T., et al.: Fear of obesity: a cause of short stature and delayed puberty. New Engl. J. Med., *309*:513, 1983.

Rabast, U., Vornberger, K. H., and Ehl, M.: Loss of weight, sodium and water in obese persons consuming a high- or low-carbohydrate diet. Ann. Nutr. Metab., *25*:341, 1981.

Ravelli, G., Stein, Z. A., and Susser, M. W.: Obesity in young men after famine exposure in utero and early infancy. New Eng. J. Med., *295*:349, 1976.

Reisin, E., et al.: Effect of weight loss without salt restriction on the reduction of blood pressure in overweight hypertensive patients. New Eng. J. Med., *298*:1, 1978.

Sorensen, T. I. A., et al.: Reduced intellectual performance in extreme overweight. Human Biol., *54*:165, 1982.

Serog, P., et al.: Effects of slimming and composition of diets on VO_2 and thyroid hormones in healthy subjects. Amer. J. Clin. Nutr., *35*:24, 1982.

Spurr, A. B., et al.: Marginal malnutrition in school-aged Colombian boys: functional consequences in maximum exercise. Amer. J. Clin. Nutr., *37*:834, 1983.

Stern, M. P., et al.: Knowledge, attitudes and behavior related to obesity and dieting in Mexican Americans and Anglos: the San Antonio heart study. Amer. J. Epidem., *115*:917, 1982.

Stewart, A. L., and Brook, R. H.: Effects of being overweight. Am. J. Public Health, *73:* 171, 1983.

Stunkard, A. J.: *Obesity.* Philadelphia, W. B. Saunders, 1980.

Sukhatme, P. V., and Margen, S.: Autoregulatory homeostatic nature of energy balance. Amer. J. Clin. Nutr., *35*:355, 1982.

Weele, S. L., and Campbell, R. G.: Normal thermic effect of glucose in obese women. Amer. J. Clin. Nutr., *37*:87, 1983.

Womersley, J., and Durnin, J. V. G. A.: A comparison of the skinfold method with extent of 'overweight' and various height-weight relationships in the assessment of obesity. Brit. J. Nutr., *38*:271, 1977.

Woo, R., Garrow, J. S., and Pi-Sunyer, F. X.: Voluntary food intake during prolonged exercise in obese women. Amer. J. Clin. Nutr., *36*:478, 1982.

Chapter 8 Vitamins

History and Reviews

Goodhart, R. S., and Shils, M. E. (eds.): *Modern Nutrition in Health and Disease.* 6th Ed. Philadelphia, Lea and Febiger, 1980 (pp. 142–294 on vitamins).

György, P.: Reminiscences on the discovery and significance of some of the B vitamins. Nutr. Rev., *34*:141, 1976.

Herbert, V., and Barrett, S.: *Vitamins and "Health" Foods: The Great American Hustle.* Philadelphia, G. F. Stickley Co., 1981.

Lepkovsky, S.: The water-soluble vitamins. Ann. Rev. Biochem., *9*:383, 1940.

Medical Research Council: *Vitamins: A Survey of Present Knowledge,* Special Reports Series No. 167. London, H. M. Stationery Office, 1932.

Rosenberg, H. R.: *Chemistry and Physiology of the Vitamins.* New York, Interscience Publishers, 1942.

Sebrell, W. H., Jr., and Harris, R. S. (eds.): *The Vitamins.* 3 vols. New York, Academic Press, 1954.

Seidell, A.: The chemistry of vitamins. Science, *60*:439, 1924.

Vitamin Losses in Food

Augustin, J., et al.: Vitamin retention during preparation and holding of mashed potatoes made from commercially dehydrated flakes and granules, J. Food Sci., *47*:274, 1982.

Dudek, J. A., and Elkins, E. R., Jr.: Nutrient composition of historical canned food samples. J. Food Sci., *48*:654, 1983 (vitamin C and carotene in over-40-year-old canned foods).

Holmes, Z. A., et al.: Vitamin retention during home drying of vegetables and fruits. Home Econ. Res. J., 7:259, 1979.

Koehler, H. H., and Hard, M. M.: Vitamin contents of pre-prepared foods sampled from a hospital food service line. J. Amer. Dietet. Assoc., *82*:622, 1983 (on thiamin, riboflavin, and vitamin C).

Lee C. Y., Massey, L. M., Jr., and Van Buren, J. P.: Effects of post-harvest handling and processing on vitamin contents of peas. J. Food Sci., *47*:961, 1982.

Van Buren, J. P., Lee, C. Y., and Massey, L. M., Jr.: Variation of vitamin concentration and retention in canned snap beans from three processing plants during two years. J. Food Sci., *47*:1545, 1982.

Other Readings (including "megavitamins" and vitamin intakes)

Allington, J. K., Matthews, M. E., and Johnson, N. E.: Nutritive value of food served calculated from food purchased in 14 nursing homes. J. Amer. Dietet. Assoc., *82*:377, 1983.

Arnold, L. E., et al.: Megavitamins for minimal brain dysfunction—a placebo-controlled study. J. Amer. Med. Assoc., *240*:2642, 1978.

Bootman, J. L., and Wertheimer, A. I.: Patterns of vitamin usage in a sample of university students. J. Amer. Dietet. Assoc., *77*(July):58, 1980.

Can vitamins help prevent cancer? Consumer Rept., *48*:243, 1983.

Committee on Nutrition: Vitamin and mineral supplement needs in normal children in the United States. Pediatrics, *66*:1015, 1980.

Dubnick, M. A., and Rucker, R. B.: Dietary supplements and health aids—a critical evaluation. Part I—Vitamins and minerals. J. Nutr. Educ., *15*:47, 1983 (on excessive supplementation).

El Nakah, A., et al., A vitamin profile of heroin addiction. Amer. J. Public Health, *69*:1058, 1979.

Gray, G. E., et al.: Dietary intake and nutrient supplement use in a Southern California retirement community. Amer. J. Clin. Nutr. *38*:122, 1983.

Herbert, V.: Will questionable nutrition overwhelm nutrition science? Amer. J. Clin. Nutr., *34*:2848, 1981.

Kershner, J., and Hawke, W.: Megavitamins and learning disorders: a controlled double-blind experiment. J. Nutr., *109*:819, 1979.

Pao, E. M.: and Mickle, S. J.: Problem nutrients in the United States. Food Tech., *35*(Sept.):58, 1981.

Rao, D. A., et al.: Nutritional status of women attending family planning clinics. J. Amer. Dietet. Assoc., *81*:682, 1982 (on vitamin A, folacin, and riboflavin).

Raskind, M.: Nutrition and cognitive function in the elderly. J. Amer. Med. Assoc., *249*:2939, 1983 (an editorial on the apparent lack of effectiveness of high levels of vitamins in senility). Also see Goodwin, J. S., et al., J. Amer. Med. Assoc., *249*:2917, 1983, on "subclinical" malnutrition in some elderly individuals.

Rudman, D. and Williams, P. J.: Megadose vitamins—use and misuse. New Eng. J. Med., *309*:488 (editorial), 1983.

Sabry, J. H., Chorostecki, D. J., and Woolcott, F. M.: Nutrient content of diets of businessmen: relation to body weight status, age, and education. J. Canad. Dietet. Assoc., *43*:216, 1982.

Chapter 9 Vitamins A, D, E, and K

Fat-soluble Vitamins: General

Bieri, J. G., and McKenna, M. C.: Expressing dietary values for fat-soluble vitamins: changes in concepts and terminology. Amer. J. Clin. Nutr., *34*:289, 1981.

Bonjour, J. P.: Vitamins and alcoholism: vitamin D, vitamin E, and vitamin K. Internat. J. Vit. Nutr. Res., *51*:307, 1981.

Fat-soluble vitamins. Dairy Council Dig., *53*:13, 1982.

Hollander, D.: Intestinal absorption of vitamins A, E, D, and K. J. Lab. Clin. Med., *97*:449, 1981.

Vitamin A: Reviews and History

(Also see refs. 1–3, 5–8, 10, and 17, this chapter.)

Bauernfeind, J. C.: Vitamin A—technology and applications. World Rev. Nutr. Dietet., *41*:110, 1983.

DeLuca, L. M., and Shapiro, S. S.(eds.): Modulation of cellular interactions by vitamin A and derivatives (retinoids). Ann. N.Y Acad. Sci., *359*:1–431, 1981.

Ganguly, J., et al.: Systemic mode of action of vitamin A. Vit. Horm., *38*:1, 1980.

Goodman, D. S. (Chairman): Vitamin A and retinoids: recent advances. Fed. Proc., *38*:2501–2543, 1979.

Goodman, D. S.: Vitamin A metabolism. Fed. Proc., *39*:2716, 1980.

Lui, N. S. T., and Roels, D. A.: Vitamin A and carotene (Chap. 6). In *Modern Nutrition in Health and Disease.*

6th Ed. Goodhart, R. S., and Shils, M. E. (eds.): Philadelphia, Lea and Febiger, 1980.

Sharman, I. M. (Chairman): Vitamin A in nutrition and disease (a symposium). Proc. Nutr. Soc., *42*:1–101 (9 papers), 1983.

Wolf, G.: Vitamin A. In Alfin-Slater, R. B., and Kritchevsky, D. (eds.): *Nutrition and the Adult-Micronutrients.* Vol. 3A in the series Human Nutrition: A Comprehensive Treatise. New York, Plenum Press, 1980, p. 97.

Zile, M. H., and Cullum, M. E.: The function of vitamin A: current concepts. Proc. Soc. Exp. Biol. Med., *172*:139, 1983.

Vitamin A and the Eye

Menon, K., and Vijayaraghavan, K.: Sequelae of severe xerophthalmia—a follow-up study. Amer. J. Clin. Nutr., *33*:218, 1979.

Pettiss, S. T.: Planning for the control of xerophthalmia. Assignment Child. (U.N.), *53/54*:77, 1981.

Solon, F., et al.: An evaluation of strategies to control vitamin A Indeficiency in the Philippines. Amer. J. Clin. Nutr., *32*:1445, 1979.

Tarwotjo, I., et al.: Interactions of community nutritional status and xeropthalmia in Indonesia. Amer. J. Clin. Nutr., *37*:645, 1983.

Underwood, B. A.: Hypovitaminosis A and its control. Bull. World Health Org., *56*:525, 1978.

Venkatasamy, G., Cobby, M. and Pirie, A: Rehabilitation of xeropthalmic children. Trop. Geogr. Med., *31*:149, 1979.

Vijayaraghavan, K., and Rao, N. P.: An evaluation of the national prophylaxis programme against blindness due to vitamin A deficiency. Nutr. Rept. Internat., *25*:531, 1982.

WHO/UNICEF/SAID: *Control of Vitamin A deficiency and xerophthalmia.* World Health Org. Tech. Rept. Ser. No. 672, 1982.

Carotenoids and Vitamin A

Bauernfeind, J. C. (ed.): *Carotenoids as Colorants and Vitamin A Precursors.* New York: Academic Press, 1981.

Emodi, A., Johnson, L., and Mix J.: Carotenoids in bakery products. Cereal Foods World, *25*:316, 1980.

Goodwin, T. W.: Nature and distribution of carotenoids. Food Chemistry, *5*:3, 1980.

Klein, B. P., and Perry, A. K.: Ascorbic acid and vitamin A activity in selected vegetables from different geographical areas of the United States. J. Food Sci., *47*:941, 1982.

Lee, C. Y., McCoon, P. E., and LeBowitz, J. M.: Vitamin A value of sweet corn. J. Agric. Food Chem., *29*:1294, 1981.

Maeda, E. E., and Salunkhe, D. K.: Retention of ascorbic acid and total carotene in solar dried vegetables. J. Food Sci., *46*:1288, 1981.

Simpson, K. L., and Chichester, C. O.: Metabolism and nutritional significance of carotenoids. Ann. Rev. Nutr., *1*:351, 1981.

Vitamin A: Other Readings

Arroyave, G., Mejia, L. A., and Aguilar, J. R.: The effect of vitamin A fortification of sugar on the serum vitamin A levels of preschool Guatemalan children: a longitudinal evaluation. Amer. J. Clin. Nutr., *34*:41, 1981.

Bonjour, J. P.: Vitamins and alcoholism. Vitamin A. Internat. J. Vit. Nutr. Res., *51*:166, 1981.

Cumming, F. J., and Briggs, M. H.: Changes in plasma vitamin A in lactating and non-lactating oral contraceptive users. Brit. J. Obst. Gyn., *90*:73, 1983.

Depression of serum levels of retinol and retinol binding protein during infection. Nutr. Rev., *39*:165, 1981.

Garfield, E.: Acne vulgaris—the adolescent's albatross. Current Contents—Life Sci., *25*(2): 5, 1982.

Hennekens, C. H., et al.: Vitamin A and risk of cancer. J. Nutr. Educ., *14*:135, 1982.

Leo, M. A., and Lieber, C. S.: Interaction of ethanol with vitamin A. Alcoholism: Clin. Exp. Res., *7*:15, 1983.

Mejia, L. A., et al.: Vitamin A deficiency and anemia in central American children. Amer. J. Clin. Nutr., *30*:1175, 1977.

Peto, R., et al.: Can dietary beta-carotene materially reduce human cancer rates?. Nature, *290*:201, 1981.

Pochi, P. E.: Hormones, retinoids, and acne. New Eng. J. Med., *308*:1024, 1983.

Rossi, G. C., Bendrick, C. J., and Wolf, G.: *In vivo* synthesis of lipid-linked oligosaccharides in the livers of normal and vitamin A-deficient rats. J. Biol. Chem., *256*:8341, 1981.

Wolback, S. B., and Howe, P. R.: Tissue changes following deprivation of fat-soluble A vitamin. Nutr. Rev., *36*:16, 1978.

Zile, M. H., Bunge, E. C., and DeLuca, H. F.: DNA labeling of rat epithelial tissues in vitamin A deficiency. J. Nutr., *111*:777, 1981.

Vitamin D: Reviews

(Also see refs. 1, 8, 10, and 43–55, this chapter.)

Bonjour, J. P.: Vitamins and alcoholism. X. Vitamin D. Internat. J. Vit. Nutr. Res., *51*:307, 1981.

Bronner, F. Chairman: Vitamin D and membrane structure and function. Fed. Proc., *41*;60–84 (5 papers), 1982.

DeLuca, H. F.: *Vitamin D.* Berlin, Springer Verlag, 1979.

Fraser, D. R.: Biochemical and clinical aspects of vitamin D function. Brit. Med. Bull., *37*:37, 1981; The physiological economy of vitamin D. Lancet *1*:969, 1983.

Harrison, H. E.: Vitamin D, the parathyroid and the kidney. The Johns Hopkins Med. J., *144*:180, 1979.

Norman, A. W.: *Vitamin D—The Calcium Homeostatic Steroid Hormone.* New York, Academic Press, 1979.

Smith, R.: Rickets and osteomalacia. Human Nutr.: Clin. Nutr., *36C*:115, 1982.

Stern, P. H.: The D vitamins and bone. Pharm. Rev., *32*:47, 1980.

Vitamin D: Other Readings

Charles, M. A., et al.: Regulation of calcium-binding protein messenger RNA by 1,25-dihydroxycholecalciferol. Calcif. Tissue Int., *33*:15, 1981.

Dilling, L. A.: Growth and nutrition of preschool Indian children in Manitoba. I. Vitamin D deficiency. Canad. J. Pub. Health, *69*:248, 1978.

Gilman, S. C., Biersner, R. J., and Bondi, K. R.: Effect of a 68-day submarine patrol on serum 25-hydroxyvitamin D levels in healthy men. Internat. J. Vit. Nutr. Res., *51*:63, 1981.

Holmes, R. P., and Kummerow, F. A.: The vitamin D status of elderly Americans. Amer. J. Clin. Nutr. *38*:335, 1983. (Letter to editor. Also see responses by Omdahl, J. L., and Garry, P. J., p. 338; and Parfitt, A. M. p. 339).

Mason, R. S., et al.: Vitamin D metabolism in hypophosphatemic rickets. Amer. J. Dis. Children, *136*:907, 1982.

Paterson, C. R.: Vitamin D deficiency rickets simulating child abuse. J. Pediatr. Orthoped., *1*:423, 1981.

Reeve L., et al.: Studies on the site of 1,25-dihydroxyvitamin D_3 synthesis *in vivo.* J. Biol. Chem., *258*:3615, 1983.

Sedrani, S. H. et al.; Sunlight and vitamin D status in normal Saudi subjects. Amer. J. Clin. Nutr., *38*:129, 1983.

Slovik, D. M., et al.: Deficient production of 1,25-dihydroxyvitamin D in elderly osteoporotic patients. New Eng. J. Med., *305*:372, 1981.

Tjellesen, L., and Christiansen, C.: Vitamin D metabolites in normal subjects during one year. A longitudinal study. Scand. J. Clin. Lab. Invest., *43*:85, 1983.

Vitamin E: Reviews and History

(Also see refs. 1, 8, and 56–75, this chapter.)

Bell, E. F., and Filer, L. J.: The role of vitamin E in the nutrition of premature infants. Amer. J. Clin. Nutr., *34*:414, 1981.

Combs, G. F.: Assessment of vitamin E status in animals and man. Proc. Nutr. Soc., *40*:187, 1981.

Drake, J. R., and Fitch, C. D.: Status of vitamin E as an erythropoietic factor. Amer. J. Clin. Nutr., *33*:2386, 1980.

Horwitt, M. K. (ed.): Symposium: Vitamin E, biochemistry, nutritional requirements and clinical studies (22 papers). Part I (939) and Part II (1105). Amer. J. Clin. Nutr., *27*:939, 1974.

Horwitt, M. K.: Therapeutic uses of vitamin E in medicine. Nutr. Rev., *38*:105, 1980.

Horwitt, M. L.: *Vitamin E* (Chapter 6B). In Goodhart, R. S., and Shils, M. E.: *Modern Nutrition in Health and Disease.* 6th Ed. Philadelphia, Lee and Febiger, 1980, p. 181.

Lubin, B., and Machlin, L. J. (eds.): Vitamin E: biochemical, hematological, and clinical aspects. Ann. N.Y. Acad. Sci., *393*:1–505, 1982.

Mason, K. E.: The first decades of vitamin E. Fed. Proc., *36*:1906, 1977.

Parrish, D. B.: Determination of vitamin E in foods—a review. Crit. Rev. Food Sci. Nutr., *13*:161, 1980.

Scott, M. L.: Advances in our understanding of vitamin E. Fed. Proc., *39*:2736, 1980.

Vitamin E: Other Readings

DeLumen, B. O., and Fiad, S.: Tocopherols of winged bean *(Psophocarpus tetragonolobus)* oil. J. Agric. Food Chem., *30*:50, 1982.

Desai, I. D., et al.: Vitamin E status of agricultural migrant workers in southern Brazil. Amer. J. Clin. Nutr., *33*:2669, 1980.

Farrell, P. M., et al.: Plasma tocopherol levels and tocopherol-lipid relationships in a normal population of children as compared to healthy adults. Amer. J. Clin. Nutr., *31*:1720, 1978.

Harman, D.: The aging process. Proc. Nat. Acad. Sci., *78*:7124, 1981.

Howard, D. R., Rundell, C. A., and Batsakis, J. G.: Vitamin E does not modify HDL-cholesterol. Amer. Soc. Clin. Path., *77*:86, 1982.

Johnson, G. J., et al.: High-dose vitamin E does not decrease the rate of chronic hemolysis in glucose-6-phosphate dehydrogenase deficiency. New Eng. J. Med., *308*:1014, 1983.

Neville, H. E., et al.: Ultrastructural and histochemical abnormalities of skeletal muscle in patients with chronic vitamin E deficiency. Neurology, *33*:483, 1983 (patients aged 5 to 11).

Posin, C. I., et al.: Human biochemical response to ozone and vitamin E. J. Tox. Environ. Health, *5*:1049, 1979.

Vitamin K: Reviews and History

(Also see refs 1, 8, and 76–79, this chapter.)

Almquist, H. J.: The early history of vitamin K. Amer. J. Clin. Nutr., *28*:656, 1975.

Corrigan, J. J., Jr.: The vitamin K-dependent proteins. Adv. Pediatrics, *28*:57, 1981.

Dam, H.: Historical survey and introduction. Vit. Horm., *24*:295, 1966.

Gallop, P. M., Lian, J. B., and Hauschka, P. V.: Carboxylated calcium-binding proteins and vitamin K. New Eng. J. Med., *302*:1460, 1980.

Intestinal microflora, injury and vitamin K deficiency. Nutr. Rev., *38*:341, 1980.

Liebman, H. A., Furie, B. C., and Furie, B., Hepatic vitamin K-dependent carboxylation of blood-clotting proteins., Hepatology, *2*:488, 1982.

Suttie, J. W., The metabolic role of vitamin K. Fed. Proc., *39*:2730, 1980.

Vitamin K: Other Readings

Bell, R. G., Vitamin K activity and metabolism of vitamin K-1 epoxide-1,4-diol. J. Nutr., *112*:287, 1982.

Bertina, R. M., et al.: New method for the rapid detection of vitamin K deficiency. Clin. Chim. Acta, *105*:93, 1980.

Dubois, J., et. al.: Vitamin K-dependent carboxylation. J. Biol. Chem., *258*:7897, 1983.

Goldsmith, G. H., et al.: Studies on a family with combined functional deficiencies of vitamin K-dependent coagulation factors. J. Clin. Invest., *69*:1253, 1982.

Israels, L. G., et al.: Vitamin K as a regulator of benzo(a)pyrene metabolism, mutagenesis, and carcinogenesis. J. Clin. Invest., *71*:1130, 1983.

Krasinski, S., et al.: Subclinical vitamin K deficiency in patients with inflammatory bowel disease and/or malabsorption disorders. Amer. J. Clin. Nutr., *37*:698(abst.), 1983.

O'Conner, M. E., et al.: Vitamin K deficiency and breast feeding. Amer. J. Dis. Children, *137*:601, 1983.

Poser, J. W., et al.: Isolation and sequence of the vitamin K-dependent protein from human bone. J. Biol. Chem., *255*:8685, 1980.

Shearer, M. J., et al.: Plasma vitamin K-1, in mothers and their newborn babies. Lancet, *2*:460, 1982.

Wallin, R., and Hutson, S.: Vitamin K-dependent carboxylation. J. Biol. Chem., *257*:1583, 1982.

Chapter 10 Vitamin B Complex I

Vitamin B Complex: General

(Also see Supplementary Reading, Chapters 8 and 11.)

Augustin, J., et al.: B vitamin content of selected cereals and baked products. Cereal Foods World, *27*:159, 1982. (Also see J. Food Sci., *47*:274, 1981.)

Bamji, M. S., and Prema, K.: Enzymatic riboflavin and pyridoxine deficiencies in young Indian women suffering from different grades of glossitis. Nutr. Rept. Internat., *24*:649, 1981 (India).

Bamji, M. S., et al.: Impact of long term, low dose B-complex vitamin supplements on vitamin status and psychomotor performance of rural school boys. Nutr. Res., *2*:147, 1982 (on riboflavin, B-6, and folacin in India).

Bonjour, J. P.: Vitamins and alcoholism. V. Riboflavin, VI. Niacin, VII. Pantothenic Acid, and VIII. Biotin. Internat. J. Vit. Nutr. Res., *50*:425, 1980.

Dong, M. H., et al.: Thiamin, riboflavin, and vitamin B-6 contents of selected foods as served. J. Amer. Dietet. Assoc., *76*:156, 1980.

Langohr, H. D., Petruch, F., and Schroth, G.: Vitamin B-1, B-2, and B-6 deficiency in neurological disorders. J. Neurol., *225*:95, 1981.

Lewis, C. M., and King, J. C.: Effect of oral contraceptive agents on thiamin, riboflavin and pantothenic acid status in young women. Amer. J. Clin. Nutr., *33*:832, 1980.

Nail, P. A., Thomas, M. R., and Eakin, R.: The effect of thiamin and riboflavin supplementation on the level of those vitamins in human breast milk and urine. Amer. J. Clin. Nutr., *33*:198, 1980.

Riboflavin and thiamine binding proteins: their physiological significance and hormonal specificity. Nutr. Rev., *37*:261, 1979.

Rose, R. C.: Transport and metabolism of water-soluble vitamins in intestine. Amer. J. Physiol., *240*:G97, 1981.

Thurnham, D. I.: Red cell enzyme tests of vitamin status: do marginal deficiencies have any physiological significance? Proc. Nutr. Soc., *40*:155, 1981.

Thiamin: Reviews and History

Butterworth, R. F.: Neurotransmitter function in thiamine-deficiency encephalopathy. Neurochem. Internat., *4*:449, 1982.

Guggenheim, K. Y.: Beriberi (Chap. 9). In *Nutrition and Nutritional Diseases: The Evolution of Concepts,* Lexington, Mass., D. C. Heath and Co., 1981.

Gubler, C. J., Fujiwara, M., and Dreyfus, P. M.: *Thiamine.* London, John Wiley and Sons, 1976.

Iber, F. L., et al.: Thiamin in the elderly—relation to alcoholism and to neurological degenerative disease. Amer. J. Clin. Nutr., *36*:1067, 1982.

Jansen, B. C. P.: Early nutritional researches on beriberi leading to the discovery of vitamin B-1. Nutr. Abstr. Rev., *26*:1, 1956.

McCormick, D. B., and Wright, L. D.: Thiamin: phosphates and analogues.

Methods Enzymol, *62*:51–120 (19 papers), 1979.

Sable, H. Z., and Gubler, C. J. (eds.): Thiamin: twenty years of progress. Ann. N.Y. Acad. Sci., *378*:1–472, 1982.

Zuidema, J. J.: Beriberi. Trop. Geogr. Med., *32*:195, 1980.

Thiamin: General Readings

(Also see references 1–19, this chapter.)

Hoyumpa, A. M., Jr., et al.: Dual system of intestinal thiamine transport in humans. J. Lab. Clin. Med., *99*:701, 1982.

Kawai, C., et al.: Reappearance of beriberi heart disease in Japan: a study of 23 cases. Amer. J. Med., *69*:383, 1980.

Khan, M. A., Klein, B. P., and Lee, F. V.: Thiamin content of freshly prepared and leftover Italian spaghetti served in a university cafeteria foodservice. J. Food Sci., *47*:2093, 1982.

Price, J.: The taste of thiamin-fortified beer. J. Food Nutr., *38*:67, 1981.

Sauberlich, H. E., et al.: Thiamin requirement of the adult human. Amer. J. Clin. Nutr., *32*:2237, 1979.

Skjöldebrand, C., et al.: Prediction of thiamin content in convective heated meat products. J. Food Tech., (UK), *18*:61, 1983.

Thiamin and wound repair. Nutr. Rev., *40*:316, 1982.

Vir, S. C., Love, A. H. G., and Thompson, W.: Thiamin status during pregnancy. Internat. J. Vit. Nutr. Res., *50*:131, 1980.

Whyte, K. F., et al.: Excessive beer consumption and beri-beri. Scottish Med. J., *27*:288, 1982.

Witt, E. D., and Goldmanrakic, P. S.: Intermittent thiamine deficiency in the rhesus monkey. 2. Evidence for memory loss. Ann. Neurol., *13*:396, 1983.

Riboflavin: Status in Other Countries

Ajayi, O. A.: Riboflavin status in Nigerian blood donors. Nutr. Rept. Internat., *25*:485, 1982.

Bates, C. J., et al.: Riboflavin status in infants born in rural Gambia, and the effect of a weaning food supplement. Trans. Royal Soc. Trop. Med. Hyg., *76*:253, 1982.

Buzina, R., et al.: The effects of riboflavin administration on iron metabolism parameters in a school-going population. Internat. J. Vit. Nutr. Res., *49*:136, 1979 Yugoslavia.

Mobarhan, S., et al.: Riboflavin status among rural children in Southern Italy. Human Nutr.: Clin. Nutr., *36C*:71, 1982.

Powers, H. J., and Thurnham, D. I.: Riboflavin deficiency in man: effects on haemoglobin and reduced glutathione in erythrocytes of different ages. Brit. J. Nutr., *46*:257, 1981 (U.K.).

Vir, S. C., et al.: Riboflavin status during pregnancy. Amer. J. Clin. Nutr., *34*:2699, 1981 (Ireland).

Riboflavin: General

(Also see references 20–39, this chapter.)

Ashoor, S. H., et al.: HPLC determination of riboflavin in eggs and dairy products. J. Food Sci., *48*:92, 1983.

Belko, A. Z., et al.: Effects of exercise on riboflavin requirements of young women. Amer. J. Clin. Nutr., *37*:509, 1983.

Hirano, M., et al.: Congenital methaemoglobinaemia due to NADH methaemoglobin reductase deficiency: successful treatment with oral riboflavin. Brit. J. Haematol., *47*:353, 1981.

Roe, D. A., et al.: Factors affecting riboflavin requirements of oral contraceptive users and nonusers. Amer. J. Clin. Nutr., *35*:495, 1982.

Pantothenic acid

(Also see references 40–50, this chapter.)

Hoppner, K., and Lampi, B.: Total pantothenic acid in breakfast cereals. Nutr. Rept. Internat., *25*:245, 1982.

Johnston, L., Vaughan, L., and Fox, H. M.: Pantothenic acid content of human milk. Amer. J. Clin. Nutr., *34*:2205, 1981.

Southern, L. L., and Baker, D. H.: Bioavailable pantothenic acid in cereal grains and soybean meal. J. Anim. Sci., *53*:403, 1981.

Unver. B., Kies, C., and Fox, H. M.: Niacin/pantothenic acid/protein interrelationships affecting the nutritive values of winter wheat for humans. Nutr. Rept. Internat., *23*:841, 1981.

Niacin: Reviews and History

(Also see references 6, 7, 33, and 51.)

Covian, F. G.: Vitamin deficiencies during the Spanish Civil War in Madrid: a reminiscence. Acta Vitaminol. Enzymol. *4*:99, 1982.

Etheridge, E. W.: *The Butterfly Caste: A Social History of Pellagra in the South.* Westport, Conn., Greenwood Publishing Co., 1972.

Goldsmith, G. A.: Niacin: antipellagra factor, hypocholesterolemic agent. J. Amer. Med. Assoc., *194*:167, 1965.

Gopalan, C., and Kamala, S. J. R.: Pellagra and amino acid imbalance. Vit. Horm. *33*:505, 1975.

Handler, P.: The status of American science. Lab. Anim. Sci., *30*:466, 1980 (on development of niacin enrichment programs).

McCormick, D. B., and Wright, L. D.(eds): Nicotinic acid: analogs and coenzymes. In Methods and Enzymology, Vitamins and Coenzymes, Pt.E., *66*:3–208 (30 papers), 1980.

Roe, D. A.: *A Plague of Corn: The Social History of Pellagra.* Ithaca, N.Y., Cornell University Press, 1973.

Stratigos, J. D., and Katsambas, A. D.: Pellagra: "a reappraisal." Acta. Vitaminol. Enzymol., *4*:115, 1982.

Sydenstricker, V. P.: The history of pellagra; its recognition as a disorder of nutrition and its conquest. Amer. J. Clin. Nutr., *6*:409, 1958.

Niacin: General Readings

(Also see references 51–59, this chapter.)

Bartlett, P. C., Morris, J. G., Jr., and Spengler, J.: Food-borne illness associated with niacin: report of an outbreak linked to excessive niacin in enriched cornmeal. Public Health Rept., *97*:258, 1982.

Bender, D. A., Magboul, B. I., and Wynick, D.: Probable mechanisms of regulation of the utilization of dietary tryptophan, nicotinamide and nicotinic acid as precursors of nicotinamide nucleotides in the rat. Brit. J. Nutr., *48*:119, 1982.

Décombaz, J., and Roux, L.: Nicotinic acid increases glycogen utilization in exercise and reduces endurance. Internat. J. Vit. Nutr. Res., *52*:221, 1982.

Grundy, S. M., et al.: Influence of nicotinic acid on metabolism of cholesterol and triglycerides in man. J. Lipid Res., *22*:24, 1981.

Patterson, D. J., et al.: Niacin hepatitis. Southern Med. J., *76*:240, 1983 (on niacin toxicity).

Thomas, R. H. M., Payne, C. M. E. R., and Black, M. M.: Isoniazid-induced pellagra. Brit. Med. J., *283*:287, 1981.

Yovos, J. G., et al.: Effects of nicotinic acid therapy on plasma lipoproteins. J. Clin. Endocrin. Metab., *54*:1210, 1982.

Chapter 11 Vitamin B Complex II

Newer Vitamins: Reviews and General Reading

(Also see reviews listed for Chapters 1, 8, and 10, and refs. 1, 2, 12, 14, 19, this chapter.)

Bonjour, J. P.: Vitamins and alcoholism. II. Folate and vitamin B_{12}. Internat. J. Vit. Nutr. Res., *50*:96, 1980.

Butte, N. F., Calloway, D. H., and Van Duzen, J. L.: Nutritional assessment of pregnant and lactating Navajo women. Amer. J. Clin. Nutr., *34*:2216, 1981 (including biotin and folacin).

Cattan, D., et al.: Effect of folate deficiency on vitamin B-12 absorption. Ann. Nutr. Metab., *26*:367, 1982.

Holmes, Z. A., et al.: Vitamin retention during home

drying of vegetables and fruits. Home Econ. Res. J., *7*:258, 1979.

Lindenbaum, J.: Folate and vitamin B_{12} deficiencies in alcoholism. Seminars Hematol, *17*:119, 1980.

Shane, B., and Stokstad, E. L. R.: The interrelationships among folate, vitamin B-12, and methionine metabolism. Adv. Nutr. Res., *5*:133, 1983.

Sneed, S. M., Zane, C., and Thomas, M. R.: The effects of ascorbic acid, vitamin B_6, vitamin B_{12}, and folic acid supplementation on the breast milk and maternal nutritional status of low socioeconomic lactating women. Amer. J. Clin. Nutr., *34*:1338, 1981.

Shojania, A. M.: Oral contraceptives: effects on folate and vitamin B_{12} metabolism. Canad. Med. Assoc. J., *126*:244, 1982.

Vitamin B-6

(Also see refs. 1–14, this chapter.)

Bapurao, S., Raman, L., and Tulpule, P. G.: Biochemical assessment of vitamin B_6 nutritional status in pregnant women with orolingual manifestations. Amer. J. Clin. Nutr., *36*:581, 1982.

Bapurao, S., and Tulpule, P. G.: Vitamin B-6 content of some Indian foods and regional diets. Indian J. Nutr. Dietet., *18*:9, 1981.

Boers, G. H. J., et al.: Pyridoxine treatment does not prevent homocystinemia after methionine loading in adult homocystinuria patients. Metabolism, *32*:390, 1983.

Bonjour, J. P.: Vitamins and Alcoholism. III. Vitamin B_6. Internat. J. Vit. Nutr. Res., *50*:215, 1980.

El Nakah, A., et al.: A vitamin profile of heroin addiction. Amer. J. Public Health, *69*:1058, 1979.

Leklem, J. E., and Reynolds, R. D. (eds.): *Methods in Vitamin B-6 Nutrition, Analysis and Status Assessment.* New York, Plenum Press, 1981.

Moretti, C., et al.: Pyridoxine (B6) suppresses the rise in prolactin and increases the rise in growth hormone induced by exercise. New Eng. J. Med., *307*:444, 1982.

Schaltenbrand, W. E., et al.: Effect of megavitamin treatment on mental performance and vitamin B-6 metabolism in mentally retarded adults. Fed. Proc. *42*:1065(abstr.), 1983 (no effect found).

Schaumburg, H., et al.: Sensory neuropathy from pyridoxine abuse—a new megavitamin syndrome. New Eng. J. Med., *309*:445, 1983.

Tryfiates, G. P., Morris H. P., and Sonidis, G. P.: Vitamin B_6 and cancer (review). Anticancer Res. *1*:263, 1981.

Biotin

(Also see refs. 15–19, this chapter.)

Bonjour, J. P.: Vitamins and alcoholism. VIII. Biotin. Internat. J. Vit. Nutr. Res., *50*:425, 1980.

Bonjour, J. P.: Biotin-dependent enzymes in inborn errors of metabolism in humans. World Rev. Nutr. Dietet. *38*:1, 1981.

Goldsmith, S. J., et al.: Biotin content of human milk during early lactational stages. Nutr. Res., *2*:579, 1982.

Hood, R. L., and Johnson, A. R.: Supplementation of infant formulations with biotin. Nutr. Rept. Internat., *21*:727, 1980.

Levenson, J. L.: Biotin-responsive depression during hyperalimentation. J. Parenter. Ent. Nutr., *7*:181, 1983.

Simmins, P.H., and Brooks, P.H.: Supplementary biotin for sows: effects on reproductive characteristics. Veterinary Rec., *112*:425, 1983.

Sweetman, L., et al.: Clinical and metabolic abnormalities in a boy with dietary deficiency of biotin. Pediatrics, *68*:553, 1981.

Swick, H. M., and Kien, C. L.: Biotin deficiency with neurologic and cutaneous manifestations but without organic aciduria. J. Pediatr., *103*:265, 1983 (also see p. 233).

Vesely, D. L.: Biotin enhances guanylate cyclase activity. Science, *216*:1329, 1982.

Whitehead, C. C.: The assessment of biotin status in man and animals. Proc. Nutr. Soc., *40*:165, 1981.

Folacin: General

(Also see refs. 20–29, this chapter.)

Brody, T., Watson, J. E., and Stokstad, E. L. R.: Folate pentaglutamate and folate hexaglutamate mediated one-carbon metabolism. Biochemistry, *21*:276, 1982.

Ek, J., and Magnus, E.: Plasma and red cell folate values and folate requirements in formula-fed term infants. J. Pediatr., *100*:738, 1982.

Further studies of acute folic acid deficiency developing during total parenteral nutrition. Nutr. Rev., *41*:51, 1982.

Gestation-related changes in folate status of mothers and their infants. Nutr. Rev., *40*:235, 1982.

Russell R. M., et al.: Increased urinery excretion and prolonged turnover time of folic acid during ethanol ingestion. Amer. J. Clin. Nutr., *38*:64, 1983 (in alcoholics).

Serum folate binders are not correlated to folate nutritional status. Nutr. Rev., *40*:23, 1982.

Tamura, T., Yoshimura, Y., and Arakawa, T.: Human milk folate and folate status in lactating mothers and their infants. Amer. J. Clin. Nutr., *33*:193, 1980.

Folacin: Distribution in Foods

(Also see Supplementary Readings, Chapter 8)

Chen, T-S., et al.: Folacin content of tea. J. Amer. Dietet. Assoc., *82*:627, 1983.

Chen, T-S., and Saad, S.: Folic acid in Egyptian vegetables: the effect of drying method and storage on the folacin content of mulukhiyah. Ecol. Food Nutr., *10*:249, 1981.

Colman, N.: Addition of folic acid to staple foods as a selective nutrition intervention strategy. Nutr. Rev., *40*:225, 1982.

Hoppner, K., and Lampi, B.: Total folacin activity in breakfast cereals, Nutr. Rept. Internat., *26*:495, 1982.

Hoppner, K., and Lampi, B.: Seasonal variation of folacin levels in market fluid milks. Canad. Inst. Food Sci. Tech. J., *14*:218, 1981.

Keagy, P. M., and Oace, S. M.: Development of a folacin bioassay in rats. J. Nutr., *112*:87, 1982.

Leichter, J.: Folate content in the solid and liquid portions of canned vegetables. Canad. Inst. Food Sci. Tech. J., *13*:33, 1980.

Mnkeni, A. P., and Beveridge, T.: Thermal destruction of pteroylglutamic acid in buffer and model food systems. J. Food Sci., *47*:2038, 1982 (also see same authors: J. Food Sci., *48*:595, 1983, and Day, B.P.F., and Gregory, J. F., III: J. Food Sci., *48*:581, 1983).

Mullin, W. J., Wood, D. F., and Howsam, S. G.: Some factors affecting folacin content of spinach, Swiss chard, broccoli and brussels sprouts. Nutr. Rept. Internat., *26*:7, 1982.

Nik-Daud, N. I., and Bender, A. E.: The content and stability of folic acid in foods. Proc. Nutr. Soc., *42*:118A (abst.), 1983.

Ristow, K. A., Gregory J. F., III, and Damron, B. L.: Thermal processing effects on folacin bioavailability in liquid model food systems, liver and cabbage. J. Agric. Food Chem., *30*:801, 1982.

Vitamin B-12

(Also see refs. 30–40, this chapter.)

Bailey, L. B., et al.: Vitamin B_{12} status of elderly persons from urban low-income households. J. Amer. Geriatr. Soc., *28*:276, 1980.

Carmel, R.: Megaloblastic anemia—vitamin B-12 and folate. In *Current Hematology*. Vol. 2. New York, John Wiley & Sons, Inc., 1983, pp. 243–281.

Contribution of the microflora of the small intestine to the vitamin B_{12} nutriture of man. Nutr. Rev., *38*:274, 1980.

Dolphin, D. (ed.): *B_{12}*. Vols. I and II. New York, Wiley-Interscience, 1982.

Herbert, V., and Drivas, G.: *Spirulina* and vitamin B_{12}. J. Amer. Med. Assoc., *248*:3096, 1982.

Kampmeier, R. H.: Pernicious anemia. Southern Med. J., *76*:151, 1983 (a history of dietary treatment).

Matthews, D. M., and Linnell, J. C.: Cobalamin deficiency and related disorders in infancy and childhood. Europ. J. Pediatr., *138*:6, 1982.

Samson, R. R., and McClelland, D. B. L.: Vitamin B_{12} in human colostrum and milk. Acta Paediat. Scand., *69*:93, 1980.

Tin-May-Than, et al.: The effect of vitamin B_{12} on physical performance capacity. Brit. J. Nutr., *40*:269, 1978.

Watson, W. S., et al.: The effect of megadose ascorbic acid ingestion on the absorption and retention of vitamin B_{12} in man. Scottish Med. J., *27*:240, 1982.

Vegetarianism

(Also see refs. 34–37, this chapter.)

Abdulla, M., et al.: Nutrient intake and health status of vegans. Chemical analyses of diets using the duplicate portion sampling technique. Amer. J. Clin. Nutr., *34*:2464, 1981.

Anderson, B. M., Gibson, R. S., and Sabry, J. H.: The iron and zinc status of long-term vegetarian women. Amer. J. Clin. Nutr., *34*:1042, 1981 (also see same authors: J. Amer. Dietet. Assoc., *82*:246, 1983, on copper, manganese, and selenium in vegetarians).

Burr, M. L., and Sweetnam, P. M.: Vegetarianism, dietary fiber, and mortality. Amer. J. Clin. Nutr., *36*:873, 1982.

Campbell, M., Lofters, W. S., and Gibbs, W. N.: Rastafarianism and the vegans syndrome. Brit. Med. J., *285*:1617, 1982.

Christoffel, K.: A pediatric perspective on vegetarian nutrition. Clin. Pediat., *20*:632, 1981.

Dwyer, J. T.: Vegetarian diets in pregnancy and lactation: recent studies of North Americans. J. Canad. Dietet. Assoc., *44*:26, 1983.

Ganapathy, S. N., et al.: Trace minerals, amino acids, and plasma proteins in adult men fed wheat diets. J. Amer. Dietet. Assoc., *78*:490, 1981.

Gray, G., et al.: Diet and hormone levels in Seventh-Day Adventist teenage girls. Prev. Med., *11*:103, 1982.

Gross, J., and Freifeld, K.: My child, the vegetarian. Family Health, *13*:34, 1981.

King, J. C., Stein, T., and Doyle, M.: Effect of vegetarianism on the zinc status of pregnant women. Amer. J. Clin. Nutr., *34*:1049, 1981.

Lehman, H. S., and Hurnik, J. F.: On an alleged moral basis of vegetarianism. Appl. Animal Ethol., *6*:205, 1980.

Murphy, M. F.: Vitamin B-12 deficiency due to a low-cholesterol diet in a vegetarian. Ann. Int. Med., *94*:57, 1981.

Read, M. H., and Thomas, D. C.: Nutrient and food supplement practices of lacto-ovo vegetarians. J. Amer. Dietet. Assoc., *82*:401, 1983.

Rouse, I. L., Armstrong, B. K., and Beilin, L. J.: Vegetarian diet, lifestyle and blood pressure in two religious populations. Clin. Exper. Pharm. Physiol., *9*:327, 1982.

Shultz, T. D., and Leklem, J. E.: Nutrient intake and hormonal status of premenopausal Seventh-Day Adventists and premenopausal nonvegetarians. Nutr. Cancer, *4*:247, 1983.

Shultz, T. D., and Leklem, J. E.: Dietary status of seventh-day adventists and nonvegetarians. J. Amer. Dietet. Assoc., *83*:27, 1983.

Choline

(Also see refs. 41–43, this chapter.)

Barak, A. J., and Tuma, D. J.: Betaine, metabolic by-product or vital methylating agent? Life Sci., *32*:771, 1983.

Barbeau, A., Growden, J. H., and Wurtman, R. J. (eds.): *Choline and Lecithin in Brain Disorders.* New York Raven Press, 1980.

Corkin, S., et al. (eds.): *Alzheimer's Disease: A Report of Progress in Research.* Aging, Vol. 19. New York, Raven Press, 1982 (see chapters by various authors on choline, pp. 35, 45, 193, 287 to 451).

Rosenberg, G. S., and Davis, K. L.: The use of cholinergic precursors in neuropsychiatric diseases. Amer. J. Clin. Nutr., *36*:709, 1982.

Scott, J. M., et al.: Pathogenesis of subacute combined degeneration: a result of methyl group deficiency. Lancet, *2*:334, 1981.

Smolin, L. A., Benevenga, N. J., and Berlow, S.: The use of betaine for the treatment of homocystinuria. J. Pediatr. *99*:467, 1981. (Also see Wilcken, D. E. L., et al.: New Eng. J. Med., *309*:448, 1983, on same topic).

Wood, J. L., and Allison, R. G.: Effect of consumption of choline and lecithin on neurological and cardiovascular systems. Fed. Proc., *41*:3015, 1982.

Inositol

(Also see refs. 44–46, this chapter.)

Andersen, D. B., and Holub, B. J.: Myo-inositol-responsive liver lipid accumulation in the rat. J. Nutr., *110*:488, 1980.

Beach, D. C., and Flick, P. K.: Early effect of myo-inositol deficiency on fatty acid synthetic enzymes of rat liver. Biochim. Biophys. Acta, *711*:452, 1982.

Burton, L. E., and Wells, W. W.: Myo-inositol deficiency: studies on the mechanism of lactation-dependent fatty liver formation in the rat. J. Nutr., *109*:1483, 1979.

Chu, S. W., and Geyer, R. P.: Myo-inositol action on gerbil intestine association of phosphatidylinositol metabolism with lipid clearance. Biochim. Biophys. Acta, *10*:63, 1982.

Carnitine

(Also see ref. 47, this chapter.)

Hahn, P.: Carnitine in the perinatal period of mammals. Nutr. Res., *2*:201, 1982.

Hahn, P., Allardyce, D. B., and Frohlich, J.: Plasma carnitine levels during total parenteral nutrition of adult surgical patients. Amer. J. Clin. Nutr., *36*:569, 1982. (Also see discussion of this paper in same journal, *38*:339, 1983).

Penn, D., Schmidt-Sommerfeld, E., and Wolf, H.: Carnitine deficiency in premature infants receiving total parenteral nutrition. Early Human Develop. *4*:23, 1980 (also see Acta Paediatr. Scand., Supplement 296, 1982 and J. Pediatr., *102*:931, 1983).

Sandor, A., et al.: On carnitine content of the human breast milk. Pediatr. Res., *16*:89, 1982.

Tripp, M., et al.: Systemic carnitine deficiency presenting as familial endocardial fibroelastosis: a treatable cardiomyopathy. New Eng. J. Med., *305*:385, 1981.

Worthley, L. I. G., et al.: Carnitine deficiency with hyperbilirubinemia, generalized skeletal muscle weakness and reactive hypoglycemia in a patient on long-term total parenteral nutrition: treatment with intravenous L-carnitine. J. Parenter. Ent. Nutr., *7*:176, 1983.

Taurine

(Also see ref. 48, this chapter.)

Hayes, K. C.: Nutritional problems in cats: taurine deficiency and vitamin A excess. Canad. Vet. J., *23*:2, 1982.

Järvenpää, A., et al.: Milk protein quantity and quality in the term infant. II. Effects on acidic and netural amino acids. Pediatrics, *70*:221, 1982 (taurine in infants).

O'Donnell J. A., III, Rogers, Q. R., and Morris, J. G.: Effect of diet on plasma taurine in the cat. J. Nutr., *111*:1111, 1981.

Rana, S. K., and Sanders, T. A. B.: A comparison of breast-milk taurine concentrations in vegans and omnivores. Proc. Nutr. Soc, *42*:(abst.), 1983.

Growth factors

(Also see ref. 49, this chapter.)

Cohen, S. S.: Polyamines in eukaryotic systems. Fed. Proc., *41*:3061, 1982 (5 papers).

Hase, Y., et al.: A case of tetrahydrobiopterin deficiency due to a defective synthesis of dihydrobiopterin. J. Inher. Metab. Dis., *5*:81, 1982.

LeWitt, P. A., et al.: Treatment of dystonia with tetrahydrobiopterin. New Eng. J. Med., *303*:157, 1983.

Russell, D. H.: Clinical relevance of polyamines. CRC Crit. Rev. Clin. Lab. Sci., *18*:261, 1983.

Nonnutritive Substances: Pangamic acid (vitamin "B-15")

B-15 fails court test. FDA Consumer, *15*(Feb.):32, 1981.

Check, W. A.: Vitamin B_{15}—whatever it is, it won't help. J. Amer. Med. Assoc., *243*:2473, 1980.

Dohn, G. L., Debnath, S., and Frisell, W. R.: Effects of commercial preparations of pangamic acid (B_{15}) on exercised rats. Biochem. Med., *28*:77, 1982.

Girandola, R. N., Wiswell, R. A., and Bulbulian, R.: Effects of pangamic acid (B-15) ingestion on metabolic response to exercise. Biochem. Med., *24*:218, 1980 (no effect seen).

Gray, M. E., and Titlow, L. W.: The effect of pangamic acid on maximal treadmill performance. Med. Sci. Sports Exercise, *14*:424, 1982 (no effect in humans).

Herbert, V.: Pangamic acid ("vitamin B_{15}"). Amer. J. Clin. Nutr., *32*:1534, 1979.

Nonnutritive Substances: Laetrile

Herbert, V.: The vitamin craze. Arch. Inter. Med., *140*:173, 1980 (on "megavitamins" and how to evaluate claims).

Kalyanaraman, U. P., et al.: Neuromyopathy of cyanide intoxication due to "laetrile" (Amygdalin). Cancer, *51*:2126, 1983.

Moertel, C. G., et al.: A clinical trial of amygdalin (laetrile) in the treatment of human cancer. New Eng. J. Med., *306*:201, 1982.

Rauws, A. G., Olling, M., and Timmerman, A.: The pharmacokinetics of amygdalin. Arch. Toxicol., *49*:311, 1982.

Relman, A. S.: Closing the books on laetrile. New Eng. J. Med., *306*:236, 1982 (also see *307*:118 and 1340, 1982 for letters by various authors.)

Sun, M.: Laetrile brush fire is out, scientists hope. Science, *212*:758, 1981.

Chapter 12 Vitamin C

Vitamin C: Reviews and History

(Also see refs. 1–3 and 19–27, this chapter.)

Beeuwkes, A. M.: The prevalence of scurvy among voyagers to America, 1493–1600. J. Amer. Dietet. Assoc., *24*:300, 1948.

Chatterjee, I. B.: Ascorbic acid metabolism. World Rev. Nutr. Dietet., *30*:69, 1978.

Counsell, J. N., and Hornig, D. H. (eds.): *Vitamin C (Ascorbic Acid)*. Englewood, N.J., Applied Science Publishers Inc., 1982.

Dickman, S. R.: The search for the specific factor in scurvy. Perspect. Biol. Med., *24*:382, 1981.

Ginter, E.: Chronic marginal vitamin C deficiency: biochemistry and pathophysiology. World Rev. Nutr. Dietet., *33*:104, 1979.

Hanck, A. (ed.): Vitamin C: new clinical applications in immunology, lipid metabolism and cancer. Internat. J. Vit. Nutr. Res., Supplement 23, 1982.

Hanck, A., and Ritzel, G. (eds): Vitamin C: recent advances and aspects in virus diseases, cancer and lipid metabolism. Internat. J. Vit. Nutr. Res., Supplement 19, 1979.

Hess, A. F.: Recent advances in knowledge of scurvy and the antiscorbutic vitamin. J. Amer. Med. Assoc., *98*:1429, 1932.

Hodges, R. E.: Vitamin C. In Alfin-Slater, R. B., and Kritchevsky, D. (eds): *Human Nutrition: A Comprehensive Treatise*. Vol. *3A*. New York, Plenum Press, 1980 (also see Hodges, R. E.: Vitamin C and cancer. Nutr. Rev., *40*:289, 1982).

Irwin, M. I., and Hutchins, B. K.: A conspectus of research on vitamin C requirements of man. J. Nutr. *106*:821, 1976.

Kasa, R. M.: Vitamin C: from scurvy to the common cold. Amer. J. Med. Tech., *49*:23, 1983.

King, C. G.: The isolation of vitamin C from lemon juice. Fed. Proc., *38*:2681, 1979.

Lind, J.: A treatise of the scurvy. Nutr. Rev., *41*:155, 1983 (a reprint of several pages of the classic report of 1753).

Lorenz, A. J.: The conquest of scurvy. J. Amer. Dietet. Assoc., *30*:665, 1954.

Nagy, S.: Vitamin C contents of citrus fruit and their products: a review. J. Agric. Food Chem., *28*:8, 1980.

Schorah, C. J.: The level of vitamin C reserves required in man: toward a solution to the controversy. Proc. Nutr. Soc., *40*:147, 1981.

Schrauzer, G. N.: Vitamin C: conservative human requirements and aspects of overdosage. Internat. Rev. Biochem., *27*:167, 1979.

*Stability of Vitamin C in Foods**

(Also see Supplementary Reading for Chapter 8 and Chapter 10, ref. 14.)

Abou-Fadel, O. S., and Miller, L. T.: (green beans and cherries). J. Food Sci., *48*:920, 1983.

Ajayi, S. O., Oderinde, S. F., and Osibanjo, O.: (fresh leafy vegetables). Food Chem., *5*:243, 1980.

Albach, R. F., and Murray, A. J.: (orange puree). J. Agric. Food Chem., *31*:653, 1983.

Augustin, J., et al.: (potato products). J. Food Sci., *46*:1697, 1981; J. Food Sci., *47*:274, 1982.

Boushell, R., and Potter, N. N.: (frozen french fried potatoes). J. Food Sci., *45*:1207, 1980.

Dennison, D. B., and Kirk, J. R.: (effect of trace minerals). J. Food Sci., *47*:1198, 1982.

Gutheil, R. A., Price, L. G., and Swanson, B. G.: (home-grown tomatoes). J. Food Protect., *43*:366, 1980.

Hallberg, L., et al.: (prolonged warming). Amer. J. Clin. Nutr., *36*:846, 1982.

Klein, B. P., Juo, C. H. Y., and Boyd, G.: (microwave, spinach). J. Food Sci., *46*:640, 1981.

Lathrop, P. J., and Leung, H. K.: (green peas). J. Food Sci., *45*:995, 1980; J. Food Sci., *45*:152, 1980.

Mabesa, L. B., and Baldwin, R. E.: (microwave, peas). J. Food Sci., *44*:932, 1979.

Maeda, E. E., and Salunkhe, D. K.: (solar dried vegetables). J. Food Sci., *46*:1288, 1981.

Massaioli, D., and Haddad, P. R.: (orange juice). Food Tech. Aust., *33*:136, 1981.

Reynolds, P., and Phillips, J. A.: (orange juice and beverages). Home Econ. Res. J., *9*:251, 1981.

Rao, M. A., et al.: (canned peas). J. Food Sci., *46*:636, 1981.

Selman, J. D., and Rolfe, E. J.: (peas). J. Food Tech., *17*:219, 1982.

Skelton, M. M., and Craig, J. A.: (home-canned tomatoes). J. Food Sci., *43*:1043, 1978 (also see Stone, M. B., et al.: Qual. Plantarum: Plant Foods. Human Nutr., *31*:327, 1982.)

Sumner, J. L., Eu, S. L., and Dhillon, A. S.: (frozen vegetables and meals-on-wheels). G. Food Nutr., *40*(1):43, 1983.

*High Levels and Potential Toxicity of Vitamin C**

(Also see refs. 2, 3, 8, 29, this chapter, and refs. 22, 24, 25, Chapter 8.)

Baker, H., Pauling, L., and Frank, O.: (effect on absorption of other vitamins). Nutr. Rept. Internat., *23*:669, 1981.

Barrett, S.: (vitamin C and colds). Environ. Nutr., *6*(5):1, 1983.

Buzzard, I. M., et al.: (blood lipid relationship). Amer. J. Clin. Nutr., *36*:94, 1982.

*In order to conserve space, full titles are not given in this section.

Ekvall, S., Chen, I. W., and Bozian, R.: (vitamin B-12 relation). Amer. J. Clin. Nutr., *34*:1356, 1981.

Finley, E. B., and Cerklewski, F. L.: (copper status of young men). Amer. J. Clin. Nutr., *37*:553, 1983.

Herbert, V.: (iron overload). New Eng. J. Med., *304*:1108 (letter), 1981.

Hughes, C., Dutton, S., and Truswell, A. S.: (urinary oxalate). J. Human Nutr., *35*:274, 1981.

Jaffe, R. M., et al.: (detection of blood in urine is inhibited). Amer. J. Clin. Path., *72*:468, 1979.

McLaren, C. J., et al.: (iron overload). Aust. New Zeal. J. Med., *12*:187, 1982 (also see Cook, J. D., et al.: Amer. J. Clin. Nutr., *37*:709 (abstr)., 1983).

Mitch, W. E., et al.: (uric acid). Clin. Pharm. Therap., *29*:318, 1981.

Moser, U., and Hornig, D.: (relation to oxalate formation). Trends Pharm. Sci., *3*:480, 1982.

Schmidt, K. H., et al.: (urinary oxalate). Amer. J. Clin. Nutr., *34*:305, 1981.

Shultz, T. D., and Leklem, T. D.: (vitamin B-6 metabolism). Amer. J. Clin. Nutr., *35*:1400, 1982.

Sutton, J. L. et al.: (nitrogeneous components of urine and lack of effect on urinary stones). Human Nutr.:Appl. Nutr., *37A*:136, 1983.

Vitamin C: General

Florencio, C. A.: Effects of iron and ascorbic acid supplementation on hemoglobin level and work efficiency of anemic women. J. Occup. Med., *23*:699, 1981.

Geraci, J. R., and Smith, T. G.: Vitamin C in the diet of Inuit hunters from Holman, Northwest Territories. Arctic, *32*:135, 1979.

Kallner, A., Hartmann, D., and Hornig, D.: Steady-state turnover and body pool of ascorbic acid in man. Amer. J. Clin. Nutr., *32*:530, 1979.

Klein, B. P., and Perry, A. K.: Ascorbic acid and vitamin A activity in selected vegetables from different geographical areas of the United States. J. Food Sci., *47*:941, 1982.

Murad, S., et al.: Regulation of collagen synthesis by ascorbic acid. Proc. Nat. Acad. Sci., *78*:2879, 1981.

Sasaki, R., et al.: Ascorbate radical and ascorbic acid level in human serum and age. J. Gerontology, *38*:26, 1983.

Shier, N. W., Heinrichs, T. H., and Hart, W.: Effects of diet on urinary l-ascorbic acid in the human. J. Food Sci., *47*:334, 1982.

Snook, J. T., et al.: Supplementation frequency and ascorbic acid status in adult males. Amer. J. Clin. Nutr., *37*:532, 1983.

Som, S., et al.: Ascorbic acid metabolism in diabetes mellitus. Metabolism, *30*:572, 1981.

Springer, N. S.,: Ascorbic acid status of children with developmental disabilities. J. Amer. Diet. Assoc., *75*:425, 1979.

Weininger, J., and King, J. C.: Effect of oral contraceptive agents on ascorbic acid metabolism in the rhesus monkey. Amer. J. Clin. Nutr., *35*:1408, 1982 (also see *37*:329 and 330 (letters), 1983).

Yung, S., Mayersohn, M., and Robinson, J. B.: Ascorbic acid absorption in humans: a comparison among several dosage forms. J. Pharm. Sci., *71*:282, 1982.

Chapter 13 Water and Minerals

Water

Andersson, B., Leksell, L. G., and Rundgren, M.: Regulation of water intake. Ann. Rev. Nutr., *2*:73, 1982.

Fitzsimons, J. T.: *The Physiology of Thirst and Sodium Appetite.* New York, Cambridge University Press, 1979.

Grander, D. N., et al.: The microcirculation and fluid transport in digestive organs. Fed. Proc., *42*:1667, 1983.

Gilles, M. E., and Paulin, H. V.: Variability of mineral intakes from drinking water. Internat. J. Epidemiol., *12*:45, 1983.

Haring, B. S. A., and Van Delft, W.: Changes in the mineral composition of food as a result of cooking in "hard" and "soft" waters. Arch. Environ. Health, *36* (No. 1):33, 1981.

Kleeman, C. R., and Fichman, M. P.: The clinical physiology of water metabolism. New Eng. J. Med., *277*:1300, 1967.

Masironi, R., and Shaper, A. G.: Epidemiological studies of health effects of water from different sources. Ann. Rev. Nutr., *1*:375, 1981.

Miller, R. W.: Carcinogens in drinking water. Pediatrics, *57*:462, 1976.

Rolls, B. F. et al: Thirst following water deprivation in humans. Amer. J. Physiol., *239*:R476, 1980.

Sonneborn, M., et al: Health effects of inorganic drinking water constituents, including hardness, iodide, and fluoride. CRC Crit. Rev. Environ. Control., *13*:1, 1983.

Wold, R. S.: Water—our critical nutrient. Nutr. Digest, *1*(1):7, 1983.

Minerals

Asimov, I.: *The Search for the Elements.* New York, Fawcet Publishing Co., 1966.

Beisel, W. R.: Single nutrients and immunity: minerals and trace elements. Amer. J. Clin. Nutr., *35*:442, 1982.

Davies, N. T.: Anti-nutrient factors affecting mineral utilization. Proc. Nutr. Soc., *38*:121, 1979.

De Portela, M. L.: Review of present knowledge on the evaluation of nutritional status with regard to mineral elements. Archivos Latinoamer. Nutr., *32*:429, 1982.

Dubick, M. A., and Rucker, R. B.: Dietary supplements and health aids—a critical evaluation. Part 1—vitamins and minerals. J. Nutr. Educ., *15*:47, 1983.

Fox, M. R., and Tao, S. H.: Mineral content of human tissues from a nutrition perspective. Fed. Proc., *40*:2130, 1981.

Frieden, E.: The chemical elements of life. Sci. Amer., *227*:52, 1972.

Greger, J. L., et al.: Calcium, magnesium, phosphorus,

copper, and manganese balance in adolescent females. Amer. J. Clin. Nutr., *31*:117, 1978.

Hamilton, E. I.: An overview: the chemical elements, nutrition, disease, and the health of man. Fed. Proc., *40*:2126, 1981.

Harland, B. F., et al.: Calcium, phosphorus, iron, iodine, and zinc in the "Total Diet". J. Amer. Dietet. Assoc., *47*:16, 1980.

Kelsay, J. L., and Prather, E. S.: Mineral balances of human subjects consuming spinach in a low-fiber diet and in a diet containing fruits and vegetables. Amer. J. Clin. Nutr. *38*:12, 1983.

Kramer, L., Spencer, H., and Osis, D.: Zinc and mineral content of weight reducing diets. Amer. J. Clin. Nutr., *34*:1372, 1981.

Mahalko, J. R., et al.: Effect of a moderate increase in dietary protein on the retention and excretion of Ca, Cu, Fe, Mg, P, and Zn by adult males. Amer. J. Clin. Nutr., *37*:8, 1983.

Mahoney, A. W.: Mineral contents of selected cereals and baked products. Cereal Foods World, *27*:147, 1982.

Newberne, P. M.: Disease states and tissue mineral elements in man. Fed. Proc., *40*:2134, 1981.

Rosenberg, I. H., and Solomons, N. W.: Biological availability of minerals and trace elements: a nutritional overview. Amer. J. Clin. Nutr., *35*:781, 1982.

Schrauzer, G. N.: Trace elements in carcinogenesis. In Draper, H. H. (ed.): *Advances in Nutritional Research.* Vol 2. New York, Plenum Publ. Co., 1979.

Walker, M. A., and Page, L.: Nutritive content of college meals. III. Mineral elements. J. Amer. Dietet. Assoc., *70*:260, 1977.

Chapter 14 The Electrolytes and Acid-Base Balance

Electrolytes: General

Arbogast, K. K.: *Exchange Lists and Diet Patterns.* New York, Van Nostrand Reinhold Company, 1980 (on modified electrolyte diets).

Fregly, M. J.: Sodium and potassium. Ann. Rev. Nutr. *1*:69, 1981.

Marsh, A. C., and Koons, P. C.: The sodium and potassium content of selected vegetables. J. Amer. Dietet. Assoc., *83*:24, 1983.

Li, A. K. C., Wills, M. R., and Hanson, G. C.: *Fluid, Electrolytes, Acid-Base and Nutrition.* London, Academic Press, 1980.

MacGregor, G. A.: Dietary sodium and potassium intake and blood pressure, Lancet, *1*:750, 1983 (a review).

Meneely, G. R., and Battarbee, H. D.: Sodium and potassium. Nutr. Rev., *34*:225, 1976.

Voors, A. W., et al.: Relation between ingested potassium and sodium balance in young Blacks and whites. Amer. J. Clin. Nutr., *37*:583, 1983.

White, P. L., and Crocco, S. C. (eds.): *Sodium and Potassium in Food and Drugs.* Monroe, Wis., American Medical Association (Department of Foods and Nutrition), 1980.

Sodium: General

Aloia, J. F., et al.: Sodium excess in postmenopausal osteoporosis, Metabolism, *32*:359, 1983.

Bertino, M., et al.: Long-term reduction in dietary sodium alters the taste of salt. Amer. J. Clin. Nutr., *36*:1134, 1982.

De Araya, C. A., et al: Sodium and potassium content in some Chilean foods. Arch. Latimoamer. Nutr., *31*:146, 1981.

Denton, D.: *The Hunger for Salt.* New York, Springer-Verlag, 1982.

Kare, M. R., Fregley, M. J., and Bernard, R. A. (eds.): *Biological and Behavioral Aspects of Salt Intake.* New York, Academic Press Inc., 1980.

Kerr, C. M., Reisinger, K. S., and Plankey, F. W.: Sodium concentration of homemade baby foods. Pediatrics, *62*:331, 1978.

Khan, M. A.: Sodium intake from meals and snacks consumed by college students. J. Amer. Dietet. Assoc., *82*:664, 1983.

Khan, M. A., and Martin, J. A.: Salt content of selected snack foods. J. Food Sci., *48*:656, 1983.

Morgan, K. J., and Bundy, K. T.: Food sources of sodium in teenagers' snacks. Cereal Foods World, *26*:69, 1981 (also see Morgan, K. J., and Zabik, M. E.: Consumption of salted snack foods by U.S. teenagers, Mich. State Univ. Research Rept. 439, 1982.)

Multhauf, R. P.: *Neptune's Gift: A History of Salt.* Baltimore, the Johns Hopkins University Press, 1978.

Ranhotra, G. S. et al.: Sodium in commercially produced frozen pizzas. Cereal Chem., *60*:325, 1983.

Various authors, in a series of 5 papers on Sodium content of foods and health aspects. Food Tech., *37*(7):45–73, 1983.

Vermeulen, R. T., et al.: Effect of water rinsing on sodium content of selected foods. J. Amer. Dietet Assoc., *82*:394, 1983.

Vitiello, M. V., et al.: Sodium-restricted diet increases nightime plasma norepinephrine and impairs sleep patterns in man. J. Clin. Endocrin. Metab., *56*:553, 1983.

Sodium and High Blood Pressure

Altschul, A. M., and Grommet, J. K.: Sodium intake and sodium sensitivity. Nutr. Rev., *38*:393, 1980.

Carruthers, S. G.: Nutrition and hypertension. J. Canad. Dietet. Assoc., *41*:274, 1980.

Fregly, M. S., and Kare, M. R. (eds.): *Role of Salt in Cardiovascular Hypertension* (Nutrition Foundation Monograph). New York, Academic Press, 1982.

Gillum, R. R., et al.: Nonpharmacologic therapy in hypertension. Amer. Heart J., *105*:128, 1983 (on weight reduction and sodium restriction).

Grommet, J. K., and Altschul, A. M.: Dietary sodium and hypertension. Nutr. Update (John Wiley and Co.), *1*:55, 1983.

Jeffery, R. W., et al.: Weight and sodium reduction for the prevention of hypertension: a comparison of group treatment and individual counseling. Amer. J. Public Health, *73*:691, 1983.

Light, K. C., et al.: Psychological stress induces sodium and fluid retention in men at high risk for hypertension. Science, *220*:429, 1983.

McCarron, D. A.: Dietary Sodium and high blood pressure. Nutr. News, *45*(2):5, 1982.

McCarron, D. A., Filer, J., and Van Itallie, T.: Current perspectives in hypertension (a symposium). Hypertension, *4* (Supplement, Sept.):III–1, 1982.

McCarron, D. A., and Kochen, T. A. (eds.): Nutrition and blood pressure control: current status of dietary factors and hypertension. Ann. Int. Med., *98*(No. 5, Part 2):701–804, 1983 (a symposium).

Salt and high blood pressure. Consumer Repts., *44*:147, 1979.

Silman, A. J., et al.: Evaluation of the effectiveness of a low sodium diet in the treatment of mild to moderate hypertension. Lancet, *1*:1179, 1983.

Potassium

Bay, W. H., and Hartman, J. A.: High potassium in low-sodium soups. New Eng. J. Med., *308*:1166, 1983.

Bia, M. J., and Defronzo, R. A.: Extrarenal potassium homeostasis. Amer. J. Physiol., *240*:F257, 1981.

Costill, D. L., Cote, R., and Fink, W. J.: Dietary potassium and heavy exercise. Amer. J. Clin. Nutr., *36*:266, 1982.

Harrington, J. T., et al.: Our national obsession with potassium. Amer. J. Med., *73*:155, 1982.

Kolata, G.: Should hypertensives take potassium? Science, *218*:361, 1982.

Lane, H. W., and Cerda, J. J.: Potassium requirements and exercise. J. Amer. Dietet. Assoc., *73*:64, 1978.

Lane, H. W., et al.: Effects of physical activity on human potassium metabolism in a hot and humid environment. Amer. J. Clin. Nutr., *31*:838, 1978.

Langford, H. G.: Potassium in hypertension. Post Grad. Med., *73*:227, 1983.

Sweadner, K. J., and Goldin, S. M.: Active transport of sodium and potassium ions. New Eng. J. Med., *302*:777, 1980.

Chloride

Forte, J. G., Machen, T. E., and Obrink, K. J.: Mechanisms of gastric H^+ and Cl^- transport. Ann. Rev. Physiol., *42*:111, 1980.

Hawker, P. C., Mashiter, K. E., and Turnberg, L. A.: Mechanisms of transport of Na, Cl, and K in the human colon. Gastroenterology, *74*:1241, 1978.

Hill, I. D., and Bowie, M. D.: Chloride deficiency syndrome due to chloride-deficient breast milk. Arch. Dis. Childhood, *58*:224, 1983.

Holliday, M. A.: Alkalosis in infancy and commercial formulas. Pediatrics, *65*:639, 1980.

Rodriguez-Soriano, J., et al.: Biochemical features of dietary chloride deficiency syndrome: a comparative study of 30 cases. J. Pediatr., *103*:209, 1983.

Simopoulos, A. P., and Bartter, F. C.: The metabolic consequences of chloride deficiency. Nutr. Rev., *38*:201, 1980.

Acid-Base Balance

Barzel, U. S.: Osteoporosis in young men. Arch. Inter. Med., *142*:2079, 1982.

Burton, R. F.: Acid and base excretion: assessment and relationships to diet and urine composition. Comp. Biochem. Physiol., *66A*:371, 1980.

Davis, G. R., et al.: Evaluation of chloride/bicarbonate exchange in the human colon in vivo. J. Clin. Invest., *71*:201, 1983.

Gonick, H. C., Goldberg, G., and Mulcare, D.: Reexamination of the acid-ash content of several diets. Amer. J. Clin. Nutr., *21*:898, 1968.

Graham, D. Y., et al.: Why do apparently healthy people use antacid tablets? Amer. J. Gastroent., *78*:257, 1983.

Kappy, M. S., and Morrow, G.: A diagnostic approach to metabolic acidosis in children. Pediatrics, *65*:351, 1980.

Masoro, E. J.: An overview of hydrogen ion regulation. Arch. Inter. Med., *142*:1019, 1982.

Moore, A., Ansell, C., and Barrie, H.: Metaolic acidosis and infant feeding. Brit. Med. J., *1*:129, 1977.

Schwartz, A. B. (ed.: *Acid-Base and Electrolyte Balance.* New York, Grune and Stratton, 1977.

Spencer, H., and Kramer, L.: Antacid-induced calcium loss. Arch. Intern. Med., *143*:657, 1983.

Stewart, P. A.: *How To Understand Acid-Base.* New York, Elsevier North Holland, Inc., 1981.

Chapter 15 Calcium, Phosphorus, and Magnesium

Reviews and General Reading

(Also see Supplementary readings for Chapters 1, 8, and 13.)

Avioli, L. V.: Calcium and Osteoporosis. Ann. Rev. Nutr., *4*:(in press), 1984.

Bronner, F., and Coburn, J. W.: *Disorders of Mineral Metabolism.* Vols. 2 and 3. New York, Academic Press, 1981 and 1982 (on calcium, phosphorus, and magnesium).

Godara, R., Kaur, A. P., and Bhat, C. M.: Effect of cellulose incorporation in a low fiber diet on fecal excretion and serum levels of calcium, phosphorus and iron in adolescent girls. Amer. J. Clin. Nutr., *34*:1083, 1981.

Harland, B. F., et al.: Calcium, phosphorus, iron, iodine and zinc in the "Total Diet." J. Amer. Dietet. Assoc., *47*:16, 1980.

Licata, A. A., et al.: Adverse effects of liquid protein fast on the handling of magnesium, calcium, and phosphorus. Amer. J. Med., *71*:767, 1981.

McCarron, D.A.: Calcium and magnesium nutrition in human hypertension. Ann. Int. Med., *98* (No 5, part 2):800, 1983.

Scythes, C. A., Gibson, R. S., and Draper, H. H.: Dietary calcium and phosphorus intakes of a sample of Canadian pre-menopausal women consuming self-selected diets. Nutr. Res., *2*:385, 1982.

Spencer, H., et al.: Effect of phosphorus on the absorption of calcium and on the calcium balance in man. J. Nutr., *108*:447, 1978 (also see Spencer, H., et al.: Amer. J. Clin. Nutr., *37*:924, 1983).

Srivastava, U., et al.: Proximate composition and nutrient content of university meals. Nutr. Rep. Internat., *24*:1139, 1981 (also see *18*:313, 1978).

Zemel, M. B., and Linkswiler, H. M.: Calcium metabolism in the young adult male as affected by level and form of phosphorus intake and level of calcium intake. J. Nutr., *111*:315, 1981.

Calcium

Allen, L. H.: Calcium bioavailability and absorption: a review. Amer. J. Clin. Nutr., *35*:783, 1982.

Allen, L. H.: The role of nutrition in the onset and treatment of metabolic bone disease. Nutr. Update, *1*:263, 1983.

Aloia, J. F.: Exercise and skeletal health. J. Amer. Geriatr. Soc., *29*:104, 1981.

Altchuler, S. I.: Dietary protein and calcium loss; A review. Nutr. Res., *2*:193, 1982.

Belizan, J. M., et al.: Reduction of blood pressure with calcium supplementation in young adults. J. Amer. Med. Assoc., *249*:1161, 1983.

Calmodulin. Brit. Med. J., *281*:1510, 1980 (editorial).

Gallagher, J. C., and Riggs, B. L.: Current concepts in nutrition: nutrition and bone disease. New Eng. J. Med., *298*:193, 1978 (also see *309*:29, 1983).

Garn, S. M., Solomon, M. A., and Griedl, J.: Calcium intake and bone quality in the elderly. Ecol. Food Nutr., *10*:131, 1981.

Heaney, R. P.: Calcium intake requirement and bone mass in the elderly. J. Lab. Clin Med., *100*:309, 1982 (editorial).

Heaney, R. P., et al.: Calcium nutrition and bone health in the elderly. Amer. J. Clin. Nutr., *36*:986, 1982 (also see Nutr. Rev., *41*:86, 1983).

Hecht, A., and Stephenson, M.: Calcium, more than just the strong stuff of bones. FDA Consumer, *15*:14, 1981.

Hillyard, C. J., et al.: Katacalcin: a new plasma calcium-lowering hormone. Lancet, *1*:846, 1983.

Llinás, R. R.: Calcium in synaptic transmission. Sci., Amer., *247*:56, 1982.

Marcus, R.: The relationship of dietary calcium to the maintenance of skeletal integrity in man—an interface of endrocrinology and nutrition. Metabolism, *31*:93, 1982.

Marie, P. J., et al.: Histological osteomalacia due to dietary calcium deficiency in children. New Eng. J. Med., *307*:584, 1982.

Means, A. R., and Dedman, J. R.: Calmodulin—an intracellular calcium receptor. Nature, *285*:73, 1980.

Osteoporosis and calcium balance. Nutr. Rev., *41*:83, 1983.

Sabry, J. H., Chorostecki, D. J., and Woolcott, D. M.: Nutrient content of diets of businessmen: relation to body weight status, age, and education. J. Canad. Dietet. Assoc., *43*:216, 1982.

Talmage, R. V., et al.: Evidence for an important physiological role for calcitonin. Proc. Nat. Acad. Sci., *77*:609, 1980.

Vogel, J. M., and Whittle, M. W.: Bone mineral changes: the second manned Skylab mission. Aviat. Space Environ. Med., *47*:396, 1976.

Wright, G. L., and Rakin, G. O.: Concentrations of ionic and total calcium in plasma of four models of hypertension. Amer. J. Physiol., *243*:H365, 1982.

Phosphorus

Chudley, A. E., Ninan, A., and Young, G. B.: Neurologic signs and hypophosphatemia with total parenteral nutrition. Canad. Med. Assoc. J., *125*:604, 1981.

Corbridge, D. E. C.: *Phosphorus: An Outline of Its Chemistry, Biochemistry and Technology*. New York, North-Holland, 1977.

Greengard, P.: Phosphorylated proteins as physiological effectors. Science, *199*:146, 1978.

Knochel, J. P.: Hypophosphatemia in the alcoholic. Arch. Inter. Med., *140*:613, 1980.

Massey, L. K., and Strang, M. M.: Soft drink consumption, phosphorus intake, and osteoporosis. J. Amer. Dietet. Assoc., *80*:581, 1982.

Zemel, M. B., et al.: Effects of calcium, ortho- and polyphosphates on calcium, zinc, iron, and copper bioavailability in man. Fed. Proc., *42*:397 (abstr.), 1983.

Ziegler, E. E., et al.: Effect of varying phosphorus intake on mineral balance of infants. Fed. Proc., *42*:397 (abstr). 1983.

Magnesium

Abraham, G. E., and Lubran, M. M.: Serum and red cell magnesium levels in patients with premenstrual tension. Amer. J. Clin. Nutr., *34*:2364, 1981.

Aikawa, J. K.: Biochemistry and physiology of magnesium. World Rev. Nutr. Dietet., *28*:112, 1978.

Allington, J. K., Matthews, M. E., and Johnson, N. E.: Nutritive value of food served calculated from food purchased in 14 nursing homes. J. Amer. Dietet. Assoc., *82*:377, 1983 (magnesium below RDA levels in 13 homes).

Altura, B. M., Altura, B. T., and Carella, A.: Magnesium deficiency—induced spasms of umbilical vessels: relation to preeclampsia, hypertension, and growth retardation. Science, *221*:376, 1983.

Classen, H. G.: Stress and magnesium. Artery, *9*:182, 1981.

Dyckner, T., and Wester, P. O.: Effect of magnesium on blood pressure. Brit. Med. J., *286*:1847, 1983.

Greger, J. L., et al.: Dietary intake and nutritional status in regard to magnesium of adolescent females. Nutr. Rept. Internat., *20*:235, 1979 (also see Greger, J. L., et al.: Nutr. Res., *1*:315, 1981).

Greger, J. L., Marhefka, S., and Geissler, A. H.: Magnesium content of selected foods. J. Food Sci., *43*:1610, 1978.

Lukaski, H. C., et al.: Maximum oxygen consumption

as related to magnesium, copper, and zinc nutriture. Amer. J. Clin. Nutr., *37*:407, 1983 (in male athletes).

Moore, M. J.: Liquid protein diets and electrolyte deficiency. J. Amer. Med. Assoc., *241*:1464, 1979.

Ranholtra, G. S.: Bioavailability of magnesium in cereal-based foods. Cereal Foods World, *28*:349, 1983.

Rude, R. K., and Singer, F. R.: Magnesium deficiency and excess. Ann. Rev. Med., *32*:245, 1981.

Schwartz, R., Spencer, H., and Jones, J.: Human magnesium absorption from leafy vegetables intrinsically labelled with stable Mg. Fed. Proc., *42*:826 (abstr.), 1983.

Seelig, M. S.: *Magnesium Deficiency in the Pathogenesis of Disease.* New York, Plenum Publishing Co., 1980.

Seelig, M. S.: Magnesium requirements in human nutrition. Contemporary Nutrition (General Mills), 7 (Jan.):1, 1982.

Sheehan, J., and White, A.: Diuretic-associated hypomagnesaemia. Brit. Med. J., *285*:1157, 1982.

Swales, J. D.: Magnesium deficiency and diuretics. Brit. Med. J., *285*:1377, 1982.

Chapter 16 The Trace Elements Iron, Iodine, Copper, and Manganese

Trace Elements: Reviews

(Also see refs. 2–7, 22, 33, 41, and 42, this chapter, and supplementary readings for Chapter 13.)

Bronner, F., and Coburn, J. W.: *Disorders of Mineral Metabolism.* Vol. I *(Trace Minerals).* New York, Academic Press, 1981.

Casey, C. E., and Hambidge, K. M.: Trace element deficiencies in man. Adv. Nutr. Res., *3*:20, 1980.

DiSilvestro, R. A., and Cousins, R. J.: Physiological ligands for copper and zinc. Ann. Rev. Nutr., *3*:261, 1983.

Dubick M. A., and Rucker, R. B.: Dietary supplements and health aids—a critical evaluation. Part I: vitamins and minerals. J. Nutr. Educ., *15*:47, 1983 (on toxicity or misuse of bone meal, dolomite, chromium, selenium, and zinc).

Gawthorne, J. M., Howell, J. M., and White, C. L. (eds.): *Trace Element Metabolism in Man and Animals.* Berlin/New York, Springer Verlag, 1982.

Lecos, C.: Tracking trace minerals. FDA Consumer, *17*(No. 6):16, 1983 (a review of essential trace minerals).

Lönnerdal, B., Keen, C. L., and Hurley, L. S.: Iron, copper, zinc, and manganese in milk. Ann. Rev. Nutr., *1*:149, 1981.

McClain, C. J.: Trace metal abnormalities in adults during hyperalimentation. J. Parenter. Ent. Nutr., *5*:424, 1981.

Prasad, A. S. (ed.): *Clinical, Biochemical, and Nutritonal Aspects of Trace Elements.* Current Topics in Nutrition and disease, Vol. 6. New York, Alan R. Liss, Inc., 1982.

Prasad, A. S.: An update on trace minerals in human nutrition. Nutr. News (National Dairy Council), *46*(April):5, 1983.

Ragan, H. A. (chm.), et al.: Biological availability of trace elements—animal models/human health. Sci. Total Environ., *28*:317-455, 1983 (14 papers from a symposium, on iron, zinc, nickel, chromium, selenium, etc.).

Sandstead, H. H.: Trace element interactions. J. Lab. Clin. Med., *98*:457, 1981.

Sarkler, B. (ed.): *Biological Aspects of Metals and Metal-related Diseases.* New York: Raven Press, 1983 (21 chapters on iron, copper, zinc, nickel, manganese, aluminum, lead, etc.).

Spivey-Fox, M. R., and Tao, S.-H.: Mineral content of human tissues from a nutrition perspective. Fed. Proc., *40*:2130, 1981.

Trace elements in human nutrition. Dairy Council Dig., *53*(1):1, 1982.

Trace Elements: General

(Also see refs. 1–10, 35, and 42, this chapter.)

Danford, D. E., Smith, J. C., Jr., and Huber, A. M.: Pica and mineral status in the mentally retarded. Amer. J. Clin. Nutr., *35*:958, 1982.

Gibson, R. S., Anderson, B. M., and Sabry, J. H.: The trace metel status of a group of post-menopausal vegetarians. J. Amer. Dietet. Assoc., *82*:246, 1983 (on copper, manganese, and selenium).

Kirkpatrick, D. C., et al.: The trace element content of Canadian baby foods and estimation of trace element intake by infants. Canad. Instit. Food Sci. Tech. J., *13*:154, 1980.

Lönnerdal, B., et al.: Zinc and copper binding proteins in human milk. Amer. J. Clin. Nutr., *36*:1170, 1982.

Mahalko, J. R., et al.: Effect of a moderate increase in dietary protein on the retention and excretion of Ca, Cu, Fe, Mg, P, and Zn by adult males. Amer. J. Clin. Nutr.: *37*:8, 1983 (moderate increase had little effect).

Patterson, K. Y., et al.: Zinc, copper, and manganese in self-chosen diets of healthy adult subjects living at home. Fed. Proc., *42*:1305 (abstr.), 1983.

Rao, C. N., and Rao, B. S. N.: Copper, manganese and cobalt balances in Indian adult men and estimation of daily requirement of copper and manganese. Nutr. Rept. Internat., *26*: 1113, 1982.

Turnlund, J., Costa, F., and Margen, S.: Zinc, copper, and iron balance in elderly men. Amer. J. Clin. Nutr., *34*:2641, 1981.

Umoren, J., and Kies, C.: Menstrual blood losses of iron, zinc, copper and magnesium in adult female subjects. Nutr. Rept. Internat., *26*:717, 1982.

Trace Elements: Availability

Bodwell, C. E.: Effects of soy protein on iron and zinc utilization in humans. Cereal Foods World, *28*:342, 1983.

Fairweather-Tait, S. J.: The availability or minerals in

food with particular reference to iron. J. Roy. Soc. Health, *2*:74, 1983.

Forbes, R. M., and Erdman, J. W., Jr.: Bioavailability of trace mineral elements. Ann. Rev. Nutr., *3*:213, 1983.

Greger, J. L., and Snedeker, S. M.: Effect of dietary protein and phosphorus levels on the utilization of zinc, copper and manganese by adult males. J. Nutr., *110*:2243, 1980.

Kelsay, J. L.: Effect of diet fiber level on bowel function and trace mineral balances of human subjects. Cereal Chem., *58*:2, 1981.

Shah, B. G.: Chelating agents and bioavailability of minerals. Nutr. Res., *1*:617, 1981.

Snedeker, S. M., Smith, S. A., and Greger, J. L.: Effect of dietary calcium and phosphorus levels on the utilization of iron, copper, and zinc by adult males. J. Nutr., *112*:136, 1982.

Vuori, E., et al.: The effects of the dietary intakes of copper, iron, manganese, and zinc on the trace element content of human milk. Amer. J. Clin. Nutr., *33*:227, 1980.

Young, V. R., and Janghorbani, M.: Legumes and mineral absorption, with special reference to soybean proteins. J. Plant Foods, *4*:57, 1982.

"Organic" Foods

Aldrich, S. R. (Chairman), Task Force of Council for Agricultural Science and Technology (Ames, Iowa): *Organic and Conventional Farming Compared,* Report No. 84, 1980.

Andrews, W. H., et al.: Bacteriological survey of sixty health foods. Appl. Environ. Microb., *37*:559, 1979.

Carter, L. J.: Organic farming becomes "legitimate." Science, *209*:254, 1980.

Hansen, H.: Comparison of chemical composition and taste of biodynamically and conventionally grown vegetables. Qual. Plantarum: Plant Foods Human Nutr., *30*:203, 1981.

It's natural! It's organic! Or is it? Consumer Rept., *45*:410, 1980.

Jolley, L. W., and Raguse, C. A.: Responses of annual range grasses and legumes to comparable applications of manurial and inorganic fertilizers. J. Range Mang., *34*:297, 1981.

Knorr, Dietrich: Natural and organic foods: definitions, quality and problems. Cereal Foods World, *27*:163, 1982.

Lockeretz, W., Shearer, G., and Kohl, D. H.: Organic farming in the corn belt. Science, *211*:540, 1981.

Price, C. C., and Brown, J.: Organic certification programs. National Food Rev. (U.S.D.A.-NFR-15), summer, p. 31, 1981.

Iron: Reviews

Bothwell, T. H., et al.: *Iron Metabolism in Man.* Oxford, Blackwell Scientific Publications, 1980.

Conrad, M. E., and Barton, J. C.: Factors affecting iron balance. Amer. J. Hemat., *10*:199, 1981 (192 refs.).

Dallman, P. R., Siimes, M. A., and Stekel, A.: Iron deficiency in infancy and childhood. Amer. J. Clin. Nutr., *33*:86, 1980.

Finch, C. A., and Huebers, H.: Perspective in iron metabolism. New Eng. J. Med., *306*:1520, 1982 (also see *307*:1405, 1982).

Jacobs, A., and Worwood, M. (eds.): *Iron in Biochemistry and Medicine.* II. London, Academic Press, 1980.

Oppenheimer, S., and Hendrickse, R.: The clinical effects of iron deficiency and iron supplementation. Nutr. Abst. Rev., *53*:585, 1983 (a review with 170 references).

Pollitt, E, and Leibel, R. L. (eds.): *Iron Deficiency: Brain Biochemistry and Behavior.* New York, Raven Press, 1982.

Rao, B. S. N.: Physiology of iron absorption and supplementation. Brit. Med. Bull., *37*:25, 1981.

Weinberg, E. D.: Iron and neoplasia. Biol. Tr. Elem. Res., *3*:55, 1981.

Iron Status: Determination and Intervention

(Also see refs. 10–16, this chapter.)

Brault-Dubuc, M., et al.: Iron status of French-Canadian children: a three year follow-up study. Human Nutr.: Applied Nutr., *37C*:210, 1983 (3 to 36 months of age).

Hershko, C., et al.: Diagnosis of iron deficiency anemia in a rural population of children. Amer. J. Clin. Nutr., *34*:1600, 1981.

Jagannathan, S. N., and Stoner, G.: A case against accepting women for blood donation as frequently as men. Fed. Proc., *42*:1182 (abst.), 1983.

Liebman, M., et al.: The iron status of black and white female adolescents from eight southern states, Amer. J. Clin. Nutr., *38*:109, 1983.

McEndree, L. S., Kies, C. V., and Fox, H. M.: Iron intake and iron nutritional status of lacto-ovo-vegetarian and omnivore students. Nutr. Rept. Internat., *27*:199, 1983.

Monsen, E. R., et al: Iron balance in superdonors, Transfusion, *23*:221, 1983.

Rafalski, H., Ponomarenko, W., and Szyler, I.: Effect of iron-fortified bread roll on hematological indices and clinical symptoms in menstruating women. Human Nutr.: Appl. Nutr., *36A*:208, 1982.

Schifman, R. B., et al.: RBC zinc protoporphyrin to screen blood donors for iron deficiency anemia. J. Amer. Med. Assoc., *248*:2012, 1982.

Simon, T. L., Garry, P. J., and Hooper, E. M.: Iron stores in blood donors. J. Amer. Med. Assoc., *245*:2038, 1981.

Singer, J. D., et al.: Diet and iron status, a study of relationships. U.S. Dept. Health and Human Services, Publicat. No. (PHS) 83-1679, 1983.

Iron Availability

(Also see ref. 21, this chapter.)

Cook, J. D., Morck, T. A., and Lynch, S. R.: The inhibitory effect of soy products on nonheme iron absorption in man. Amer. J. Clin. Nutr., *34*:2622, 1981.

Fairweather-Tait, S. J.: Studies on the availability of iron in potatoes. Brit. J. Nutr., *50*:15, 1983 (also see *50*:51, 1983, on ferric orthophosphate absorption).

Garry, P. J., et al.: Iron absorption from human milk and formula with and without iron supplementation. Pediatr. Res., *15*:822, 1981.

Gillooly, M., et al.: The effects of organic acids, phytates and polyphenols on the absorption of iron from vegetables. Brit. J. Nutr., *49*:331, 1983.

Hallberg, L., et al.: Iron absorption from some Asian meals containing contamination iron. Amer. J. Clin. Nutr., *37*:272, 1983.

Hallberg, L., and Rossander, L.: Absorption of iron from Western-type lunch and dinner meals. Amer. J. Clin. Nutr., *35*:502, 1982.

Hallberg, L., and Rossander, L.: Effect of different drinks on the absorption of non-heme iron from composite meals. Human Nutr.: Applied Nutr., *36A*:116, 1982.

MacPhail, A. P., et al.: Factors affecting the absorption of iron from Fe(III)EDTA. Brit. J. Nutr., *45*:215, 1981 (on iron chelate).

Morck, T. A., and Cook, J. D.: Factors affecting the bioavailability of dietary iron. Cereal Foods World, *26*:667, 1981.

Morck, T. A., et al.: Iron availability from infant food supplements. Amer. J. Clin. Nutr., *34*:2630, 1981.

Morck, T. A., Lynch, S. R., and Cook, J. D.: Inhibition of food iron absorption by coffee. Amer. J. Clin. Nutr., *37*:416, 1983.

Ranhotra, G. S., et al.: Bioavailability of iron in iron-fortified fluid milk. J. Food Sci., *46*:1342, 1981.

Schricker, B. R., and Miller, D. D.: In vitro estimation of relative iron availability in breads and meals containing different forms of fortification iron. J. Food Sci., *47*:723, 1982.

Skikne, B. S., Lynch, S. R., and Cook, J. D.: Role of gastric acid in food iron absorption. Gastroenterology, *81*:1068, 1981.

Van Campen, D. R., and Welch, R. M.: Availability to rats of iron from spinach—effects of oxalic acid. J. Nutr., *110*:1618, 1980.

Yeung, D. L., et al.: Iron intake of infants: the importance of infant cereals. Canad. Med. Assoc. J., *125*:999, 1981.

Ascorbic Acid and Iron Absorption

(Also see ref. 21, this chapter.).

Hallberg, L., et al.: Deleterious effects of prolonged warming of meals on ascorbic acid content and iron absorption. Amer. J. Clin. Nutr., *36*:846, 1982.

Morck, T. A., Lynch, S. R., and Cook, J. D.: Reduction of the soy-induced inhibition of nonheme iron absorption. Amer. J. Clin. Nutr., *36*:219, 1982.

Nienhuis, A. W.: Vitamin C and iron. New Eng. J. Med., *304*:170, 1981.

Nojeim, S. J., and Clydesdale, F. M.: Effect of pH and ascorbic acid on iron valence in model systems and in foods. J. Food Sci., *46*:606, 1981.

Rathee, S., and Pradhan, K.: Effect of ascorbic acid on availability of iron from an egg-based whole day diet of college girls. Ind. J. Nutr. Dietet., *17*:90, 1980.

Effect of Fiber on Iron Availability

Camire, A. L., and Clydesdale, F. M.: Interactions of soluble iron with wheat bran. J. Food Sci., *47*:1296, 1982.

Faraji, B., Reinhold, J. G., and Abadi, P.: Human studies of iron absorption from fiber-rich Iranian flat breads. Nutr. Rept. Internat., *23*:267, 1981.

Garcia-Lopez, S., and Wyatt, C. J.: Effect of fiber in corn tortillas and cooked beans on iron availability. J. Agric. Food Chem., *30*:724, 1982.

Ranhotra, G. S., et al.: Iranian flat breads: relative bioavailability of iron. Cereal Chem., *58*:471, 1981.

Reinhold, J. G., et al.: Binding of iron by fiber of wheat and maize. Amer. J. Clin. Nutr., *34*:1384, 1981.

Simpson, K. M., Morris, E. R., and Cook, J. D.: The inhibitory effect of bran on iron absorption in man. Amer. J. Clin. Nutr., *34*:1469, 1981.

Iron, Physical Fitness, and Work Performance

Ehn, L., et al.: Iron status in athletes involved in intense physical activity. Med. Sci. Sports Exercise, *12*:61, 1980.

Hunding, A., et al.: Runner's anemia and iron deficiency. Acta Med. Scand., *209*:315, 1981.

Florencio, C. A.: Effects of iron and ascorbic acid supplementation on hemoglobin level and work efficiency of anemic women. J. Occup. Med., *23*:699, 1981.

Koziol, B., et al.: Changes in work tolerance associated with metabolic and physiological adjustment to moderate and severe iron deficiency anemia. Amer. J. Clin. Nutr., *36*:830, 1982.

Paulev, P., et al.: Dermal excretion of iron in intensely training athletes. Clin. Chim. Acta, *127*:19, 1983.

Plowman, S. A., and McSwegin, P. C.: The effects of iron supplementation on female cross country runners. J. Sports Med., *21*:407, 1981.

Iron: General Readings

(Also see refs. 2–22, this chapter.)

Iron deficiency and intestinal absorption of sugars. Nutr. Rev., *40*:205, 1982.

Lozoff, B., et al.: The effects of short-term oral iron therapy on developmental deficits in iron-deficient anemic infants. J. Pediatr., *100*:351, 1982 (also see *101*:948, 1982 and *103*:339, 1983).

Owen, G., et al.: Iron nutriture of infants exclusively breast-fed the first five months. J. Pediatr., *99*:237, 1981.

Rector, W. G., Jr., et al.: Non-hematologic effects of chronic iron deficiency. Medicine, *61*:382, 1982.

Stockman, J. A., III: Infections and iron. Amer. J. Dis. Children, *135*:18, 1981.

Tucker, D. M., and Sandstead, H. H.: Spectral electroencephalographic correlates of iron status: tired blood revisited. Physiol. Behavior, *26*:439, 1981.

Walter, T., Kovalskys, J., and Stekel, A.: Effect of mild iron deficiency on infant mental development scores. J. Pediatr. *102*:519, 1983.

Iodine

Allegrini, M., Pennington, J. A. T., and Tanner, J. T.: Total diet study: determination of iodine intake. J. Amer. Dietet. Assoc., *83*:18, 1983.

Bleichrodt, N., et al.: Effects of iodine deficiency on mental and psychomotor abilities. Amer. J. Phys. Anthro., *53*:55, 1980.

Bruhn, J. C., et al.: Sources and content of iodine in California dairy products. J. Food Protect. *46*:41, 1983.

Dietary goitrogens. Lancet, *1*:1394, 1982 (also see letters on this topic and cretinism in Lancet, *2*:552, 1982 and Gaitan, E., et al.: J. Clin. Endocrin. Metab., *56*:767, 1983 [on environmental goitrogens]).

Emrich, D., et al.: Influence of increasing iodine intake on thyroid function in euthyroid and hyperthyroid states. J. Clin. Endocrin. Metab., *54*:1236, 1982.

Ermans, A. M., et al. (eds): *Role of cassava in the etiology of endemic goitre and cretinism.* New York, UNIPUB, 1980.

Fischer, P. W. F., and L'Abbé, M.: Iodine in iodized table salt and in sea salt. Canad. Instit. Food Sci. Tech. J., *13*:103, 1980.

Gaitan, J. E., et al.: Defective thyroidal iodine concentration in protein-calorie malnutrition. J. Clin. Endocrin. Metab., *57*:327, 1983.

Hershman, J. M., et al.: Endemic goiter in Vietnam. J. Clin. Endocrin. Metab., *57*:243, 1983.

Koutras, D. A.: Clinical aspects of excess iodine in iodine deficiency. J. Molec. Med., *4*:139, 1980 (part of a special issue on thyroid and iodine—25 articles).

Maberly, G. F., et al.: Effect of iodination of a village water-supply on goitre size and thyroid function. Lancet, *2*:1270, 1981.

Matovinovic, J.: Endemic goiter and cretinism at the dawn of the third millennium. Ann. Rev. Nutr., *3*:341, 1983.

Nunez, J., and Pommier, J.: Formation of thyroid hormones. Vit. Horm., *39*:175, 1982.

Stanbury, J. B., and Hetzel, B. S. (eds.): *Endemic Goiter and Endemic Cretinism.* New York, John Wiley and Sons, 1980.

Tai, M., et al.: The present status of endemic goitre and endemic cretinism in China. Food Nutr. Bull., *4*(No. 4): 13, 1982.

Vorherr, H., et al.: Vaginal absorption of povidone-iodine. J. Amer. Med. Assoc., *244*:2628, 1980 (an active ingredient in certain contraceptives).

Wenlock, R. W., et al.: Trace nutrients 4–iodine in British food. Brit. J. Nutr., *47*:381, 1982.

Wolinsky, I., et al.: Iodination of salt. Baroda J. Nutr., 7:1, 1980.

Copper: Reviews

(Also see refs 2–4, 22, and 31, this chapter.)

Ize-Lamache, L., et al.: Zinc and copper abnormalities in fasting patients undergoing total parenteral nutrition. Arch. Invest. Med. (Mexico), *12*:241, 1981.

Solomons, N W.: On the assessment of zinc and copper nutriture in man. Amer. J. Clin. Nutr., *32*:856, 1979.

Walravens, P. A.: Nutritional importance of copper and zinc in neonates and infants. Clin. Chem., *26*:185, 1980.

Copper: General Readings

(Also see refs. 28–39, this chapter.)

Anand, S., et al.: Copper status of Indian pregnant women of low socio-economic group and its effect on the outcome of pregnancy. Internat. J. Vit. Nutr. Res., *51*:410, 1981.

Castillo-Durán, C., et al.: Controlled trial of copper supplementation during the recovery from marasmus. Amer. J. Clin. Nutr., *37*:898, 1983.

Copper metabolism in premature and low-birth-weight neonates. Nutr. Rev., *39*:333, 1981.

Epstein, O., et al.: Hair copper in primary biliary cirrhosis. Amer. J. Clin. Nutr., *33*:965, 1980.

Feller, D. J., O'Dell, B. L., and Bylund, D. B.: Alternations in neurotransmitter receptor binding in discrete areas of the copper-deficient rat brain. J. Neurochem., *38*:519, 1982.

Finley, E. B., and Cerklewski, F. L.: Influence of ascorbic acid supplementation on copper status in young adult men. Amer. J. Clin. Nutr., *37*:553, 1983 (high vitamin C reduces copper status).

Kenney, M. A.: Copper nutrition of 4-year-old children of two races. Nutr. Rept. Internat., *27*:1227, 1983 (Mexican-Americans and blacks).

Lukasewycz, O. A., and Prohaska, J. R.: Immunization against transplantable leukemia impaired in copper-deficient mice. J. Nat. Cancer Inst., *69*:489, 1982.

Milne, D. B., Omaye, S. T., and Amos, W. H.: Effect of ascorbic acid on copper and cholesterol in adult cynomolgus monkeys fed a diet marginal in copper. Amer. J. Clin. Nutr., *34*:2389, 1981.

Nishi, Y., et al.: Copper deficiency associated with alkali therapy in a patient with renal tubular acidosis. J. Pediatr., *98*:81, 1981.

Prohaska, J. R., and Heller, L. J.: Mechanical properties of the copper-deficient rat heart. J. Nutr., *112*:2142, 1982.

Shike, M., et al.: Copper metabolism and requirements in total parenteral nutrition. Gastroenterology, *81*:290, 1981.

Tanaka, Y., et al.: Nutritional copper deficiency in a Japanese infant on formula. J. Pediatr., *96*:255, 1980.

Turnlund, J. R., et al.: Copper absorption in elderly men determined by using stable ^{65}Cu. Amer. J. Clin. Nutr., *36*:587, 1982 (also see Amer. J. Clin. Nutr. *37*:716(abstr.), 1983 for effect of cellulose and phytate).

Vir, S. C., et al.: Serum and hair concentrations of copper during pregnancy. Amer. J. Clin. Nutr., *34*:2382, 1981.

Copper-Zinc Relationships

Burke, D. M., et al.: Copper and zinc utilization in elderly adults. J. Gerontology, *36*:558, 1981.

Freeland-Graves, J. H., et al.: Effect of dietary Zn/Cu ratios on cholesterol and HDL-cholesterol levels in women. Nutr. Rept. Internat., *22*:285, 1980.

Holden, J. M., Wolf, W. R., and Mertz, W.: Zinc and copper in self-selected diets. J. Amer. Dietet. Assoc., *75*:23, 1979.

Ritchey, S. J.: Interrelationships among protein, zinc, and copper in human nutrition. Cereal Chem., *58*:18, 1981.

Taper, L. J., Hinners, M. L., and Ritchey, S. J.: Effects of zinc intake on copper balance in adult females. Amer. J. Clin. Nutr., *33*:1077, 1980.

Manganese

(Also see refs. 41 and 42 this chapter.)

Chan, W-Y., Bates, J. M., Jr., and Rennert, O. M.: Comparative studies of manganese binding in human breast milk, bovine milk and infant formula. J. Nutr., *112*:642, 1982.

Hatano, S., et al.: Erythrocyte manganese concentration in healthy Japanese children, adults, and the elderly, and in cord blood. Amer. J. Clin. Nutr., *37*:457, 1983.

Rognstad, R.: Manganese effects on gluconeogenesis. J. Biol. Chem., *256*:1608, 1981.

Wenlock, R. W., Buss, D. H., and Dixon, E. J.: Trace nutrients 2. Manganese in British food. Brit. J. Nutr., *41*:253, 1979.

Chapter 17 The Newer Trace Elements

Newer Trace Elements: Reviews and Books

(Also see Supplementary Readings, Chapter 16.)

Clark, M. J., et al. (eds.): *Copper, Molybdenum and Vanadium in Biological Systems.* Berlin, Springer-Verlag, 1983.

Freifeld, K., and Englemayer, S.: Hair analysis—are you being scalped? Health, *15*(No. 7):33, 1983.

Golden, M. H. N.: Review article: trace elements in human nutrition. Human Nutr.: Clin. Nutr., *36C:*185, 1982.

Golden, M. H. N., and Golden, B. E.: Trace elements: potential importance in human nutrition with particular reference to zinc and vanadium. Brit. Med. Bull., *37*:31, 1981.

Hackler, L. R. (Chairman): Symposium: impact of foods on trace mineral availability and metabolism. Cereal Chem., *58:*1–26, (5 papers), 1981.

Nielsen, F. H.: Trace elements. Ann. Rev. Nutr., *4:* (in press), 1984.

Schrauzer, G. N.: Trace elements in carcinogenesis. Adv. Nutr. Res., *2:*219, 1979.

Turnlund, J. R.: Bioavailability of selected minerals in cereal products. Cereal Foods World, *27:*152, 1982.

Zinc: Books and Reviews

Nriagu, J. O. (ed.): *Zinc in the Environment, Part 2: Health Effects.* New York, John Wiley and Sons, Inc., 1980.

Prasad, A. S., et al.: *Clinical Applications of Recent Advances in Zinc Metabolism.* New York, Alan R. Liss, Inc., 1982 (11 chapters).

Prasad, A. S.: Clinical, biochemical, and nutritional spectrum of zinc deficiency in human subjects: an update. Nutr. Rev., *41:*197, 1983 (also see pp. 209, 211, 217, and 221).

Roth, H. -P. and Kirchgessner, M.: Zn metalloenzyme activities. World Rev. Nutr. Dietet., *34:*144, 1980.

Solomons, N. W.: Recent progress in zinc nutrition research, Nutr. Update, *1:*123, 1983.

Zinc: Absorption and Availability

Casey, C. E., Walravens, P. A., and Hambidge, K. M.: Availability of zinc: loading tests with human milk, cow's milk, and infant formulas. Pediatrics, *68:*394, 1981.

Faridi, H. A., et al.: Iranian flat breads: relative availability of zinc. J. Food Sci., *48:*107, 1983.

Franz, K. B., et al.: Relative bioavailability of zinc from selected cereals and legumes using rat growth. J. Nutr. *110:*2272, 1980.

Hogarth, F. W.: Should zinc be added to textured vegetable protein? J. Human Nutr., *35:*379, 1981.

Matseshe, J. W., et al.: Recovery of dietary iron and zinc from the proximal intestine of healthy man: studies of different meals and supplements. Amer. J. Clin. Nutr., *33:*1946, 1980.

Rendleman, J. A., and Grobe, C. A.: Cereal complexes: binding zinc by bran and components of bran. Cereal Chem., *59:*310, 1982.

Young, V. R., and Janghorbani, M.: Soy proteins in human diets in relation to bioavailability of iron and zinc: a brief overview. Cereal Chem., *58:*12, 1981.

Zinc: General Reading

Bettger, W. J., and O'Dell, B. L.: A critical physiological role of zinc in the structure and function of biomembranes. Life Sciences, *28:*1425, 1981 (a review—171 refs.).

Collipp, P. J., et al.: Zinc deficiency: improvement in growth and growth hormone levels with oral zinc therapy. Ann. Nutr. Metab., *26:*287, 1982.

Cossack, Z. T., and Prasad, A. S.: Effect of protein source on the bioavailability of zinc in human subjects. Nutr. Res., *3:*23, 1983.

Dorea, J. D., et al.: Nutritional status and zinc nutriture in infants and children in a poor urban community of Brazil. Ecol. Food Nutr., *12:*1, 1982.

Flint, D. M., et al.: Zinc and protein status in the elderly. J. Human Nutr., *35:*287, 1981.

Ghavami-Maibodi, S. Z., et al.: Effect of oral zinc supplements on growth, hormonal levels, and zinc in healthy short children. Ann. Nutr. Metab., *27:*214, 1983 (in East Meadow, N.Y.).

Golden, B. E., and Golden, M. H. N.: Plasma zinc, rate of weight gain, and the energy cost of tissue deposition in children recovering from severe malnutrition on a cow's milk or soya protein based diet. Amer. J. Clin, Nutr., *34:*892, 1981 (Also see *34:*900, 1981).

Hambidge, K. M., et al.: Zinc nutritional status during pregnancy: a longitudinal study. Amer. J. Clin. Nutr. *37:*429, 1983 (in Colorado).

Rothbaum, R. J., et al.: Serum alkaline phosphatase and zinc undernutrition in infants with chronic diarrhea. Amer. J. Clin. Nutr., *35:*595, 1982.

Srivastava, U. S., Nadeau, M. H., and Carbonneau, N.: Mineral intakes of university students: zinc content. J. Canad. Dietet. Assoc., *38:*302, 1977.

Welsh, S. O., and Marston, R. M.: Zinc levels of the U.S. food supply—1909–1980. Food Tech., *36*(No. 1):70, 1982 (before processing and cooking).

Fluorine

(Also see refs. 61–75, this chapter.)

Allukian, M., Steinhurst, J., and Dunning, J. M.: Community organization and a regional approach to fluoridation of the greater Boston area. J. Amer. Dent. Assoc., *102:*491, 1981.

Clark, N., and Corbin, S.: The evolution of standards for naturally occurring fluorides: an example of scientific due process. Public Health Rept., *98:*53, 1983.

Hefti, A., and Marthaler, T. M.: Bone fluoride concentrations after 16 years of drinking water fluoridation. Caries Res., *15:*85, 1981.

Horowitz, H. S., et al.: A program of self-administered fluorides in a rural school system. Commun. Dent. Oral Epidem., *8:*173, 1980.

Maheshwari, U. R., et al.: Fluoride balance studies in healthy men during bed rest with and without a fluoride supplement. Amer. J. Clin. Nutr., *36:*211, 1982 (also see *34:*2679, 1981).

Siegel, C., and Gutgesell, M. E.: Fluoride supplementation in Harris County, Texas. Amer. J. Dis. Children, *136:*61, 1982.

Spencer, H., Osis, D., and Lender, M.: Studies of fluoride metabolism in man. A review and report of original data. Sci. Total Environ., *17:*1, 1981.

Taves, D. R.: Dietary intake of fluoride: ashed (total fluoride) v. unashed (inorganic fluoride) analysis of individual foods. Brit. J. Nutr. *49:*295, 1983 (93 food items in Rochester, N. Y.).

Cobalt

(Also see general readings for Chapters 13, 16, and 17.)

Taylor, A., and Marks, V.: Cobalt: a review. J. Human Nutr., *32:*165, 1978.

Molybdenum

(Also see refs. 76–80, this chapter.)

Coughlan, M. P. (ed.): *Molybdenum and Molybdenum Containing Enzymes.* Oxford, Permagon Press, 1980.

Fan, W.: Studies of the etiologic relationship of molybdenum deficiency to Keshan disease. Acta Nutrimenta Sinica, *4:*275, 1982 (in China).

Nell, J. A., and Annison, E. F.: Molybdenum requirements of chickens. Brit. Poult. Sci., *21:*183, 1980.

Newton, W. E., and Otsuka, S. (eds.): *Molybdenum Chemistry of Biological Significance.* New York, Plenum Press, 1980.

Selenium

(Also see refs. 81–91, this chapter.)

Burk, R. F.: Biological activity of selenium. Ann. Rev. Nutr., *3:*53, 1983.

Combs, G. F., Jr., and Combs, S. B.: The nutritional biochemistry of selenium. Ann. Rev. Nutr., *4:* in press, 1984.

Committee on Selenium: *Selenium in Nutrition.* Washington, D. C., National Academy Press, 1983.

Greger, J. L., and Marcus, R. E.: Effect of dietary protein, phosphorus, and sulfur amino acids on selenium metabolism of adult males. Ann. Nutr. Metab., *25:*97, 1981.

Lane, H. W., et al.: Selenium content of selected foods. J. Amer. Dietet. Assoc., *82:*24, 1983.

Levander, O. A.: Recent developments in selenium nutrition. Nutr. Update, *1:*147, 1983.

Palmer, I. S., et al.: Selenium intake and urinary excretion in persons living near a high selenium area. J. Amer. Dietet. Assoc., *82:*511, 1983 (in South Dakota).

Salonen, J. T., et al.: Association between cardiovascular death and myocardial infarction and serum selenium in a matched-pair longitudinal study. Lancet, *2:*175, 1982.

Shultz, T. D., and Leklem, J. E.: Selenium status of vegetarians, nonvegetarians, and hormone-dependent cancer subjects. Amer. J. Clin. Nutr., *37:*114, 1983.

Willett, W. C., et al.: Prediagnostic serum selenium and risk of cancer. Lancet, *2:*130, 1983 (a large cooperative study in the U.S.).

Young, V. R., et al.: Selenium bioavailability with reference to human nutrition. Amer. J. Clin. Nutr., *35:*1076, 1982.

Chromium

(Also see refs. 92–97, this chapter.)

Anderson, R. A., and Bryden, N. A.: Concentration, insulin potentiation, and absorption of chromium in beer. J. Agric. Food Chem., *31:*308, 1983.

Anderson, R. A., et al.: Effect of exercise (running) on serum glucose, insulin, glucagon, and chromium excretion. Diabetes, *31:*212, 1982 (also see Anderson, R. A., et al.: Amer. J. Clin. Nutr., *36:*1184, 1982).

Kumpulainen, J. T., et al.: Determination of chromium in selected United States diets. J. Agric. Food Chem., *27:*490, 1979.

Kumpulainen, J., et al.: Dietary chromium intake of lactating Finnish mothers: effect on the Cr content of their breast milk. Brit. J. Nutr., *44:*257, 1980.

Kumpulainen, J., and Vuori, E.: Longitudinal study of chromium in human milk. Amer. J. Clin. Nutr., *33:*2299, 1980.

Lim, T. H., et al.: Kinetics of trace element chromium (III) in the human body. Amer. J. Physiol., *244:*R445, 1983.

Liu, V. J. K., and Abernathy, R. P.: Chromium and insulin in young subjects with normal glucose tolerance. Amer. J. Clin. Nutr., *35:*661, 1982.

Mertz. W.: Chromium: an essential micronutrient. Contemp. Nutr. (General Mills), *7*(March):1, 1982.

Nickel

(Also see ref. 98, this chapter, and general readings.)

Solomons, N. W., et al.: Bioavailability of nickel in man: effects of foods and chemically-defined dietary constituents on the absorption of inorganic nickel. J. Nutr., *112:*39, 1982.

Spears, J. W., et al.: Nickel depletion in the neonatal pig. Fed. Proc., *42:*819 (abstr.) 1983.

Thauer, R. K., et al.: Three new nickel enzymes from anaerobic bacteria. Naturwissenschaften, *70:*60, 1983.

Vanadium

(Also see refs. 99–101, this chapter.)

Bond, G. H., and Hudgins, P. M.: Inhibition of red cell CA^{2+}-ATPase by vanadate. Biochim. Biophys. Acta, *600:*781, 1980.

Byrne, A. R., and Kosta, L.: Vanadium in foods and in human body fluids and tissues. Sci. Total Environ., *10:*17, 1978.

Grantham, J. J.: The renal sodium pump and vanadate, Amer. J. Physiol., *239:*F97, 1980.

Myron, D. R., et al.: Vanadium content of selected foods as determined by flameless atomic absorption spectroscopy. J. Agric. Food Chem., *25:*297, 1977.

Nielsen, F. H., and Uthus, E. O.: Interactions among vanadium, iron and cystine in the rat. Fed. Proc., *42:*819 (abstr.), 1983.

Nutritional oedema, albumin, and vanadate. Lancet, *1:*646, 1981.

Vanadium, vitamin C and depression. Nutr. Rev., *40:*293, 1982.

Silicon

(Also see refs. 102–104, this chapter.)

Carlisle, E. M.: The nutritional essentiality of silicon. Nutr. Rev., *40:*193, 1982.

Silicon and bone formation. Nutr. Rev., *38:*194, 1980.

Silicon overdosage in man. Nutr. Rev., *40:*208, 1982.

Lead

(Also see refs. 107, 108, this chapter.)

Annest, J. L.: Chronological trend in blood lead levels between 1976 and 1980. New Eng. J. Med., *308:*1373, 1983.

Bellinger, D. C., et al.: Lead and the relationship between maternal and child intelligence. J. Pediatr., *102:*523, 1983.

Biddle, G. N.: Toxicology of lead (a review). J. Assoc. Off. Anal. Chem., *65:*947, 1982.

Charney, E., Sayre, J., and Coulter, M.: Increased lead absorption in inner city children: where does the lead come from? Pediatrics, *65:*226, 1980.

40% of all cans will be lead-free by end of 1983, Moore predicts. Food Chem. News., *25*(April 11):13, 1983.

Hunt, T. H., et al.: Childhood lead poisoning and inadequate child care. Amer. J. Dis. Children, *136:*538, 1982.

Little, P., Fleming, R. G., and Heard, M. J.: Uptake of lead by vegetable foodstuffs during cooking. Sci. Total Environ., *17:*111, 1981.

Mahaffey, K. R.: Nutritional factors in lead poisoning. Nutr. Rev., *39:*353, 1981 (also see *40:*255, 1982).

Marlowe, M., et al.: Increased lead burdens and trace-mineral status in mentally retarded children. J. Special Educ., *16:*87, 1982 (also see Behav. Disord., *7:*163, 1982).

Nriagu, J. O.: Saturnine gout among Roman aristocrats. Did lead poisoning contribute to the fall of the Empire? New Eng. J. Med., *308:*660, 1983 (also see 309: 431, 1983).

Schaffner, R. M.: Lead in canned foods. Food Tech., *35*(12):60, 1981.

Tin

Ferretti, G. A., Tanzer, J. M., and Tinanoff, N.: The effect of fluoride and stannous ions on *Streptococcus mutans.* Caries Res., *16:*298, 1982.

Greger, J. L., and Baier, M.: Tin and iron content of canned and bottled foods. J. Food Sci., *46:*1751, 1981.

Johnson, M. A., and Greger, J. L.: Effects of dietary tin on tin and calcium metabolism of adult males. Amer. J. Clin. Nutr., *35:*655, 1982; also see Amer. J. Clin. Nutr., *35:*1332, 1982 (on tin, copper, iron, manganese, and magnesium).

Nonessential Toxic Elements

Armstrong, B. G., and Kazantzis, G.: The mortality of cadmium workers. Lancet, *1:*1425, 1983 (6995 men studied in U.K.).

Carmichael, N. G., et al.: Teratogenicity, toxicity and perinatal effects of cadmium (a review). Human Tox., *1:*155, 1982.

Caster, W. O., and Wang, M.: Dietary aluminum and Alzheimer's disease—a review. Sci. Total Environ., *17:*31, 1981 (also see Nutr. Rev., *38:*242, 1980).

Cornatzer, W. E., et al.: Effect of arsenic deprivation on phosphatidylcholine biosynthesis in liver microsomes in the rat. Nutr. Rept. Internat., *27:*821, 1983.

Hutton, M.: Sources of cadmium in the environment.

Ecotoxicol. Environ. Safety, *7:*9, 1983 (part of a series of 17 papers on cadmium).

Klein, G. L., et al.: Aluminum loading during total parenteral nutrition. Amer. J. Clin. Nutr., *35:*1425, 1982.

Lydiard, R., and Gelenberg, A. J.: Hazards and adverse effects of lithium. Ann. Rev. Med., *33:*327, 1982 (also see p. 355 on the role of lithium in medicine—a review).

Ott, S. M., et al.: Aluminum is associated with low bone formation in patients receiving chronic parenteral nutrition. Ann. Int. Med., *96:*910, 1983.

Perry, H. M., Jr., and Kopp, S. J.: Does cadmium contribute to human hypertension? Sci. Total Environ., *26:*223, 1983 (also see Science, *217:*837, 1982).

Ryan, J. A., Pahren, H. R., and Lucas, J. B.: Controlling cadmium in the human food chain: a review and rationale based on health effects. Environ. Res., *28:*241, 1982.

Skoryna, S. C.: Effects of oral supplementation with stable strontium. Canad. Med. J., *125:*703, 1981.

Chapter 18 Food: Our Source of Nutrients and Nonnutrients

*Books and Reviews**

(Also see Supplementary Readings for Chapter 1 and refs. 1, 4, 11–20, 22–26, Chapter 18.)

Altschul, A. M., and Wilcke, H. L. (eds.): *New Protein Foods.* 4 vols. New York, Academic Press, 1981.

Hawthorn, J.: *Foundations of Food Science.* San Francisco, Freeman and Co., 1981.

Hayes, J. (ed.): *Food—from Farm to Table: The 1982 Yearbook of Agriculture.* Washington, D. C., USDA, 1982 (44 chapters on food economics, marketing, and buying).

Hayes, J. (ed.): *Will There Be Enough Food? The 1981 Yearbook of Agriculture.* Washington, D. C., USDA, 1981 (30 chapters on food production, marketing, and food export and aid to other countries).

Robinson, R.: *The Organic Constituents of Higher Plants.* Amherst, Mass., Cordus Press, 1983.

Schwimmer, S.: *Source Book of Food Enzymology.* Westport, Conn., Avi Publishing Co., 1981.

Stewart, G. T., and Amerine, M. A.: *Introduction to Food Science and Technology.* New York, Academic Press, 1982.

*The above list is only a small sampling of the several hundreds of books and reviews on some aspects of foods published each year. For more recent listings see the book review sections of such reliable journals as *Food Technology, Nutrition Abstracts and Reviews, Canadian Institute of Food Science and Technology Journal, Journal of Nutrition Education, Journal of the American Dietetic Association,* and the *Journal of the Canadian Dietetic Association.* No attempt is made here to list popular books on health foods, most of which are unreliable. Any that are listed are exceptions and are considered reliable.

Tyler, V. E.: *The Honest Herbal.* Philadelphia, Penn., George F. Stickley Co., 1982.

Welsh, S. O., and Marston, R. M.: Review of trends in food use in the United States, 1909 to 1980. J. Amer. Dietet. Assoc., *81:*120, 1982.

Food Processing and Preservation: Heating and Canning

(Also see refs. 3–7, this chapter.)

Food Tech., *37*(April):92–142, 1983. (On retort pouches—pp. 92 and 123; freezing—pp. 103 and 110; irradiation—p. 117; and aseptic canning—pp. 128 and 138. Also see other recent issues of Food Technology for additional readings on this and other practical topics dealing with food processing.)

Lecos, C.: Old milk stays fresh in aseptic package. FDA Consumer, *16:*7, 1982 (also see Jelen, J.: J. Food Protect., *45:*878, 1982).

Pflug, I. J., Davidson, P. M., and Holcomb, R. G.: Incidence of canned food spoilage at the retail level. J. Food Protect., *44:*682, 1981 (also see pp. 686 and 692).

Seigle, N.: Retort pouches: an overview. Nat. Food Rev. (USDA), *NFR* 18 (Spring):5, 1982.

Microwave Cooking

(Also see ref. 5, this chapter.)

Cremer, M. L.: Sensory quality and energy use for scrambled eggs and beef patties heated in institutional microwave and convection ovens. J. Food Sci., *47*:871, 1982.

Fruin, J. T., and Guthertz, L. S.: Survival of bacteria in food cooked by microwave oven, conventional oven and slow cookers. J. Food Protect., *45*:695, 1982.

Glasscock, S. J., et al.: Microwave blanching of vegetables for frozen storage. Home Econ. Res. J., *11*:149, 1982.

Tsen, C. C.: Microwave energy for bread baking and its effect on the nutritive value of bread: a review. J. Food Protect., *43*:638, 1980.

Zimmermann, W. J.: Evaluation of microwave cooking procedures and ovens for devitalizing Trichinae in pork roasts. J. Food Sci., *48*:856, 1983.

Food Irradiation

(Also see ref. 10, this chapter.)

Expert Panel on Food Safety and Nutrition of the Institute of Food Technology: Radiation preservation of foods. Food Tech., *37*(Feb.):55, 1983.

Black, E. F., and Libby, L. M.: Commercial food irradiation. Bull. Atomic Sci., *39*(6):48, 1983.

Food Tech., *37*(Feb.):38–61, 1983 (on food irradiation, including legal aspects, pp. 38 and 44; USDA program, p. 46; and other aspects, pp. 48 and 55).

Food Packaging

Anthony, S., Jr.: Package development. Cereal Foods World, *27*:264, 1982.

Bourland, C. T., et al.: Space shuttle food package development. Food Tech., *36*(Sept.):38, 1982.
Keeping food fresh. Consumer Rept., *48*:139, 1983.
McKernan, B. J.: Developments in rigid metal containers for food. Food Tech., *37*(April):134, 1983.

Processing and Nutritive Value

(Also see Chapters 8–12 and refs. 3–10, this chapter.)

Blumenberg, L. S., Snider, S., and Vollmar, E. K.: Quality of green beans and energy required for high temperature processing. Home Econ. Res. J., *11*:143, 1982 (ascorbic acid retention).
Drew, F., and Rhee, K. S.: Energy use, cost, and product quality in preserving vegetables at home by canning, freezing, and dehydration. J. Food Sci., *45*:1561, 1980 (ascorbic acid and carotene retention).
Dudek, J. A., and Elkins, E. R., Jr.: Nutrient composition of historical canned food samples. J. Food Sci., *48*:654, 1983.
Haytowitz, D. B., and Matthews, R. H.: Effect of cooking on nutrient retention of legumes. Cereal Foods World, *28*:362, 1983.
Maeda, E. E., and Salunkhe, D. K.: Retention of ascorbic acid and total carotene in solar dried vegetables. J. Food Sci., *46*:1288, 1981.
Mazza, G., Hung, J., and Dench, M. J.: Processing/nutritional quality changes in potato tubers during growth and long term storage. Canad. Instit. Food Sci. Tech. J., *16*(1):39, 1983.
Reynolds, P., and Phillips, J. A.: Vitamin C retention in orange juice, imitation orange juice, and orange beverage from frozen concentrates. Home Econ. Res. J., *9*:251, 1981.

Food Preservation: General

(Also see refs. 3–11.)

Erickson, L. E.: Recent developments in intermediate moisture foods. J. Food Protect., *45*(April):484, 1982.
Extending the shelf life of fresh foods by combining controlled atmospheres and refrigeration (symposium). Food Tech., *34*(March):44–71, 1980.
Hertzberg, R., Vaughan, B., and Greene, J.: *Putting Food By*, 3rd ed. Marion, Ohio, Consumers Union, 1982.
Thorne, S.: *Developments in Food Preservation I.* Englewood, N. J., 1982.

Microbial Contamination of Food

(Also see refs. 14–19, this chapter.)

Ballintine, C. L., and Herndon, M. L.: Who, why, when and where of food poisons (and what to do about them). FDA Consumer, *16*(July–Aug):24, 1982.
Bryan, F. L.: Epidemiology of milk-borne diseases. J. Food Protect., *46*(7):637, 1983.
Bryan, F. L.: Foodborne disease risk assessment of foodservice establishments in a community. J. Food Protect., *45*(1):93, 1982.
Bryan, F. L., et al.: Hazard analyses of fried, boiled and steamed Cantonese-style foods. J. Food Protect., *45*(5):410, 1982 (also see p. 422 on Chinese-style roast pork, and p. 430 on Hawaiian-style foods).
Center for Disease Control, Public Health Service: *Foodborne Disease Surveillance.* Atlanta, Georgia, Centers for Disease Control, USDHHS, 1983.
Current problems in botulism of interest to the food industry (symposium). Food Tech., *36* (Dec.):85–118, 1982 (also see pp. 58–77 on food microbiology topics).
Kornacki, J. L., and Marth, E. H.: Foodborne illness caused by Escherichia coli: a review. J. Food Protect., *45*:1051, 1982.
Pizzo, P. A., Purvis, D. S., and Waters, C.: Microbiological evaluation of food items. J. Amer. Dietet. Assoc., *81*:272, 1982.
Schwab, A. H., et al.: Microbiological quality of some spices and herbs in retail markets. Appl. Environ. Microb., *44*:627, 1982.
Stewart, A. W.: Effect of cooking on bacteriological populations of "soul foods." J. Food Protect., *46*:19, 1983.
Wehr, H. M.: Attitudes and policies of governmental agencies on microbial criteria for foods—an update. Food Tech., *36*(Sept.):45, 1982.

Nonnutrients and Toxins in Food: Reviews

(Also see refs. 11–25, this chapter.)

Fairweather, F. A. (chairman): Nutrition and toxicology. Proc. Nutr. Soc., *40*:47–94, 1981 (a symposium with 5 articles on various topics).
Foster, E. M.: Food safety: problems of the past and perspectives of the future. J. Food Protect., *45*:658, 1982.
Jelinek, C.: Occurrence and methods of control of chemical contaminants in foods. Environ. Health Persp., *39*:143, 1981.
Ory, R. L. (ed.): *Antinutrients and Natural Toxicants in Foods.* Westport, Conn., Food and Nutrition Press, 1981.
Roy, D. N.: Toxic amino acids and proteins from Lathyrus plants and other leguminous species: a literature review. Nutr. Abstr. Rev.—Series A, *51*:691, 1981.
Wurtman, R. J., and Wurtman, J. J.: *Nutrition and the Brain. Vol. 4: Toxic Effects of Food Constituents on the Brain.* New York, Raven Press, 1979.

Nonnutrients in Food

(Also see Table 18–4, refs. 4 and 12, this chapter, and current issues of J. Food Sci. and J. Agric. Food Chem.).

Anderson, K., et al.: Nitrate and nitrite excretion of humans as influenced by addition of spinach to free-choice diets. Nutr. Rept. Internat., *27*:77, 1983.
Bressani, R., et al.: Tannin in common beans. J. Food Sci., *48*:1000, 1983.
Carlson, D. G., et al.: Glucosinolates in crucifer vegetables: turnips and rutabagas. J. Agric. Food Chem., *29*:1235, 1981.

Coleman, E. C., et al.: Isolation and identification of volatile compounds from baked potatoes. J. Agric. Food Chem., *29*:42, 1981 (228 compounds identified).

Lichtenberger, L. M., et al.: Importance of dietary amines in meal-induced gastrin release. Amer. J. Physiol., *243*:G341, 1982.

Reddy, N. R., et al.: Phytates in legumes and cereals. Adv. Food Res., *28*:1, 1982.

Toxins in Foods

(Also see Table 18–5, and refs. 4, and 13–21, this chapter.)

Brunton, J. (chairman): Safety assessment of drug residues in food-producing animals (symposium). J. Environ. Path. Toxicol., *3*(5–6): 3–139 (13 papers), 1980.

Craun, G. F., et al.: Methaemoglobin levels in young children consuming high-nitrate well water in the United States. Internat. J. Epidem., *10*:309, 1981.

Fisher, T. F.: Plastic food containers (questions and answers). J. Amer. Med. Assoc., *249*:1650, 1983.

Hurst, W. J., et al.: Biogenic amines in chocolate—a review. Nutr. Rept. Internat., *26*:1081, 1982.

Huxtable, R. J.: Herbal teas and toxins: novel aspects of pyrrolizidine poisoning in the United States. Perspect. Biol. Med., *24*:1, 1980.

Roberts, H. J.: Potential toxicity due to dolomite and bonemeal. Southern Med. J., *76*:556, 1983.

Smith, T. A., et al.: Some non-nutritional nitrogenous constituents of foods. Food Chem. *6*:167–263 (7 papers), 1981 (mainly toxic substances).

Food Allergy

(Also see Chapter 23.)

Buckley, R. H., and Metcalfe, D.: Food allergy. J. Amer. Med. Assoc., *248*:2627, 1982.

Food sensitivity. Diary Council Dig., *54*(2):1, 1983.

Pearson, D. J., et al.: Food allergy: how much in the mind? Lancet, *1*:1259, 1983.

Wilson, C. W. M. (chairman): Food allergies in man (symposium) Proc. Nutr. Soc., *42*:213–257 (6 papers), 1983.

Suspected Cancer-Producing Substances and Mutagens in Foods: Books and Reviews

(Also see refs. 15, 19–25, this chapter.)

Hilker, D. M.: Carcinogens occurring naturally in food. Nutr. Cancer, *2*:217, 1981.

Hirono, I.: Natural carcinogenic products of plant origin. CRC Crit. Rev. Toxicol., *8*:235, 1981.

Mutagens in cooked and processed foods (symposium). Food Tech., *36*:48–65, 1982.

Sandler, R. S.: Diet and cancer: Food additives, coffee and alcohol. Nutr. Cancer, *4*:273, 1983.

Suspected Cancer-Producing Substances and Mutagens in Foods: Research Articles

BHA and BHT—positive and negative effects in test conditions (also see Shirai, et al. and food additive listings): Food Cosmet. Toxicol., *19*:147, 1981 (no cancer effects in rats); Toxicology, *21*:95, 1981 (tumors in mouse lungs); Cancer Letters, *14*:219, 1981 (inhibition of mammary tumor in mice); Nutr. Rev., *40*:189, 1982 (a review of BHT on drug metabolism); Bull. Environ. Contam. Toxicol., *29*:115, 1982 (tumor production of BHT in mouse fibroblasts); Environ. Mutagenesis, *5*:353, 1983 (a review); Cancer Res., *41*:4309, 1981, and *42*:1199, 1982; and Carcinogenesis, *3*:15, 1982, and *4*:131, 1983 (the last four references are on the inhibitory effect of BHA on benzopyrene metabolism, a carcinogen).

Bjeldanes, L. F., et al.: Effects of meat composition and cooking conditions on mutagen formation in fried ground beef. J. Agric. Food Chem., *31*:18, 1983.

Bjeldanes, L. F., et al.: Mutagens from the cooking of food, II and III. Food Chem. Toxicol., 20:357 and 369, 1982.

Results of mutagenicity testing, using bacteria, of food-related substances: Cancer Res., *43*:1467, 1983 (beef extracts); Food Chem. Toxicol., *20*:531, 1982 (extracts of soy sauce and beef used in Chinese cooking); Food Chem. Toxicol., *20*:383, 1982 (smoke condensates—mainly negative effects); Cancer, *47*:889, 1981 (nitrite-induced mutagens from human feces); J. Agric. Food Chem., *30*:937, 1982 (dried and salted stored fish); Environ. Mutagenesis, *3*:401, 1981 (72 flavonoids and related substances); J. Amer. Oil Chem. Soc., *60*:576, 1983 (general lack of mutagens in normal deep-fat fried potatoes, onion rings, and fish).

Shirai, T., et al.: Lack of carcinogenicity of butylated hydroxytoluene on long-term administration to $B6C3F_1$ mice. Food Chem. Toxicol., *20*:861, 1982.

Spingarn, N. E., et al.: Formation of mutagens in cooked foods. IV. Effect of fat content in fried beef patties. Cancer Letters, *12*:93, 1981.

Stich, H. F., et al.: Clastogenic activity of dried fruits. Cancer Letters, *12*:1, 1981.

Sugimura, T.: Mutagens, carcinogens and tumor promoters in our daily food. Cancer, *49*:1970, 1982.

Anti-Mutagenicity Activity of Foods

Aspry, K. E., and Bjeldanes, L. F.: Effects of dietary broccoli and butylated hydroxyanisole on liver-mediated metabolism of benzo(a)pyrene. Food Chem. Toxicol., *21*(2):133, 1983.

Joner, P. E., and Dommarsnes, K.: Effects of herbal and ordinary teas on the mutagenicity of benzo(a)pyrene in the Ames test. Acta Agric. Scand., *33*:53, 1983.

Moorman, W. F. B., et al.: Physical properties of dietary fiber and binding of mutagens. J. Food Sci., *48*:1010, 1983.

Nishioka, H., et al.: Human saliva inactivates mutagenicity of carcinogens. Mutation Res., *85*:323, 1981.

Reddy, G. V., et al.: Antitumor activity of yogurt components. J. Food Protect., *46*:8, 1983.

Suwa, Y., et al.: Sulfite suppresses the mutagenic property of coffee. Mutation Res., *102*:383, 1983.

Coffee and Caffeine: Reviews and Popular Articles

(Also see ref. 21, this chapter.)

Benarde, M. A., and Weiss, W.: Coffee consumption and pancreatic cancer. Brit. Med. J., *284*:400, 1982 (no direct relationship found). Also see *285*:214, 1982.

Caffeine: what it does, and how to consume less. Consumer Rept., *46*:595 and 597, 1981 (includes a table of amounts of caffeine in popular foods).

Clark, M., et al.: Is caffeine bad for you? Newsweek (July 19):62, 1982.

Curatolo, P. W., and Robertson, D.: The health consequences of caffeine. Ann. Inter. Med., *98*:641, 1983 (a review).

Feinstein, A. R., et al.: Coffee and pancreatic cancer: the problems of etiologic science and epidemiologic case-control research. J. Amer. Med. Assoc., *246*:957, 1981 (editorial review).

Lecos, C.: Caution light on caffeine. FDA Consumer, *14*(Oct.):6, 1980.

Mosher, B. A.: The Health Effects of Coffee. 2nd Ed. Summit, N. J., American Council on Science and Health, 1983.

Coffee and Caffeine: Cancer and Breast Disease

Ernster, V. L., et al.: Effects of caffeine-free diet on benign breast disease: a randomized trial. Surgery, *91*:263, 1982 (little difference, if any, noted).

Lawson, D. H., et al.: Coffee and tea consumption and breast disease. Surgery, *90*:801, 1981 (little or no relationship found).

MacMahon, B., et al.: Coffee and cancer of the pancreas. New Eng. J. Med., *304*:630, 1981 (also see same issue, p. 1604; Brit. Med. J., *283*:1355, 1981 and *284*:400, 1982; and Lancet, *2*:92, 415, 474, and 689, 1981, for discussion of this paper).

Marrett, L. D., et al.: Coffee drinking and bladder cancer in Connecticut. Amer. J. Epidem., *117*:113, 1983 (some relationship found).

Marshall, J., et al.: Caffeine consumption and benign breast disease: a case-control comparison. Amer. J. Public Health, *72*:610, 1982 (no effect seen).

General Studies of Coffee and Caffeine

Cameron, P., and Boehmer, J.: And coffee too. Internat. J. Addict., *17*:569, 1982.

Cherek, D. R., et al.: Effects of caffeine on human aggressive behavior. Psychiatr. Res., *8*:137, 1983.

Cines, B. M., and Rozin, P.: Some aspects of the liking for hot coffee and coffee flavor. Appetite: J. Intake Res., *3*:23, 1982.

Dobmeyer, D. J., et al.: The arrhythmogenic effects of caffeine in human beings. New Eng. J. Med., *308*:814, 1983 (coffee avoidance by persons with abnormal heart rhythms).

Gilliland, K., and Andress, D,: Ad lib caffeine consumption, symptoms of caffeinism, and academic performance. Amer. J. Psychiatry, *138*:512, 1981.

Gordon, N. F., et al.: Effects of caffeine ingestion on thermoregulatory and myocardial function during endurance performance. South Afric. Med. J., *62*:644, 1982.

Medeiros, D. M.: Caffeinated beverage consumption and blood pressure in Mississippi young adults. Nutr. Rept. Internat., *26*:563, 1982.

Murray, S. S., et al.: Coffee consumption and mortality from ischemic heart disease and other causes. Amer. J. Epidem., *113*:661, 1981.

Rosenberg, L., et al.: Selected birth defects in relation to caffeine-containing beverages. J. Amer. Med. Assoc., *247*:1429, 1982.

Thelle, D. S., et al.: The Tromso heart study—does coffee raise serum cholesterol? New Eng. J. Med., *308*:1454, 1983.

Food Additives: Reviews and General Reading

(Also see refs. 4, 11, 14, 18, and 22–26, this chapter.)

Expert Panel on Food Safety and Nutrition and the Committee on Public Information: *Monosodium Glutamate (MSG)*. Chicago, Instit. of Food Technology, 1980.

Gunnison, A. F.: Sulphite toxicity: a critical review of in vitro and in vivo data. Food Cosmet. Toxicol., *19*:667, 1981.

Hall, R. L., and Merwin, E. J.: The role of flavors. Food Techl., *35*(June):46, 1981.

Middlekauff, R. D.: Food and color additives: where do we go from here? Cereal Foods World, *26*(June):273, 1981.

Smith, J. L., and Palumbo, S. A.: Microorganisms as food additives. J. Food Protect., *44*:936, 1981.

Wintermantel, J.: If it isn't needed, don't use it. Cereal Foods World, *26*:631, 1981.

Nonnutritive and Nutritive Sweeteners

Arnold, D. L.: Two-generation saccharin bioassays. Environ. Health Perspect., *50*(April):27, 1983.

FDA Consumer, *15*(May):27, 1981; *15*(Sept.):8, 1981; and *16*(June):10, 1982 (various authors on nonnutritive sweeteners).

Horwitz, D. L., and Bauer-Nehrling, J. K.: Can aspartame meet our expectations? J. Amer. Dietet. Assoc., *83*:142, 1983.

Howe, G. R., and Burch, J. D.: Artificial sweeteners in relation to the epidemiology of bladder cancer. Nutr. Cancer, *2*:213, 1981.

Morrison, A. S., et al.: Artificial sweeteners and bladder cancer in Manchester, U. K., and Nagoya, Japan. Brit. J. Cancer, *45*:332, 1982 (no risk found with saccharin).

Rose, D. J., and Anderson, J. J. B.: Sweeteners in our society. World Rev. Nutr. Dietet., *41*:200, 1983.

Silverman, D. J., et al.: Artificial sweeteners and lower urinary tract cancer. Amer. J. Epidem., *117*:326, 1983.

Walker, A. M., et al.: An independent analysis of the National Cancer Institute study on nonnutritive sweeteners and bladder cancer. Amer. J. Public Health, *72*:376, 1982.

Widespread use of aspartame stymied by its high cost. Chem. Eng. News, *61*(June 13), 1983.

Wurtman, R. J.: Neurochemical changes following high-dose aspartame with dietary carbohydrates. New Eng. J. Med., *309*:429, 1983.

Nitrates and Nitrites in Food

An assessment of nitrite for the prevention of botulism (symposium). Food Tech., *34*(May):228–254 (6 papers), 1980.

Boddé, T.: Nitrite report stirs little controversy: alternatives being explored. Bioscience, *32*:90, 1982.

Green, L. C., et al.: Nitrate biosynthesis in man. Proc. Nat. Acad. Sci., *78*:7764, 1981.

Kurzer, M. S., and Calloway, D. H.: Nitrate and nitrogen balances in men. Amer. J. Clin. Nutr., *34*:1305, 1981.

Marriott, N. G., et al.: Use of nitrite and nitrite-sparing agents in meats: review. J. Food Protect., *44*:881, 1981.

BHA and BHT in Food

(Also see page A.65.)

Babich, H.: Butylated hydroxytoluene (BHT): a review. Environ. Res., *29*:1, 1982.

Deschner, E. E., and Wattenberg, L. W.: The proliferative effect of dietary butylated hydroxyanisole on methylazoxymethanol treated colonic mucosa. Cancer Letters, *16*:197, 1982.

Hansen, E. V., et al.: Study on toxicity of butylated hydroxyanisole (BHA) in pregnant gilts and their foetuses. Toxicology, *23*:79, 1982 (no defects noticed in reproduction data).

Vorhees, C. V., et al.: Developmental neurobehavioral toxicity of butylated hydroxyanisole (BHA) in rats. Neurobehav. Toxicol. Teratol., *3*:321, 1981 (high levels of BHA not as toxic as BHT).

Food Colors and Hypersensitivity

Expert Panel on Food Safety and Nutrition and the Committee on Public Information: *Food Colors*. Chicago, Institute of Food Technology, 1980.

Francis, F. J.: Natural food colorants. Cereal Foods World, *26*:565, 1981.

Lipton, M. A., and Mayo, J. P.: Diet and hyperkinesis—an update. J. Amer. Dietet. Assoc., *83*:132, 1983.

Little, A. C.: The eyes have it. J. Amer. Dietet. Assoc., 77:688, 1980 (on food colors).

Silbergeld, E. K., and Anderson, S. M.: Artificial food colors and childhood behavior disorders. Bull. N.Y. Acad. Med., *58*:275, 1982.

Weiss, B.: The behavioral toxicity of food additives. Nutr. Update, *1*:21, 1983.

Food Safety: Risk and Benefits

Campbell, T. C.: Chemical carcinogens and human risk assessment. Fed. Proc., *39*:2467, 1980.

Clydesdale, F. M.: Nutritional consequences of technology. J. Food Protect., *45*(9):859, 1982.

Foster, E. M.: Is there a food safety crisis? Food Technol., *36*(Aug.):82, 1982.

Goldblith, S. A. (chairman): Risk versus benefits: the future of food safety (symposium). Nutr. Rev., *38*:33 (3 papers), 1980.

Gray, J. I., and Morton, I. D.: Some toxic compounds produced in food by cooking and processing. J. Human Nutr., *35*:5, 1981 (160 references).

Hutt, P. B.: Regulating carcinogenic food contaminants. Cereal Foods World, *26*(Feb.):81, 1981.

Lecos, C.: Determining when a food poses a hazard. FDA Consumer, *17*(June):25, 1983.

Possible mechanisms of thresholds for carcinogens and other toxic substances. J. Amer. College Toxicol., *2*:1–321 (23 papers), 1983.

Food Enrichment

(Also see ref. 26, this chapter.)

Emodi, A. S., and Scialpi, L.: Quality of bread fortified with ten micronutrients. Cereal Chem., *57*:1, 1980.

Quick, J. A., and Murphy, E. W.: *Fortification of Foods: A Review.* Washington D.C., Information Division, Food Safety and Inspection Service, USDA, pp. 1–39, 1982.

Food Regulations and Food Purchasing

(Also see refs. 27–32, and current issues of FDA Consumer and National Food Review.)

Blanciforti, L.: Expenditures on nutritious foods. National Food Rev. (USDA), *NFR 17*:18, Winter 1982.

Food spending and income. National Food Rev. (USDA), *NFR 22*:21, Spring 1983.

Government to consider simpler nutrition labels. Consumer Rept., *48*:108, 1983.

Morgan, K. J., et al.: Household size and the cost of nutritionally equivalent diets. Amer. J. Public Health, *73*:530, 1983.

Schaus, E. E., and Briggs, G. M.: Economical foods—based on the number of USRDA nutrients purchased for one dollar. J. Nutr. Educ., *15:*130, 1983.

Senauer, B.: The current status of food and nutrition policy and the food programs Amer. J. Agric. Econ., *64*:1009, 1982.

The 75th anniversary issue of the FDA. FDA Consumer, *15*:4–64, 1981 (food safety, labels, etc.).

Stephenson, M. G.: FDA view of nutrition regulations. Cereal Foods World, *28*:143, 1983.

Wallerstein, M. B.: Dynamics of food policy formulation in the USA. Food Policy, 7:229, 1982.

Whitfield, R. A.: A nutritional analysis of the food stamp program. Amer. J. Public Health, 72:793, 1982.

Wills, R. L., and Mentzer, R. L.: The effect of generics on the food market structure. Nat. Food Rev. (USDA), *NFR 18*:7, Spring 1982.

Quality of Specific Foods

Cala, R. F., Morgan, K. J., and Zabik, M. E.: The contribution of children's snacks to total dietary intakes. Home Econ. Res. J., *10*:150, 1981.

Consumer information in Consumer Reports on: frozen pot pies, *46*:555, 1981; fish 'n chips, *47*:237, 1982;

frozen fried chicken, *47*:362, 1982; breads, *47*:438, 1982; 'fruit' drinks, *47*:456, 1982; peanut butter, *47*:522, 1982; coffee, *48*:110, 1983; beer, *48*:342, 1983; tomato and vegetable juices, *48*:499, 1983; yogurt, *48*:386, 1983; ketchup, *48*:552, 1983.

Douglass, J. S., and Matthews, R. M.: Nutrient content of pasta products. Cereal Foods World, *27*:558, 1982.

Dunkley, W. L. (chairman): Our industry today—reducing fat in milk and dairy products. J. Dairy Sci., *65*:442 (11 papers) 1982.

Fenner, L.: The spices of life. FDA Consumer, *17*(6):10, 1983.

Food. 3. Eating the Moderate Fat and Cholesterol Way. Chicago, American Dietetic Association, 1982.

Hopkins, H.: All you knead to know about bread. FDA Consumer, *16*(Feb.):16, 1982.

Kinsman, D. M.: A fresh look at processed meats. Food Nutr. News, *53*(5):1, 1982.

Snack foods. Cereal Foods World, *28*:284–305, 1983 (industry and consumer viewpoints).

Chapter 19 Food Beliefs and Eating Patterns

Dwyer, J. T., et al.: The 'new' vegetarians: group affiliation and dietary strictures related to attitudes and life style. J. Amer. Dietet. Assoc., *64*:376, 1974.

Farb, T. P., and Armelagos, G.: *Consuming Passions: The Anthropology of Eating.* Boston, Houghton Mifflin, 1980.

Freedman, R. L.: *Human Food Uses. A Cross-cultural, Comprehensive Annotated Bibliography.* Westport, Conn., Greenwood Press, 1981.

Greene, L. S. (ed.): *Malnutrition, Behavior and Social Organization.* New York, Academic Press, 1977.

Haas, J. D., and Harrison, G. G.: Nutritional anthropology and biological adaptation. Ann. Rev. Anthropol., *6*:69, 1977.

Harrison, G. G., Rathje, W. L., and Hughes, W. W.: Food waste behavior in an urban population. J. Nutr. Educ., 7:13, 1973.

Harwood, A.: The hot-cold theory of disease. Implications for treatment of Puerto Rican patients. J. Amer. Med. Assoc., *216*:1153, 1971.

Hertzler, A. A., Wenkam, N., and Standal, B.: Classifying cultural food habits and meanings. J. Amer. Dietet. Assoc., *80*:421, 1982.

Jarvis, W. T.: Food faddism, cultism, and quackery. Ann. Rev. Nutr., *3*:35, 1983.

Jelliffee, E. F. P., and Jelliffe, D. B.: *Adverse Effects of Food.* New York, Plenum, 1982.

King, S.: Eating behaviour and attitudes to food, nutrition and health. Brit. Nutr. Foundation, Nutr. Bull., 7(2):89, 1982.

Onuoha, G. B. I.: The changing scene of food habits and beliefs among the Mbaise people of Nigeria. Ecol. Food Nutr., *11*:245, 1982.

Robson, J. R. K.: Contribution of anthropology to the assessment of nutritional status. Symposium. Fed. Proc., *37*:47, 1978.

Root, W., and De Rochement, R.: *Eating in America: A History.* New York, Ecco Press, 1976.

Sanjur, D.: *Social and Cultural Perspectives in Nutrition.* Englewood Cliffs, N.J., Prentice-Hall, 1982.

Simoons, F. J.: *Eat Not This Flesh. Food Avoidance in the Old World.* Madison, Univ. of Wisconsin Press, 1967.

Snow, L. F., and Johnson, S. M.: Folklore, food, female reproductive cycle. Ecol. Food Nutr., 7:41, 1978.

Yeung, D. L., Cheung, W. Y., and Sabry, J. H.: The hot-cold food concept in Chinese culture and its application in a Canadian-Chinese community. J. Canad. Dietet. Assoc., *34*:1, 1973.

Chapter 20 Applied Nutrition

Ahlstrom, A., and Rasanen, L.: Review of food grouping systems in nutrition education. J. Nutr. Educ., *5*:13, 1973 (international).

Allen, D. E., Patterson, Z. J., and Warren, G. L.: Nutrition, family commensality, and academic performance among high school youth. J. Home Econ., *62*:333, 1970.

American Academy of Pediatrics: Nutritional aspects of vegetarianism, health foods and fad diets. Pediatrics, *59*:460, 1977.

Anderson, B. M., Gibson, R. S., and Sabry, J. H.: The iron and zinc status of long-term vegetarian women. Amer. J. Clin. Nutr., *34*:1042, 1981.

Beaton, G. H., et al.: Sources of variance in 24-hour dietary recall data: implications for nutrition study design and interpretation. Carbohydrate sources, vitamins and minerals. Amer. J. Clin. Nutr., *37*:986, 1983.

Dwyer, J. T., et al.: Nutritional status of vegetarian children. Amer. J. Clin. Nutr., *35*:204, 1982.

Food and Nutrition Board: *Proposed System for Assessing Changing Food Consumption Patterns and Their Effect on Nutrient Intake and Health.* Washington, D.C., National Academy of Science, 1981.

Garn, S. M., Clark, D. C., and Guire, K. E.: Husband-wife similarities in hemoglobin levels. Ecol. Food Nutr., *5*:47, 1976.

Gillespie, A. H., and Roderuck, C. E.: A method for developing a nutrient guide. Home Econ. Res. J., *11*:21, 1982.

Hegsted, D. M.: What is a healthful diet? Primary Care, *9*:445, 1982.

Hertzler, A. A., and Anderson, H. L.: Food guides in the United States. J. Amer. Dietet. Assoc., *64*:19, 1974.

Jankelson, O. M., et al.: Effect of coffee on glucose tolerance and circulating insulin in men with maturity-onset diabetes. Lancet, *1*:527, 1967.

King, J. C., et al.: Evaluation and modifcation of the basic four food guide. J. Nutr. Educ., *10*:27, 1978.

Lansky, D., and Brownell, K. D.: Estimates of food quantity and calories: errors in self-report among obese patients. Amer. J. Clin. Nutr., *35*:727, 1982.

Marrs, D. C.: Milk drinking by the elderly of three races. J. Amer. Dietet. Assoc., *72*:495, 1978.

Ohlson, M. A., and Harper, L. J.: Longitudinal studies of food intake and weight of women from ages 18 to 56 years. J. Amer. Dietet. Assoc., *69*:626, 1976.

Pao, E. M.: Changes in American food consumption patterns and their nutritional significance. Food Tech., *35*:43, 1981.

Patten, S. E.: Nutrition and the elderly: a cultural perspective. Geriatrics, *37*:141, 1982.

Pollitt, E., Leibel, R. L., and Greenfield, D.: Brief fasting, stress, and cognition in children. Amer. J. Clin. Nutr., *24*:1526, 1981.

Ross, M. H.: Dietary behavior and longevity. Nutr. Rev., *35*:257, 1977.

Saraswathi, G., Umpathy, K. P., and Renukadevi, B. C.: Effect of selected breakfast items on blood sugar level and its relationship to choice reaction time and span of attention during late morning hours in college women. Indian J. Nutr. Dietet., *18*:209, 1981.

Schutz, H. G., et al.: Food supplement usage in seven western states. Amer. J. Clin. Nutr., *36*:897, 1982.

Siegel, R. K.: Herbal intoxication: psychoactive effects from herbal cigarettes, tea and capsules. J. Amer. Med. Assoc., *236*:473, 1976.

Swenerton, H., and Dunkley, W. L.: Recent activities of public agencies to assure healthful diets for Americans. J. Dairy Sci., *65*:484, 1982. Symposium: Assessment of nutritional status. Amer. J. Clin. Nutr., *35*(supplement):1112, 1982.

Welsh, S. O., and Marston, R. M.: Review of trends in food use in the United States, 1909–1980. J. Amer. Dietet. Assoc., *81*:120, 1982.

Wretlind, A.: Standards for nutritional adequacy of the diet: European and WHO/FAO viewpoints. Amer. J. Clin. Nutr., *36*:366, 1982.

Chapter 21 Nutrition, Sports, and Physical Activity

Ahlborg, G., et al.: Substrate turnover during prolonged exercise in man: splanchnic and leg metabolism of glucose, free fatty acids, and amino acids. J. Clin. Invest., *53*:1080, 1974.

Anderson, H. T., and Barkue, H.: Iron deficiency and muscular work performance. Scand. J. Lab. Clin. Invest., *25*(supplement):114, 1970.

Baecke, J. A. H., Burema, J., and Frijters, J. E. R.: A short questionnaire for the measurement of habitual physical activity in epidemiological studies. Amer. J. Clin. Nutr., *36*:936, 1982.

Bortz, W. M., et al.: Catecholamines, depamine, and endorphin levels during extreme exercise. New Eng. J. Med., *305*:466, 1981.

Brooks, G. A., and Gaesser, G. A.: End points of lactate and glucose metabolism after exhausting exercise. J. Appl. Physiol., *49*:1057, 1980.

Chavez, A., Martinez, C., and Bourges, H.: Nutrition and development of infants from poor rural areas. 2. Nutritional level and physical activity. Nutr. Rept. Internat., *5*:139, 1972.

Davies, C. T. M.: Physiological responses to exercise in East African children. 2. The effects of schistosomiasis, anemia and malnutrition. J. Trop. Pediatr., *19*:115, 1973.

Emiola, M., and O'Shea, J. P.: Effects of physical activity and nutrition on bone density measured by radiographic techniques. Nutr. Rept. Internat., *17*:669, 1978.

Folkens, C. H., et al.: Physical fitness training and mental health. Amer. Psychol., *36*:373, 1981.

Frisch, R. E., et al.: Delayed menarche and amenorrhea of college athletes in relation to age of onset of training. J. Amer. Med. Assoc., *246*:1559, 1981.

Garlaschi, C., et al.: Effect of physical exercise on secretion of growth hormone, glucagon, and cortisol in obese and diabetic children. Diabetes, *24*:758, 1975.

Hirsch, E., Ball, E., and Godkin, L.: Sex differences in the effect of voluntary activity on sucrose-induced obesity. Physiol. Behavior, *29*:253, 1982.

Ingram, D. K., Reynolds, M. A., and Goodrick, C. L.: Relationship of sex, exercise, and growth rate to life span in the Wistar rat: a multivariate correlational approach. Gerontology, *28*:23, 1982.

Jetté, M., et al.: The nutritional and metabolic effects of a carbohydrate-rich diet in a glycogen supercompensation training regimen. Amer. J. Clin. Nutr., *32*:2140, 1978.

Johnson, C. C., et al.: Diet and exercise in middle-aged men. J. Amer. Dietet. Assoc., *81*:695, 1982.

Liebman, M., et al.: Effects of coarse wheat bran fiber and exercise on plasma lipids and lipoproteins in moderately overweight men. Amer. J. Clin. Nutr., *36*:71, 1983.

Lopes, J., et al.: Skeletal muscle function in malnutrition. Amer. J. Clin. Nutr., *36*:602, 1982.

Marable, N. L., et al.: Urinary nitrogen excretion as influenced by muscle building exercise programs and protein intake variation. Nutr. Rept. Internat., *19*:795, 1979.

Mayer, J., and Bullen, B.: Nutrition and athletic performance. Physiol. Rev., *40*:369, 1960.

Millward, D. J., et al.: Effect of exercise on protein metabolism in humans as explored with stable isotopes. Fed. Proc., *41*:2686, 1982.

Parizkova, J.: *Nutrition, Physical Fitness and Health.* Internat. Series on Sports Sciences. Vol. 7. Baltimore, University Park Press, 1978.

Ransford, C. P.: A role for amines in the antidepressant effect of exercise: a review. Med. Sci. Sports Exercise, *14*:1, 1982.

Rebar, R. W., and Cumming, D. C.: Reproductive function in women athletes. J. Amer. Med. Assoc., *246*:1590, 1981.

Richard, D., et al.: Role of exercise-training in the prevention of hyperinsulinemia caused by high energy diet. J. Nutr., *112*:1756, 1982.

Salonen, J. T., Tuomilehto, J., and Puska, P.: The relation of physical activity to changes in serum cholesterol and body weight in a three-year follow-up of population sample. Scand. J. Med., *9*:109, 1981.

Sidney, K. H., et al.: Endurance training and body composition of the elderly. Amer. J. Clin. Nutr., *30*:326, 1977.

Smith, M. P., et al.: Exercise intensity, dietary intake, and high-density lipoprotein cholesterol in young female competitive swimmers. Amer. J. Clin. Nutr., *36*:251, 1982.

Smith, N. J.: Gaining and losing weight in athletics. J. Amer. Med. Assoc., *236*:149, 1976.

Tsai, A. C., Bach, J., and Borer, K. T.: Somatic, endocrine and serum lipid changes during detraining in adult hamsters. Amer. J. Clin. Nutr., *34*: 373, 1981.

Westerman, R.: Fluid and electrolyte replacement in sweating athletes. J. Amer. Med. Assoc., *212*:1713, 1970.

Woo, R., Garrow, J. S., and Pi-Sunyer, F. X.: Effect of exercise on spontaneous calorie intake in obesity. Amer. J. Clin. Nutr., *36*:470, 1982.

Young, V. R., and Torun, B.: Physical activity: impact on protein and amino acid metabolism and implications for nutritional requirements. In Harper, A. E., and Davis, G. U. (eds.): *Nutrition in Health and Disease and International Development* (The XII International Congress of Nutrition, San Diego, California). New York, Alan R. Liss, Inc., 1981.

Chapter 22 Nutrition, Pregnancy, and Lactation

Bwesey, R. G., and Watson, M. L.: The effect of sodium restriction during gestation on offspring brain development in rats. Amer. J. Clin. Nutr., *37*:43, 1983.

Chan, G. M., et al.: Growth and bone mineralization of normal breast-fed infants and the effects of lactation on maternal bone mineral status. Amer. J. Clin. Nutr., *36*:438, 1982.

Cherry, F. F., et al.: Plasma zinc in hypertension/toxemia and other reproductive variables in adolescent pregnancy. Amer. J. Clin. Nutr., *34*:2367. 1981.

Committee on Nutrition of Mother and Preschool Child, NRC: *Alternative Dietary Practices and Nutritional Abuses in Pregnancy.* Washington, D.C., National Academy Press, 1982.

Danford, D. E.: Pica and nutrition. Ann. Rev. Nutr., *2*:303, 1982.

Delgado, H., et al.: Nutrition and length of gestation. Nutr. Res., *2*:117, 1982.

Doyle, W., et al.: Dietary survey during pregnancy in a low socio-economic group. Human Nutr.: Appl. Nutr., *36A*:95, 1982.

Garn, S. M., Hoff, K., and McCabe, K. D.: Is there nutritional mediation of the "smoking effect" on the fetus? Amer. J. Clin. Nutr., *32*:1181, 1979.

Glenn, F. B., Glenn, W. D., and Duncan, R. C.: Fluoride tablet supplementation during pregnancy for caries immunity: a study of offspring produced. Amer. J. Obst. Gyn., *153*:560, 1982.

Goldfarb, J., and Tibbetts, E.: *Breastfeeding Handbook. A Practical Reference for Physicians, Nurses and Other Health Professionals.* Hillside, N.J. Enslow, 1981.

Groisser, D. S., Rosso, P., and Winick, M.: Coffee consumption during pregnancy: subsequent behavioral abnormalities of the offspring. J. Nutr., *112*:829, 1982.

Hicks, L. E., Langham, R. A., and Takenaka, J.: Cognitive and health measures following early nutritional supplementation: a sibling study. Amer. J. Public Health, *72*:1110, 1982.

Hingson, R., et al.: Effects of maternal drinking and marijuana use on fetal growth and development. Pediatrics, *70*:539, 1982.

Hytten, F. E., and Leitch, I.: *The Physiology of Human Pregnancy.* 2nd Ed. Philadelphia, J. B. Lippincott, 1971.

King, J. C., Stein, T., and Doyle, M.: Effect of vegetarianism on the zinc status of pregnant women. Amer. Clin. Nutr., *34*:1049, 1981.

Linn, S., et al.: No association between coffee consumption and adverse outcomes of pregnancy. New Eng. J. Med., *306*:141, 1982 (see discussion of this and other papers in letters to the editor New Eng. J. Med., *306*:1548–1550, 1982.)

Lonnerdal, B., Forsum, E., and Hambraeus, L.: A longitudinal study of the protein, nitrogen, and lactose contents of human milk from Swedish well-nourished mothers. Amer. J. Clin. Nutr., *29*:1127, 1976.

Naismith, D. J., Richardson, D. P., and Pritchard, A. E.: The utilization of protein and energy during lactation in the rat with particular regard to the use of fat accumulated in pregnancy. Brit. J. Nutr., *48*:433, 1982.

Nongovernmental Organization on UNICEF: Symposium. Women and breastfeeding: promotion, support, and community action. New York, 866 United Nations Plaza, 1981.

Pau, M-Y., and Milner, J. A.: Effect of arginine deficiency on mammary gland development in the rat. J. Nutr., *112*:1827, 1982.

Pereira, M., et al.: Effects of prenatal nutritional supplementation on the placenta: report of a randomized controlled trial. Amer. J. Clin. Nutr., *36*:229, 1982.

Picone, T. A., et al.: Pregnancy outcome in North American women. II. Effects of diet, cigarette smoking, stress, and weight gain on placentas, and on neonatal physical and behavioral characteristics. Amer. J. Clin. Nutr., *36*:1214, 1982.

Raman, L., et al.: Effect of calcium supplementation to undernourished mothers during pregnancy on the bone density of neonates. Amer. J. Clin. Nutr., *31*:466, 1978.

Ruth, R. E., and Goldsmith, S. K.: Interaction between zinc deprivation and acute ethanol intoxication during pregnancy in rats. J. Nutr., *111*:2034, 1981.

Saner, G,: Urinary chromium excretion during pregnancy and its relationship with intravenous glucose loading. Amer. J. Clin. Nutr., *34*:1676, 1981.

Schuster, K., Bailey, L. B., and Mahan, C. S.: Vitamin B_6 status of low-income adolescent and adult pregnant women and the condition of their infants at birth. Amer. J. Clin. Nutr., *34*:1731, 1981.

Tracy. T., and Miller, G. L.: Obstetric problems of the massively obese. Obst. Gyn., *33*:204, 1969.

Widdowson, E. M., and Cowen, J.: The effect of protein deficiency and calorie deficiency on the reproduction of rats. Brit. J. Nutr., *27*:85, 1972.

Wynn, M., and Wynn, A.: The importance of maternal nutrition in the weeks before and after conception. Birth, *9*:39, 1982.

Chapter 23 Nutrition in Infancy and Childhood

History and Review

Anderson, S. A., Chinn, H. I., and Fisher, K. D.: History and current status of infant formulas. Amer. J. Clin. Nutr., *35*:381, 1982.

Ashworth, A., et al.: Infant and young child feeding—an annotated bibliography. Early Human Develop., *6*(Suppl):S1–S165, 1982.

Baer, M. T.: Nutrition and development disabilities. Nutr. Update, *1*:179, 1983.

Briggs, C.: Recent developments in infant feeding and nutrition. Nutr. Update, *1*:227, 1983.

Cohen, S. A.: *Happy Babies, Happy Kids.* New York, Delilah Books, 1982 (see review in Amer. J. Dis. Children, *137*:93, 1983).

Jelliffe, D. B., and Jelliffe, E. F. P.: *Human Milk in the Modern World.* Oxford, Oxford University Press, 1978.

Lebenthal, E., et al.: Impact of development of the gastrointestinal tract on infant feeding. J. Pediatr., *102*:1, 1983.

Radbill, S. X.: Infant feeding through the ages. Clin. Pediatr., *20*:613, 1981.

Suskind, R. M. (ed.): *Textbook of Pediatric Nutrition.* New York: Raven Press, 1981.

Tsang, R. C., and Nichols, B. L. (eds.): *Nutrition and Child Health: Perspectives for the 1980s.* New York: Alan R. Liss, Inc. 1981.

Whitehead, R. G.: Nutritional aspects of human lactation. Lancet, *1*:167, 1983.

Winick, M.: *Growing Up Healthy: A Parent's Guide to Good Nutrition.* New York, William Morrow & Co., 1982 (see review in Amer. J. Dis. Children, *137*:93, 1983).

Nutrition and Growth

Costom, B. H.: Effect of a comprehensive nutritional program on the growth and ponderosity of infants. Clin. Pediatr., *22*:105, 1983.

Ernst, J. A., et al.: Growth outcome of the very low-birth-weight infant at one year. J. Amer. Dietet. Assoc., *82*:44, 1983.

Falkner, F., and Tanner, J. M., (eds.): *Human Growth: Vol. III: Neurobiology and Nutrition.* London: Bailliere Tindall, 1979.

Ferris, A. G., et al.: The effect of diet on weight gain in infancy. Amer. J. Clin. Nutr., *33*:2635, 1980.

Graham, G. G. et al.: Later growth of malnourished infants and children. Amer. J. Dis. Children, *136*:348, 1982.

Hammill, P. V., et al.: Physical growth: National Center for Health Statistics percentiles. Amer. J. Clin. Nutr., *32*:607, 1979.

Morris, A. M., et al.: Anthropomorphic measurements of 3, 4, 5 and 6 year old girls and boys. Growth, *44*:253, 1980.

Roche, A. F., and Himes, J. H.: Incremental growth charts. Amer. J. Clin. Nutr., *33*:2041, 1982.

Spurr, G. B., et al.: Marginal malnutrition in school-aged Colombian boys: anthropometry and maturation. Amer. J. Clin. Nutr., *37*:119, 1983.

Breast-Feeding: General

Bloom, K., et al.: Breast versus formula feeding. Acta Paediatr. Scand. *Suppl. 300*: 1–26, (3 papers), 1982.

Brown, R. E.: Breast-feeding and family planning: a review of the relationships. Amer. J. Clin. Nutr., *35*:162, 1982.

Goldman, A. S., et al.: Immunologic factors in human milk during the first year of lactation. J. Pediatr., *100*:563, 1982.

Hilden, J., et al.: Contraceptives and the new trend in breast-feeding—a causal connection? J. Trop. Pediatr., *29*:40, 1983.

Kaplowitz, D. D., and Olson, C. M.: The effect of an education program on the decision to breastfeed. J. Nutr. Educ., *15*:61, 1983.

La Leche League International: *The Womanly Art of Breastfeeding.* Franklin Park, Illinois, 1981.

Lawrence, R. A.: *Breast Feeding: A Guide for the Medical Profession.* St. Louis, C. V. Mosby, 1980.

Lawrence, R. A.: Practices and attitudes toward breast-feeding among medical professionals. Pediatrics, *70*:912, 1982.

Martinez, G. A., and Nalezienski, J. P.: 1980 update: The recent trend in breast-feeding. Pediatrics, *67*:260, 1981.

Myres, A. W.: Breast-feeding: a Canadian perspective on a global priority. Canad. Med. Assoc. J., *125*:1078, 1981.

Ogra, P. L., and Greene, H. L.: Human milk and breastfeeding—an update on the state of the art. Pediatr. Res., *16*:266, 1982.

Paine, R., and Coble, R. J.: Breast-feeding and infant health in a rural U.S. community. Amer. J. Dis. Child., *136*:36, 1982.

Popkin, B. M., et al.: Breast-feeding patterns in low-income countries. Science, *218*:1088, 1982.

Roberts, C. C., et al: Adequate bone mineralization in breast-fed infants. J. Pediatr., *99*:192, 1981.

Weinstein, L.: Breast milk—a natural resource. Amer. J. Obst. Gyn., *136*:973, 1980.

Welch, R. M., and Findlay, J. W. A.: Excretion of drugs in human milk. Drug Metabolism Rev., *12*:261, 1981.

Welsh, J. K., and May, J. T.: Anti-infective properties of breastmilk. J. Pediatr., *94*:1, 1979.

Young, H. B., et al.: Milk and lactation: Some social and developmental correlates among 1000 infants. Pediatrics, *69*:169, 1982.

Committee Reports

Breast-feeding: a commentary of the Canadian Pediatric Society and the American Academy of Pediatrics. Pediatrics, *62*:591, 1978.

Committee on Nutrition, American Academy of Pediatrics: Nutrition and lactation. Pediatrics, *68*:435, 1981.

Committee on Nutrition, American Academy of Pediatrics: The promotion of breast feeding. Pediatrics, *69*:654, 1982.

Infant feeding: General

Andrew, E. M., Clancy, K. L., and Katz, M.: Infant feeding practices of families belonging to a prepaid group practice health plan. Pediatrics, *65*:978, 1980.

Andrew, E. M., Clancy, K. L., and Katz, M. Sources of kilocalories and micronutrients in the infant diet. J. Amer. Dietet. Assoc., *79*:131, 1981.

Barness, L. A.: Who gives nutritional advice? Who follows it? Pediatrics, *65*:1045, 1980.

Cala, R. F., Morgan, K. J., and Zabik, M. E.: The contribution of children's snacks to total dietary intakes. Home Econ. Res. J., *10*:150, 1981.

Child nutrition programs update (U.S.). Dairy Council Digest, *53*(6):31, 1982.

Farris, R. P., et al.: Influence of milk source on serum lipids and lipoproteins during the first year of life: Bogalusa Heart Study. Amer. J. Clin. Nutr., *35*:42, 1982.

Fomon, S. J., et al.: Recommendations for feeding normal infants. Pediatrics, *63*:52, 1979.

Foman, S. J. et al.: Sweetness of diet and food consumption by infants. Proc. Soc. Exp. Biol. Med., *173*:190, 1983.

McBeath, W. H.: Taster's choice boycott. Amer. J. Public Health, *73*:640, 1983 (editorial on policies of advertising infant foods).

Myres, A. W., Pediatric nutrition topics. J. Canad. Dietet. Assoc., *43*:284 (4 papers), 1982.

Pao, E. M., Himes, J. M., and Roche, A. F.: Milk intakes and feeding patterns of breast-fed infants. J. Amer. Dietet. Assoc., 77:540, 1980.

Pollitt, E., and Wirtz, S.: Mother-infant feeding interaction and weight gain in the first month of life. J. Amer. Diet. Assoc., *78*:596, 1981.

Roy, S., III.: Perspectives on adverse effects of milks and infant formulas used in infant feeding. J. Amer. Dietet. Assoc., *82*:373, 1983.

Sandström, B., et al.: Zinc absorption from human milk, cow's milk, and infant formulas. Amer. J. Dis. Children, *137*:726, 1983.

Sarett, H. P., et al.: Decisions on breast-feeding or formula feeding and trends in infant-feeding practices. Amer. J. Dis. Children, *137*:719, 1983.

Ziegler, E. E., and Foman, S. J.: Lactose enhances mineral absorption in infancy. J. Pediatr. Gastro. Nutr., *2*:288, 1983.

Infant Feeding: Committee Reports and Miscellaneous

Committee on Nutrition, Academy of Pediatrics: On the feeding of supplemental foods to infants. Pediatrics, *65*:1178, 1980.

Committee on Nutrition, American Academy of Pediatrics: The use of whole cow's milk in infancy. Pediatrics, 72:253, 1983.

Infant formula regulation and infant food problems (symposium). J. Assoc. Off. Anal. Chem., *65*:1471–1509 (10 papers), 1982 (including analysis and nutritional adequacy).

WHO/UNICEF statement on infant and young child feeding. WHO Chronicle, *33*:435, 1979.

Nutrient Requirements and Intakes: General

Bruhn, J. C., and Franke, A. A.: Iodine in human milk. J. Dairy Sci., *66*:1396, 1983.

Casey, C. E., Walravens, P. A., and Hambidge, K. M.: Availability of zinc: loading tests with human milk, cow's milk and infant formulas. Pediatrics, *68*:394, 1981.

Feeley, R. M., et al.: Calcium, phosphorus, and magnesium contents of human milk during early lactation. J. Pediatr. Gastro. Nutr., *2*:262, 1983.

Finberg, L.: Human milk feeding and vitamin D supplementation—1981. J. Pediatr., *99*:228, 1981 (editorial).

Garza, C., et al.: Changes in the nutrient composition of human milk during gradual weaning. Amer. J. Clin. Nutr., *37*:61, 1983.

Harzer, G., et al.: Changing patterns of human milk lipids in the course of the lactation and during the day. Amer. J. Clin. Nutr., *37*:612, 1983. (Also see Bitman, J., et al.: Amer. J. Clin. Nutr., *38*:300, 1983.)

Johnston, L., Vaughan, L., and Fox, H. M.: Pantothenic acid content of human milk. Amer. J. Clin. Nutr., *34*:2205, 1981.

Lönnerdal, B., et al.: Iron, zinc, copper, and manganese in infant formulas. Amer. J. Dis. Children, *137*:443, 1983.

Mackillop, F. M., and Durnin, J. V. G. A.: The energy and nutrient intake of a random sample (305) of infants. Human Nutr.: Appl. Nutr., *36A*:405, 1982.

Matoth, Y., et al.: Folate nutrition and growth in infancy. Arch. Dis. Childhood, *54*:699, 1979.

Morck, T. A., et al.: Iron availability from infant food supplements. Amer. J. Clin. Nutr., *34*:2630, 1981.

Reeve, L. E., et al.: Vitamin D of human milk: identification of biologically active forms. Amer. J. Clin. Nutr., *36*:122, 1982.

Sadowitz, P. D., and Oski, F. A.: Iron status and infant feeding practices in an urban ambulatory center. Pediatrics, 72:33, 1983.

Walter, T., et al.: Effect of mild iron deficiency on infant mental development scores. J. Pediatr., *102*:519, 1983 (also see *101*:948, 1982).

Whitehead, R. G., Paul, A. A., and Cole, T. J.: A critical analysis of measured food energy intakes during infancy and early childhood in comparison with current international recommendations. J. Human Nutr., *35*:339, 1981.

Yeung, D. L., et al.: Food and nutrient intake of infants during the first 18 months of life. Nutr. Res., *2*:3, 1982.

Committee Reports and Miscellaneous

Clinical memorandum—nutritional vitamin B12 deficiency in infants. Amer. J. Dis. Children, *135*:556, 1981.

Committee on Nutrition, American Academy of Pediatrics: Pediatrics, *53*:115, 1974 (salt intake); *58*:765, 1976 (iron supplementation); *62*:408, 1978 (zinc); *63*:150, 1979 (fluoride supplements); *66*:1015, 1980 (vitamin and mineral supplements).

Overnutrition and Obesity in Children

Archibald, E. H., et al.: Effect of a weight-reducing high-protein diet on the body composition of obese adolescents. Amer. J. Dis. Children, *137*:658, 1983.

Coates, T. O., and Thoresen, C. E.: Treating obesity in children and adolescents: a review. Amer. J. Public Health, *68*:143, 1978.

Crawford, P. B., Hankin, J. H., and Huanemann, R. L.: Environmental factors associated with preschool obesity. III. Dietary intakes, eating patterns, and anthropometric measuresments. J. Amer. Dietet. Assoc., *72*:589, 1978 (also see *64*:480, 488, 1974).

Dietz, W. H., Jr.: Obesity in infants, children, and adolescents in the United States. Nutr. Res., *1*:117, 289, 1981 (a series of reviews).

Epstein, L. H., et al.: Effects of weight loss on fitness in obese children. Amer. J. Dis. Children, *137*:654, 1983.

Kramer, M. S.: Do breastfeeding and delayed introduction of solid foods protect against subsequent obesity? J. Pediatr., *98*:883, 1981.

Food Allergy and Sensitivity

(Also see Supplementary Readings, Chapter 18.)

Denny, F. W. (chairman): National Institutes of Health consensus development conference: statement on defined diets and childhood hyperactivity. Amer. J. Clin. Nutr., *37*:161, 1983.

Gray, G. E., and Gray, L. K.: Diet and juvenile delinquency. Nutr. Today, *18*:14, 1983 (no support for a direct relationship).

Gruskay, F. L.: Comparison of breast, cow, and soy feedings in the prevention of onset of allergic disease—a 15 year prospective study. Clin. Pediatr., *21*:486, 1982.

Kolata, G.: Consensus on diets and hyperactivity. Science, *215*:958, 1982.

Stare, F. J., Whelan, E. M., and Sheridan, M.: Diet and hyperactivity: is there a relationship? Pediatrics, *66*:521, 1980.

Weiss, B.: The behavioral toxicity of food additives. Nutr. Update, *1*:21, 1983 (in children).

Vegetarianism

(Also see Chapters 10, 16, 17, and 22.)

Christoffel, K.: A pediatric perspective on vegetarian nutrition. Clin. Pediatr., *20*:632, 1981.

Committee on Nutrition, American Academy of Pediatrics: nutritional aspects of vegetarianism, health foods, and fad diets. Pediatrics, *59*:460, 1977.

Shinwell, E. D., and Gorodischer, R.: Totally vegetarian diets and infant nutrition. Pediatrics, *70*:582, 1982.

Malnutrition in Infants and Children

Ashworth, A.: International differences in infant mortality and the impact of malnutrition: a review. Human Nutr.: Clin. Nutr., *36C*:7, 1982.

Aykroyd, W. R.: Nutrition and mortality in infancy and early childhood: past and present relationships. Amer. J. Clin. Nutr. *24*:480, 1971.

Baxter, D. H.: Malnutrition and learning—a bibliography. School Food Serv. Res. Rev., 7(1):50, 1983.

Beardslee, W. R., et al.: The effects of infantile malnutrition on behavioral development, a follow-up study. Amer. J. Clin. Nutr. *35*:1437, 1982.

Committee on International Nutrition Programs, Food and Nutrition Board: *Immune Response of the Malnourished Child.* Washington, D.C., The National Research Council, 1976.

Dorea, J. G.: Nutritional status and zinc nutriture in infants and children in a poor urban community of Brazil. Ecol. Food Nutr., *12*:1, 1982.

Fabius, R. J., et al.: Malnutrition associated with a formula of barley water, corn syrup, and whole milk. Amer. J. Dis. Children, *135*:615, 1981.

Ghosh, S., and Brown, R. E.: Weaning foods in developing countries. Amer. J. Clin. Nutr., *32*:1984, 1981 (letters).

Guthrie, G. M., et al.: Early termination of breastfeeding among Philippine urban poor. Ecol. Food Nutr., *12*:195, 1983.

Jackson, R. L.: Longterm consequences of suboptimal nutritional practices in early life: some important benefits of breast feeding. Pediatr. Clin. North Amer., *24*:63, 1977.

Omolulu, A.: Breast-feeding practice and breast milk intake in rural Nigeria. Human Nutr.: Applied Nutr., *36A*: 445,1982.

Read, M. S., and Felson, D.: *Malnutrition, Learning and Behavior.* National Institute of Child Health and Human Development, Dept. of Health, Education, and Welfare Pub. No. (NIH) 76–1036, April 1976.

Somogyi, J. C., and Haenel, H.: Nutrition in early childhood and its effects in later life. Biblio. Nutr. Dieta, No. 31, 1982 (a symposium, 14 papers).

Waterlow, J. C.: Childhood malnutrition–the global problem. Proc. Nutr. Soc., *38*:1, 1979.

Winick, M.: *Malnutrition and Brain Development.* New York, Oxford Univ. Press, Inc., 1976.

Child Nutrition Programs and School Lunch

Akin, J. S., et al.: Impact of the school lunch program on nutrient intakes of school children. School Food Serv. Res. Rev., 7(1), 13, 1983.

Anon.: Child nutrition programs update (U.S.) Dairy Council Digest, *53*(6):31, 1982.

Hiemstra, S. J.: National school lunch program trends. School Food Serv. Res. Rev., 7(1), 6, 1983.

Keyser, D. L., Vaden, A. G., and Dayton, A. D.: Factors affecting participation in child nutrition programs. School Food Serv. Res. Rev., 7(1):29, 1983 (Also see pages 38 and 41 for information on day-care centers—nutritional aspects).

School lunch: America's no. 1 energy source. School Food Service J., *36*:31, 1982.

School lunch: how it has changed. School Food Service J., *36*:22, 1982.

Journals for Additional Reading

(See current issues of these major examples of peer-reviewed journals for recent information on infant and/or child nutrition.)

Acta Paediatrics Scandinavica
American Journal of Clinical Nutrition
American Journal of Diseases of Children
American Journal of Public Health
Archives of Diseases in Childhood (U.K.)
Assignment Children (U.K.)
Biology of the Neonate (Switzerland)
British Medical Journal
Canadian Medical Journal
Early Human Development (Netherlands)
European J. of Pediatrics (West Germany)
Journal of Dentistry for Children
Journal of Pediatric Gastroenterology and Nutrition (Vol. 3 in 1984)
Journal of Pediatrics
Journal of the American Medical Association
Journal of Tropical Pediatrics (U.K.)
Lancet (U.K.)
New England Journal of Medicine
Pediatrics
Pediatric Research
Public Health Reports
School Food Service Research Review

Chapter 24 Dental Health, Nutrition, and Diet

Reviews and General Reading

Diet and Dental Health, A Study of Relationships: United States, 1971–74. Vital and Health Statistics Series 11, No. 225. PHS 82–1675. Washington, D.C., National Center for Health Statistics, 1982.

Imfield, T. N.: *Identification of Low Caries Risk Dietary Components.* Basel, Switz., S. Karger, 1983.

Newbrun, E.: Sugar and dental caries: a review of human studies. Science, *217*:418, 1982.

Randolph, P. M.: *Diet, Nutrition and Dentistry.* St. Louis, C. V. Mosby Co., 1980.

Schoen, M. H., and Freed, J. R.: Prevention of dental disease: caries and periodontal disease. Ann. Rev. Public Health, *2*:1981.

Screebny, L. M.: Sugar and human dental decay. World Rev. Nutr. Dietet., *40*:19, 1982.

Dental Caries and Sugars

Clancy, K. L., et al.: Snack food intake of adolescents and caries development. J. Dent. Res., *45*:568, 1977.

Lauder, N. M., and Valentine, A. D.: Diet and dental caries. J. Human Nutr., *34*:158, 1980.

Leveille, G. A., and Coccodrilli, G. D.: Cariogenicity of foods: current concepts. Food Tech., *36*(Sept.):93, 1982.

Newbrun, E., and Frostell, G.: Sugar restriction and substitution for caries prevention. Caries Res., *12*(Suppl): 65, 1978.

Screebny, L. M.: Cereal availability and dental caries. Commun. Dent. Oral Epidem., *11*:148, 1983.

Fluoridation

Andrus, P. L.: The role of fluoride in the prevention of dental caries. Texas Med., *78*:57, 1982.

Boriskin, J. M., and Fine, J. I.: Fluoridation election victory: a case study for dentistry in effective political action. J. Amer. Dent. Assoc., *102*:486, 1981.

Burt, B.: The epidemiological basis for water fluoridation in the prevention of dental caries. J. Public Health Policy, Dec. 1982, p. 391.

Clark, N., and Corbin, S.: The evolution of standards for naturally occurring fluorides. Public Health Rept., *98*:53, 1983.

Ekstrand, J., et al.: Plasma fluoride concentrations in pre-school children after ingestion of fluoride tablets and toothpaste. Caries Res., *17*:379, 1979.

Evans, C. A.: Challenges to the adoption of community water fluoridation. Fam. Comm. Health, *3*:33, 1980.

Heifetz, S. B.: Alternative methods of delivering fluorides: an update. In Horowitz, A. M., and Thomas, H. B. (eds.): *Dental Caries Prevention in Public Health Programs.* USDHHS, NIH Publ. No. 81–2235:25, 1981.

Horowitz, A. M.: *Preventing Tooth Decay: A Guide for Implementing Self-Applied Fluorides in School Settings.* Bethesda, Md., National Institute Dental Research, USDHHS, NIH Publ. No. 82–1196, 1982.

Horotwitz, H. S.: The future of self-applied fluorides. J. Public Health Dent., *41*:255, 1981 (also see *40*:268, 1980).

Leverett, D. S.: Fluorides and dental caries. Science, *220*:146, 1983 (also see Science, *217*:26, 1982 and letters to editor, *220*:142 and 144, 1983).

Margolis, F. J., et al.: Fluoride supplements for children. Amer. J. Dis. Child., *134*:865, 1980.

Myers, H. M.: Dose-response relationship between water fluoride levels and the category of questionable dental fluorosis. Commun. Dent. Oral Epidem., *11*:109, 1983.

Rebich, T., Jr.: The St. Regis environmental health issue: assessment of dental defects. J. Amer. Dental Assoc., *106*:630, 1983(reported dental fluorosis in Native American children).

Periodontal Disease

Firestone, A. R.: Effect of increasing contact time of sucrose solution or powdered sucrose on plaque pH in vivo. J. Dental Res., *61*:1243, 1982.

Jacobs, H. H.: Nutrition and the development of oral tissues. J. Amer. Dietet. Assoc., *83*:50, 1983.

Stahl, S. S.: Nutritional influences on periodontal disease. World Rev. Nutr. Dietet., *13*:277, 1971.

Stamm, J. W.: Methods for the prevention of periodontal diseases. Fam. Comm. Health *3*:41, 1980.

Other References on Dental Health

Kovar, M. G.: Health status of U.S. children and use of medical care. Pub. Health Rep., *97*:3, 1982.

Lehner, T., Russel, M. W., and Caldwell, J.: Immunisation with a purified protein from streptococcus mutans against dental caries in rhesus monkeys. Lancet, *1*:995, 1980.

Mueninghoff, L. A., and Johnson, M. H.: Erosion: a case caused by unusual diet. J. Amer. Dent. Assoc., *104:*51, 1982.

Schachtele, C. F.: Changing perspectives on the role of diet in dental caries formation. Nutr. News, *45*(4): 13, 1982.

Winter, G. B.: Maternal nutritional requirements in relation to the subsequent development of teeth in children. J. Human Nutr., *30:*93, 1976.

Chapter 25 Malnutrition—A Global Perspective

Abalu, G. O. I.: Solving Africa's food problem. Food Policy, 7:247, 1982.

Austin, J. E. (ed.): *Global Malnutrition and Cereal Fortification.* Cambridge, Mass., Ballinger Publ. Co., 1979.

Baldwin, R. L.: *Animals, Feed, Food and People.* Boulder, Colo., Westview Press, 1980.

Beal, V. A., and Laus, M. J.: Proceedings: Symposium on dietary data collection, analysis, and significance. Mass. Agric. Expt. Stat. Res. Bull., No. 675, 1982.

Beaton, G. H.: Evaluation of nutrition interventions: methodological considerations. Amer. J. Clin. Nutr., *35*:000, 1982.

Berb, A.: *The Nutrition Factor: Its role in National Development.* Washington, D.C., Brookings Institution, 1973.

Berg, A. (ed.): *Malnourished People: A Policy View.* Washington, D.C., World Bank, 1981.

Brown, R. E.: *Starving Children: The Tyranny of Hunger.* New York, Springer Publ. Co., 1977.

Caliendo. A. *Nutrition and the World Food Crisis.* New York, Macmillan, 1979.

Carloni, A. S.: Sex disparities in the distribution of food within rural households. Food Nutr., 7:3, 1981.

Chavez, A., and Martinez, C.: *Growing Up in a Developing Community?* Mexico, Instituto Nacional de la Nutricion, 1982.

FAO/WHO: Food and nutrition strategies in national development. 9th Rept., Joint FAO/WHO Expert Committee on Nutr., FAO Nutr. Meetings Rept. Ser. No. 56, Rome, 1976.

Francois, P., Périssé, J., and Kamoun, A.: A Tunisian case study. The effects of household size and income on the probability of energy inadequacy. Food Nutr., *8*:32, 1982.

Garn, S. M., Hopkins, P. J., and Ryan, A. S.: Differential fatness gain of low income boys and girls. Amer. J. Clin. Nutr., *34*:1465, 1981.

Gebre-Medhin, M., and Vahlquist, B.: Famine in Ethiopia—the period 1973–75. Nutr. Rev., *35*:194, 1977.

Hakim, P., and Solimano, G.: *Development, Reform and Malnutrition in Chile.* Cambridge, Mass., MIT Press, 1978.

Hulse, J. H.: Food science and nutrition: the gulf between rich and poor. Science, *216*:1291, 1982.

Joy, J. L.: Food and nutrition planning. J. Agric. Econ., *24*:165, 1973.

Kent, G.: Food trade: the poor feed the rich. Food Nutr. Bull., *4*(4):24, 1982.

Kirk, D., and Eliason, E. K.: *Food and People.* San Francisco, Boyd and Fraser, 1983.

Kloth, T. I., et al.: Sehel nutrition survey, 1974. Amer. J. Epidem., *103*:383, 1976.

Levinson, F. J.: Toward success in combatting malnutrition: an assessment of what works. Food Nutr. Bull., *4*(3):23, 1982.

Lunven, P.: The nutritional consequences of agricultural and rural development projects. Food Nutr. Bull., *4*(3):17, 1981.

Mittendorf, H. J., an Hertag, O.: Marketing costs and margins for major food items in developing countries. Food Nutr., *8*:27, 1982.

Overholt, C., et al.: The effects of nutritional supplementation on the diets of low-income families at risk of malnutrition. Amer. J. Clin. Nutr., *36*:1153, 1982.

Pariser, E. R., et al.: *Fish Protein Concentrate: Panacea for Protein Malnutrition?* Cambridge, Mass., MIT Press, 1978.

Plucknett, F. L., and Smith, N. J. H.: Agricultural research and third world food production. Science, *217*:215, 1982.

Pollitt, E.: Child poverty in South America: reflections on its magnitude, and the basic-need development approach. Archivos Latinoamer. Nutr., *31*:235, 1981.

Popkin, B. M., and Solon, F. S.: Income, time, the working mother and child nutriture. Environ. Child Health, *22*:156, 1976.

Satyanarayana, K., et al.: Effect of nutritional deprivation in early childhood on later growth—a community study without intervention. Amer. J. Clin. Nutr., *34*:1636, 1981.

Seltzer, M (ed.): *Home Economics and Agriculture in Third World Countries.* St. Paul, Minn., Univ. of Minnesota, 1980.

Smil, V.: Energy flows in the developing world. Amer. Scientist, *67*:522, 1979.

Symposium: Impact of infection on nutritional status. Amer. J. Clin. Nutr., *30*:1203, 1977.

Symposium: Protein-energy malnutrition. Proc. Nutr. Soc., *38*:1, 1979.

Transaction: Articles—food crisis? Society, *17*(6):18, 1980.

Tripp, R. B.: Farmers and traders. Some economic determinants of nutritional status in northern Ghana. Food Nutr., *8*:3, 1982.

Walker, A. R. P., and Walker, B. F.: Recommended dietary allowances and third world populations. Amer. J. Clin. Nutr., *34*:2319, 1981.

Underwood, B. A. (ed.): *Nutrition Intervention Strategies in National Development.* New York, Academic Press, 1982.

WHO: Nutritional surveillance. Report of the Joint FAO/UNICEF/WHO Expert Committee on Methodology of Nutritional Surveillance. WHO Tech. Rept. Ser. no. 593, Geneva, 1976.

WHO: The role of the health sector in food and nutrition. Tech. Rept. Ser. No. 607, Geneva, 1981.

Winikoff, B.: *Nutrition and National Policy.* Cambridge, Mass., MIT Press, 1978.

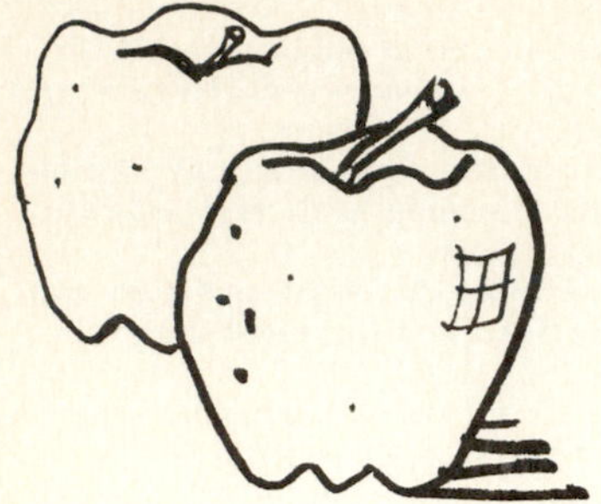

Index

Page numbers in *italics* refer to illustrations and tables. For nutrient values of many foods not listed in index, see Appendix Table 2.

Estimated Safe and Adequate Daily Dietary Intakes of Additional Selected Vitamins and Minerals[a] (1980–RDA)

	Age (years)	Vitamins: Vitamin K (μg)	Vitamins: Biotin (μg)	Vitamins: Pantothenic Acid (mg)	Trace Elements[b]: Copper (mg)	Trace Elements[b]: Manganese (mg)	Trace Elements[b]: Fluoride (mg)	Trace Elements[b]: Chromium (mg)	Trace Elements[b]: Selenium (mg)	Trace Elements[b]: Molybdenum (mg)	Electrolytes: Sodium (mg)	Electrolytes: Potassium (mg)	Electrolytes: Chloride (mg)
Infants	0–0.5	12	35	2	0.5–0.7	0.5–0.7	0.1–0.5	0.01–0.04	0.01–0.04	0.03–0.06	115–350	350–925	275–700
	0.5–1	10–20	50	3	0.7–1.0	0.7–1.0	0.2–1.0	0.02–0.06	0.02–0.06	0.04–0.08	250–750	425–1275	400–1200
Children and Adolescents	1–3	15–30	65	3	1.0–1.5	1.0–1.5	0.5–1.5	0.02–0.08	0.02–0.08	0.05–0.1	325–975	550–1650	500–1500
	4–6	20–40	85	3–4	1.5–2.0	1.5–2.0	1.0–2.5	0.03–0.12	0.03–0.12	0.06–0.15	450–1350	775–2325	700–2100
	7–10	30–60	120	4–5	2.0–2.5	2.0–3.0	1.5–2.5	0.05–0.2	0.05–0.2	0.1–0.3	600–1800	1000–3000	925–2775
	11+	50–100	100–200	4–7	2.0–3.0	2.5–5.0	1.5–2.5	0.05–0.2	0.05–0.2	0.15–0.5	900–2700	1525–4575	1400–4200
Adults		70–140	100–200	4–7	2.0–3.0	2.5–5.0	1.5–4.0	0.05–0.2	0.05–0.2	0.15–0.5	1100–3300	1875–5625	1700–5100

[a]Because there is less information on which to base allowances, these figures are not given in the main table of the RDA and are provided here in the form of ranges of recommended intakes.

[b]Since the toxic levels for many trace elements may be only several times usual intakes, the upper levels for the trace elements given in this table should not be habitually exceeded.

(Reproduced from: Recommended Dietary Allowances, Ninth Edition [1980], with the permission of the National Academy of Sciences, Washington, D.C.)